FOOD SAFETY 1993

Food Research Institute

Department of Food Microbiology and Toxicology
University of Wisconsin–Madison
Madison, Wisconsin

prepared by
M. Ellin Doyle
Carol E. Steinhart
Barbara A. Cochrane

Marcel Dekker, Inc. New York•Basel•Hong Kong

ISBN: 0-8247-9156-8

The publisher offers discounts on this book when ordered in bulk quantities. For more information, write to Special Sales/Professional Marketing at the address below.

This book is printed on acid-free paper.

MARCEL DEKKER, INC.
270 Madison Avenue, New York, New York 10016

Current printing (last digit):
10 9 8 7 6 5 4 3 2 1

PRINTED IN THE UNITED STATES OF AMERICA

Preface

Food Safety 1993 is a comprehensive summary of the literature on food safety and foodborne illness published during the latter half of 1991 and the first half of 1992. The journals covered by the *Life Sciences* and *Agriculture, Biology & Environmental Sciences* editions of *Current Contents* were surveyed. Articles from over 550 sources are included in this volume. Such a comprehensive volume would not have been possible without the extensive library resources of the University of Wisconsin–Madison.

We have included as broad a range of articles as we deemed possible. Some sections in Part I, DIET AND HEALTH, include primarily research papers covering epidemiological and intervention studies in humans and experimental studies with primates. The sheer volume of work on rodents precludes inclusion of any but a few of the most salient papers. Coverage of pesticides has also been limited in the interest of producing a manageable volume. Readers should note that some food components are covered in more than one section of this volume. For example, articles on dietary fiber and on n-3 fatty acids are present in several sections of DIET AND HEALTH, while selenium, which can have both beneficial and toxic effects, is included in both DIET AND HEALTH and in Chapter 8, INDIRECT ADDITIVES, RESIDUES, AND CONTAMINANTS.

While we have made every effort to assure accuracy, we encourage readers to consult the original publications for specific information.

Foodborne viruses are reviewed annually by Dr. Dean O. Cliver of the Food Research Institute and form a valuable addition to our annotated bibliography of food safety literature.

Contents

3   DIET AND CARDIOVASCULAR DISEASE

4   OTHER EFFECTS OF DIET

5   MEASUREMENT AND BIOAVAILABILITY OF FOOD COMPONENTS

PART II: SAFETY OF FOOD COMPONENTS

6   ASSESSMENT OF FOOD SAFETY

7   INTENTIONAL (DIRECT) ADDITIVES

8   INDIRECT ADDITIVES, RESIDUES, AND CONTAMINANTS

9   NATURALLY OCCURRING TOXICANTS AND FOOD CONSTITUENTS OF TOXICOLOGICAL INTEREST

PART III: FOODBORNE MICROBIAL ILLNESS

10   MYCOTOXINS

11   FOODBORNE BACTERIAL INTOXICATIONS AND INFECTIONS

12   FOODBORNE PARASITES

APPENDIX

FOOD- AND WATER-ASSOCIATED VIRUSES

Part I: Diet and Health

1

Overview

General historical and epidemiological studies
Fatty acids
Carbohydrates and fiber
Minerals
Oxidant defense
Special foods and diets

GENERAL HISTORICAL AND EPIDEMIOLOGICAL STUDIES

In 1987, more than 70% of deaths in the USA could be attributed to seven causes with dietary associations: heart disease, cancers, stroke, alcohol-related events, diabetes, liver disease, and atherosclerosis (*1*). Two additional prevalent causes of morbidity, osteoporosis and diverticular disease, are also diet-related. The author discusses some widespread nutritional beliefs and dietary practices of consumers that are based on misconceptions and inadequate guidelines. These are related to fallacies in traditional thinking such as "tunnel vision medicine," which emphasizes particular diseases; "tunnel vision nutrition," which emphasizes the associated dietary parameter(s); and the inane exhortation to eat a variety of foods (who doesn't?) rather than specified proportions of these foods.

The report of a World Health Organization study group considers historical and social aspects of the diet–health relationship (*2*). Only relatively recently has the food supply of some societies become secure enough to permit indulgence in preferred foods. When this happened, the link between diet and disease began to appear. Recognizing that diet-related disease is as likely due to excesses as to deficiencies, the study group suggested safe ranges of intakes for worldwide prevention of chronic disease. Developing countries are urged not to imitate food-system practices and policies based on outmoded nutritional knowledge, which wealthy nations are now having such difficulty altering. Nevertheless, in virtually every developing country, diet-related chronic disease is becoming a new health problem as traditional diets are abandoned.

Papers at a symposium on dietary habits and disease patterns in Europe considered methodological questions, epidemiology of ischemic heart disease (IHD), and changes in types of fats produced and consumed (*3*). Although differences between northern and southern states in food intake and incidence of IHD are real, comparisons are complicated because nutrient intake shows a normal distribution whereas distribution of specific foods is skewed. A surprising finding in IHD studies was that the largest (negative) correlation was with plasma vitamin E and there was no correlation with either total plasma cholesterol or blood pressure in the midrange of values. IHD mortality in 19 countries was strongly correlated with consumption of dairy fat excluding cheese. Changes in farming practices and food processing have introduced *trans* and branched-chain fatty acids into the diet, whose effects are not yet known.

Three papers discuss relationships between the Mediterranean diet and health, based on the International Cooperative Study on the Epidemiology of Coronary Heart Disease ("Seven Countries Study") and follow-up investigations (*4–6*). The "Mediterranean diet" is a fairly specific diet eaten in coastal areas of a few countries. It is characterized by relatively high amounts of fish, olive oil, fruit, and vegetables and low amounts of meat and animal fat. Populations adhering to this diet have lower mortality rates from all causes, coronary heart disease (CHD), and cancer. The ratio of monounsaturated to saturated fatty acids explains nearly two-thirds of the variance in the all-cause death rate (*4*); and because oleic acid accounts for almost all of the monounsaturated fat, it becomes the dietary item of major interest. Since monounsaturates appear to be neutral with respect to CHD risk factors and moderate consumption of oily fish is protective, partial replacement of saturated with monounsaturated fatty acids and inclusion of one or two meals of fatty fish weekly would give considerable flexibility in planning acceptable, healthful diets (*5*). However, disturbing changes have been documented, population by population, in traditional Mediterranean diets (*4,6*). There is a trend toward greater intake of meat, dairy products, fat, sugar, and total energy and a decreased intake of dry legumes. The main determinants of this are urbanization, income, and inadequate nutritional education. Through timely educational intervention, the decrease in legume consumption seems to have been halted in some places, but the other influences are beyond control of public health services.

Germany provides a laboratory for learning what happens when genetically similar people are artificially and randomly divided, live under different conditions for nearly 30 years, and then are reunited (*7*). In 1989, most major causes of mortality in German men and women were nutrition-related and some differences between East and West were apparent: deaths from IHD, arteriosclerosis, and hypertension were more common in the East, whereas the mortality rate from breast, colon, lung, and pancreatic cancer was higher among women in the West. The most notable differences in diet were a very large cabbage intake in East Germany (which may have been protective against cancer), a relatively small intake of citrus fruit, and differences in the amounts and types of alcoholic beverages consumed. In East Germany and eastern Europe generally diets were quite different from those in the West, and a trend toward a more Western diet is now expected. Nutritionists and epidemiologists are poised to assess the effects.

A large, 17-year cohort study in Japan revealed close associations between diet and mortality from major causes (*8*). In men, frequent consumption of green and yellow vegetables reduced risk of death from all causes, "other" heart diseases, all cancers, liver cirrhosis, and cancer of the stomach, lung, and prostate. In women, green and yellow vegetables reduced mortality from all causes, other heart diseases, all cancers, and stomach cancer. The protective effect against lung and cervical cancer was greatest among heavy smokers, suggesting a crucial role for the antioxidant constituents; the vegetables' fiber is likely important in lowering risks from certain other diseases. Lower mortality from many causes, especially IHD, other heart disease, and cerebrovascular disease, was observed in persons who ate fish daily. The effect was independent of smoking and compatible with the idea that certain fatty acids in fish reduce risk for these diseases. Risk for breast cancer was elevated to western levels in women who ate meat daily. Among all persons who ate meat daily, daily consumption of green and yellow vegetables afforded some protection against many diseases. Again, this suggests the importance of fiber in a high-fat diet. High grain consumption was negatively associated with death from all causes and from diabetes, IHD, and cerebrovascular disease.

Like geographic studies, occupational epidemiology can yield insights into diet and health. In the U.S. restaurant industry, where alcohol and high-fat foods are readily available and exposure to tobacco smoke is likely, elevated proportionate mortality ratios were found among subsets of restaurant workers for chronic liver disease and cirrhosis, alcoholism, diabetes mellitus, and certain cancers associated with alcohol and/or smoking (*9*).

A persistent problem in firmly establishing specific links between diet and health has been the difficulty of measuring usual dietary intake. The Food and Agricultural Organization, World Health Organization, and other groups sponsored a critical assessment of common types of dietary surveys, their pitfalls and application to various kinds of studies (*10*). New data provide information on actual intake not only of macronutrients and micronutrients but also of additives and contaminants. Comparison of these figures with recommended dietary intakes and maximum residue limits provides insights into margins of safety. Other problems that plague the assessment of whether a dietary component really alters the risk of disease include the long latent period of chronic and degenerative diseases, the multiplicity of their risk factors, the relatively small population-wide differences in exposures and risks, and the complexity of diet; however, difficulties of dietary assessment are inherent in all of these (*11*). This paper discusses public health implications of a population-based approach to dietary modification and limitations to the high-risk approach. From a public health perspective, small changes in diet for everyone will have a greater impact on morbidity and mortality than large changes in the diet of high-risk individuals.

Relatively few of the thousands of food items available are selected by an individual and prepared according to cultural and personal preferences (*12*). From this process, on a population basis, emerge patterns in food use that may be associated with disease risk. In a case–control study of diet and cancer in western New York, Randall et al. extracted seven dietary patterns by principal components analysis and studied their association with five health-related behaviors (trimming fat from meat, use of discretionary fats, choice of cooking fat, alcohol intake, and cigarette smoking). They found that, compared to men, women were more likely to trim fat from meat, consumed less alcohol, and had lower exposure to smoking; and their dietary patterns were more independent of the fats used. Several eating patterns were positively associated with total fat intake but differed in their associations with high-risk behaviors. The authors' long-range goal in understanding dietary patterns and high-risk behaviors is to develop targeted interventions to reduce risks, particularly of cancer at specific sites. An example of such an intervention is provided in a paper on the nutritional implications of cigarette smoking (13). Not only do many smokers consume an inadequate diet; smoking itself produces nutrient imbalances, which are reviewed. Arguments for giving persons who do not stop smoking dietary advice to ameliorate the harmful effects of smoking are discussed.

A second look at "positive family history" as a risk factor for chronic disease (14) revealed that diet is an important potential confounder to be considered in evaluating the relative importance of genetic and environmental influences. Even among adult siblings living apart in different countries, there were statistically significant sibling correlations for most measures of dietary intake. This demonstrates the need to incorporate dietary variables in genetic models of chronic disease.

Many dietary habits and preferences may have evolutionary roots. Some of these were addressed in a discussion of foraging strategies and the "natural" diets of primates (15). Papers were under the major topics of foraging and dietary strategies of nonhuman primates, evolution of hominid foraging and diet, food of hunter–gatherers, and the history of human diets. Foley and Lee discussed the large energy cost of the human brain and its implications for diet and feeding behavior (16). They argue that the slow rate of development and prolonged period of immaturity within the genus *Homo* indicates that mothers were under energetic and time-budget constraints for which dietary adjustment could only partly compensate. They suggest that evolution of large brains within *Homo* required increased foraging efficiency, consumption of large amounts of high-quality food, and

life-history changes, and thus depended on ecological conditions. A separate review explores the idea that lipid availability determines the limits of brain growth, just as protein is important to body, and minerals to skeletal, growth (17). It suggests that rather than "evolving a large brain," *Homo sapiens* found a way to avoid *losing* relative brain capacity as most other species apparently did when they evolved larger bodies. The large-brained marine mammals are an exception, notable because these animals had access to ample docosahexaenoic acid (DHA). An explanation for big brains based on nutrient flow is outlined. Biochemical and physiological evidence is presented to support the theory that *Homo sapiens* evolved, not on the savannah, but at the land–water interface where the availability of marine lipids had a pivotal role.

Dietary changes accompanied changes in subsistence practices beginning about 12,000 years ago in the Near East and Mediterranean region (18). It is assumed that energy-rich plant foods were substituted for energy-poor ones and consumption of animal foods plummeted. Skeletal pathologies indicative of anemia and osteoporosis are associated with the transition from hunting and gathering to agriculture. Modeling studies of possible diets of adult males during the transition indicated that protein deficiency was likely only if people suffered from chronic energy deficiency and ate no meat; calcium deficiency was possible in an agrarian system if there was at least moderate chronic energy deficiency; but anemia was unlikely to have been due to deficiency of iron in the diet.

Effects of recent rapid changes from the hunter–gatherer lifestyle to a western diet and lifestyle have been amply documented. The traditional diet of Australian aborigines protected against the obesity, non-insulin-dependent diabetes mellitus (NIDDM), and cardiovascular disease that are now rampant in westernized aborigine communities (19). With westernization, hunter–gatherer food preferences and eating behaviors were retained but the availability of energy-rich foods was no longer limited and minimal energy was involved in their procurement. As a result, behaviors, preferences, and genetic traits that favored survival under feast-and-famine conditions in the traditional lifestyle became maladaptive. A review of NIDDM in developing populations further highlights the genetic link (*20*). Micronesians, Polynesians, American Indians, and Australian aborigines have a higher-than-average genetic susceptibility to NIDDM, which is apparently unmasked by obesity, reduced physical activity, dietary change, and stress. It has been proposed that in traditional feast-and-famine societies a "thrifty genotype" promoted survival through maximum metabolic efficiency, whereas the same genotype wreaks havoc in modernized feast-only societies.

A dietary survey in 1987–1988 found that adult Alaska Natives (Eskimos, Indians, and Aleuts) consumed more energy, protein, fat, carbohydrate, iron, and vitamins A and C but less calcium and alcohol than the general adult population of the USA (*21*). They ate six times more fish but less fruits and vegetables. Large seasonal variations in diet persist, and Alaska Natives still rely on traditional foods and eating practices, which may protect against chronic diseases and counteract the effects of their high-fat diet. Although past rates of heart disease, cancer, and diabetes have been lower in Alaska Natives than in whites in the USA, they are now increasing. The continuing uniqueness of the Native Alaskan diet offers opportunity to better understand the relationship between diet and specific diseases, formulate dietary advice that recognizes an individual's risk of developing specific diseases, and establish nutrition surveillance systems that identify detrimental dietary changes in time to take appropriate action.

A survey of contemporary human diets emphasized excesses and deficiencies, rather than ways in which satisfactory mixtures can be achieved (*22*). At the same time, the author emphasized that with adequate nutritional information, humans can frequently still "forage" for a variety of foods that supply all the nutrients they require.

FATTY ACIDS

A brief review summarized evidence for the relationship of dietary fat to heart disease, cancer, and diseases for which obesity is a risk factor (*23*).

Other reviews considered the roles of polyunsaturated fatty acids (PUFAs) (*24*), n–3 fatty acids (*25*), and tropical oils (*26*) in nutrition and health. In mammals, palmitoleic, oleic, linoleic, and linolenic acids are desaturated and elongated to form four families of long-chain highly unsaturated fatty acids (*24*). When incorporated into the phospholipids of cell membranes, these PUFAs influence membrane fluidity—which determines membrane permeability and the behavior of membrane-bound enzymes and receptors. PUFAs also give rise to the eicosanoids, which influence many cellular processes. Because mammals cannot synthesize linoleic and linolenic acids, a dietary source is required. Intake of 1–2% of calories as linoleate and 0.2–0.5% as linolenate is considered adequate for humans. n–3 and n–6 PUFAs are metabolically and functionally distinct and frequently have opposing physiological functions (*25*). Therefore their balance is important for health, homeostasis, and normal development. Human evolution probably occurred in the context of relatively low amounts of dietary n–3 and n–6 fatty acids in roughly a 1:1 ratio; agribusiness, agriculture, and the technology of the vegetable oil industry have unbalanced this critical ratio in modern diets. An extensive review (179 references) defended the place of palm oil in a healthful diet and identified some drawbacks of current labeling laws (*26*). Laboratory and clinical trials with palm oil are discussed in terms of its structure; biochemistry; constituents; effects on sterol metabolism, thrombus formation, and carcinogenesis; and the anomalous behavior of stearic acid, which fails to increase plasma cholesterol levels according to predictions.

Two important roles of dietary fatty acids are as modulators of cytokine synthesis (*27*) and determinants of membrane structure and cell function (*28*). In these capacities they have sweeping effects on health. Cytokines are protein mediators serving as communication signals between cells (*27*). They include the interleukins and tumor necrosis factor. Their synthesis and perhaps functions are modulated by dietary PUFAs through changes in metabolites of arachidonic acid (AA) and eicosapentaenoic acid (EPA). Because cytokines are mediators of both defense and disease, playing key roles in the interrelationships among nutrition, the immune system, and disease, dietary manipulation of n–3 PUFAs for a specific function should be undertaken only with consideration of the implications for other functions and disease states. As constituents of the cell membrane, dietary fatty acids determine not only membrane properties and functions, but the activity of enzymes that synthesize membrane constituents, hormone-activated functions, and even the expression of activity in the cell nucleus *(28)*. The effects of dietary fatty acids on the function of various cell and tissue types, and consequences for health and disease, are reviewed.

Dietary *trans* fatty acids can impair synthesis of 20- and 22-carbon PUFAs and reduce growth in experimental animals, but it has been difficult to document adverse effects in humans. Investigators in Germany analyzed the fatty acids in plasma of 29 4-day-old premature infants *(29)*. Because enteral feeding was not yet fully established in these infants, it was assumed that the composition of plasma lipids reflected intrauterine nutrition and metabolism. *Trans*-octadecenoic acid and total *trans* fatty acids were not related to precursor linoleic and α-linolenic acids, but they did correlate inversely with n–3 and n–6 PUFAs and to the product:substrate ratio of long-chain PUFA synthesis. They were also inversely correlated to birth weight (but not to gestational age). This study revealed a possible alteration of essential fatty acid metabolism and reduction of early growth by *trans* isomers in humans. The data cast doubt on the safety of dietary *trans* fatty acids for pregnant and lactating women and newborns.

Although humans elongate and desaturate α-linolenic acid (18:3n–3) much more slowly than rodents, in both the major function of α-linolenic acid has been assumed to be production of longer-chain n–3 fatty acids. However, neither humans nor rodents convert the major part of dietary α-linolenic acid to longer-chain PUFAs and both oxidize a substantial portion of it even in the total absence of dietary 20:5n–3 and 22:6n–3 fatty acids. Canadian scientists asked whether 18:3n–3 itself has important functions and its oxidation is biologically useful rather than merely "wasteful" *(30)*. From this perspective, their review found numerous indications for beneficial effects of the 18:3n–3 molecule per se. In addition, β-oxidation provides acetate for de novo synthesis of long-chain fatty acids and cholesterol. While it may seem implausible that an essential nutrient should be degraded for this "purpose" or that supplies of acetate for lipid synthesis could be limiting, our incomplete understanding of human evolution and early human development cannot rule out this possibility. Further, in exercise performance studies, oxidation of serum 18:3n–3 is specifically associated with the caffeine-induced delay in exhaustion. The authors conclude that 18:3n–3 has significant roles not only as a precursor fatty acid but in its own right.

The types of n–6 PUFAs in the diet may be more important than the total amount *(31)*. In rats, the amount of dietary linoleic acid (18:2n–6) had relatively little effect on the arachidonic acid (20:4n–6) content of tissue phospholipids, whereas only small amounts of dietary arachidonic acid sharply increased the arachidonic acid in tissue phospholipids. The effect may be even greater in humans, with their more limited desaturase activities. Perhaps more attention should be paid to the arachidonic acid content of diets, which in the USA is estimated as 170 mg daily but could easily be three times that value.

A comprehensive investigation determined the effects of well-defined lipid-supplemented diets on the fatty acid composition of various tissues, organs, and blood components in the common marmoset monkey (*Callithrix jacchus*) *(32)*. Heart and skeletal muscle had similar fatty acid profiles and responded similarly to dietary change, indicating that a skeletal muscle biopsy might have considerable diagnostic value if results in the marmoset also apply to humans. Plasma and red blood cell fatty acids reflected the composition of dietary fat, whereas platelet fatty acids reflected metabolism of dietary fat. Kidney and liver profiles are similar and related to plasma profiles, suggesting another potentially useful diagnostic correlation. Brain and aorta differed significantly from other tissues. The authors conclude that the lipid metabolism of the common marmoset recommends this species as a model for studies of lipid nutrition.

The cholesterol controversy

The relationship between plasma cholesterol (or, alternatively, *lowering* of plasma cholesterol) and mortality has generated some new analyses and a lot of debate (*33–69*). The interest arises because despite the clear relationship between CHD mortality and blood cholesterol level, results of trials to lower cholesterol are often equivocal and there is evidence that low cholesterol levels are associated with increased mortality from other causes. From the Whitehall Study, Davey Smith et al. concluded that the inverse associations seen in some cohort studies between plasma cholesterol level and mortality from certain causes may be due to other characteristics that place subjects with low cholesterol at increased risk of death (*33*). For example, relatively low cholesterol levels were more common among subjects who had been recently widowed, were in lower employment grades, had disease at baseline, or had recent or unexplained weight loss. A reader protested that it is premature to attribute these observations to sociodemographic or other confounding factors (*34*), when increased mortality from neoplastic and nonneoplastic pulmonary disease could result from impairment of pulmonary immune function by low cholesterol levels. Davey Smith defended his original interpretation (*35*). In another analysis, Davey Smith and Pekkanen found that mortality was higher for intervention groups in drug studies of cholesterol reduction but lower for intervention groups in dietary studies (*36*). Although the dietary intervention trials were weak in design, size, and length of follow up and the apparent difference in outcome between drug and dietary trials was not definitive, the authors cited other evidence for the safety and efficacy of dietary lowering of cholesterol. They concluded that if cholesterol lowering becomes a public health goal, dietary change is probably safer and certainly more cost-effective than widespread drug treatment. This is in contrast to Oliver's gloomy conclusions from a Finnish study that inexplicably found more cardiac deaths, nonfatal myocardial infarctions, deaths associated with violence, and deaths from all causes in intervention groups 10 y after the end of a multiple-intervention

trial (*37*). From this, Oliver concluded that multiple interventions in middle-aged men may do more harm than good and that CHD is not readily amenable to control except when rigorous and specific interventions are targeted at the few persons most at risk. These two reports (*36,37*) engendered a storm of correspondence (*38–46*). One reader thought it irresponsible to abandon lifestyle strategies on evidence as flimsy as the Finnish study, when a 23% drop in death rate among 35- to 74-year-old British men during the last decade coincides with changes in lifestyle and indicates that something is working (*38*). Others (*39–42*) pointed out weaknesses of these studies and warned of the dangers and ethical problems of not treating persons at high risk for CHD (*39,40*), or suggested that better results are obtained with newer cholesterol-lowering drugs such as simvastatin and lovastatin (*41*). Truswell pointed out that mortality patterns have been changing in different ways in different countries, and when contrasting trends are examined dietary change is the variable most consistently associated with trends in mortality (*42*). Another reader stressed that lifestyle interventions may change behavior, but not necessarily in a healthy direction: treating people who do not feel sick may lead to a variety of symptoms, including those of depression (*43*). To illustrate the intangibles, he cited a study of Italian Americans. The older subjects, obese smokers, had an unusually low incidence of heart disease. The younger generation tended not to smoke, ate a low-fat diet, held fast-track jobs, broke from community ties, and had an increased incidence of heart disease. One letter pointed out alleged misinterpretations of the Finnish study (*44*). Another applauded the suggested moratorium on use of cholesterol-lowering drugs on the grounds that even in high-risk groups the chance of having a myocardial infarction in a given 5-year period is small, so that treatment would expose many persons to the disadvantages of drug treatment with little probability of their realizing the advantages (*45*). A problem with the publicity that the cholesterol controversy has received is that people often draw erroneous conclusions from news reports, frustrating efforts of public health departments and physicians (*46*). Davey

Smith and Pekkanen (*47*) and Oliver (*48*) responded to these comments. The former emphasized that in the primary prevention of disease even a small adverse effect can outweigh any benefits and reiterated their belief that use of cholesterol-lowering drugs may be justified for primary prevention only in patients with severe familial hyperlipidemias.

Ramsay et al. reviewed 16 published trials of dietary reduction of serum cholesterol (*49*). When the step 1 diet was the intervention, net reduction in serum cholesterol was from 0% to 4% over 6 months to 6 years; reductions of 0.6–2.0% over 5–10 years were achieved through population education; combined population and individual dietary advice resulted in changes of from −2.1% to +1.0% over 4–10 years. For most adults, this response was too small to have clinical significance. Cholesterol reductions of 6.5–15.5% were achieved with more rigorous diets, but these diets were considered unpalatable to some degree. The authors believe it is unrealistic to depend on diet to reduce cholesterol concentrations in most adults. They warn against seeking out healthy people and turning them into patients by prescribing drugs when a step 1 diet fails to have the desired effect. Readers reported that the problem is not with the diet but with adherence to it (*50*). In their study of 30 young, healthy subjects, a moderately stringent diet (total fat 26 en%) was well accepted and brought about an 11–12% reduction in total serum cholesterol; it likely had other beneficial effects as well. An even larger effect would be anticipated in hypercholesterolemic subjects. Evans called attention to his own study published in 1972, in which an average cholesterol reduction of 22% was achieved in highly motivated hypercholesterolemic subjects through a program that educated the spouse who did the shopping and cooking, specified what to eat as well as what to avoid, and provided a book of tempting recipes (*51*). Complicating the picture, according to another reader, are the single-minded emphasis on cholesterol reduction and the self-serving interests of the "cholesterol industry" and some dietary experts who have much at stake in the controversy (*52*). The interpretation and analysis of Ramsay et al. were disputed by another reader (*53*). Ramsay et al. responded to all comments (*54*).

Two editorials and an invited letter addressed the puzzling relationship between cholesterol and violent death (*55–57*). In summarizing, Katz submits that "While we are not at a point where those of us with low serum cholesterol levels should eat a bit of extra saturated fat to reduce the risk of violent death, we should remain open-minded" and accept the challenge to solve the enigma (*55*). The issue is whether "excessive" cholesterol reduction might in some people produce membrane malfunction through unbalanced reduction of membrane cholesterol, and if it does, what would the malfunction and its clinical manifestations be (*56*). Oliver hypothesizes that the increase in plasma cholesterol levels in middle-aged men is partly adaptive, and interfering with it might be harmful. Some aging cells, for example, may lose their ability to adapt their receptor systems and cholesterol synthesis to changes in plasma phospholipids. The complex mechanisms regulating lipid peroxidation might also be disturbed. For cholesterol reduction to affect behavior, the cholesterol content of the brain (particularly of brain cell membranes) would have to be altered and this would have to alter neurological function (*57*). The available data, summarized by Mason et al., suggest that both may be true. Cholesterol is freely exchanged between serum and biological membranes (*58*). Engelberg proposes that reduction of serum cholesterol decreases the cholesterol content of brain cell membranes, which lowers lipid microviscosity and decreases the exposure of serotonin receptors on the membrane surface, which decreases the uptake of serotonin from blood and relaxes serotonin's inhibition of impulsive behavior. This idea needs to be tested, but existing information on cholesterol, serotonin, and behavior indicate that such an investigation would be fruitful. Some readers were intrigued by this hypothesis and offered further support for it (*59,60*); others advanced arguments to discredit it (*61–63*). Salter proposed an alternative hypothesis related to overall intake of dietary fat (*61*).

Some correspondence addressed a paper by Wysowski and Gross (*Arch. Intern. Med.* 150:2169–2172, 1990), who "explained away" the apparent excess of suicides and violent deaths in cholesterol-lowering trials by examining and accounting for these deaths case by case. Muldoon et al. (*64*) and Vasan (*65*) disputed the claim that the observed excess was "small" and due largely to alcoholism and psychiatric conditions present in some subjects when they entered the studies. It is not surprising that unnatural deaths associated with treatment occurred in the most susceptible persons, such as those with a drinking problem or mood swings; this does not rule out a role for cholesterol lowering in these deaths. That no plausible biological mechanism has been confirmed is a reason to search for one, not to deny its possibility. Wysowski and Gross defended their conclusions largely by citing poor compliance, dropouts, and coexistence of alcoholism and other problems (*66,67*).

Rossouw et al. reported that reanalysis of data on excess nonmedical deaths in secondary prevention trials failed to find an excess from either nonmedical causes or cancer (*68*). Secondary prevention trials differ from primary prevention trials in that more than 80% of deaths are from cardiovascular causes. Therefore a treatment that lowers cardiovascular mortality would be expected to reduce overall mortality.

Finally, after reviewing the literature on the cholesterol debate, Epstein concluded that there is no cause–effect association between low serum cholesterol or cholesterol lowering and risk of cancer, except perhaps at very low cholesterol levels (*69*). Nevertheless, more information is needed on the apparent increase in cancer mortality among men with very low levels of serum cholesterol that was seen in prospective epidemiological studies. However, there is a strong inverse relationship between noncardiovascular, noncancer mortality and serum cholesterol in intervention studies, and it is urgent to find the reasons for this. Epstein suspects that the association, though real, is not causal—that the explanation will be found in confounding factors or some factor independently linked to both low lipid levels and, for example, aggressiveness. The accuracy of death certification also needs to be verified for cases of noncardiovascular death because in cardiovascular studies other causes of death would be less carefully documented.

CARBOHYDRATES AND FIBER

A Nestlé Nutrition Workshop addressed topics such as historical, political, and economic aspects of sugar; and the biochemistry, metabolism, and physiologic and pathologic effects of various carbohydrates (*70*). Würsch's contribution and the ensuing discussion reviewed dietary fiber and unabsorbed carbohydrates in terms of their chemical and physical properties, metabolic and physiologic effects, and how these are altered by food technology (*71*). The metabolism of carbohydrates by the bacterial flora of the large intestine was discussed, especially with respect to production and fate of short-chain fatty acids. The role of undigestible carbohydrate in cancer prevention and cholesterol metabolism was reviewed.

The variety and complexity of dietary fibers pose many problems for investigators (*72*). Fibers are inevitably altered during isolation and purification, making data on individual fibers almost irrelevant to ordinary people eating whole foods outside the setting of a clinical trial. Whole high-fiber plant foods also supply many bioactive substances in addition to fiber. In assessing the health effects of such foods it also is necessary to consider that when people eat more high-fiber foods they eat less of something else. These problems have caused great confusion among scientists and the public. At the very least, it is necessary to distinguish clearly between the effects of high-fiber whole foods and fiber concentrates. Public perceptions of fiber in foods are especially diverse, partly because the layperson's concept of fiber as "roughage" long predates scientific uses of the term (*73*). The existence of a variety of terms used in a variety of ways makes fiber a vague concept for the public. Additional education about fiber in foods is recommended so people can make more rational food choices.

Individual fibers also have diverse effects. In rats, lactose acts like dietary fiber when it enters the cecum and colon (*74*). Its effects on nitrogen excretion and influence on the growth, metabolism, and species distribution of intestinal microorganisms was discussed. Beans provide beneficial dietary fiber. Two papers briefly reviewed the chemistry and physiological effects of soy fiber (*75*) and the classification and physiological effects of fibers with emphasis on that from dry beans (*76*). Both papers mentioned protective effects against various diseases, and other nutritional and economic benefits.

MINERALS

A publication from an international symposium on trace elements in man and animals contains sections on the metabolism of individual elements (including their bioavailability, essentiality, and toxicity); dietary requirements and intake of trace elements; roles of these elements in health, disease, infection and immunity, genetics, endocrinology, and calcium metabolism; soil–plant–animal relationships; and analytical methods (*77*). Papers from an international symposium on calcium-regulating hormones, body functions, and kidney were published in the *Contributions to Nephrology* series (*78*). Sections in this volume cover the role of calcium-regulating hormones in the relationship between calcium and hypertension, and the relationship between calcium and hypertension, arteriosclerosis, renal diseases, diabetes mellitus, and aging. Still another symposium addressed the role of calcium in cancer, hypertension and cardiovascular disease, and osteoporosis (*79*). This symposium identified important areas for future research. It is necessary to know whether a strategy for preventing or treating one condition will be beneficial or detrimental in terms of something else (must I trade one disease for another?). Studies of the comorbidity of diseases (e.g., osteoporosis and colon cancer, kidney stone formation and hypertension or colon cancer, or hypertension and stomach cancer) are needed. Nutrient–nutrient interactions, such as between fat and calcium, need further study. People eat food, not nutrients: food is a complex combination of nutrients that interact with each other and nonnutrient food constituents. A very interesting question is the significance of defective diet at different stages of life. To what extent is it possible (or impossible) to "make up for" a poor diet during one stage by proper attention to nutrition during another?

OXIDANT DEFENSE

While depending on oxidative metabolism for life, aerobic organisms must defend themselves against oxidative damage. Bermond comprehensively reviewed the biological oxidative environment, biological antioxidant systems (the different types of food antioxidants and their protective mechanisms), risk situations for oxidative damage and diseases related to these situations, and safety of antioxidant substances (*80*; 301 references). The overview of a symposium on antioxidants in health and disease summarizes the types of life-sustaining roles of oxygen and free radicals and then deals with selected aspects of the antioxidant control system, chiefly lipid-soluble and nonenzymatic factors (*81*). A paper in this symposium reviews the antioxidant properties of carotenoids, verified by studies using carotenoids with no pro-vitamin A activity (*82*). In a model system using soybean lipoxygenase for enzymatic generation of peroxyl radicals, the authors found that β-carotene inhibits oxidation of linoleic acid and formation of the hydroperoxide product. They discussed the bleaching of β-carotene by soybean lipoxygenase and its possible significance. From a different approach, Tee reviewed carotenoids and retinoids in human nutrition (*83*; 237 references). The history of these substances is traced from the earliest documented recognition of vitamin A deficiency at least 3500 years ago in Egypt and China. Their structure, nomenclature, physical and chemical properties, biosynthesis and metabolism, occurrence, and functions are discussed. Epidemiological, clinical, and laboratory studies of the role of carotenoids and retinoids in different diseases are reviewed, including results in some primary prevention and treatment trials.

Lipid peroxidation is a deteriorative reaction associated with aging, lung injury, alcoholic liver disease, atherosclerosis, initiation and promotion of cancer, and some degenerative diseases. Like carotenoids, vitamin E protects against free radical–induced damage to cellular lipids. Odeleye et al. designed experiments with rats to stimulate production of free radicals by feeding ethanol, test whether increasing dietary PUFAs during ethanol feeding would increase the levels of damaging lipid peroxidation products, and evaluate the effects of vitamin E on these processes (*84*). Vitamin E supplementation sharply reduced ethane exhalation (a measure of lipid peroxidation) in rats fed ethanol, cod liver oil, or both. Significant reduction of hepatic lipid peroxidation products in vitamin E–fed rats was also demonstrated. Palozza and Krinsky exposed hexane solutions of rat liver microsomal lipids to a radical initiator to study the mechanisms by which α-tocopherol and β-carotene inhibit radical-initiated peroxidation (*85*). A lag phase in formation of conjugated dienes occurred with concentrations of the initiator <4 mM, suggesting inhibition by endogenous antioxidants, presumably tocopherols. At 4 mM initiator, diene production was linear for at least 120 min. Under these conditions, both α-tocopherol and β-carotene produced a concentration-dependent lag in diene production, which presumably represented the time required to deplete the antioxidant. Their effects were additive. After the lag, diene formation resumed at a rate comparable to that in the absence of antioxidant. Similar results were obtained when formation of malondialdehyde was monitored. β-Carotene also appeared to protect endogenous tocopherols from radical-initiated destruction in this system. The results support the idea that the chain-propagating peroxyl radical is trapped by these antioxidants.

Restricted energy intake is another form of oxidant defense, as discussed in a brief review (*86*). In particular, dietary restriction can protect against damage to DNA from free radicals (*87*). 8-Hydroxy-deoxyguanosine (8-OH-dG) was measured as an indicator of oxidative damage in nuclear and mitochondrial DNA of rats fed ad libitum (controls) or fed 60% of the amount eaten by controls. Levels of 8-OH-dG hydroxydeoxyguanosine were twice as high in mitochondrial as in nuclear DNA, supporting the idea that mitochondria are exposed to greater oxidative stress because they are the major cellular site of free radical production. Dietary restriction significantly reduced 8-OH-dG in nuclei by ~30% and in mitochondria by >20%.

Radiation induces cellular damage through peroxidative effects. In mice, long-term consumption (in drinking water) of the major phenolic constituent of green tea prevented radiation-induced increase of lipid peroxides in liver and significantly prolonged life after lethal whole-body X-irradiation (*88*). The effect on survival was much less than would be predicted from the near-total prevention of radiation-induced hepatic lipid peroxidation, indicating that other factors are also involved in radiation-induced injury and death. The protective substance is (–)-epigallocatechin 3-*O*-gallate, which accounts for up to 10% of the dry weight of unfermented *Thea sinensis* or 8.7 g/kg of fresh leaves. Oolong tea (semifermented *Camellia sinensis*) contains only one-tenth this amount; black tea (fermented *Camellia sinensis*) contains still less.

SPECIAL FOODS AND DIETS

A volume in the *Advances in Meat Research* series was devoted to topics concerning meat and health (*89*). These included content and effects of fatty acids from meat, the relationship between blood cholesterol and dietary cholesterol, meat and cancer, toxic substances produced during processing and cooking, residues and pathogens in meat and meat products, nutrients provided by meat, and recent advances in meat technology. Meat from wild animals and aquatic sources is not discussed. An overview of the volume provides historical background on procurement, preservation, and consumption of meat and discusses current patterns and trends in meat consumption (*90*). Health concerns are briefly mentioned.

Grundy asks whether red meat has a place in healthy diets (*91*). Although it contains saturated fats and fairly large amounts of cholesterol, lean red meat is less hypercholesterolemic than widely believed. If consumption of red meat does not exceed 6 ounces per day, intake of cholesterol can easily be kept below the recommended limit. In pigs, both types and amounts of fat can be altered by dietary manipulation; but it is not possible in practice to significantly modify the fatty acid composition of beef. The association between meat intake and risk for CHD and various cancers is discussed. One explanation for a meat–cancer connection lies in meat's fat content; hence the best advice might be, eat lean meat and trim the fat. However, people who eat a lot of meat are likely to eat less of other things that might protect against disease. Data on young adults from the CARDIA study, conducted in 1985 and 1986, showed that frequent meat-eaters tended to drink more alcohol than infrequent meat-eaters; and their diet contained more energy, fat, and protein, and less carbohydrate, starch, fiber, vitamins A and C, and calcium (*92*). Overall, young adults who ate meat infrequently also differed in other dietary and lifestyle practices that could be expected to have an influence on their health.

The consequences of vegetarianism for nutrition and health were reviewed by Dwyer (*93*). She discussed the range of eating styles compatible with health, nutrient deficiencies that may arise on vegetarian diets, and the relationship of vegetarianism to risk factors for degenerative and other diseases, particularly with respect to the life cycle. In Finland, 42 omnivorous adults and 28 lactovegetarians participated in a 7-month study to evaluate the effects of a low-fat lactovegetarian diet on health parameters (*94*). Twenty-one of the omnivorous subjects switched to a lactovegetarian diet; all other subjects maintained their customary diets. The lactovegetarian diet had a favorable effect on serum concentrations of cholesterol and retinol, but effects on serum apolipoproteins A-1, B, and C-II, α-tocopherol, and triglycerides were minimal and no group showed changes in weight, body mass index, defecation frequency, or maximal oxygen intake during the study. However, the "new" lactovegetarians reported changes in their perceived health. These were more pronounced during the first two months, but throughout the study subjects reported enhanced alertness and less constipation. Serum concentrations of 25-hydroxy-vitamin D fluctuated with the seasons; the wintertime reduction was greatest in subjects on the lactovegetarian diet.

In discussing the promise of biotechnology and the safety evaluation of novel foods, Miller pointed out that "we are talking about the regulation of homeostasis at the molecular level" (*95*). Specifically, he is referring to the role of diet in regulating activation, deactivation, and detoxification of xenobiotics and the impact of xenobiotics on the availability and utilization of nutrients. This involves a very complex, multifactorial set of events and places enormous responsibility on those who evaluate the wholesomeness and safety of the food supply. Miller states that a new discipline is required for evaluation of wholesomeness; the fragmented disciplines of nutrition, toxicology, microbiology, etc. are no longer equal to the task.

Microalgae and cyanobacteria are drawing increasing intention as food and food supplements (*96*). Food-grade microalgae are already used as a source of colorants and to extend shelf life. They are constituents of pastas, snack foods, candy, gum, and beverages and are available as supplements because of their putative health benefits. This review summarizes the considerable nutritional and economic advantages of cultivated microalgae and their promise for developed and developing countries. Some common genera, such as *Chlorella, Scenedesmus,* and *Spirulina* (cyanobacteria) are considered individually. Possible risks and negative effects are mentioned. Although the miraculous claims sometimes made for these tiny organisms may be overenthusiastic, microalgae have potential to provide not only economic and nutritious food but also a source of new compounds of nutritional and biological interest.

LITERATURE CITED

1. Lachance, P.A. Diet–health relationship. In *Food Safety Assessment,* J.W. Finley, S.F. Robinson, and D.J. Armstrong (eds.). Washington, DC, American Chemical Society. *ACS Symp. Ser.* 484:278–296 (1992).

2. Diet, nutrition and the prevention of chronic diseases. A report of the WHO Study Group on Diet, Nutrition and Prevention of Noncommunicable Diseases. (Excerpted from executive summary of report by

the editors of *Nutrition Reviews*). *Nutr. Rev.* 49:291–301 (1991).

3. Ulbricht, T. Dietary habits and disease patterns across Europe. *Food Policy* (Oct.):425–426 (1991).

4. Buzina, R., K. Suboticanec, and M. Saric. Diet patterns and health problems: diet in southern Europe. *Ann. Nutr. Metab.* 35(Suppl. 1):32–40 (1991).

5. Sanders, T.A.B. The Mediterranean diet: fish and olives, oil on troubled waters. *Proc. Nutr. Soc.* 50:513–517 (1991).

6. Fidanza, F. The Mediterranean Italian diet: keys to contemporary thinking. *Proc. Nutr. Soc.* 50:519–526 (1991).

7. Kohlmeier, L., and R. Dortschy. Diet and disease in East and West Germany. *Proc. Nutr. Soc.* 50:719–727 (1991).

8. Hirayama, T. Diet and mortality. In *Life-Style and Mortality: A Large-Scale Census-Based Cohort Study in Japan.* Basel, Karger. *Contrib. Epidemiol. Biostat.* 6:93–95 (1990).

9. Burnett, C., J. Gittleman, and N. Lalich. Preventable mortality in the restaurant industry. (Abstract.) *Am. J. Epidemiol.* 134:743 (1991).

10. Evers, S. Diet–disease relationships: public health perspectives. *Prog. Food Nutr. Sci.* 15:61–83 (1991).

11. Macdonald, I. (ed.). *Monitoring Dietary Intakes.* New York, Springer-Verlag. *ILSI Monographs* (1991).

12. Randall, E., J.R. Marshall, S. Graham, and J. Brasure. High-risk health behaviors associated with various dietary patterns. *Nutr. Cancer* 16:135–151 (1991).

13. Preston, A.M. Cigarette smoking—nutritional implications. *Prog. Food Nutr. Sci.* 15:183–217 (1991).

14. Sellers, T.A., L.H. Kushi, and J.D. Potter. Can dietary intake patterns account for the familial aggregation of disease? Evidence from adult siblings living apart. *Genet. Epidemiol.* 8:105–112 (1991).

15. Widdowson, E.M., and A. Whiten (eds.). *Foraging Strategies and Natural Diet of Monkeys, Apes and Humans. Phil. Trans. R. Soc. Lond. B* 334:159–295 (1991).

16. Foley, R.A., and P.C. Lee. Ecology and energetics of encephalization in hominid evolution. *Phil. Trans. Roy. Soc. Lond. B* 334:223–232 (1991).

17. Crawford, M.A. The role of dietary fatty acids in biology: their place in the evolution of the human brain. *Nutr. Rev.* 50:3–11 (1992).

18. Ulijaszek, S.J. Human dietary change. *Phil. Trans. Roy. Soc. Lond. B* 334:271–279 (1991).

19. O'Dea, K. Traditional diet and food preferences of Australian aboriginal hunter–gatherers. *Phil. Trans. Roy. Soc. Lond. B* 334:233–241 (1991).

20. Zimmet, P., S. Serjeantson, G. Dowse, et al. Diabetes mellitus and cardiovascular disease in developing populations: hunter–gatherers in the fast lane. In *Sugars in Nutrition.* M. Gracey, N. Kretchmer, and E. Rossi (eds.) New York, Vevey/Raven Press, Ltd. *Nestlé Nutrition Workshop Series* 25:197–212 (1991).

21. Nobmann, E.D., T. Byers, A.P. Lanier, et al. The diet of Alaska Native adults: 1987–1988. *Am. J. Clin. Nutr.* 55:1024–1032 (1992).

22. Widdowson, E.M. Contemporary human diets and their relation to health and growth: overview and conclusions. *Phil. Trans. Roy. Soc. Lond. B* 334:289–295 (1991).

23. Bray, G.A. A health and nutritional perspective on fat, cholesterol, and risks to health. *Adv. Appl. Biotechnol.* 12:13–19 (1991).

24. Sardesai, V.M. Nutritional role of polyunsaturated fatty acids. *J. Nutr. Biochem.* 3:154–166 (1992).

25. Simopoulos, A.P. Omega-3 fatty acids in health and disease and in growth and development. *Am. J. Clin. Nutr.* 54:438–463 (1991).

26. Elson, C.E. Tropical oils: nutritional and scientific issues. *Crit. Rev. Food Sci. Nutr.* 31:79–102 (1992).

27. Meydani, S.N. Modulation of cytokine production by dietary polyunsaturated fatty acids. *Proc. Soc. Exp. Biol. Med.* 200:189–193 (1992).

28. Clandinin, M.T., S. Cheema, C.J. Field, et al. Dietary fat: exogenous determination of membrane structure and cell function. *FASEB J.* 5:2761–2769 (1991).

29. Koletzko, B. *Trans* fatty acids may impair biosynthesis of long-chain polyunsaturates and growth in man. *Acta Pædiatrica* 81:302–306 (1992).

30. Cunnane, S.C., Z.-Y. Chen, J. Yang, et al. α-Linolenic acid in humans: direct functional role or dietary precursor? *Nutrition* 7:437–439 (1991).

31. Whelan, J., K.S. Broughton, M.E. Surette, and J.E. Kinsella. Dietary arachidonic and linoleic acids: comparative effects on tissue lipids. *Lipids* 27:85–88 (1992).

32. Charnock, J.S., M.Y. Abeywardena, V.M. Poletti, and P.L. McLennan. Differences in fatty acid composition of various tissues of the marmoset monkey (*Callithrix jacchus*) after different lipid supplemented diets. *Comp. Biochem. Physiol.* 101A:387–393 (1992).

33. Davey Smith, G., M.J. Shipley, M.G. Marmot, and G. Rose. Plasma cholesterol concentration and mortality. *JAMA* 267:70–76 (1992).

34. Goldstein, M.R. Cholesterol and noncardiac mortality. (Letter.) *JAMA* 267:2740–2741 (1992).

35. Davey Smith, G. Cholesterol and noncardiac mortality. (Reply.) *JAMA* 267:2741 (1992).

36. Davey Smith, G., and J. Pekkanen. Should there be a moratorium on the use of cholesterol lowering drugs? *Br. Med. J.* 304:431–434 (1992).

37. Oliver, M.F. Doubts about preventing coronary heart disease. *Br. Med. J.* 304:393–394 (1992).

38. O'Connor, M. The cholesterol controversy. (Letter.) *Br. Med. J.* 304:711 (1992).

39. Reckless, J.P.D. The cholesterol controversy. (Letter.) *Br. Med. J.* 304:712 (1992).

40. Winder, T. The cholesterol controversy. (Letter.) *Br. Med. J.* 304:712–713 (1992).

41. Tobert, J.A. The cholesterol controversy. (Letter.) *Br. Med. J.* 304:712 (1992).

42. Truswell, A.S. The cholesterol controversy. (Letter.) *Br. Med. J.* 304:912–913 (1992).

43. Thomas, P. The cholesterol controversy. (Letter.) *Br. Med. J.* 304:912 (1992).

44. Ryan, M.F., A. Moran, and A.F. Jones. The cholesterol controversy. (Letter.) *Br. Med. J.* 304:711–712 (1992).

45. Ryabinski, E.A. The cholesterol controversy. (Letter.) *Br. Med. J.* 304:712 (1992).

46. Polanska, A.I. The cholesterol controversy. (Letter.) *Br. Med. J.* 304:712 (1992).

47. Davey Smith, G., and J. Pekkanen. The cholesterol controversy. (Reply.) *Br. Med. J.* 304:913 (1992).

48. Oliver, M.F. The cholesterol controversy. (Reply.) *Br. Med. J.* 304:913 (1992).

49. Ramsay, L.E., W.W. Yeo, and P.R. Jackson. Dietary reduction of serum cholesterol concentration: time to think again. *Br. Med. J.* 303:953–957 (1991).

50. Marckmann, P., and B. Sandstrom. Dietary reduction of serum cholesterol concentration. (Letter.) *Br. Med. J.* 303:1331–1332 (1991).

51. Evans, D.W. Dietary reduction of serum cholesterol concentration. (Letter.) *Br. Med. J.* 303:1332 (1991).

52. Skrabanek, P. Dietary reduction of serum cholesterol concentration. (Letter.) *Br. Med. J.* 303:1332 (1991).

53. Thompson, G.R. Dietary reduction of serum cholesterol concentration. (Letter.) *Br. Med. J.* 303:1332 (1991).

54. Ramsay, L.E., W.W. Yeo, and P.R. Jackson. Dietary reduction of serum cholesterol concentration. (Reply.) *Br. Med. J.* 303:1332–1333 (1991); *Br. Med. J.* 303:1551 (1991).

55. Katz, A.M. Cholesterol and violent death. *J. Mol. Cell Cardiol.* 23:1343–1344 (1991).

56. Oliver, M.F. Might reduction of plasma cholesterol imperil cell physiology? (Letter.) *J. Mol. Cell Cardiol.* 23:1335–1337 (1991).

57. Mason, R.P., L.G. Herbette, and D.I. Silverman. Can altering serum cholesterol affect neurologic function? *J. Mol. Cell Cardiol.* 23:1339–1342 (1991).

58. Engelberg, H. Low serum cholesterol and suicide. *Lancet* 339:727–728 (1992).

59. Barradas, M.A., D.P. Mikhailidis, and A.F. Winder. Low serum cholesterol and suicide. (Letter.) *Lancet* 339:1168 (1992).

60. Oliver, M.F. Low serum cholesterol and suicide. (Letter.) *Lancet* 339:1168–1169 (1992).

61. Salter, M. Low serum cholesterol and suicide. (Letter.) *Lancet* 339:1169 (1992).

62. Severs, N.J. Low serum cholesterol and suicide. (Letter.) *Lancet* 339:1001 (1992).

63. Brunner, E., G. Davey Smith, J. Pilgrim, and M. Marmot. Low serum cholesterol and suicide. (Letter.) *Lancet* 339:1001–1002 (1992).

64. Muldoon, M.F., S.B. Manuck, and K.A. Matthews. Does cholesterol lowering increase non–illness-related mortality? (Letter.) *Arch. Intern. Med.* 151:1453 (1991).

65. Vasan, R.S. Lowering cholesterol and death due to accidents, suicides: unresolved issues. (Letter.) *Arch. Intern. Med.* 152:414 (1992).

66. Wysowski, D.K., and T.P. Gross. Lowering cholesterol and death due to accidents, suicides: unresolved issues. (Reply.) *Arch. Intern. Med.* 152:414,417 (1992).

67. Wysowski, D.K., and T.P. Gross. Does cholesterol lowering increase non–illness-related mortality? (Reply.) *Arch. Intern. Med.* 151:1453–1454 (1991).

68. Rossouw, J.E., P.L. Canner, and S.B. Hulley. Deaths from injury, violence, and suicide in secondary prevention trials of cholesterol lowering. (Letter.) *New Engl. J. Med.* 325:1813 (1991).

69. Epstein, F.H. Low serum cholesterol, cancer and other noncardiovascular disorders. *Atherosclerosis* 94:1–12 (1992).

70. Gracey, M., N. Kretchmer, and E. Rossi (eds.). *Sugars in Nutrition.* New York, Raven Press. *Nestlé Nutrition Workshop Series* 25 (1991).

71. Würsch, P. Dietary fiber and unabsorbed carbohydrates. In *Sugars in Nutrition.* M. Gracey et al. (eds.). *Nestlé Nutrition Workshop Series* 25:153–168 (1991).

72. Spiller, G.A. Beyond dietary fiber. *Am. J. Clin. Nutr.* 54:615–617 (1991).

73. Sobal, J., and C.M. Cassidy. Public perceptions of fiber in foods. *Ecol. Food Nutr.* 26:303–312 (1991).

74. Schulze, J., and H.-J. Zunft. Lactose—ein potentieller Ballaststoff. Zur Regulierung ihrer microökologischen Wirksamkeit im Intestinaltrakt. 3. Mitt. Ballaststoffwirkung der Lactose also Folge microbieller Aktivität. *Nahrung* 35:903–920 (1991).

75. Slavin, J. Nutritional benefits of soy protein and soy fiber. *J. Am. Diet. Assoc.* 91:816–819 (1991).

76. Hughes, J.S. Potential contribution of dry bean dietary fiber to health. *Food Technol.* 45(9):122–126 (1991).

77. Momcilovic, B. (ed.). Seventh International Symposium on Trace Elements in Man and Animals. *Trace Elements in Man and Animals* 7 (1991).

78. Moril, H. (ed.). *Calcium-Regulating Hormones. I. Role in Disease and Ageing.* Contrib. Nephrol. 90 (1991).

79. Rivlin, R.S. Summary and conclusions: areas for further study. *Am. J. Clin. Nutr.* 54:288S–290S (1991).

80. Bermond, P. Biological effects of food antioxidants. In *Food Antioxidants.* B.J.F. Hudson (ed.). New York, Elsevier Applied Science. Elsevier Applied Food Science Series. Pp. 193–251 (1990).

81. Olson, J.A., and S. Kobayashi. Antioxidants in health and disease: overview. *Proc. Soc. Exp. Biol. Med.* 200:245–247 (1992).

82. Canfield, L.M., J.W. Forage, and J.G. Valenzuela. Carotenoids as cellular antioxidants. *Proc. Soc. Exp. Biol. Med.* 200:260–265 (1992).

83. Tee, E-S. Carotenoids and retinoids in human nutrition. *Crit. Rev. Food Sci. Nutr.* 31:103–163 (1992).

84. Odeleye, O.E., C.D. Eskelson, R.R. Watson, et al. Vitamin E reduction of lipid peroxidation products in rats fed cod liver oil and ethanol. *Alcohol* 8:273–277 (1991).

85. Palozza, P., and N.I. Krinsky. The inhibition of radical-initiated peroxidation of microsomal lipids by both α-tocopherol and β-carotene. *Free Rad. Biol. Med.* 11:407–414 (1991).

86. Anonymous. Energy intake restriction and oxidant defense. *Nutr. Rev.* 49:278–280 (1991).

87. Chung, M.H., H. Kasai, S. Nishimura, and B.P. Yu. Protection of DNA damage by dietary restriction. *Free Rad. Biol. Med.* 12:523–525 (1992).

88. Uchida, S., M. Ozaki, K. Suzuki, and M. Shikita. Radioprotective effects of (–)-epigallocatechin 3-*O*-gallate (green-tea tannin) in mice. *Life Sci.* 50:147–152 (1992).

89. Pearson, A.M., and T.R. Dutson (eds.). *Meat and Health. Adv. Meat Res.* 6 (1990).

90. Briggs, G.M., and B.S. Schweigert. An overview of meat in the diet. *Adv. Meat Res.* 6:1–20 (1990).

91. Grundy, S.M. Does red meat have a role in healthy diets? In *Biotechnology for Control of Growth and Product Quality in Meat Production: Implications and Acceptability.* P. van der Wal, G.M. Wever, and F.J. van der Wilt (eds.). Proceedings of an International Symposium, Washington, DC, 5–7 Dec. 1990. Wageningen, Pudoc. Pp. 195–203 (1991).

92. Slattery, M.L., D.R. Jacobs, Jr., J.E. Hilner, et al. Meat consumption and its associations with other diet and health factors in young adults: the CARDIA study. *Am. J. Clin. Nutr.* 54:930–935 (1991).

93. Dwyer, J.T. Nutritional consequences of vegetarianism. *Annu. Rev. Nutr.* 11:61–91 (1991).

94. Mäenpää, P., A. Karinpää, M. Jauhiainen, et al. Effects of low-fat lactovegetarian diet on health parameters of adult subjects. *Ecol. Food Nutr.* 25:255–267 (1991).

95. Miller, S.A. Novel foods: safety and nutrition. *Food Technol.* 46(3):114–117 (1992).

96. Kay, R.A. Microalgae as food and supplement. *Crit. Rev. Food Sci. Nutr.* 30:555–573 (1991).

2

Diet and Cancer

Overview
Epidemiology
Clinical and laboratory studies

OVERVIEW

The link between diet and cancer is firmly established in principle. Milner reviewed the information about nutrients and nonnutrients whose effects on carcinogenesis have been verified, particularly those for which mechanisms of action can be explored (*1*). At the same time he emphasized that the overall diet, not a single dietary component, is what can turn events toward or away from cancer. A corollary of this is that when cancer occurs, the dietary culprit is unlikely to be a contaminant or carcinogen taken out of the context of the total diet. This idea was underscored in a historical look at interest in the link between diet and cancer (*2*). According to traditional wisdom, malignancies arise from exposure to carcinogens, which were therefore the main target for research. But the list of chemical carcinogens grew so fast and so large that it became impossible to identify which ones pose a significant hazard, let alone to know what to do about it. Meanwhile, epidemiologists were proposing "life-style" hypotheses emphasizing dietary pattern. According to this line of thinking, the overall diet modulates the influence of a host of carcinogenic and anticarcinogenic agents.

The proceedings of a conference on nutrition and cancer were published as a supplement to *Cancer Research* (*3*). Sessions at this conference were devoted to fats and energy, micronutrients and microconstituents, diet-associated carcinogens and mutagens, and mechanisms and risk assessment. In his keynote address, Doll spoke of the emergence of consensus among epidemiologists that diet might be responsible for 30–60% of cancers in developed countries—and that reduction of this effect would require decreasing consumption of fat, increasing consumption of fruits, vegetables, fibers, and certain micronutrients, and perhaps improving methods of food preservation (*4*). He reviewed dietary trends and trends in cancer incidence and mortality, with examples for specific countries and cancer sites. His conclusions are encouraging: dietary changes that might reduce risk of fatal cancer by 20–60% are practicable, and such changes have probably already contributed to recent reductions in

the incidence of cancers of the stomach, colon, rectum, gallbladder, ovary, and endometrium. Participants in a panel discussion looked to future lines of inquiry that might be productive given the new perspective on diet and cancer (*5*).

A lively article highlighted some recent reviews of issues related to cancer and diet (*6*). The author rationalized the discrepant findings of a study linking meat consumption with colon cancer in North American nurses and a case–control study in Japan that demonstrated an inverse relationship. Other dietary and nondietary factors varied so greatly between studies that it was pointless to consider the results out of their context. Reviews of fiber, cereals, sugar, and even hot peppers were touched on.

Another review discussed the mechanisms of neoplastic conversion and the subsequent growth and development of neoplastic cells (*7*). Cancers of specific sites were considered in terms of mechanisms, geography, and nutritional traditions. One of a pair of complementary tables summarized causes of cancer in North America: lifestyle (related to tobacco, diet, alcohol, sun, mycotoxin, and hepatitis B virus); transplacental chemicals; occupational; cryptogenic (viruses?); iatrogenic; multifactorial; and unspecified. The other listed specific actions that would promote health and lower risk of various chronic diseases.

In an important initiative, the National Cancer Institute signed agreements with the Food and Drug Administration (FDA) and private companies and institutions to test foods for cancer prevention (*8*). The goal is to exploit the protective properties of natural phytochemicals by incorporating them into new fortified food products. The first studies will use fractions from citrus fruits, garlic, flaxseed, soybeans, and the parsley–carrot–celery family of vegetables. Later studies will be based on the most promising candidates from the initial groups plus cruciferous and solanaceous vegetables and combinations. Safety studies in animals will be followed by intervention trials in people at high risk for cancer. A positive outcome from these studies has been anticipated by several food companies that have already begun their own "designer food" projects. Meanwhile, epidemiologists from seven European countries have launched a prospective 5-year (or longer) dietary study in which more than 250,000 people will keep detailed food diaries and provide blood samples for analysis (9). In conjunction with this the effect of hormone replacement therapy will be studied in Great Britain.

It is important to know how the public perceives the role of dietary and other environmental factors in the causation and prevention of cancer, to maximize the impact of public health programs (10). A postal survey in South Australia revealed a relatively high degree of awareness and acceptance of lifestyle factors as determinants of cancer risk. This awareness extended with few differences to all sociodemographic groups. The roles of diet and cigarette smoking were widely recognized, but the importance of pollution of the food supply was overestimated relative to nutrient imbalance. In this setting, the most effective public health efforts would most likely be ones directed at skill transfer and removal of barriers to change.

In discussing the future of nutrition research in cancer prevention, Greenwald first reviewed the role of specific dietary factors in cancer risk (11). He then described ongoing and proposed research programs, with emphasis on the extramural programs of the National Cancer Institute. Dietary guidelines developed by various organizations and government agencies were summarized. The author then identified gaps in knowledge, named some important areas for future research, and discussed changes in the food supply that have implications for health.

A volume in a series on nutrition dealt with the subject of vitamins and cancer prevention (12). The book is based on presentations at the Gladys Emerson Memorial symposium held at UCLA on 2–3 March 1989. Approaches range from basic laboratory research to clinical studies to preliminary studies of vitamin deficiency in cancer patients. Chapters address the role of specific vitamins in preventing or treating cancer and the mechanisms by which vitamins protect against neoplasia. Of particular interest are discussions of folate, 1,25-dihydroxyvitamin D_3, and coenzyme Q_{10}. A conference at the National Institutes of Health, September 1990, was devoted

to the biologic functions of ascorbic acid and its relation to cancer (13). Presentations considered vitamin C in relation to free radical scavenging, regulation of cellular and enzymatic function, the immune system, malignant transformation and growth of tumor cells, therapeutic applications, and dietary requirements.

Although a link between cancer and high consumption of red meat is frequently taken as proved, Kritchevsky's review suggests that a cause–effect relationship is far from established (14). For example, in the USA between 1940 and 1970 per capita meat consumption more than doubled, while cancer mortality was virtually unchanged. Further, risk of colon cancer did not show the socioeconomic gradient exhibited by meat consumption. Overall, 6 of 11 case–control studies of colon cancer found a positive association with meat consumption, 1 found a negative association, and 4 found none. Nor have epidemiologic studies of other types of cancer yielded convincing evidence that simply deleting beef (or meat) from the typical American diet would substantially reduce cancer risk. Having established this point, Kritchevsky reviewed animal and clinical studies of meat components, specifically protein, fat, and cholesterol. Again, results are inconclusive and sometimes surprising. Protein and fat may merely reflect the real culprit, affluence, which is manifested in excessive energy consumption and insufficient energy expenditure. Evidence for this is reviewed.

While evidence accumulates for a protective effect of wheat (15) and other fiber against cancer, the FDA has hesitated to allow health claims for fiber in nutrition labeling (16). Nevertheless, they do endorse dietary guidelines recommending daily intake of 25 g of dietary fiber. While the distinction between health claims and dietary guidelines may be important in some circles, it should not obscure the message that fiber is a crucial constituent of a healthful diet.

A discussion of the "fat hypothesis" and cancer evaluated results of laboratory, clinical, and epidemiological studies (17). It concludes that although many lines of investigation converge upon fat as the main culprit in carcinogenesis, it is nearly impossible to control for the multitude of confounding factors. The authors believe that as the picture becomes more complex, more evidence points against the fat hypothesis than toward it. Further, they point out that after the key gene changes in carcinogenesis are known, nutrition's impact on the incidence and repair of DNA damage must still be understood.

Messina and Messina reviewed the use of soy foods and their potential role in cancer prevention (*18*). One of the sacred crops of ancient China, soybeans contain several substances with anticarcinogenic activity. Among these, protease inhibitors and phytic acid have traditionally been considered "antinutrients" but are beginning to be viewed in a positive light. Increasingly, the importance of nonnutrient phytochemicals is being recognized, and soybeans are rich in them.

A lead article in *Science* discusses possibilities for the primary prevention of cancer (*19*). We are at "the threshold of an era when many of the most prevalent human cancers can, to a significant extent, be prevented through lifestyle changes or medical interventions." This bold statement is defended by a review of trends in incidence and mortality rates of major cancers and analysis of why these changes have occurred.

EPIDEMIOLOGY

Cancer epidemiologists are eager to exploit Europe's opportunities to understand the causes of cancer (*20*). Each of some two dozen nations has its own distinctive cuisine, customs, climate, genetic makeup, and cancer rates; these factors frequently vary regionally within a country, as well. Europe's largest epidemiological database is being established at the International Agency for Research on Cancer in Lyons, France. A wide range of prospective studies are in the planning stage. Some patterns have already been identified: for example, south-to-north gradients in death rates for all cancers, lung, breast, and colon cancer, and malignant melanoma. The rarer cancers of the liver, esophagus, larynx, and buccal cavity are more frequent in the south.

In epidemiology, case–control and cohort studies can be viewed as alternative conceptualizations of the same problem (*21*). Although two major types of bias, selection and recall, occur more frequently in the former, case–control studies are generally more manageable in terms of size and cost. The authors weighed the advantages and disadvantages of case–control studies on the role of nutrition in cancer etiology and discussed several studies done in Athens. For colorectal, stomach, breast, and lung cancer, diverticulosis, and cholelithiasis, high vegetable intake was generally protective, whereas evidence for other food groups and constituents was variable and less convincing.

Difficulties in interpreting cancer incidence and mortality data were discussed by Doll (*22*). Mortality data have historically been more complete and reliable than incidence data, but the correlation between incidence and mortality has become progressively weaker since about 1960, when rapid progress in cancer treatment began. With the establishment of comprehensive tumor registries and screening programs, incidence data have become more complete, but as a result much of the "increase" in cancer incidence may be more apparent than real. Although this paper was a general epidemiologic assessment of progress against cancer, Doll's points apply to studies of nutrition and cancer and he specifically considered changes possibly related to fat consumption. Noting that fat disappearance statistics in several countries parallel decreases in incidence of colon cancer, he proposed other factors that could account for at least part of the change. These include a trend to classify cancers of the colorectal junction as rectal rather than colonic, increased consumption of nondigestible carbohydrates and perhaps cruciferous vegetables, and widespread use of prophylactic colectomy for familial adenomatous polyposis. Reduced incidence of ovarian and endometrial cancer could be due at least in part to use of newer combined steroid contraceptives. If reduced intake of saturated fat has had a beneficial influence on incidence of breast and prostate cancers, this has been masked by other factors (such as widespread screening programs) causing these cancers to be recorded more often.

Cross-cultural epidemiologic cancer research in Hawaii has been facilitated by the Hawaii Tumor Registry (*23*). Descriptive studies reveal wide ethnic diversity in cancer incidence and survival, which correlates with culture and lifestyle, particularly dietary practices. Incidence rates are presented for men and women by site and ethnicity. These data are discussed in terms of diet and compared with populations in the respective homelands. Similar studies in Argentina found that mortality rates from gastric cancer were higher in most countries of origin than in the respective Argentinean immigrants and were lowest of all in native-born Argentineans (*24*). In contrast, mortality from esophageal cancer was higher in Argentina than in Europe. Only Uruguay and Germany had higher mortality rates than Argentina for breast and colon cancer, and migrants' risk for these cancers converged toward that of Argentinean natives. Risk for liver cancer was somewhat lower in South American migrants to Argentina. Differences existed for cancers of other sites as well. When variation in the reliability of death certification and other confounding factors and biases were considered, dietary variables—most notably meat, fat, and beer consumption—remained an important probable influence.

The lifestyle of Seventh-Day Adventists (particularly in its emphasis on vegetarianism and abstinence from biblical "unclean" foods, drugs, alcohol, tobacco, and caffeine-containing beverages) is regarded as protective against cancer. In Norway, where the incidence of cancer is generally low, the standardized incidence ratio (SIR) for Seventh-Day Adventists (compared with the general population) did not differ significantly from unity (*25*). For lung and other respiratory cancers and "other unspecified diagnoses" the SIR was somewhat lower for Seventh-Day Adventists; for cancer of the uterine corpus and "other female genital" cancers it was higher. Incidence rates in relatively new members tended to exceed rates for long-time members, but the study did not distinguish between religiously active and inactive Adventists. A possible conclusion from this study is that the main factors in cancer etiology in Norway are different from the factors in which Seventh-Day Adventists differ from the general population.

A study in western New York state looked at the role of putative cancer risk factors embedded in dietary patterns (*26*). Seven dietary patterns were identified in men and seven in women. Associations were examined between them and intakes of alcohol, energy, total fat, and dietary fiber, type of fat, and smoking. In men, alcohol use correlated with smoking and high-fat dietary patterns incorporating numerous sources of saturated fat. Alcohol use in women was unrelated to smoking or to intake of fat or total energy. Thus men and women showed distinctive eating styles that exposed them differentially to putative cancer risks. Additive effects were clearer for men than for women.

A prospective study of women in Sweden suggested that nonprotein energy intake was a positive risk factor for cancer (*27*). Dietary fat did not fully explain the increased risk associated with energy intake. While there was a possible negative association between relative protein intake and all-site cancer, the conclusion that energy intake from nonprotein sources is a determinant of cancer was better supported by the data.

In a series of hospital-based case–control studies in northern Italy, relative cancer risks were determined by tertile of vegetable and fruit consumption, based on a food-frequency questionnaire (*28*). More than 8000 cancer patients and 6000 controls participated in these studies. Corrections were made for age, sex, area of residence, education, and smoking. Vegetables consistently protected against epithelial cancers, relative risk in the upper tertile ranging from 0.2 for esophagus, liver, and larynx to 0.7 for breast. Vegetables afforded no protection against nonepithelial lymphoid neoplasms. High fruit consumption protected strongly against cancers of the upper digestive and respiratory tract; with sites lower in the digestive tract the protection became progressively weaker. Protection was significant for liver, pancreas, prostate, and urinary sites but not for rectum, breast, thyroid, or female genital cancers. There was no protective effect of fruit against lymphomas or myelomas.

Because xanthophylls, as well as β-carotene, may protect against smoking-related cancers, Japanese investigators determined the relationship between serum xanthophyll levels and consumption of cigarettes, alcohol, and certain foods in healthy inhabitants of Japan (*29*). Women had significantly higher intake than men of milk, pulses, green and other vegetables, and fruit. Serum zeaxanthin and β-carotene concentrations were positively correlated with intake of green vegetables, eggs, and milk for both sexes; serum levels of β-cryptoxanthin were correlated with intake of fruit, milk, pulses, and green vegetables for men and fruit for women. By stepwise multiple regression analysis, β-cryptoxanthin and β-carotene concentrations were inversely associated with cigarette and alcohol consumption.

Although the Italian studies (described in *28*) showed no overall relationship between tea drinking and cancer risk (*30*), Chinese green tea may afford protection against smoking-related cancers (*31*). The micronucleus test is a standard genotoxicological assay. Analysis of matched-pair data for healthy smokers and nonsmokers showed that smoking significantly increases micronucleus formation in peripheral-blood lymphocytes. Alcohol increases micronucleus formation in smokers still further, whereas tea decreases the micronucleus formation induced by smoking.

The frequent finding of an association between low blood cholesterol levels and increased cancer risk is of considerable concern in light of efforts to reduce cholesterol to prevent heart disease. Kritchevsky evaluated results of the National Health and Nutrition Survey Epidemiologic Follow-up Study, which reported one of the strongest relationships between low cholesterol and increased cancer risk (*32*). He compared diets of participants who developed cancer and those who did not. His theory was that if diet could account for the lower cholesterol levels of the cancer patients then dietary manipulations to reduce cholesterol must be reconsidered—whereas if diet did not explain the difference, other hypotheses for the association would have to be sought. Besides a 24-hour dietary recall measure taken at baseline, information on participants' smoking habits, alcohol consumption, education, family income, height, weight, and body fat distribution was also available. Dietary fat and cholesterol consumption were directly associated with cancer occurrence in men but inversely associated

in women. However, in men, diet could not explain the blood cholesterol–cancer relation. Whatever mechanism linked low blood cholesterol and high dietary cholesterol to cancer, it appeared to be related to the body's hormonal or metabolic milieu, and the distribution of body fat was involved. Men with peripheral adiposity who developed cancer tended to consume less cholesterol than those who did not, whereas the opposite was true for men with central adiposity. Among women who had peripheral adiposity, cancer was directly associated with serum cholesterol; for central adiposity the association was inverse. Kritchevsky suggested that some inconsistencies in the literature may be explained by differing proportions of central adiposity in study populations.

In Finland, investigators looked for associations between serum concentrations of α-tocopherol, β-carotene, retinol, retinol-binding protein, and selenium and the subsequent occurrence of cancers of low incidence (lip, oral cavity, pharynx, larynx, esophagus, liver, kidney, gallbladder, urinary bladder, brain, and skin) (*33*). Nearly 40,000 adults participated in the nested case–control study. Although several sites showed a trend toward elevated cancer risk and low levels of the serum variables, the association reached statistical significance only for bladder cancer and retinol-binding protein (p = .05) and for melanoma and α-tocopherol and β-carotene (p's <.01). Because the total number of these cancers was small (115), no firm conclusions could be drawn from the results. A similar study compared case–control differences in prediagnostic serum levels of retinol, β-carotene, vitamin E, and selenium for 10 cancer sites in 10 study populations (*34*). Low levels of β-carotene were most likely to be associated with subsequent cancer, but there were marked differences in the strength of the association according to site. A low level of retinol did not appear to be an important risk factor for cancer at any site. Prediagnostic levels of vitamin E and selenium were generally lower in case-patients than in controls, but the differences were seldom greater than 10%. The relative specificity of particular antioxidants for protection at particular sites, the advantages of dose–response studies over case–control studies, and the problem of amassing sufficient data for the rarer sites were discussed. The authors suggest that a measure of total serum antioxidant activity be developed to supplement data on individual substances. For squamous cell skin cancer, these authors found that case-patients had higher median micronutrient levels than controls for all micronutrients but selenium (35). If levels above the median are considered high, case-patients were more likely than their matched controls to have high levels of retinol, vitamin E, lycopene, total carotenoids, and retinol-binding protein. Selenium was inversely associated with risk of squamous cell skin cancer; no association was seen for β-carotene. Although these results provide some evidence for a protective role for selenium, they do not support an anticancer role for the other micronutrients.

High intake of fruits, vegetables, and carotenoids and high levels of β-carotene in the blood are consistently associated with reduced risk of lung cancer and frequently with reduced risk of certain other cancers, as well. The simplest explanation, but not the only one, is that β-carotene is protective. Other carotenoids, other constituents of the fruits and vegetables, or dietary patterns tightly linked with frequent vegetable and fruit consumption could also be invoked to explain the results. A group of investigators from the National Cancer Institute and elsewhere are conducting a comprehensive study to identify dietary patterns that are highly correlated with fruit and vegetable intake and to develop and test a liquid chromatographic method for recovery and resolution of the common carotenoids in blood (36). They are also considering the individual carotenoid composition of foods when analyzing relationships between diet and cancer prospectively and retrospectively. Repeatedly, they find stronger associations with intake of foods (total vegetables, dark green vegetables, yellow-orange vegetables, fruit) than with estimated intake of carotenoids. Two possibilities, which the authors plan to investigate further, are that intake of food groups rich in β-carotene is a better measure of β-carotene intake than is an approximate index of the hydrocarbon carotenoids, or that the protective agent is one or more other constituents of these foods.

Block reviewed the epidemiologic evidence for a protective effect of vitamin C against cancer (37). She found it to be very strong for 11 cancers of epithelial origin, but not for 4 hormone-dependent cancers. All 8 studies that reported a vitamin C index in cancer of the oral cavity, larynx, or esophagus found a significantly higher risk associated with low intake. Of 11 lung cancer studies that specifically mentioned vitamin C, 5 found a significant protective effect, 4 found a nonsignificant protective effect, and 2 found no effect. Five of 6 studies that examined the risk of pancreatic cancer in relation to either vitamin C or fruit intake found significant protection. All 7 studies on vitamin C intake and risk of stomach cancer found a significant protective effect. Vitamin C appears more strongly and consistently protective against rectal cancer than against colon cancer, but some protection against colon cancer is observed. When the diets of pregnant women were investigated in a study of childhood brain tumors, low intake of vitamin C was significantly associated with a threefold increase in risk of brain tumors in the offspring.

Although vitamin C does not afford significant protection against hormone-dependent cancers, a study in Japan suggested that dietary phytoestrogens may (38). Certain lignans and isoflavonoids in the traditional Japanese diet are converted by the intestinal microflora to weakly estrogenic substances exhibiting a variety of antiestrogenic, antiproliferative, antiviral, cytotoxic, and growth-inhibiting effects. By stimulating the production of sex hormone–binding globulin in the liver they may influence the biological activity of sex hormones. Urinary excretion of these substances was studied in 10 women and 9 men living in a rural Japanese village, who ate the typical low-fat Japanese diet based on rice, soy products, fish, and vegetables. Urinary excretion of lignans was low, but excretion of isoflavonoids was very high and correlated with consumption of soybean products. It has been suggested that the low mortality rates from breast and prostate cancer in Japan are related to the high intake of soybean products.

Colorectal cancer

The expression "colorectal cancer" refers nonspecifically to three cancers with distinctive epidemiologic and etiologic features. Failure to distinguish among these is the source of much confusion in the literature. Weisburger reviewed the epidemiology, causes, mechanisms, and prevention of cancers of the proximal and distal colon and rectum (*39*). He cited findings from animal studies, geographical epidemiology, studies of migrants and subpopulations that adhere to distinctive traditions, and time trends. The roles of activity, iatrogenic factors, associated diseases, sex, and genetic elements were considered. Genotoxic and nongenotoxic mechanisms of carcinogenesis were explained and protective factors were discussed.

The evolution of colorectal cancer from normal mucosa is driven multifactorially (*40*). Inheritance and diet are critical; physical activity, alcohol consumption, and body composition are also involved. Dietary influences come into play at each stage of the multistage carcinogenic process, but their effect may depend on genetic factors. Definitive understanding of the relationships between diet, inheritance, and colorectal cancer await the results of large prospective, randomized intervention studies such as have recently been initiated in Europe and the USA. Giovannucci et al. reported one of the few studies of the relationship of diet to risk of colorectal adenomas, which are early precursors of cancer (*41*). Using data from food-frequency questionnaires completed by 7284 male health professionals who had had a colonoscopy or sigmoidoscopy, they determined relative risk of adenoma by quintile of nutrient intake. After adjustment for total energy, risk of colorectal adenoma was positively associated with intake of saturated fat and with the ratio of red meat to fish and chicken intakes, and inversely associated with intake of all sources of dietary fiber. Because adenomatous polyps frequently appear 10 years or more before the clinical diagnosis of cancer, this study links dietary factors with events very early in the transition from normal mucosa to malignancy.

Disagreements over the relative roles of different dietary factors in development of colon cancer frequently originate in the high correlations between nutrients and the ways in which researchers try to compensate for these correlations (*42*). This paper described and applied a set of diagnostic tools for assessing the magnitude of collinearity in epidemiologic data, reviewed four methods for addressing collinearity problems in multivariate regression models, and evaluated the results from application of each method to data from a case–control study of diet and colon cancer. Although the study addressed only the potential collinearity problems between total fat and total caloric intake, similar difficulties would arise for total protein and total caloric intake. The fundamental problem with multicollinear nutrient data is that they contain insufficient information to discriminate the influence of highly correlated nutrients. Therefore the epidemiologist must impose constraints on the data to address analytical problems associated with collinearity; how to do this is a critical element of the procedures described in this paper.

Another problem in comparing case–control studies of colorectal cancer relates to the type of dietary information used—retrospective versus original (*43*). To evaluate the seriousness of this, participants in a cohort study who had filled out a dietary questionnaire in 1967 (original information) were asked to fill out a similar questionnaire in 1987, with reference to their dietary habits in 1967 (retrospective information). All 50 surviving subjects who had had a diagnosis of colorectal cancer completed the questionnaire in 1987, as did 150 controls selected at random from original participants who did not have colorectal cancer. Case-subjects and controls had a similar tendency to misestimate their previous food intake, and this tendency was closely related to changes in consumption during the intervening years. Subjects whose dietary habits had not changed appreciably provided retrospective information that agreed well with the original. However, compared with controls, case-subjects tended to underestimate their previous consumption of coffee and sweets and overestimate their consumption of eggs, fruits, and vegetables when their original estimate had been "high." When the original estimate was "low," case-subjects more frequently overestimated previous consumption of fruits and vegetables, whereas controls overestimated previous consumption of potatoes and milk. When changes in dietary habits were analyzed, case-subjects and controls showed similar changes.

A case–control study of the relationship of diet to occurrence of colorectal cancer in Athens, Greece, characterized a high-risk diet as high in protein, saturated fat, and cholesterol, and low in vegetables—the opposite of a low-risk diet (*44*). However, case–subjects had substantially and highly significantly lower serum levels of total cholesterol and high-density lipoprotein (HDL) cholesterol than controls. Thus, again, diet could not explain serum cholesterol values (see *32*). Alternative explanations for this well known paradox are discussed in terms of the data from this study.

A case–control study in Sweden found a positive association between colorectal cancer and usual meat consumption during the previous five years (*45*). High total meat intake, frequent consumption of brown gravy, and preference for a heavily browned meat surface each independently increased the risk; and the risk was greater for rectal than for colon cancer. Surprisingly, consumption of boiled meat was associated with greater risk than consumption of meat fried lightly. Although it has been known for some time that carcinogens are formed when meat is cooked at high temperatures, this is one of the few epidemiologic studies to consider the method of cooking.

In a prospective study of nearly 90,000 women, Willett et al. found an association between intake of red meat and colon cancer (see Chapter 2, *Food Safety 1991*, reference 27). Numerous readers have commented on this study (*46–53*). It was noted that the authors failed to distinguish between cancers of the proximal and distal colon, which are thought to have different pathogenetic mechanisms and whose relative incidence in women varies with age (*46*). Nor was the possibility of hereditary nonpolyposis colorectal cancer considered in the data analysis. In lumping beef, pork, lamb, and processed meat products such as bacon and sausage into the category "red meat," the authors failed to account for the huge range of fat content and possible role of other constituents, especially in processed meats (*47*). They also did not discuss other aspects of "healthy" and "unhealthy" lifestyles that tend to be associated with healthy and unhealthy diets (*48*). A practitioner of family and sports medicine was concerned that active women and girls already at risk for iron deficiency might turn away from the best source of iron available to them, when the only significant risk was associated with consumption of more than a quarter of a pound of red meat daily (*49*). Estimates of dietary fiber used in this study may have been less than ideal and could have had a major effect on conclusions from the study (*50*). The possibility of a detection bias was suggested (*51*): high meat consumption would cause more positive tests for occult blood in the stool, and investigation of these could yield some incidental diagnoses of colon cancer. Willett et al. explained why this was unlikely in their study (*54*). In response to another comment (*52*), they explained why they did not analyze total mortality in their relatively young population. Finally, a reader looked at the 2:1 risk ratio for colon cancer in meat eaters compared with fish eaters from a different perspective (*53*). Meat eaters had an incidence of colon cancer of 0.113%, whereas the incidence in fish eaters was 0.056%. The writer questioned whether the 0.059% difference in these rates is seriously worth worrying about. Willett et al. argued that it is (*54*), considering the young age of the study population and the short duration of follow-up.

A case–control study of diet and colon cancer was conducted in Argentina, where the usual diet is high in red meat (*55*). One hundred and ten case-patients were matched on age and sex with 220 neighborhood controls. Analysis of information on food consumption during the 5-year period ending 6 months before interview showed a highly protective effect of dietary fiber and some evidence for a protective effect of niacin. Total energy consumption increased relative risk by a factor of 1.84 per 1000 calories.

In a hospital-based study in northeastern Italy, subjects completed a questionnaire giving the frequency of consumption of specific food items before onset of the problem leading to the current hospitalization (*56*). Analysis of data for 123 cases of colon cancer, 125 cases of rectal cancer, and 699 controls revealed a protective effect for fiber- and vegetable-rich diets. Frequent consumption of refined starchy foods, eggs, cheese, or red meat was a risk factor. Some foods had differential effects on the odds ratios for colon and rectal cancer. For most subjects, a substantial proportion of dietary fiber was supplied by vegetables. Although the study could not determine whether risk was modified by fiber itself, a fiber component, a particular fiber type, or associated micronutrients, failure to find an association with fruit intake seems to argue against a protective role for micronutrients such as vitamin C and β-carotene. Refined carbohydrate products, a risk factor in this study, comprised a larger fraction of the diet than they do in the USA. Somewhat different results were obtained from a hospital-based case–control study in China, where the usual diet is quite unlike the usual Italian diet (57). Here, increased risk of colorectal cancer was associated with low intake of green vegetables, chives and celery, meat, eggs, grain, and soybean products. Results were similar but not identical for men and women and for colon and rectal cancer. The findings for meat were interesting in this population whose meat consumption is generally low. The greater risk associated with low meat consumption suggests that there is an optimal amount of meat, greater than zero, in a healthy diet.

A dietary study of hospitalized colorectal cancer patients in Majorca, with age- and sex-matched hospital and population controls, found that risk of colorectal cancer increases with increasing intake of total calories and cholesterol and decreases with increasing intake of pulses and folic acid (58). Of the three main components of total energy, protein (mainly animal) and carbohydrate were associated with risk; no significant effect of lipids or saturated fats was found.

Although adenomatous polyps are precursors of colorectal cancer, it is not known what proportion of colorectal cancers originate from such polyps or what proportion of polyps become cancerous. Furthermore, little is known about the etiology of adenomatous polyps beyond the fact that there is a genetic predisposition to them. An Australian case–control study tested the hypothesis that diet and alcohol consumption play a role in development of adenomatous colorectal polyps and that dietary risk factors are similar to those for colorectal cancer (59). Case and control groups had similar family histories of colorectal cancer. Subjects with adenomatous polyps had a significantly lower intake

of fiber and vegetables than controls; men with polyps were also characterized by a higher intake of beef, milk, and beer. Results were less clear in a study of exercise, diet, and adenomatous polyps in Japanese self-defense officials (60). The men, mostly in their early 50s, were given a comprehensive retirement health examination (including a colonoscopy) and a self-administered questionnaire addressing dietary and other habits. Leisure time spent doing strenuous activities was inversely related to the risk of polyps, but dietary relationships were merely suggestive. A nonsignificant decrease in risk was associated with frequent consumption of rice, green tea, and instant coffee. No association was seen for fruits, vegetables, meat, fish, or several other food items. In a Swedish study, low physical activity at work and in leisure time was associated with increased risk for colon but not rectal cancer (61). This study also found that frequent intake of meat, brown gravy, heavily browned fried meat, fish, and eggs was associated with increased colorectal cancer risk, as was high intake of fat or protein. A high intake of dietary fiber decreased risk at most colorectal sites.

A study in New York City of diet and the recurrence of colorectal adenomatous polyps found no associations for men (62). For women, however, significantly increased odds ratios were found for high versus low quartiles of beef, cheese, total fat, and saturated fat consumption. Decreased odds ratios were associated with high fish, carbohydrate, and fiber consumption. Marginal effects were seen for total energy and vitamin A intake. Two ongoing studies are sharpening the focus on fiber's role in the recurrence of adenomatous polyps (63). In one, patients are taught a low-fat, high-fiber, high-fruit, high-vegetable dietary pattern after having polyps removed. In the other, similar subjects are given a high-fiber supplement but otherwise retain their customary dietary pattern. Together these studies should indicate whether the key is fiber or another dietary component or components. The responses of men and women to modified diets may differ (64). After polypectomy, 201 subjects in Toronto were randomized to diet-counseling and control groups. After 12 months, fat consumption averaged 25% of energy in the counsel group and 33% in controls; fiber consumption was 35 and 16 g, respectively. Women who received counseling had a reduced rate of polyp recurrence, associated with reduced levels of serum cholesterol and fecal bile acids. Men, however, had an increased rate of recurrence, associated with decreased serum cholesterol but increased fecal bile acids.

Although a relationship between dietary fiber and development of cancers of the gastrointestinal tract seems fairly certain, the mechanisms and intermediates involved are not well understood. Klurfeld reviewed carcinogenetic mechanisms mediated by dietary fiber (65). The role of fecal bile acids has been studied most extensively, but incongruities in human studies have not been resolved. Bacterial degradation of dietary fiber to short-chain fatty acids seems important, but the most readily fermentable fibers are no more protective than fibers refractive to fermentation. Promising topics for study include physical characteristics of the feces, aqueous-phase bile acids, alterations in mucins, mutagenicity of intestinal contents, changes in mucosal cytokinetics, enzyme activity (e.g., ornithine decarboxylase and aryl hydrocarbon hydroxylase), neurogenic effects of bulk and short-chain fatty acids, local and systemic gut hormones and growth factors, transit time, pH, and availability of energy.

A large case–control study of dietary fiber and colorectal cancer conducted at SUNY–Buffalo added to the evidence for sex and site differences in response to fiber components (66). High intakes of total vegetable fiber, cellulose, hemicellulose, and lignin were associated with increased risk of sigmoid colon cancer in women, but there was no association with risk at other subsites in women or at any site in men. The various fiber components appeared to have somewhat different effects in women, but strong correlations between the components made it difficult to analyze these results. This study could not draw any conclusions about cereal fiber, but a Swedish study did (67). A dietary survey of 41 colorectal cancer patients, 41 matched controls, and 801 hospital and population controls found that, per unit of energy, the habitual diet of cancer patients contained less cereal fiber ($p < .001$) as well as less riboflavin, calcium, and phosphorus.

Overall, cancer patients consumed more fat, protein, carbohydrate, and total energy and less cereal fiber than matched controls, but these differences were not statistically significant. High alcohol consumption was correlated with increased risk ($p < .05$). High intakes of calcium or cereal fiber, relative to energy, were associated with reduced risk of colon cancer; a similar association was found for intake of total fiber or cereal fiber and risk of rectal cancer.

One factor in the positive correlation between latitude and death rate from colon cancer may be intensity and duration of exposure to sunlight, with consequent effects on vitamin D and calcium metabolism. To investigate this, laboratory, clinical, and epidemiologic studies were reviewed (68). Patterns of fat, fiber, fruit, and vegetable consumption do not readily explain the geographic pattern of colon-cancer mortality in the USA. However, at high latitudes, serum concentrations of vitamin D metabolites tend to be low and absorption of calcium may be poorer, especially in the elderly. Further, in animal studies, dietary supplementation with calcium and (or) vitamin D partly protects against colon tumors induced by a high-fat diet. All lines of evidence suggest to the authors that substantial reductions in rates of colon cancer could be achieved in many parts of the world by optimizing intake of calcium and vitamin D. The usual cautions regarding vitamin D toxicity are still warranted, and additional precautions are necessary for persons at risk for certain types of renal stones. Safe and effective ranges of calcium and vitamin D consumption for specific populations in the context of geography and culture need to be established worldwide.

A carefully reasoned review of admittedly meager data concluded that intestinal exposure to ingested iron may be an important determinant of colorectal cancer risk in humans (69). Iron has been associated with both initiation and promotion of tumors. Differences in intake of iron and substances such as phytate that affect its bioavailability may explain differences in colon-cancer risk between high- and low-risk countries and within the USA. The review touches on iron's role in nutrition and metabolism; the complex system of iron absorption, transport, and storage that maintains adequate supplies while protecting against toxicity; the global nonproblem of iron deficiency if the root causes of anemia are controlled; the consequences of iron overload; and the rationale and experimental evidence for iron's role in colorectal cancer.

The relationship between folate intake and risk of colorectal cancer was assessed in a case–control study at SUNY-Buffalo (70). Again, a differential effect was seen according to site. While folate (controlled for total energy intake) was not consistently associated with colon cancer risk, risk of rectal cancer was reduced in the highest category of intake. For men in the highest quartile, the effect was highly significant (p <.001). The authors propose that the folate content of fruits and vegetables partly explains their protective effect. Folate has not been systematically studied in this regard, and in light of the depressed folate status in some segments of the U.S. population such investigations appear warranted.

Observations that ownership or use of a refrigerator reduces risk of gastric cancer were not initially extended to cancer at other sites. Another study from SUNY-Buffalo measured the magnitude of the "refrigerator effect" on cancers at other gastrointestinal sites (71). Case-patients were matched with age-, sex-, and neighborhood-matched controls and interviewed regarding their usual diet, smoking and drinking history, and years of refrigerator ownership. No effects were found for cancer of the mouth or esophagus. For men but not women, refrigerator use was strongly protective against stomach cancer, weakly protective against colon cancer, and possibly weakly protective against rectal cancer.

Gastric and esophageal cancer

A hospital-based case–control study of stomach cancer in high- and low-risk areas of the Federal Republic of Germany identified several possible diet-related risk factors (72). In addition to material collected from the case–control study, data on traditional habits going as far back as 1910 were analyzed. From the historical data, use of vegetables and legumes was associated with the low-risk area, whereas mashed potato, cabbage, and farinaceous dishes were dominant in the high-risk area. Cultivation and use of tomatoes began relatively late in the high-risk area. The traditional wood used for smoking in the low-risk area was beech; various woods, including spruce, were used in the high-risk area. From the case–control study, low intake of vitamin C, noncentralized water supply, refrigerator use for <25 y, and use of spruce wood for smoking meat at home were associated with increased risk of gastric cancer. These associations applied to both individuals and regions. A similar study in two Belgian provinces with contrasting gastric-cancer mortality rates identified other dietary risk factors (73). Consumption of most raw or cooked vegetables and fresh fruit (especially apples) was protective, as was consumption of lean meat. Increased risk was associated with meal and flour products, including white bread, and sugar. In contrast to other vegetables, beans increased risk for gastric cancer; this, however, may support the findings for carbohydrate-rich foods. Most sources of fat did not show a clear effect, but oils with a high ratio of polyunsaturated to saturated fatty acids were associated with decreased risk.

Another case–control study was conducted in four provinces of Spain (74). One was a low-risk area; the others had relatively high rates of gastric cancer. From 15 hospitals, 354 cases of confirmed gastric adenocarcinoma were selected, along with a control for each from the same hospital matched by age, sex, and area of residence. Information on diet was obtained from dietary histories and frequency questionnaires. Increased risk was associated with habitual consumption of preserved fish, cold cuts, and oily fruits. Cooked green vegetables, fresh noncitrus fruit, and dried fruit were protective. Effects were additive: high intakes of a protective and a risky food group canceled each other, whereas intake of two protective food groups enhanced protection, and conversely. This observation may have practical implications for public health campaigns, because efforts to get people to eat more of something are generally more successful than exhortations to eat less of something. Preference for salty foods and addition of salt at the table were not associated with risk.

In Italy, gastric cancers in high- and low-risk areas may differ by histologic type (*75*). When 923 tumors were categorized according to the Lauren classification, intestinal types outnumbered diffuse by 3:1 in the high-risk north-central region, whereas the two types were equally abundant in low-risk areas. Intestinal types were also more common at older ages and in men. However, diet-related risks for the two types were similar: increased risk was associated with high intake of meat, dried or salted fish, seasoned cheeses, and traditional soups, whereas heavy consumption of fresh fruits and vegetables was protective. Indices for specific nutrients associated with the food groups showed the same risk patterns as the foods. Occurrence of both histologic types was inversely associated with socioeconomic status but unrelated to cigarette smoking. Thus, despite other differences, the intestinal and diffuse types of gastric carcinoma appear to share common etiologic factors. Sixty-eight of the 923 tumors occurred in the gastric cardia (*76*). Compared with other gastric cancers, these were more common in men than in women and had a greater tendency to be associated with a family history of this cancer. Dietary risk factors were the same as for gastric cancer in general, considering the limited data for the cardia site. However, the proportion of cardia tumors in this study is much smaller than that reported by countries where sharp increases in the incidence of cancers of the cardia and lower esophagus have recently been noted, suggesting a need for research on environmental and host determinants of this emergent tumor.

Fresh fruits were significantly protective against gastric cancer in a smaller case–control study in rural Leon, Spain (*77*). Consumption of home-made sausages or home-cured meats conferred some risk, which reached statistical significance if the meats were smoked. There was a nonsignificant protective effect from consumption of fresh vegetables.

A prospective study of gastric cancer mortality in a cohort of initially healthy high-risk men suggested that excess gastric cancer risk in the North Central USA is partly due to foreign birth or having an immigrant parent from Scandinavia or Germany, where risk is also high (*78*). An association between low educational attainment and laboring or semiskilled occupations was found only for foreign-born and first-generation Americans. The strongest risk factor in this study was cigarette smoking, and it was dose-related; risk was also increased among pipe smokers and men who used smokeless tobacco. No excess risk was associated with drinking alcohol. When dietary factors were examined, none of the 7 food groups (meats, fish, dairy, breads, fruits, vegetables, cruciferous vegetables) was significantly associated with risk, but several of the 35 individual food items were risk factors: salted fish, bacon, milk, cooked cereal, and apples. One explanation offered for the surprising association between apple consumption and increased risk was that quantities of apples were customarily stored in conditions under which they could become moldy. Patulin, a mycotoxin contaminant found in apple products, induces sarcomas in rats at the injection site.

Kashmir has a nonmigrant population of Muslims, Hindus, and Sikhs with distinctive personal and dietary habits (*79*). Overall its rate of esophagogastric cancer is very high, but the rate among Hindus is relatively low. Muslims and most Hindus do not drink alcohol, whereas alcohol consumption is common among Sikh men. Smoking is common among Hindu and Muslim men, and Muslims frequently use snuff; Sikhs do not smoke. Up to 10 cups per day of salted tea, boiling hot, is drunk by Muslims; Hindus drink 2–4 cups per day of green tea boiled with spices. Most Kashmiries have an adequate intake of locally grown fruit. Their staple diet is boiled rice and a boiled leafy cruciferous vegetable. Most of them eat lamb. Other special food items are dried and pickled vegetables, sun-dried and smoked fish, red chilies, lotus stem, other local vegetables, mixed spice cake, saffron, and mawal (*Celosia argentea*, a vegetable food colorant). Because of the large number of gastric (966) and esophageal (1515) cancers diagnosed during the three-year study in a valley whose population is ~2.9 million, a study of dietary risk factors seems important.

Rapid social changes in Hong Kong during the past 20 years have produced considerable heterogeneity in exposure to possible etiologic factors for esophageal cancer, enhancing the likelihood of detecting both risk factors and protective factors for this tumor in a population whose risk is high by international standards (*80*). In a study of 400 patients hospitalized for esophageal cancer and 1598 hospital and clinic controls, interviewers questioned subjects about sociodemographic characteristics, smoking, drinking, tea and coffee consumption, and personal and family medical history. A food-frequency questionnaire inquired about past and recent consumption of 22 food items. The following significant risk factors were identified by multivariate analysis: tobacco smoking, alcohol drinking, preference for high-temperature drinks and soups, infrequent consumption of green vegetables or citrus fruits, and consumption of pickled vegetables. Assuming that risk is multiplicative, the combined attributable risk due to these exposures was 89%. In preliminary analyses, protective trends were seen for carrots, tomatoes, and noncitrus fruits; low educational attainment and eating salted fish increased risk. Support was given to the assumption of multiplicative risk by a modeling study in Italy (*81*). In this study of 211 men with esophageal cancer and 712 controls, an additive model was inadequate for describing relative risk, but the data fitted a multiplicative model. Major risk factors were alcohol and tobacco consumption and a low β-carotene index. Retinol index had no association with risk. Case-patients were less educated and of lower social class than controls. The use of statistical modeling in studies such as this is discussed. In Transkei, extensive inquiries were made into the diet and social habits of 100 esophageal cancer patients and 100 controls (*82*). Regression analysis identified smoking, use of traditional medicines, and consumption of black nightshade (*Solanum nigrum*) as significant risk factors. Drinking traditional beer was not a risk factor. The findings are discussed in terms of the rapid increase in incidence of esophageal cancer in Transkei since 1950, which has accompanied population expansion, reduced availability of milk, meat, sorghum, and millet, and greater dependence on corn and perhaps wild vegetables.

Breast cancer

Adams briefly reviewed the literature on relationships between hormones, fat, and breast cancer (*83*). He made the following points: (i) Japanese women have a much lower incidence of breast cancer than Americans, but the difference disappears within two generations when they migrate to the USA; (ii) positive association between breast cancer risk and intake of saturated fats is repeatedly seen in postmenopausal women; a similar association exists between breast cancer risk and body mass index, again only for postmenopausal women; and (iii) hormones, particularly estrogens, are thought to act as promoters of breast carcinogenesis. Experiments with rodents support observations in humans. When hormone profiles of American and Japanese women were compared, dehydroepiandrosterone sulfate (DHEAS) concentrations were significantly higher in the blood of Americans. An estrogen, 5-androstene-3β,17β-diol, is formed peripherally from this and in Western women it reaches biologically active levels. Urinary metabolites of DHEAS, 11-deoxy-17-ketosteroids, were also higher in American women. This demonstrates a positive correlation between DHEAS, its metabolites, and incidence of breast cancer and leads Adams to hypothesize a direct link between diet, secretion of hormones (especially DHEAS), and development of breast cancer. He suggests that diet and body fat provide fatty acids that act directly or indirectly on the mammary gland and augment prolactin and DHEAS secretion, generating a hormonal environment conducive to tumorigenesis. However, a study of hormone levels in vegetarian and nonvegetarian teenaged girls produced the opposite results and conclusions (*84*). When hormone levels of vegetarian (Seventh-Day Adventist) and nonvegetarian girls in the Chicago area were compared, vegetarians had somewhat *higher* DHEAS luteal and follicular levels than nonvegetarians, with a significant difference in the luteal phase of the menstrual cycle. The authors cited other evidence for an *inverse* relationship between DHEAS levels and breast cancer risk. Vegetarians in this study ingested significantly less total fat, saturated fat, sucrose, cholesterol, protein, and caffeine and significantly more unsaturated fat and fiber than nonvegetarians, but none of these nutrients was associated with DHEAS. Nevertheless, the link between a vegetarian diet and DHEAS suggests how low-fat diets during adolescence may reduce subsequent breast cancer risk.

A review by Rose uses evidence from epidemiologic and animal studies to suggest how dietary fiber may modify the putative adverse influence of fat (*85*). The mechanisms by which fiber protects against breast cancer probably involve estrogen metabolism and bioactivity through effects of fiber on the enterohepatic circulation of estrogens, enhanced fecal excretion of estrogens, and actions of fiber-associated phytoestrogens. Phytoestrogens have weak estrogenic activity, but by competing with more potent estrogens for receptor binding sites they may exert a net antiestrogenic effect. Thus a diet rich in phytoestrogens might downregulate estrogen bioactivity and protect against breast cancer.

A case–control study in Moscow found that dietary factors are more important for postmenopausal than premenopausal breast cancer (*86*). A decreased risk for postmenopausal breast cancer was associated with high intakes of cellulose, monosaccharides and disaccharides, vitamin C, β-carotene, and polyunsaturated fatty acids (PUFAs). High protein intake was a risk factor with a very high odds ratio but also very wide confidence limits. Alcohol was a risk factor for both premenopausal and postmenopausal women, but it reached significance only in the postmenopausal group. Other differences between premenopausal and postmenopausal case-patients and controls were discussed.

The role of diet in breast cancer development was evaluated in an Australian case–control study (*87*). Groups of 100 patients with breast cancer, benign epithelial hyperplasia, or fibrocystic disease and roughly 200 control subjects participated. Cancer patients and controls were matched by age and electoral district. Patients with fibrocystic disease were matched to those with benign epithelial hyperplasia, and these groups shared the same controls. The authors hypothesized that dietary patterns of the group with fibrocystic disease (not considered a risk factor for cancer) would resemble

dietary patterns of controls, whereas patients with benign epithelial hyperplasia (a probable precursor of malignancy) were expected to resemble cancer patients in their dietary patterns. The results supported this hypothesis. Consumption of red meat, "savory meals," or starches increased risk of hyperplasia and neoplasia, whereas consumption of chicken and fish or fruit was protective.

A prospective case–cohort study conducted on the island of Guernsey found plasma selenium concentration to be at most a weak indicator of breast cancer risk (*88*). However, only a limited and moderate range of selenium exposures and a relatively short time span (10 years) were considered.

An epidemiological study of postmenopausal breast cancer in western New York confirmed that risk increases with a family history of breast cancer, a history of benign breast disease, high body mass (Quetelet) index, and age at first pregnancy and decreases with number of children and pregnancies (*89*). After adjustment for confounding factors, risk was highest among women with the lowest consumption of carotene or substances correlated with consumption of carotene. Risk was not associated with retinol ingestion or with fat intake, whether in terms of quantity or proportion of total energy intake.

In extending to 8 years the follow-up of nearly 90,000 women enrolled in a health study, Willett et al. found no evidence to suggest a major adverse influence of total or saturated fat intake by middle-aged women on breast cancer risk (*90*). However, in this same study population, consumption of vitamin A (including supplements) and vitamin E showed inverse relationships with breast cancer risk (*91*). The association was significant for vitamin A but nonsignificant for vitamin E; both associations were slightly stronger for premenopausal than for postmenopausal women. No association was seen for vitamin C.

Death rates from breast cancer in southern Italy are low, but in northern Italy they have recently approached rates in the USA (*92*). Distinctive dietary patterns are found in these three areas. Southern Italy has the lowest consumption of meat, milk, and cheese and the highest consumption of fish, bread and baked goods, pastas, and vegetables.

Northern Italy has the highest consumption of cheese and fruits and the lowest consumption of fish. The USA has the highest consumption of meat, milk, and eggs and the lowest consumption of bread and baked goods and pastas. High consumption of olive oil characterizes southern Italy, whereas butter intake in northern Italy is three times higher than in the south and is similar to that in the USA. Vegetable oils other than olive oil were little used in Italy before 1970; since then they have come to represent more than one-third of the fats in both north and south.

In a case–control study of breast cancer in Argentina, where the mortality rate for this disease is high, information was obtained on demographic, socioeconomic, and reproductive variables, frequency of consumption of 40 food items, and methods of cooking (93). After nondietary risk factors were controlled for, weak positive associations were found between breast cancer risk and intake of beef, fried foods, and >3 eggs per week. The most likely reason for failure to find strong associations with dietary factors was lack of sufficient heterogeneity in nutritional exposures within the study population. The authors had expected to find a stronger relationship between breast cancer risk and beef consumption. Failure to find one may mean that none exists; however, beef consumption was high (generally >4 times per week) in both case and control groups.

Evidence is accumulating that diet can influence survival of cancer patients as well as the initial development of their disease. However, a study of breast cancer patients in Denmark found no prognostic significance for reproductive or hormonal risk factors, dietary variables, alcohol consumption, or smoking (94).

Lung and laryngeal cancer

Although smoking and drinking alcohol are established risk factors for both lung and laryngeal cancer, dietary factors related to laryngeal cancer risk have been less frequently examined. A case–control study of laryngeal cancer in white men in western New York analyzed the interaction of diet with smoking and alcohol (95). Case-patients consumed significantly more fat and kilocalories than controls; their intake of carotenoids and vitamin C tended to be less. Beer, hard liquor, and total alcohol intake were strongly associated with risk; wine intake was generally low and was not associated with risk. Cigarette smoking was also a major risk factor but use of cigars and pipes was not. There were dietary interactions with smoking and drinking. High intake of carotenoids was most protective for light smokers, whereas risk associated with high intake of fat was greatest for heavy smokers. The relationship between carotenoid intake and risk was similar at high and low fat intakes, and conversely. High retinol intake was positively associated with risk in heavy drinkers; there was no interaction between retinol and carotenoids. When odds ratios were calculated for 129 individual foods, seven raw vegetables were significantly protective, whereas risk was positively associated with intake of mayonnaise, milk, doughnuts, veal, cooked peas, and cooked cauliflower. High total intake of raw vegetables was protective; high intake of milk and milk products increased risk. Overall, smoking was the overwhelming risk factor for laryngeal cancer. Dietary variables could modulate the effect of smoking, but their effect was much weaker.

A case–control study of laryngeal cancer in Shanghai again found cigarette smoking to be the most important risk factor (96). There was no dose-related effect of alcohol drinking on risk, but amounts of alcohol consumed were generally low. High intake of vegetables and fruits, particularly dark yellow and *Allium* vegetables (garlic and onions), was protective; high intake of liver, salted fish, meat and eggs, and deep-fried foods increased risk. Some occupational risks were also identified, and elevated risk was linked to long-term use of kerosene stoves in cooking.

A prospective study of 4538 Finnish men evaluated the relationship between dietary cholesterol and fatty acids and lung cancer risk (97). During 20 years of follow-up, 117 cases of lung cancer were diagnosed. Intake of total and saturated fats was nonsignificantly related to risk, but no increased risk was associated with cholesterol intake. As with laryngeal cancer, the effect of fat was dwarfed by the risk associated with smoking and was mainly seen in smokers. In comparing populations whose dietary habits differ widely, however, the importance of diet is more readily seen. American men have a much higher lung cancer mortality rate than Japanese (72.2 vs. 38.2 per 100,000 in 1985) (*98*). Nevertheless, the proportion of smokers is higher in Japan that in the USA, and although the Japanese tend to begin smoking at a later age they smoke more cigarettes per day. There are no important differences in inhalation patterns and type of cigarette smoked. Differences and changes in consumption of fruits and vegetables in the two countries are too small to affect lung cancer mortality, but the difference in fat consumption is striking: in 1950 and 1985, respectively, 40% and 43.5% (USA) vs. 7.9% and 24.5% (Japan). The authors summarized mechanisms by which fat is thought to promote cancer through actions on endocrine, autocrine, and immune systems, oncogenes, gut bacteria, membrane structure, and lipid peroxides.

There were several reports that high intake of fruits and vegetables protects against lung cancer (*99–101*). When the relationship between dietary antioxidants and risk of lung cancer was examined in the Finnish cohort described in reference *97*, nonsignificant protective effects were found for carotenoids, vitamin E, and vitamin C in nonsmokers (*99*). In the total cohort, margarine and fruit were significantly protective, although again the effect was stronger in nonsmokers. The relative risk for the lowest quartile of margarine intake, compared with the highest, was 4.0 (p <.001) and for fruits was 1.8 (p = .05). The authors suggest that food sources rich in carotenoids, vitamin C, and vitamin E have other constituents with independent protective effects against lung cancer. A nested case–control study in a cohort of 41,837 women in the Iowa Women's Health Study found that the 101 case-patients consumed significantly less tomatoes, green leafy vegetables, fruit, and all fruits and vegetables (*100*). The associations did not differ by smoking status, and no association was found with intake of β-carotene. Among tin miners of the Yunnan Province, China, exposure to radon and arsenic increases risk of lung cancer (*101*). To learn whether diet affects this risk, 183 miners with newly diagnosed lung cancer and 183

age-matched occupational controls were interviewed about their usual diet and smoking history. Miners who reported a low intake of yellow and light-green vegetables or tomatoes were at significantly greater risk for lung cancer after adjustment for radon, arsenic, and smoking. There was a monotonic relationship between quartile of intake and odds ratio for lung cancer.

Because of reports associating dietary cholesterol with lung cancer incidence, a cohort of 1878 middle-aged men who in 1958 were employed by the Western Electric Company in Chicago was followed for 24 years, to determine whether cholesterol intake was related to lung cancer in that population (*102*). After adjustment for smoking, age, and intake of β-carotene and fat, the relative risk of lung cancer associated with a 500 mg/day increment of dietary cholesterol was 1.9. The association persisted after adjustment for serum cholesterol and dietary fat. Moreover, it seemed to be specific to cholesterol from eggs. Mean values for dietary cholesterol from eggs and other sources were 238 and 491 mg/day, respectively, but 11 other foods or food groups that could provide appreciable amounts of cholesterol were not significantly associated with lung cancer risk. One interpretation of these results is that something associated with eggs besides cholesterol is a risk factor for lung cancer. However, reanalysis of data from a case–control study in Hawaii to look for an "egg effect" failed to corroborate the findings of the Western Electric study (*103*). There was a significant positive trend of the odds ratio with increasing consumption of total cholesterol and cholesterol from sources other than eggs for men but not women.

The mortality rates of lung cancer were greater in the north of Italy than in the south in 1980 and 1982, although the proportions of smokers, surveyed in 1977, were similar (*104*). Information on dietary habits derived from annual surveys conducted from 1960 through 1965 showed that the diet in southern Italy contained less saturated and polyunsaturated fat and more foods of plant origin than the diet in northern Italy.

The lung cancer rate among men in Gejiu City, Yunnan Province, China, is one of the highest in the world (*105*). In this tin-mining community, rice is the dietary staple and bean curd is the primary source of additional protein. A case–control study of diet and lung cancer risk was conducted because it was thought that in this situation the simplicity and relative homogeneity of the diet might serve to highlight links between diet and lung cancer. Where possible, each case-subject was matched with a miner control and a Gejiu City control and was queried about usual frequency of intake of 31 food items and food groups. Case-subjects ate rice and noodles somewhat more often than controls, but ate most other items less often. The differences were significant for bean curd, meat (pork), eggs, fresh greens, tomatoes, dark-green leafy vegetables, light-green vegetables, bananas, oranges, and apples. Intake of pork, eggs, and the three fruits was directly related to income and education, which were inversely related to lung cancer risk. Case–control differences nevertheless persisted across income and education strata. By regression analysis, results were similar across duration categories of underground mining exposure. Nonsmokers were too few to permit evaluation of dietary associations in this group. The results provide further evidence that fruits and vegetables are protective against lung cancer but do not support the theory that β-carotene is specifically responsible for the effect.

In addition to protecting against lung cancer, fruits and vegetables may lengthen survival of lung cancer patients (*106*). Analysis of records from the Hawaii Tumor Registry showed covariate-adjusted median survival times for women of 33, 21, 15, and 18 months from the highest to the lowest quartiles of vegetable intake. There was also a significant trend for fruit intake and survival in women. High consumption of tomatoes or oranges significantly improved survival in men; broccoli and perhaps tomatoes were beneficial in women. No associations were found for consumption of specific micronutrients or of other carotene-rich foods.

To confirm findings of a cohort study in which an excess of lung cancer occurred among certain groups of meat industry workers, a nested case–control study of lung cancer in the meat industry was undertaken (*107*). It confirmed the existence of excess risk of lung cancer throughout the meat industry. Risk increased with duration of employment in the meat industry. The major risk factors for meat handlers compared to workers in non-meat industries were contact with raw meat for ≥5 y, contact with raw meat in abattoirs, and contact with raw meat in supermarkets. However, workers having contact with raw meat in meat-packing plants and supermarkets were not at significantly higher risk than workers in these departments who did not have direct contact with meat, suggesting that other occupational risk factors may be involved, such as exposure to fumes from heat-sealing plastic during wrapping.

Pancreatic cancer

An investigation of excess pancreatic cancer mortality among workers in a chemical manufacturing plant failed to find an association with alcohol consumption or any dietary factor, other than an inconsistent association with decaffeinated coffee (*108*). However, other studies have identified possible diet–pancreatic cancer relationships (*109–113*). Case–control studies were conducted in Adelaide, Australia; Montreal and Toronto, Canada; Utrecht, The Netherlands; and Opole, Poland (*109*). These five populations have moderate-to-high rates of pancreatic cancer and distinctive dietary practices (not specified). Comprehensive diet histories were compiled using a common protocol and questionnaire. Positive dose-related associations were consistently found for intake of carbohydrates and cholesterol, and negative associations for intake of dietary fiber and vitamin C. There was no association with weight or body mass index. In Adelaide, case-subjects consumed more boiled eggs, omelettes, and sweet and fatty food items than controls (*110*). They consumed less of certain vegetables, fruits, and several nutrients derived principally from plant foods. Pancreatic cancer was not associated with coffee drinking. In Opole, the association between pancreatic cancer and cholesterol intake (but not serum cholesterol) was particularly strong (*111*). There was a strong inverse association with vitamin C intake and weak inverse associations with retinol and fiber. The data suggested an inverse association between pancreatic cancer and intake of PUFAs and positive associations with carbohydrate and perhaps protein.

In Utrecht, after controlling for confounding factors, significant inverse dose-related effects were seen for vegetables, particularly cruciferous vegetables (*112*). Positive dose–response gradients were found for consumption of eggs and fish. Low-fiber vegetables were more strongly protective than high-fiber vegetables in directly interviewed subjects, pointing to protective elements in addition to fiber. Vitamin C was protective in women but not in men. Consumption of beer, spirits, red wine, and fortified wine was not related to risk for pancreatic cancer in Utrecht; there was an inverse relationship for white wine consumption, but only a small number of subjects were involved (*113*). There was no association with lifetime consumption of tea or instant coffee, caffeinated or decaffeinated; an inverse relationship with lifetime total coffee consumption failed to reach significance ($p <.06$).

Prostate cancer

A review by Abraham et al. addressed major topics in the epidemiology of prostate cancer (*114*). Blacks in the USA have the highest mortality rates in the world for this cancer. They are followed by whites in Norway, Switzerland, and Sweden. The lowest mortality rates occur among Asians in Singapore, Japan, and Hong Kong. However, the incidence of prostate cancer has been rising in Japan, where major dietary changes have occurred in the last 30 y. Further, the incidence of the disease is positively correlated with that of other diet-related cancers and is much higher in Japanese immigrants to Hawaii. Studies on the relationships between prostate cancer and intake of fats and vitamin A and carotenoids are summarized in text and tables. Although evidence for an adverse effect of fat from cohort studies is not as strong or consistent as from case–control studies, such an effect is supported by limited animal data. For effects of β-carotene, other carotenoids, or fruits and vegetables, the data are equivocal. A protective effect of carotenoids is seen principally in the context of a low-fat diet; it is also possible that some fruits contain risk-enhancing factors. Reports of a link between cadmium and cancer risk pertain mostly to occupational exposure. Insufficient data are available on other dietary components.

Rates of prostate cancer are very low in Third World countries in populations that maintain a traditional lifestyle, but they rise in urban populations where lifestyles are in transition (*115*). Information on risk factors for these populations is meager; neither smoking nor alcohol consumption seems to be involved. A case–control study among blacks in Soweto, South Africa, found that high consumption of fat, meat, or eggs increased risk, whereas high consumption of fruits or vegetables was protective. Specific foods that afforded protection were carrots, cabbage, and spinach; dietary fiber was also protective. Employment in an occupation that permitted ready access to a Western diet increased risk. No associations were seen for anthropometry, education, social class, smoking, and drinking.

A case–control study in northern Italy identified high milk consumption as a significant risk factor for prostate cancer (*116*). This agrees with most previous reports. Surprisingly, however, no consistent associations were found for cheese or butter intake, other sources of animal fat, or total fat.

Bladder cancer

A case–control study of diet and bladder cancer in men was conducted in five regions of Spain (*117*). Each of 432 case-patients was matched with one hospital and one community control. The average dietary pattern was typical for Mediterranean populations. Subjects in the highest quartile of intake of saturated fat were at significantly increased risk for bladder cancer. Smaller risks associated with high intake of monounsaturated fats and calcium and a protective effect of iron disappeared after correcting for saturated fat. Vitamin E remained slightly protective after correction for saturated fat. No association was seen for intake of retinol, vitamin C, total vitamin A, or carotene. Tobacco smoking and occupational exposures were major risk factors but failed to explain all cases of bladder cancer in this study. Smoking and occupational exposures were also the major risk factors for bladder cancer in a German study (*118*). A significant twofold increase in risk was associated with heavy coffee consumption in men and women and with beer and total fluid consumption in men. Chronic urinary tract infection and family history of bladder cancer were also risk factors. For men, frequent consumption of high-fat meals was a significant risk factor. Frequent consumption of canned foods increased risk for both men and women. Dietary, smoking, family history, and medical history variables did not interact with risk attributable to occupational exposure.

Cancer of the uterine cervix

American Indian women in the Southwest have high rates of cervical dysplasia and cervical cancer but low rates of cancer at other sites (*119*). A pilot case–control study in this population evaluated the relationship between cytological abnormalities and dietary intake of various micronutrients. Forty-two women with cervical dysplasia and 58 with normal cytology provided 24-h dietary recall information. Although no differences between case-subjects and controls were statistically significant, women whose intake of vitamin C, vitamin E, or folacin was low were at higher risk for cervical dysplasia. Whereas many epidemiological investigations suggest a protective role for dietary vitamin A, β-carotene, or other carotenoids, a study in the Netherlands failed to detect such a role for β-carotene in the etiology of cervical dysplasia (*120*). Subjects were 257 women with cervical dysplasia and 705 population controls who were thought to be free of dysplasia but were not examined cytologically when they entered the study. Information on diet and other risk factors was obtained by postal questionnaire. There was no indication that β-carotene protects against development of cervical dysplasia. In fact, there was a slightly higher risk of dysplasia in women with the highest intake of β-carotene. Nor could a relationship be shown with dietary retinol. Fiber and vitamin C were weakly but nonsignificantly protective.

A case–control study at major cancer treatment centers in Costa Rica, Panama, Mexico City, and Bogota, Colombia investigated dietary (*121*) and serological (*122*) indicators of risk for invasive cervical cancer. After adjustment for confounding factors, women in the highest quartiles of fruit and fruit juice consumption were at slightly lower risk. Vegetables, foods of animal origin, folacin-rich foods, complex carbohydrates, and legumes were not associated with risk. Based on nutrient indices, significant trends of decreasing risk were found for vitamin C, β-carotene, and other carotenoids. However, adjustment for vitamin C intake attenuated the effect of β-carotene. For cancer patients, serologic investigations were restricted to those with stage I and II disease, to minimize the effects of disease on serum markers. Case-patients and controls did not differ significantly in serum levels of retinol, cryptoxanthin, lycopene, α-carotene, lutein, or α-tocopherol. The mean level of β-carotene was somewhat lower in cancer patients; that of γ-tocopherol was higher, especially in stage II patients. After adjustment for confounding factors, a significant trend of decreasing risk was found for serum β-carotene. The unexpected findings for γ-tocopherol might represent an alteration caused by the disease process, but no evidence for a disease effect was seen for the other markers. The general concordance between dietary and serum data suggests that β-carotene has a protective role in the etiology of cervical cancer and demonstrates the discriminatory value of simultaneously analyzing blood and dietary indicators.

Ovarian cancer

Although many "ovarian cancer families" have been identified since epidemiologists began to look for them and by far the greatest risk is for a woman from such a family who has a first-degree relative with this disease, dietary and other factors are also involved. Piver et al. reviewed the epidemiology and etiology of ovarian cancer (*123*). The highest incidence is in industrialized countries, with the notable exception of Japan. Moreover, Japanese women born in the USA have rates of ovarian cancer approaching those of white American women. This implicates lifestyle or environmental factors. In several studies, high intake of animal fat has been associated with ovarian cancer, whereas there is no association with use of coffee, alcohol, or tobacco. One case–control study found yogurt and cottage cheese to be the only regularly used foods associated with increased risk. At the same time, cancer patients had a lesser ability to metabolize the galactose component of lactose (milk sugar). In general, countries with the greatest per capita milk consumption and the largest percentage of women with impaired ability to metabolize galactose have the highest incidence of ovarian cancer. Together these observations imply that exposure of ovaries to galactose increases their risk of developing malignant tumors. When whole milk and low-fat or skim milk were considered separately, however, the increased risk from high milk consumption could apparently be attributed to the milk's fat content. Another study found no difference between cancer patients and controls in frequency of consuming dairy foods or amount of lactose consumed (*124*). Eating carrots reduced risk; and after adjustment for body mass, smoking, and lactose consumption, regression analysis revealed a significant protective effect of β-carotene.

Use of oral contraceptives appears to be protective against ovarian cancer but may interact with dietary factors. Harlow et al. conducted a case–control study of the influence of diet on the association between ovarian cancer risk and use of oral contraceptives (*125*). The association between oral contraceptive use and ovarian cancer was modified by various nutrients; protective effects were largely confined to women with greater than median consumption of calories, carbohydrates, protein, animal fat, or lactose. Among women who ingested ≤11 g/day of lactose, use of oral contraceptives for ≥3 months was associated with a nonsignificant increase in risk; whereas for those who consumed >11 g/day of lactose, use of oral contraceptives for ≥3 months significantly decreased risk. Within this group the association was strongest for >4 years of oral contraceptive use and >2 years of use after age 30. While this study raises more questions than it answers, it does generate several testable hypotheses concerning causation of ovarian cancer. These were discussed in a commentary by Mettlin (*126*). In response, Cramer and Harlow elaborated on their proposed model for pathogenesis of ovarian cancer (*127*). They also discussed the difficulties in discriminating lactose effects from animal fat effects in most previous studies, or the failure of investigators to address this problem at all (*128*). They emphasized the value of measuring blood activity of

galactose-1-phosphate uridyl transferase ("transferase"), a key enzyme in galactose metabolism. Cramer and Harlow found that the ratio of dietary lactose to transferase activity was the strongest variable associated with ovarian cancer risk.

Thyroid cancer

A pooled analysis was conducted of four similarly designed case–control studies of risk factors for thyroid cancer in Switzerland and northern Italy (*129*). Odds ratios were <1.0 for high intakes of most vegetables and fruits; significant trends were observed for carrots, green salad, and citrus fruits. Fish and raw ham were also protective. Odds ratios were >1.0 for high consumption of several types of starchy foods, cheese, butter, oils other than olive, poultry, cooked ham, and sausages. These findings are discussed in terms of possible mechanisms for the protective or risk-enhancing effects. In particular it is noted that goiter is endemic in several of the study areas, which might explain why fish (an iodine source) was protective in this study but not in some others. Overall, mechanisms involving iodine were invoked. The authors suggested that nutritional goitrogens could have the same effect as iodine deficiency by directly affecting thyroid function, inhibiting iodine uptake by the thyroid, or increasing its renal excretion.

Risk factors for fetal or embryonic cells

A study of nutrition during pregnancy and its relationship to pregnancy estrogens was conducted in Greece, to help explain how nongenetic prenatal factors influence cancer risk in offspring (*130*). Total estrogens, estradiol, and estriol were determined in blood samples taken from 141 women during their 26th and 31st weeks of pregnancy. No food group or nutrient was significantly associated with any hormone at both sampling times. Fairly consistent findings were positive associations between potato consumption and most hormone levels and a negative association between vitamin A intake and estradiol and total estrogens. Weight gain up to the 31st week was nonsignificantly associated with total estrogens and estradiol. Although this study permits only tentative conclusions, it suggests that quantitative aspects of diet as reflected by weight gain are more important than dietary composition in influencing the level of pregnancy estrogens and, through this mechanism, the occurrence of gonadal germ cell tumors and conditions associated with them.

CLINICAL AND LABORATORY STUDIES

Vitamins and antioxidants

Oxidative damage to DNA is pivotal in carcinogenesis, aging, and degenerative disease processes. Simic and Bergtold reviewed the rationale for using biomarkers as an index of genetic damage and evaluated thymidine glycol and 8-hydroxydeoxyguanosine as urinary biomarkers (*131*). Levels of these markers were monitored in one man and one woman throughout four controlled dietary cycles. Within the high- and low-calorie cycles, different types of food were fed for 10-day periods while keeping total calories constant. Concentrations of biomarkers were lower in the calorie-restricted diets. With high-calorie diets lacking fruits and vegetables, marker levels were roughly three times higher than with high-calorie diets rich in fruits and vegetables. The authors attributed these differences to plant antioxidants, although the experiments were not designed to identify the dietary component responsible for observed effects. Responses of the subjects were qualitatively similar, but quantitative results depended on both diet and individual reactions. Therefore, because interindividual variation in urinary biomarker levels is great, population averages might obscure significant trends in individuals. The authors recommend assay of urinary biomarkers to assess the carcinogenic or anticarcinogenic properties of diets, specific foods, or individual food components and to evaluate individual responses to nutritional regimens.

The effect of supplementation with vitamins A, C, and E on cell kinetics was evaluated in 41 patients who had undergone polypectomy for colorectal adenomas (*132*). Twenty received vitamin supplements and 21 received placebo. Six biopsy specimens were taken from each subject before treatment and after 3 and 6 months of treatment, for determination of the thymidine labeling index and Φh. (Φh is the ratio of the number of labeled cells in the upper 40% of the crypt to the total number of labeled cells in the crypt. It is an indicator of abnormal expansion of the proliferative compartment and is considered an intermediate marker of cancer risk.) The placebo group showed no significant change in cell kinetics, whereas patients receiving vitamins showed a progressive decline in Φh ($p < .05$ after 3 months and $p < .01$ after 6 months). The thymidine labeling index decreased significantly in the 40% of the crypt near the mucosal surface. Thus vitamins A, C, and E can reduce abnormalities in cell kinetics that may indicate a precancerous condition.

CAROTENOIDS AND RETINOIDS. The ability of β-carotene and canthaxanthin to protect against chemical carcinogenesis was evaluated in a mouse model of bladder cancer (*133*). Mice receiving supplemental β-carotene before and after exposure to the carcinogen developed significantly fewer tumors than unsupplemented mice; canthaxanthin, a carotenoid with no provitamin A activity, was not protective. These results suggest that in this model, the protective effect is not a general property of carotenoids but may result from conversion of carotenoids to retinoids.

The breast carcinogen 7,12-dimethylbenz[*a*]anthracene (DMBA) is thought to act via a free radical mechanism. The effects of dietary kelp (the brown alga *Laminaria religiosa*) on lipid peroxidation and glutathione peroxidase activity were evaluated in livers of rats treated with DMBA (*134*). In both short-term (2 weeks) and long-term (28 weeks) experiments, levels of lipid peroxides were similar in untreated controls and rats receiving DMBA plus kelp, and were significantly lower than levels in rats treated with DMBA alone. In the long-term experiment, glutathione peroxidase activity was lowest in DMBA-treated rats and highest in untreated controls, whereas in the short-term experiment activity was highest in DMBA-treated rats and similar in the other two groups. Thus dietary kelp protected against the lipid peroxidation induced by DMBA; the short-term burst of peroxidase activity may have been induced by the excess peroxides. Kelp is rich in antioxidants, particularly β-carotene; fiber constituents probably also offer protection, by inhibiting DMBA absorption through the intestinal tract. β-Carotene also protected against preneoplastic hepatic lesions in a rat model (*135*). Administration of β-carotene throughout the experiment significantly reduced the incidence, multiplicity, total number and size, and average focal area of hepatocyte nodules induced by a single injection of diethylnitrosamine (initiation) followed by five doses of 2-acetylaminofluorene (promotion). β-Carotene was also protective when administered only before initiation, but not when administered only during promotion. This suggests that the inhibitory effects are exerted primarily during the initiation phase of hepatocarcinogenesis. By linear regression analysis there was a positive relationship between hepatic concentration of β-carotene and number of nodules, but an inverse relationship between hepatic concentration of total vitamin A and number of nodules.

The frequency of chromosome aberrations was evaluated in bone marrow cells of mice treated with β-carotene (0–200 mg/kg) by gavage for 5 days before administration of cyclophosphamide (*136*). Significant protective effect was seen at doses of 5–25 mg/kg after 24 and 32 h, but not after 16 h. The authors propose that the lack of a dose–response relationship was due to the changing balance of mechanisms that inhibit activation of promutagens and stimulate enzymatic detoxification.

β-Carotene, administered orally to mice, reduced new blood vessel formation in the tumor cell–induced angiogenesis assay and increased new blood vessel formation in the lymphocyte-induced angiogenesis assay (*137*). Hairless mice were X-irradiated and then injected intradermally with normal human lymphocytes, HeLa cells, nontumorigenic SKv cells, or tumorigenic SKv keratinocytes. Three days later the new blood vessels growing into the injection site were counted. β-Carotene-treated mice showed significantly less angiogenesis

than controls in response to both of the tumor-cell lines; there was no difference in response to the nontumorigenic SKv cells. These results suggest that the anticarcinogenic effect of β-carotene is due partly to inhibition of angiogenesis within the tumor mass and partly to stimulation of the immune response.

Dietary palm oil carotenes and tocotrienols inhibited formation of viral-induced lymphomas and DMBA-induced skin cancers in female hairless mice in a dose-related way (*138*). The carotenes and tocotrienols appeared to act by different mechanisms: tocotrienols delayed the appearance of lymphomas but did not affect the ultimate extent of tumor development, whereas palm oil carotenes not only delayed the appearance of lymphomas but caused their subsequent regression. Palm oil carotenes completely inhibited development of epithelial papillomas at all concentrations tested, whereas tocotrienols were only partially inhibitory and synthetic carotene was completely inhibitory only at the highest concentration tested. However, another dietary carotene, canthaxanthin, had adverse effects in a female C3H/HeN mouse model of ultraviolet B-induced skin cancer (*139*). When they were 5 weeks old, mice were started on diets containing canthaxanthin, retinyl palmitate, neither, or both. At 18 weeks, part of each dietary group began a 28-week course of ultraviolet irradiation. Canthaxanthin reduced the number of several classes of T lymphocytes, while significantly decreasing tumor-free survival. Retinyl palmitate enhanced or had no effect on these cell populations and reversed or ameliorated the effects of canthaxanthin. The authors concluded that dietary retinyl palmitate and canthaxanthin modulate host T-cell immune response within a growing tumor and may affect tumorigenicity.

The mechanism for the cancer chemopreventive action of carotenoids was sought in their effect on gap junctional communication and lipid peroxidation in C3H/10T1/2 cells (*140*). Dose-related increases in gap junctional intercellular communication were observed with the following order of potency: β-carotene > canthaxanthin > lutein > lycopene > α-carotene. Methyl-bixin was inactive at 10^{-5} M, the highest concentration tested. α-Tocopherol was marginally active. These activities were strongly correlated with the ability to inhibit methylcholanthrene-induced neoplastic transformation. However, the capacity of carotenoids and α-tocopherol to inhibit lipid peroxidation was consistent neither with their ability to inhibit neoplastic transformation nor with their ability to increase junctional communication. In this system, carotenoid-enhanced intercellular communication seems to provide a mechanism for chemoprevention; the data also imply that carotenoids and retinoids function in an analogous manner independent of the carotenoid's provitamin A status.

Vitamin A affords protection against lung cancer, but inadequate intake of this vitamin is prevalent. Interactions between dietary fat and vitamin A were examined in a mouse model of *N*-nitroso-diethylamine-induced lung cancer (*141*). A fat-deficient diet nonsignificantly reduced tumor incidence (7 of 23 mice, vs. 9 of 23 untreated controls), whereas a vitamin A–deficient diet increased tumor incidence to 22 of 23 mice and tumor burden from 3.7 to 6.8. The fat-deficient diet ameliorated the effects of vitamin A deficiency, reducing tumor incidence to 13 of 23 mice and tumor burden to 4.0. Though the study was not designed to detect a protective effect of vitamin A with a high-fat diet, it did demonstrate a protective role for a low-fat diet in vitamin A deficiency. It is noteworthy that animals initially had substantial body stores of vitamin A and showed no visible signs of deficiency during the experiment. Since fat deficiency reduces vitamin A stores, high intake of vitamin A in a very-low-fat diet might augment protection.

Retinoic acid strongly inhibits growth of T-47D human breast cancer cells in vitro (*142*). Synergistic inhibition was observed when cells were treated with retinoic acid and 1,25-dihydroxyvitamin D_3 or an antiestrogen (4-hydroxytamoxifen, 4-hydroxy-clomiphene, or LY117018), but retinoic acid did not affect estradiol-stimulated growth. Concentrations of vitamin D receptors and estrogen receptors were unaffected by inhibitory concentrations of retinoic acid. Thus retinoic acid appears to inhibit proliferation of breast cancer cells directly and to interact with 1,25-dihydroxyvitamin D_3 and

antiestrogens through a mechanism that does not involve receptors.

VITAMIN C. To distinguish between hormonal and chemical mechanisms of estrogen-induced carcinogenesis, Liehr studied the effect of vitamin C on hormone-induced tumor formation and hormone-dependent growth in the Syrian hamster renal-tumor model (*143*). In male hamsters treated with estradiol or diethylstilbestrol (DES), vitamin C decreased incidence of renal tumors by ~50% but had no effect on hormone-dependent tumor growth. It also reduced the concentration of the genotoxic quinone metabolite of DES and its DNA adducts. From these results, Liehr postulated that vitamin C acts by reducing the metabolic oxidation of estrogens and proposed a chemical model for estrogen-induced carcinogenesis (via oxidation to quinones and formation of DNA adducts, rather than hormonal regulation of growth).

Based on the finding that a combination of dehydroascorbic acid and vitamin B-12 inhibits mitosis of tumor cells in mice, these substances were injected into mice with implanted Ehrlich ascites tumor and leukemia and their effect on survival was evaluated (*144*). All tumor-bearing controls were dead by day 19, but more than half of the vitamin-treated mice were still alive on day 60. In vitro, neither dehydroascorbate nor vitamin B-12 alone affected mitosis; together they inhibited mitosis in leukemia and ascites cells but not in normal cells. Dehydroascorbate was more effective than ascorbate. When vitamin B-12 is combined with vitamin C, the cobalt of the B-12 attaches covalently to a carbon in vitamin C. Cobalt acetate and cobalt sulfate, combined with ascorbate, inhibited mitosis as effectively as the combination with vitamin B-12, indicating that cobalt is the critical moiety of B-12 in this system and the active material is cobalt ascorbate.

Dietary L-ascorbate delayed the appearance and reduced the incidence of spontaneous mammary tumors in RIII mice in a dose-related manner, and also significantly delayed onset and reduced incidence of ultraviolet light–induced skin tumors in hairless mice (*145*). However, the meaning of these findings in terms of human cancers is questionable because the doses of vitamin C used were very high and also because the response of rodents, which synthesize vitamin C endogenously, may differ from that of humans.

Daily oral administration of vitamin C to mice and rats significantly reduced DNA, RNA, and protein synthesis in 3-methylcholanthrene-induced basal cell and squamous cell carcinomas (*146*). The effect was related to dose and plasma concentration of vitamin C. In mice bearing B16 melanoma, supplemental vitamin C alone somewhat inhibited tumor growth and increased survival (*147*). Its major effects, however, were to enhance the benefits of levodopa methylester chemotherapy and augment the antimetastatic activity of tyrosine- and phenylalanine-restricted diets. Dehydroascorbic acid, in contrast, increased tumor growth and decreased survival. In animals receiving vitamin C but no chemotherapy, two distinct populations of mice became apparent after 19 days: tumors in one were refractory to inhibition by vitamin C, whereas tumors in the other were inhibited until 31 days, after which they grew slowly.

The multiple effects of ascorbic acid on cell metabolism complicate efforts to explain its antitumor activity, but some clues came from in vitro studies of ascorbate's inhibition of chemical transformation in C3H/10T1/2 cells (*148*). Ascorbate reduced the NADH:NAD$^+$ ratio. In decreasing order of activity and in a dose-dependent manner, ascorbate, isoascorbate, and dehydroascorbate stimulated matrix collagen and glycoprotein synthesis; this activity was related to ability to inhibit methylcholanthrene-induced transformation. In untransformed cells, ascorbate and to a lesser extent dehydroascorbate reduced total lipids, enhanced release of lipids into the medium, and altered ratios between various lipid fractions. Together these results suggest that inhibition of transformation by ascorbate, isoascorbate, and dehydroascorbate involves regulation of the redox potential, glycoproteins, and lipids in C3H/10T1/2 cells. A study in mice with implanted human mammary tumors further suggests that the antitumor activity of ascorbate is related to its chemical properties rather than its role as a vitamin (*149*). Administered in water or food, D-isoascorbic acid and ascorbic acid had similar

inhibitory effects, in the presence of traces of copper III, on growth of subrenal tumor implants. This raises the possibility that certain oxidation or degradation products of these isomers are the active antineoplastic agents in this model.

It is not clear what experiments in rodents and cell culture mean for people; but one retrospective analysis of survival in patients with incurable cancer suggests they mean something (*150*). Examination of computerized records of all cancer patients attending three district hospitals in Scotland during a 4.5-year period identified 1826 patients who had reached an incurable stage. Of these, 294 had received supplemental ascorbate at some time in their illness. The mean survival time of ascorbate-supplemented patients was 343 days, nearly double the 180-day survival of the 1532 unsupplemented patients. Although these results are inconclusive because of the nature of the study, they would seem to justify further blinded, controlled trials.

TOCOPHEROLS AND TOCOTRIENOLS. Compared with nonsmokers, smokers show an increased respiratory burst reaction (RBR) of peripheral blood neutrophilic granulocytes. The RBR involves the NADPH–oxidase system, which generates superoxide anions, and myeloperoxidase, which generates hypochlorous acid. The superoxide anion can undergo dismutation to oxygen and peroxide. Because this can cause oxidative stress, the effect of antioxidants on the RBR of smokers was estimated by the luminol reaction (*151*). After 10 days of supplementation with 200 μg of L-seleno-methionine and 1000 mg of vitamin E, the RBR of the smokers was reduced by 20–75% and was statistically no different from that of the nonsmokers. Other studies suggest that the usual daily intake of vitamin E from foods is insufficient to counteract free radical formation related to smoking. The author suggests that smokers use relatively high amounts of antioxidants to counter the pathological processes associated with smoking. Strenuous physical exercise also increases oxidative reactions and lipid peroxidation in lung tissue in animals (*152*). Groups of control rats and rats given selenium and vitamin E supplements were exposed to one bout of swimming until exhaustion. In lung tissue of controls, this induced increased activity of superoxide dismutase, selenium-dependent glutathione peroxidase, and glutathione *S*-transferase, presumably in response to enhanced formation of superoxide anions and peroxides. In antioxidant-supplemented groups, these enzyme activities were significantly lower than in controls both before and after exercise, indicating reduced generation of oxygen free radicals. The effects of vitamin E and selenium were additive.

Palm oil differs substantially from other fats and oils in fatty acid composition, minor constituents, and structure of its triglycerides. In the DMBA-induced rat mammary tumor model, palm oil was less tumorigenic than corn oil, soybean oil, beef tallow, or lard (*153*). However, palm oil stripped of its tocopherols and tocotrienols enhanced tumorigenesis and addition of 1000 ppm of the tocotrienol-rich fraction to diets of rats fed corn oil slightly reduced tumorigenesis. In this system, therefore, part of the favorable effects of dietary palm oil are attributable to its tocotrienol constituents, which can partially protect against the cancer-promoting effects of corn oil.

Fat

Henderson discussed the rationale for large and small randomized human intervention trials to investigate causal relations between diet and disease and associated questions (*154*). She considered the questions that could appropriately be addressed in such trials, focusing on dietary fat intervention trials for cancer prevention. She described the complementary high-risk and public health strategies for community-wide primary prevention of disease. Metabolic studies in conjunction with dietary interventions can detect changes in biomarkers, monitor compliance, and provide short-term surrogate endpoint measures that reduce cost and improve the reliability of studies. Another type of dietary trial tests interventions to produce long-term changes in dietary behavior in individuals and population-wide. All trials must be designed to limit exposure of low- or average-risk persons to interventions that may have adverse effects; it thus becomes important to distinguish between an intervention meant to lower risk in high-risk

individuals and one that may lower the overall rate of disease in a community.

One index of cancer susceptibility is the level of adenosine diphosphate ribosyl transferase (ADPRT) in peripheral blood mononuclear leukocytes (*155*). This enzyme has been inversely linked to risk for cancers of the lung, colon, and breast and to conditions that predispose to cancer, such as colorectal polyps. A double-blinded trial was conducted to learn whether fatty acids modify levels of ADPRT. After two baseline measurements, 47 women were assigned to take capsules of soybean lecithin (*n*-6; 7.2 g daily) or fish oil concentrate (*n*-3, 1.5 g daily), with ADPRT determinations 4 and 6 weeks after beginning the capsules. After 6 weeks, ADPRT had decreased slightly with lecithin treatment and increased with fish oil. For the 39 subjects who complied well with the protocol, ADPRT was 21% higher in the fish oil group than in the lecithin group. Thus the balance between *n*-3 and *n*-6 fatty acids can modulate ADPRT, and low-dose fatty acid supplementation can alter the enzyme to a degree consistent with altering susceptibility to cancer.

When eicosapentaenoate (EPA) or docosahexaenoate (DHA) was added to the tissue culture medium, transformation of irradiated C3H/10T1/2 cells was reduced (*156*). Similarly, EPA and DHA reduced formation of transformed foci in C3H/10T1/2 and NIH/3T3 cells transfected with the *ras* oncogene. Cells grown with EPA or DHA produced much less prostaglandin E upon challenge, indicating suppression of changes in arachidonate production or utilization that occur during transformation. EPA and DHA caused extensive remodeling of the molecular species of the four phospholipid classes examined. The authors consider various mechanisms by which *n*-3 fatty acids might inhibit transformation and propose that the protective effect stems from changes in the composition of fatty acids released from phospholipids by the action of phospholipases, the result of which is interference with arachidonate metabolism.

BREAST CANCER. Welsch reviewed the relationship between dietary fat and experimental mammary tumorigenesis in rodents (*157*). Spontaneous, induced, and transplanted tumors and metastasis were considered in relation to amount and type of dietary fat and the question of fat vs. calories. Most evidence suggests that the influence of fat is stronger during the promotion phase than during the initiation phase of tumorigenesis, though fat consumption during any period of life may affect tumor development. Threshold effects for total fat and types of fat were discussed, including possible protective effects. Although a low-fat, high-calorie diet reportedly induced rat breast tumors more than a high-fat, low-calorie diet, other evidence supports the idea that enhancement of mammary tumorigenesis by a high-fat diet is a function of the fat, not the calories. The level of exercise also interacts with fat and energy consumption; intense exercise to exhaustion enhances tumorigenesis. Limited data show that the quantitative and qualitative influences of dietary fat on development of human breast carcinomas in immunodeficient mice parallel those on rodent tumors.

The effects of palm oil, soybean oil, and hydrogenated soybean oil on DMBA-induced rat mammary tumors were compared at two levels of fat intake (*158*). With 5% dietary fat, rats fed palm oil had the lowest incidence of tumors and rats fed soybean oil had the highest. With 20% fat, tumor incidence in the palm oil and soybean oil groups was the same and higher than in the hydrogenated oil group, but tumor multiplicity, mean tumor weight, and tumor burden were least in the palm oil group. These data suggest that palm oil is less active than the other oils in promoting DMBA-induced mammary tumors in rats. They also suggest that hydrogenated soybean oil is a less potent promoter than regular soybean oil, in agreement with studies showing a less potent effect for saturated fatty acids and *trans* fatty acids, which in some ways behave as if they were saturated. The tumor-promoting effects of diets high in linoleic acid were confirmed in female SENCAR mice (*159*). Mice were fed diets containing 15% fat, with 0.8, 4.5, or 8.4% as linoleic acid. Mammary tumors were induced by intragastric administration of DMBA. Tumor incidence during the first 15 weeks was directly related and latency to 40% incidence was inversely related to level of dietary linoleic acid. High dietary linoleic acid was associated specifically with increased incidence of the adenosquamous carcinoma histologic type. When MDA-MB-435 human breast cancer cells were transplanted into nude mice fed 5 and 23% corn oil diets, incidence of primary tumors was slightly higher in the high-fat group (*160*). However, a strong effect on metastasis was seen. Of the mice with palpable primary tumors, 18 of 27 in the high-fat group had macroscopic lung metastases, compared with only 8 of 21 in the low-fat group.

A study of the association between plasma lipids and breast cancer was conducted among 196 patients at a breast clinic and two physicians' offices in Buffalo, NY (*161*). Subjects completed a health questionnaire and donated a fasting blood sample before undergoing diagnostic breast biopsy. The 83 women found to have breast cancer had significantly higher plasma triglyceride levels than the 113 who did not have cancer. Further, women with elevated triglyceride or cholesterol levels had lower β-carotene levels. Both high and low cholesterol levels were associated with cancer, but in different ways. Women with more advanced stages of cancer had lower cholesterol levels, consistent with other findings that the metabolic effects of breast cancer may lower plasma cholesterol. These data are compatible with the hypothesis that plasma triglycerides and β-carotene (or related dietary factors) play an etiologic role in breast cancer.

From surveying experimental and epidemiological data, Carroll and Parenteau developed a mechanism linking dietary fat and breast cancer (*162*). They propose that the effects of dietary fat on mammary carcinogenesis are largely mediated by its effects on the adipose tissue of the mammary gland, which influence the growth potential of the mammary parenchyma. High-fat diets encourage energy storage and may promote breast cancer by increasing the amount of adipose tissue in the mammary gland. This would facilitate the transfer of PUFAs, eicosanoids, estrogens, or other growth-promoting substances from adipose to glandular tissue. Low-fat diets would have the opposite effect, reducing exposure of glandular tissue to growth-promoting substances. A similar review of the data and consideration of changes in the management of patients with localized breast cancer led others to outline the rationale for evaluating reduction of dietary fat as adjuvant therapy in postmenopausal breast cancer (*163*). Eight lines of reasoning support the argument that such trials would be timely and of great importance. (1) Epidemiological data show major differences in stage-by-stage survival of patients with localized breast cancer between countries with low-fat and high-fat diets. (2) Relationships have been demonstrated between fat intake and factors prognostic of clinical outcome (e.g., lymph node involvement or estrogen receptor status of tumor) in patients with breast cancer. (3) Weight gain and obesity are consistently associated with increased risk of breast cancer recurrence. (4) Animal experiments provide abundant evidence for the adverse influence of fat on breast tumor growth and metastasis. (5) Linoleic acid promotes growth of human breast cancer cells in vitro. (6) Plausible mechanisms have been advanced to explain how fat intake mediates breast cancer growth and metastasis. (7) Studies have demonstrated good compliance with dietary fat reduction regimens, making dietary intervention practical. (8) A large enough population is available for definitive assessment of dietary interventions.

SKIN CANCER. Reasoning from rat models of breast and pancreatic tumors, investigators hypothesized that high intake of linoleic acid would also enhance phorbol ester's promotion of DMBA-induced skin tumors in SENCAR mice (*164*). Results were unexpected. At dietary linoleic acid levels of 0.8–8.4% with total fat held at 15%, there was a strong inverse relation ($r = -.92$) between linoleate and papilloma number but no relation with papilloma incidence. Moreover, at the highest levels of linoleate the cumulative incidence of carcinomas lagged behind that at the lowest for up to 30 weeks; at intermediate levels incidence was increased, reaching 100% at 41 weeks compared with 69 and 68% at the lowest and highest linoleate levels, respectively. The fatty acid composition of epidermal phospholipids reflected dietary linoleate levels and epidermal prostaglandin E_2 concentration was inversely related to linoleate. Because incidence of mammary tumors showed a dose–response relationship to dietary linoleic acid, the authors concluded that the effects of linoleate are target-specific. Also using

this SENCAR mouse model, other workers investigated the effects of diet and calorie restriction (*165*). Both total diet restriction and carbohydrate-plus-fat calorie restriction inhibited development of papillomas and carcinomas during the tumor promotion phase but not during initiation; calorie restriction was somewhat more effective. When high- and low-fat isocaloric diets were tested, high fat fed during initiation reduced development of papillomas but not carcinomas; high fat fed during and after promotion enhanced numbers of papillomas and development of carcinomas. However, a high-fat diet fed after DMBA initiation, without phorbol ester promotion, did not cause tumors, indicating that the diet enhanced phorbol promotion but was not itself a promoter. Epidermal protein kinase C activity was increased by a high-fat diet and decreased by calorie restriction. Calorie restriction also altered turnover of inositol lipids.

Locniskar et al., using the same model, compared the effects of 5 and 10% dietary corn oil (*166*). The level of corn oil influenced the fatty acid composition of epidermal phospholipids and altered prostaglandin E_2 levels but had only modest effects on skin tumorigenesis. These investigators also compared the effects of fish, coconut, and corn oil in diets containing 10% fat. When the diets were fed before and during the initiation phase only (mice switched to 5% corn oil diet before phorbol ester promotion), there were no significant effects on final papilloma incidence, yield, or size (*167*). However, when fed during promotion by benzoyl peroxide, the diets did differentially affect tumor promotion (*168*): contrary to expectations, saturated fat (coconut oil) caused the highest numbers of papillomas and incidence of carcinomas, whereas the corn oil diet resulted in the fewest papillomas and lowest incidence of carcinomas. Hyperplastic epidermal changes did not reflect promoting activity, nor was induction of ornithine decarboxylase activity correlated with the tumor response. Thus, although dietary fat did modulate tumor promotion by benzoyl peroxide, the mechanism remains unclear. The effects of these diets on events elicited by phorbol ester was examined (*169*). Fatty acid composition of epidermal phospholipids reflected the fatty acid composition of the diet. The fish oil diet reduced prostaglandin E production in epidermal homogenates, elevated epidermal hyperplasia, and altered the subcellular distribution of protein kinase C in the epidermis. Thus diets rich in *n*-3 fatty acids modulate phorbol ester–elicited events in mouse skin to a greater extent than diets containing high proportions of saturated or *n*-6 fatty acids. However, the influence of dietary fat on these events does not reflect the apparent promotion-enhancing activity of the fats, leaving the mechanism for the latter still unexplained.

Changes in membrane composition, eicosanoid metabolism, and immunoresponsiveness were examined to learn how *n*-6 and *n*-3 fatty acids modulate ultraviolet-induced carcinogenesis in hairless mice (*170*). The fatty acid composition of epidermis, plasma, and red blood cells reflected dietary fatty acids, and epidermal capacity to metabolize arachidonic acid was closely related to dietary intake of *n*-6 fatty acids. Animals fed *n*-3 fatty acids had strikingly lower levels of prostaglandin E_2, even when fed supplementary *n*-6 fatty acids. Irradiated mice fed *n*-3 fatty acids had a reduced inflammatory response and delayed hypersensitivity to dinitrochlorobenze.

COLON CANCER. A metaanalysis examined 14 studies of colon carcinogenesis in rats for relationships between the type and quantity of dietary fat and incidence of carcinoma, controlling for calorie consumption (*171*). There was a strong positive correlation between fat intake and incidence of colon carcinoma for Fischer 344 rats but not Sprague-Dawley rats. For both strains, regression coefficients were positive for saturated and polyunsaturated fat and negative for monounsaturated fat. However, the only highly significant coefficient was for polyunsaturated fat in Fischer rats ($p <.01$). Further analysis showed that the strong association between total fat calories and colon carcinoma in Fischer rats was affected very little by control for total calories. The analysis suggests a protective effect of *n*-3 fatty acids, whereas *n*-6 PUFA appears to be a risk factor for Fischer (but perhaps not for Sprague-Dawley) rats.

Both type and amount of dietary fat affect antioxidant mechanisms in the colonic mucosa of the rat without producing overt oxidative tissue damage (*172*). Animals were fed diets with 5 or 20% corn oil, or 19% menhaden oil or beef tallow supplemented with 1% corn oil. Total glutathione and activities of catalase, glutathione peroxidase, superoxide dismutase, glutathione-*S*-transferase, and glutathione reductase were measured in homogenates of the colonic mucosa. The high-fat diets depressed glutathione peroxidase activity; low-fat and menhaden oil diets increased catalase and glutathione-*S*-transferase activity. However, ornithine decarboxylase activity was not induced by the high-fat diets and thiobarbituric acid–reacting substances were virtually undetectable.

In rats, high- and low-fat diets with PUFA-to-saturated fatty acid ratios of 1.2 and 0.3 did not affect total cholesterol, total phospholipids, or distribution of phospholipid classes in colonic mucosal cells (*173*). Diets high in fat or with a high PUFA-to-saturated fatty acid ratio increased the PUFA content of mucosal cell phospholipids at the expense of monounsaturated fatty acids. Levels of lipid peroxides, expressed as nmol/mg of protein, were higher in membrane fractions of rats fed high-fat diets; higher peroxide levels, expressed per nanomol of phospholipid, occurred in mucosal cells of rats fed diets with a high PUFA-to-saturated fatty acid ratio. Although an influence of dietary fat on peroxide levels was clearly shown, it was not clear whether the amount or the nature of the fat was responsible.

The effects of 12% dietary perilla oil (rich in α-linolenic acid), safflower oil, and palm oil on chemically induced colon carcinogenesis in rats were compared (*174*). Serum and mucosal fatty acid compositions reflected the fatty acid composition of the diet. After 10 weeks, concentrations of fecal bile acids did not differ significantly between groups. However, deoxycholic acid–induced activity of ornithine decarboxylase in the colonic mucosa was significantly lower at 10 weeks in the group fed perilla oil; and at 35 weeks, the incidence of colon cancer was also significantly lower in the perilla oil group. Apparently the protective effect of perilla oil results from decreased sensitivity of the mucosa to tumor promoters arising from the altered fatty acid composition in epithelial cell membranes, not from a decrease of promoters such as bile acids.

The effect of 0 and 1.25% dietary cholesterol on initiation and promotion of chemically induced preneoplastic colonic lesions was examined in two mouse strains that differ in their cholesterol metabolism (*175*). In both strains, cholesterol increased the number of aberrant crypt foci, enhanced cell proliferation, and altered the proliferative pattern and crypt morphometrics in the colonic epithelium. Genetic differences in cholesterol metabolism did not influence the results.

The hypothesis that diet-induced colonic epithelial hyperproliferation is caused by increased bile acids and luminal lytic activity in the colon was tested in rats (*176*). A new method was also developed to quantify hemolysis in the presence of fecal water, measuring iron release by atomic absorption spectrophotometry; this is taken as a measure of lytic activity. Rats were fed diets supplemented with different levels of cholesterol plus deoxycholate. In a dose-dependent manner, steroid feeding increased both total fecal and soluble bile acid concentrations, lytic activity of fecal water, and colonic proliferation. Lytic activity was strongly correlated with proliferation ($r = .85$, $p < .001$).

Another way in which dietary fat could influence colon carcinogenesis is by affecting liver microsomal metabolism of colon-specific carcinogens (*177*). To test this idea, Sprague-Dawley rats were fed a 5% corn oil diet or a 20% corn oil, menhaden oil, or beef tallow diet for up to 9 months. After 2 weeks on the test diets, some rats in each group were given weekly injections of the colon carcinogen 1,2-dimethylhydrazine dihydrochloride. Liver microsomes were assayed for N-demethylase activity for aminopyrine and the carcinogen. High-fat diets, especially fish oil, elevated the activity of aminopyrine demethylase, reflecting the cytochrome P450IIB isozyme. Exposure to 1,2-dimethylhydrazine dihydrochloride enhanced activity of the P450IIE isozyme, especially with a beef tallow diet. Therefore multiple forms of P450 are affected by high-fat diets and this effect depends on the fatty acid composition of the dietary lipid.

PANCREATIC CANCER. Mammals cannot convert stearic and oleic acids to fatty acids of the n-3 or the n-6 series. Oleic acid promotes carcinogenesis in some models, whereas stearic acid is inhibitory. The effect of diets with 20% stearic or oleic acid on pancreatic fatty acids and chemically induced preneoplastic lesions was studied in weanling male rats (*178*). Pancreatic lipids reflected dietary lipid composition, but oleic acid feeding reduced the relative content of other fatty acids more than did stearic acid feeding. The number and volumetric indices of atypical acinar cell nodules were evaluated at 26 weeks. The main finding was that unsaturated fat (oleic acid) promoted chemically induced pancreatic carcinogenesis whereas saturated fat (stearic acid) did not.

LUNG CANCER. The effects of EPA and DHA on growth of a human lung carcinoma was studied in athymic Balb-C mice (*179*). Experimental diets were basal diet, basal diet supplemented with EPA and DHA at two levels, and basal diet supplemented with palmitic acid isocaloric with the EPA/DHA diets. Some animals were started on the diets after their tumors had reached a designated size; others began the diets before tumors were implanted. In both types of experiment, dietary EPA/DHA strongly inhibited tumor growth; 40% of mice fed EPA/DHA before tumor implantation were tumor-free when the experiment was terminated. The fatty acid composition of neutral and polar lipids in the liver and tumor reflected the dietary intake of n-3 fatty acids. In the EPA/DHA group tumor levels of prostaglandin E_2 were reduced 7.4-fold. This may be a factor in the inhibition of tumor growth.

Fiber and carbohydrate

One explanation for the generally lower cancer incidence among vegetarians is that they have a lower burden of carcinogens than their omnivorous counterparts. Urinary mutagenicity is an index of this burden. To test the hypothesis that different levels of mutagens are excreted in the urine of ovolacto-vegetarians and persons eating a mixed Western diet, 63 men ate strictly controlled Western or vegetarian diets with limited energy supply and a defined balance of protein, fat, and carbohydrate (*180*). Substantial urinary mutagenicity was found in both groups and there was no difference between groups for any parameter. Moreover, there was considerable variation within groups despite the careful control of the diets. The authors suggest that individual differences in absorption, metabolism, and excretion patterns are of sufficient magnitude to mask group differences. Laboratory experiments, however, do find effects of fiber on metabolism and excretion of mutagens (*181*). Rats were fed a diet containing no fiber, sorghum fiber, wheat fiber, or pectin to which a radiolabeled food carcinogen, MeIQx, was added. Urine and feces were collected for analysis of radioactivity and mutagenicity. Fiber increased fecal radioactivity and mutagenicity with a corresponding decrease in urinary parameters. Diets containing fiber, especially insoluble sorghum and wheat bran, protected the large bowel by diluting MeIQx and shortening its transit time; in addition, the kidneys of rats fed sorghum and wheat bran retained less radioactivity than kidneys of rats in the pectin and control groups. However, none of the fibers affected retention of MeIQx in the liver, and DNA adduct formation in liver and kidney did not differ significantly between groups.

BREAST CANCER. Because estrogens appear to be involved in development of breast cancer and dietary fiber is protective, Rose et al. determined the effect of wheat, oat, and corn bran on serum estrogen concentrations in 62 premenopausal women (*182*). After 2 months on a diet supplemented with one of these brans to provide ~30 g/day of fiber, the group supplemented with wheat bran had significantly reduced serum estrone and estradiol levels; there was no change in progesterone or sex hormone–binding globulin. Oat and corn brans did not affect serum estrogens. These results suggest that the favorable effect of fiber on breast cancer risk is partly due to its effect on the concentrations and bioavailability of circulating estrogens. In an in vitro system, 17β-estradiol bound to various fibers more strongly than did estrone, estriol, or estrone-3-glucuronide (*183*). Cholestyramine and lignin bound nearly all the estrogen in the medium; other fibers that bound >80% of the estrogens were linseed, oats, barley chaff, and wheat bran. Corn, rye, and white wheat flour had a relatively low affinity for estrogens. When tested for

digestibility in pigs, fibers with the highest percentage of lignin had the lowest digestibility and the highest affinity for estrogens.

Studies with female rats evaluated the effect of wheat bran on chemically induced breast tumor development, plasma estrogen levels, and estrogen excretion (*184*). Experimental diets contained 11% fiber based on wheat bran and 0.5% fiber based on white wheat flour. When rats were treated with *N*-nitrosomethylurea to induce mammary tumors, tumor incidence and latency were similar in the two dietary groups, although tumor weight and multiplicity were somewhat lower in the high-fiber group. In untreated females, fecal excretion of free and conjugated estrogens was roughly 3 times greater in the high-fiber group and urinary excretion was lower. Diet had no effect on plasma concentrations of total estrone throughout the estrus cycle or on unconjugated 17β-estradiol during the basal part of the cycle; during the peak of the cycle, plasma 17β-estradiol was more elevated in the high-fiber group than in the low-fiber group. The authors concluded that dietary wheat bran interrupts the enterohepatic circulation of estrogens without significantly affecting plasma levels. Dietary fiber also influenced excretion of radiolabeled estrogen injected into male rats (*185*). Rats fed a diet with 11.6% wheat bran excreted roughly twice as much radiolabel in the feces during the first day after injection as rats fed 2%- or <1%-fiber diets, whereas urinary excretion was significantly higher in rats on the two low-fiber diets. Even when the intestinal microflora is adapted to the experimental diets, wheat bran still accelerates fecal excretion of labeled compounds. Again, the authors tentatively attribute this to interruption of the enterohepatic circulation of estrogens.

COLON CANCER. Bleyl reviewed the two-step (initiation, promotion) theory of the etiology and pathogenesis of colon cancer, with emphasis on the role of dietary fiber (*186*). He discussed exogenous (e.g., dietary carcinogens) and endogenous (e.g., bile acid metabolism) factors and the effect of fiber on gastrointestinal function and colon carcinogenesis. Data from animal experiments support the conclusion that dietary fiber acts only during the promotion stage and that the "protective effect" is a delay in promotion. The various effects of fiber are specific to particular plant fibers.

Several studies in humans addressed the effects of dietary fiber on colonic markers of cancer risk (187–190). Oat, corn, and wheat bran modified colonic bacterial enzymes and bile acids in distinctive ways in premenopausal women (187). For 8 weeks, subjects ate their customary diets supplemented with one of the brans to increase total fiber intake to ~30 g/day. Stools were collected before and after the period of fiber supplementation for determination of four bacterial enzymes, bile acids, and neutral sterols. Wheat bran decreased concentrations of fecal deoxycholic acid, lithocholic acid, 12-ketolithocholic acid, and neutral sterols and activities of all bacterial enzymes. Oat bran did not affect secondary bile acids or 7α-dehydroxylase but decreased the other bacterial enzymes. Corn bran increased 7α-dehydroxylase, lithocholic acid, and cholesterol and decreased deoxycholic acid coprostanol and cholestenone levels and nitroreductase and azoreductase activity. In a study of postpolypectomy and nonpolyp subjects, diets were supplemented with oat or wheat bran to learn whether these fibers modify putative risk factors for colon cancer (188). Biopsies taken before and after the intervention showed no change in thymidine labeling index of colonic crypt cells, thymidine labeling pattern, or incidence of nuclear aberrations. However, oat bran significantly reduced fecal pH by 0.23 ± 0.07 units and wheat bran increased fecal butyrate concentrations. These results did not demonstrate an advantage of one fiber over the other. As another measure of colon cancer risk, urinary and fecal mutagenicity was measured in healthy adults before and 3 months after they switched from a well-balanced mixed diet to a lactovegetarian diet (189). With the lactovegetarian diet there was a lower intake of protein and fat and higher intake of carbohydrate, fiber, calcium, and vitamin C. Total fecal mutagenic activity was not affected by diet, but the concentration of direct-acting mutagens decreased after the dietary change; this might be explained by a dilution mechanism resulting from increased fiber intake. Both concentration and amount of urinary promutagens

decreased on the lactovegetarian diet. In another dietary study, 9 subjects adopted an extreme, uncooked vegan diet for 1 month and then resumed a conventional diet; 9 controls maintained their conventional diet (190). Fecal choloylglycine and activities of hydrolase, β-glucuronidase, and β-glucosidase decreased significantly during the first week of the vegan diet and then remained constant throughout the remainder of the vegan period, returning to initial levels within 2 weeks after the conventional diet was resumed. Daily urinary output and serum concentrations of phenol and p-cresol also decreased during the vegan dietary period. Thus this extreme vegan diet caused a decrease in certain bacterial enzymes and toxic products that are considered risk factors for colon cancer.

Konjac mannan is a glucomannan frequently used in traditional Japanese foods. When fed to Fischer 344 rats it significantly reduced fecal β-glucuronidase, nitroreductase, and azoreductase activities and production of phenol and indole (191). In male C3H/He mice bearing human intestinal flora, it reduced fecal activities of β-glucuronidase and nitroreductase and production of p-cresol and indole. Konjac mannan feeding produced only slight changes in composition of the intestinal microflora.

Dietary fiber attenuated the tumor-promoting activity of a high-fat diet in nude mice bearing human colon cancer HT29 or WiDr xenografts (192). Although somewhat different results were obtained with the two cell lines, the high-fat, no-fiber diet generally enhanced tumor volume, weight, and protein content. It enhanced DNA content in tumors of the HT29 group and ornithine decarboxylase activity in tumors of the WiDr group. Since these tumors were remote from the large intestine, the authors believe the observed effects could be due to a circulating trophic factor.

The effect of oat, rye, and barley bran and sugar-beet fiber on bile acid metabolism was studied in rats in the context of high- and low-fat diets (193). All types of fiber significantly increased fecal output and reduced concentrations of bile acids. With rye bran, however, the total output of fecal bile acids was increased; and oat bran slightly but significantly increased the pool of bile acids in the small intestine. The dietary fat level (5 or 20% corn oil) did not affect these parameters. Results for sugar-beet fiber were unexpected because about 50% of this fiber is soluble. This and the effect of rye bran illustrate the limitations of fiber analysis in predicting physiological effects of a fiber source.

Various fibers have distinct patterns of effects in different regions of the rat colon (*194*). Oat bran and guar gum (highly fermentable fibers) were compared with wheat bran in their effects on the luminal environment. With the low-fiber control, guar, and oat bran diets there was a falling gradient of short-chain fatty acids and pH along the large bowel. With wheat bran, total short-chain fatty acid levels in fresh feces were three times those with the other diets, and fecal butyrate concentrations and pH were maintained at cecal values in the distal large bowel. Slowly fermented fibers appear to have the greatest effect on the distal environment. The effect of wheat bran on butyrate concentration is notable because butyrate has putative antitumor activity.

The effects of high-risk (high-fat, low-fiber, low-calcium) and low-risk (low-fat, high-fiber, high-calcium) diets on formation of aberrant crypt foci and colon tumors were studied in male rats (*195*). After 4 weeks, half of the rats in each dietary group were injected with azoxymethane and half with saline. After 6 weeks, half of the rats in each dietary/injection group were crossed over to the other diet for 6 weeks. The number of aberrant crypt foci in azoxymethane-treated rats decreased in the order high-risk/high-risk > low-risk/high-risk > high-risk/low-risk > low-risk/low-risk. Among saline controls, only the high-risk/high-risk group developed foci, and these were fewer than in azoxymethane-treated groups. When part of the azoxymethane-treated rats were continued on their respective diets for an additional 14 weeks, 92% of rats on the high-risk diet developed tumors, compared with 33% of those crossed over to the low-risk diet. No tumors developed in saline-injected rats. The authors claim that theirs is the first study to demonstrate a linear relationship between formation of aberrant crypt foci and subsequent development of colon tumors in the same group of experimental animals.

The incidence of 1,2-dimethylhydrazine-induced colon cancer in rats was influenced by supplementation with soluble dietary fibers (*196*). Rats were maintained on a basal diet supplemented with 5% cellulose during an 8-week initiation phase, then subdivided into groups receiving no fiber, 10% pectin, 10% guar gum, or 5% pectin + 5% guar gum. Supplementation with 10% pectin or guar gum significantly suppressed cancer incidence but the pectin–guar gum combination did not. The effect was restricted to the descending colon, which had the highest incidence of tumors in all dietary groups.

One way in which dietary fiber protects against colon cancer may be by adsorbing mutagens or carcinogens. Two in vitro studies demonstrated the ability of potato (*197*) and taro (*198*) fiber to adsorb the hydrophobic mutagen 1,8-dinitropyrene. Cell walls from potato skins strongly adsorbed the mutagen, whereas cell walls from the fleshy part of the tuber adsorbed only weakly. Pectic polysaccharides in the flesh walls appeared responsible for maintaining the mutagen in solution. Competition between soluble and insoluble fiber components may have important implications for the distribution and availability of hydrophobic mutagens in the alimentary tract. Whereas dicotyledonous plants and cereal grains provide nearly all the fiber in European diets, non-grain monocotyledonous plants (banana, yam, pineapple, coconut, taro) are the staple fiber sources in Polynesian diets. Preparations of unlignified cell walls from three edible parts of taro (*Colocasia esculenta*) were tested for their mutagen-binding ability. Although the walls of grasses and grains (Poaceae) are frequently assumed to be typical of monocotyledons, this study showed that taro cell walls have monosaccharide compositions and mutagen-binding properties more similar to those of dicotyledons and that there may be important differences in the major dietary fibers of European and South Pacific food plants.

The growth of dimethylhydrazine-induced dysplastic crypt foci was studied in female rats in the context of a high-fat, low-fiber, low-calcium diet with 46% carbohydrate as corn starch or sucrose (*199*). Under these conditions, starch reduced proliferative activity in the colon as measured by the thymidine labeling index. Starch-fed rats also had a smaller number of dysplastic crypts per focus.

Dietary restriction

To determine the effects of diet on benzo[a]pyrene metabolism in hepatocytes, rats were fed control, high-fat, or food-restricted diets (200). Hepatocytes were then isolated and incubated with benzo[a]pyrene. The triacylglycerol content of hepatocytes was proportional to dietary fat and calories, whereas the rate of benzo[a]pyrene metabolism was inversely related to triacylglycerol content. The metabolic changes occurred without changes in activity of the relevant microsomal enzymes as determined in microsomal preparations. The authors suggest that diet modulates benzo[a]pyrene metabolism by inducing changes in intracellular triacylglycerol, particularly in lipid droplets, thus altering access of benzo[a]pyrene to enzyme binding-sites. Innovative experiments by the same group further evaluated the effects of food restriction on hepatic metabolism of benzo[a]pyrene (201). Rats were fed ad libitum or given 65% of the food eaten by the ad libitum group for 3 weeks. Benzo[a]pyrene was then infused directly into their livers; the livers were removed, a small lobe was excised for analysis, and the remaining parts were transplanted into naive rats. In this way, any observed effects of food restriction were effects specifically on the liver, rather than on some other physiological or biochemical process. Food restriction roughly doubled polar metabolites of benzo[a]pyrene in blood of donors and quadrupled metabolites in liver. Four hours after transplantation, polar metabolites in the blood and transplanted liver of hosts were 2 to 3 times as high in animals that received livers from food-restricted donors. Rates of monooxygenation and glucuronidation in intact cells were also about twice as high in livers from food-restricted rats. These findings support the conclusions of the previous study (200). The authors further hypothesize that food restriction enhances the supply of cofactors that stimulate benzo[a]pyrene metabolism.

The effects of dietary fat, protein, and energy intake on initiation and promotion of azoxymethane-induced cancers were examined in 3×3 factorial experiments (202). In the initiation experiment, rats were fed experimental diets (8, 16, or 32% of energy from casein with 12, 24, or 48% of energy

from corn oil) during the initiation period and then switched to a control diet during the promotion period; in the promotion experiment, the experimental diets were fed during promotion. Low-protein diets during initiation were highly significantly associated with risk of renal and mesenchymal malignancies; high-protein diets during initiation nonsignificantly increased risk of polypoid adenocarcinoma of the colon. No other relationships were seen between diet and carcinogenesis in either phase. However, multiple logistic regression analysis combining results of the two experiments found that ad libitum energy intake was significantly associated with intestinal carcinogenesis, the risk increasing by $6.2 \pm 2.6\%$ for each additional kilocalorie consumed. The lowest quintile of rats consumed 60 kcal/day, whereas the highest averaged 74 kcal/day. This corresponded to more than a doubling of risk. Another combined analysis of several studies found that energy intake was the most important determinant of fatal neoplastic disease in male Fischer 344 rats (203). Particular attention was given to leukemia and pituitary adenoma, the most common fatal neoplasms in this strain. The only dietary manipulation that depressed mortality rate due to neoplasia involved reduction in energy intake; reduction of mineral, protein, or fat intake without an accompanying reduction in energy had at most a marginal effect.

Protein

One effect of low protein intake is to increase thermogenesis (the proportion of energy intake expended as heat). At the same time, protein restriction reduces the development of aflatoxin B_1–induced hepatocellular γ-glutamyl transpeptidase–positive (GGT+) foci and tumors in male Fischer 344 rats (204). The association between thermogenesis and development of GGT+ foci was studied in rats treated with aflatoxin and then fed diets containing 4, 8, 12, 16, or 22% protein for 6 weeks. Development of GGT+ foci was sharply reduced in animals fed 4 and 8% protein, yet calorie consumption per 100 g of body weight was greater. Urinary norepinephrine and dopamine and rate of norepinephrine turnover in brown adipose tissue were also elevated in these animals. There was a negative trend in oxygen consumption with increasing levels of dietary protein. Thus inhibited development of GGT+ foci at low levels of protein intake is associated with several indicators of increased thermogenesis. The same research group evaluated the potential of remodeled preneoplastic foci in aflatoxin B_1–treated rats to renew growth in response to reexposure to high dietary protein (*205*). All animals were fed a 20% casein diet during initiation. One group was maintained on this diet for 4 additional 3-week feeding periods (designated 20:20:20:20); another was switched to a 5% casein diet (5:5:5:5). Other groups were switched to alternating high- and low-protein dietary regimens. Subgroups of rats were killed after each 3-week period. Development of GGT+ foci was suppressed throughout the promotion period in animals fed 5% casein and enhanced in animals fed 20% casein. Rats on 20:5 and 20:20:5 regimens showed regression of foci to the level seen under 5:5 and 5:5:5 regimens, respectively. The remodeled foci, however, retained potential for an even greater growth rate upon reintroduction of the high-casein diet: development of foci was significantly greater in the 20:5:20 and 20:20:5:20 groups than in the 5:5:20 and 5:5:5:20 groups, respectively. Thus development of foci stimulated by early exposure to a high-protein diet could be reversed and held in check by a low-protein diet; but upon reexposure to promoter, development resumed at a greater rate than upon first exposure.

Methyl deficiency

Beyond the realization that choline-deficient diets are carcinogenic for rats, little is known of the carcinogenic mechanism. Review of studies of hepatocarcinogenesis in rodents fed choline-deficient and -sufficient diets suggested a nutritional model of hepatocarcinogenesis (*206*). It is based on the following observations, among others: (i) choline deficiency initially leads to deposition of fat in hepatocytes and their subsequent death, which triggers compensatory regeneration; (ii) animals fed a choline-deficient diet followed by a choline-sufficient diet have a higher rate of hepatocarcino-

genesis than animals fed only the deficient diet; and (iii) c-*myc* gene amplification appears universal in this model of hepatocarcinogenesis, but the number of excess copies per tumor cell is greater when choline is refed after deficiency and some adjacent nontumor tissue also shows gene amplification. The authors propose that repeated cycles of cell injury, death, and regeneration produce the gene alterations required for initiation, promotion, and transformation of liver cells; that choline deficiency can cause this chain of events; but that lack of choline hampers, or restoration of choline facilitates, some cellular event or events that enhance tumorigenesis.

A study in male Fischer rats supported the hypothesis that methyl-deficient diets are carcinogenic at least partly because they induce hypomethylation of DNA and accompanying changes in regulation of gene expression (*207*). By Northern blot analysis, livers of rats given methyl-deficient diets or the hepatocarcinogen 2-acetylaminofluorene had significantly elevated levels of c-*fos* and c-*myc* mRNA and somewhat elevated c-Ha-*ras* mRNA, compared to controls. Concomitantly, there were sharp decreases in levels of mRNAs for epidermal growth factor and its receptor. The appearance of hypomethylated DNA in livers of methyl-deficient rats coincided with the changes in these mRNAs. Further investigation indicated that depletion of *S*-adenosylmethionine pools was responsible for the DNA hypomethylation, which caused changes in expression of genes with key roles in growth regulation (*208*). Changes in DNA methylation and gene expression were gradually reversed after restoration of an adequate diet. The authors suggest that although human diets are unlikely to be as severely methyl-deficient as the experimental diet, many are borderline; and effects of such diets may be exacerbated by consumption of mycotoxins or therapeutic agents, or by substance abuse. Thus it is plausible that interactions of marginally methyl-deficient diets, contaminants, and drugs could contribute to cancer in humans through the mechanism of altered DNA methylation and aberrant gene expression.

Breast cancer in rats is also influenced by dietary sources of methyl groups (*209,210*). Female

Sprague–Dawley rats were weaned to a 20% casein diet supplemented with DL-methionine and injected with *N*-nitrosomethylurea when they were 7 weeks old (*209*). Five weeks later they were divided into groups fed isocaloric, isoprotein diets with casein, soybean protein, or soybean protein plus methionine. The soybean protein diet with its low methionine content significantly repressed the incidence and growth of mammary tumors; methionine supplementation increased tumor incidence but not mean tumor weight. In contrast, in a model of DMBA-induced mammary tumorigenesis, supplementation of a basal diet with DL-methionine had no effect on induction and growth of adenocarcinoma but cancer cells were more highly differentiated in the supplemented group (*210*).

Minerals

CALCIUM. Welberg et al. reviewed epidemiological, animal, in vitro, and clinical evidence that calcium protects against colon cancer (*211*). Amid all the positive findings, however, they observed that calcium supplementation increases proliferation of epithelial cells in the sigmoid colon of patients with adenomatous polyps. This finding warrants follow-up study. Lipkin reviewed diseases of the gastrointestinal tract that lead to increased frequencies of cancer (*212*). These were discussed in terms of the effects of calcium on proliferation and differentiation of gastrointestinal cells and tumor occurrence in rodent models and human subjects.

Thymidine labeling index (LI), mitotic index (MI), nuclear aberration (NA), and intraductal proliferation (IDP) are early markers of mammary cancer risk; the LI in colonic epithelial cells is a similar marker for colon cancer. Effects of dietary phytic acid and minerals on these markers were assessed in mice (*213*). Phytate supplementation reduced LI and NA in the mammary gland; iron or calcium supplementation increased the colon LI and all mammary markers; phytate reversed the effects of minerals. Significant relationships were also found between the various markers.

Among the mechanisms suggested for calcium's protective action against colon cancer is the chelation of fatty acids and bile salts in the small intestine to form nontoxic calcium soaps. Calcium may also act on the colonic mucosa. Effects of dietary calcium on fecal concentrations of free fatty acids and free bile acids were measured in Sprague–Dawley rats (*214*). Compared with rats fed a control diet, rats whose intake of calcium was tripled had 33% lower concentrations of fecal free bile acids and 117% higher concentrations of fecal free fatty acids. When rat colonic explants were cultured at three levels of calcium, the rate of crypt cell production was inversely related to calcium concentration.

Because dietary factors influence colorectal cancer risk and modulate both fecal mutagenicity and fecapentaene concentrations, these fecal parameters were evaluated in ovolactovegetarian and omnivorous subjects (*215*). Counter to expectations, the predominant fecapentaenes were excreted in higher concentrations by the vegetarians. Nutrient intake accounted for only 22% of fecapentaene excretion; dietary calcium was the most significant factor positively correlated with this. Although fecapentaenes are considered strong fecal mutagens, only 1 of 20 samples was significantly mutagenic for *Salmonella typhimurium* TA100. Furthermore, aqueous extracts of feces from omnivores and vegetarians were equally mutagenic, although extracts from omnivores contained no detectable fecapentaenes. The authors postulate that increased excretion of fecapentaenes results in decreased exposure to them, and therein lies reduction of colon cancer risk. The relationships between diet and fecapentaene excretion were complex, however, and no mutagenicity was attributable to these compounds.

A review of the modulating effects of calcium on colon cancer in animal models and high-risk human subjects concluded that dietary fat is in some way an etiologic factor in colon carcinogenesis (*216*). Under conditions of basic colonic pH, fatty acids and bile acids can cause cell loss and compensatory hyperproliferation. Calcium may reduce lipid damage by complexing with fat to form harmless calcium soaps. Definitive conclusions about the ability of calcium to prevent colon cancer in humans await the results of ongoing clinical trials.

Four elevated-risk features of the Western diet are high fat, high phosphorus, low calcium, and low vitamin D contents. A study in rats and mice examined the effects on colonic hyperproliferation of increasing dietary calcium while maintaining the other high-risk elements (*217*). At a calcium level corresponding to the median intake for an adult in the USA, there were significantly increased numbers of proliferating cells in crypt columns in the sigmoid colon of mice and rats and in the ascending colon of mice. With high calcium intake, hyperproliferation was only slightly greater than in animals fed a nonstressful diet.

There is evidence that calcium and vitamin D together modulate colon carcinogenesis (*218–220*). This subject was reviewed by Newmark and Lipkin (*218*). Having shown that calcium supplementation of a vitamin D–sufficient diet reduced the size and multiplicity of dimethylhydrazine-induced colon tumors (*219*), investigators examined relationships between dietary calcium and vitamin D in terms of K-*ras* and H-*ras* mutations (*220*). Rats were fed a control diet or calcium-supplemented diets either deficient or sufficient in vitamin D. DNA from dimethylhydrazine-induced tumors was amplified and examined for *ras* oncogene point mutations. About one-third of the tumors from control and vitamin D–deficient animals had K-*ras* guanine-to-adenine mutations; no K-*ras* mutations were found in tumors from calcium-supplemented, vitamin D–sufficient animals; no H-*ras* mutations were detected in tumors from any dietary group. Altering K-*ras* mutations may be one way in which calcium and vitamin D status influence colon carcinogenesis in this model.

The activity of ornithine decarboxylase, the rate-limiting enzyme in biosynthesis of polyamines, is greatly elevated in colon carcinomas and it is sometimes considered an index of cancer risk. An age-related increase in basal rectal mucosal ornithine decarboxylase activity was found in patients with adenomatous polyps; the increase could be suppressed by calcium supplementation (*221*). Although tyrosine kinase activity was unaffected by calcium, concentrations of phosphotyrosine membrane proteins with M_r 40,000–60,000 and 80,000–100,000 were suppressed in patients whose ornithine decarboxylase activity was suppressed. No nonpolyp controls were studied.

However, Paraskava questioned the safety of calcium supplementation to prevent colon cancer in high-risk patients (*222*). Citing observations that calcium inhibits proliferation of normal colonic epithelium but colorectal cancers and adenomas are relatively refractory to calcium, the author suggests that reduced response to calcium occurs early in tumor development before cells become malignant. It is therefore possible that while inhibiting growth of normal epithelium, calcium could promote selective outgrowth of abnormal cells.

No effects of dietary calcium or vitamin D were seen in a mouse model of DMBA-induced, phorbol ester–promoted skin tumors (*223*). Nor, however, were serum levels of calcium affected by the various diet regimens.

Because calcium seems to inhibit the promotion of colon cancer by dietary fat and interactions between calcium, phosphorus, and vitamin D have been reported, Carroll et al. investigated these interactions in a breast cancer model (*224*). After initiation of tumors by DMBA, rats were switched to a high-fat diet in which levels of calcium, phosphorus, and vitamin D were systematically varied. Overall, the results indicated that vitamin D is protective at low levels of calcium and phosphorus, whereas high amounts of phosphorus increase risk at low levels of calcium and vitamin D.

CADMIUM. Most interest in cadmium has been in cadmium as a carcinogen, but anticarcinogenic activity has also been observed. Lung and liver tumors were initiated by diethylnitrosamine in B6C3F1 mice, after which 0, 500, or 1000 ppm of cadmium was supplied in drinking water for 50 weeks (*225*). The low level of spontaneous tumors in these animals was not affected by cadmium, but at 1000 ppm cadmium, incidence of diethylnitrosamine-initiated tumors was reduced to control levels; 500 ppm cadmium had an intermediate effect. When administered subcutaneously during initiation and followed by sodium barbital promotion, cadmium again suppressed tumor formation. However, it did not reduce the size of tumors that did form, indicating that what was modified was the population of cells available for promotion, not the promotion process itself. The authors suggest that cadmium is specifically toxic for previously initiated lung and liver cells.

SODIUM CHLORIDE. The effects of NaCl on lipid peroxidation in gastric mucosa and urine were assessed in rats (226). Animals were fed diets supplemented with 0–4.0% NaCl for 5 weeks; some rats given 0 or 4% NaCl were also given 20 ppm of indomethacin in their drinking water. There was a dose-related and closely correlated increase of malondialdehyde in urine and gastric mucosa. At 2 and 4% NaCl, proliferation of fundic mucosal cells was also significantly increased. All these effects were suppressed by indomethacin. Thus NaCl, a gastric tumor promoter, enhances lipid peroxidation and cell proliferation in the gastric mucosa.

SELENIUM. Yu et al. reported further findings (see *Food Safety 1991* Chapter 2, reference *185*) in intervention trials with selenium supplementation in Chinese populations at high risk for liver cancer (227). Five townships with initially similar high rates of primary liver cancer were studied; four served as controls, while the fifth used table salt fortified with 15 ppm of anhydrous sodium selenite. In the fifth year of the study, control townships had age-adjusted incidence rates of liver cancer ranging from 42.7 to 58.9 per 100,000, compared with 27.5/ 100,000 in the experimental township. A second trial evaluated selenized yeast supplements vs. placebo for 4 years in carriers of the hepatitis B virus surface antigen. Incidence of liver cancer was 4.4% in the placebo group and 0% in the selenium-supplement group. Unscheduled DNA synthesis and occurrence of micronuclei were also significantly less in the supplemented subjects. A third trial was conducted in members of families with a high incidence of primary liver cancer. Again, supplementation with selenized yeast significantly reduced liver cancer incidence, unscheduled DNA synthesis, and micronucleus formation.

Selenium supplementation before and during initiation with DMBA was tightly correlated in a dose-related way with reduction in rat mammary tumors ($r = -.99$) (228). When selenium feeding

(4 µg/g) was continued through the promotion phase final tumor incidence was further reduced to 5%. Supplementation for 2 weeks sharply reduced the occurrence of DMBA–DNA adducts, which correlated positively with final tumor incidence ($r = .99$).

Orotic acid

Visek reviewed information on nitrogen-stimulated orotic acid synthesis and nucleotide imbalance, with special reference to effects of dietary orotic acid, including tumor promotion (229). Whereas these studies documented tumor-promoting effects of orotic acid, another paper reported dose-related mitoinhibitory effects in isolated rat hepatocytes (230). Rats were subjected to various manipulations that induce proliferation of liver cells. Hepatocytes were then isolated and cultured in the presence of different levels of orotic acid. Orotic acid inhibited DNA synthesis even when added 24 hours after the hepatocytes were primed with transforming growth factor α. This indicates that the target site is not at the level of the growth-factor receptor or early receptor-mediated events. There is evidence that orotic acid increases the pool of uridine nucleotides and decreases the pool of adenosine nucleotides, inhibiting the expression of the ribonucleoside diphosphate reductase gene and consequently inhibiting mitosis. Nucleotide imbalance is invoked as a mechanism for both promoting (229) and inhibitory (230) effects.

Anticarcinogens and antimutagens

To evaluate the SOS chromotest for detection of antimutagens, bacteria were treated with a variety of mutagens and known antimutagens were added simultaneously or after mutagen treatment (231). The time of adding the antimutagen was critical for some substances; and some substances inhibited only certain mutagens. Overall, the test was very useful for detection of antimutagens.

Many major and minor dietary components modulate the effects of mutagens and carcinogens. Piero et al. studied the influence of main dietary components on genotoxicity of food mutagens (232). Variations of type and amount of fat altered the genotoxic activity of a variety of indirectly active dietary mutagens by interfering with or enhancing activation processes. Type, amount, and timing of fat intake also act on the promotion phase. Other main dietary components including starch, cellulose, and calcium interact with dietary fat. Wattenberg reviewed animal studies on the inhibition of carcinogenesis by minor dietary constituents (*233*). These substances act as blocking agents by preventing carcinogens from reaching or reacting with critical target sites, as suppressing agents by preventing or interrupting the neoplastic process in cells that otherwise would become malignant, or both. Examples of the action of various types of blocking and suppressing agents are given.

With the large and growing number of dietary anticarcinogens that have been identified, the idea of "designer" foods and ingredients for cancer prevention is timely (*234,235*). Pariza discussed the promise and potential problems of designer foods, emphasizing the complexity of the scientific and regulatory issues involved (*234*). He presented a hypothetical example of a designer fat substitute, drawing partly from his own work on conjugated linoleic acid. Meanwhile, the National Cancer Institute has launched a five-year "Designer Foods" initiative to study, evaluate, and develop experimental foods for cancer prevention (*235*). In tables, diagrams, and text Caragay summarized the foods and phytochemicals of interest and the steps in carcinogenesis at which they might act.

Studies on the effects of 250 plant constituents on phorbol ester–induced inflammation have identified critical structural features associated with activity (*236*). The double bond at the 2,3 positions of flavonoids, the alkyl group at C-4 of sterols and triterpenes, and the methylene-dioxyl group at the 2,3 positions of the berberine structure are involved in inhibition of tumor promotion. Induction of epidermal ornithine decarboxylase activity by phorbol ester was inhibited by cepharanthine, sitosterol, lupan-type triterpene derivatives, and flavonoid aglycones.

In vivo and in vitro studies of dietary phytoestrogens and breast cancer suggested possible mechanisms for their action (*237*). Data were reported for 30 postmenopausal women in the Finlandia study (11 omnivores, 10 vegetarians, and 9 apparently healthy women who had been treated for breast cancer by surgical removal of the breast). Vegetarians had plasma levels of sex hormone–binding globulin at least twice as high as omnivores and breast cancer patients; they also had significantly higher urinary excretion of lignans, isoflavonoids, diphenols, and enterolactone. There were significant negative correlations between sex hormone–binding globulin and urinary estrone and 16α-hydroxyestrone. These observations and results from binding and in vitro cell culture studies suggest that lignans and isoflavonoids affect sex hormone metabolism and carcinogenesis by altering plasma levels of sex hormone–binding globulin, resulting in decreased uptake and activity of these steroids and inhibition of growth of hormone-dependent cancers.

***ALLIUM* VEGETABLES.** Allixin is a bioactive compound (a "phytoalexin" or "stress compound") produced by garlic. Because it inhibited the promotion of skin tumors by phorbol ester in a mouse model, its possible antimutagenic activity was of interest (*238*). In the *S. typhimurium* TA100/rat liver S9 system, allixin showed a dose-related inhibition of aflatoxin B_1-induced Histidine$^+$ revertants. At 75 µg/mL it inhibited aflatoxin B_1 binding to calf thymus DNA and reduced formation of DNA adducts. It also inhibited formation of organosoluble metabolites and glutathione conjugates of aflatoxin. At least some of these effects may be mediated through inhibition of microsomal P450 enzymes. A derivative of aged garlic extract, *S*-allyl cysteine, inhibited growth of LA-N-5 human neuroblastoma cells in vitro, with half-maximal response at ~600 µg/mL (*239*). However, this compound was unable to induce differentiation in neuroblastoma cells or to potentiate the effects of retinoic acid and 8-bromo-cAMP, agents that do promote differentiation of these cells.

Another component of garlic oil, diallyl sulfide, inhibits the metabolic activation of carcinogenic nitrosamines such as 4-(methylnitrosamino)-1-(3-pyridyl)-1-butanone (*240*). Female A/J mice were pretreated with diallyl sulfide and then given a single dose of the carcinogen. Some mice were killed immediately to assess microsomal metabolism of the carcinogen. Oxidative metabolites in diallyl sulfide–treated mice were reduced by as much as 90% in the lung; they were also sharply reduced in liver microsomes. At 16 weeks, 100% of the controls had lung tumors, compared to 38% of treated animals; tumor multiplicity was 7.2 vs. 0.6 tumors/mouse in the respective groups. Other investigators studied the effects of diallyl sulfide on benzo[*a*]pyrene-induced carcinogenesis in the mouse, to elucidate the mechanism of its antineoplastic activity (*241*). Diallyl sulfide increased activity of glutathione *S*-transferase (which detoxifies a variety of electrophilic xenobiotics, including some harmful metabolites of benzo[*a*]pyrene) by up to 60% in the stomach; this resulted from new enzyme synthesis. Pulmonary glutathione *S*-transferase activity also increased, but not in a dose-related way. Increases in activity of glutathione peroxidase, another detoxification enzyme, were even greater in stomach and lungs and were dose-related. No effect on glutathione-dependent enzymes was seen in liver or kidney. The results suggest that diallyl sulfide and perhaps other organosulfur compounds exert an antineoplastic effect by modulating glutathione-dependent detoxification enzymes. With the rat liver S9 fraction as the metabolic activation system, diallyl sulfide and ajoene (another organosulfur compound from garlic) inhibited aflatoxin B_1 binding to calf thymus DNA and aflatoxin–DNA adduct formation (*242*). This was correlated with an inhibition of microsomal cytochrome P450-dependent aflatoxin metabolism, as the two compounds also decreased formation of water-soluble and organosoluble aflatoxin B_1 metabolites. However, these authors did not find any effect of diallyl sulfide or ajoene on glutathione *S*-transferase activity.

CRUCIFEROUS VEGETABLES. Compounds in cruciferous vegetables also induce enzymes of xenobiotic metabolism, affording protection against carcinogens and other toxic electrophilic compounds. Quinone reductase is one of these enzymes. By monitoring quinone reductase induction in cultured murine hepatoma cells as an assay for anticarcinogens, investigators isolated and identified (–)-1-isothiocyanato-(4*R*)-(methylsulfinyl)butane (sulforaphane) as a potent phase II enzyme inducer in broccoli (*Brassica oleracea italica*) (*243*). To identify the structural features responsible for the activity, the authors synthesized and tested racemic sulforaphane and several analogues differing in the oxidation state of the sulfur and the number of methylene groups. The presence of oxygen on sulfur enhanced potency. Sulforaphane and its sulfide and sulfone derivatives induced both quinone reductase and glutathione *S*-transferase activities in several mouse tissues.

Vegetables of the genus *Brassica* also contain an indolylmethyl glucosinolate known as glucobrassicin (*244*). From this is generated, by a thioglucosidase-mediated autolytic process, indole-3-carbinol. In the stomach indole-3-carbinol forms a variety of condensation products, which are responsible for some of the alterations in carcinogen metabolism observed in animals fed *Brassica* plant foods or indole-3-carbinol itself. The chemistry, pharmacology, and antineoplastic activity of these substances are discussed. There are other actions of indole-3-carbinol as well. In 12 healthy men and women, ingestion of 6–7 mg/day of indole-3-carbinol for 7 days increased 2-hydroxylation of estradiol by ~50% (*245*). Urinary excretion of 2-hydroxyestrone was significantly increased relative to excretion of estriol, confirming the induction of 2-hydroxylation. Thus indole-3-carbinol alters endogenous estrogen metabolism toward increased production of catechol estrogen, providing one explanation for how eating cruciferous vegetables reduces cancer risk. This research group further studied the effects of dietary indole-3-carbinol on estradiol metabolism in a spontaneous mammary tumor mouse model (*246*). Indole-3-carbinol increased the cytochrome P450 content of hepatic microsomes and the level of estradiol 2-hydroxylation up to 5-fold. After 8 months, mice fed 500 or 2000 ppm of indole-3-carbinol had significantly lower tumor incidence and multiplicity than controls and tumor latency was prolonged at the higher dose. The authors concluded that indole-3-carbinol induces P450-dependent estrogen metabolism and is chemopreventive in their mammary tumor model. The protective effect may result from increased

2-hydroxylation and inactivation of endogenous estrogens.

TEA. The polyphenols in green tea (*Camellia sinensis*) have antigenotoxic activity and protect mice against skin tumors induced by ultraviolet B radiation (*247*). Female SKH-1 hairless mice were given plain drinking water or drinking water supplemented with 0.1% (w/v) green tea polyphenols throughout the study. Another group was treated with four topical applications of the polyphenols. Eight days after the start of these treatments, the mice began a 25-week protocol of ultraviolet B exposure. Drinking water supplementation lowered tumor incidence and multiplicity (p <.01) and increased tumor latency (p <.05); topical application of polyphenols afforded some protection, but less than ingested polyphenols. At concentrations in drinking water similar to those in some beverages, green tea polyphenols also protected mice against skin tumors induced according to other protocols (*248*): (i) ultraviolet B irradiation followed by treatment with phorbol ester; (ii) treatment with 7,12-dimethylbenz[*a*]anthracene followed by irradiation; (iii) initiation with 7,12-dimethylbenz[*a*]anthracene and promotion with phorbol ester. Tumor incidence and multiplicity were both reduced.

N-Nitrosodiethylamine induces forestomach and lung tumors in >90% of treated A/J mice (*249*). When a green tea infusion was the sole source of liquid throughout the experiment, pulmonary tumor incidence was decreased by 44% and multiplicity by 60%; forestomach incidence was decreased by 26% and multiplicity by 63%. Treatment with a single 103 mg/kg dose of 4-(methylnitrosamino)-1-(3-pyridyl)-1-butanone produced pulmonary adenomas in nearly all mice, at a multiplicity of 9.3/mouse after 16 weeks. A 0.6% extract of decaffeinated green or black tea given during carcinogen treatment decreased tumor multiplicity by ~65%; when given after carcinogen treatment until the end of the experiment, the green tea extract decreased tumor incidence and multiplicity by 30 and 85%, respectively. Black tea extract given after carcinogen treatment decreased multiplicity by 63% but did not influence tumor incidence. In a rat model of chemical carcinogenesis, the polyphenol

fraction of green tea inhibited formation of colon tumors (*250*). After tumor induction by azoxymethane, experimental groups were given 0.01 or 0.1% polyphenols in drinking water throughout the promotion period, weeks 11–26. Tumor incidence and multiplicity were significantly lower in the two polyphenol-treated groups than in controls, but at these dosages no effect of dose was observed. These experiments show that tea polyphenols are effective when given during either initiation (*249*) or promotion (*249,250*).

QUERCETIN. Quercetin is a flavonoid widespread in fruits and vegetables. Its antiproliferative activity on normal bone marrow and leukemic blast cells was tested in an in vitro clonogenic assay (*251*). All 4 acute lymphoid leukemias and 12 of 14 acute myeloid leukemias tested were highly sensitive to quercetin, showing >50% growth inhibition at a concentration of 2×10^{-6} M. Normal bone marrow cells were inhibited <50% at a quercetin concentration of 2×10^{-5} M. When normal bone marrow was depleted in CD34+ cells, the remaining population was highly sensitive to 2×10^{-5} M quercetin, whereas the isolated CD34+ progenitors were fully resistant. These findings suggest that quercetin can inhibit growth of many leukemias without suppressing normal hematopoiesis.

Quercetin also inhibits colonic neoplasia (*252,253*). In in vitro studies, quercetin at concentrations between 10^{-9} and 10^{-6} M reversibly inhibited proliferation of three human colon cancer cell lines in a dose-dependent manner (*252*). The inhibition was due to blocking in the G_0/G_1 phase of the cell cycle. In a whole-cell assay with 17β-[^{3}H]estradiol as a tracer, the authors demonstrated that the inhibitory potential of quercetin and several related flavonols was directly correlated with their affinity for type-II estrogen binding sites. This mechanism may also be operative in vivo. Dietary quercetin (0.1, 0.5, and 2.0%) and rutin (1.0 and 4.0%) were fed to mice to assess their ability to inhibit azoxymethanol-induced colon tumors (*253*). In mice not treated with the carcinogen, quercetin and rutin had no effect on proliferative parameters in the colonic epithelium. In carcinogen-treated mice, 2% quercetin and 4% rutin significantly reduced hyperproliferation and inhibited the shift of S-phase cells to the middle and upper portion of crypts. These mice also had significantly fewer carcinogen-induced focal areas of dysplasia. Regardless of treatment, tumors were most frequent in the distal colon. Quercetin and rutin both reduced tumor incidence, but for rutin this effect was not statistically significant.

ELLAGIC ACID. Ellagic acid is a plant phenol found in certain fruits and nuts, particularly strawberries. It has antimutagenic and anticarcinogenic activities. When added to mouse liver microsomes, it increasingly inhibited NADPH-dependent lipid peroxidation up to a concentration of 2×10^{-3} M (*254*). Maximum inhibition (70%) of ascorbate-dependent lipid peroxidation occurred at an ellagic concentration of 10^{-3} M. Consistent with these results, feeding of ellagic acid to mice significantly depressed microsomal NADPH- and ascorbate-dependent lipid peroxidation. In addition, feeding caused significant increases in levels of reduced glutathione and glutathione reductase in liver and lungs, but no change in catalase or superoxide dismutase activity.

Ellagic acid also inhibits xenobiotic metabolism by cytochrome P450IIE1. This effect was examined using hydroxylation of 4-nitrophenol to monitor catalytic activity in a rat liver S9 fraction (*255*). In addition, the effect of ellagic acid on mutagenicity of *N*-nitrosodimethylamine was studied in a system using *S. typhimurium* TA100 and rat liver S9. Both experiments demonstrated ellagic acid's inhibition of cytochrome P450IIE1-mediated metabolism, which may account at least partly for its antimutagenic effects.

A lyophilized extract of *Quercus actissima* significantly retarded oxidation of refined, bleached, and deodorized lard and fish oil (*256*). The authors postulated that ellagic acid contributed to the antioxidative action of this extract.

LIPIDS AND MODIFIED LIPIDS. Antitumor effects of lipids and lipid derivatives have been reported. In mice bearing a transplanted colon carcinoma, daily administration of EPA by gavage beginning after tumors became palpable delayed progression of tumor growth (*257*). The effect was dose-related, with a maximum response at 1.25–2.5 g/kg of EPA. At this dosage, host body-weight was maintained, degradation of skeletal muscle was reduced, and survival time was roughly doubled. γ-Linoleic acid has a less pronounced effect, and only at a dose of 5 mg/kg at which there was some toxicity. Other studies have shown that DHA has no activity in this system.

Conjugated dienoic derivatives of linoleic acid (CLA) are a newly recognized class of anticarcinogenic fatty acids. This is of great interest because, as Pariza points out (*258*), linoleic acid itself is the only fatty acid that has clearly been shown to *enhance* cancer risk in rodents. Pariza reviewed his studies of the various activities and food sources of CLA. CLA is most abundant in dairy products and meat of ruminants and less abundant in meat of nonruminants; plant oils and eggs are poor sources. The most active form is the *cis*-9,*trans*-11 isomer. When CLA is ingested, all isomers subsequently appear in triglycerides, whereas only the *cis*-9,*trans*-11 isomer is found in phospholipid (*259*). CLA is an effective antioxidant in vitro and in vivo. Dietary CLA is incorporated into phospholipids of liver microsomes, rendering them more resistant to oxidation than microsomes from control animals. In vitro, CLA shifts benzo[*a*]pyrene metabolism in mouse fibroblasts away from activation and toward detoxification, again suggesting an antioxidant effect. A hypothetical antioxidative mechanism is presented. One further effect of CLA is inhibition of the ornithine decarboxylase response to phorbol ester.

When rats were fed 0.5, 1.0, or 1.5% CLA beginning before treatment with benz[*a*]anthracene and continuing to the end of the experiment, the total number of mammary adenocarcinomas was reduced by 32, 56, and 60%, respectively (*260*). Tumor incidence and cumulative tumor weight were also reduced. Because CLA suppresses peroxidation of fatty acids in the test tube, endogenous lipid peroxidation products in liver and mammary gland were measured. Lipid peroxidation was suppressed in mammary gland but not in liver. However, maximum antioxidant activity was achieved at a much lower CLA dosage than that for maximum antitumor activity, indicating that some other anticarcinogenic mechanism was involved.

2-Amino-3-methylimidazo[4,5-*f*]quinoline (IQ) is a carcinogen formed in grilled ground beef. IQ–DNA adduct formation was measured in mice treated with IQ after 45 days of daily CLA administration by gavage (*261*). CLA inhibited adduct formation in livers of both male and female mice and in kidney, lung, and large intestine of females. There was no effect in stomach or small intestine. Liver, lung, and stomach are considered IQ target organs; large intestine, small intestine, and kidney are nontarget organs. Thus CLA activity in this system varies with the organ and irrespective of whether the organ is an IQ target.

The in vitro effects of physiologic concentrations of CLA and β-carotene were evaluated for human malignant melanoma, colorectal, and breast cancer cell lines (*262*). In melanoma and breast cancer cells, CLA caused significant dose- and time-dependent mortality; colon cancer cells were also inhibited, but not in a dose-related way at the concentrations tested. β-Carotene inhibited only breast cancer cells. Incorporation of tritium-labeled leucine, thymidine, and uridine was significantly reduced in breast cancer cells treated with CLA; only incorporation of labeled leucine was reduced in melanoma and colon cancer cells.

PROTEASE INHIBITORS. Feeding of diets with soybeans, supplemental ascorbate, or both enhanced cellular and humoral immunity in rats in the presence of dibutylamine and sodium nitrite, precursors of the carcinogen dibutylnitrosamine (*263*). In the spleen lymphocyte transformation test, dibutylamine/nitrite treatment alone decreased blastogenesis, whereas feeding soybeans and/or ascorbate with or without dibutylamine/nitrite treatment significantly increased blastogenesis over levels in untreated controls fed a basal diet. Similarly, in the spleen lymphocyte migration inhibition test, inhibition activity was lower than control levels in treated mice not receiving dietary supplements and higher in diet-supplemented mice whether or not they were treated. Treated mice exhibited significant decrease in percentage of rosette-forming cells; this percentage was increased by supplemented diets and again,

the effect of dibutylamine/nitrite treatment was reversed. Total serum proteins and individual fractions, including γ-globulin, were significantly reduced by treatment and this was prevented by soybean and/or ascorbate feeding. The reduction in serum proteins is attributable to the toxicity and carcinogenicity of the dibutylnitrosamine formed in vivo by animals treated with the precursors. Although the mechanism for the effect of soybeans was not explored, the authors implied that protease inhibitors were involved.

The soybean-derived Bowman–Birk protease inhibitor suppresses carcinogenesis in vitro and in vivo. To discover a mechanism for this, its effect on expression of oncogenes in colon of irradiated and nonirradiated rats was explored (*264*). Standard dot and Northern blot analysis of cellular RNA demonstrated that the Bowman–Birk protease inhibitor prevented radiation-induced overexpression of c-*myc* and c-*fos* without affecting their normal expression. It did not affect radiation-induced overexpression or normal expression of c-Ha-*ras* and c-EGFR or normal expression of c-actin. Thus the inhibitor selectively suppressed overexpression of c-*myc* and c-*fos* while not affecting crypt proliferation; by implication, a protease is involved in the enhanced expression of these genes. The Bowman–Birk protease inhibitor also suppressed *N*-nitrosomethylbenzylamine-induced esophageal carcinogenesis in rats (*265*). Lesions were produced by injection of the carcinogen. Some rats were fed the protease inhibitor throughout the experiment. The inhibitor reduced the frequency of papillomas and carcinomas by 45%. The frequency of five features characteristic of preneoplastic esophageal lesions was also significantly reduced, the greatest reduction being in occurrence of lesions with simple hyperplasia.

To learn how the Bowman–Birk inhibitor prevents development of lung tumors in the mouse, its effect on protease activity in selected mouse tissues was determined (*266*). After a single injection of the purified inhibitor, hydrolysis of a synthetic substrate was sharply reduced in lung homogenates; smaller but still significant reductions were seen in liver and kidney homogenates. Maximal inhibition in lung (44%) occurred 2 hours after injection, but not until after 4 hours in kidney and 16 hours in liver. Inhibition was dose-related whether purified Bowman–Birk inhibitor was injected in vivo or added to an in vitro lung homogenate system. The inhibitor had no significant influence on the disposition of benzo[*a*]pyrene in mice although it did decrease activities of hepatic cytochrome P450 and P450-dependent monooxygenases. The authors concluded that the chemopreventive effects of Bowman–Birk inhibitor on lung tumors in mice are most likely mediated through protease inhibition in the target organ rather than by a nonspecific effect on carcinogen metabolism and disposition.

A protease inhibitor from pigeon pea (*Cajanus cajan*) was isolated, purified, and partially characterized (*267*). It markedly reduced aflatoxin B_1-induced β-galactosidase activity in *Escherichia coli* PQ37, regardless of the order in which protease inhibitor and aflatoxin were added to the medium. This suggests that the inhibition was due to action on the protease produced in response to aflatoxin-induced DNA damage in the bacteria. The results are consistent with the hypothesis that protease inhibitors suppress growth of transformed cells by inhibiting a protease-like activity required for unrestrained growth.

FLAXSEED LIGNANS. Lignans have antimitotic, antioxidant, weak estrogenic, and antiestrogenic properties, and flaxseed is an exceptionally abundant source of mammalian lignan precursors (*268*). A short-term feeding trial in female rats addressed the question of whether supplementing a high-fat, tumor-promoting diet with flaxseed flour or defatted flaxseed meal could reduce the risk for mammary cancer as indicated by some early markers for mammary carcinogenesis. The fat content of all diets was 20%. After 4 weeks, flaxseed supplementation reduced mammary gland epithelial cell proliferation by 39–55% and nuclear aberrations by 59–66%. These effects were accompanied by increased urinary excretion of lignans, reflecting the ability of flaxseed to supply lignan precursors. With a similar protocol, flaxseed supplementation also suppressed early markers of colon carcinogenesis in male rats (*269*). The numbers of aberrant crypts and foci were reduced by 41–53% and 48–57%, respectively, in the descending colon of supplemented

groups, and the [^{3}H]thymidine labeling index was somewhat lower. Again, urinary excretion of lignans was strikingly increased (10- to 40-fold). In a clinical study, flaxseed consumption for 6 weeks increased urinary lignan excretion (enterodiol and enterolactone) 7- to 28-fold in six healthy young men (*270*). There were no significant changes in plasma levels of total testosterone, free testosterone, or sex hormone–binding globulin. Although it has been postulated that dietary lignans inhibit hormone-dependent carcinogenesis by modulating the hormonal environment, short-term flaxseed consumption did not alter the hormonal milieu.

NATURAL FOODS AND MEDICINES. Extracts of sesame, chestnut, dad-lily, laver, red date, green tea, kelp, and bamboo shoot were tested by Ames test procedures for antimutagenic activity in *S. typhimurium* TA98 and TA100 (*271*). All of them significantly reduced the number of revertants induced by aflatoxin B_1 or metabolic extracts from *Aspergillus versicolor* or *Aspergillus ochraceus*, although results varied somewhat with the *Salmonella* strain and the mutagen tested.

Feeding of an Ayurvedic food supplement (M-4) significantly reduced the number and size of metastatic lung nodules in female mice bearing transplanted Lewis lung carcinomas (*272*). Differences in tumor morphology were also seen. In particular, tumor cells of M-4-treated mice had slightly smaller nuclei and much more cytoplasm than tumor cells of untreated mice and appeared more differentiated. This type of food supplement has been used in India for thousands of years to enhance health. M-4 itself has been reported effective in preventing or treating cancer and atherosclerosis. It contains Indian gull nut (*Terminalia chebula*), Indian gooseberry (*Emblica officinalis*), dried pepper catkins (*Piper longum*), Indian pennywort (*Hydrocotyle asiatica*), nutgrass (*Cyperus rotundus*), white sandlewood (*Santalum album*), butterfly pea (*Clitoria ternatea*), shoeflower (*Hibiscus rosa-sinensis*), aloewood (*Aquilaria agallocha*), licorice (*Glycyrrhiza glabra*), cardamom (*Elettaria cardamomum*), cinnamon (*Cinnamomum zeylanicum*), turmeric (*Curcuma longa*), ghee (clarified butter), and sugar. The results of this mouse study indicate that there is some biological basis for use of this ancient preparation.

Water extracts from 107 vegetables and 60 mushrooms were examined for antimutagenic activity in an Ames-type assay using *S. typhimurium* TA98 (*273*). Extracts of lemonbalm (*Melissa officinalis*), thyme (*Thymus vulgaris*), butterbur flower (*Petasites japonicus*), momijigasa (*Cacalia delphiniifolia*), oregano (*Origanum vulgare*), field horsetail (*Equisetum arvense*), shiroza (*Chenopodium album*), gyojaninniku (*Allium victorialis* var. *platyphyllum*), and tarragon (*Artemisia dracunculus*) most strongly inhibited the mutagenicity of Trp-P-1. Extracts from 37 other plants also reduced revertants by at least 50%. Many of the plants belonged to the families Compositae, Labiatae, Cruciferae, and Umbelliferae. Of the mushrooms, *Volvariella volvacea* var. *volvacea*, *Armillariella mella*, *Meripilus giganteus*, *Russula nigricans*, *Cantharellus cibarius*, *Laetiperus sulphureus* var. *miniatus*, *Collybia maculata*, *Lactarius volemus*, *Grifola frondosa*, *Morchella esculenta* var. *esculenta*, and *Naematoloma sublateritium* had substantial antimutagenic activity.

Extracts of lettuce and chard were administered to male Balb/C mice simultaneously with benzo[*a*]pyrene, by gastric intubation (*274*). When urine samples were tested for mutagenicity by the Ames test, urine from benzo[*a*]pyrene-treated rats produced up to 4 times the number of revertants that were induced by urine from controls. Urine from animals given extracts from either vegetable reduced the number of benzo[*a*]pyrene-induced revertants to control levels. Referring to papers by others, the authors postulate that the effect is largely attributable to chlorophyll.

A number of polysaccharides with antitumor activity isolated from different sources have the same basic β-1,3-glucan structure. However, an antitumor rice bran polysaccharide is an α-1,6-glucan with 5% branching at the 3-positions of glucose in the backbone (*275*). The primary structure is very similar to that of B512 dextran, which has neither antitumor nor immunostimulating activity. To reveal the structural characteristics responsible for the antitumor activity of rice bran polysaccharide it was partially hydrolyzed with formic acid, partially degraded ultrasonically, or passed through a strongly acidic ion exchange resin. The M_r is ~10^6 as determined by gel permeation chromatography, but a change in apparent molecular weight that occurs upon passage through the ion exchange resin indicates that the substance is a molecular aggregate. Degradation products with M_r >10^4 retained in vivo antitumor activity against Meth-A fibrosarcoma in mice and in vitro stimulatory effects on macrophages to induce tumoricidal activity and interleukin 1 production. Smaller particles were virtually inactive. Thus the polysaccharide is characteristically an aggregate, but aggregation is not necessary for its antitumor activity.

Of the major population groups in Singapore, Malays and Indians have a lower rate of gastric and colorectal carcinoma and peptic ulcer than Chinese; they also eat more chili (*276*). An active constituent of chili, capsaicin, protects against gastric mucosal injury in some models; and since chili accelerates gastrointestinal transit it might inhibit colon carcinogenesis. Sprague–Dawley rats were fed 0, 100, or 200 mg of chili powder daily; some rats in each dietary group received subcutaneous injections of azoxymethane weekly for 6 weeks as well. The number, size, and location of benign and malignant duodenal and colonic tumors in carcinogen-treated animals were not affected by chili intake. In the dietary controls, mucosal contents of nucleic acid and protein were higher in chili-fed animals but the rate of crypt cell production was unaffected. Thus chili did not affect carcinogenesis or mucosal proliferation but moderately increased mucosal mass.

Betel leaves (*Piper betle* L.) are prescribed for many ailments in traditional Asian Indian medicine and are an ingredient of a chew called "pan" (*277*). Antimutagenic and anticarcinogenic activities of betel leaf extract have been reported. The effect of betel leaf extract and some of its constituents (eugenol, hydroxychavicol, β-carotene, and α-tocopherol) on benzo[*a*]pyrene-induced forestomach tumors in mice was evaluated. On a molar basis, maximum protection was afforded by β-carotene and α-tocopherol. All substances except β-carotene increased levels of reduced glutathione in liver, whereas all except eugenol enhanced glutathione *S*-transferase activity. There was a wide range of α–tocopherol and β-carotene contents in fresh betel leaves from different sources.

In some cultures, ginseng is commonly used to protect against stress, the common cold, and inflammatory diseases (*278*). To see if ginseng has antimutagenic properties as well, a preparation from a ginseng callus tissue culture, known as bioginseng, was tested. When added to culture medium for Chinese hamster cells at concentrations of 10 and 100 μg/mL, the bioginseng preparation stimulated cell proliferation and decreased the frequency of sister chromatid exchanges, indicating antimutagenic activity. At 1000 μg/mL the bioginseng was weakly cytotoxic. Addition of mitomycin C to the culture medium caused a 4-fold increase in number of cells with chromosomal aberrations; addition of bioginseng before or with the mutagen halved the frequency of mutagen-induced aberrations. Bioginseng also reduced the number of cells with chromosomal aberrations induced by nitroso-methylurea in mice with Ehrlich's ascites tumors. The authors attribute these effects to bioginseng's activity as an antioxidant and free-radical scavenger.

Licorice (*Glycyrrhiza glabra* L.) has been used as a sweetening agent and as a drug in traditional Chinese medicine. Some of its constituents and their derivatives reportedly have antiinflammatory, antiviral, and anticarcinogenic activity (*279*). Three compounds in licorice (extract 348, carbenoxolone, and glycyrrhetinic acid) inhibited aflatoxin B_1-induced, S9-mediated mutagenesis in *S. typhimurium* TA100 in a dose-dependent manner. They also sharply inhibited aflatoxin B_1 binding to calf thymus DNA and significantly decreased its activation to mutagenic and carcinogenic metabolites. However, the authors urge caution in the use of licorice as a cancer preventative or for its other reputed health benefits because high doses and extended use have also produced harmful effects.

Nagasawa et al. reported further studies of the chemopreventive role of motherwort (*Leonurus sibiricus* L.), an herbal medicine, against preneoplastic and neoplastic lesions of the mammary gland and uterus in multiparous GR/A mice (*280*). Extracts of motherwort were separated on ion exchange resins into adsorbed and nonadsorbed fractions. The two fractions suppressed incidence

and growth of palpable spontaneous mammary tumors to a similar extent. Neither fraction alone affected pregnancy-dependent mammary tumors, mammary hyperplastic alveolar nodules, or uterine adenomyosis. The complete motherwort extract, however, promoted pregnancy-dependent mammary tumors and inhibited hyperplastic alveolar nodules and adenomyosis. It appears that the motherwort extract contains multiple active components, some of which work synergistically.

Rats can be partially protected from the hepatotoxicity of aflatoxin B_1 by crocetin, a natural carotenoid (*281*). Groups of rats were given 25 μg of aflatoxin B_1 in DMSO 5 times per week for 9 weeks, 0.1 mg/day of crocetin in DMSO for 10 weeks, both aflatoxin and crocetin, DMSO only, or no treatment. After 45 weeks, no liver lesions were found in the controls or the crocetin group. Three aflatoxin-treated rats died before the end of the experiment. Of the 10 that remained alive, all had liver lesions. Eight of 13 rats receiving both aflatoxin and crocetin had lesions. Aflatoxin treatment alone increased serum activities of four liver enzymes and levels of bilirubin. With simultaneous administration of crocetin all these values were normal except for γ-glutamyl transpeptidase, whose activity remained slightly elevated. This work demonstrated an anticarcinogenic activity of crocetin during initiation, corroborating findings with other antioxidants. Having previously shown that crocetin enhances hepatic glutathione *S*-transferase activity in rats, the authors postulate that rat liver has an inducible glutathione *S*-transferase that decreases formation of aflatoxin–DNA adducts.

β-Myrcene is a monoterpene found in many essential oils and has a long history of use in perfumes, as a food additive, and in folk medicine (*282*). Its effect on mutagen-induced sister chromatid exchanges was studied in Chinese hamster V79 cells and human hepatic tumor (HTC) cells. In V79 cells, β-myrcene effectively inhibited sister chromatid exchanges induced by cyclophosphamide and aflatoxin B_1 in a dose-dependent manner but had no effect on induction by benzo[*a*]pyrene and DMBA. It also inhibited cyclophosphamide-induced sister chromatid exchanges in HTC cells, which are able to activate cyclophosphamide to its biologically active metabolites. These results are compatible with the idea that β-myrcene affects the genotoxicity of indirect-acting mutagens by inhibiting certain forms of cytochrome P450 enzymes that activate premutagens such as cyclophosphamide and aflatoxin B_1.

Biochanin A, an isoflavone from red clover (*Trifolium pratense* L.), was discovered while screening plant extracts for potential antimutagenic and anticarcinogenic blocking agents. The mechanisms by which biochanin A inhibits metabolic activation of benzo[*a*]pyrene were studied in hamster embryo cell cultures (*283*). Biochanin A inhibited both the metabolic oxidation of benzo[*a*]pyrene and the glucuronidation of its metabolites. It also inhibited oxidation of the carcinogen by rat liver S9 fraction and decreased formation of DNA adducts in hamster embryo cells. In a V79 cell–mediated mutation assay, it reduced the number of benzo[*a*]pyrene-induced mutants in a dose-dependent way. Thus several lines of evidence indicate that biochanin A inhibits metabolic activation of benzo[*a*]pyrene.

The anticarcinogenic activities of three limonoid glucosides from oranges were tested in the hamster buccal pouch model of carcinogenesis (*284*). After an initial treatment with limonin 17-β-D-glucopyranoside, nomilin 17-β-D-glucopyranoside, or nomilinic acid 17-β-D-glucopyranoside, buccal pouches were painted on alternate days, five times a week, with the limonoid glucoside and with DMBA dissolved in mineral oil. Controls were painted with mineral oil and water or mineral oil and one of the limonoids. After 15 weeks, most of the carcinogen-treated animals had multiple tumors, regardless of limonoid treatment. However, limonin 17-β-D-glucopyranoside treatment roughly halved the average tumor burden and average tumor mass and nonsignificantly reduced the total number of tumors. The authors discuss the implications of these findings for citrus fruits in terms of biochemical and flavor changes during ripening and structure–anticarcinogenicity relationships among the limonoids.

Catechol, a naturally occurring phenolic antioxidant, strongly promotes *N*-methyl-*N'*-nitro-*N*-nitrosoguanidine–initiated carcinogenesis in the rat forestomach and glandular stomach (*285*). It and its analogs hydroquinone and resorcinol are present in cigarette smoke; catechol is also found in onions, crude beet sugar, oxidative hair dyes, and coffee. Although not mutagenic in the Ames test, catechol and hydroquinone induce sister chromatid exchanges and delay cell division in human lymphocytes. However, all three compounds exhibited anticarcinogenic activity in a female Syrian golden hamster model of pancreatic cancer. Tumors were initiated with *N*-nitrosobis(2-oxopropyl)amine, after which animals were maintained on a basal diet or basal diet with catechol, hydroquinone, or resorcinol. After 20 weeks there was a reduced incidence of neoplastic and preneoplastic pancreatic lesions in all antioxidant-treated groups. The results suggest a weak inhibitory activity on pancreatic carcinogenesis for this class of compounds, perhaps through a common mechanism.

Emodin is a biologically active anthraquinone produced especially in the Polygonaceae and Rhamnaceae and certain fungi (*286*). Although hepatotoxic, cytotoxic, and mutagenic activities have been described, antimutagenic effects were reported from China. *Rheum palmatum* and *Polygonum cuspidatum* (used as laxatives and anticancer drugs in traditional Chinese medicine) and their active component emodin induced dose-dependent decreases in the mutagenicity of three cooked-food mutagens in *S. typhimurium* TA98. Emodin reduced the mutagenicity of IQ by directly inhibiting hepatic microsomal activation and not by interacting with proximate IQ metabolites or modifying DNA repair in the bacterial cell.

Pariza's research group has studied the anticarcinogenic activity of Japanese-style fermented soy sauce (shoyu) (*287,288*). First they established that soy sauce has anticarcinogenic activity in a mouse model of forestomach neoplasia (*287*). Female mice were fed a diet containing 0–30% soy sauce for two weeks after which they were treated with benzo[*a*]pyrene. Soy sauce caused a significant dose-dependent reduction in forestomach neoplasms after 23 weeks; the maximal effect occurred with a 20% soy sauce diet. Nitrite at up to 500 ppm in drinking water did not influence the number of neoplasms in any group. Unexpectedly, soy sauce induced ornithine decarboxylase activity. A solution of sodium chloride corresponding to the concentration of salt in the soy sauce also induced the enzyme, to a lesser extent. Soy sauce contains considerable antioxidant activity, which was partially purified by ethyl acetate extraction (*288*). The ethyl acetate fraction also contained flavor and aroma compounds; the amino-carbonyl color compounds remained in the larger, ethyl acetate–insoluble fraction. Both fractions inhibited benzo[*a*]pyrene-induced forestomach neoplasia when fed after exposure to the carcinogen. The soluble fraction was partially characterized by high-performance liquid chromatography. A major flavor/aroma component is 4-hydroxy-2(or 5)-ethyl-5(or 2)-methyl-3(2H)-furanone, which accounted for a considerable part of soy sauce's antioxidant activity and effectively inhibited benzo[*a*]pyrene-induced neoplasia in the mouse forestomach.

SPICES. The main coloring component of turmeric, curcumin, has antioxidative, antimutagenic, and anticarcinogenic activity in animals (*289*). When 1.5 g/day of turmeric was given to 22 healthy men for 30 days, it reduced the urinary excretion of mutagens in smokers to 49–60% of the baseline level, depending on the test strain and use of the S9 fraction. It did not alter mutagenicity in nonsmokers, and did not affect serum aspartate aminotransferase and alanine aminotransferase activity, levels of glucose or creatinine, or lipid profiles in either group. In mouse models of DMBA-induced skin tumorigenesis and benzo[*a*]pyrene-induced forestomach neoplasia, 2% dietary turmeric significantly suppressed both types of tumor (*290*). A 5% turmeric diet for 7 days decreased hepatic cytochrome b_5 and P450 levels by 38%, and increased hepatic glutathione *S*-transferase activity by 32% and glutathione levels by 12%, suggesting that the protective effect is at least partly exerted through effects on these substances. Curcumin itself is a mixture of phenolic compounds. When the effects of individual curcumins were studied in these mouse models, curcumin I inhibited forestomach tumors in female Swiss mice and curcumin III inhibited skin tumors in female Swiss bald mice (*291*). Curcumin I also inhibited DMBA-initiated, phorbol ester–promoted skin tumors in female Swiss mice. In vitro, both compounds had dose-dependent

cytotoxicity against human chronic myeloid leukemia and both reduced binding of carcinogen to calf thymus DNA. Dietary curcumin I significantly decreased hepatic glutathione *S*-transferase activity and increased glutathione content in livers of male Swiss mice. This group of experiments shows that curcumins inhibit cancer during initiation, promotion, and progression stages.

The effects of 0.5–2.0% dietary cloves on hepatic cytochromes and enzymes were monitored for 30 days in Swiss albino mice (*292*). Cloves consistently enhanced glutathione *S*-transferase activity and levels of cytochrome b_5 and acid-soluble sulfhydryl compounds. Cytochrome P450 and radiation-induced malondialdehyde levels were significantly reduced in all groups after 30 days. Although aryl hydrocarbon hydroxylase activity was unaffected, DT-diaphorase activity was increased by the 1.0 and 2.0% clove diets after 30 days. In an in vivo bone marrow assay for micronucleus formation, dietary cloves had no effect alone or on DMBA-induced genotoxicity. Similar studies revealed a possible enzymatic basis for the anticarcinogenic and antioxidative effects of dietary mace (*Myristica fragrans* Houtt.) (*293*). Male Swiss albino mice were fed 0.5, 1.0, or 2.0% mace for up to 30 days. Mace supplements enhanced glutathione *S*-transferase, DT-diaphorase, cytochrome b_5, cytochrome P450, and sulfhydryl levels and decreased radiation-induced malondialdehyde levels in a dose- and time-dependent manner. Aryl hydrocarbon hydroxylase was slightly increased at the highest dosage after 20 days. No induction of micronuclei or modulation of DMBA-induction of genotoxicity was seen in the bone marrow micronucleus assay. As for cloves, the results indicate simultaneous enhancement of major phase I and phase II enzymes accompanied by a larger glutathione *S*-transferase–glutathione pool and resistance to radiation-induced liver damage.

Dietary supplementation with 1% extracts of rosemary (*Rosmarinus officinalis* L.) decreased incidence of DMBA-induced mammary tumors in rats by 47% (*294*). One percent and 0.5% extracts also inhibited in vivo binding of DMBA to mammary epithelial cell DNA by 42%. Formation of two major DMBA–DNA adducts was selectively reduced.

Through bioassay-guided fractionation, the bioactive compound myristicin was isolated from parsley (*Petroselinum sativum* Hoffm.) leaf oil (*295*). It had high potency as an inducer of glutathione *S*-transferase in mouse liver and small-intestinal mucosa. To begin to establish structure–function relationships, the olefinic bond of myristicin was reduced by catalytic hydrogenation to yield dihydromyristicin. This compound retained high potency in the liver and small-intestine assays, showing that the isolated double bond is not necessary for enzyme-inducing activity.

Nigella sativa seeds and saffron (*Crocus sativus*) are commonly used as spices and in treatment of disease by traditional Asian Indian medicine (*296*). Topical application of *N. sativa* and saffron extracts was inhibitory in a two-stage initiation–promotion model of skin carcinogenesis in mice. One treatment, after application of DMBA and before a series of twice-weekly applications of croton oil, reduced papilloma incidence from 90% (controls) to 77% for *N. sativa* and 50% for saffron groups. Papilloma multiplicity was also significantly reduced. Intraperitoneal administration of *N. sativa* extract and oral feeding of saffron 30 days after 20-methylcholanthrene injections reduced incidence of soft-tissue sarcomas from 100% to 33 and 10%, respectively.

MAILLARD BROWNING PRODUCTS. The Maillard reaction of amino acids with sugars occurs during food processing, cooking, and storage. The antimutagenicity of Maillard reaction products was studied in model systems employing fructose, glucose, and xylose as sugars and arginine, glycine, lysine, and tryptophan as amino acids (*297*). Xylose–amino acid combinations had the strongest reducing power and antioxidant activity and fructose–amino acid combinations the weakest. No reaction product showed mutagenicity or toxicity in *S. typhimurium* TA98 in the presence of S9. Most Maillard reaction products, especially those with xylose or tryptophan in combination, strongly inhibited mutagenicity of IQ, 3-amino-1,4-dimethyl-5*H*-pyridol-(4,3-*b*)indole, and 2-amino-6-methyl-dipyridol(1,2-*a*:3′,2′-*d*)imidazole; the exceptions were fructose–glycine and fructose–arginine, which increased the mutagenicity of 3-amino-1,4-dimethyl-5*H*-pyridol-(4,3-*b*)indole. Mutagenicity of benzo[*a*]pyrene was moderately inhibited in most cases but was increased by the Maillard reaction product of glucose–arginine. Mutagenicity of aflatoxin B$_1$ was greatly increased by all reaction products except that of xylose–tryptophan. Antimutagenic effects correlated well with antioxidative activity and reducing power. It appears that in some cases Maillard reaction products have a bifunctional property of comutagenicity and antimutagenicity.

The final products of the Maillard reaction are called melanoidins. The absorption and distribution of two kinds of melanoidins formed between glucose and glycine were studied in rats and their antimutagenicity in an *S. typhimurium* assay was evaluated (*298*). Seven hours after oral administration, 12.8% of a ^{14}C-labeled melanoidin of M_r ~800 was absorbed and distributed in liver, kidney, urine, blood, and breath (as CO_2). Less than 1% of the melanoidin of M_r 3000 was absorbed. Eighty percent of the low-molecular-weight melanoidin was bound to protein in the plasma. This protein-bound form significantly inhibited the mutagenicity of Trp-P-1 in *Salmonella*, and the authors suggested that it may have similar antimutagenic activity in vivo.

CAFFEINE. Welsch's research group has been investigating the effect of chronic caffeine consumption on development and growth of mammary carcinomas in rats. They have now reported the influence of caffeine on DMBA-induced benign and carcinomatous mammary tumors induced by DMBA (*299,300*) and *N*-methyl-*N*-nitrosourea (*300*). Four models were used in the first study (*299*): a single administration of DMBA to young virgin rats, young ovariectomized estrogen-treated virgin rats, old virgin rats, and old rats that had raised one litter. Caffeine was given in drinking water (500 mg/L) beginning 3–31 days after DMBA treatment. Caffeine significantly reduced the incidence of benign mammary fibroadenomas in all three virgin rat models and nonsignificantly in the parous rat model. In ovariectomized estrogen-treated rats, caffeine also significantly reduced the incidence of mammary gland cysts. It had no significant effect on incidence or total number of mammary carcinomas in either group of young rats, whereas in both parous and virgin old rats it significantly reduced the total number of mammary carcinomas. The second study attempted to temporally characterize the action of caffeine (*300*). In initiation studies caffeine was given from 30 days before until 4 days after carcinogen treatment; in promotion studies, it was given from 3–4 days after carcinogen treatment until the end of the experiment. Caffeine consumption during the initiation phase reduced the mean number of DMBA-induced mammary carcinomas by 50% and benign tumors by 28%; during promotion it reduced the mean number of benign tumors by 57% but had no significant influence on number of carcinomas. Virtually all of the *N*-methyl-*N*-nitrosourea-induced tumors were carcinomas, and caffeine had no effect on tumorigenesis with this carcinogen. These results suggest that caffeine is affecting the activation of DMBA, although no pronounced effect of caffeine on urinary excretion of tritiated DMBA was detected. Further study of the differing effects of different carcinogens in various rat models should help to explain the inconsistent and sometimes contradictory observations on the influence of caffeine on benign and malignant breast disease in humans.

Various mechanisms have been proposed for the anticarcinogenic effects of caffeine. Investigators in India examined caffeine's effects on carcinogen-activating and -detoxifying enzymes in mice (*301*). Administered in drinking water or intragastrically, caffeine increased hepatic and pulmonary levels of cytochrome P450 in a dose-dependent manner. There was also a dose-related increase in hepatic arylhydrocarbon hydroxylase activity; intragastric administration was more effective than oral ingestion. Only intragastrically administered caffeine enhanced pulmonary arylhydrocarbon hydroxylase activity. Hepatic glutathione-*S*-transferase activity and levels of reduced glutathione were roughly doubled at the highest caffeine dosage; pulmonary glutathione-*S*-transferase activity was also sharply increased. These effects might explain the anticarcinogenic activity of caffeine.

PROBIOTICS. The colonic flora plays key roles in colonic carcinogenesis. A study was undertaken to reveal the effect of bifidobacteria on 1,2-dimethylhydrazine-induced colon cancer in mice (*302*). Colonization and selective proliferation were achieved by oral administration of indigenous bifidobacteria and a bifidogenic diet (5% Neosugar). After a 2-week adaptation to the experimental and control diets, mice received 6 weekly injections of carcinogen. The incidence of aberrant crypts and foci was nearly 50% lower 38 weeks after the last injection in animals treated with bifidobacteria. The aberrance that did occur in the bifidobacteria-treated group tended to be more confined to the distal colon. The authors attribute the effects of the bifidobacteria to their acidifying action.

The antimutagenicity of milk cultured with various lactic acid bacteria was evaluated against *N*-methyl-*N'*-nitro-*N*-nitrosoguanidine in an *S. typhimurium* TA100 system (*303*). Working cells of 71 strains belonging to the genera *Lactobacillus, Streptococcus, Lactococcus,* and *Bifidobacterium* were tested at the beginning of the stationary phase (after 18 h of incubation). Milk cultured with *Lactobacillus acidophilus* LA106 suppressed mutagen-induced mutations by 77%; four other *L. acidophilus* strains suppressed mutation by >50%. The two strains of *Lactobacillus casei* ssp. *casei* tested were also highly antimutagenic, suppressing 57 and 61% of mutagen-induced mutations. One strain each of *Lactobacillus helveticus, Lactobacillus delbrueckii* ssp. *bulgaricus,* and *Streptococcus salivarius* ssp. *salivarius* were >50% inhibitory. All 71 strains suppressed mutation to some extent. Possible mechanisms for this activity were discussed.

Propionic acid bacteria also exhibit antimutagenic activity (*304*). Dialysates of four strains were tested in the Ames test, using sodium azide as the mutagen. All four (*Propionibacterium pentosaceum, Propionibacterium acnes,* and 2 strains of *Propionibacterium shermanii*) significantly reduced the incidence of sodium azide–induced revertants. Inhibition was enhanced if the dialysate and mutagen were coincubated for 20 min before the assay. The antimutagenic activity of *P. shermanii* was in the protein fraction. Three major molecular-weight peaks were separated, and the activity toward sodium azide was found in the second and third peaks.

Literature Cited

1. Milner, J.A. Diet and carcinogenesis. In *Food Safety Assessment*. J.W. Finley, S.F. Robinson, and D.J. Armstrong (eds.). *ACS Symp. Series* 484:297–315 (1992).

2. Cottrell, R.C. Dietary patterns and cancer. *Ann. Nutr. Metab.* 35(Suppl. 1):98–102 (1991).

3. Visek, W.J. (ed.) *Proceedings of the Conference on Nutrition and Cancer*. Atlanta, GA, 17–19 April 1991. *Cancer Res.* 52(Suppl.) (1992).

4. Doll, R. The lessons of life: keynote address to the Nutrition and Cancer Conference. *Cancer Res.* 52(Suppl.):2024S–2029S (1992).

5. Conney, A.H., R.H. Adamson, R.W. Hart, et al. Panel discussion: Nutrition and Cancer Conference. *Cancer Res.* 52(Suppl.):2124S–2125S (1992).

6. Jones, J.M. Cancer and diet—the controversy continues. *Cereal Foods World* 36:832–833 (1991).

7. Weisburger, J.H. Carcinogenesis in our food and cancer prevention. *Adv. Exp. Med. Biol.* 289:137–152 (1991).

8. Reynolds, T. Agreements signed to test foods for cancer prevention. *J. Natl. Cancer Inst.* 83:1050–1052 (1991).

9. Cherfas, J. Europeans launch diet, cancer study. *Science* 254:1448–1449 (1991).

10. Baghurst, K.I., P.A. Baghurst, and S.J. Record. Public perceptions of the role of dietary and other environmental factors in cancer causation or prevention. *J. Epidemiol. Commun. Health* 46:120–126 (1992).

11. Greenwald, P. The future of nutrition research in cancer prevention. In *Vitamins and Cancer Prevention*. S.A. Laidlaw and M.E. Swendseid (eds.). *Contemp. Issues in Clin. Nutr.* 14:111–127 (1991).

12. Laidlaw, S.A., and M.E. Swendseid (eds.). *Vitamins and Cancer Prevention. Contemp. Issues in Clin. Nutr.* 14 (1991).

13. Block, G., D.E. Henson, and M. Levine (eds.). *Ascorbic Acid: Biologic Functions and Relation to Cancer*. Proceedings of conference. Bethesda, MD, 10–12 Sept. 1990. *Am. J. Clin. Nutr.* 54(Suppl.) (1991).

14. Kritchevsky, D. Meat and cancer. In *Meat and Health*. A.M. Pearson and T.R. Dutson (eds.). *Adv. Meat Res.* 6:89–103 (1990).

15. Crossette, L.B. Evidence of protective effects of wheat fiber grows. *J. Natl. Cancer Inst.* 83:1614–1615 (1991).

16. Taylor, E., and K. Smigel. FDA proposes fat, cancer health claim; hesitates on fiber. *J. Natl. Cancer Inst.* 83:1618–1619 (1991).

17. Philip, W., T. James, and A. Ralph. Dietary fats and cancer. *Nutr. Res.* 12(Suppl. 1):S147–S158 (1992).

18. Messina, M., and V. Messina. Increasing use of soyfoods and their potential role in cancer prevention. *J. Am. Diet. Assoc.* 91:836–840 (1991).

19. Henderson, B.E., R.K. Ross, and M.C. Pike. Toward the primary prevention of cancer. *Science* 254:1131–1138 (1991).

20. Balter, M. Europe: as many cancers as cuisines. *Science* 254:1114–1115 (1991).

21. Trichopoulos, D., A. Tzonou, K. Katsouyanni, and A. Trichopoulou. Diet and cancer: the role of case–control studies. *Ann. Nutr. Metab.* 35(Suppl. 1):89–92 (1991).

22. Doll, R. Progress against cancer: an epidemiologic assessment. *Am. J. Epidemiol.* 134:675–688 (1991).

23. Goodman, M.T., and G.N. Stemmermann. Cancer registration and incidence in Hawaii. *Eur. J. Cancer* 27:1701–1706 (1991).

24. Matos, E.L., M. Khlat, D.I. Loria, et al. Cancer in migrants to Argentina. *Int. J. Cancer* 49:805–811 (1991).

25. Fønnebø, V., and A. Helseth. Cancer incidence in Norwegian Seventh-Day Adventists 1961 to 1986. *Cancer* 68:666–671 (1991).

26. Randall, E., J. Marshall, and S. Graham. Putative cancer risks inherent in dietary patterns of males and females in Western New York. (Abstract.) *Am. J. Epidemiol.* 134:763 (1991).

27. Lissner, L., Ø. Helgesson, C. Bengtsson, et al. Energy and protein intake in relation to cancer incidence among Swedish women. (Abstract.) *Am. J. Epidemiol.* 134:763 (1991).

28. Negri, E., C. La Vecchia, S. Franceschi, et al. Vegetable and fruit consumption and cancer risk. *Int. J. Cancer* 48:350–354 (1991).

29. Ito, Y., R. Sasaki, S. Suzuki, and K. Aoki. Relationship between serum xanthophyll levels and the consumption of cigarettes, alcohol or foods in healthy inhabitants of Japan. *Int. J. Epidemiol.* 20:615–620 (1991).

30. La Vecchia, C., E. Negri, S. Franceschi, et al. Tea consumption and cancer risk. *Nutr. Cancer* 17:27–31 (1992).

31. Xue, K.-X., S. Wang, G.-J. Ma, et al. Micronucleus formation in peripheral-blood lymphocytes from smokers and the influence of alcohol- and tea-drinking habits. *Int. J. Cancer* 50:702–705 (1992).

32. Kritchevsky, S.B. Dietary lipids and the low blood cholesterol–cancer association. *Am. J. Epidemiol.* 135:509–520 (1992).

33. Knekt, P., A. Aromaa, J. Maatela, et al. Serum micronutrients and risk of cancers of low incidence in Finland. *Am. J. Epidemiol.* 134:356–361 (1991).

34. Comstock, G.W., T.L. Bush, and K. Helzlsouer. Serum retinol, beta-carotene, vitamin E, and selenium as related to subsequent cancer of specific sites. *Am. J. Epidemiol.* 135:115–121 (1992).

35. Alberg, T., T. Bush, K. Helzlsouer, and G.W. Comstock. Prediagnostic serum retinol, carotenoids, vitamin E, and selenium and subsequent risk of squamous cell skin cancer. (Abstract.) *Am. J. Epidemiol.* 134:764 (1991).

36. Ziegler, R.G., A.F. Subar, N.E. Craft, et al. Does β-carotene explain why reduced cancer risk is associated with vegetable and fruit intake? *Cancer Res.* 52(Suppl.):2060S–2066S (1992).

37. Block, G. Epidemiologic evidence regarding vitamin C and cancer. *Am. J. Clin. Nutr.* 54:1310S–1314S (1991).

38. Adlercreutz, H., H. Honjo, A. Higashi, et al. Urinary excretion of lignans and isoflavonoid phytoestrogens in Japanese men and women consuming a traditional Japanese diet. *Am. J. Clin. Nutr.* 54:1093–1100 (1991).

39. Weisburger, J.H. Causes, relevant mechanisms, and prevention of large bowel cancer. *Semin. Oncol.* 18:316–336 (1991).

40. Winawer, S.J., and M. Shike. Dietary factors in colorectal cancer and their possible effects on earlier stages of hyperproliferation and adenoma formation. *J. Natl. Cancer Inst.* 84:74–75 (1992).

41. Giovannucci, E., M.J. Stampfer, G. Colditz, et al. Relationship of diet to risk of colorectal adenoma in men. *J. Natl. Cancer Inst.* 84:91–98 (1992).

42. Smith, K.R., M.L. Slattery, and T.K. French. Collinear nutrients and the risk of colon cancer. *J. Clin. Epidemiol.* 44:715–723 (1991).

43. Hammar, N., and S.E. Norell. Retrospective versus original information on diet among cases of colorectal cancer and controls. *Int. J. Epidemiol.* 20:621–627 (1991).

44. Trichopoulou, A., A. Tzonou, C.C. Hsieh, et al. High protein, saturated fat and cholesterol diet, and low levels of serum lipids in colorectal cancer. *Int. J. Cancer* 51:386–389 (1992).

45. de Verdier, M.G., U. Hagman, R.K. Peters, et al. Meat, cooking methods and colorectal cancer: a case–referent study in Stockholm. *Int. J. Cancer* 49:520–525 (1991).

46. Bufill, J.A. Relation of meat, fat, and fiber intake to the risk of colon cancer in women. (Letter.) *New Engl. J. Med.* 326:199 (1992).

47. Graham, S., and M. Swanson. Relation of meat, fat, and fiber intake to the risk of colon cancer in women. (Letter.) *New Engl. J. Med.* 326:199–200 (1992).

48. Bland, J.S. Relation of meat, fat, and fiber intake to the risk of colon cancer in women. (Letter.) *New Engl. J. Med.* 326:200 (1992).

49. Loosli, A.R. Relation of meat, fat, and fiber intake to the risk of colon cancer in women. (Letter.) *New Engl. J. Med.* 326:200 (1992).

50. Calvert, R.J., and L. Prosky. Relation of meat, fat, and fiber intake to the risk of colon cancer in women. (Letter.) *New Engl. J. Med.* 326:200–201 (1992).

51. Acheson, L. Relation of meat, fat, and fiber intake to the risk of colon cancer in women. (Letter.) *New Engl. J. Med.* 326:201 (1992).

52. White, R.R. Relation of meat, fat, and fiber intake to the risk of colon cancer in women. (Letter.) *New Engl. J. Med.* 326:201 (1992).

53. Baldwin, R. Relation of meat, fat, and fiber intake to the risk of colon cancer in women. (Letter.) *New Engl. J. Med.* 326:201 (1992).

54. Willett, W.C., M.J. Stampfer, G.A. Colditz, et al. Relation of meat, fat, and fiber intake to the risk of colon cancer in women. (Reply.) *New Engl. J. Med.* 326:201–202 (1992).

55. Iscovich, J., K.A. L'Abbé, R. Castelleto, et al. Colon cancer in Argentina: risk from fiber and nutrients. (Abstract.) *Am. J. Epidemiol.* 134:745 (1991).

56. Bidoli, E. S. Franceschi, R. Talamini, et al. Food consumption and cancer of the colon and rectum in north-eastern Italy. *Int. J. Cancer* 50:223–229 (1992).

57. Hu, J., Y. Liu, Y. Yu, et al. Diet and cancer of the colon and rectum: a case–control study in China. *Int. J. Epidemiol.* 20:362–367 (1991).

58. Benito, E., A. Stiggelbout, F.X. Bosch, et al. Nutritional factors in colorectal cancer risk: a case–control study in Majorca. *Int. J. Cancer* 49:161–167 (1991).

59. Kune, G.A., S. Kune, A. Read, et al. Colorectal polyps, diet, alcohol, and family history of colorectal cancer: a case–control study. *Nutr. Cancer* 16:25–30 (1991).

60. Kono, S., K. Shinchi, N. Ikeda, et al. Physical activity, dietary habits and adenomatous polyps of the sigmoid colon: a study of self-defense officials in Japan. *J. Clin. Epidemiol.* 44:1255–1261 (1991).

61. de Verdier, M.G., U. Hagman, S. Norell, et al. Diet, body mass, physical activity, and colorectal cancer. (Abstract.) *Am. J. Epidemiol.* 134:746 (1991).

62. Neugut, A.I., W.C. Lee, G.C. Garbowski, et al. Diet and recurrence of colorectal adenomatous polyps: a case–control study. (Abstract.) *Am. J. Epidemiol.* 134:746 (1991).

63. Smigel, K. Fewer colon polyps found in men with high-fiber, low-fat diets. *J. Natl. Cancer Inst.* 84:80–81 (1992).

64. McKeown-Eyssen, G. Recurrence of colorectal polyps: a randomized trial of a low fat high fiber diet. (Abstract.) *Am. J. Epidemiol.* 134:746 (1991).

65. Klurfeld, D.M. Dietary fiber-mediated mechanisms in carcinogenesis. *Cancer Res.* 52(Suppl.):2055S–2059S (1992).

66. Xing, X., J. Marshall, F. Freudenheim, et al. Dietary fiber components and colorectal cancer. (Abstract.) *Am. J. Epidemiol.* 134:746 (1991).

67. Arbman, G., O. Axelson, A.-B. Ericsson-Begodzki, et al. Cereal fiber, calcium, and colorectal cancer. *Cancer* 69:2042–2048 (1992).

68. Garland, C.F., F.C. Garland, and E.D. Gorham. Can colon cancer incidence and death rates be reduced with calcium and vitamin D? *Am. J. Clin. Nutr.* 54:193S–201S (1991).

69. Nelson, R.L. Dietary iron and colorectal cancer risk. *Free Rad. Biol. Med.* 12:161–168 (1992).

70. Freudenheim, J.L., S. Graham, J.R. Marshall, et al. Folate intake and carcinogenesis of the colon and rectum. *Int. J. Epidemiol.* 20:368–374 (1991).

71. Freudenheim, J.L., S. Graham, J.R. Marshall, et al. Refrigeration and cancer in the gastrointestinal tract. (Abstract.) *Am. J. Epidemiol.* 134:744–745 (1991).

72. Boeing, H., and R. Frentzel-Beyme. Regional risk factors for stomach cancer in the FRG. *Environ. Health Perspect.* 84:83–89 (1991).

73. Tuyns, A.J., R. Kaaks, M. Haelterman, and E. Riboli. Diet and gastric cancer. A case–control study in Belgium. *Int. J. Cancer* 51:1–6 (1992).

74. González, C.A., J.M. Sanz, G. Marcos, et al. Dietary factors and stomach cancer in Spain: a multicentre case–control study. *Int. J. Cancer* 49:513–519 (1991).

75. Buiatti, E., D. Palli, S. Bianchi, et al. A case–control study of gastric cancer and diet in Italy. III. Risk patterns by histologic type. *Int. J. Cancer* 48:369–374 (1991).

76. Palli, D., S. Bianchi, A. Decarli, et al. A case–control study of cancers of the gastric cardia in Italy. *Br. J. Cancer* 65:263–266 (1992).

77. Sanchez-Diez, A., R. Hernandez-Mejia, and A. Cueto-Espinar. Study of the relation between diet and gastric cancer in a rural area of the province of Leon, Spain. *Eur. J. Epidemiol.* 8:233–237 (1992).

78. Kneller, R.W., J.K. McLaughlin, E. Bjelke, et al. A cohort study of stomach cancer in a high-risk American population. *Cancer* 68:672–678 (1991).

79. Khuroo, M.S., S.A. Zarger, R. Mahajan, and M.A. Banday. High incidence of oesophageal and gastric cancer in Kashmir in a population with special personal and dietary habits. *Gut* 33:11–15 (1992).

80. Cheng, K.K., N.E. Day, S.W. Duffy, et al. Pickled vegetables in the aetiology of oesophageal cancer in Hong Kong Chinese. *Lancet* 339:1314–1319 (1992).

81. Valsecchi, M.G. Modelling the relative risk of esophageal cancer in a case–control study. *J. Clin. Epidemiol.* 45:347–355 (1992).

82. Sammon, A.M. A case–control study of diet and social factors in cancer of the esophagus in Transkei. *Cancer* 69:860–865 (1992).

83. Adams, J.B. Human breast cancer: concerted role of diet, prolactin and adrenal C_{19}-Δ^5-steroids in tumorigenesis. *Int. J. Cancer* 50:854–858 (1992).

84. Persky, V.W., R.T. Chatterton, L.V. Van Horn, et al. Hormone levels in vegetarian and nonvegetarian

teenage girls: potential implications for breast cancer risk. *Cancer Res.* 52:578–583 (1992).

85. Rose, D.P. Dietary fiber, phytoestrogens, and breast cancer. *Nutrition* 8:47–51 (1992).

86. Zaridze, D., Y. Lifanova, D. Maximovitch, et al. Diet, alcohol consumption and reproductive factors in a case–control study of breast cancer in Moscow. *Int. J. Cancer* 48:493–501 (1991).

87. Ingram, D.M., E. Nottage, and T. Roberts. The role of diet in the development of breast cancer: a case–control study of patients with breast cancer, benign epithelial hyperplasia and fibrocystic disease of the breast. *Br. J. Cancer* 64:187–191 (1991).

88. Overvad, K., D.Y. Wang, J. Olsen, et al. Selenium in human mammary carcinogenesis: a case–cohort study. *Eur. J. Cancer* 27:900–902 (1991).

89. Graham, S., R. Hellmann, J. Marshall, et al. Nutritional epidemiology of postmenopausal breast cancer in western New York. *Am. J. Epidemiol.* 134:552–566 (1991).

90. Willett, W.C., D.J. Hunter, M.J. Stampfer, et al. Dietary fat and breast cancer: an 8-year follow-up. (Abstract.) *Am. J. Epidemiol.* 134:715 (1991).

91. Hunter, D.J., M.J. Stampfer, G.A. Colditz, et al. A prospective study of consumption of vitamins A, C, and E and breast cancer risk. (Abstract.) *Am. J. Epidemiol.* 134:715 (1991).

92. Taioli, E., A. Nicolosi, and E.L. Wynder. Dietary habits and breast cancer: a comparative study of United States and Italian data. *Nutr. Cancer* 16:259–265 (1991).

93. Matos, E.L., D.B. Thomas, N. Sobel, and D. Vuoto. Breast cancer in Argentina: case–control study with special reference to meat eating habits. *Neoplasma* 38:357–366 (1991).

94. Ewertz, M., S. Gillanders, L. Meyer, and K. Zedeler. Survival of breast cancer patients in relation to factors which affect the risk of developing breast cancer. *Int. J. Cancer* 49:526–530 (1991).

95. Freudenheim, J.L., S. Graham, T.E. Byers, et al. Diet, smoking, and alcohol in cancer of the larynx: a case–control study. *Nutr. Cancer* 17:33–45 (1992).

96. Zheng, W., W.J. Blot, X.-O. Shu, et al. Risk factors for laryngeal cancer among males in Shanghai, China. (Abstract.) *Am. J. Epidemiol.* 134:725 (1991).

97. Knekt, P., R. Seppänen, R. Järvinen, et al. Dietary cholesterol, fatty acids, and the risk of lung cancer among men. *Nutr. Cancer* 15:267–275 (1991).

98. Wynder, E.L., E. Taioli, and Y. Fujita. Ecologic study of lung cancer risk factors in the U.S. and Japan, with special reference to smoking and diet. *Jpn. J. Cancer Res.* 83:418–423 (1992).

99. Knekt, P., R. Järvinen, R. Seppänen, et al. Dietary antioxidants and the risk of lung cancer. *Am. J. Epidemiol.* 134:471–479 (1991).

100. Steinmetz, K.A., J.D. Potter, and A.R. Folsum. Lung cancer, vegetables, and fruit: the Iowa Women's Health Study. (Abstract.) *Am. J. Epidemiol.* 134:725 (1991).

101. Forman, M.R., S.X. Yao, B.I. Graubard, et al. The effect of dietary intake of fruits and vegetables on the odds ratio of lung cancer among Yunnan tin miners. (Abstract.) *Am. J. Epidemiol.* 134:725 (1991).

102. Shekelle, R.B., A.H. Rossof, and J. Stamier. Dietary cholesterol and incidence of lung cancer: the Western Electric study. *Am. J. Epidemiol.* 134:480–484 (1991).

103. Goodman, M.T. Dietary cholesterol and incidence of lung cancer: the Western Electric study. (Letter.) *Am. J. Epidemiol.* 134:543–544 (1991).

104. Taioli, E., A. Nicolosi, and E.L. Wynder. Possible role of diet as a host factor in the aetiology of tobacco-induced lung cancer: an ecological study in southern and northern Italy. *Int. J. Epidemiol.* 20:611–614 (1991).

105. Swanson, C.A., B.L. Mao, J.Y. Li, et al. Dietary determinants of lung-cancer risk: results from a case–control study in Yunnan Province, China. *Int. J. Cancer* 50:876–880 (1992).

106. Goodman, M.T., L.N. Kolonel, L.R. Wilkens, et al. Dietary factors in lung cancer prognosis. *Eur. J. Cancer* 28:495–501 (1992).

107. Johnson, E.S. Nested case–control study of lung cancer in the meat industry. *J. Natl. Cancer Inst.* 83:1337–1339 (1991).

108. Garabrant, D.H., J. Held, B. Langholz, et al. DDT and related compounds and risk of pancreatic cancer. *J. Natl. Cancer Inst.* 84:764–771 (1992).

109. Howe, G.R., P. Ghadirian, H.B. Bueno de Mesquita, et al. A collaborative case–control study of nutrient intake and pancreatic cancer within the SEARCH programme. *Int. J. Cancer* 51:365–372 (1992).

110. Baghurst, P.A., A.J. McMichael, A.H. Slavotinek, et al. A case–control study of diet and cancer of the pancreas. *Am. J. Epidemiol.* 134:176–179 (1991).

111. Zatonski, W., K. Przewozniak, G.R. Howe, et al. Nutritional factors and pancreatic cancer: a case–control study from south-west Poland. *Int. J. Cancer* 48:390–394 (1991).

112. Bueno de Mesquita, H.B., P. Maisonneuve, S. Runia, and C.J. Moerman. Intake of foods and nutrients and cancer of the exocrine pancreas: a population-based case–control study in the Netherlands. *Int. J. Cancer* 48:540–549 (1991).

113. Bueno de Mesquita, H.B., P. Maisonneuve, C.J. Moerman, et al. Lifetime consumption of alcoholic beverages, tea and coffee and exocrine carcinoma of the pancreas: a population-based case–control study in The Netherlands. *Int. J. Cancer* 50:514–522 (1992).

114. Abraham, M., Y. Nomura, and L.N. Kolonel. Prostate cancer: a current perspective. *Am. J. Epidemiol.* 134:200–227 (1991).

115. Walker, A.R.P., B.F. Walker, N.G. Tsotetsi, et al. Case–control study of prostate cancer in black patients in Soweto, South Africa. *Br. J. Cancer* 65:438–441 (1992).

116. La Vecchia, C., E. Negri, B. D'Avanzo, et al. Dairy products and the risk of prostatic cancer. *Oncology* 48:406–410 (1991).

117. Riboli, E., C.A. González, G.López-Abente, et al. Diet and bladder cancer in Spain: a multi-centre case–control study. *Int. J. Cancer* 49:214–219 (1991).

118. Kunze, E., J. Chang-Claude, and R. Frentzel-Beyme. Life style and occupational risk factors for bladder cancer in Germany. *Cancer* 69:1776–1790 (1992).

119. Buckley, D.I., R.S. McPherson, C.Q. North, and T.M. Becker. Dietary micronutrients and cervical dysplasia in southwestern American Indian women. *Nutr. Cancer* 17:179–185 (1992).

120. de Vet, H.C.W., P.G. Knipschild, M.E.C. Grol, et al. The role of beta-carotene and other dietary factors in the aetiology of cervical dysplasia: results of a case–control study. *Int. J. Epidemiol.* 20:603–610 (1991).

121. Herrero, R., N. Potischman, L.A. Brinton, et al. A case–control study of nutrient status and invasive cervical cancer. I. Dietary indicators. *Am. J. Epidemiol.* 134:1335–1346 (1991).

122. Potischman, N., R. Herrero, L.A. Brinton, et al. A case–control study of nutrient status and invasive cervical cancer. II. Serologic indicators. *Am. J. Epidemiol.* 134:1347–1355 (1991).

123. Piver, M.S., T.R. Baker, M. Piedmonte, and A.M. Sandecki. Epidemiology and etiology of ovarian cancer. *Semin. Oncol.* 18:177–185 (1991).

124. Engle, A., J.E. Muscat, and R.E. Harris. Nutritional risk factors and ovarian cancer. *Nutr. Cancer* 15:239–247 (1991).

125. Harlow, B.S., D.W. Cramer, J. Geller, et al. The influence of lactose consumption on the association of oral contraceptive use and ovarian cancer risk. *Am. J. Epidemiol.* 134:445–453 (1991).

126. Mettlin, C.J. Progress in the nutritional epidemiology of ovary cancer. *Am. J. Epidemiol.* 134:457–459 (1991).

127. Cramer, D.W., and B.L. Harlow. Progress in the nutritional epidemiology of ovary cancer. *Am. J. Epidemiol.* 134:460–461 (1991).

128. Cramer, D.W., and B.L. Harlow. Commentary: re: "A case–control study of milk drinking and ovarian cancer risk." *Am. J. Epidemiol.* 134:454–456 (1991).

129. Franceschi, S., F. Levi, E. Negri, et al. Diet and thyroid cancer: a pooled analysis of four European case–control studies. *Int. J. Cancer* 48:395–398 (1991).

130. Petridou, E., K. Katsouyanni, C. Hsieh, et al. Diet, pregnancy estrogens and their possible relevance to cancer risk in the offspring. *Oncology* 49:127–132 (1992).

131. Simic, M.G., and D.S. Bergtold. Dietary modulation of DNA damage in humans. *Mutat. Res.* 250:17–24 (1991).

132. Paganelli, G.M., G. Biasco, G. Brandi, et al. Effect of vitamin A, C, and E supplementation on rectal cell proliferation in patients with colorectal adenomas. *J. Natl. Cancer Inst.* 84:47–51 (1992).

133. Mathews-Roth, M.M., N. Lausen, G. Drouin, et al. Effects of carotenoid administration on bladder cancer prevention. *Oncology* 48:177–179 (1991).

134. Maruyama, H., K. Watanabe, and I. Yamamoto. Effect of dietary kelp on lipid peroxidation and glutathione peroxidase activity in livers of rats given breast carcinogen DMBA. *Nutr. Cancer* 15:221–228 (1991).

135. Moreno, F.S., M.B.S.L. Rizzi, M.L.Z. Dagli, and M.V.C. Penteado. Inhibitory effects of β-carotene

on preneoplastic lesions induced in Wistar rats by the resistant hepatocyte model. *Carcinogenesis* 12:1817–1822 (1991).

136. Salvadori, D.M.F., L.R. Ribeiro, M.D.M. Oliveira, et al. The protective effect of β-carotene on genotoxicity induced by cyclophosphamide. *Mutat. Res.* 265:237–244 (1992).

137. Szmurlo, A., M. Marczak, L. Rudnicka, et al. Beta-carotene in prevention of cutaneous carcinogenesis. *Acta Dermatol. Venereol. (Stockh.)* 71:528–530 (1991).

138. Tan, B. Antitumor effects of palm carotenes and tocotrienols in HRS/J hairless female mice. *Nutr. Res.* 12(Suppl. 1):S163–S173 (1992).

139. Rybski, J.A., T.M. Grogan, M. Aickin, and H.L. Gensler. Reduction of murine cutaneous UVB-induced tumor-infiltrating T lymphocytes by dietary canthaxanthin. *J. Invest. Dermatol.* 97:892–897 (1991).

140. Zhang, L.-X., R.V. Cooney, and J.S. Bertram. Carotenoids enhance gap junctional communication and inhibit lipid peroxidation in C3H/10T1/2 cells: relationship to their cancer chemopreventive action. *Carcinogenesis* 12:2109–2114 (1991).

141. Khanduja, K.L., I.B. Koul, R.K. Gandhi, et al. Effect of combined deficiency of fat and vitamin A on *N*-nitrosodiethylamine-induced lung carcinogenesis in mice. *Cancer Lett.* 62:57–62 (1992).

142. Koga, M., and R.L. Sutherland. Retinoic acid acts synergistically with 1,25-dihydroxyvitamin D_3 or antioestrogen to inhibit T-47D human breast cancer cell proliferation. *J. Steroid Biochem. Mol. Biol.* 39:455–460 (1991).

143. Liehr, J.G. Vitamin C reduces the incidence and severity of renal tumors induced by estradiol or diethylstilbestrol. *Am. J. Clin. Nutr.* 54:1256S–1260S (1991).

144. Poydock, M.E. Effect of combined ascorbic acid and B-12 on survival of mice with implanted Ehrlich carcinoma and L1210 leukemia. *Am. J. Clin. Nutr.* 54:1261S–1265S (1991).

145. Pauling, L. Effect of ascorbic acid on incidence of spontaneous mammary tumors and UV-light–induced skin tumors in mice. *Am. J. Clin. Nutr.* 54:1252S–1255S (1991).

146. Lupulescu, A. Vitamin C inhibits DNA, RNA and protein synthesis in epithelial neoplastic cells. *Int. J. Vit. Nutr. Res.* 61:125–129 (1991).

147. Meadows, G.G., H.F. Pierson, and R.M. Abdallah. Ascorbate in the treatment of experimental transplanted melanoma. *Am. J. Clin. Nutr.* 54:1284S–1291S (1991).

148. Ibric, L.L.V., A.R. Peterson, and A. Sevanian. Mechanisms of ascorbic acid–induced inhibition of chemical transformation in C3H/10T1/2 cells. *Am. J. Clin. Nutr.* 54:1236S–1240S (1991).

149. Tsao, C.S. Inhibiting effect of ascorbic acid on the growth of human mammary tumor xenografts. *Am. J. Clin. Nutr.* 54:1274S–1280S (1991).

150. Cameron, E., and A. Campbell. Innovation vs. quality control: an 'unpublishable' clinical trial of supplemental ascorbate in incurable cancer. *Med. Hypoth.* 36:185–189 (1991).

151. Clausen, J. The influence of selenium and vitamin E on the enhanced respiratory burst reaction in smokers. *Biol. Trace Elem. Res.* 31:281–291 (1991).

152. Veera Reddy, K., Charles Kumar, T., M. Prasad, and P. Reddanna. Exercise-induced oxidant stress in the lung tissue: role of dietary supplementation of vitamin E and selenium. *Biochem. Int.* 26:863–871 (1992).

153. Nesaretnam, K., H.T. Khor, J. Ganeson, et al. The effect of vitamin E tocotrienols from palm oil on chemically-induced mammary carcinogenesis in female rats. *Nutr. Res.* 12:63–75 (1992).

154. Henderson, M.M. Role of intervention trials in research on nutrition and cancer. *Cancer Res.* 52(Suppl.):2030S–2034S (1992).

155. Roush, G.C., R.W. Pero, J. Powell, et al. Modulation of the cancer susceptibility measure, adenosine diphosphate ribosyl transferase (ADPRT), by differences in low-dose *n*-3 and *n*-6 fatty acids. *Nutr. Cancer* 16:197–207 (1991).

156. Takahashi, M., M. Przetakiewicz, A. Ong, et al. Effect of ω3 and ω6 fatty acids on transformation of cultured cells by irradiation and transfection. *Cancer Res.* 52:154–162 (1992).

157. Welsch, C. Relationship between dietary fat and experimental mammary tumorigenesis: a review and critique. *Cancer Res.* 52(Suppl.):2040S–1048S (1992).

158. Kritchevsky, D., M.M. Weber, and D.M. Klurfeld. Influence of different fats (soybean oil, palm olein or hydrogenated soybean oil) on chemically-induced mammary tumors in rats. *Nutr. Res.* 12(Suppl. 1):S175–S179 (1992).

159. Fischer, S.M., C.J. Conti, M. Locniskar, et al. The effect of dietary fat on the rapid development of mammary tumors induced by 7,12-dimethylbenz(*a*)anthracene in SENCAR mice. *Cancer Res.* 52:662–666 (1992).

160. Rose, D.P., J.M. Connolly, and C.L. Meschter. Effect of dietary fat on human breast cancer growth and lung metastasis in nude mice. *J. Natl. Cancer Inst.* 83:1491–1495 (1991).

161. Potischman, N., C.E. McCulloch, T. Byers, et al. Associations between breast cancer, plasma triglycerides, and cholesterol. *Nutr. Cancer* 15:205–215 (1991).

162. Carroll, K.K., and H.I. Parenteau. A proposed mechanism for effects of diet on mammary cancer. *Nutr. Cancer* 16:79–83 (1991).

163. Chlebowski, R.T., D. Rose, I.M. Buzzard, et al. Adjuvant dietary fat intake reduction in postmenopausal breast cancer patient management. *Breast Cancer Res. Treatment* 20:73–84 (1991).

164. Fischer, S.M., J. Leyton, M.L. Lee, et al. Differential effects of dietary linoleic acid on mouse skin-tumor promotion and mammary carcinogenesis. *Cancer Res.* 52(Suppl.):2049S–2054S (1992).

165. Birt, D.F., E.S. Kris, M. Choe, and J.C. Pelling. Dietary energy and fat effects on tumor promotion. *Cancer Res.* 52(Suppl.):2035S–2039S (1992).

166. Locniskar, M., M.A. Belury, A.G. Cumberland, et al. The effect of the level of dietary corn oil on mouse skin carcinogenesis. *Nutr. Cancer* 16:1–11 (1991).

167. Locniskar, M., M.A. Belury, A.G. Cumberland, et al. The effect of various dietary fats on skin tumor initiation. *Nutr. Cancer* 16:189–196 (1991).

168. Locniskar, M., M.A. Belury, A.G. Cumberland, et al. The effect of dietary lipid on skin tumor promotion by benzoyl peroxide: comparison of fish, coconut and corn oil. *Carcinogenesis* 12:1023–1028 (1991).

169. Belury, M.A., J. Leyton, K.E. Patrick, et al. Modulation of phorbol ester-elicited events in mouse epidermis by dietary *n*–3 and *n*–6 fatty acids. *Prostaglandins Leukotrienes Essential Fatty Acids* 44:19–26 (1991).

170. Fischer, M.A., and H.S. Black. Modification of membrane composition, eicosanoid metabolism, and immunoresponsiveness by dietary omega-3 and omega-6 fatty acid sources, modulators of ultraviolet-carcinogenesis. *Photochem. Photobiol.* 54:381–387 (1991).

171. Zhao, L.P., L.H. Kushi, R.D. Klein, and R.L. Prentice. Quantitative review of studies of dietary fat and rat colon carcinoma. *Nutr. Cancer* 15:169–177 (1991).

172. Kuratko, C., and B.C. Pence. Changes in colonic antioxidant status in rats during long-term feeding of different high fat diets. *J. Nutr.* 121:1562–1569 (1991).

173. Turini, M.E., A.B.R. Thomson, and M.T. Clandinin. Lipid composition and peroxide levels of mucosal cells in the rat large intestine in relation to dietary fat. *Lipids* 26:431–440 (1991).

174. Narisawa, T., M. Takahashi, H. Kotanagi, et al. Inhibitory effect of dietary perilla oil rich in the *n*–3 polyunsaturated fatty acid α-linolenic acid on colon carcinogenesis in rats. *Jpn. J. Cancer Res.* 82:1089–1096 (1991).

175. Rao, A.V., S.A. Janezic, D. Friday, and C.W. Kendall. Dietary cholesterol enhances the induction and development of colonic preneoplastic lesions in C57BL/6J and BALB/cJ mice treated with azoxymethane. *Cancer Lett.* 63:249–257 (1992).

176. Lapré, J.A., and R. Van der Meer. Diet-induced increase of colonic bile acids stimulates lytic activity of fecal water and proliferation of colonic cells. *Carcinogenesis* 13:41–44 (1992).

177. Pence, B.C., S.-Y. Tsai, and B.C. Richard. Effects of dietary fat on hepatic microsomal metabolism of 1,2-dimethylhydrazine. *Cancer Lett.* 59:225–229 (1991).

178. Khoo, D.E., B. Flaks, H. Oztas, et al. Effects of dietary fatty acids on the early stages of neoplastic induction in the rat pancreas. Changes in fatty acid composition and development of atypical acinar cell nodules. *Int. J. Exp. Pathol.* 72:571–580 (1991).

179. de Bravo, M.G., R.J. de Antueno, J. Toledo, et al. Effects of an eicosapentaenoic and docosahexaenoic acid concentrate on a human lung carcinoma grown in nude mice. *Lipids* 26:866–870 (1991).

180. Edenharder, R., M. Mitschke, and K. Jung. Urinary mutagenicity in vegetarians and people on a mixed-Western diet. *Zbl. Hyg.* 192:494–508 (1992).

181. Sjödin, P., M. Nyman, L.L. Nielsen, et al. Effect of dietary fiber on the disposition and excretion of a food carcinogen (2-^{14}C-labeled MeIQx) in rats. *Nutr. Cancer* 17:139–151 (1992).

182. Rose, D.P., M. Goldman, J.M. Connolly, and L.E. Strong. High-fiber diet reduces serum estrogen

concentrations in premenopausal women. *Am. J. Clin. Nutr.* 54:520–525 (1991).

183. Arts, C.J.M., C.A.R.L. Govers, H. van den Berg, et al. In vitro binding of estrogens by dietary fiber and the in vivo apparent digestibility tested in pigs. *J. Steroid Biochem. Mol. Biol.* 38:621–628 (1991).

184. Arts, C.J.M., A.Th.H.J. de Bie, H. van den Berg, et al. Influence of wheat bran on NMU-induced mammary tumor development, plasma estrogen levels and estrogen excretion in female rats. *J. Steroid Biochem. Mol. Biol.* 39:193–202 (1991).

185. Arts, C.J.M., C.A.R.L. Govers, H. van den Berg, et al. Effect of wheat bran on excretion of radioactively labeled estradiol-17β and estrone-glucuronide injected intravenously in male rats. *J. Steroid Biochem. Mol. Biol.* 42:103–111 (1992).

186. Bleyl, D.W.R. Ballaststoffstudie. Wirkungen auf Coloncarcinogenese. *Nahrung* 35:767–781 (1991).

187. Reddy, B.S., A. Engle, B. Simi, and M. Goldman. Effect of dietary fiber on colonic bacterial enzymes and bile acids in relation to colon cancer. *Gastroenterology* 102:1475–1482 (1992).

188. Kashtan, H., H.S. Stern, D.J.A. Jenkins, et al. Colonic fermentation and markers of colorectal-cancer risk. *Am. J. Clin. Nutr.* 55:723–728 (1992).

189. Johansson, G., A. Holmén, L. Persson, et al. The effect of a shift from a mixed diet to a lacto-vegetarian diet on human urinary and fecal mutagenic activity. *Carcinogenesis* 13:153–157 (1992).

190. Ling, W.H., and O. Hänninen. Shifting from a conventional diet to an uncooked vegan diet reversibly alters fecal hydrolytic activities in humans. *J. Nutr.* 122:924–930 (1992).

191. Fujiwara, S., T. Hirota, H. Nakazato, et al. Effect of konjac mannan on intestinal microbial metabolism in mice bearing human flora and in conventional F344 rats. *Food Chem. Toxicol.* 29:601–606 (1991).

192. McGarrity, T.J., L.P. Peiffer, S.T. Kramer, and J.P. Smith. Effects of fat and fiber on human colon cancer xenografted to athymic nude mice. *Digest. Dis. Sci.* 36:1606–1610 (1991).

193. Gallaher, D.D., P.L. Locket, and C.M. Gallaher. Bile acid metabolism in rats fed two levels of corn oil and brans of oat, rye and barley and sugar beet fiber. *J. Nutr.* 122:473–481 (1992).

194. McIntyre, A. G.P. Young, T. Taranto, et al. Different fibers have different regional effects on luminal contents of rat colon. *Gastroenterology* 101:1274–1281 (1991).

195. Shivapurkar, N., Z. Tang, and O. Alabaster. The effect of high-risk and low-risk diets on aberrant crypt and colonic tumor formation in Fischer-344 rats. *Carcinogenesis* 13:887–890 (1992).

196. Heitman, D.W., W.E. Hardman, and I.L. Cameron. Dietary supplementation with pectin and guar gum on 1,2-dimethylhydrazine-induced colon carcinogenesis in rats. *Carcinogenesis* 13:815–818 (1992).

197. Harris, P.J., A.M. Roberton, H.J. Hollands, and L.R. Ferguson. Adsorption of a hydrophobic mutagen to dietary fibre from the skin and flesh of potato tubers. *Mutat. Res.* 260:203–213 (1991).

198. Ferguson, L.R., A.M. Roberton, R.J. McKenzie, et al. Adsorption of a hydrophobic mutagen to dietary fiber from taro (*Colocasia esculenta*), an important food plant of the South Pacific. *Nutr. Cancer* 17:85–95 (1992).

199. Caderni, G., F. Bianchini, A. Mancina, et al. Effect of dietary carbohydrates on the growth of dysplastic crypt foci in the colon of rats treated with 1,2-dimethylhydrazine. *Cancer Res.* 51:3721–3725 (1991).

200. Zaleski, J., G.Y. Kwei, R.G. Thurman, and F.C. Kauffman. Suppression of benzo[*a*]pyrene metabolism by accumulation of triacylglycerols in rat hepatocytes: effect of high-fat and food-restricted diets. *Carcinogenesis* 12:2073–2079 (1991).

201. Wall, K.L., W. Gao, W. Qu, et al. Food restriction increases detoxification of polycyclic aromatic hydrocarbons in the rat. *Carcinogenesis* 13:519–523 (1992).

202. Clinton, S.K., P.B. Imrey, H.J. Mangian, et al. The combined effects of dietary fat, protein, and energy intake on azoxymethane-induced intestinal and renal carcinogenesis. *Cancer Res.* 52:857–865 (1992).

203. Shimokawa, I., B.P. Yu, and E.J. Masoro. Influence of diet on fatal neoplastic disease in male Fischer 344 rats. *J. Gerontol.* 46:B338–B323 (1991).

204. Horio, F., L.D. Youngman, R.C. Bell, and T.C. Campbell. Thermogenesis, low-protein diets, and decreased development of AFB$_1$-induced preneoplastic foci in rat liver. *Nutr. Cancer* 16:31–41 (1991).

205. Youngman, L.D., and T.C. Campbell. High protein intake promotes the growth of hepatic preneoplastic foci in Fischer #344 rats: evidence that early remodeled foci retain the potential for future growth. *J. Nutr.* 121:1454–1461 (1991).

206. Lombardi, B., N. Chandar, and J. Locker. Nutritional model of hepatocarcinogenesis: rats fed choline-devoid diet. *Digest. Dis. Sci.* 36:979–984 (1991).

207. Dizik, M, J.K. Christman, and E. Wainfan. Alterations in expression and methylation of specific genes in livers of rats fed a cancer promoting methyl-deficient diet. *Carcinogenesis* 12:1307–1312 (1991).

208. Wainfan, E., and L.A. Poirier. Methyl groups in carcinogenesis: effects on DNA methylation and gene expression. *Cancer Res.* 52(Suppl.):2071S–2077S (1992).

209. Hawrylewicz, E.J., H.H. Huang, and W.H. Blair. Dietary soybean isolate and methionine supplementation affect mammary tumor progression in rats. *J. Nutr.* 121:1693–1698 (1991).

210. Torsten, U., D. Senger, and H.K. Weitzel. Influence of diet on breast cancer size and morphology in rats treated with DMBA. *Arch. Gynecol. Obstet.* 249:51–58 (1991).

211. Welberg, J.W.M., J.H. Kleibeuker, R. Van der Meer, et al. Calcium and the prevention of colon cancer. *J. Gastroenterol.* 26(Suppl. 188):52–59 (1991).

212. Lipkin, M. Application of intermediate biomarkers to studies of cancer prevention in the gastrointestinal tract: introduction and perspective. *Am. J. Clin. Nutr.* 54:188S–192S (1991).

213. Thompson, L.U., and L. Zhang. Phytic acid and minerals: effect on early markers of risk for mammary and colon carcinogenesis. *Carcinogenesis* 12:2041–2045 (1991).

214. Appleton, G.V.N., R.W. Owen, E.E. Wheeler, et al. Effect of dietary calcium on the colonic luminal environment. *Gut* 32:1374–1377 (1991).

215. de Kok, T.M.C.M., A. van Faassen, R.A. Bausch-Goldbohm, et al. Fecapentaene excretion and fecal mutagenicity in relation to nutrient intake and fecal parameters in humans on omnivorous and vegetarian diets. *Cancer Lett.* 62:11–21 (1992).

216. Wargovich, M.J., P.M. Lynch, and B. Levin. Modulating effects of calcium in animal models of colon carcinogenesis and short-term studies in subjects at increased risk for colon cancer. *Am. J. Clin. Nutr.* 54:202S–205S (1991).

217. Newmark, H.L., M. Lipkin, and N. Maheshwari. Colonic hyperproliferation induced in rats and mice by nutritional-stress diets containing four components of a human Western-style diet (series 2). *Am. J. Clin. Nutr.* 54:209S–214S (1991).

218. Newmark, H.L., and M. Lipkin. Calcium, vitamin D, and colon cancer. *Cancer Res.* 52:2067S–2070S (1992).

219. Sitrin, M.D., A.G. Halline, C. Abrahams, and T.A. Brasitus. Dietary calcium and vitamin D modulate 1,2-dimethylhydrazine-induced colonic carcinogenesis in the rat. *Cancer Res.* 51:5608–5613 (1991).

220. Llor, X., R.F. Jacoby, B.-B. Teng, et al. K-*ras* mutations in 1,2-dimethylhydrazine-induced colonic tumors: effects of supplemental dietary calcium and vitamin D deficiency. *Cancer Res.* 51:4305–4309 (1991).

221. Lans, J.I., R. Jaszewski, F.L. Arlow, et al. Supplemental calcium suppresses colonic mucosal ornithine decarboxylase activity in elderly patients with adenomatous polyps. *Cancer Res.* 51:3416–3419 (1991).

222. Paraskava, C. Colorectal cancer and dietary intervention. (Letter.) *Lancet* 339:869–870 (19920.

223. Pence, B.C., B.C. Richard, R.S. Lawlis, and C.N. Kuratko. Effects of dietary calcium and vitamin D_3 on tumor promotion in mouse skin. *Nutr. Cancer* 16:171–181 (1991).

224. Carroll, K.K., E.A. Jacobson, L.A. Eckel, and H.L. Newmark. Calcium and carcinogenesis of the mammary gland. *Am. J. Clin. Nutr.* 54:206S–208S (1991).

225. Waalkes, M.P., B.A. Diwan, C.M. Weghorst, et al. Anticarcinogenic effects of cadmium in B6C3F1 mouse liver and lung. *Toxicol. Appl. Pharmacol.* 110:327–335 (1991).

226. Takahashi, M., T. Hasegawa, F. Furukawa, et al. Enhanced lipid peroxidation in rat gastric mucosa caused by NaCl. *Carcinogenesis* 12:2201–2204 (1991).

227. Yu, S.-Y., Y.-J. Zhu, W.-G. Li, et al. A preliminary report on the intervention trials of primary liver cancer in high-risk populations with nutritional supplementation of selenium in China. *Biol. Trace Elem. Res.* 29:289–294 (1991).

228. Liu, J., K. Gilbert, H.M. Parker, et al. Inhibition of 7,12-dimethylbenz[*a*]anthracene-induced mammary tumors and DNA adducts by dietary selenite. *Cancer Res.* 51:4613–4617 (1991).

229. Visek, W.J. Nitrogen-stimulated orotic acid synthesis and nucleotide imbalance. *Cancer Res.* 52(Suppl.):2082S–2084S (1992).

230. Manjeshwar, S., A. Sheikh, G. Pichiri-Coni, et al. Orotic acid, nucleotide-pool imbalance, and liver-tumor promotion: a possible mechanism for the mitoinhibitory effects of orotic acid in isolated rat hepatocytes. *Cancer Res.* 52(Suppl.):2078S–2081S (1992).

231. Sato, T., K. Chikazawa, H. Yamamori, et al. Evaluation of the SOS chromotest for the detection of antimutagens. *Environ. Molec. Mutagen.* 17:258–263 (1991).

232. Piero, D., C. Giovanna, and B. Franca. Modulation of the genotoxicity of food mutagens by main dietary components. In *New Horizons in Biological Dosimetry.* B.L. Gledhill and F. Mauro (eds.). *Prog. Clin. Biol. Res.* 372:49–58 (1991).

233. Wattenberg, L.W. Inhibition of carcinogenesis by minor dietary constituents. *Cancer Res.* 52(Suppl.):2085S–2091S (1992).

234. Pariza, M.W. Designer foods: effects on development of cancer. *J. Natl. Cancer Inst. Monogr.* 12:105–107 (1992).

235. Caragay, A.B. Cancer-preventive foods and ingredients. *Food Technol.* 46(4):65–68 (1992).

236. Yasukawa, K., M. Takido, M. Akasu, et al. Inhibitory effects of plant constituents on tumor promotion during carcinogenesis. *J. Pharmacobio-Dyn.* 15:S-3 (1992).

237. Adlercreutz, H., Y. Mousavi, J. Clark, et al. Dietary phytoestrogens and cancer: in vitro and in vivo studies. *J. Steroid Biochem. Mol. Biol.* 41:331–337 (1992).

238. Yamasaki, T., R.W. Teel, and B.H.S. Lau. Effect of allixin, a phytoalexin produced by garlic, on mutagenesis, DNA-binding and metabolism of aflatoxin B_1. *Cancer Lett.* 59:89–94 (1991).

239. Welch, C., L. Wuarin, and N. Sidell. Antiproliferative effect of the garlic compound S-allyl cysteine on human neuroblastoma cells in vitro. *Cancer Lett.* 63:211–219 (1992).

240. Hong, J.-Y., Z.Y. Wang, T.J. Smith, et al. Inhibitory effects of diallyl sulfide on the metabolism and tumorigenicity of the tobacco-specific carcinogen 4-(methylnitrosamino)-1-(3-pyridyl)-1-butanone (NNK) in A/J mouse lung. *Carcinogenesis* 13:901–904 (1992).

241. Gudi, V.A., and S.V. Singh. Effect of diallyl sulfide, a naturally occurring anti-carcinogen, on glutathione-dependent detoxification enzymes of female CD-1 mouse tissues. *Biochem. Pharmacol.* 42:1261–1265 (1991).

242. Tadi, P.P., B.H.S. Lau, R.W. Teel, and C.E. Herrmann. Binding of aflatoxin B_1 to DNA inhibited by ajoene and diallyl sulfide. *Anticancer Res.* 11:2037–2042 (1991).

243. Zhang, Y., P. Talalay, C.-G. Cho, and G.H. Posner. A major inducer of anticarcinogenic protective enzymes from broccoli: isolation and elucidation of structure. *Proc. Natl. Acad. Sci. USA* 89:2399–2403 (1992).

244. Bradfield, C.A., and L.F. Bjeldanes. Modification of carcinogen metabolism by indolylic autolysis products of *Brassica oleraceae*. In *Nutritional and Toxicological Consequences of Food Processing.* M. Friedman (ed.). *Adv. Exp. Med. Biol.* 289:153–163 (1991).

245. Michnovicz, J.J., and H.L. Bradlow. Altered estrogen metabolism and excretion in humans following consumption of indole-3-carbinol. *Nutr. Cancer* 16:59–66 (1991).

246. Bradlow, H.L., J.J. Michnovicz, N.T. Telang, and M.P. Osborne. Effects of dietary indole-3-carbinol on estradiol metabolism and spontaneous mammary tumors in mice. *Carcinogenesis* 12:1571–1574 (1991).

247. Wang, Z.Y., R. Agarwal, D.R. Bickers, and H. Mukhtar. Protection against ultraviolet B radiation–induced photocarcinogenesis in hairless mice by green tea polyphenols. *Carcinogenesis* 12:1527–1530 (1991).

248. Wang, Z.-Y., M.-T. Huang, T. Ferraro, et al. Inhibitory effect of green tea in the drinking water on tumorigenesis by ultraviolet light and 12-O-tetradecanoylphorbol-13-acetate in the skin of SKH-1 mice. *Cancer Res.* 52:1162–1170 (1992).

249. Wang, Z.Y., J.-Y. Hong, M.-T. Huang, et al. Inhibition of N-nitrosodiethylamine- and 4-(methylnitrosamino)-1-(3-pyridyl)-1-butanone-induced tumorigenesis in A/J mice by green tea and black tea. *Cancer Res.* 52:1943–1947 (1992).

250. Yamane, T., N. Hagiwara, M. Tateishi, et al. Inhibition of azoxymethane-induced colon carcinogenesis in rat by green tea polyphenol fraction. *Jpn. J. Cancer Res.* 82:1336–1339 (1991).

251. Larocca, L.M., L. Teofili, G. Leone, et al. Antiproliferative activity of quercetin on normal bone marrow and leukaemic progenitors. *Br. J. Haematol.* 79:562–566 (1991).

252. Ranelletti, F.O., R. Ricci, L.M. Larocca, et al. Growth-inhibitory effect of quercetin and presence of type-II estrogen-binding sites in human colon-cancer cell lines and primary colorectal tumors. *Int. J. Cancer* 50:486–492 (1992).

253. Deschner, E.E., J. Ruperto, G. Wong, and H.L. Newmark. Quercetin and rutin as inhibitors of azoxymethanol-induced colonic neoplasia. *Carcinogenesis* 12:1193–1196 (1991).

254. Majid, S., K.L. Khanduja, R.K. Gandhi, et al. Influence of ellagic acid on antioxidant defense system and lipid peroxidation in mice. *Biochem. Pharmacol.* 42:1441–1445 (1991).

255. Wilson, T., M.J. Lewis, K.L. Cha, and B. Gold. The effect of ellagic acid on xenobiotic metabolism by cytochrome P-450IIE1 and nitrosodimethylamine mutagenicity. *Cancer Lett.* 61:129–134 (1992).

256. Hosono, A., T. Kishi, and H. Otani. Antioxidative effect of a leaf extract from *Quercus actissima* Carr. on lard and fish oil. *Agric. Biol. Chem.* 55:1397–1398 (1991).

257. Beck, S.A., K.L. Smith, and M.J. Tisdale. Anticachectic and antitumor effect of eicosapentaenoic acid and its effect on protein turnover. *Cancer Res.* 51:6089–6093 (1991).

258. Pariza, M.W. CLA, a new cancer inhibitor in dairy products. *Bull. IDF* 257:29–30 (1991).

259. Pariza, M.W., Y.L. Ha, H. Benjamin, et al. Formation and action of anticarcinogenic fatty acids. In *Nutritional and Toxicological Consequences of Food Processing.* M. Friedman (ed.). *Adv. Exp. Med. Biol.* 289:269–272 (1991).

260. Ip, C., S.F. Chin, J.A. Scimeca, and M.W. Pariza. Mammary cancer prevention by conjugated dienoic derivative of linoleic acid. *Cancer Res.* 51:6118–6124 (1991).

261. Zu, H.-X., and H.A.J. Schut. Inhibition of 2-amino-3-methylimidazo[4,5-*f*]quinoline–DNA adduct formation in CDF$_1$ mice by heat-altered derivatives of linoleic acid. *Food Chem. Toxicol.* 30:9–16 (1992).

262. Shultz, T.D., B.P. Chew, W.R. Seaman, and L.O. Luedecke. Inhibitory effect of conjugated dienoic derivatives of linoleic acid and β-carotene on the in vitro growth of human cancer cells. *Cancer Lett.* 63:125–133 (1992).

263. Medhat, A.M., K.S.El-D. Abdelwahaab, A.A. El Aaser, et al. Soybean and ascorbate feeding in experimental carcinogenesis: immunological studies. *Tumori* 77:372–378 (1991).

264. St. Clair, W.H., and D.K. St. Clair. Effect of the Bowman–Birk protease inhibitor on the expression of oncogenes in the irradiated rat colon. *Cancer Res.* 51:4539–4543 (1991).

265. von Hofe, E., P.M. Newberne, and A.R. Kennedy. Inhibition of *N*-nitrosomethylbenzylamine-induced esophageal neoplasms by the Bowman–Birk protease inhibitor. *Carcinogenesis* 12:2147–2150 (1991).

266. Oreffo, V.I.C., P.C. Billings, A.R. Kennedy, and H. Witschi. Acute effects of the Bowman–Birk protease inhibitor in mice. *Toxicology* 69:165–176 (1991).

267. Osowole, O.A., J.N. Tonukari, and A.O. Uwaifo. Isolation and partial characterization of pigeon pea protease inhibitor: its effect on the genotoxic action of aflatoxin B$_1$. *Biochem. Pharmacol.* 43:1880–1882 (1992).

268. Serraino, M., and L.U. Thompson. The effect of flaxseed supplementation on early risk markers for mammary carcinogenesis. *Cancer Lett.* 60:135–142 (1991).

269. Serraino, M., and L.U. Thompson. Flaxseed supplementation and early markers of colon carcinogenesis. *Cancer Lett.* 63:159–165 (1992).

270. Shultz, T.D., W.R. Bonorden, and W.R. Seaman. Effect of short-term flaxseed consumption on lignan and sex hormone metabolism in men. *Nutr.Res.* 11:1089–1100 (1991).

271. Ruan, C.-c., Y. Liang, J.-l. Liu, et al. Antimutagenic effect of eight natural foods on moldy foods in a high liver cancer incidence area. *Mutat.Res.* 279:35–40 (1992).

272. Patel, V.K., J. Wang, R.N. Shen, et al. Reduction of metastases of Lewis lung carcinoma by an Ayurvedic food supplement in mice. *Nutr. Res.* 12:51–61 (1992).

273. Ueda, S., Y. Kuwabara, N Hirai, et al. Antimutagenic capacities of different kinds of vegetables and mushrooms. (In Japanese; tables and abstract in English.) *Nippon Shokuhin Kogyo Gakkaishi* 38:507–514 (1991).

274. Pèrez, A., G. Gago. Antimutagenic activity of lettuce and chard extracts. *Nahrung* 35:369–371 (1991).

275. Tanigami, Y., S. Kusumoto, S. Nagao, et al. Partial degradation and biological activities of an

antitumor polysaccharide from rice bran. *Chem. Pharm. Bull.* 39:1782–1787 (1991).

276. Kang, J.Y., B. Alexander, F. Barker, et al. The effect of chilli ingestion on gastrointestinal mucosal proliferation and azoxymethane-induced cancer in the rat. *J. Gastroenterol. Hepatol.* 7:194–198 (1992).

277. Bhide, S.V., M.B.A. Zariwala, A.J. Amonkar, and M.A. Azuine. Chemopreventive efficacy of a betel leaf extract against benzo[a]pyrene-induced forestomach tumors in mice. *J. Ethnopharmacol.* 34:207–213 (1991).

278. Umnova, N.V., T.L. Michurina, N.I. Smirnova, et al. In vitro and in vivo studies of antimutagenic properties of bioginseng in mammalian cells. *Bull. Exp. Biol. Med.* 111:658–661 (1991).

279. Ngo, H.N., R.W. Teel, and B.H.S. Lau. Modulation of mutagenesis, DNA binding, and metabolism of aflatoxin B_1 by licorice compounds. *Nutr. Res.* 12:247–257 (1992).

280. Nagasawa, H., H. Inatomi, M. Suzuki, and T. Mori. Further study on the effects of motherwort (*Leonurus sibiricus* L) on preneoplastic and neoplastic mammary gland growth in multiparous GR/A mice. *Anticancer Res.* 12:141–143 (1992).

281. Wang, C.-J., J.-D. Hsu, and J.-K. Lin. Suppression of aflatoxin B_1-induced hepatotoxic lesions by crocetin (a natural carotenoid). *Carcinogenesis* 12:1807–1810 (1991).

282. Röscheisen, C., H. Zamith, F.J.R. Paumgartten, and G. Speit. Influence of β-myrcene on sister-chromatid exchanges induced by mutagens in V79 and HTC cells. *Mutat. Res.* 264:43–49 (1991).

283. Chae, Y.-H., S.L. Coffing, V.M. Cook, et al. Effects of biochanin A on metabolism, DNA binding and mutagenicity of benzo[a]pyrene in mammalian cell cultures. *Carcinogenesis* 12:2001–2006 (1991).

284. Miller, E.G., A.P. Gonzales-Sanders, A.M. Couvillon, et al. Inhibition of hamster buccal pouch carcinogenesis by limonin 17-β-D-glucopyranoside. *Nutr. Cancer* 17:1–7 (1992).

285. Maruyama, H., T. Amanuma, D. Nakae, et al. Effects of catechol and its analogs on pancreatic carcinogenesis initiated by *N*-nitrosobis(2-oxopropyl)amine in Syrian hamsters. *Carcinogenesis* 12:1331–1334 (1991).

286. Lee, H., and L.-J. Tsai. Effect of emodin on cooked-food mutagen activation. *Food Chem. Toxicol.* 29:765–770 (1991).

287. Benjamin, H., J. Storkson, A. Nagahara, and M.W. Pariza. Inhibition of benzo[a]pyrene-induced mouse forestomach neoplasia by dietary soy sauce. *Cancer Res.* 51:2940–2942 (1991).

288. Nagahara, A., H. Benjamin, J. Storkson, et al. Inhibition of benzo[a]pyrene-induced mouse forestomach neoplasia by a principal flavor component of Japanese-style fermented soy sauce. *Cancer Res.* 52:1754–1756 (1992).

289. Polasa, K., T.C. Raghuram, T.P. Krishna, and K. Krishnaswamy. Effect of turmeric on urinary mutagens in smokers. *Mutagenesis* 7:107–109 (1992).

290. Azuine, M.A., and S.V. Bhide. Chemopreventive effect of turmeric against stomach and skin tumors induced by chemical carcinogens in Swiss mice. *Nutr. Cancer* 17:77–83 (1992).

291. Nagabhushan, M., and S.V. Bhide. Curcumin as an inhibitor of cancer. *J. Am. Coll. Nutr.* 11:192–198 (1992).

292. Kumari, M.V.R. Modulatory influences of clove (*Caryophyllus aromaticus*, L) on hepatic detoxification systems and bone marrow genotoxicity in male Swiss albino mice. *Cancer Lett.* 60:67–73 (1991).

293. Kumari, M.V.R. Modulatory influences of mace (*Myristica fragrans*, Houtt.) on hepatic detoxification systems and bone marrow genotoxicity in male Swiss albino mice. *Nutr. Res.* 12:385–394 (1992).

294. Singletary, K.W., and J.M. Nelshoppen. Inhibition of 7,12-dimethylbenz[a]anthracene (DMBA)-induced mammary tumorigenesis and of in vivo formation of mammary DMBA-DNA adducts by rosemary extract. *Cancer Lett.* 60:169–175 (1991).

295. Zheng, G.-q., P.M. Kenney, and L.K.T. Lam. Myristicin: a potential cancer chemopreventive agent from parsley leaf oil. *J. Agric. Food Chem.* 40:107–110 (1992).

296. Salomi, M.J., S.C. Nair, and K.R. Panikkar. Inhibitory effects of *Nigella sativa* and saffron (*Crocus sativus*) on chemical carcinogenesis in mice. *Nutr. Cancer* 16:67–72 (1991).

297. Yen, G.-C., L.-C. Tsai, and J.-D. Lii. Antimutagenic effect of Maillard browning products obtained from amino acids and sugars. *Food Chem. Toxicol.* 30:127–132 (1992).

298. Lee, E.L., N.V. Chuyen, F. Hayase, and H. Kato. Absorption and distribution of [^{14}C]melanoidins in rats and the desmutagenicity of absorbed melanoidins

against Trp-P-1. *Biosci. Biotech. Biochem.* 56:21–23 (1992).

299. Wolfrom, D.M., A.R. Rao, and C.W. Welsch. Caffeine inhibits development of benign mammary gland tumors in carcinogen-treated female Sprague-Dawley rats. *Breast Cancer Res. Treatment* 19:269–275 (1991).

300. VanderPloeg, L.C., D.M. Wolfrom, and C.W. Welsch. Influence of caffeine on development of benign and carcinomatous mammary gland tumors in female rats treated with the carcinogens 7,12-dimethyl-benz(a)anthracene and N-methyl-N-nitrosourea. *Cancer Res.* 51:3399–3404 (1991).

301. Gandhi, R.K., and K.L. Khanduja. Action of caffeine in altering the carcinogen-activating and -detoxifying enzymes in mice. *J. Clin. Biochem. Nutr.* 12:19–26 (1992).

302. Koo, M., and A.V. Rao. Long-term effect of *Bifidobacteria* and neosugar on precursor lesions of colonic cancer in CF_1 mice. *Nutr. Cancer* 16:249–257 (1991).

303. Hosoda, M., H. Hashimoto, H. Morita, and M. Chiba. Antimutagenicity of milk cultured with lactic acid bacteria against N-methyl-N'-nitro-N-nitrosoguanidine. *J. Dairy Sci.* 75:976–981 (1992).

304. Vorobjeva, L.I., T.A. Cherdinceva, S.K. Abilev, and N.V. Vorobjeva. Antimutagenicity of propionic acid bacteria. *Mutat. Res.* 251:233–239 (1991).

3

Diet and Cardiovascular Disease

Overview, epidemiology, and general dietary
   studies
Effects of fiber
Effects of protein
Effects of fats
Antioxidants
Minerals
Other

OVERVIEW, EPIDEMIOLOGY, AND GENERAL DIETARY STUDIES

Herzberg summarized pathways of fatty acid and triglyceride synthesis and metabolism with respect to their regulation by major dietary components (*1*). Plasma triglycerides are derived from dietary fat and endogenous hepatic synthesis; their circulating level reflects the balance between their delivery into and removal from the plasma. Polyunsaturated fats reduce hepatic fatty acid synthesis through effects on the enzymes involved. Dietary fish oil affects both synthesis and removal of circulating triglycerides. Although its major hypotriglyceridemic effect is to reduce fatty acid synthesis and triglyceride secretion, particularly in hypertriglyceridemic persons, there is also evidence that fish oil can increase the oxidation of fatty acids in skeletal muscle and heart.

Elevated serum cholesterol level is a major link in the chain connecting diet and coronary heart disease (CHD) (*2*). A position statement for the National Heart Foundation of Australia reviewed studies of the association between diet and CHD. Key points were the following. High intake of saturated fatty acids (SFAs) is associated with elevated serum cholesterol and LDL-cholesterol and increased risk of CHD. When *n*–6 polyunsaturated fatty acids (PUFAs) are substituted for SFAs they lower serum cholesterol; *n*–3 PUFAs lower serum triglycerides, decrease platelet aggregability, and may further reduce risk of CHD by other mechanisms. Monounsaturated fatty acids (MUFAs) reduce serum cholesterol levels when substituted for SFAs. *Trans* fatty acids behave, in most cases, as SFAs. Total fat intake itself is not strongly associated with CHD but may contribute to obesity; abdominal obesity increases CHD risk. Dietary cholesterol increases serum cholesterol in some people. High alcohol intake increases blood pressure, serum triglyceride levels, and mortality from cardiovascular disease (CVD); light alcohol consumption reduces risk of CHD. Sugar consumption is not associated with CHD. High salt intake is related to hypertension in salt-sensitive people; potassium intake may be inversely related. Plant foods reduce risk of CHD through mechanisms that include lowering serum cholesterol and blood pressure.

A review in *The Lancet* discussed hypercholesterolemic and thrombogenic dietary components and protective factors (*3*). The authors derived indexes of a diet's atherogenicity and thrombogenicity, eliminating shorter-chain SFAs and stearic acid from the SFA factor and including MUFAs. The new indexes give a sometimes radically different indication of risk than the widely used PUFA/SFA (P/S), but they are in good agreement with observation.

A different perspective on diet, CVD, and CHD faults some common assumptions about risks associated with dietary fat and cholesterol and emphasizes cereal products as the mainstay of a nutritional approach to lowering risk (*4*). The role of oat products in such an approach is discussed.

Grundy emphasized the multiplicity of factors responsible for hypercholesterolemia and the complexity of their interactions (*5*). He reviewed LDL metabolism and receptor activity, including hepatic secretion of VLDL, the major lipoproteins containing apolipoprotein B (apoB). Dietary and age-related factors in borderline hypercholesterolemia were discussed, with preventive measures. Causes, treatment, and prevention of moderate and severe hypercholesterolemia were similarly considered.

A workshop on metabolic and nutritional factors in hypertension developed recommendations for treatment and prevention (*6*). The recommendations emphasize the importance of making decisions about pharmacological and nonpharmacological interventions on a case-by-case basis in the context of an overall risk assessment, which includes family history and other factors specific to the patient. Areas for further research were suggested.

Another review discussed cardiovascular risk factors and their interactions in hypertensive subjects, particularly with reference to stroke (*7*). When pharmacological interventions are used, trade-offs between side effects, efficacy, and cost must always be considered. In many cases it would be more productive to tackle lifestyle factors, including diet.

In Australia and the USA, mortality from CHD in men has been decreasing sharply since 1968–1970; in the U.K. a slower decline began in the late 1970s (*8*). Roberts considered dietary and other possible factors in this decline, concluding that change in the dietary P/S ratio is the major dietary factor. This judgment was based on analysis of food disappearance data for the three countries and the lag time between the dietary change and the beginning of decline in CHD mortality. In the future, *n*–3 PUFAs, MUFAs, and antioxidants may need to be factored in to account for continuing rate changes. A decline in ischemic heart disease (IHD) since 1970 in Iceland has similarly been tied to a reduction in risk factors (smoking, systolic blood pressure, and serum cholesterol concentration) (*9*). The fall in serum total cholesterol levels coincided with reduced consumption of dairy fat and margarine.

Hypertension is an emerging problem in many tropical countries (*10*). Among black Africans, the major consequence is an increase in stroke and cerebrovascular disease, whereas in Asians the problem is manifest predominantly in increased CHD. Urbanization and its accompanying lifestyle and dietary changes are involved in all cases. For black Africans, who tend to be more salt-sensitive than Whites and Asians, reduction of dietary salt would probably be an effective preventive measure. An interesting but probably unprovable hypothesis was discussed: that salt-sensitivity was selected for in Blacks whose ancestors were taken into slavery, because the extreme conditions on the slave ships, where great numbers of captives died, would have favored the genetically determined capacity to conserve sodium.

A report on high blood pressure concluded that prevention and control of factors related to lifestyle must be components of any strategy for dealing with the blood-pressure problem (*11*). The author believes that both population-wide and high-risk strategies are necessary because of the considerable excess CHD morbidity and mortality associated with even slight elevations of systolic blood pressure above the ideal (>120 mm Hg). Historical and cultural aspects of dietary salt consumption and results of the recent Intersalt study were discussed and other important dietary risk factors were briefly considered. The author urged high national priority for a policy commitment to a strategy for comprehensive care and primary prevention of hypertension.

Of the various nonpharmacological interventions to reduce blood pressure, weight reduction, sodium restriction, moderation of alcohol intake, and aerobic exercise have been the most effective in primary and secondary prevention (*12*). However, Kaplan pointed out methodologic difficulties that plague most short-term intervention studies, stating that none provide conclusive evidence of efficacy in preventing the complications of hypertension. For example, the extent to which increased potassium intake is responsible for the apparent effects of decreased sodium intake has not been established, nor has individual calcium sensitivity been taken into account. Blood-pressure effects of macronutrients, caffeine, smoking, alcohol intake, exercise, and relaxation were briefly mentioned.

Plasma cholesterol concentrations measured during childhood are well correlated with concentrations later in life. Lloyd contrasted the strategies of screening all children for hypercholesterolemia and of programs for dietary change (*13*). While recommending targeted screening of children in families with familial hypercholesterolemia, she emphasized the potential benefits of population-wide dietary change designed to lower plasma cholesterol, beginning with children when they are 2 years old. However, the effect of such dietary change on the health and growth of children needs to be monitored.

For a dietary subanalysis of the NHANES I Epidemiologic Followup Study, dietary intakes of sodium, potassium, calcium, and total calories were examined (*14*). Data reinforce the importance of weight control in the primary prevention of hypertension. However, no significant association was found between intake of any cation and development of hypertension in Blacks or Whites of either sex. The authors suggested that their failure to demonstrate such an association was due to imprecision of the dietary recall data and possible misclassification of hypertension status.

Weizel examined the "cholesterol story," which currently consists of "more questions than answers" for the practicing physician (*15*). The current therapeutic approach to reducing CHD mortality is based on evidence that elevated plasma cholesterol is a major risk factor. Weizel showed that in Germany 70% of fatal myocardial infarctions occur in persons older than 65 years and questioned the feasibility and even the advisability of prophylactic therapy in that age group. In contrast, a case was made for aggressive attempts at prevention in the younger at-risk group. Here the problem is to find good predictive markers, because even persons with familial hypercholesterolemia are heterogeneous with respect to CHD risk. The author summarized the role of PUFAs, MUFAs, SFAs, and *trans* fatty acids. There are responders and nonresponders to dietary therapy, and failure frequently leads to drug therapy because by then the patient expects treatment. In summary, the ideal situation for intervention occurs when a physician works with a cooperative patient who meets current criteria for high risk of CHD.

Analysis of diet–cholesterol relationships in a sample of 413 men in the Framingham study showed that dietary variables predict serum cholesterol levels independently of other CHD risk factors (*16*). Significant direct predictors of cholesterol levels were dietary fat (amount), cholesterol (mg/1000 calories), and protein (amount and percent of calories). Fat (percent of calories) and cholesterol (mg) were marginally significant. Inverse correlates were total carbohydrate (amount and percent of calories) and simple carbohydrate (percent of calories). An inverse correlation with complex carbohydrates was marginally significant.

Ninety men referred for coronary angiography to investigate findings suggestive of CHD and who had plasma cholesterol levels >6.0 mmol/L were randomized to receive usual care, dietary intervention, or dietary intervention plus cholestyramine for 3 years (*17*). The lipid-lowering diet had a fat content of 27%, SFA content of 8–10%, cholesterol content of 100 mg/1000 kcal, n–6 + n–3 PUFA content of 8%, and soluble plant fiber (chiefly pectin) content equivalent to 3.6 g of polygalacturonate per 1000 kcal. At the end of this time dietary change alone was as effective as diet plus cholestyramine in significantly retarding progression and increasing regression of coronary artery disease; the latter treatment was additionally associated with a net increase in coronary lumen diameter.

The independent and interactive effects of sodium restriction and a high-fiber, low-fat diet with a high P/S ratio were studied in 95 hypertensive subjects (*18*). Subjects followed a low-sodium diet with either high fiber and low fat or normal fat and fiber for 8 weeks. Half of each group received enteric-coated 100 mmol NaCl tablets and half received placebo. Sodium restriction significantly reduced standing and supine systolic blood pressure but had no effect on diastolic blood pressure. The low-fat, high-fiber diet had no effect on blood pressure but significantly reduced serum total cholesterol, LDL cholesterol, and HDL cholesterol. Together, salt restriction and a low-fat, high-fiber diet have greater potential than either alone to reduce CVD risk in hypertensive persons.

The Seventh-Day Adventist Church encourages vegetarianism and discourages use of drugs, tobacco, alcohol, and caffeine-containing beverages. As part of the Cardiovascular Disease Studies in Norway, coronary risk factors were compared in Seventh-Day Adventists and age-, sex-, and residence-matched controls (*19*). Serum cholesterol was significantly lower in Seventh-Day Adventists, in both men and women; blood pressure was significantly lower only in women. Ex-members of the church and members who did not comply with the recommended lifestyle had higher values for risk factors than compliant members.

In relation to a cardiovascular intervention program for adults living in Norsjö, Sweden, an investigation of CVD risk factors in 15-year-old residents was conducted (*20*). Total cholesterol concentrations exceeded 5 mmol/L in 14% of boys and 32% of girls; based on the target value of 3.9 mmol/L for 5- to 18-year-olds, 69% of the study group had high serum cholesterol. The diet of the 15-year-olds was similar to that of the adults, although individual variation was great. On average, intake of fruit, vegetables, fiber, and vitamins A, C, and B_6 was low and intake of total fat and SFAs was high. In comparison with international studies of this age group, cholesterol concentrations were lower than reported from Norway and Finland, similar to those in Holland, and higher than those in Italy.

In 1972 a major demonstration program for CHD prevention (the North Karelia Project) was undertaken in eastern Finland where the CHD mortality rate was especially high (*21*). Since an initial rapid drop in risk factor values, the rate of improvement has steadily declined. A more recent study area in southwestern Finland, where risk is lower, has shown little change. The high serum cholesterol levels in North Karelia before the project can be explained mainly by the high intake of saturated fats (23% of calories) and cholesterol (~600 mg daily). During the first 10 years of the project intake of saturated fat was reduced to 19–20% of calories and cholesterol to ~450 mg. Although use of traditional sources of saturated fats such as butter and high-fat milk has continued to decline, consumption of other dairy products such as cheese has increased, explaining the much smaller change in serum cholesterol between 1982 and 1987. During the study the dietary P/S ratio in North Karelia has increased from 0.17 to 0.30 in urban men and from 0.15 to 0.21 in rural men. Other habits and characteristics of Finns contributing to CHD risk, and changes in them, are discussed.

A study in Northern Ireland explored the relationship between patterns of food intake and nutritional health as defined by hematological and biochemical measures (*22*). Four dietary patterns were identified by principal components analysis on the correlation matrix of 41 food groups in the dietary intake inventory. The "traditional" diet was based on bread, spreading fats, tea and coffee, desserts, potatoes, milk, preserves, eggs, bacon, and vegetables; chips, alcoholic beverages, and rice and pasta were avoided. The "cosmopolitan" diet was based on fruit, vegetables, rice and pasta, egg and cheese dishes, cream, cheese, patés, breakfast cereals, fatty fish, and shellfish; "common" foods such as chips, legumes, sausages, savory pies, and beer were avoided. The "convenience food" diet was based on foods such as beer, chips, soft drinks, nuts, cheese, rice and pasta, savory pies, and cooked meat dishes. The "meat and two veg" diet was based on meat and vegetables, sauces, potatoes, wines and spirits, fish, and shellfish. A number of small but statistically significant associations were found between diet pattern and blood measurements, and somewhat different results were obtained for men and women. Total cholesterol was negatively associated with the cosmopolitan diet in women. HDL cholesterol was positively correlated with cosmopolitan and convenience diets in women, and with these plus the meat and two veg diet in men. Measures of iron status were negatively associated with the traditional diet and positively associated with the meat and two veg diet. Folate status was positively correlated with convenience and cosmopolitan diets in women. Dietary components and interactions considered responsible for these and other findings were discussed. These baseline data on diet and health indexes can be used in future epidemiological investigations.

To assess cross-cultural relations between diet and plasma lipoproteins, dietary and plasma data for urban and rural adults from the Puriscal region, Costa Rica, were compared with data for adults in the Framingham Offspring Study (*23*). Total and LDL cholesterol were significantly higher in Framingham residents than in Puriscal residents, whereas elevated triglyceride and apoB levels, low HDL cholesterol and apoA-I levels, and smaller LDL particles were more frequent among Puriscal residents. Measures for urban Puriscal residents fell between those for subjects in rural Puriscal and Framingham subjects for many of the parameters, such as intake of protein, saturated fat, and animal fat. Puriscal residents also consumed more carbohydrate than their Framingham counterparts. Adults in urban Puriscal tended to have more body fat, be more sedentary, and have a more atherogenic diet and plasma lipid profile than adults in rural Puriscal, but Puriscal residents taken together had a less atherogenic diet, plasma profile, and lifestyle than Framingham residents. A dietary evaluation of a random sample of 51 families in metropolitan San José, Costa Rica, found that the macronutrient composition of the diet met the recommendations of the U.S. National Cholesterol Education Program (*24*). However, the total dietary fiber intake of 20.3 g/day, the 12.6% of calories from sucrose, and the low P/S ratio were not within the guidelines and represent atherogenic risk factors associated with cardiovascular disease.

A study was made of CHD mortality rates and diet in 17 autonomous regions of Spain (*25*). The most consistent finding was a high negative correlation between CHD mortality and meat intake. Although not compatible with evidence that meat and animal fats promote CHD, these data do support studies showing that stearic acid reduces plasma levels of cholesterol and LDL in comparison with diets high in palmitic or oleic acid. Negative correlations between CHD mortality and consumption of total fat, olive oil, and milk were not significant when data for the Canary Islands were excluded. The difference between effects of foods and effects of individual nutrients needs to be studied.

A study of healthy adults in northern Italy found several correlations between dietary factors and risk factors for CHD (26). Compared with Italian recommendations, total energy intake conformed with guidelines but protein and fat intakes were excessive and carbohydrate intake was low. The cholesterol/SFA index, a measure of the hypercholesterolemic and atherogenic potential of the diet, was high in ~50% of the study population. However, vitamin A intake was more than adequate in 70%. In adults 10–39 years old there was a positive association between total and saturated fat, energy, and alcohol intake and values of some blood lipid parameters. For older subjects, lipid values were correlated with body mass index. Overall, values of risk factors were typical for a Western population and efforts to correct intake of fat, cholesterol, and alcohol were recommended for prevention of CHD.

Workers in India investigated the influence of a diet rich in fruits, vegetables, and cereals on blood lipids in subjects with CHD or at high risk for it (27). The cardioprotective diet had 27.5% of energy from fat, a P/S ratio of 1.38, 120 mg of cholesterol, and 26.0 g of dietary fiber per 1000 kcal; the control diet had 30% of energy from fat, a P/S ratio of 0.74, 164 mg of cholesterol, and 14.0 g of dietary fiber per 1000 kcal. After 8 weeks subjects on the intervention diet had a significant decrease in serum total cholesterol, LDL cholesterol, and triglycerides compared with baseline levels and the control group. In another Indian study, patients were randomized to one of two diets within 48 hours after acute myocardial infarction (28). In diet A, meat and eggs were replaced with fish, vegetarian meat substitutes, and nuts to achieve low levels of saturated fat, cholesterol, salt, and caffeine and high levels of soluble fiber, vitamins, and minerals. Frequent small meals were served. In diet B, patients received a typical low-calorie diet during hospitalization and later were placed on a diet prescribed by their physician. After 6 weeks, patients on diet A had a significant decrease in serum total and LDL cholesterol and triglycerides but no change in HDL cholesterol, compared with baseline levels and changes in diet group B. The more favorable lipid profile and significant decrease in body weight in group A accompanied a decrease in total cardiac events including fatal and nonfatal acute myocardial infarctions and sudden cardiac death. Total mortality did not differ between groups during the 6-week follow-up.

The traditional diet of the Tarahumara Indians of Mexico was low in fat and high in fiber and these people had a very low incidence of risk factors for CHD (29). Thirteen Tarahumara Indians ate their traditional 2700-kcal/day diet for one week and were then fed a diet typical of affluent societies: excessive calories (4100 kcal/day), total fat, saturated fat, and cholesterol. After 5 weeks of eating the affluent diet, the subjects' plasma cholesterol had increased by 31%, LDL cholesterol by 39%, HDL cholesterol by 31%, and triglycerides by 18%. All subjects gained weight, the mean increase being 3.8 kg. If sustained, these changes could increase the CHD risk of this population.

Agheli et al. reported one of the first studies of the effect of a clinically sound, hypocaloric, but not extreme diet on lipoprotein parameters in adults with type IV hypertriglyceridemia (30). Normolipidemic subjects were controls. On entry into the study, the diet of the 5 hypertriglyceridemic subjects contained 2565 ± 412 kcal. The treatment diet contained an average of 1625 kcal with 40% carbohydrate, 35% fat, 25% protein, and a P/S ratio of 1.02. The major source of carbohydrate was cereals and starchy foods containing little sugar; protein was supplied by fish, lean meat, poultry, and skim or low-fat milk or yogurt; the main fats were sunflower oil and margarine. Treatment decreased serum triglycerides by 52%, total cholesterol by 12%, free cholesterol by 30%, and all constituents of

VLDL by 58% in the hypertriglyceridemic subjects. Changes in the IDL, LDL, and HDL compartments were also seen. Only minor changes occurred in phospholipid fractions and fatty acid profiles. The results indicate that a nonextreme nutritional regimen can substantially decrease serum lipids and normalize lipoprotein composition in type IV hypertriglyceridemic subjects.

It is not known whether categories of CHD risk as defined by plasma total cholesterol concentrations apply equally to elderly and younger adults, nor is it known if the same relationships hold between dietary factors and plasma lipid parameters (*31*). To determine whether true age-related changes in dietary intake occur and if so, how they relate to concentrations of plasma lipids, the diets of 157 healthy elderly men and women were analyzed in a cross-sectional. longitudinal study. Significant decreases in intake of total fat, SFAs, PUFAs, and cholesterol occurred during the 9-year study, accompanied by significant decreases in plasma total, HDL, and LDL concentration. Ratios of total and LDL cholesterol to HDL cholesterol increased over time. The decrease in total fat and cholesterol intakes were significantly correlated with the decrease in plasma total cholesterol. In women but not men, changes in total fat, SFA, and PUFA intake over time showed significant positive correlation with changes in fasting triglyceride concentrations. These findings were discussed in terms of their interpretation and implications for the nutrition and health of the elderly.

Plasma levels of VLDL and triglycerides increase after a sudden increase in dietary carbohydrate. However, some investigators questioned whether such an increase is inevitable (*32*). Beginning with a typical American diet containing 40% fat, 45% carbohydrate, and 15% protein they decreased fat and increased carbohydrate in four increments of 5%. Each dietary period lasted 10 days and lipid parameters were monitored throughout the study. Plasma triglyceride and VLDL did not change significantly, whereas plasma total and LDL cholesterol levels were greatly reduced. HDL cholesterol also decreased. After the phased part of the study, some subjects returned to the "normal" diet during a 6-week washout period. They were then suddenly subjected to the high-carbohydrate phase 4 diet. Under this protocol, plasma triglyceride concentration increased over baseline by 47% and VLDL increased by 73%. These findings verify that sudden introduction to a high-carbohydrate, low-fat diet produces carbohydrate-induced hypertriglyceridemia, but this effect is circumvented by gradual introduction of the diet while the beneficial effects on total and LDL cholesterol still occur.

Plasma lipid and lipoprotein concentrations were compared in healthy men who ate a self-selected diet followed, in random order, by high-fat low-fiber and low-fat high-fiber diets for 10 weeks each (*33*). Test diets contained 41% fat plus 2.0 g/MJ of fiber and 19% fat plus 4.6 g/MJ of fiber, respectively. On the low-fat dietary arm of the study, total, LDL, and HDL cholesterol were 17–20% lower than on the high-fat arm; lipid changes were minor. Plasma cholesterol was reduced >0.52 mmol/L in 59% of men when the low-fat diet was compared with the self-selected diet and in 79% of men when it was compared with the high-fat diet. Marked reductions occurred within 6 weeks.

Substantial changes in serum lipid parameters were reported in 4587 adults who participated in a 3-week residential program of dietary change and daily aerobic exercise (*34*). Forty percent of the subjects had a diagnosis of CHD, 43% had hypertension, and 16% had diabetes mellitus; many had more than one diagnosis. The remaining subjects entered the program for preventive reasons. Fifteen percent of calories were derived from protein, <10% from fat, and the remainder from carbohydrate, with 35–40 g of dietary fiber per 420 kJ and 25 mg/day of cholesterol. Daily exercise was prescribed by an exercise physiologist based on the individual's assigned training heart rate; subjects also attended educational classes. Under this strict regimen total and LDL cholesterol levels were reduced by 23%, most of the change occurring during the first 2 weeks. HDL cholesterol was reduced by 16% and triglyceride levels by 33%. A small number of subjects were followed up after 18 months. Those who continued to comply with the program maintained their improved lipid status. In an editorial discussion of this paper, Grundy speculated on various explanations for the results (*35*).

He suggested that exercise played a more important role than the author credited to it and that the controlled environment reduced cholesterol levels by reducing stress; regression to the mean could explain another portion of the change. He questioned whether such a severe diet could or should be maintained over a lifetime. The relative merits of increasing carbohydrates or increasing PUFAs and MUFAs have not been determined. For these reasons and others, Grundy believes the study diet has not been shown to be superior to the National Cholesterol Education Program (NCEP) diet and is certainly less practical for the general public. The NCEP recommends a diet low in saturated fat and cholesterol, with weight loss if indicated, to correct excessive plasma cholesterol levels (36). Fruits, vegetables, cereals, nuts, and oils are substituted for eggs, meat, and butter in this diet. The hypothesis that exercise will increase HDL cholesterol levels in moderately overweight sedentary people who adopt a hypocaloric NCEP diet was tested. Adults (132 men and 132 women) were randomly assigned to control diet, hypocaloric NCEP diet, or hypocaloric NCEP diet with walking or jogging. At the end of a year, subjects in both interventions had reached or nearly reached the NCEP Step 1 dietary goals and significantly reduced their mean body fat. Men who exercised and dieted lost significantly more weight than men in the other two groups. Weight loss in the diet-only group did not significantly change HDL cholesterol levels in comparison with the control group. In contrast, plasma levels of HDL cholesterol increased significantly in men who dieted and exercised. In women who dieted and exercised, plasma HDL cholesterol was significantly higher than in the diet-only group but not different from that in the controls. An additional finding, which needs a longer follow-up for confirmation, was a significant decrease in nonfatal acute myocardial infarction in the interventions groups.

Results after one year of follow-up were presented for a previously reported short-term trial of a cardioprotective diet in patients with recent acute myocardial infarction (37). Patients with definite or possible acute myocardial infarction and unstable angina were assigned to a fat-reduced diet within 24–48 hours of infarction. Group A patients ($n = 204$) were advised to eat more fruit, vegetables, nuts, and grains, whereas group B patients ($n = 202$) were given no further dietary advice. After one year, blood lipoprotein concentrations and body weight were significantly lower in group A than in group B. The incidence of cardiac events and total mortality were also significantly lower in group A (50 vs. 82 and 21 vs. 38, respectively).

It has been suggested that the high cholesterol and SFA content of milk consumed in infancy can influence lipid metabolism throughout life. To learn whether the method of infant feeding is associated with adult serum lipid concentrations and IHD mortality, a follow-up study was conducted of men born in Hertfordshire, England, between 1911 and 1930 (38). Of 5471 subjects, 1381 had been both breast- and bottle-fed, 3733 had been breast-fed only, and 357 had been bottle-fed only; only 69% of those who were exclusively breast-fed had been weaned at 1 year, compared with 90% of breast- and bottle-fed and 94% of bottle-fed subjects. At the time of the study, 474 men had died from IHD. Standardized mortality ratios were 97 in breast-fed subjects who had not been weaned at 1 year, 95 in bottle-fed subjects, 79 in breast-fed subjects who had been weaned at 1 year, and 73 in men who had been breast- and bottle-fed. Men not weaned at 1 year and bottle-fed men had the highest serum concentrations of total cholesterol, LDL cholesterol, and apoB. The authors conclude that the age of weaning and method of infant feeding may influence adult levels of serum LDL cholesterol and IHD mortality.

A study in rhesus monkeys (*Macaca mulatta*) established that species as a model for CHD (39). In a colony of 160 monkeys fed an atherogenic diet, 14 showed electrocardiographic and echocardiographic evidence of CHD. Compared with 14 matched normal controls, these monkeys had higher arterial blood pressure, lower plasma concentrations of HDL cholesterol and apoA-I, and higher plasma concentrations of total cholesterol and LDL cholesterol. Therefore rhesus monkeys develop CHD as a consequence of coronary artery atherosclerosis and risk factors for CHD are similar to those in humans.

EFFECTS OF FIBER

Reviews

Topping reviewed the effects of soluble-fiber polysaccharides on plasma cholesterol concentration and colonic fermentation (*40*). These polysaccharides occur in natural foods and are widely used as stabilizers and thickeners by the food industry. They reduce plasma cholesterol through a mechanism involving enhanced steroid excretion and altered fat absorption; this activity may be a function of the fiber's viscosity in solution. Soluble fibers also slow small intestinal transit and nutrient absorption; and although resistant to human digestive enzymes, they are fermented to short-chain fatty acids by colonic bacteria. These acids are involved in fiber's antineoplastic activity in the colon but not in its hypocholesterolemic activity. Subjects that need investigation include the caloric yield from fiber polysaccharides and the relationships between a fiber's chemical structure and physiologic effects.

Shinnick et al. (*41*; 102 references) updated the LSRO's 1987 review of the effects of fiber on lipid levels in human serum (Life Science Research Office; *Physiological Effects and Health Consequences of Dietary Fiber*; S.M. Pilch, ed.; Fed. Am. Soc. Exp. Biol., Bethesda, MD, 1987). They critically reviewed all relevant research but emphasized results of clinical studies involving oats and oat bran. The consistent reduction of cholesterol concentrations by soluble fiber sources is independent of alterations in fat intake. In oats, the soluble fiber fraction rich in mixed-linkage β-glucans is largely responsible for this activity. Another summary traces the story of oats and cholesterol beginning with a study in Holland some 30 years ago (*42*).

Studies in human subjects

Although oat bran usually reduces plasma cholesterol levels regardless of fat intake, a trial with 40 hypercholesterolemic adults found no effect when oat bran was added to the usual diet (*43*). Using a 4 × 4 Latin square design, subjects added 0, 30, 60, or 90 g/day of oat bran to their otherwise self-selected diet for 1-month periods. This is the setting in which oat bran is most frequently used by the general public. Consumption of up to 90 g/day of oat bran did not significantly lower plasma total or LDL cholesterol in this group of hypercholesterolemic subjects who continued to eat a diet relatively high in SFAs. Two other studies, one in the context of a "typical Australian diet" (*44*) and one in the context of a lipid-lowering diet (*45*), produced disparate results. In the Australian study (*44*), mildly hypercholesterolemic men were adapted for 3 weeks to a baseline diet containing 30–34% fat and two servings per day of wheat cereal. This was followed by two 4-week treatments with an additional 18 g/day of nonstarch polysaccharide as wheat or oat bran in a randomized crossover design. Oat bran supplementation significantly lowered plasma total and LDL cholesterol, whereas wheat bran supplementation did not. Total fat and saturated fat consumption did not change throughout the study, ruling out fat displacement as a mechanism for the effect of oat bran. In the other study (*45*), hyperlipidemic subjects were stabilized on a lipid-lowering diet for at least 3 months and then oat-bran and wheat-bran breads of comparable fiber content were added to the diet for 4-week periods in a single-blind, crossover design. Both breads lowered serum cholesterol by ~4%. The authors concluded that the hypocholesterolemic effect is a general property of dietary fiber.

A recent study by Davidson et al. (*Food Safety 1991*, Chapter 3, reference 40) engendered some critical comment from readers. One letter criticized the controls (28, 56, and 84 g of oat products vs. 28 g of wheat) and suggested that observed effects were due to fat displacement (*46*). It further suggested that if the effect was a direct one of β-glucan, as Davidson et al. purported to show, then oat bran with its higher content of β-glucans should have been more effective than an equal amount of oatmeal, but in most cases it was not. A second letter questioned the statistical power claimed for the study and discussed the effect of a lower power on interpretation of the results (*47*). Davidson et al. responded to these comments, explaining their basis for ruling out a fat-displacement effect and justifying their statistical assumptions (*48*).

The hypolipidemic effects of guar gum and oat fiber were compared in hypercholesterolemic adults *(49)*. Throughout the study, subjects ate their normal diet whether or not it was fat-modified. The only adjustment was isocaloric substitution of the oat fiber supplement for part of the usual carbohydrate (the guar gum supplement did not contribute significantly to total calories). Supplements were taken in water, three times a day, before meals. Each treatment lasted 3 weeks and a crossover design was used. Both supplements reduced total and LDL cholesterol, but guar gum was significantly more effective.

Better data are needed to establish guidelines for use of soluble fibers in dietary management of hypercholesterolemia. Randomized, double-blind, placebo-controlled trials in healthy hypercholesterolemic adults were conducted with a variety of soluble dietary fibers to address this data deficiency *(50)*. Dietary fiber mixtures were prepared as powders in a carbohydrate base and mixed with water for ingestion at meal-time. Subjects maintained their customary eating and activity patterns. Acacia gum, which produces a palatable beverage of low viscosity when mixed with water, had no significant lipid-lowering effect when provided as either the major component (56%) of a mixed-fiber supplement or the sole source (15 g) of soluble fiber. When locust bean gum and pectin were substituted for acacia gum in a mixture that also contained psyllium fiber and guar gum, both the mixture and a guar gum control significantly reduced total, LDL, and HDL cholesterol but had no effect on triglycerides. To establish dose effects of the fiber mixture, subjects consumed the supplement one, two, or three times a day at meal-time. Significant dose-related trends were seen for LDL cholesterol, and this accounted for most of the effect on total cholesterol. Effects on HDL cholesterol and triglycerides were inconsistent. Results were similar for men and women and corroborated other observations that hypocholesterolemic effects are related to viscosity.

Tablets containing 7 g of a 60:30:10 mixture of beet, barley, and citrus fibers were tested for antihypertensive effects in 63 mildly hypertensive subjects *(51)*. A randomized, double-blind, placebo-controlled design was used. Subjects consumed their normal diet throughout the 3-month trial. Body weight decreased slightly in both groups, most likely because the tablets caused a feeling of satiety. The fiber supplement significantly reduced diastolic blood pressure and fasting serum insulin and triglycerides but had no effect on systolic blood pressure.

Because wheat germ has been hypotriglyceridemic and hypocholesterolemic in short-term animal and clinical studies, a long-term study was conducted in type IIa and IIb hyperlipidemic subjects *(52)*. In the initial phase, subjects consumed their customary diet for 4 weeks and took wheatgerm supplements in conjunction with their customary diet for 4 weeks, in a random crossover design. One group received raw wheat germ and another received partially defatted wheat germ. After the crossover phase subjects consumed their assigned supplements for an additional 14 weeks. In the crossover phase, raw wheat germ decreased plasma total and VLDL cholesterol and the apoB/apoA-I ratio. After 14 weeks, plasma total and LDL cholesterol, triglycerides, and the apoB/apoA-I ratio were reduced. With partially defatted wheat germ there were only transient decreases in plasma triglycerides and esterified cholesterol.

A crossover study assessed the effects of barley (soluble fiber, largely β-glucan) and wheat (insoluble fiber, largely cellulose) on plasma cholesterol concentrations in mildly hypercholesterolemic men *(53)*. Comparable barley and wheat foods were supplied as muesli, bread, spaghetti, and biscuits for the two 4-week diet periods; subjects were instructed to keep exercise, alcohol intake, and other dietary constituents constant throughout the trial. Consumption of barley was associated with significant decreases in plasma total and LDL cholesterol; HDL cholesterol, triglycerides, and glucose concentrations did not change. Wheat consumption had no favorable effects on lipid parameters. An order effect was observed: the change in plasma cholesterol was greater in subjects who ate wheat foods before barley foods. This could be a duration effect or a result of the nonsignificant hypercholesterolemic effect of the wheat foods. Similar results were obtained in another study comparing soluble fiber (from oats and dried beans) and insoluble fiber (from wheat products) in a rigorously controlled experiment conducted on a metabolic ward (*54*). Again, the soluble fiber significantly reduced total and LDL cholesterol and apoB in hypercholesterolemic men, whereas wheat bran had no effect. HDL cholesterol and apoA-I did not change in either group. Triglycerides decreased in both groups but this was significant only for oat bran. Oat bran supplements again proved superior to wheat bran in a 14-day study of 84 healthy middle-aged adults (*55*). Because this was part of a study that also examined the effects of these fibers on colorectal cancer risk, roughly half of the subjects had a history of polypectomy. Metabolically controlled, defined diets were delivered to subjects' homes. Both treatments significantly decreased concentrations of total, LDL, and HDL cholesterol and apoA-I, but the effects were greater for oat bran. In addition, oat bran significantly reduced apoB concentrations.

Ten men with primary hypercholesterolemia completed a metabolic-ward study to determine the effects of refined wheat–based bakery products on their serum lipid values (*56*). After eating a high-carbohydrate, high-fiber control diet for 7 days they switched to a diet rich in soluble fiber from bakery products for 21 days. Both diets provided 25 g of total dietary fiber per day, but the bakery diet supplied 6 g more of soluble fiber. Serum total cholesterol concentrations stabilized during the control period and then decreased 6.4% during the bakery diet. Serum LDL cholesterol, apoB-100, and the apoB-100/apoA-I ratio also decreased during the bakery diet. Thus a modest increase in soluble fiber from wheat, with total fiber held constant, favorably affected lipid parameters in hypercholesterolemic men.

To test the effects of various fibers on postprandial lipemia, 6 normolipidemic men ate a series of test meals at intervals of 7–15 days (*57*). Throughout the study they followed their typical self-selected Western diets, which were high in calories, fat, and cholesterol and low to moderate in dietary fiber. The evening before a test meal they ate a standard light meal. The five test meals were given in random order. They consisted of a basal low-fiber meal containing 70 g of fat and 756 mg of cholesterol and the basal meal enriched with 10 g of total dietary fiber as oat bran, rice bran, or wheat fiber of 4.2 g total dietary fiber as wheat germ. Added fiber induced no change in serum glucose or insulin responses to the test meal or in serum apoB and apoA-I concentrations. The serum triglyceride response was significantly lower with oat bran, wheat fiber, and wheat germ; wheat fiber also reduced chylomicron cholesterol. Cholesterolemia decreased postprandially for 6 hours; the decrease was greatest after the oat bran meal. Thus the various cereal fibers reduced postprandial lipemia to different extents.

Richter et al. reported an interaction between dietary fiber and the cholesterol-lowering drug lovastatin (*58*). When 15 g/day of pectin was added to treatment with a lipid-lowering diet and lovastatin, they unexpectedly found a sharp increase in LDL cholesterol in the first three hypercholesterolemic patients on the protocol. Levels returned to previous values for lovastatin alone after pectin supplementation was stopped. Two patients who were taking 50–100 g/day of supplemental oat bran in addition to lovastatin also experienced a rise in LDL cholesterol. The authors suggested that these fibers decrease absorption of lovastatin from the gut and recommended that patients taking lovastatin and related drugs be advised not to take pectin or oat bran at the same time. The fiber–lovastatin interaction may explain some treatment failures.

Animal studies

Baked oat bran has a higher content of insoluble fiber than unprocessed oat bran, due to its higher Klason lignin content and a shift from soluble to insoluble β-glucans (*59*). When the effects of unprocessed and baked oat bran were evaluated in rats, the two were comparable. Relative to the fiber-free control diet, both oat bran diets increased wet and dry fecal weight and decreased transit time of food; metabolizable energy and apparent digestibility of dry matter and protein decreased, but lipid digestibility was not significantly affected. Plasma total cholesterol concentration decreased with both oat bran diets and there was an inverse linear relationship between plasma cholesterol and fecal excretion of bile acids.

The hypocholesterolemic properties of whole barley (ground meal of two cultivars), oat bran, and wheat red dog were compared in chicks and rats (60). Chicks were fed the experimental diets for 10 days; rats, for 6 weeks. Oat bran and one of the barley cultivars significantly lowered total and LDL cholesterol levels in both chicks and rats without affecting HDL cholesterol. Soluble β-glucan was the strongest predictor of serum cholesterol response in both species. Beyond that, species differences were observed in the response to the various fibers, and there were differences in responses to the two barley cultivars. Somewhat different results were obtained in a long-term (29-week) study of the effects of various dietary fibers (61). Male and female rats were fed rodent lab chow or a purified diet supplemented with 4 or 14% cellulose, oat bran, hard wheat bran, soft wheat bran, or corn bran. Among the observed differences were that cholesterol levels were higher in males fed soft wheat bran than in males fed hard wheat, oat, or corn bran, and that the 4% oat bran diet induced lower levels of HDL cholesterol than the 14% wheat bran diets. In general, the various cereal brans influenced total serum lipid levels in different ways, which reflected their differing amounts and types of fiber constituents.

In a dose–response study, the hypocholesterolemic effects of diets containing 10.9–43.7% full-fat rice bran were evaluated in hamsters (62). The effects of defatted rice bran and crude rice bran oil at levels equivalent to their amount in the 43.7% rice bran diet were also evaluated. All diets were adjusted to 10% total dietary fiber with cellulose; some diets were cholesterol-free and some contained 0.3% cholesterol. Whether or not cholesterol was added, plasma cholesterol levels were significantly lower in animals fed the 43.7% full-fat rice bran diet than in those fed 10% cellulose. The effect of full-fat rice bran was dose-related. Full-fat rice bran was the only treatment that significantly lowered both plasma and liver cholesterol. Rice bran oil alone was ineffective, and recombined rice bran oil and defatted rice bran were less effective than the full-fat product.

Konjac mannan, isolated from tubers of *Amorphophallus konjac,* has been used as a food in Japan. When fed to hamsters as a 5% supplement to commercial rodent chow, it significantly decreased levels of cholesterol in serum and liver and reduced the elevation of serum cholesterol caused by cholesterol feeding (63). Although there was no direct evidence for an effect on bile acid absorption, konjac mannan feeding altered biliary bile acid composition. The proportion of chenodeoxycholic acid in biliary bile acids was significantly increased in animals fed cholesterol plus konjac mannan, providing indirect evidence that konjac mannan inhibits the intestinal absorption of bile acids.

Addition of raw wheat germ to the fat-rich diet of adult rats produced a significant dose-related reduction in plasma total, esterified, VLDL, and LDL cholesterol and plasma VLDL and LDL triglycerides (64). A diet with 3.5% raw wheat germ decreased liver triglycerides and cholesterol; it had no influence on fecal excretion of fat and bile acids, but increased the ratio of coprosterol to cholesterol. Defatted wheat germ had no effect on liver and fecal lipids but significantly increased fecal excretion of bile acids. It decreased plasma LDL cholesterol, esterified cholesterol, and triglycerides. It appears that both raw and defatted wheat germ in small quantities can alter values of plasma lipid parameters, possibly through different mechanisms.

When 12% lard, by weight, was added to the semipurified diet of male rats it lowered the production of acetic, propionic, and butyric acids in the cecum, decreased the mass of colonic bacteria, and nonsignificantly increased the liver's cholesterol level compared with a 1% lard diet(65). Addition of 3% pectin to the lard-containing diet did not counteract the intestinal changes but nonsignificantly reduced the lard-induced increase in liver cholesterol. It reduced plasma cholesterol concentrations at both levels of dietary lard.

Sprague-Dawley rats were fed diets containing 7.5% fiber as cellulose (controls), pectin, psyllium, or oat bran for 3 weeks. Half of the rats in each fiber group were also fed 0.3% cholesterol (66). Of the cholesterol-fed rats, the cellulose controls had significantly higher levels of liver cholesterol than the three experimental groups, and rats in the pectin plus cholesterol group had liver cholesterol levels as low as those in the no-cholesterol groups. Serum cholesterol levels were also lowest in the pectin group of cholesterol-fed rats. Short-chain fatty acid concentrations were measured in the hepatic portal vein. With cholesterol feeding, the oat bran group had the highest butyrate concentrations and the pectin group had the highest propionate concentrations; all fiber groups had significantly higher levels of fecal neutral sterols than the cellulose controls. Without added cholesterol only rats in the pectin group excreted more fecal neutral steroids than the controls. The authors suggest that soluble dietary fibers exert their hypocholesterolemic effect by increasing excretion of fecal neutral sterols.

When 30% sugar-beet fiber was substituted for an equivalent amount of wheat starch in a fructose-based low-fat diet for rats, numerous effects were observed (67). The cecum was significantly enlarged, concentration of volatile fatty acids was increased, and plasma triglyceride and cholesterol concentrations were reduced in both the postprandial and the postabsorptive periods. Liver lipogenesis triglyceride levels were depressed but cholesterol levels were unchanged. Fiber-fed rats were less fat than controls and adipose tissue lipogenesis was depressed postprandially. These results show that substitution of fermentable fiber for easily digested carbohydrate has multiple effects on lipid parameters and obesity.

ApoB is synthesized in liver and small intestine as an obligate component of triglyceride-rich lipoproteins (68). To find how dietary fiber acts to decrease apoB concentrations, the effect of a low-fat, 30% sugar-beet diet on expression of the intestinal apoB gene in the rat was studied. Fiber feeding markedly increased fecal bile salt and cholesterol excretion. It had no effect on jejunal apoB mRNA levels, but decreased the level of ileal apoB mRNA. No apoB mRNA was detected in the cecum in either fiber-free or fiber-fed animals. The authors concluded that dietary fiber can modulate expression of the apoB gene at the mRNA level in the intestine, and that increased fecal bile salt excretion may be involved. Results with sugar beet fiber

may not be typical. Other fibers that interact with bile salt metabolism in different ways might affect apoB expression differently.

EFFECTS OF PROTEIN

Building on evidence from protein-feeding studies, Sanchez and Hubbard hypothesize that the control of cholesterol by insulin and glucagon is regulated by dietary and plasma amino acids (69). When human subjects are fed test meals identical except for protein source, the amino acid composition of the meal influences not only postprandial levels of plasma amino acids but also levels of insulin and glucagon. Hypocholesterolemic soy protein, rich in arginine and glycine, increases postprandial levels of these amino acids and decreases the insulin/glucagon ratio. Arginine and glycine themselves are hypocholesterolemic. Hypercholesterolemic casein, with a relatively high lysine/arginine ratio, induces a high postprandial insulin/glucagon ratio. Lysine and branched-chain amino acids are hypercholesterolemic. Therefore the authors propose the insulin/glucagon ratio as an early metabolic index of the effect of dietary proteins on serum cholesterol levels and as a mechanism through which diet influences cardiovascular disease.

Milk proteins contain specific highly conserved, biologically active sequences. Among these are peptides with antithrombotic and hypotensive activity (70). These activities are based in part on functional similarities and sequence homologies between the fibrinogen γ chain and κ casein: the casein peptides combine with receptor sites to prevent binding of fibrinogen with platelets. In addition, peptide sequences that block the hydrolysis of angiotensin I by angiotensin converting enzyme (ACE) are located in β casein. These have hypotensive activity.

An enzymatic hydrolysate of α-zein, a maize endosperm protein, also has hypotensive activity (71). α-Zein was hydrolyzed by various proteases to provide peptides for evaluation of in vitro ACE-inhibitory activity and in vivo hypotensive activity in spontaneously hypertensive rats (SHR). Among the hydrolysates, thermolysin hydrolysate had the greatest ACE-inhibitory activity and also reduced systolic blood pressure in SHR after intraperitoneal or oral administration. The active peptides now need to be identified and characterized.

Subjects with mild hypercholesterolemia participated in an evaluation of the effects of mycoprotein on blood lipids (72). Mycoprotein is a high-quality protein produced by continuous fermentation culture of *Fusarium graminearum* Schwabe. The preparation has a low fat content, with unsaturated fatty acids predominating, and significant amounts of dietary fiber. One group of subjects ate cookies containing mycoprotein and one group ate nutrient-balanced cookies in which soy concentrate was substituted for the mycoprotein. After 8 weeks, total cholesterol was reduced by 0.95 mmol/L in the mycoprotein group and 0.46 mmol/L in the soy group; corresponding reductions in LDL cholesterol were 0.84 and 0.34 mmol/L. All differences were statistically significant. These results confirm those of metabolic studies showing that mycoprotein improves values of blood lipid parameters.

Fish proteins also affect lipid profiles (73). Rabbits were fed diets containing casein, soy, or fish protein with corn oil or coconut oil as the lipid. Dietary proteins and lipids exerted both independent and interactive effects on serum lipids. Compared with soy protein, casein elevated total cholesterol; compared with corn oil, coconut oil raised total and VLDL cholesterol and decreased the LDL/HDL ratio. Fish protein maintained a high level of HDL cholesterol regardless of lipid source, whereas corn oil decreased HDL cholesterol with soy and casein feeding. Similar interactions were observed in regulation of liver cholesterol levels.

A proteinaceous inhibitor of platelet aggregation, designated BM-1, has been isolated from chub mackerel (74). Eight healthy men took 6 g of BM-1 daily for 30 days, after which samples of peripheral blood platelets were isolated. Platelet aggregation in response to ADP and collagen was sharply and significantly inhibited. The BM-1 preparation contained 61.3% protein, whose amino acid composition was determined; 0.4% lipid; 0.5% carbohydrate; and 37.8% water.

Soy protein

Carroll reviewed findings of clinical studies on the hypocholesterolemic response to soy protein (75). Substitution of soy protein for animal protein or addition of soy protein to the diet has given variable results, but European investigators have generally found that it lowers serum total and LDL cholesterol in hypercholesterolemic subjects. With high-protein, low-fat diets reductions of 20% or more have been achieved. HDL cholesterol levels are little changed. In hypertriglyceridemic subjects soy protein also lowers triglyceride levels. Men and women respond similarly, but responses are sometimes greater in young subjects and subjects with normal lipid levels generally show little change. Characteristics of subjects, diet composition, and protocol are discussed as explanations for the variability of results.

Children with familial hypercholesterolemia were given a soy-protein beverage and a cow-milk beverage in a crossover study to measure effects on plasma lipoproteins (76). Each arm of the trial lasted 4 weeks, with a washout period between. Subjects ate basal diets providing 20% of energy as protein and 28% as fat with a P/M/S fatty acid ratio of 1:3:3. No changes in plasma total or LDL cholesterol or apolipoprotein were observed, but the soy beverage significantly reduced concentrations of triglyceride and VLDL cholesterol and increased HDL cholesterol. Because the genetic defect in familial hypercholesterolemia is partly manifest as a lowered concentration of HDL cholesterol, the increase in HDL cholesterol caused by soy protein may be considered clinically important and beneficial.

Beynen discussed ambiguities in interpreting studies of the dietary protein–serum cholesterol relationship (77). For example, even the purest preparations of casein and soybean protein contain up to 20% nonprotein material, which in the case of soybean includes fiber, phytosterols, phytic acid, and saponins. It is difficult to rule out these substances as being partly or entirely responsible for observed effects. Several hypotheses have been advanced to explain the apparent activity of soy protein, but a mechanism has yet to be definitively established to account for the hypocholesterolemic effects of soy preparations.

The opposite cholesterolemic effects of casein and soy protein are accentuated when cebus monkeys are fed semipurified diets supplemented with cholesterol (*78*). In a crossover experiment, the dietary protein source made little difference in plasma cholesterol parameters in the setting of a cholesterol-free diet. However, when 0.2% cholesterol was added to the diet, crossover from soy protein to casein increased total cholesterol from 7.97 ± 1.09 to 9.33 ± 1.31 mmol/L and crossover from casein to soy protein decreased cholesterol from 9.64 ± 0.58 to 7.41 ± 1.07 mmol/L. Most of the change was attributable to changes in VLDL and LDL cholesterol. These results corroborate findings of other studies in human subjects and animals. Only in rabbits are significant protein-induced changes in cholesterol noted in the absence of dietary cholesterol (for example, see reference *73*). It is also interesting that Samman failed to find an effect of fish-oil supplementation on plasma LDL parameters in endogenously hypercholesterolemic rabbits when the dietary protein was casein (*79*).

In another soy-vs.-casein study, serum lipid levels and other variables were measured in adult male rats (*80*). Casein-fed rats had higher serum levels of insulin, triglycerides, and total and HDL cholesterol and lower levels of fecal fat. Measures of adiposity also increased. Higher insulin levels and increased fat absorption may explain these results. Carrying this type of study a step further, the effect of dietary protein on the fatty acid composition of VLDL was examined (*81*). Rats were fed semipurified diets containing olive oil and either casein or soy protein. The expected effects on plasma lipid levels were seen. VLDL from casein-fed rats had relatively more oleic acid and less linoleic and arachidonic acid in the phosphatidylcholine fraction. The proportion of 5,8,11-eicosatrienoic acid (n–9) varied among the lipid classes in response to dietary protein and differences in other fatty acids were also noted. These differences appeared to influence prostanoid production. For example, when mouse peritoneal macrophages were incubated with VLDL from soy-fed animals a saturable accumulation of 6-keto-prostaglandin $F_{1\alpha}$ and thromboxane

B_2 occurred in the medium, whereas only very low levels of these substances were detected when macrophages were incubated with VLDL from casein-fed animals.

Dietary protein also affects the peroxidation of eicosapentaenoic acid (EPA) in SHR (*82*). For 4 weeks, rats were fed diets with protein supplied as casein, soy protein, or soy protein plus 0.3% methionine; half of the rats on each diet received 4% supplemental EPA. Liver glutathione peroxidase activity and glutathione levels were lower in soy-fed rats than in casein-fed rats, but addition of methionine to the soy abolished most of this difference, whether or not EPA was added to the diet. Similarly, rats fed EPA plus soy protein had higher lipid peroxide levels in liver, kidney, and testis than rats fed EPA plus casein; again, addition of methionine to the soy protein abrogated most of the difference. EPA feeding tended to produce larger changes in peroxide levels in soy-fed rats than in casein-fed rats. The authors conclude that methionine has a regulatory role in EPA utilization when fed in the context of a soy protein diet.

Experiments were performed to validate the hamster as a model for studying interactive effects of dietary protein and cholesterol on plasma lipid parameters (*83*). Results consistent with those from human studies and rat models were obtained when hamsters were fed 25% casein or soy protein diets with and without cholesterol. Differences were sharply accentuated in the presence of dietary cholesterol; but wide interanimal variability decreased the statistical significance of results.

EFFECTS OF FATS

Kromhout reviewed the often disparate results of cross-cultural, prospective, and intervention studies linking dietary fats to serum cholesterol concentrations, CVD, and general health (*84*). Advantages and disadvantages of the various approaches and reasons for discrepant findings were discussed. The Seven Countries Study showed unambiguously that dietary saturated fat is a major determinant of cross-cultural differences in serum cholesterol and CHD mortality. Dietary intervention studies establish the cholesterol-elevating effect of saturated fat. In intervention studies the beneficial effect of cholesterol-lowering is strongest for the endpoint, acute myocardial infarction, and becomes stronger the longer follow-up is continued; it can take 2 years or longer before survival curves for the intervention and control groups begin to diverge. Although the relationships between dietary fat, serum cholesterol, and CHD mortality are becoming clearer, research is needed to accurately assess intake of saturated fat, explain the effects of eating small amounts of fish, and more sharply define the relationships between different classes of fatty acids, lipoproteins, and CHD mortality.

An evaluation of the database for the "usual care" arm of the Multiple Risk Factor Intervention Trial (MRFIT) corroborated reports that n–3 fatty acids are protective against CVD (85). When the effects of PUFA intake on 10.5-year mortality rates were examined by proportional hazards regression analysis, significant inverse associations were found between both linolenic acid and fish oil fatty acids and mortality from CHD, total CVD, and all causes. Results were more significant when PUFAs were expressed as percent of total calories. There was also evidence that the composition of dietary PUFAs influences cancer mortality. Weaker, but still suggestive, relationships emerged from examination of CHD morbidity and mortality in two male cohorts from the Framingham Study (86). For 420 men aged 45–55 years, incidence of CHD was positively associated with the proportion of dietary energy contributed by total, monounsaturated, and saturated fat. These effects were at least partly independent of other established risk factors. However, in 393 men aged 56–65 years, none of the dietary lipids were associated with CHD.

Kaplan reexamined the data from six lipid intervention trials for primary prevention of CHD (87). One of his purposes was to evaluate observations that despite significant reductions in morbidity and mortality from CHD there was no decrease in overall mortality because of concomitant increases of cancer and violent deaths in treated subjects (see also Chapter 1, references 33–69). Kaplan concluded that the adverse effects seen in

these trials can neither be proved related to reduction in cholesterol levels nor disregarded as biological or statistical quirks. For both health-related and economic reasons he advised caution in advocating widespread treatment of persons with mild hypercholesterolemia.

In defense of meat and meat fats, Reiser and Shorland reviewed the role of fats in nutrition and obesity, relationships between fatty acids and thrombosis, and cholesterol homeostasis (88). They pointed out fallacies in some popular assumptions about fat, emphasizing the importance of a balanced fat intake. Steps already taken by the meat industry to reduce and modify the fat in meat animals were discussed.

Effects on plasma lipids and lipid metabolism

Norum reviewed the literature on the effects of dietary fat on blood lipids (89). The enhancement of cholesterol levels attributed to SFAs is largely due to SFAs having chains of 12, 14, and 16 carbon atoms; these increase total cholesterol predominantly by increasing LDL. MUFAs, particularly oleic acid, were formerly considered neutral in this respect; however, oleic acid is as effective as linoleic acid in lowering plasma LDL cholesterol if it is substituted for palmitic acid. Whether PUFAs and MUFAs really lower LDL cholesterol or are merely neutral depends on what substitution or comparison is made. Also discussed were effects of dietary fat on plasma triglycerides, apolipoproteins, lipoproteins, and enzymes of lipid metabolism; chylomicron metabolism; regulation of apolipoprotein gene expression; and pathways of VLDL, LDL, and HDL metabolism. Another review focused on how cholesterol and specific fatty acids interact to modulate circulating levels of LDL cholesterol and on reasons for variable individual responses to these lipids (90). Cholesterol synthesis in different species and different organs was reviewed. The concentration of plasma LDL cholesterol is determined by the rates at which VLDL is converted to LDL and LDL is removed from the plasma by receptor-dependent and -independent transport processes. Rate constants for these processes can be determined experimentally and can be used to predict how LDL cholesterol would change if one or more of the constants were altered. Modulation of LDL receptor activity was discussed. A third review also discussed mechanisms by which dietary fat composition may affect circulating cholesterol levels (*91*). Most studies have found that SFAs increase total and LDL cholesterol; PUFAs decrease total, LDL, and HDL cholesterol; and MUFAs reduce total and LDL cholesterol without affecting HDL cholesterol. Changes in fecal sterol excretion, exogenous cholesterol absorption, lipoprotein composition, and lipoprotein catabolism may accompany changes in fat intake but a direct causal relationship has not been proved. The authors considered the idea that shifts in LDL receptor-mediated transport cause the responses of circulating cholesterol to dietary fat.

A brief review considered health effects of Mediterranean diets and MUFAs (*92*). It listed nuts and oils rich in MUFAs and discussed their incorporation into a healthful diet.

An editorial by Sacks and Willett asked whether a diet that lowers LDL cholesterol inevitably lowers "good" HDL cholesterol as well (*93*). It considered some paradoxical observations on the relationship between HDL cholesterol levels and CHD risk and suggested that lowering HDL cholesterol or the HDL/LDL cholesterol ratio may actually be quite safe. As a practical alternative to traditional low-fat cholesterol-lowering diets they suggested the Mediterranean option, using MUFAs as the major dietary fats.

Although studies totally substituting one fat source for another produce experimentally valid results, they do not reflect effects of fats and oils as they are normally used (*94*). This was illustrated by findings from studies using oil mixes, with emphasis on palm oil. With background information from total substitution studies, fats should be studied by feeding at levels and in mixtures approximating their actual usage. The author also stressed the need to delineate the effects of fatty acids as a function of their abundance at different positions in individual triglycerides.

Rice bran oil is a new oil recently introduced into the Indian market. Its biochemistry and hypolipidemic action were reviewed (*95*). In fatty acid composition it resembles groundnut oil. Rich in tocopherols and tocotrienols, it has substantial antioxidative activity. Other constituents are oryzanol (a mixture of ferulic acid esters of triterpene alcohols) and squalene. The unsaponifiable fraction has a hypolipidemic, hypocholesterolemic effect in animals. One component of this fraction, cycloartenol, is structurally similar to cholesterol and may compete with it for binding sites, enhancing the excretion and metabolism of cholesterol. In cynomolgus monkeys (*Macaca fascicularis*), rice bran oil lowers serum total and LDL cholesterol and apoB (*96*). The extent of reduction was correlated with initial serum cholesterol levels and was dose-related. Further, the cholesterol-lowering ability was not explained by the oil's fatty acid composition.

Both *cis* and *trans* isomers are created when PUFAs are hydrogenated. Although the final word is not in on health effects of *trans* fatty acids, *trans* isomers tend to behave more like SFAs than like PUFAs or MUFAs and have been hypercholesterolemic in some studies. However, reviewing mixed results of studies on *cis* and *trans* fatty acids and serum lipoproteins, Katan and Mensink concluded that it is premature to condemn all partially hydrogenated vegetable oils as cholesterolemic (*97*). They stated that the hydrogenation process can be fine-tuned to produce nearly any specified mix of *cis*, *trans*, and saturated fatty acids. Moreover, margarines differ widely in composition; some of those on the European market contain no *trans* fatty acids at all, being combinations of unhydrogenated oil and saturated fat that yield a semisolid product. The authors suggested that the range of suitable replacements for butter and other animal fats may be more restricted than first was thought, but more information is needed.

STUDIES IN HUMAN SUBJECTS. Zock and Katan compared the effects of linoleic acid [*cis,cis*-C18:2(*n*–6)] and its hydrogenation products elaidic [*trans*-C18:1(*n*–9)] and stearic acids on serum lipoprotein levels in healthy, normolipidemic adults (*98*). In a multiple crossover design, each subject was give three experimental diets for 3 weeks each: a linoleate diet, which supplied 12.0% of total energy as linoleic acid, 2.8% as stearic acid, and 0.1%

as *trans* fatty acids; a stearate diet, which supplied 3.9% of energy as linoleic acid, 11.8% as stearic acid, and 0.3% as *trans* fatty acids; and a *trans* diet, which supplied 3.8% as linoleic acid, 3.0% as stearic acid, and 7.7% as monounsaturated *trans* fatty acids, largely elaidic acid. The *trans* diet significantly lowered HDL cholesterol and raised LDL cholesterol relative to the linoleate diet; these and earlier results suggest a linear dose-dependent relationship. A similar but smaller effect was seen with the stearate diet. Thus hydrogenation of linoleic acid yields two products, both of which increase LDL and decrease HDL relative to linoleic acid, and large-scale substitution of solid vegetable fats for animal fats may offer few health advantages. However, Nestel et al. did not find that elaidic acid altered HDL cholesterol in mildly hypercholesterolemic men (*99*). They compared the cholesterolemic effects of two semihardened blends of edible oils (P/M/S ratio of 0.8:1.3:1) and typical Australian dietary fat with a P/M/S ratio of 0.4:0.9:1.0. The test blends significantly lowered serum LDL cholesterol without affecting HDL cholesterol or triglycerides. The *trans* fatty acid content of the blends was 16% and was mostly elaidic acid. They concluded that so long as the linoleic acid/palmitic acid ratio in the oil blend exceeds that in the prevailing Australian diet, partial hydrogenation does not eliminate the blend's LDL-lowering potential.

The effects of rapeseed oil and sunflower seed oil on lipoprotein levels were compared in healthy adults (*100*). The rapeseed oil diet contained 16% MUFAs, 6% *n*–6 PUFAs, and 2% *n*–3 PUFAs; the sunflower oil diet contained 10% MUFAs, 13% *n*–6 PUFAs, and 0% *n*–3 PUFAs. After a baseline diet rich in saturated fats, the experimental diets were tested for 3.5 weeks each in a blinded crossover design. Both diets reduced serum total and LDL cholesterol levels but the effect was greater for the rapeseed diet. VLDL cholesterol and total, VLDL, and LDL triglycerides decreased more with sunflower oil than with rapeseed oil. Neither test diet altered HDL cholesterol levels. The rapeseed oil diet produced more favorable HDL_2/LDL cholesterol and apoA-I/apoB ratios than the sunflower oil diet.

The effects of almonds and almond oil on plasma lipid parameters were studied in moderately hypercholesterolemic subjects in the context of a diet based on grains, beans, vegetables, fruit, and low-fat milk products (*101*). During the test diet period, 100 mg/day of raw almonds was provided and almond oil was the only fat used in food preparation. There was a rapid, sustained reduction in LDL cholesterol but no change in HDL or VLDL cholesterol or triglycerides; total cholesterol fell rapidly during the first 3 weeks and then remained constant. Total fat intake increased during the experimental period, from 28 to 37% of total calories; this was due to increased consumption of MUFAs. Protein intake also increased, carbohydrate intake decreased, and the P/S ratio changed from <1.0 to >1.0. These results show that a diet containing a higher amount of fat than is generally recommended in cholesterol-lowering diets can still be hypocholesterolemic when the diet is high in plant foods and MUFAs. Somewhat different results for MUFAs were obtained in a comparison of MUFA- and PUFA-enriched diets in healthy adults who maintained their customary diets except for the oil used (*102*). Subjects were first placed on a PUFA-enriched (sunflower oil) diet for 12 weeks and then on a MUFA-enriched (olive oil) diet for 16 weeks (men) or 28 weeks (women). Both diets contained 36–37% of calories as fat. The MUFA diet did not change total cholesterol in men but increased it 9% in women; HDL cholesterol increased by 17% in men and 30% in women. The total/HDL cholesterol ratio (an index of atherogenic risk) fell significantly in both men and women. There were no changes in plasma LDL cholesterol or total triglycerides.

Changes in serum lipid and apolipoprotein concentrations were measured in men who ate diets based on 39% fat from safflower or canola oil for 8 weeks (*103*). Compared with the typical American baseline diet, both oil-based diets significantly reduced serum total and LDL cholesterol and apoB-100. There were no changes in serum triglycerides, apoA-I, or total HDL, HDL_3, or HDL_2 cholesterol. Again (see reference *101*), this study showed that LDL cholesterol levels can be lowered when fat intake remains high if SFA intake is minimized, and that high-PUFA diets do not necessarily lower HDL cholesterol. In fact, reducing total dietary fat without reducing SFAs may not alter total plasma cholesterol concentrations (*104*). When normal men were tested on an average American diet with 37% of calories from fat and 16% from SFAs, a 30%-fat diet with 9% SFAs, and a 30%-fat diet with 14% SFAs, switching from the American diet to the lower-fat diet for 7 weeks did not change total and LDL cholesterol unless this reduction was achieved by lowering SFA intake. Plasma triglycerides did not change with either reduced-fat diet.

In another high-fat dietary study, butter, beef tallow, cocoa butter, and olive oil were tested as sole fat sources in liquid test diets containing 40% of energy as fat (*105*). The study was a metabolic-ward investigation of 10 men aged 51–72 years. Diets were fed in random order for 3 weeks each. Total and LDL cholesterol concentrations decreased with diet in the order butter > beef tallow > cocoa butter > olive oil. HDL cholesterol did not change significantly. Thus, compared with olive oil, butter is unquestionably a cholesterolemic fat. Beef fat and cocoa butter were mildly hypercholesterolemic but not significantly different from each other. As indicated by fecal excretion of fatty acids, >90% of dietary oleic, palmitic, and stearic acids was absorbed.

A representative cross-sectional study among adults residing in Basel, Switzerland, found a significant association between serum levels of total cholesterol and consumption of meat and sausages (*106*). Men who ate meat or sausage daily had a mean cholesterol concentration of 6.29 mmol/L; for women this value was 6.63 mmol/L. For subjects who ate meat or sausage no more than once weekly, values were 5.66 mmol/L for men and 5.33 mmol/L for women. These associations remained significant after multiple linear regression analysis with age, sex, social status, body mass index, and consumption of whole-grain bread, yogurt or cottage cheese, eggs, and alcohol taken as possible confounding factors. HDL cholesterol was not influenced by consumption of meat and sausages.

The effects of diets relatively enriched in palm, coconut, and hydrogenated soybean oil were compared in healthy young men (*107*). Test diets contained 35% fat, 50% of which was provided by the test oil incorporated into muffins or cookies. The 9 subjects who completed the randomized crossover trial ate each diet for 3 weeks, with 2 weeks of ad libitum diet between tests. In the palm oil phase, which was the particular interest of the authors, there were no changes in total or LDL cholesterol, or apoprotein A or B. HDL cholesterol was slightly elevated and triglycerides were slightly reduced, but there were too few subjects to establish the significance of these trends. In the coconut oil phase, total and LDL cholesterol were significantly elevated. No changes occurred during the soybean oil phase. This short-term study adds to the substantial evidence that palm oil, unlike most tropical oils, is not hypercholesterolemic.

Moderate changes in amount and type of dietary fat can improve plasma cholesterol status. Twenty young women in Iowa and Nebraska participated in a study to compare the effects of a "1974 diet" (41% fat, P/S = 0.3) and a "modified diet" (30% fat, P/S = 1.0) (*108*). A modified crossover design was used, with preexperimental and postexperimental periods on a self-selected diet. Experimental diets were eaten for 28 days. An order effect was observed, which represented a carryover effect from the modified diet. When the modified diet preceded the 1974 diet, no difference in HDL and HDL_3 cholesterol was seen between the experimental diets; but when the modified diet came second these HDL values were higher than in the 1974 phase. Similarly, more neutral steroid was excreted with the 1974 diet and the difference was greater when the 1974 diet followed the self-selected diet. Five of the Nebraskan subjects were Chinese and 1 was Iranian, whereas all Iowan subjects were Caucasian; self-selected diets of the two groups differed substantially, and some differences in response to the test diets were observed. Whether these represent racial differences is not known.

The ability of long-term fairly stringent dietary modification to reduce cholesterol levels was evaluated in moderately hypercholesterolemic premenopausal women (*109*). The test diet was based on the American Heart Association's phase 3 diet, considered the most extreme low-fat diet that can be based on normal foods with the expectation of compliance by a seriously motivated subject. After eating a typical American diet for 1 month, subjects ate the test diet (21% of calories from fat, P/S = 1.8) for 5 months. The results demonstrate the importance of following changes in lipid parameters for a prolonged period. HDL cholesterol decreased by 12% during the first 2 months but had returned to 5% below baseline after 5 months. HDL_2 cholesterol decreased throughout the study, whereas HDL_3 cholesterol was 5% below baseline after 1 month but 7% above baseline after 5 months. After 5 months, total and LDL cholesterol had decreased by 7 and 11%, respectively, and total triglycerides had increased by ~30%. Plasma apoA-II, the only apolipoprotein to change, increased 15%. The greatest decreases in total, LDL, and HDL_2 cholesterol (and the only significant decreases) occurred in the leanest women. The same research group also tested the hypothesis that insulin-like growth factor I (IGF-I) modulates hepatic production and peripheral utilization of lipoproteins (110). Serum concentrations of IGF-I were inversely correlated with total and LDL cholesterol and apoB during both high- and low-fat dietary phases. IGF-I increased with reduced fat intake only in obese subjects. The authors concluded that IGF-I may be involved in regulating LDL cholesterol in moderately hypercholesterolemic women but perhaps does not play a role in the beneficial response to reduced fat intake.

ANIMAL STUDIES. After early observations that plasma cholesterol concentrations are increased by high intakes of saturated fat it became apparent that not all saturated fatty acids are equally to blame. The cholesterolemic effects of coconut, palm, soybean, and high-oleic-acid safflower oil mixtures were tested in adult cebus, squirrel, and rhesus monkeys (111). These oils were blended to obtain mixtures with P/S ratios of 0.12–1.04, which provided 30% of dietary calories. Monkeys were rotated through four 12-week dietary periods, after which they were fed a diet containing mostly lauric and palmitic acids as SFAs. Changes in plasma cholesterol were in the same direction in the three species, but cebus monkeys were most responsive and rhesus monkeys, least. All species showed a sharp decline in plasma cholesterol concentrations when 12:0 (lauric) and 14:0 (myristic) fatty acids

were replaced by 16:0 (palmitic acid). A progressive decrease in LDL cholesterol was associated with decrease in 14:0 + 16:0 fatty acids; total cholesterol decreased as 12:0 + 14.0 decreased. The lowest values for total, LDL, and LDL/HDL cholesterol and triglycerides were obtained with the diet having the highest P/S ratio. Thus palmitic acid was less hypercholesterolemic than lauric plus myristic acids; and of these two, myristic was more hypercholesterolemic than lauric. In another experiment, cebus and rhesus monkeys were fed diets relatively enriched in 18:2 (high-linoleic-acid safflower oil), 18:1 (high-oleic-acid safflower oil), or 16:0 (palm oil) fatty acids (112). In rhesus monkeys, no diet produced changes in total, LDL, or HDL cholesterol, but plasma triglyceride concentrations were directly related to the degree of saturation of the major dietary fatty acid. In cebus monkeys, total and HDL cholesterol concentrations were lower on the 18:2 diet than on 18:1 or 16:0 but LDL cholesterol and triglycerides did not change. Tracer studies of lipoprotein metabolism showed that ~64% of LDL catabolism was receptor-mediated regardless of diet, and diet did not affect apoB pool sizes or fractional catabolic rates. There were some differences in apoA-I parameters. The authors concluded that 16:0 and 18:1 have similar effects on LDL and HDL metabolism in normocholesterolemic animals and that the hypocholesterolemic effect of 18:2 results from reduction of HDL cholesterol. When data from numerous feeding studies in cebus monkeys were reanalyzed and compared with results from studies in human subjects, myristic acid again was the principal hypercholesterolemic SFA (113). Oleic acid (18:1) appeared neutral in these studies, whereas linoleic acid (18:2) was hypocholesterolemic but there was an upper limit for the effect. Effects of palmitic acid were variable in human subjects and depended on the cholesterol content of the diet. In normocholesterolemic subjects who consumed ≤300 mg/day of cholesterol, it had no effect. However, in hypercholesterolemic subjects, especially those consuming ≥400 mg/day of cholesterol, palmitic acid made a modest contribution to hypercholesterolemia.

Plasma triglyceride concentrations and HDL size and composition were evaluated in rats fed different fats (*114*). The apparent digestibility of palm oil and beef tallow was less than that of corn oil, butterfat, and coconut oil. Plasma total cholesterol levels were similar for animals fed palm oil, beef tallow, and corn oil, and higher than in animals feed butterfat or coconut oil. HDL apoA-I and apoE resided on significantly smaller particles in rats fed saturated fat than in rats fed corn oil. HDL contained less protein and more triglyceride, free cholesterol, and apoE with saturated-fat feeding. Elevated plasma and VLDL triglyceride levels were also seen in animals fed saturated fat. VLDL triglyceride concentrations were inversely correlated with the HDL modal diameter of apoE-containing lipoproteins. The authors concluded that triglyceride and HDL metabolism are interrelated and the mechanisms involved may be independent of cholesteryl ester transfer protein.

In rat intestinal microsomes, the dietary (n–6)/(n–3) ratio modulates lipid chylomicron-synthesizing enzymes (*115*). After 4 weeks of feeding n–3 PUFAs, acyl-CoA:cholesterol acyltransferase, acyl-CoA:lysophosphatidylcholine acyltransferase, and acyl-CoA:1,2-diacylglycerol acyltransferase activities were enhanced, whereas acyl-CoA:2-monoacylglycerol acyltransferase activity was not affected. Major alterations in the fatty acid composition of microsomal lipids associated with altering the dietary (n–6)/(n–3) ratio could account for the modification in membrane-bound enzyme activities. The authors proposed that high intake of n–3 PUFAs enhances the velocity of chylomicron synthesis in rats.

A study in rats examined whether the stereospecific composition of fish oil and peanut oil is involved in the lipid's digestibility and effects on lipid metabolism (*116*). Nonpurified diets containing native or randomized fish or peanut oil or beef tallow were fed. Randomization of the oils did not affect any lipid measurement. The apparent digestibility of beef tallow was the lowest of the fats fed. Apparent absorption of 18:1(n–9) and PUFAs did not depend on the fatty acid profile, but apparent absorption of 16:1(n–7) and SFAs was generally highest in rats fed fish oil. Ingestion of fish oil affected lipid parameters in the expected way. Thus the effects of these fats on plasma lipids and fatty acid profiles are due solely to their fatty acid

composition and not to positional effects of the fatty acid in the fat molecule.

A study in guinea pigs tested the hypothesis that dietary fat–mediated differences in hepatic apoB and apoE receptor number and LDL composition and size have independent effects on LDL kinetics (*117*). It found that dietary PUFAs lower plasma LDL levels partly by increasing apoB/E receptor-mediated fractional LDL turnover and decreasing apoLDL flux. The extent of dietary fat saturation also influences LDL composition and size, which independently affects LDL turnover rates in vivo.

Using a hamster model, Woollett et al. showed that SFAs and PUFAs independently regulate LDL-receptor activity and production rate (*118*). SFAs suppressed receptor-dependent LDL transport, whereas PUFAs enhanced it; the magnitude of these effects was roughly the same, although in opposite directions. Substituting PUFAs for SFAs increased receptor activity significantly more than merely reducing SFAs, indicating the independence of the two effects. In addition, SFAs caused a dose-related increase in the rate of LDL cholesterol production and raised the level of LDL cholesterol in plasma; PUFAs did not affect either of these. In further studies, these authors examined the regulatory effects of SFAs 6:0–18:0 on hepatic LDL receptor activity (*119*; also see reference *90*). Hamsters were fed diets in which fat was supplied by olive oil plus triglyceride containing a single species of SFA. The hepatic total lipid fraction became enriched in 12:0, 14:0, 16:0, and 18:0 SFAs but not in the 6:0, 8:0, and 10:0 compounds. Only the 12:0, 14:0, and 16:0 fatty acids suppressed LDL-receptor activity and increased the production rate of LDL cholesterol. The 16:0 and 18:0 compounds lowered the hepatic total cholesterol pool without altering rates of cholesterol synthesis in extrahepatic organs; thus changes in delivery of cholesterol to the liver do not explain the effect on hepatic cholesterol pool size. Since the 12:0-, 14:0-, and 16:0-mediated changes in LDL kinetics took place with no detectable alteration in external sterol balance, the regulatory effects of these SFAs appear to occur through change in an intrahepatic regulatory pool of sterol.

Another study in hamsters compared the responses of serum, liver, and heart lipids to dietary palm oil, palm oil triglycerides, coconut oil, and olive oil (*120*). Like palm oil, the palm oil triglyceride fraction was not hypercholesterolemic. Nor did increasing oleic acid and decreasing palmitic acid intake improve the lipidemic response. Compared with coconut oil, all three of these dietary fats lowered serum total and LDL cholesterol levels without affecting HDL cholesterol. However, palm oil, palm oil triglycerides, and olive oil increased hepatic total cholesterol and cholesteryl ester without affecting heart total cholesterol and cholesteryl ester, whereas coconut oil increased these heart lipids. Thus the different dietary fats may cause a redistribution of cholesterol pools between plasma and tissues.

Dietary cholesterol

STUDIES IN HUMAN SUBJECTS. Hopkins performed a metaanalysis of 27 studies of the effects of dietary cholesterol on serum cholesterol in humans (*121*). This was the first such analysis to include baseline intake of cholesterol, which ranged from 0 to >>300 mg/day. The effect of different P/S ratios was also considered. The hyperbolic equation

$$y = 1.22(e^{-0.00384x_0})(1 - e^{-0.00136x}),$$

where y is the change in serum cholesterol in mmol/L, x is added dietary cholesterol in mg/day, and x_0 is baseline dietary cholesterol in mg/day, gave a good fit to the data ($p < .0005$, $r = .617$). Genetic and other factors involved in individual variability were discussed and a hypothetical model of responsiveness to dietary cholesterol was presented. A reanalysis by McNamara of data from 68 studies with 1490 participants found that a 100-mg/day increase in dietary cholesterol raised plasma cholesterol levels by an average of 2.3 mg/dL, independent of the amount of dietary cholesterol fed, dietary fat quality or quantity, and baseline plasma cholesterol level (*122*). Findings from the 68 studies were remarkably consistent, even with major differences in experimental design, diet composition, amount of cholesterol fed, and characteristics of the subjects. The observed change was much smaller than the changes calculated using the formulas of Keys (6.8 mg/dL per 100 mg/day of

dietary cholesterol) and Hegsted (9.6 mg/dL per 100 mg/day). In fact, McNamara argued that the change is so small as to be virtually undetectable against the background of the large normal variation in cholesterol levels. In considering the safety and efficacy of cholesterol-lowering diets for the public in general, he observed that losing 5 kg of body weight would lower endogenous cholesterol production by ~100 mg/day and would have a more favorable impact on blood cholesterol and health in general than reducing dietary intake by a similar amount. However, in the roughly 30% of the population whose rate of endogenous cholesterol synthesis does not adequately compensate for exogenous cholesterol, dietary reduction remains important.

To test the hypothesis that apoE phenotype modulates the response to a cholesterol-rich diet, a feeding experiment was conducted among 36 normolipidemic students with apoE phenotypes E3/2, E3/3, E4/3, and E4/4 (*123*). After a baseline period during which subjects ate their regular diets, omitting eggs, they supplemented this diet with 3 egg yolks per day for 3 weeks and then returned to the baseline diet. Baseline levels of plasma lipids and apoB did not differ between phenotypes. After the cholesterol-rich diet there were modest increases in total cholesterol of 13, 18, and 12% in the E3/2, E3/3, and E4/3 groups, respectively; the E4/4 group had nearly a 30% increase. The E4/4 group also had stronger responses of LDL cholesterol and apoB. The small number of subjects in this trial precludes definitive conclusions from the results.

Another egg-feeding experiment in healthy young men found that egg intake did not alter plasma lipoprotein and coagulation profiles (*124*). During the baseline phase subjects ate 3 eggs per week for 2 months. This was followed by a 5-month experimental phase in which one group continued to eat 3 eggs per week and two groups ate 7 or 14 eggs per week. The mean coefficients of variation in total plasma cholesterol were 5.4–7.4% in the three groups and were greater than the mean changes of 0.2–5.6% in plasma cholesterol from baseline to the end of the experiment. In these subjects, within a reasonable range of intake, eggs did not influence CHD risk markers.

The remarkable case of a normocholesterolemic 88-year-old man who ate 25 eggs a day (see *Food Safety 1991*, Chapter 3, reference *120*) prompted a review and discussion of physiological responses to increased dietary cholesterol (*125*). Metabolically, this man adapted three ways: by reducing endogenous cholesterol synthesis, sharply reducing fractional absorption of dietary cholesterol, and doubling the normal rate of bile acid synthesis. This indicates that in some individuals intestinal cholesterol absorption and hepatic bile acid synthesis can be regulated over an enormous range to compensate for changes in dietary cholesterol. The mechanisms involved and individual variations in response to dietary cholesterol were discussed.

The influence of dietary fat, cholesterol, and total energy on serum lipids was tested in healthy men who took part in four annual 8-day cross-country ski trips in the Swedish mountains (*126*). A different one of the following diets was consumed on each trip: standard, low-energy, high-cholesterol, and high-fat plus high-cholesterol. With all diets, serum triglycerides and VLDL-LDL cholesterol decreased as expected. However, HDL cholesterol and the HDL/total cholesterol ratio increased only with the two high-cholesterol diets. Thus vigorous physical exercise decreases VLDL-LDL cholesterol regardless of diet, but the cholesterol content of the diet determines the response of the HDL cholesterol fraction.

The effects of a cholesterol-free diet were studied for 1 year in 22 healthy Japanese men who were trainees at a Zen temple (*127*). The major changes in serum cholesterol occurred within two weeks after the Zen diet regimen was begun. Total and LDL cholesterol and apoB fell by 10.4, 12.8, and 11.7%, respectively; the cholesterol/lipid ratio in LDL also decreased, and serum triglycerides increased from 54 to 75 mg/dL. Thus even in normocholesterolemic subjects whose initial diet was low in fat and cholesterol, the switch to a cholesterol-free diet with very little saturated fat and a high P/S ratio caused further significant and sustained reduction in serum cholesterol.

ANIMAL STUDIES (MONKEYS). Groups of cebus monkeys were fed diets with corn oil and coconut oil with and without added cholesterol (*128*). Plasma lipoproteins and apolipoproteins and hepatic lipids and apoA-I, apoB, apoE, and LDL receptor mRNAs were measured. In monkeys fed corn oil, dietary cholesterol had no effect on values of any parameter. Animals fed coconut oil without cholesterol had elevated values for all plasma parameters; liver cholesteryl ester and triglyceride levels were also increased but there were no changes in mRNA. When cholesterol was added to the coconut oil diet, plasma parameters had higher values, as did hepatic triglycerides and apoA-I and apoB mRNAs; hepatic LDL receptor mRNA levels were significantly decreased. Liver triglyceride content and free and esterified cholesterol levels were positively correlated with apoA-I and apoB mRNA levels and negatively correlated with LDL receptor mRNA level. Although hepatic apoA-I mRNA and plasma apoA-I were positively correlated, there was no relationship between hepatic apoB mRNA and plasma apoB, suggesting that hepatic apoA-I mRNA is an important determinant of circulating apoA-I but this relationship does not hold for apoB. The data suggest that a diet high in SFAs and cholesterol increases hepatic accumulation of triglycerides and cholesterol, which suppress hepatic LDL receptor mRNA. The authors hypothesize that triglycerides act on apoA-I and apoB mRNAs, whereas cholesterol acts on apoE mRNA.

Selective breeding has produced baboons whose plasma levels of HDL_1, LDL, and VLDL are elevated when they eat a diet enriched in cholesterol and saturated fat (*129*). Their slower cholesteryl ester transfer could account for the increased HDL_1 but not for the LDL and VLDL. To reveal the mechanism for the LDL–VLDL effect, baboons of the high HDL_1 phenotype were fed lard or corn oil diets with high or low cholesterol in a crossover design. The lard diet increased hepatic apoE mRNA and decreased hepatic LDL receptor and HMG-CoA synthase mRNA levels. The amount of hepatic apoA-I message was related to apoA-I concentrations in plasma and HDL and with cholesterol concentration in HDL fractions. As in reference *128*, however, there was no such relationship between plasma apoB and its hepatic message. Further, despite high levels of HDL_1 and VLDL+LDL, baboons with the high HDL$_1$ phenotype had elevated levels of mRNA for LDL receptors and HMG-CoA synthase. This study raises additional questions about the pathophysiology of VLDL and LDL accumulation in animals with the high HDL$_1$ phenotype.

To determine the effect of MUFAs and n–3 PUFAs on cholesterol absorption, African green monkeys were fed diets enriched in lard, oleic-acid-rich safflower oil, or fish oil at two levels of dietary cholesterol (*130*). Initial challenge with lard and high cholesterol distinguished high and low responders to dietary cholesterol. These groups of animals were evenly distributed between the high- and low-cholesterol regimens. Animals fed high-cholesterol diets consistently had higher total and LDL cholesterol levels and a lower percentage of cholesterol absorption than animals fed low-cholesterol diets; HDL cholesterol was not affected by dietary cholesterol levels. With fish oil, total, LDL, and HDL cholesterol levels were lower than with lard or safflower oil. With high-cholesterol diets, the percentage of cholesterol absorbed was significantly lower in animals fed safflower or fish oil than in animals fed lard.

Another factor in the variability of response to high-fat, high-cholesterol diets could be the distribution of body fat (*131*). Studies in male cynomolgus monkeys demonstrated a negative relationship between predominance of central body fat and the response to cholesterol feeding. This suggests a relationship between central obesity and the metabolic variables that have commonly been attributed to total obesity.

Feeding studies in rhesus monkeys suggested that dietary cholesterol increases serum bile acid levels via an increase in the intestinal bile acid pool, which results from increased hepatic production of bile acids and their excretion into the bile (*132*). Feeding triparanol to inhibit endogenous synthesis of cholesterol had no effect on serum bile acid levels in either high or low responders to dietary cholesterol. However, feeding plant sterols to high responders reduced serum bile acids when the diet also contained large amounts of cholesterol.

ANIMAL STUDIES (RODENTS). The effect of phytosterols in rats (*133*) was similar to that in

monkeys (*132*). Wistar rats were fed diets containing a cholesterol overload, with or without added phytosterols (24 or 96 mg/day). The cholesterol overload sharply increased VLDL and LDL cholesterol. Phytosterols reduced this effect in a dose-related way.

In rats, cholesterol feeding caused a dose-related increase in plasma and hepatic concentrations of triglycerides and cholesteryl esters (*134*). Plasma LDL and VLDL lipids were elevated, whereas HDL lipids were reduced. Hepatic secretion of VLDL triglyceride phospholipid, free cholesterol, and cholesteryl ester increased in proportion to dietary cholesterol in experiments in which triglyceride synthesis was stimulated by oleic acid. Secretion of VLDL protein and apoB were also increased. These and other findings suggest that the changes resulting from cholesterol feeding are partly due to increased hepatic secretion of all VLDL lipids and apoB. VLDL particles are assembled without modification of the surface lipid ratios, but they contain a greater proportion of cholesteryl esters than triglyceride in the core, because of the stimulated transport of cholesteryl ester from the expanded hepatic pool. Fatty acids and cholesterol can stimulate hepatic VLDL formation, but the composition of the VLDL will vary according to the specific stimulus.

On both high-cholesterol and cholesterol-free diets, male rats fed crude or refined palm oil had significantly lower levels of serum total and LDL cholesterol and triglycerides than rats fed refined groundnut oil (*135*). Hepatic microsomal HMG-CoA levels were regulated by exogenous cholesterol in all dietary groups, but HMG-CoA reductase levels were lower in the palm oil groups than in the groundnut oil group and fecal excretion of bile acids and neutral sterols was higher in the palm oil groups. This again demonstrates the hypocholesterolemic effect of palm oil and shows that it cannot be attributed to β-carotene, which has been removed from the refined product.

Rats hypersensitive to dietary cholesterol were fed cholesterol-enriched diets containing different fats (*136*). Serum cholesterol concentrations did not change when PUFAs were substituted for SFAs of plant origin, but tended to decrease with an increase in amount of dietary fat. A palm oil–corn oil mixture produced lower liver cholesterol concentrations than lard at both 12 and 22% dietary fat. There was no fat-related difference in fecal steroid excretion or fatty acid composition of serum and liver phospholipids. With zymosan injection, serum triglycerides were reduced in the palm oil–corn oil group and liver cholesterol was reduced in the lard group. Thus immunological stimulation appears to alter lipid metabolism in response to the type of dietary saturated fat.

When fed moderate levels of cholesterol, Syrian hamsters demonstrated a dose-related increase in LDL cholesterol levels in response to dietary n–3 PUFAs (*137*). This could be partly explained by a concomitant decrease in hepatic LDL-receptor binding. However, the reduction in HDL cholesterol with n–3 PUFA feeding was independent of dietary cholesterol content.

Dietary fish and fish oil

REVIEWS AND STUDIES IN HUMAN SUBJECTS. Many cross-cultural, cohort, and case–control studies and randomized clinical trials indicate that fish oil and fatty fish confer protection against CVD (*138*). Although studies of each type suffer from characteristic methodologic and interpretational problems, together they compensate for some individual weaknesses and provide complementary data. Effects on blood pressure, clotting, extent of atherosclerotic lesions, blood lipids, cardiac arrhythmias, and infarct size have been reported. For some effects, a modest amount of fatty fish in the diet is sufficient; for others, pharmacologic doses of n–3 fatty acids are required. The evidence for a relationship between n–3 fatty acids and heart disease was also reviewed from the viewpoint of regulating health claims for n–3 PUFA preparations (*139*). Endpoints (risk factors) for assessing this association were discussed. The relative importance of changes in various surrogate markers of CHD risk must be evaluated so that any health claim truly represents a benefit to the general population and is safe for all.

A study was made of residents of Tromsø, Norway, to determine relationships between fish consumption (fatty and lean) and lipid variables (*140*). There was a dose-related association between fish consumption and plasma n–3, n–6, and n–9 fatty acids. Plasma EPA was a better index of fish consumption than docosahexaenoic acid (DHA). Multivariate analysis controlling for anthropometric and lifestyle factors showed an inverse correlation between EPA and triglycerides and positive correlations between EPA and HDL cholesterol and apoA-I. DHA did not correlate with triglycerides and was inversely associated with HDL cholesterol and apoA-I. EPA (but not DHA) in platelet phospholipids was associated with lower triglyceride and higher HDL cholesterol levels. These results indicate that habitual consumption of small amounts of fish has biological effects and that EPA and DHA have different relations with lipoprotein metabolism. In another study, consumption of fish with moderate amounts of n–3 PUFAs had an undesirable effect on LDL cholesterol and apoB concentrations in normotriglyceridemic young men (*141*). Diets containing 200 g of Dover sole, Chinook salmon, or sablefish were fed for 18 days in a three-period crossover design. Compared with the sole and prestudy diets, salmon and sablefish increased apoB and LDL cholesterol levels. The amount of EPA in platelet fatty acids increased in the order prestudy < sole < sablefish < salmon; total serum cholesterol increased on the sablefish diet, decreased on the salmon diet, and did not change on the sole diet. The authors emphasized that even though some markers of CHD risk may be adversely affected, the net influence of fish and fish oils depends on the balance between beneficial and harmful effects.

Jacotot reviewed the effect of n–3 PUFAs on plasma lipids and apoproteins and on VLDL, chylomicron, LDL, and HDL metabolism (*142*). Fish oil is particularly effective in reducing plasma triglycerides in types IV and V hyperlipidemia, which are related to increased VLDL. The significance of this for preventing CHD is unclear, however, as type IV hypertriglyceridemia is associated with relatively insignificant atherosclerosis. Jacotot believes that the importance of fish oils for the secondary hyperlipidemia associated with diabetes, chronic renal failure, and organ transplants could be considerable and should be further investigated.

Horrobin views the benefits of fish oil (n–3 PUFAs) with some reservations (*143*). If animals are made deficient in essential fatty acids (EFAs), refeeding the *n*–6 series causes rapid and striking improvement in symptoms, whereas refeeding *n*–3 EFAs has few desirable effects and may make things worse; there is "simply no contest when it comes to assessing the relative importance of the *n*–3 and the *n*–6 EFAs." Fatty acids in each series interfere with the metabolism of those in the other, but *n*–3 EFAs do this more effectively. In Westerners, high doses of fish oil sharply reduce levels of dihomogamma-linoleic acid (DGLA), a metabolite of linoleic acid that has many desirable actions. It is noteworthy that Eskimos (whose extremely low rate of CVD first called attention to the benefits of a fatty fish diet) have high plasma levels of both EPA and DGLA. This suggests that their fatty acid metabolism differs from Westerners' and the same diet might have different effects in different populations. Further, there is a consistent tendency for fish oil to raise cholesterol and for *n*–6 EFAs to lower it slightly, although fish oil indisputably has the greater hypotriglyceridemic effect. Quantitatively, comparison of EPA, which has passed the rate-limiting desaturation steps, with linoleic acid, which has not, is unreasonable; a more valid comparison would be with γ-linoleic acid or DGLA. To prevent and treat CVD and inflammatory processes an intervention that raises both EPA and DGLA would be ideal; in any case, EPA should not be raised at the expense of DGLA.

High doses of EPA ethyl ester were administered to subjects for 12 weeks while they remained on ad libitum diets (*144*). Effects on plasma lipoprotein subfractions and activities of lecithin:cholesterol acyltransferase and lipid transfer protein were assessed. Lipid transfer protein activity increased by 25% after 4 weeks and 32% after 12 weeks. Significant decreases occurred in plasma total cholesterol, triglycerides, and apoB; in VLDL-associated cholesterol, triglycerides, phospholipids, apoB, apoC-II, and apoC-III; and in LDL_1-associated cholesterol, phospholipids, and apoB. The authors discussed evidence that reducing values of LDL_1 parameters is important for preventing atherosclerosis.

Thirty subjects with primary hypertriglyceridemia were randomized to receive capsules of oleic acid (placebo) or low- or high-dose fish oil for 6 weeks (*145*). Triglyceride levels fell in both fish-oil groups, but there were no significant changes in total, LDL, or HDL cholesterol, apoB, or LDL apoB. High-dose fish oil significantly lowered lipoprotein(a) levels, and if only subjects with lipoprotein(a) levels >10 mg/dL were analyzed, there were significant declines in both fish-oil groups. Plasma concentration of lipoprotein(a) is a marker for CHD risk, and the authors suggest that the response of lipoprotein(a) to fish oil might differ between normolipidemic and hyperlipidemic subjects. In subjects with type III or IV hyperlipidemia, a 12-week regimen of 6 g/day of *n*–3 PUFAs sharply lowered total and VLDL triglycerides and VLDL apoB (*146*). β-VLDL was also reduced in type III (dysbetalipoproteinemic) subjects. Reduction in VLDL was associated with a significant elevation of LDL, which in a few individuals might attenuate the beneficial effect on VLDL and β-VLDL. As others have done, these authors emphasized that the interactive effect of these pathways on overall cardiovascular risk is not well understood.

In connection with a larger study to assess the effect of fish oil on psoriasis and atopic dermatitis, effects on physical properties and metabolism of LDL were evaluated in 12 treated subjects and 11 controls (*147*). Participants received 6 g/day of corn oil or ethyl esters of *n*–3 PUFAs for 6 months. The concentration of LDL cholesteryl esters and the amount of lipids per milligram of LDL protein were lower in the fish-oil group, whereas LDL apoB was significantly increased. The expected changes in fatty acid composition of the various fractions were observed. Differential scanning calorimetric studies, circular dichroism spectral studies, ^{13}C NMR spectroscopic studies, and other tests were also carried out on LDL fractions from the two groups. Although the marine *n*–3 PUFAs induced some changes in the lipid moiety of LDL, these changes had no measurable effect on LDL metabolism.

By suppressing *n*–6 PUFA metabolism, *n*–3 PUFAs change the products of arachidonate cyclooxygenation; however, effects on synthesis of prostaglandin E_2, most potent of mammalian prostaglandins, are not well characterized. To test the hypothesis that fish oil alters prostaglandin E biosynthesis, the influence of fish oil supplementation on urinary excretion of the major prostaglandin E metabolite was measured in 36 healthy men (*148*). For 10-week periods, subjects ate a basal diet supplemented sequentially with 15 g/day of fat approximating the basal dietary fat in composition, 15 g/day of fish oil concentrate, and 15 g/day of fish oil concentrate with 200 mg/day of α-tocopherol. Although individual responses varied widely, there was an average 14% reduction in prostaglandin E metabolite after fish oil supplementation, with no further change at the end of the fish oil plus α-tocopherol period. Seven subjects had a decrease >30%; one showed first a substantial increase followed by a decrease during α-tocopherol supplementation. The authors cautioned that in view of the critical regulatory roles attributed to prostaglandin E, much more should be learned about prostaglandin E_2 and E_3 biology, the consequences of a long-term diet-induced reduction of prostaglandin E synthesis, and the pharmacology of marine lipids before prolonged use of fish-oil supplements is widely recommended.

Still another possibly detrimental effect of *n*-3 PUFAs was demonstrated in healthy male medical students (*149*). A "usual" basal diet was developed from a dietary history questionnaire. Three diets were prescribed for 3-week periods in a crossover design: basal diet with butter, basal diet with margarine, and basal diet with butter and 6 g/day of MaxEPA. Lipoprotein and apolipoprotein subfractions, hemostasis indexes, and plasminogen-activator inhibitor activity were evaluated. With MaxEPA supplementation serum triglycerides and VLDL were lower and HDL_2 cholesterol was higher; there was a significant decrease in platelet aggregation, as well. These results are desirable in terms of CVD risk. However, LDL cholesterol and plasminogen-activator inhibitor activity increased significantly and the increases were correlated. This result could be undesirable.

In normolipidemic men, supplementation with 6 g/day of a formulation of *n*-3 fatty acid ethyl esters for 6 weeks increased HDL_2 cholesterol by 74% and decreased HDL_3 by 19%; the HDL_2 to HDL_3 mass ratio increased from 0.30 to 0.47 (*150*). Both HDL cholesterol fractions became enriched in cholesteryl ester and triglycerides and depleted in free cholesterol and phospholipids. Thus a putatively protective HDL subfraction was increased by this treatment even though there was no change in total HDL cholesterol content. In considering the hypotriglyceridemic activity of *n*-3 PUFAs in relation to effects on HDL, the authors discussed the possibility that *n*-3 fatty acids act as fraudulent substrates of β-oxidation. Alternatively, these fatty acids may be preferentially incorporated into HDL.

Human hepatoma HepG2 cells were used to study the effect of LDL from subjects taking an EPA/DHA supplement on LDL receptor activity and LDL-receptor mRNA abundance (*151*). Lipid parameters in the subjects were also measured. Compared to baseline LDL, fish-oil LDL reduced LDL receptor activity in HepG2 cells. Scatchard analysis showed that the reduction was due to a decrease in number of receptors, not to a decrease in binding affinity. LDL-receptor mRNA and apoA mRNA were also reduced by fish-oil LDL. Free cholesterol was reduced but cholesteryl esters were increased in HepG2 cells incubated with fish-oil LDL. The results show that moderate supplementation with EPA and DHA (~2.5% of total calories) in normal adults produces a more buoyant LDL particle enriched in cholesteryl esters of *n*-3 fatty acids. These LDL particles depress LDL receptor activity and LDL receptor mRNA abundance in HepG2 cells, apparently because of their *n*-3 PUFA content rather than changes in mass lipid transport.

A further consequence of fish-oil supplementation in healthy adults is reduction of selenium content in serum and erythrocytes, increase in glutathione peroxidase activity in erythrocytes and platelets, and decrease in glutathione concentration in erythrocytes (*152*). This suggests that fish oil impairs some key mechanism of defense against peroxidative damage in blood cells and that similar effects could also occur in other cells. The authors hypothesize that enrichment of erythrocyte and platelet membranes with PUFAs generates increased amounts of lipid peroxides, allosterically activating glutathione peroxidase; with time this damages the integrity of the enzyme molecule, resulting in release of selenium. They suggest that selenium status be assessed before and during PUFA supplementation, and that selenium supplements should be given only when serum or erythrocyte levels are reduced.

STUDIES IN ANIMALS. When pigs were fed a fish-oil supplement to an atherogenic diet, reductions in serum thromboxane B_2, prostacyclin (measured as its major metabolite $PGF_{1\alpha}$), and leukotriene B_4 were observed (*153*). Compared with the low-fat, low-cholesterol mash diet, the atherogenic diet itself reduced the levels of several eicosanoids; supplementation with fish oil augmented these reductions, suggesting inhibition of both the cyclooxygenase and the lipoxygenase pathways. One explanation for the antiatherogenic effect of fish oil invokes reduced recruitment of monocytes and proliferation of smooth muscle cells.

The mechanism by which n–3 PUFAs lower plasma triglycerides was investigated in rats (*154*). Animals were fed semipurified diets with 10% fish oil or olive oil, or a nonpurified low-fat diet for 15 days. Hepatic triglyceride output was estimated after inhibition of lipoprotein lipase by Triton WR 1339. Rats fed the low-fat and fish-oil diets had lower rates of triglyceride formation than rats fed olive oil. However, the three groups removed intraarterially administered chylomicrons labeled with [1-^{14}C]oleate and [$9,10(n)$-^{3}H]triolein from the plasma at identical rates. Hepatic radioactivity and fat content were lowest in rats fed fish oil, indicating preferential metabolism of n–3 fatty acids in the liver. Chylomicrons from donor rats fed fish oil containing [^{14}C]cholesterol and rats fed olive oil containing [^{3}H]cholesterol were removed at similar rates when infused together. Thus the slower formation of plasma VLDL triglycerides appears to result from increased hepatic oxidation of fatty acids and consequent decreased plasma triglyceride concentrations.

Fish oil alters cholesterol transport and metabolic pathways in rat liver, resulting in more rapid disposition of plasma-derived cholesterol into the bile (*155*). [^{3}H]Cholesteryl oleate–labeled unilamellar liposomes were injected to label intrahepatic cholesterol pools, and plasma and bile were collected. Compared with corn oil, fish oil lowered plasma cholesterol by 38% and triglycerides by 69%. This was accompanied by a 28% increase in

bile acid pool size, a 4-fold increase in the cholic acid/chenodeoxycholic acid ratio in bile, accelerated excretion of endocytosed free cholesterol into bile, accelerated incorporation of endocytosed cholesterol into bile acids, increased bile acid–independent bile flow, and a 3-fold increase in hepatic alkaline phosphatase activity.

The ratio of n–3 to n–6 PUFAs, not the amount of dietary n–3 PUFAs, determines the degree to which eicosanoid biosynthesis from arachidonic acid is inhibited in rats (*156*). At constant n–3/n–6 ratios, the amount of dietary fat had no effect on eicosanoid synthesis. Both linolenic acid and menhaden oil suppressed arachidonic acid concentrations in liver, platelet, and lung phospholipids and also suppressed synthesis of thromboxane B_2 and 6-keto-$PGF_{1\alpha}$.

Dietary fish oil reduces adipose tissue trophic growth in rats in addition to its well known hypotriglyceridemic effect and reduction of lipogenesis. To understand the metabolic basis for this, the response of fat pad mass, fat cell size, fat cell lipolysis, and lipoprotein binding to adipocyte plasma membranes to fish-oil feeding was measured in adolescent male rats (*157*). Feeding 20% MaxEPA as the sole dietary fat significantly reduced plasma triglyceride levels and epididymal and perirenal fat pad mass. Isoproterenol-stimulated lipolysis was significantly higher in rats fed fish oil than in pair-fed controls given 20% lard. MaxEPA feeding also produced a 2- to 3-fold reduction in adipocyte volume but did not change in fat cell number. Plasma membranes of epididymal adipocytes from MaxEPA-fed rats bound less HDL_1, probably as a result of reduced fat-cell size or altered membrane structure. If the same effects occur in people, they may be relevant to obesity and CVD risk. To the extent that coronary risk is related to visceral fat mass, an n–3 PUFA–mediated reduction in central adiposity could contribute to the cardioprotective action of these fatty acids.

Agemaki (*Sinonovacula constricta*) is a popular shellfish in western Japan (*158*). Shellfish are generally considered undesirable because of their high cholesterol content, but when mice were fed cholesterol-free or cholesterol-enriched diets with and without 5% freeze-dried agemaki, diets containing agemaki lowered the concentrations of plasma and liver cholesterol and plasma triglycerides under both cholesterol regimens. The agemaki contained substantial amounts of $n-3$ PUFAs and plant sterols, which may have been responsible for this effect.

Lipoprotein and apolipoprotein synthesis and metabolism

STUDIES IN HUMANS AND MONKEYS. High plasma concentrations of lipoprotein(a) are considered a risk factor for acute myocardial infarction and a marker of CHD. However, some studies continue to indicate that lipoprotein(a) levels are refractory to modification by dietary lipids (*159–161*). The effect of short-term $n-3$ PUFA supplementation on plasma concentrations of lipoprotein(a) was evaluated in healthy men and groups of subjects at high risk for CHD (subjects with angina pectoris, diabetes, hyperlipidemia, or hypertension) (*159*). Effects of long-term supplementation were also monitored in healthy subjects. Although there were large individual differences in lipoprotein(a) levels at the beginning of the study and large individual responses to $n-3$ PUFA supplementation, no significant change was seen in any group regardless of dose or duration of supplementation. After long-term supplementation there was a significant decrease in lipoprotein(a) in subjects whose initial level was >20 mg/dL. Normolipidemic men were studied under dietary regimens that altered the amount of cholesterol and the type and amount of dietary fat (*160*). Although correlated changes were observed in LDL cholesterol and apoB, there was no associated lipoprotein(a) response to any diet. Nor was there any correlation between baseline lipoprotein(a) level and dietary response, unlike the results in reference *159*. Thus, at least in normolipidemic men, determinants of plasma lipoprotein(a) are different from determinants of LDL. In a third study, clinically healthy adults were selected for a broad range of serum lipoprotein(a) levels (3–94 mg/dL) (*161*). They were treated with placebo or capsules containing EPA + DHA in a crossover design, with different groups receiving low, medium, and high doses. ApoA was measured as an indicator of lipoprotein(a). Again, no effect of $n-3$ PUFAs was seen regardless of baseline levels of lipoprotein(a), although there was a dose-related reduction in triglyceride levels.

In contrast to the frequent finding that circulating lipoprotein(a) level, which is primarily under genetic control, is not modified by diet, Hornstra et al. found that dietary palm oil lowered serum lipoprotein(a) in normocholesterolemic men (*162*). Thirty-eight subjects participated in a crossover trial consisting of two 6-week periods. A "normal Dutch diet" was the control; palm oil was used as the major fat in similar foods for the test diet. All but 6 had a decrease in lipoprotein(a) after the palm-oil diet; overall, palm oil was associated with a highly significant reduction of ~10%. There was no order effect. Use of palm oil as the major dietary lipid did not change levels of triglycerides, total cholesterol, or total HDL cholesterol, although there were significant increases in HDL_2 cholesterol and $apoA_1$ and decreases in LDL and IDL trilycerides and apoB.

Three isocaloric diets progressively enriched in MUFAs at the expense of PUFAs were tested in normolipidemic men, to look for effects of diet on apoA-I-containing lipoprotein particles (*163*). Oleic acid significantly increased total, LDL, and HDL cholesterol, triglycerides, phospholipids, apoA-I, apoA-II, apoB, lipoprotein A-I, and lipoprotein A-I–A-II, in most cases in a dose-related manner. Subjects varied considerably in their levels of lipoprotein A-I particles, and when they were separated into groups with high, medium, and low levels there were significant differences in levels of apoA-I and HDL cholesterol. Among other differences, the high lipoprotein A-I group had the lowest mean body mass index and the highest concentration of HDL-associated apoC-III. Thus in this normolipidemic population the level of lipoprotein A-I particles seemed to be positively associated with protection against coronary artery disease. Overall, a dietary P/M ratio of 1.0 appeared optimal. This had the same beneficial effect on LDL cholesterol as the PUFA-rich diet without concomitantly reducing HDL cholesterol.

The mechanisms by which dietary fatty acids and cholesterol modulate plasma HDL cholesterol, apoA-I levels and kinetics, and hepatic apoA-I mRNA were investigated in cebus monkeys (*Cebus albifrons*) (*164*). Compared with corn oil, coconut oil elevated plasma total, VLDL + LDL, and HDL cholesterol and apoA-I. Addition of dietary cholesterol had no effect on these parameters in coconut oil–fed animals but increased their values in the corn oil group. The apoA-I fractional catabolic rate was decreased and the production rate increased in the coconut oil groups and cholesterol enhanced this effect. The decreased apoA-I fractional catabolic rate was associated with an increased HDL core-lipid to surface ratio. Liver apoA-I mRNA was elevated in the coconut oil groups, but this was not affected by dietary cholesterol. The lack of parallel effects of fat and cholesterol suggests that fat influences the level of hepatic apoA-I message, whereas cholesterol affects apoA-I production rate by a mechanism not related to the hepatic message.

RODENT STUDIES. Ten strains of inbred mice were studied to determine how dietary fat and cholesterol regulate LDL receptor and apoB (*165*). High-fat diets with cholesterol increased plasma total, VLDL, and LDL cholesterol and apoB in all 10 strains. VLDL and LDL became enriched in cholesterol and the proportion of total cholesterol transported in these fractions rose at the expense of HDL. Beyond this there were marked quantitative differences between strains with respect to lipid and lipoprotein concentrations and composition and distribution of cholesterol in response to high-fat and high-cholesterol diets. In three strains selected for detailed study, all high-fat and cholesterol-enriched diets suppressed hepatic LDL-receptor mRNA transcription. However, LDL-receptor mRNA levels in liver and intestine were decreased only by cholesterol-containing diets. Thus, whereas dietary cholesterol operated at the transcriptional level to decrease message levels, dietary fat inhibited transcription but at the same time enhanced mRNA stability. There were no consistent diet-induced changes in hepatic apoB mRNA levels, although high-fat diets increased apoB mRNA transcription. In the intestine, apoB message levels increased modestly but significantly on high-fat diets. It appears that molecular regulation of apoB and LDL-receptor

is affected differently by fatty acids and cholesterol and the regulation is tissue-specific. In similar studies the same research group found that dietary fat and cholesterol also differ in their regulatory effects on apoA-I and apoA-II gene expression and plasma concentrations of various HDL components in inbred mice (*166*). Differences were seen at the transcriptional and post-transcriptional levels and between the three mouse strains.

In rats, hepatic expression of the apoA-I gene is up-regulated by a MUFA-rich diet (*167*). This finding is interesting in view of the results reported in reference *163*. With the control chow diet, dietary cholesterol had no effect on hepatic apoA-I mRNA. All experimental groups were give 0.1% cholesterol, with fat supplied by coconut, corn, or olive oil. Levels of hepatic apoA-I mRNA increased in the order control = coconut oil < corn oil < olive oil.

Endogenous lipid peroxidation

After 4 weeks of ingesting 10 g/day of MaxEPA, peroxidation of plasma lipoproteins was highly significantly enhanced in both smokers and nonsmokers, as measured by thiobarbituric acid–reactive substances and metabolism of conditioned LDL by macrophages (*168*). In smokers, a fish-oil effect was evident both before and 90 min after smoking. Supplementation with 400 mg/day of vitamin E abrogated the effect of fish oil in nonsmokers but only partially counteracted it in smokers, although smokers and nonsmokers did not differ in baseline levels of vitamin E in serum or LDL. These results argue against indiscriminate fish oil supplementation in the population at large.

MUFAs may provide a dietary means to decrease susceptibility of LDL to oxidation while not increasing LDL cholesterol concentrations (*169,170*). When LDL from healthy, normolipidemic subjects eating an oleate-rich diet was compared with LDL from subjects eating a linoleate-rich diet, generation of thiobarbituric acid–reactive substances was significantly lower in LDL from the oleate group; and after incubation with endothelial cells, LDL from the oleate group underwent less degradation by macrophages (*169*). At the same time, the oleate diet maintained the baseline level of HDL cholesterol. These results support the contention that replacing SFAs with MUFAs offers more advantages than replacement with PUFAs. A crossover study comparing PUFA- and MUFA-enriched diets in normal men produced similar results (*170*). Both diets lowered plasma total and LDL cholesterol and neither affected the antioxidant content of plasma LDL. However, the oleate-rich diet increased the resistance of LDL to lipid peroxidation as measured by rate of oxygen consumption after challenge with a free-radical initiator.

Relative to PUFAs, MUFAs also reduced the susceptibility of VLDL + LDL to peroxidation in rats (*171*). However, in this study, an olive oil diet was more effective than a triolein diet. The authors hypothesized that a better balance between unsaturated fatty acids and other unspecified natural antioxidants gave the greater protective capacity to olive oil.

Weanling rats were fed diets containing equal amounts of SFAs, MUFAs, and PUFAs, but with different n–3/n–6 ratios (*172*). The control diet contained lard and corn oil. Diets enriched in n–3 reduced total and HDL cholesterol and platelet thromboxane B_2 levels. In the group fed menhaden oil, manganese superoxide dismutase (SOD) activity was reduced in heart, and copper–zinc SOD was decreased in liver and aorta. These changes were greater in females than in males. As assessed by thiobarbituric acid–reactive substances in heart, liver, and urine, lipid peroxidation was increased by n–3 PUFAs, again, more in females than in males. These and other results suggest that increased lipid peroxidation occurs in specific target tissues where high amounts of n–3 fatty acids are incorporated and where the activity of protective enzymes is not increased correspondingly.

Atherosclerosis and coronary heart disease

Frederick Stare reviewed his own lifetime of research, including 50 years of his and other work at Harvard in nutrition, atherosclerosis, and CVD (*173*). Three other reviews discussed the role of n-3 and n-6 fatty acids in CHD with special emphasis on intervention studies in humans (*174*), and the role of fish oil in prevention (*175*) and risk (*176*) of atherosclerosis. The first reviewer concluded that n-3 PUFAs probably protect against CHD but their mode of action is uncertain; an effect on serum cholesterol is unlikely to be relevant (*174*). The cholesterol-lowering effect of the n-6 fatty acids, on the other hand, probably is clinically important, although only linoleic acid has been investigated in detail. Support for a role for fish oils in inhibiting atherosclerosis is based on epidemiologic, animal, and in vitro studies and studies with clinical end points in humans (*175*). Fish oils have diverse effects on platelets, endothelial cells, monocytes, prostaglandin and leukotriene metabolism, and blood lipids. Studies using fish oil to inhibit postangioplasty restenosis have produced inconclusive and inconsistent results. The reviewers concluded that there is enough support for the hypothesis that n-3 fatty acids inhibit atherosclerosis to justify its further study in human subjects. The modification of atherosclerosis risk factors by n-3 PUFAs was covered briefly in the third review (*176*). In one other short review, the effects of dietary cholesterol, SFAs, MUFAs, and PUFAs on plasma lipids and atherosclerosis were summarized (*177*). Dietary cholesterol is significantly related to CHD risk independent of any effect on serum cholesterol, indicating some other mode of action such as a direct effect on arterial walls or influence on chylomicron metabolism. As a family, SFAs increase serum cholesterol concentrations but the magnitude of the effect varies from fatty acid to fatty acid; stearic acid, which can be desaturated to oleic acid, may decrease cholesterol concentration. Although PUFAs beneficially influence CHD risk factors, they have numerous immunologic and metabolic activities, some of which may be undesirable. MUFAs, when substituted for SFAs, decrease LDL cholesterol as efficiently as PUFAs without concomitantly decreasing HDL cholesterol; they may also reduce blood pressure. Unlike a high-carbohydrate diet, they do not cause hypertriglyceridemia. Their overall metabolic impact may be superior to that of PUFAs.

Analyzing the diet–heart issue from the perspective of the dietary role of dairy products, reviewers concluded that the balance of dietary components, not the type of fat, is involved in development of atherosclerosis (*178*). They stressed the susceptibility of PUFAs to oxidative degradation and the role of oxidized lipids in formation of atherosclerotic plaques. They warned of nutrition-related disorders that might arise if dairy products were eliminated from the diet.

A fish oil–feeding experiment was conducted in 11 patients scheduled for removal of obstructive atherosclerotic plaques, to measure incorporation of dietary DHA and EPA into advanced lesions (*179*). Relative to their plasma concentrations, more DHA than EPA was deposited in plaques. Further, whereas the level of PUFAs in plasma plateaued after 3 weeks of fish-oil feeding, their level in plaques continued to increase linearly. Thus changes in the plasma fatty acid profile are rapidly reflected by substantial changes in plaque fatty acids. The clinical implications of this need to be considered. Another indication of the role of DHA in atherosclerosis came from analysis of adipose tissue biopsies and segments of coronary arteries sampled from 40 consecutive autopsies (*180*). The degree of coronary artery disease was inversely related to the DHA content of periumbilical adipose tissue.

It has been suggested that insulin resistance in the absence of overt diabetes underlies several risk factors for coronary artery disease. Because hyperinsulinemia is a consequence of insulin resistance, investigators studied fasting insulin concentrations in nondiabetic men with coronary artery disease (*181*). They found that intake of SFAs, which is correlated with risk of atherosclerosis, was also positively associated with fasting insulin concentrations independently of body mass index.

Two studies on effects of dietary fat on plasma lipoproteins and apolipoproteins in African green monkeys (*Cercopithecus aethiops* ssp. *pygerythrus* and *C. aethiops* ssp. *aethiops*) were reported (*182*). Effects of SFAs and *n–*3 and *n–*6 PUFAs on plasma LDL size and composition were summarized, with reference to the significance of cholesteryl ester content. The extent of aortic atherosclerosis was determined, to see if oxidation of LDL lipids resulting from PUFA feeding was important in initiating or exacerbating atherosclerosis. On the contrary, the percent of stenosis was less in the *n–*6 PUFA-fed than in SFA-fed animals and the percent of

surface covered with fatty streaks was less with *n-*3 PUFAs than with SFAs. Although the studies supported the hypothesis that enlargement of LDL particle size and enrichment of LDL particles with cholesteryl oleate are atherogenic, they failed to establish the mechanism of LDL-induced atherosclerosis. Dietary PUFAs appear more likely to have beneficial than detrimental effects on development of atherosclerosis.

Kritchevsky reviewed dietary fat studies in rabbit models of atherosclerosis (*183*). In rabbits, the severity of atherosclerosis is related to the level of fat saturation regardless of whether cholesterol is included in the diet. Cocoa butter is less atherogenic than might be expected, probably due to its high stearic acid content. Peanut oil is surprisingly atherogenic; this is a function of its triglyceride structure, as randomization of the oil significantly reduces its atherogenicity.

Greenberg reported that dietary fish oil inhibits development of atherosclerosis in most animal models and has been shown to inhibit intimal proliferation in vein grafts in dogs (*184*). His review summarized results of the graft studies and work with several rabbit, pig, and nonhuman primate models. Although significant changes in lipid and lipoprotein concentrations and profiles are consistently observed, they do not account for the full extent of fish oil's antiatherogenic activity. Effects on platelet–vessel wall interactions and various cytokines and growth factors also appear to be involved.

In rabbits, cholesterol feeding produced parallel qualitative and quantitative changes in plasma and aortic tissue levels of cholesterol oxides (*185*). Hypercholesterolemic plasma and aorta contained several oxysterols not found in normal plasma or tissue. Although some of the cholesterol oxides may represent oxidized cholesterol products derived from the food, endogenous formation of cholesterol oxides also occurs via a free-radical mechanism.

The hypothesis that *n–*6 PUFAs have the same antiatherogenic effect as *n–*3 PUFAs in the context of a high-cholesterol high-SFA diet was tested in pigs by raising the P/S ratio with fish oil or corn oil (*186*). The fish-oil supplement reduced time-weighted average plasma cholesterol levels by 30% and shifted terminal lipoprotein patterns from predominantly apoB and apoE particles to particles containing only apoB. Atherogenesis was reduced as judged by several morphometric criteria. None of these changes occurred to any significant degree with the corn oil supplement.

Ischemic heart disease

In the U.K., several marine oils are hydrogenated to produce margarine. To learn whether *trans* fatty acids formed during this process are associated with death from IHD, the fatty acid compositions of fat specimens collected during autopsy were determined (*187*). Samples were from 136 men who died of IHD and 95 controls who died from unrelated causes. IHD specimens were significantly enriched in 16:1 *trans* isomers and had a higher ratio of 16:1 *trans* to "higher" (C_{20} plus C_{22}) fatty acids than control specimens. This is what would be expected if case subjects had eaten more margarine produced from highly unsaturated marine oils such as anchovy, pilchard, sardine, or menhaden, which require greater hydrogenation than the less unsaturated herring oil. The isomeric PUFAs are thought to obstruct or compete with utilization of native PUFAs.

The diets of 365 subjects with IHD, hyperlipidemia, or strong family history of heart attacks were supplemented with fish-oil concentrate for 4 years, with no further dietary modification (*188*). Serum triglyceride levels in hypertriglyceridemic subjects fell by >1 mmol/L during the first month and remained at this level; levels in normotriglyceridemic subjects dropped slightly. Similarly, serum total cholesterol fell in the first month in hypercholesterolemic subjects, and remained fairly constant thereafter; there was no change in subjects with a concentration <6.5 mmol/L at baseline; and HDL cholesterol rose in both groups. There was a progressive decline in plasma fibrinogen throughout the study. The mean reinfarction rate in patients receiving conventional treatment was nearly 7 times the rate in patients given conventional treatment plus *n*–3 PUFAs. No clinical chemistry or hematological parameters were adversely affected by the fish oil.

One evaluation of fish oil supplementation to prevent restenosis after coronary angioplasty found no effect at a dose of 3 g/day (*189*). After 6 months the incidence of restenosis was 32% in 58 subjects treated with fish oil, aspirin, and calcium blockers and 27% in 49 subjects receiving only aspirin and calcium blockers. However, another trial using a dose of 15 g/day for 6 months found a 22–36% restenosis rate (depending on the criteria used to define restenosis) in the fish-oil group compared with 40-53% in the control group receiving olive-oil placebo (*190*). A dietary assessment revealed that a higher usual consumption of *n*–3 PUFAs was also associated with a lower frequency of restenosis. Results for dietary and supplemental *n*–3 PUFAs were of similar magnitude, however, and it is difficult to explain how similar effects could be attributed to such different amounts of the same substances.

Myocardial perfusion may improve and stenotic lesions may regress in patients on a regimen of low-fat, low-cholesterol diet and physical exercise (*191*). Compared with patients receiving "usual care," the intervention group had a greater frequency of regression (7/18 vs. 1/12). The significant reduction in stress-induced myocardial ischemia in this group, which was not limited to subjects showing regression of lesions, was thought to result from the program of regular physical exercise.

The effects of *n*–3 and *n*-6 PUFAs on myocardial ischemic damage has been extensively studied in rats (*192–197*). Ischemic arrhythmia was induced in male hooded Wistar rats by occlusion of the coronary artery, after 44 weeks of feeding various lipid-modified diets (*192*). Complete substitution of *n*–6 for saturated fatty acids sharply reduced the number of ventricular premature beats, and the incidence and severity of ventricular tachycardia and ventricular fibrillation. However, supplementing a SFA-containing diet with modest amounts of *n*–6 PUFAs had no effect, whereas including a comparable amount of fish oil completely prevented ventricular fibrillation. The mixed diets contained similar proportions of SFAs, MUFAs, and PUFAs, with only the type of PUFA varying. Thus the benefits conferred by *n*–3 PUFAs on the mechanical performance of the heart were direct, not due to coincidental changes in other dietary fatty acids.

The ability of *n*-6 PUFAs to protect against reperfusion-induced arrhythmias after myocardial ischemia was studied in an open-chest rat model (*193*). Animals were fed 12% linoleic acid in their food pellets for 4 weeks. They were then anesthetized and subjected to 6 or 12 min of myocardial ischemia by coronary artery ligation, followed by reperfusion. This produced severe dysrhythmias in all control animals. Linoleic acid–fed rats had a much lower incidence of ventricular fibrillation after both 6 and 12 min of ischemia; incidence of other arrhythmias was also reduced, during the period of ischemia as well as during reperfusion. There are also microcirculatory manifestations of reperfusion failure after transient ischemia (*194*). Lehr et al. investigated whether pharmacologic and dietary treatment to inhibit postischemic leukocyte–endothelial interaction would preserve normal capillary perfusion after ischemia and reperfusion. Functional capillary density decreased 40% from baseline in control animals 30 min after reperfusion; this was associated with a very marked increase in capillary heterogeneity. Slight recovery had occurred by 24 hours postinfusion. In contrast, animals fed 5% fish oil for 4 weeks before the experiments and animals treated with MK-886 to inhibit leukotriene biosynthesis had no loss of functional capillary density throughout the ischemia, reperfusion, and postreperfusion periods; normal capillary perfusion was also preserved. Although dietary fish oil has a variety of activities, the similarity of results with fish oil and MK-886 suggests that in this experiment fish oil inhibited endogenous leukotriene synthesis, which prevented postischemic leukocyte–endothelium interaction. In another rat model, Paulson et al. compared effects of 15 weeks of fish oil and corn oil feeding on myocardial low-flow ischemic–reperfusion injury in isolated working hearts of Wistar Kyoto and stroke-prone SHR (*195*). Recovery of cardiac contractile performance was significantly better in fish oil groups than in corn oil groups, regardless of strain. The beneficial effects were primarily on the heart's pumping capacity, as measured by aortic flow. These results provide further evidence

that dietary fish oil can reduce the mortality risk from CVD.

In contrast, long-term feeding of α-linolenic acid enhanced ischemic vulnerability in SHR (*196*). This was manifest as decreased activity of myocardial enzymes such as creatine kinase and aspartate aminotransferase and an elevation of plasma enzymes. The higher level of thiobarbituric acid–reactive substances in heart tissue and plasma of linolenic acid–fed rats suggests that increased lipid peroxidation contributes to this vulnerability. When large amounts of substrate are made available for free radical–induced lipid peroxidation (as through α-linolenate feeding), dietary antioxidants may not be sufficient for protection in this strain of rat, which is known to have defects in antioxidative defense mechanisms.

When rats were fed a low-fat diet with a P/S ratio of 1.2 and *n*-6/*n*-3 ratio of 5.0, 0.05–1.0% dietary cholesterol had no effect on plasma cholesterol concentrations but did cause a dose-dependent increase in liver cholesterol (*197*). A dietary cholesterol level of 0.2% had the maximum effect on the indexes examined in these rats. Δ6-Desaturase activity in liver microsomes, linoleate desaturation index in liver phosphatidylcholine, and production of prostaglandin by the aorta and thromboxane A_2 by platelets all decreased with cholesterol feeding. Thus dietary cholesterol had a characteristic influence on lipid parameters even when given in a diet otherwise protective against atherosclerosis.

Blood pressure

Although obesity, alcohol intake, and dietary sodium, potassium, and magnesium are generally considered the major nongenetic determinants of blood pressure, fatty acids and antioxidants are also factors in the etiology of hypertension (*198*). Cross-sectional population studies and clinical trials have generally shown that *n*–3 PUFAs lower blood pressure; the effects of SFAs and *n*–6 PUFAs have been inconsistent, and the effect of MUFAs is not known. The Kuopio Ischaemic Heart Disease Risk Factor Study found that dietary intake of SFAs was positively associated and linolenic acid intake negatively associated with resting blood pressure in 722 healthy Finnish men. There are also inverse associations between blood levels of vitamin C and blood pressure and between selenium status and blood pressure, but these associations have not been shown to be causal.

Kenny believes that the case for fish oil is less firmly established than indicated in reference *198* (*199*). For example, the same population of Greenland Eskimos who are famous for their low incidence of CHD also have a high incidence of stroke, and this has not been explained. Other problems with the theory that fish oil protects against CHD via a hypotensive effect were presented. The author advanced a hypothesis to explain how fish oil could reduce hypertension in some subjects while having an adverse effect in others. Dietary fish oil enhances the α-adrenergic pressor effect and decreases the vascular response to angiotensin. Thus the effect of fish oil would depend on whether hypertension was mediated by catecholamines or increased sympathetic drive, or by the vascular effects of angiotensin. A diet rich in marine oils and fish may retard atherogenesis and reduce blood pressure in persons with high renin levels, but at the same time increase arterial pressure and enhance the response to catecholamine-mediated pressor stimuli.

Singer summarized evidence showing that individual PUFAs have qualitatively and quantitatively different effects in hypertension and hyperlipidemia (*200*). For example, 18:2n–6 fatty acid lowers total and LDL cholesterol; n–3 fatty acids also lower serum triglycerides; and long-chain n–3 PUFAs are more effective than 18:3n–3. In a clinical trial, ingestion of sunflower or linseed oil decreased systolic blood pressure during a psychophysiological stress test in patients with mild essential hypertension. The hypolipidemic and hypotensive effects of 18:2n–6 and 18:3n–3 indicate significant activity of dietary C_{18} PUFAs themselves, in addition to their being desaturated and elongated to form long-chain PUFAs and their role in eicosanoid biosynthesis.

Eggs can be enriched in n–3 PUFAs by feeding fish oils to laying hens. Such enriched eggs were tested for their effects on lipid and lipoprotein levels and blood pressure in heathy adults (*201*). In a crossover design, subjects ate four normal eggs per day or four PUFA-enriched eggs per day for 4-week periods. Mean plasma cholesterol level increased during the normal-egg phase but was unchanged by PUFA-enriched eggs. Plasma triglycerides increased with control eggs and decreased with PUFA-enriched eggs. Control eggs did not change blood pressure, but there was an order effect on the influence of n–3 eggs on blood pressure: when n–3 eggs were eaten during the first test phase, both systolic and diastolic blood pressure were lowered, whereas only systolic pressure was significantly decreased when n–3 eggs were eaten during the second test phase.

The effect of dietary fatty acids on blood pressure and urinary excretion of eicosanoids and sodium was measured in women (see reference *108* for diets and study design) (*202*). As in the former study, the order of test diets influenced the results. When the self-selected diet was followed first by a 30% fat diet with P/S = 1 and then by a 40% fat diet with P/S = 0.3, no effect on urinary eicosanoids was seen; with the reverse order of test diets, eicosanoids fell on the high-fat diet and returned to baseline on the modified diet. Diet did not affect diastolic blood pressure, but systolic blood pressure was decreased when the modified diet came first. The change from self-selected to experimental diet did not explain the order effect, and the authors suggested that linoleate is depleted from tissues more slowly than it is replenished. Sodium excretion was significantly enhanced by the high-fat diet when it followed the modified diet.

The effects of low-dose n–3 PUFA supplementation on blood pressure were evaluated in a randomized, double-blind, controlled two-period crossover study in hypertensive patients (*203*). There was a 4-week washout period between phases. Fish-oil supplementation was associated with significant reductions from baseline for supine diastolic and sitting systolic blood pressure, whereas safflower oil supplementation was not associated with significant change in any blood pressure parameter. An order effect was observed for sitting diastolic and sitting mean arterial blood pressure: fish oil significantly reduced these measures during the first test period.

In a crossover study evaluating the effects of fish oil supplementation and sodium restriction on blood pressure in normotensive elderly subjects, neither fish oil nor sodium restriction alone caused significant reduction in any blood pressure parameter (*204*). However, the combination of fish oil and sodium restriction for 4 weeks significantly reduced systolic, diastolic, and mean arterial blood pressure. Other groups of subjects treated for 4-week periods with sunflower oil with and without sodium restriction showed no significant changes in blood pressure. Another study by the same authors tested these treatments in a larger number of normotensive elderly adults (*205*). Each group received only one of the four treatments: sunflower oil or fish oil, with or without sodium restriction. Systolic blood pressure fell in the sodium-restricted sunflower oil group but there was only a transient fall in diastolic blood pressure. Fish oil alone produced only a small change in blood pressure, but in combination with sodium restriction it substantially reduced both systolic and diastolic blood pressure. As in the previous study (*204*), fish oil and sodium restriction interacted to lower blood pressure, the effect being most obvious for diastolic blood pressure.

Experiments in rats also show an interactive effect of fish oil and sodium on blood pressure (*206,207*). Using stroke-prone SHR, Howe et al. showed that the beneficial effect of fish oil on blood pressure was nullified by increasing dietary sodium (*206*). Observations after ganglion blockade indicated that the antihypertensive effect of fish oil probably does not result from reduction in sympathetic vascular tone. In further studies comparing stroke-prone SHR and normotensive rats, this research group showed that fish oil reduced blood pressure in hypertensive but not in normotensive rats (*207*). There was a further decrease when dietary sodium was restricted. The antihypertensive effect of fish oil did not depend on neurally mediated vasoconstriction but was associated with reduced basal resistance in the mesenteric artery. Further, when stroke-prone SHR were fed fish oil from the age of 4 weeks, the development of hypertension was delayed (*208*). Again, the authors observed that dietary fish oil depressed the contractile responses mediated by sympathetic nerve stimulation in a mesenteric vascular bed preparation.

A long-term feeding study comparing the effects of menhaden oil and a corn-oil control in SHR found no effect on blood pressure after 12 or 18 months (*209*). However, rats fed menhaden oil had significantly less aortic arteriosclerosis, myocardial damage, and renal interstitial fibrosis and lower plasma levels of triglycerides and cholesterol than controls. This indicates that menhaden oil lessens hypertensive damage to the renal and cardiovascular systems.

A diet rich in linseed oil (10% by weight, with 61.2% α-linolenic acid) had multiple effects on the cardiovascular system in SHR (*210*). Systolic blood pressure fell by 59 mm Hg after 20–25 days. The viscous and elastic components of viscosity were reduced at various shear rates, and the aggregation index was decreased. The decreased viscosity could improve flow conditions in the microcirculation, leading to a better oxygen supply. When SHR were injected twice daily with γ-linolenic acid, their systolic blood pressure became stabilized in the normotensive range after 2 weeks (*211*). Withdrawal of treatment increased systolic blood pressure from 140 to 165 mm Hg within one day; after 1 week it was stabilized at 191 mm Hg. Aspirin alone had no effect on blood pressure, but a combination of aspirin and γ-linolenic acid nullified the hypotensive effect of the fatty acid.

Use of the immunosuppressive drug cyclosporine has sharply increased the incidence of hypertension in transplant recipients. This is frequently accompanied by renal toxicity. In an attempt to counteract these effects, the influence of dietary fatty acids on cyclosporine-induced hypertension was examined in borderline hypertensive rats (*212*). Safflower oil (providing linoleic acid), evening primrose oil (γ-linolenic acid), and fish oil were fed. Both evening primrose oil and fish oil prevented the hypertensive response to 0.1 mg/kg/day of cyclosporine; with 10.0 mg/kg/day of cyclosporine, evening primrose oil was protective but fish oil had no significant effect. Evening primrose oil prevented the cyclosporine-induced reduction in glomerular filtration rate and fish oil diminished this cyclosporine effect. Fish oil also nonsignificantly reduced the elevation in renovascular resistance. Thus dietary fatty acids can ameliorate the effects of cyclosporine on blood pressure and the kidney.

Effects of dietary lipids on platelets

Platelet reactivity plays a major role in myocardial infarction, independently of serum lipids, blood pressure, or smoking (*213*). Moreover, the tendency of platelets to aggregate is diet-dependent and the major dietary determinant is fat. n–3 PUFAs are the only fatty acids that can decrease platelet reactivity; however, even a regular high intake of these does not completely protect against the harmful effect of SFAs. From the standpoint of protecting against thrombosis and myocardial infarction, the ideal diet should have an n–3/n–6 ratio of ~1:6 and a P/S ratio of 0.5–0.7. Sufficient antioxidants should be ingested to stabilize the unsaturated fatty acids. A research group in Denmark has studied the Greenland Eskimos extensively to learn how their diet protects them from ischemic heart disease (*214*). One observation was that fatty acid profiles of Greenlanders are strikingly different from those of Danes. Further, in Greenlanders, EPA is a major precursor of platelet prostanoids, at the expense of arachidonic acid. The dietary n–3 PUFAs shift the balance in platelets between proaggregatory thromboxane and antiaggregatory prostacyclin in an antiaggregatory direction. These differences between Greenlanders and Danes were mirrored by differences between Japanese fishermen and Japanese farmers.

French researchers have found that EPA and DHA influence platelet aggregation by entirely different mechanisms, and DHA is the more potent (*215*). EPA is released from phospholipid subclasses in the same way as endogenous arachidonic acid, with which it competes for the formation of thromboxane A_2. DHA, in contrast, is not released but is transferred from phosphatidylcholine to phosphatidylethanolamine during platelet activation. DHA decreases thromboxane formation from arachidonic acid, thromboxane-induced aggregation, and specific binding of thromboxane to platelet membranes. The metabolism of DHA at the membrane phospholipid level probably explains most of its biological activity in platelets.

Until recently, aspirin was the only substance known to protect against myocardial infarction. Because fish oil has now been shown to produce similar results, the combined effects of aspirin and fish oil were studied in patients with clinically stable but advanced coronary artery disease (*216*). Fish oil suppressed thromboxane B_2 production (an index of thromboxane A_2) by 38%, but aspirin virtually abolished it. However, aspirin also inhibited prostaglandin I_2 (prostacyclin) production and fish oil could not entirely compensate for this. The authors believe that the decrease in prostacyclin with moderate doses of aspirin ($\leq$325 mg/day) is accounted for by loss of prostaglandin endoperoxide substrates, which is an unavoidable consequence of the aspirin-induced inactivation of platelet cyclooxygenase. Endothelial cell cyclooxygenase, in contrast, is minimally affected because endothelial cells can rapidly replenish their enzyme. Aspirin did not negate the effects of n–3 PUFAs on the eicosanoid profile. An accompanying editorial discussed these findings (*217*).

The influence of fish (as opposed to fish oil supplements) on platelet function and fatty acid composition was reported by four research groups (*218–221*). One study in healthy young men compared diets containing catfish and salmon (*218*). Although there were minor differences in results for the two groups, the direction of change was the same: bleeding time and clotting time were prolonged; platelet count decreased and fibrinogen concentration increased slightly; EPA and DHA were incorporated into platelet phospholipids. Another study compared the effects of incorporating 200 g/day of salmon, sablefish, and Dover sole into a Western diet in a three-way crossover design (*219*). Again, subjects were healthy young men. The salmon and sablefish content of n–3 fatty acids was nearly twice as great as the content in sole, and the n–6/n–3 ratio was consequently much lower. These differences were reflected in platelet fatty acid profiles. Bleeding time increased moderately during the salmon diet; collagen-stimulated platelet aggregation increased with sablefish. With both salmon and sablefish, ADP-stimulated platelet aggregation increased and thromboxane B_2 concentration decreased. Finnish workers studied the effects of fish diet and exercise, separately and together, in healthy young women (*220*). The fish diet produced changes in the fatty acid composition of platelets and erythrocyte ghosts, but the magnitude of change was less than previously observed in young men. Both exercise and fish diet slightly decreased serum triglycerides, and the effects were additive. Parameters of prostanoid metabolism and platelet function were unchanged. However physical fitness, measured by maximum oxygen uptake and maximum exercise intensity, was inversely correlated with serum triglycerides, total and LDL cholesterol, and platelet aggregation. The results suggest sex differences in the efficiency with which *n*–3 PUFAs modify lipid metabolism. An Australian study of healthy men evaluated the effects of a control diet, a lean fish diet, and a lean fish diet supplemented with fish oil in a three-way crossover design (*221*). Both fish diets reduced the number of circulating neutrophils and enhanced the fibrinolytic potential, but the effects of the diet with fish oil were greater. The fish-plus-oil diet also reduced the platelet count. At least some of the effects were thought to be eicosanoid-mediated. The authors concluded that a practical amount of lean fish can improve some hematological parameters involved in the etiology of CVD.

In an in vitro study, platelets from healthy young men were incubated with EPA, DHA, linoleic acid, and various mixtures of these fatty acids, with and without α-tocopherol (*222*). Incubation mixtures including DHA or EPA exhibited reduced platelet aggregation in response to collagen. α-Tocopherol had little influence on this. No consistent relationship was seen between thromboxane synthesis and platelet aggregation.

Because a high plasma level of lipoprotein(a) is a risk factor for atherosclerosis and may play a subtle role in fibrinolysis, the effects of fish oil on platelet aggregability and membrane fluidity were studied in groups of normolipidemic subjects with normal and elevated lipoprotein(a) concentrations (*223*). The same responses of plasma triglycerides, platelet aggregation, and thromboxane production were seen in both groups before and after fish-oil supplementation. Fluorescent probe analysis revealed no differences in membrane fluidity between platelets from high- and low-lipoprotein(a) normolipidemic subjects, but there were differences between these and platelets from subjects with types IIB and IV hyperlipidemia. These results indicate that lipoprotein(a) level does not influence in vitro behavior of platelets from normolipidemic subjects.

The effects of fish oil hydroxy fatty acids on cellular lipoxygenases and platelet aggregation were studied in platelets from humans and rats (*224*). When added to the incubation medium with human platelets, the hydroxy fatty acids strongly inhibited the 12-lipoxygenase pathway and also inhibited the cyclooxygenase pathway, but to a much lesser extent. The 5-lipoxygenase pathway in polymorphonucleocytes, which leads to leukotriene production, was also less sensitive to inhibition than the 12-lipoxygenase pathway. In rats, dietary EPA and DHA led to formation of hydroxylated metabolites that inhibited platelet aggregation and regulated lipoxygenase activity in both platelets and polymorphonucleocytes.

Trans isomers of 20:5*n*–3 and 22:6*n*–3 fatty acids were isolated from rats fed heated linseed oil and compared with the corresponding *cis* isomers in their ability to inhibit arachidonic acid metabolism in human platelets (*225*). Although *cis* and *trans* isomers appeared to have similar modes of action, different amounts were required for maximum effectiveness.

The effect of diets with different fatty acid composition on fatty acid profiles and prostaglandin synthesis by platelets and cultured endothelial cells was examined (*226*) (see reference *108* for description of subjects, diets, and study design). Plasma parameters, platelet fatty acid composition, and erythrocyte phospholipids responded to the change from self-selected to controlled diets, but as in the companion studies (*108,202*), order effects were seen. Overall, the results indicated that increasing dietary linoleic acid from 4.8 to 7.6% of calories decreases synthesis of prostacyclin and prostaglandin E_2 by human endothelial cells and that dietary supplementation with linoleic acid has a longer carryover effect than dietary reduction. Changes in plasma fatty acids and prostaglandin synthesis were correlated with platelet thromboxane B_2 synthesis.

The MRC Diet and Reinfarction Trial found a reduction in all-cause mortality of 29% over a 2-year period in men advised to eat fatty fish at least twice a week; no benefit could be attributed to reduction of fat intake, but there was a trend toward reduced mortality as the P/S ratio increased (*227*). Platelet activity was assessed in a subsample of participants in that trial. Platelets from men whose diet had a P/S ratio >0.5 showed decreased secondary ADP-stimulated aggregation in platelet-rich plasma and decreased ADP-stimulated aggregation in whole blood. With other results from the MRC Diet and Reinfarction Trial, these observations suggest a role for platelet activity in the relationship between diet and ischemic heart disease.

An 11-week metabolic study was conducted in healthy men to determine the effects of diets providing fats mainly as saturated fats, canola oil, or safflower oil on platelet function and fatty acid composition (*228*). Fatty acids in platelet phospholipids reflected the composition of the dietary fat. After three weeks, both PUFA diets reduced platelet aggregation; canola oil increased lag time to aggregation and decreased ATP secretion when collagen was used as agonist. There were strong associations between thromboxane B_2 in platelet-poor plasma and various measures of platelet function in whole blood from subjects eating the canola-oil diet. However, these effects were only temporary: platelet aggregation returned to baseline values by 8 weeks after the oil-based diets were initiated. The authors suggest that 8 weeks is too long for observing acute effects of diet and perhaps too short for long-term effects to become evident.

Dietary borage oil (rich in γ-linolenic acid) markedly but reversibly increased the DGLA content of all phospholipid classes except sphingomyelin in platelets of healthy men (*229*). However, sphingomyelins became enriched in nervonic acid during the borage oil phase of the trial. Other changes in fatty acid composition were also observed, although the relative abundance of the phospholipid classes did not change. Phospholipid arachidonic levels did not change, probably reflecting the low activity of $\Delta 5$ desaturase in human platelets and a limited exchange of arachidonate-containing phospholipid between plasma and

platelets. The physiological significance of these changes has not been investigated.

When a portion of dietary linoleic acid was replaced by oleic acid in healthy men, the thresholds of ADP- and collagen-stimulated platelet aggregation were lower in the oleic acid group (*230*). This difference became significant after 63 days and continued to increase throughout the 92-day experiment. Thus increasing dietary linoleic acid at the expense of oleic acid may favorably change platelet aggregation even when total and saturated fat are unchanged, indicating that relatively minor dietary modifications and substitutions can have beneficial effects on platelet aggregation.

Unexpectedly, rapeseed- and sunflower-oil diets enhanced in vitro platelet aggregation and thromboxane production in healthy men, compared with milk-fat and habitual diets (*231*). Most differences between the oil diets and the milk-fat or habitual diets were highly significant. Platelet aggregation was not correlated with changes in platelet fatty acid composition. This study was well controlled, and the experimental diets differed only in their fatty acid composition. Because dietary unsaturated fatty acids generally have antithrombotic effects, the relationship between in vivo and in vitro platelet aggregation clearly needs further study.

Three studies in rats addressed the effect of dietary fat on platelet aggregation (*232–234*). One trial compared the effect of fish oils having different EPA/arachidonic acid ratios in otherwise identical diets (*232*). Only the oil with the higher ratio significantly lowered platelet aggregability and in vitro thromboxane production, presumably reflecting replacement of arachidonic acid with EPA in phospholipid fractions. The antithrombotic potential of the oils represented a combination of low arachidonic acid content and high EPA/arachidonic acid ratio. When diets high in MUFAs, *n*–6 PUFAs, and *n*–3 PUFAs were fed to rats, the respective arachidonate contents in platelet phospholipids were 91, 79, and 51%, respectively, of values with the high-SFA control diet (*233*). In the presence of $CaCl_2$, collagen- and thrombin-induced aggregation of washed platelets was lowest for the saturated-fat group despite a high production of thromboxane B_2. In contrast, although the *n*–3 PUFA diet caused platelets to aggregate actively, thromboxane B_2 production was low. When indomethacin-treated platelets were activated with the thromboxane A_2 analogue U46619, a second agonist was required for aggregation. Such U46619-induced aggregation was greater in arachidonate-poor platelets than in arachidonate-rich platelets. The authors concluded that diet modifies the ability of platelets to react with thromboxane A_2 in such a way that a decrease in substrate-limited generation of thromboxane A_2 is compensated for by an increased response to thromboxane, and conversely. They suggest that the altered response is due to altered transduction of the thromboxane signal. A third study in rat platelets indicated that membrane fatty acid composition at least partly controls phospholipase A_2 activity, which releases arachidonic acid from membrane phospholipids and is required for thromboxane synthesis (*234*). Rats were fed diets containing 30% of energy as mixtures of beef tallow and corn oil to supply 3.0–9.0% of energy as linoleic acid. Cholesterol was added to equalize the cholesterol content of all diets. Phospholipase A_2 activity and thromboxane synthesis were correlated and decreased as dietary linoleic acid increased from 4.5 to 9.0%. Platelet fatty acid composition also reflected the linoleate content of the diet. Other factors may also operate at lower linoleate concentrations.

Effects of dietary lipids on erythrocytes

Investigators warned that a crossover design is inappropriate for studies of variables that may be influenced by altered membrane fatty acid composition: for example, in fish-oil feeding experiments (*235*). They found that erythrocyte EPA did not return to baseline until 18 weeks after the end of a 6-week diet regimen based on 200 g/day of lean fish plus 5 g/day of fish oil, and after 18 weeks DHA was still elevated. Because an 18-week washout period is prohibitive, a parallel design becomes mandatory.

Many dietary studies using fish and fish oil involve large doses for a relatively short time. However, a Finnish study showed that similar changes can result from much smaller amounts given over a longer time (*236*). Five groups of young men were offered 0.5 (control), 1, 2, 3, or 5 meals per week containing freshwater fish or Baltic herring. The average numbers of fish meals per week actually eaten by the respective experimental groups were 0.9, 1.5, 2.3, and 3.8. In all major glycerophospholipid classes the ratio of n–3 to n–6 fatty acids in erythrocyte ghosts increased in a dose-dependent manner throughout the 12-week study. The rate and magnitude of change varied: changes in phosphatidylcholine occurred rapidly but were small and the rate of change decreased after 5 weeks, whereas changes in phosphatidylserine were large and the rate of change remained relatively constant even after 12 weeks. Significant changes were seen with as few as 1.5 fish meals per week.

Marmoset monkeys were fed four diets containing 14.3–15.3% fat: a reference diet (32% fat as linoleic acid) with and without EPA and an atherogenic diet (7% of fat as linoleic acid, plus 0.2% cholesterol) with and without EPA (*237*). Analysis of erythrocyte membrane phospholipids found an inverse relationship between dietary 18:2n–6 fatty acid and incorporation of 20:5n–3 regardless of whether the major dietary n–3 fatty acid was 18:3n-3 (α-linolenate) or 20:5n–3. For most dietary treatments, the equation of Lands et al. satisfactorily predicted the observed results for n–3, n–6, and n–9 PUFAs of 20 or 22 carbons; n–6 was poorly predicted for the atherogenic diets. More 20:5n–3 was incorporated into phosphatidylethanolamine than into phosphatidylcholine.

The effects of linoleic acid supplementation on blood pressure and kinetics of erythrocyte sodium transport were studied in 20 middle-aged adults (*238*). Dietary intervention consisted of substituting soybean oil, soy milk, and soy lecithin for SFAs for 2 months. Eight subjects had mild essential hypertension and low baseline levels of linoleic acid in erythrocyte membrane. These "responders" to the soy diet had significant decreases in systolic blood pressure, diastolic blood pressure, and heart rate, and increases in membrane linoleic acid content and apparent affinity for internal hydrogen. The only significant changes in nonresponders were an increase in Hill's number and a decrease in lithium–sodium exchange.

Four papers reported effects of dietary fats on various properties of rat erythrocytes (*239–242*).

Weanling rats were fed diets containing 20% groundnut, coconut, safflower, or mustard oil for 4 months and the lipid composition of erythrocyte membranes and activities of membrane-bound enzymes were evaluated (*239*). Fatty acid composition reflected the dietary fatty acids and influenced enzyme activities. Activities of all enzymes assayed except Mg^{2+}-ATPase were elevated in the mustard oil group; Ca^{2+},Mg^{2+}-ATPase was lowest in the safflower oil group. In another study, dietary *n*–3 PUFAs increased osmotic resistance of erythrocytes by 25–45% at salt concentrations of 0.37–0.44% (*240*). There was no change in phospholipid or cholesterol content of membranes, but the phosphatidylethanolamine fraction was slightly decreased and the phosphatidylserine fraction slightly increased after *n*–3 feeding. The major change was an increase of EPA, primarily at the expense of linoleic acid. The authors suggest that both fatty acid composition and the nature of the phospholipid polar head group may influence the osmotic fragility of erythrocytes. When ethanol was chronically administered to rats it decreased the arachidonic acid content of erythrocyte membranes (*241*). This effect was prevented by concomitant dietary administration of evening primrose oil, and the oil alone elevated membrane arachidonate. A similar effect of ethanol in liver membranes, with an increase in palmitic acid, was not reversed by evening primrose oil. The authors concluded that *n*–6 PUFAs are particularly sensitive to ethanol, which may inhibit the $\Delta6$ desaturase; the protective effect of evening primrose oil in erythrocytes could possibly help alleviate withdrawal symptoms in alcoholics. Finally the effects of high-α-linolenate (18:3*n*–3) and high-linoleate (18:2*n*–6) diets on hemolysis and lipid peroxidation were compared in rat erythrocytes (*242*). Rates of hemolysis were similar in N_2 and O_2 atmospheres. No significant amounts of conjugated dienes were detected during the incubations, nor were changes in fatty acid composition observed, indicating that hemolysis occurred in the absence of significant lipid peroxidation. When a free radical initiator was used to stimulate hemolysis, conjugated dienes formed and P/S ratios decreased; again, however, there was no difference between the dietary groups. Thus hemolysis can occur without involving lipid peroxidation, but it is accelerated by free radicals through lipid peroxidation. Although α-linolenic acid auto-oxidizes several times faster than linoleic acid, this difference is not reflected in rates of hemolysis and auto-oxidation in rat erythrocytes.

In rabbits, supplementation of a conventional diet with fish oil elevated *n*–3 PUFAs in erythrocytes while decreasing oleic and linoleic acids (*243*). Oxidative stress induced by cumene hydroperoxide increased overall fatty acid peroxidation in erythrocytes from the fish oil group, and this was accompanied by decreased hemolysis. The authors propose that *n*–3 PUFAs act as an oxidizable buffer, preventing oxidative damage to membrane proteins and allowing oxidation of fatty acids to occur until a critical level of intact phospholipid remains in the erythrocyte membrane.

Effects of dietary lipids on vascular tissue

A symposium on fish oil and blood-vessel wall interactions was held in Spain in 1990 (*244*). Several papers presented at this symposium are summarized elsewhere in this chapter (*142,176,184,188, 213–215,245,254*). Boulanger et al. discussed the effect of *n*–3 PUFAs on endothelium-dependent relaxations and production of nonprostanoid relaxing factors by endothelial cells (*245*). Production of nonprostanoid relaxing factors is augmented in pigs by feeding cod liver oil or EPA; enhanced release of relaxing factors also occurs in endothelial cells cultured with EPA. The relaxing factor specifically affected seems to be not nitric oxide but some other unidentified substance. The improvement in endothelium-dependent relaxations in hypercholesterolemic and atherosclerotic blood vessels upon fish-oil feeding could explain part of the beneficial effect of *n*–3 PUFAs on CVD risk.

Leukocyte–endothelium interaction after injection of oxidized human LDL was assessed in hamsters fed a control diet and a diet supplemented with fish oil (*246*). In controls, oxidized LDL elicited a rolling and sticking of leukocytes to the endothelium of arterioles and postcapillary venules, which peaked 15 min after injection (from 3 ± 1 to

91 ± 25 cells/mm^2 in arterioles and from 13 ± 6 to 150 ± 46 cells/mm^2 in venules). In the fish oil group the corresponding values after 15 min were 15 ± 7 and 20 ± 5 cells/mm^2. Thus inhibition of the leukocyte–endothelium interaction may be yet another mechanism by which fish oil is protective against experimental and clinical atherosclerosis.

In cultured smooth muscle cells from the rat aorta, fish oil and EPA attenuated the effects of various vasoactive agonists on cytosolic calcium concentration and eicosanoid production (247). These may represent beneficial effects of fish oil on atherosclerosis and hypertension.

Dietary treatment of atherosclerosis also normalizes vascular responses of the eye in a primate model (248). Normal cynomolgus monkeys and atherosclerotic monkeys fed atherogenic and regression diets were tested for blood flow to the retina after serotonin infusion. Serotonin had little effect in normal monkeys, but it reduced blood flow to the retina by ~80% in monkeys eating the atherogenic diet. Atherosclerotic monkeys eating the regression diet were similar to the controls in their lack of response to serotonin.

To study the long-term effect of short-term high-cholesterol diets in early life on arterial wall thickness and vascular reactivity, groups of young rabbits were fed cholesterol-free or high-cholesterol diets for 3 weeks, or a high-cholesterol diet for 3 weeks followed by a cholesterol-free diet for 13 weeks (249). Controls showed no change in intimal-plus-medial wall thickness, whereas this value increased from 0.55 to 0.88 μm in cholesterol-fed groups and the change persisted after 13 weeks on the recovery diet. Median arterial blood pressure was not affected by diet. However, there was a dose-related rise in blood pressure after intravenous administration of noradrenaline; this was significantly greater in both cholesterol-fed groups. These results demonstrate prolonged structural and functional vessel wall abnormalities after a short-term diet-induced increase in serum cholesterol, which might predispose the animals to chronic hypertension or atherosclerosis.

The profile of C_{20} PUFAs in vascular tissue and platelets can be modified by diets enriched in C_{18} n–3 and n–6 PUFAs (250). Rats were fed purified diets containing sesame, borage, or linseed-plus-safflower oil for 7 weeks. The diets supplied comparable amounts of 18:2n–6. As expected, sesame oil increased levels of 18:1n–9, borage oil increased 18:3n–6, and linseed plus safflower oil increased 18:3n–3 in aortic tissue and platelets. Borage oil also increased the elongated 20:3n–6 and 20:4n–6 fatty acids, and linseed plus safflower oil increased 20:5n–3 and 22:6n–3 elongation products. Using the same dietary regimens, groups of rats were exposed to ethanol vapor during the final 6 days of feeding (251). This produced a moderate blood ethanol level (118 $\pm$ 6.6 mg/dL). No significant changes were seen in the aortic fatty acid content. The most marked of various changes seen in platelets was a decrease in 20:4n–6 upon ethanol exposure. This was prevented by the borage oil diet.

To understand the role of changes intrinsic to the blood vessel in ischemic injury and vascular occlusion, the effect of dietary fish oil on vascular contractility in preanoxic and postanoxic aortic rings was evaluated (252). Groups of rats were fed 20% menhaden oil or beef tallow supplemented with 3% corn oil, or 23% corn oil. Under both preanoxic and postanoxic conditions, aortic rings from rats fed fish or corn oil contracted less than rings from tallow-fed rats. The greatest relaxation response to acetylcholine was seen in rings from rats fed fish oil. The authors speculate that these vascular effects of fish-oil feeding may increase blood flow to ischemic and reperfused tissues in vivo.

Experiments in cynomolgus monkeys suggested a novel mechanism for fish oil's protective effect against atherosclerosis (253). The effect of dietary isocaloric substitution of fish oil for lard on the binding of LDL to arterial proteoglycans was examined in a crossover design having two 15-week periods of atherogenic diet separated by a 6-week washout. During each phase, LDL was isolated, characterized physically and chemically, and tested for ability to interact in vitro with arterial proteoglycans. LDL particles differed in size and chemical composition during the two diet periods. Binding to proteoglycans was greater in lard-fed animals regardless of which diet was fed first. Thus diet-induced changes in LDL particles alter in vitro interactions with artery wall proteoglycans.

Other effects of dietary lipids on the cardiovascular system

Studies in normolipidemic and hyperlipidemic men <55 years old and normolipidemic men >55 years old demonstrated effects of fatty acids on peripheral capillary blood flow (*254*). Among the younger normolipidemic subjects, nailfold capillary blood cell velocity was higher in the group receiving fish oil capsules than in the olive oil group. Hyperlipidemic men responded to both $n–3$ and $n–6$ PUFAs with increased capillary blood cell velocities. After a 1-month washout, serum lipid profiles had returned to baseline but increased capillary blood flow persisted. Bran supplements had no effect on blood flow. Older normolipidemic men had significantly increased blood flow velocities after supplementation with $n–3$ fatty acids plus vitamin E, but $n–3$ PUFAs alone nonsignificantly reduced blood flow. The author proposed that PUFAs increase peripheral capillary blood flow by altering vascular tone and blood viscosity when antioxidant status is adequate, but with insufficient antioxidants $n–3$ PUFAs can be detrimental.

Hamsters were used to study the mechanism by which dietary fish oil protects against ischemia–reperfusion injury (*255*). The microcirculation in striated muscle was measured by fluorescence microscopy in awake animals, using the dorsal skinfold chamber preparation. In controls, 4 hours of ischemia caused adherence of fluorescently stained leukocytes to the endothelium of postcapillary venules, capillary obstruction, and breakdown of endothelial integrity. Four weeks of a fish oil–enriched diet before testing markedly reduced these manifestations of ischemia–reperfusion injury. Fish oil feeding caused displacement of arachidonic acid by EPA and consequent increase of leukotriene B_5 at the expense of the potent adhesion-promoting leukotriene B_4. Preservation of microvascular perfusion is probably one beneficial effect of $n–3$ PUFAs.

Dietary fish oil supplements in rabbits increased plasma levels of $n–3$ PUFAs, increased $n–3$ incorporation into platelets, and reduced thromboxane B_2 formation (*256*). In the brain, fish oil selectively affected cerebral arteriolar reactivity, which

normally depends on cyclooxygenase metabolism of arachidonic acid and formation of vasoactive oxygen radicals. Thus dietary $n–3$ PUFAs might reduce pathophysiological responses to acute hypertension or traumatic brain injury.

A critical examination of the literature on the effects of lipids on membrane proteins (138 references) found evidence against a role for fluidity (*257*). A mathematical analysis of viscosity-dependent effects was presented, motion in phospholipid bilayers was reviewed, and the mechanisms and dynamics of protein motion were considered in detail. Experimental observations on effects of solvent viscosity on rates of reactions catalyzed by water-soluble enzymes and on membrane protein reactions were summarized. The latter studies provided no evidence favoring the idea that phospholipids influence ATPase activity through order or viscosity effects. The only lipid requirement for proper function of a protein in a biological membrane is apparently that lipids be in the liquid crystalline phase, which is the case at physiological temperatures when the lipids contain one saturated and one unsaturated chain; this is assured by the specificity of the phospholipases. Beyond this, fluidity of the lipid bilayer is not an important determinant of activity for the proteins studied.

Studies in rats (*258*) and marmoset monkeys (*259*) found effects of dietary fats on membrane lipid composition and enzyme activity in the heart. Cardiac sarcolemma was analyzed from groups of rats fed diets containing 20% groundnut, coconut, safflower, or mustard oil for 16 weeks (*258*). The fatty acid composition of membrane lipids reflected dietary fatty acids. ATPase activity was highest in the coconut oil group, whereas acetylcholinesterase activity was highest in the mustard oil group. There were no differences in 5'-nucleotidase activity, cholesterol/phospholipid molar ratio, or sialic acid content. Cholesterol and phospholipid contents and lipid/protein ratio were lowest in the group fed groundnut oil. It appears that modification of the sarcolemmal membrane fatty acid composition modulates activities of sarcolemmal enzymes that regulate cardiac function. In the marmoset, dietary 20:5$n–3$ and its elongation product 22:5$n–3$ were extensively incorporated into the phosphatidylcholine and phosphatidylethanolamine of cardiac membranes (*259*). However, these changes in membrane composition did not affect basal membrane-associated adenylate cyclase activity or its responsiveness to various agonists. Thus, by whatever mechanisms *n*–3 PUFAs affect cardiovascular function, effects on the cardiac β-adrenergic receptor–catecholamine-stimulated adenylate cyclase system are unlikely to be involved.

Modulation of lipid metabolism and hemostasis by dietary lipids was studied in normal young adults using a crossover design (*260*). After stabilization on a reduced-cholesterol "modified Western diet," there were 23-day periods of MUFA- and PUFA-rich diets. Reduction of dietary cholesterol decreased factor VIIc and fibrinogen and increased fibrinolysis; both test diets decreased serum total and LDL cholesterol but had no anticoagulatory or pro-fibrinolytic effects. In this study the PUFA-rich diet contained 10% unspecified PUFAs. Another study in young adults added fish oil capsules to the subjects' usual diet for 21 days and found an unexpected effect on fibrinolysis (*261*). The concentration of plasminogen activator inhibitor type-1 was increased in all subjects; mean levels rose from 14.4 ± 4.4 ng/mL before supplementation to 23.7 ± 10.2 ng/mL after. No significant changes occurred in tissue-type or urokinase-type plasminogen activator. The authors concluded that if fish-oil supplementation decreases risk of CHD it is not because of *increased* fibrinolytic activity but in spite of *decreased* fibrinolytic capacity.

Studies in mice fed normal and atherogenic high-fat diets demonstrated significant in vitro effects of the atherogenic diet on several macrophage activities (*262*). Phagocytosis of aggregated LDL was only slightly inhibited by the high-fat diet, although phorbol myristate acetate–induced production of reactive oxygen species was significantly reduced. Cytotoxic activity of the macrophages was less in the high-fat group when cells were stimulated with lipopolysaccharide or macrophage-activating factor. The receptors or recognition structures for both of these response modifiers are in the plasma membrane. In contrast, *N*-acetylmuramyl-L-alanyl-D-isoglutamine was equally effective in both groups; the receptor for this immunomodulator is in the cytoplasm. Thus a high-fat diet appears to affect the interaction of immunomodulators with membrane receptors. The results also suggest that if similar effects occur in vivo, the necrotic areas seen in atherosclerotic lesions in these animals must result from mechanisms other than enhanced free radical release. Perhaps dying macrophages in these lesions release agents cytotoxic to underlying smooth muscle cells.

ANTIOXIDANTS

Steinberg briefly reviewed the strengths and weaknesses of the "oxidative modification" hypothesis of atherogenesis (*263*). A diagrammatic representation of the hypothesis showed the ways in which oxidized LDL is potentially more atherogenic than native LDL. Although there is enough evidence supporting the hypothesis to warrant further study, in vivo evidence is limited. Clinical trials have lacked the rigorous design and control needed to firmly establish the effectiveness of antioxidative therapy. Nor can epidemiologic investigations establish causal relationships. The author discussed the difficulties of designing and conducting a definitive clinical trial.

Plasma antioxidants, indexes of lipid peroxidation, and CHD risk factors were assessed in a Scottish population, with reference to present and past smoking habits (*264*). There were no differences between current smokers, past smokers, and nonsmokers in intake or plasma concentrations of vitamin A, vitamin E, or carotenoids. Smoking decreased plasma glutathione peroxidase activity and increased levels of conjugated dienes, indicating a sustained oxidative load. Plasma vitamin C was lowest in current smokers and highest in non-smokers, despite comparable dietary intakes of this vitamin in the three groups. Current and past smokers had higher plasma levels of LDL and triglycerides. The authors suggest that inadequate antioxidant status and sustained free-radical load exacerbates the oxidation of LDL and increases its atherogenic properties in smokers and others at increased risk for CHD.

Tocopherols and vitamin E

Evidence for a therapeutic effect of vitamin E in the pathogenesis of spontaneous atherosclerosis was comprehensively reviewed by Janero (*265*). Development of vessel lesions in animal models and probably in humans represents interactions between injury to the vessel wall and responses to injury by vascular tissue and blood components; vascular endothelial and smooth muscle cells, circulating monocytes and resident macrophages, and the amount and nature of lipoproteins are involved. Although there is compelling in vitro evidence that vitamin E acts on cells and lipoproteins involved in pathogenesis of spontaneous atherosclerosis and vitamin E is probably the major (perhaps only) lipid-soluble, chain-breaking antioxidant, there is little evidence that the processes affected by vitamin E are important in spontaneous atherogenesis or that vitamin E has the same effects in vivo as in vitro. Pharmacologic investigation in nutritional and hyperlipidemic animal models is needed to establish an antiatherogenic role of vitamin E in spontaneous atherogenesis, and its mechanistic basis.

The antioxidant component of atherogenic risk was evaluated in 79 healthy adult vegetarians and 79 age- and sex-matched controls (*266*). Among vegetarians, mean plasma α-tocopherol was 714 $\pm$ 46 μg/dL for men and 725 $\pm$ 24 μg/dL for women; cholesterol values were 122 $\pm$ 5 and 138 $\pm$ 3 mg/dL for men and women, respectively. Corresponding values among omnivores were 928 $\pm$ 38 and 883 $\pm$ 23 μg/dL for α-tocopherol and 206 $\pm$ 6 and 188 $\pm$ 4 mg/dL for cholesterol. However, vegetarians had a significantly higher tocopherol/cholesterol molar ratio. They also had a more favorable plasma fatty acid profile, and the linoleic/oleic acid ratio correlated well with the α-tocopherol/cholesterol ratio. The LDL fraction, which transports the bulk of tocopherol, may be better protected against peroxidation in vegetarians.

After a 6-week stabilization period during which dietary intake of fat was modified, the effects of Palmvitee (a tocotrienol- and α-tocopherol-rich fraction of palm oil) and vitamin E–depleted palm oil were compared in hypercholesterolemic subjects (*267*). The number of Palmvitee and placebo capsules taken per day was increased by 1 capsule every 4 weeks to a maximum of 4, with three different dose levels per capsule. Although serum vitamin E, total tocopherol, and total tocotrienol increased in a dose-related way in the Palmvitee group, there were no significant changes in serum lipids or changes in lipids predicted by serum vitamin E status. Nor were there changes in plasma prostaglandins or platelet function. Thus serum responses to supplemental tocopherols and tocotrienols were not accompanied by other changes in coronary risk factors. Although vitamin E supplementation did not alter LDL or lipid levels in this or another study (*268*), the resistance of LDL to oxidation could be increased by dietary supplementation. Twelve clinically healthy young adults were given daily dosages of 0, 150, 225, 800, or 1200 IU of α-tocopherol for 21 days (*268*). α-Tocopherol in plasma and LDL increased in a tightly correlated dose-related manner, while γ-tocopherol decreased. The resistance of LDL against copper-mediated oxidation (measured as lag time to oxidation) was higher during vitamin E supplementation but varied considerably between subjects. A further study of copper-mediated LDL oxidation in smokers and nonsmokers also showed a protective effect of vitamin E but not β-carotene (*269*). Ingestion of 1000 IU/day of D,L-α-tocopherol for 1 week increased plasma and LDL concentrations of vitamin E 3.0-fold and 2.4-fold, respectively, in nonsmoking men; resistance of LDL to oxidation increased directly with vitamin E concentration. However, although β-carotene supplementation strongly increased β-carotene levels in plasma and LDL of smokers, it had no significant effect on resistance of LDL to oxidation in either smokers or nonsmokers. Further, smoking did not alter the oxidation resistance of LDL.

A double-blind, placebo-controlled trial of vitamin E supplementation to prevent restenosis after percutaneous transluminal coronary angioplasty found less restenosis in the treatment group (*270*). The overall incidence of restenosis (defined by abnormal angiogram, thallium test, or exercise stress test) was 50% in controls and 35% in the treatment group. The difference failed to reach statistical significance (p = .06) because only 100 patients completed the protocol.

Steiner discussed the influence of vitamin E on platelet function in humans (*271*). In vitro, vitamin E inhibits platelet aggregation and release, but ex vivo aggregation studies have not shown an effect of dietary vitamin E supplementation. The discrepant results are probably due to the maximum levels of vitamin E attainable in platelets and plasma. Studies of α-tocopherol supplementation and platelet adhesion in a laminar flow chamber using platelet-rich plasma showed major inhibition at doses as low as 200 IU/day. Reduced adherence to collagen, fibrinogen, and fibronectin were demonstrated and this was accompanied by morphologic differences in tocopherol-enriched platelets that did adhere to adhesive surfaces. The reason for the shape change is not known, but it may be involved in the vitamin E–induced reduction of platelet adhesiveness.

Atherosclerosis was monitored for 36 months in groups of cynomolgus monkeys eating basal and atherogenic diets (*272*). Some monkeys fed the atherogenic diet received α-tocopherol supplements from the beginning of the study; some were given α-tocopherol only after atherosclerosis was established by ultrasound evaluation; and others received no supplementation throughout the study. Animals eating the basal diet remained disease-free. Animals in the prevention group (supplemented with α-tocopherol throughout the study) had an average of 61% stenosis in the common carotid arteries; animals in the regression group (given α-tocopherol after documentation of atherosclerosis) had an average of 18% stenosis; and unsupplemented animals had 87% stenosis. Histopathologic changes tended to be greater in untreated monkeys. Plasma tocopherol levels were inversely correlated with percent stenosis as shown by ultrasound.

Dietary supplementation with vitamin E protected heart tissue from oxidant stress during exhaustive endurance exercise in rats (*273*). Unsupplemented exercised rats showed increased generation of free radicals in the myocardium; free radical–mediated lipid peroxidation measured as malondialdehyde production was greater in both exercised and sedentary unsupplemented rats. Vitamin E supplementation completely abolished free radical production in exercised rats and suppressed malondialdehyde production in both sedentary and exercised animals. The protective effect was not mediated through enhancement of antioxidant enzymes (superoxide dismutase, catalase, or glutathione peroxidase).

Vitamin C

Simon reviewed the evidence for a protective role of vitamin C against CVD, beginning with pioneering work on the atherosclerosis of scurvy in the guinea pig (*274*). In humans, most evidence is observational or correlational; experimental trials frequently show a reduction in serum cholesterol only for hypercholesterolemic persons with low serum vitamin C levels. There are also data suggesting a synergistic effect between vitamins C and E in lipid peroxidation and effects of vitamin C on hemostasis and several serum lipid parameters. Gender, cigarette smoking, diabetes, hypertension, aging, pregnancy, and use of oral estrogen-containing contraceptives are CVD risk factors related to vitamin C. Thus although no evidence conclusively links vitamin C with CVD, many observations suggest a relationship.

Epidemiological studies found a strong relationship between elevated blood pressure and low intakes or low blood levels of vitamin C in three population samples from the Boston area: elderly adults, young and middle-aged adults, and elderly Chinese-Americans (*275,276*). Associated with each 30 μmol/L increase in plasma ascorbic acid was a 3.7–9.5% increase in HDL cholesterol, a 4.1% decrease in LDL cholesterol, and a 1.9–5.5% decrease in blood pressure. Even though the results were statistically significant independent of other variables that affect blood pressure, the investigators concluded only that a *diet* high in vitamin C was related to blood pressure and the observations were not necessarily due to vitamin C itself. Another reviewer called for definitive clinical studies to learn whether vitamin C has a physiological effect on blood pressure, citing evidence from epidemiology, two small intervention trials, and work with animal models (*277*). He pointed out that vitamin C has many roles unrelated to preventing scurvy, and the diet of our ancestors probably contained 10 times the current recommended intake of vitamin C, or more.

When human blood plasma and LDL were exposed to various oxidative challenges, ascorbic acid protected lipids against any detectable peroxidation by intercepting oxidants before they could do any oxidative damage (278). It was superior in this respect to other water-soluble plasma antioxidants as well as to α-tocopherol, ubiquinol-10, lycopene, and β-carotene. Of the lipid-soluble antioxidants, ubiquinol-10 was the most effective in the experimental system. In cardiac tissue from marginally ascorbic acid–deficient guinea pigs, ascorbic acid also protected against oxidative damage (279). The damage observed was not due to a lack of enzymatic scavengers of reactive oxygen species or to reduction in glutathione transferase activity, although the level of glutathione decreased considerably. Thiobarbituric acid–reactive substances accumulated, fluorescent pigment was formed, and cardiac microsomal membranes lost their structural integrity. If these observations can be extrapolated to people, they indicate that chronic subclinical ascorbic acid deficiency can cause progressive oxidative damage that could eventually lead to degenerative heart disease.

Other

Gerster reviewed the potential of β-carotene in preventing CVD (280). She covered the epidemiology and causes of CVD, the role of oxidative processes and antioxidant defense systems in CVD, and the known properties and actions of β-carotene. Although findings related to β-carotene are inconsistent and inconclusive, some are encouraging. For example, preliminary results from the Physicians' Health Study indicated that patients with stable angina pectoris who took 50 mg of β-carotene every other day for at least 2 years experienced only half as many cardiovascular events as patients who took placebo. Whether this was due to antioxidant effects or to an increase in plasma HDL was not known.

Multivariate analysis of factors related to the plasma fatty acid profile in healthy adults indicated that antioxidant micronutrients should be measured when PUFA metabolism is studied (281). The strongest finding was a relationship between fatty acid composition of phospholipids and serum selenium concentration: serum selenium was inversely related to percentage of SFAs and directly related to percentage of essential fatty acids and long-chain *n*–6 PUFAs. It was the only variable predictive of the unsaturation index of plasma phospholipids.

Smith pointed out that current preoccupation with cholesterol's role as villain ignores its essentiality in life processes (282). Also ignored is the ubiquity of oxidized cholesterol derivatives (which are implicated in atherosclerosis) in human blood and various tissues. As an alternative to viewing these oxysterols as agents of injury to the aorta, Smith suggested that oxysterols oxidized in the B ring are evidence of past interception of blood and tissue oxidants by cholesterol as an ordinary feature of oxygen metabolism. Such interception, followed by hepatic metabolism of the oxysterol and subsequent biliary secretion and fecal excretion, would constitute an in vivo antioxidant system. In this context, whether cholesterol and oxysterols cause or exacerbate atherosclerosis is not yet understood. Smith did not claim elevated plasma levels to be beneficial for this reason, or deny the associations of elevated plasma cholesterol levels with disease. He merely focused attention on possible benefits derived from cholesterol in the blood.

MINERALS

Kotchen et al. reviewed the role of nutrition in preventing hypertension (283). The strongest associations in both adolescents and adults were between blood pressure and body weight, and changes in blood pressure over time were correlated with weight change. Smaller correlations were found between salt intake and blood pressure, and salt-restriction trials have demonstrated small but significant effects. Individuals varied in their sensitivity to salt and there was some evidence of gender differences. Trials in children and infants have given inconsistent results. The reviewers concluded that avoidance of salt excess is appropriate but it is premature to recommend rigorous salt restriction for the entire population.

Karppanen reviewed the mechanism by which mineral elements influence blood pressure, and the interactions between sodium, calcium, potassium, and magnesium in their effects on blood pressure (*284*). In hypertensive patients treated with drugs, restriction of sodium and supplementation with potassium and magnesium reduce the drug dosage needed to control hypertension. Replacement of common table salt with a commercial mixture containing 65% NaCl, 25% KCl, and 10% $MgCl_2$ had antihypertensive effects in trials with Japanese and Finnish patients; addition of *l*-lysine HCl improved the taste. In another short review of the relationship between dietary cations and blood pressure, Kesteloot concluded that mole for mole, potassium is 2.5 times more effective in lowering blood pressure than sodium is in raising it (*285*). However, the effect of calcium was considered still controversial: intervention studies suggest an antihypertensive effect, whereas serum and urinary calcium levels correlate positively with blood pressure. More data are needed before magnesium can be evaluated, and there may also be interactions with dietary phosphorus, protein, and fat. McCarron and Luft warned that failure to appreciate the interactions among dietary cations and anions and the heterogeneity of the blood pressure response could produce unexpected and perhaps undesired effects when salt intake is manipulated (*286*).

Magnesium

Marier reviewed trends in dietary magnesium intake during the 20th century, discussing losses due to refining, processing, and preparation of foods (*287*). The magnesium status of specific populations and subgroups gives evidence that inadequate metabolic magnesium status is widespread in the modern world, ranging from borderline adequacy to 50% of the recommended intake. The "water factor" hypothesis evolved to account for epidemiological observations on the mortality rate from cerebrovascular disease, CVD, and all causes. Hard water can contribute roughly 25% of the total

intake of magnesium in parts of the USA; in a Canadian survey, the magnesium content of drinking water provided the strongest correlation (inverse) of any waterborne mineral with CVD and all-cause mortality. The cardioprotective effect of waterborne magnesium has also been observed in South Africa, Poland, and the former Soviet Union, making it a global phenomenon.

In a randomized, single-blind, controlled study, one group of subjects ate their usual diet while another group ate a magnesium- and potassium-enriched diet (*288*). By the end of 6 weeks the high-mineral group had experienced significant decreases in serum total and LDL cholesterol and triglycerides. This was accompanied by a significant increase in serum magnesium. However, the diets differed importantly in other respects as well, particularly in fiber and cholesterol content.

In young Wistar rats, administration of 15% ethanol in drinking water caused hypertension and a decreased magnesium concentration in erythrocytes, aorta, and skeletal muscle (*289*). Magnesium supplementation (1% MgO in chow) prevented these effects of alcohol. The half-life of norepinephrine in the heart and spleen was also increased by magnesium. Blood pressure was positively correlated with intracellular calcium concentration and extracellular fluid volume, and negatively with magnesium in erythrocytes, aorta, and skeletal muscle and the ouabain-sensitive ^{22}Na efflux rate constant. The results suggested that magnesium's hypotensive effect was via decreased sympathetic nervous activity and decreased intracellular sodium concentration caused by activation of the sodium pump.

Potassium

A randomized, controlled, year-long trial showed that increasing dietary potassium with natural foods while minimizing overall dietary change reduced the need for antihypertensive drugs in a group of hypertensive outpatients (*290*). The intervention diet was tailored for each patient, based on consumption of a specified number of "equivalent potassium rations." Control patients ate their customary diet but this was monitored throughout the study. During the year, drug therapy was incrementally reduced according to a fixed protocol, provided that blood pressure remained below 160/95 mm Hg. By the end of the study, blood pressure could be controlled using <50% of the initial dosage in 81% of patients in the intervention group but in only 29% of controls. Average drug consumption was 24% of the baseline level in the intervention group and 60% in controls.

To see whether potassium itself or the chloride salt was responsible for reducing blood pressure in earlier trials, 12 hypertensive patients were treated daily for 8 weeks each with placebo and a mixture containing 60 mmol of potassium citrate and 60 mmol of potassium bicarbonate (*291*). No changes in blood pressure or heart rate were observed. Although KCl was not tested in this crossover trial, the authors suggested that salts of potassium other than chloride may not have a hypotensive effect; and since most of the potassium in potassium-rich foods in not in chloride form it may be ineffective in lowering blood pressure.

A potassium-, magnesium-, and *l*-lysine-enriched salt alternative was tested in rats (*292*). It was given at 1.75 times the level of regular salt to provide the same amount of NaCl as the controls received. Regular salt caused pronounced left ventricular hypertrophy in both SHR and Wistar-Kyoto rats, but increased blood pressure only in the spontaneously hypertensive strain. The salt alternative did not increase blood pressure in either strain; it did not cause ventricular hypertrophy in Wistar-Kyoto rats, and caused only a slight degree of hypertrophy in SHR. The NaCl-induced volume load remained normal in the salt alternative groups. Another study showed that dietary potassium determines the degree of NaCl sensitivity in Charles River SHR (*293*). On a 2/1% high-potassium diet they were resistant to NaCl-induced rises in blood pressure and increased mortality.

Calcium

McCarron argued that there is a threshold for the calcium–blood pressure relationship, whose set point is influenced by demographic, lifestyle, nutritional, and clinical variables (*294,295*). He hypothesized that the relatively high prevalence of

hypertension in certain segments of the population reflects an altered set of this threshold. Epidemiologic observations in numerous ethnic groups, men and women, young and old, consistently show an independent, inverse relationship between dietary calcium intake and blood pressure. Analysis of the NHANES I database indicated a threshold of daily calcium intake at 400–600 mg, below which risk of hypertension increased; there was also evidence of a second threshold at ~1200 mg/day. An average set point seems to be 700–800 mg. The strength of the relationship varies, however. Moreover, some intervention trials have shown an antihypertensive effect of calcium and others have not. If observations in animals can be extrapolated to people, high-risk groups suffering from disordered calcium metabolism may require more calcium than normal individuals to achieve a lowering of blood pressure. McCarron suggested that supplemental calcium holds most promise as an antihypertensive agent in Blacks, Japanese, alcoholics, diabetics, salt-sensitive subjects, pregnant women, and the elderly.

Parallel studies in salt-loaded, borderline hypertensive human subjects and DOCA salt-treated rats assessed the effects of oral calcium supplementation on salt-induced increases in blood pressure and sodium metabolism (*296*). In the clinical study, each dietary period lasted 1 week. On a high-salt diet, the percent increase in mean blood pressure was smaller in subjects receiving 2160 mg/day of calcium than in those receiving 250 mg/day. Calcium loading also produced smaller weight gain, greater urinary sodium excretion, and increased magnesium in erythrocytes. Increased calcium intake also attenuated the blood pressure increase in rats, increased urinary sodium excretion, decreased intracellular and extracellular sodium retention, and normalized enhanced sympathetic nervous activity.

A 28-year follow-up study of calcium intake and CVD and CHD mortality in Dutch civil servants showed at most a weak inverse association between calcium intake and mortality (*297*). Because dietary patterns were stable and major calcium sources were included when the original data were collected in the 1950s, the authors do not believe this finding can be explained by misclassification of calcium intake.

Analysis of data from the Framingham Children's Study found an inverse relationship between dietary calcium and systolic blood pressure in 3- to 6-year-old children, but no relationship with diastolic pressure (298). Calcium intake ranged from 4.9 to 19.6 mmol per 4200 kJ, and mean systolic blood pressure ranged from 73 to 129 mm Hg. Multiple linear regression analysis adjusted for effects of sex, height, body mass index, and heart rate showed a decrement of 2.27 mm Hg for each 2.5 mmol increment of calcium intake.

A clinical trial was undertaken in 1194 nulliparous women to determine the effects of a 2 g/day calcium supplement on the incidence of gestational hypertension and preeclampsia (299). The rate of hypertensive disorders of pregnancy was 9.8% in the calcium group and 14.8% in the placebo group; the risk was lower throughout pregnancy, but particularly after the 28th week, in the calcium group. Another study randomly assigned normotensive and hypertensive pregnant women to receive 1 g/day of calcium or placebo (300). Calcium significantly lowered diastolic blood pressure in the hypertensive subjects.

Countering all these studies showing beneficial effects of increased calcium intake on blood pressure, Seely asked whether excessive calcium intake in prosperous countries might be a major cause of coronary artery disease and the hypertension of old age (301). He argued that calcium was early implicated as a cause of "hardening of the arteries," but was later overlooked in the preoccupation with cholesterol. Now calcium channel blockers are widely used antihypertensive drugs; many people "take calcium supplements with one hand and calcium antagonists with the other," the right hand truly not knowing what the left is doing. Seely calculated calcium requirements for various age groups, compared these with calcium intake in advanced and poorer countries, and discussed indicators that a high intake of calcium is harmful. He concluded that reduction of dietary calcium to ~300–400 mg/day, the quantity consumed in many third-world countries, could bring many long-term benefits. However, in calculating the "requirement"

Seely did not consider fecal excretion and bioavailability of various forms of dietary calcium, except for a brief mention of phytate.

High oral calcium had opposite effects in two genetic models of salt-induced hypertension (302). In female stroke-prone SHR, mean arterial pressure was 137 mm Hg in rats given 2% calcium and 175 mm Hg in rats given 0.4% calcium, whereas 2% calcium aggravated salt-induced hypertension in female Dahl salt-sensitive rats (141 vs. 124 mm Hg). The disparate effects may stem from differential actions of oral calcium on vascular responsiveness to exogenous vasoconstrictors in these models. The mechanisms of the calcium effect were addressed in two other studies using the SHR model (303,304). In one, 4-week-old SHR and Wistar-Kyoto rats were divided into calcium-supplemented and control groups (303). After 3 weeks, the calcium group of SHR had reduced blood pressure, pressor response to norepinephrine in isolated mesenteric artery, and platelet cytosolic free calcium compared with distilled water controls. No differences were seen between groups of Wistar-Kyoto rats. The authors concluded that in SHR, calcium supplementation reduces blood pressure by reducing sympathetic nerve activity and vascular tone. The second study tested the hypothesis that in salt-sensitive SHR, calcium prevents NaCl-induced hypertension by a sympatholytic mechanism and increases diuretic and natriuretic responses to acute volume loading (304). Calcium supplementation attenuated the hypertensive effect of a high-NaCl diet in salt-sensitive SHR but did not affect blood pressure in salt-resistant SHR or Wistar-Kyoto controls. It prevented salt-induced increase in plasma norepinephrine concentration and decrease in anterior hypothalamic norepinephrine turnover in the sensitive rats. It also prevented exaggerated hypotensive and bradycardic responses to microinjection of clonidine into the anterior hypothalamus, and up-regulation of α_2-adrenoceptor number in the anterior hypothalamus. These findings support the idea that calcium acts through a sympatholytic mechanism. The study also suggested that a calcium-induced enhancement of natriuretic and diuretic responses to a volume load in sensitive SHR fed a high-salt diet contributes to the observed changes.

Because erythrocyte sodium transport is altered during the pathogenesis of hypertension in SHR and calcium protects against increases in blood pressure, the effect of 0.1, 0.6, and 4.0% dietary calcium on sodium ion transport systems was evaluated (*305*). Calcium had no effect on blood pressure in Wistar-Kyoto control rats, but there was an indirect dose-related association between calcium and blood pressure in SHR rats. Calcium intake was inversely related to sodium levels in erythrocytes and directly related to the activity of the sodium pump in SHR; passive sodium permeability and sodium–potassium cotransport were not affected.

Interactive effects of dietary sodium and calcium were studied in stroke-prone SHR fed low (0.3%) and high (3.1%) levels of sodium in combination with low (0.2%) and high (2.0%) levels of calcium (*306*). Blood pressure was higher in the low-calcium–high-sodium group than in the other groups. This group also had higher basal and ionomycin-stimulated calcium concentrations in platelets and lymphocytes. The high-sodium diet was associated with elevated erythrocyte sodium levels regardless of dietary calcium, but had little effect on levels of ionized calcium in the blood. These results demonstrate interactive effects of dietary sodium and calcium on blood pressure and cellular calcium handling in the SHR model of genetic hypertension.

Sodium chloride

Folkow critically reviewed studies on salt and hypertension, drawing parallels between rats and humans in their tolerance to a range of salt intakes, mechanisms involved in this, and genetic differences in salt tolerance (*307*). Risks at the high end of the intake spectrum are well known in both species; risks at the low end have begun to be evaluated in rats. Salt sensitivity in humans may reflect the benefit, in some environments, of mechanisms favoring salt conservation. The set point of salt balance in "salt conservers" predisposes them to hypertension when salt is freely available. Folkow concluded that research should be directed toward identification and analysis of salt-sensitive groups and individuals so as to interfere as little as possible

with the lifestyle of the great majority of salt-resistant persons.

An international symposium on "Sodium Restriction as a Public Health Measure for the General Population" was held in Bonn in October 1990 (*308*). Several papers from the symposium are summarized in this section. Epidemiologic studies and sodium-reduction trials consistently show a relationship between blood pressure and urinary sodium excretion (*309*). Taken together, controlled studies show that a decrement of 70–75 mmol/day in sodium excretion is associated with a 4.9 mm Hg decrease in systolic pressure and 2.6 mm Hg in diastolic pressure in hypertensive subjects; corresponding values for normotensive subjects are 1.7 and 1.0 mm Hg. Similar analysis of within-population epidemiologic studies showed a 100-mmol decrement in sodium excretion to be associated with a 3.7 mm Hg decrease in systolic and a 2.0 mm Hg decrease in diastolic blood pressure. Results from Intersalt were discussed. Epidemiologic studies further show that a decrease of 2–3 mm Hg in average blood pressure decreases CHD mortality rates by 4–5% and stroke mortality by 6–8%. A second review also summarized circumstantial and direct evidence that high salt consumption predisposes individuals and populations to hypertension (*310*). Additive effects on blood pressure are obtained with sodium restriction, diuretics, and other drugs such as beta-blockers and angiotensin converting enzyme inhibitors. Another author, however, questioned whether Intersalt's conclusions are applicable to the German population (*311*). Determinants of individual blood pressure and epidemiologic determinants that influence the entire population distribution may be quite different. Knowledge of the latter could be used to develop population-wide prevention strategies with great potential to reduce CVD morbidity and mortality. However, this author's study of Intersalt evidence did not permit the conclusion that general salt restriction was warranted. In contrast, there were consistent, quantitatively relevant individual and population associations between body mass index and blood pressure, suggesting that weight reduction would be a pragmatic public health measure for the German population. A skeptic from the U.K. (*312*) reviewed evidence for a link between salt intake and blood pressure, concluding that any program to reduce salt intake by the general public would produce extremely small benefits in terms of blood pressure, especially as possible adverse effects have not been examined.

Watt addressed questions of the nature and importance of salt sensitivity (*313*). Although genetic and acquired models of salt sensitivity in animals give credence to the existence of salt sensitivity in people, they do not prove it. Watt discussed the need to define salt sensitivity in people in terms of one or more characteristics that confer it, and to test the effect of sodium intake on blood pressure using a rigorous study design with adequate statistical power. The literature was reviewed in this light, with the conclusion that salt sensitivity is a powerful idea for which there is little direct evidence— and none to permit a targeted approach to prevention and treatment of hypertension. The observation that sodium restriction lowers blood pressure in hypertensive subjects is evidence for acquired salt sensitivity, without necessarily having causal significance. Other workers proposed a mechanism for salt sensitivity in human subjects (*314*). They postulated simultaneous up-regulation of α_2 adrenoceptors and down-regulation of β_2 adrenoceptors when salt-sensitive subjects eat a high-salt diet. Such an increase in the operative α_2/β_2 adrenoceptor ratio would not occur in resistant subjects. The increased ratio in sensitive persons would likely lead to increased central sympathetic outflow, through receptor changes in certain brain structures, and to enhanced end-organ response in resistance vessels and the kidney. This would increase vasoconstriction and sodium reabsorption. Long-term follow-up of salt-sensitive normotensive subjects to show whether they develop essential hypertension would test this hypothesis.

Blaustein and Hamlyn reviewed the pathogenesis of essential hypertension, reexamining the hypothesis that an endogenous digitalis-like substance and sodium–calcium exchange are involved (*315*). They discussed the roles of salt and the kidneys, interactions between the cardiovascular system and kidneys, how natriuretic hormones restore and maintain normal plasma volume, and evidence for involvement of a humoral agent with digitalis-like properties. They then presented a diagrammatic model of the pathogenesis of essential hypertension involving sodium intake, kidney and cardiovascular function, volume effects, sympathetic neurons, and the digitalis-like substance. The model is still incomplete, but it suggests directions for future research.

Law et al. responded to criticism of their metaanalyses showing that the association between salt intake and blood pressure is large and of substantial public health importance (*316*; see *Food Safety 1991,* Chapter 3, references *278* and *279*). Observed blood pressure decreases in individual sodium restriction trials were remarkably close to predicted values, for trials that varied widely according to age of subjects, extent of salt restriction, blood pressure at baseline, and extent of blood pressure reduction. Equally close agreement between observed and predicted amounts of blood pressure reduction were obtained considering only trials that were double-blinded, ruled out order effects, and presented diets identical except for salt content. The results of their analysis were consistent with results from Intersalt and indicated a substantial reduction in mortality from a simple dietary change. In the following article in the same journal, Swales examined the role of metaanalysis in the salt–blood pressure debate (*317*). Although the apparent power of a metaanalysis is greater than that of the component studies, the likelihood that systematic errors in published reports will lead to misleading conclusions is also greater. Several sources of serious error were discussed: publication bias (negative results are less often published), quality of data, linearity or nonlinearity of the relationship, and the assumptions underlying dietary advice for the general population.

Effects of a moderately low-salt diet were evaluated in 20 hypertensive subjects (*318*). All subjects followed a salt-restricted diet for two 9-week periods, separated by a 1-week washout. During the "low-sodium" diet subjects were given lactose capsules, and during the "normal-sodium" diet they received supplementary salt capsules. The study was double-blinded and the order of diets randomized. The low-sodium diet caused a drop in blood pressure, which was accompanied by decreased peripheral resistance in carotid and forearm circulation. Brachial artery diameter was also increased. This change was not related to blood pressure changes but was related to age, and was negatively correlated with baseline intracellular sodium content. The increase in diameter of the brachial artery but not the carotid with salt restriction suggests varying salt dependence among arteries.

Reduced β-adrenoceptor responsiveness is common in the elderly (*319*). Because sodium restriction corrects this defect in hypertensive subjects, Feldman studied the effect of dietary salt on vascular and lymphocyte β-adrenergic responsiveness in older normotensive subjects (aged 57 ± 2 years). With a high-sodium diet (400 meq/day), the older subjects showed reduced maximal isoproterenol-mediated vasodilation compared with young normotensive subjects previously studied; but with a low-sodium diet, maximal isoproterenol-mediated vasodilation was significantly increased in the elderly. The low-sodium diet significantly reduced blood pressure and mean arterial pressure was inversely correlated with the extent of stimulated vasodilation. These results show that sodium restriction corrects the aging-related defect in vascular and lymphocyte β-adrenergic responsiveness and suggests a role for diet modification in adrenergic regulation of vascular tone in the elderly.

Behavioral stress and a high-salt diet increase blood pressure additively in nonhuman primates (*320*). Four adult baboons were exposed to daily conflict-type stress for 2 weeks, 3 weeks of stress plus high dietary sodium, and finally two 2-week periods of stress plus sodium plus antihypertensive drug therapy. Two baboons served as nonstressed controls and ate a normal diet. In all 4 experimental animals, stress alone raised the blood pressure and the increase was roughly doubled during the phase of stress plus high salt. Water intake, urine osmolality, and sodium excretion increased and levels of serum sodium, plasma renin activity, and plasma vasopressin decreased; there was no change in urinary excretion of norepinephrine or epinephrine. The hypertension was resistant to oral atenolol hydrochloride and hydrochlorothiazide, two antihypertensive drugs in common clinical use.

Investigators in India reported a "summer salt" phenomenon: some hypertensive patients were able to discontinue or decrease use of their antihypertensive medication during the summer, only to restart it again in winter (*321*). This suggested that nondietary factors in sodium balance can influence blood pressure—for example, increased loss of salt through sweat during hot months.

To verify reported adverse effects of salt restriction on lipid and glucose metabolism, 147 nonobese normotensive adults were enrolled in a single-blind crossover trial of low-sodium (20 mmol/day) and high-sodium (300 mmol/day) diets (*322*). Each phase lasted 7 days. Sodium restriction reduced mean arterial pressure an average of 7.5 mm Hg in 17% of subjects, had no effect in 67%, and raised mean arterial pressure by an average of 6.0 mm Hg in 16%. In sensitive, resistant, and reverse-reactor groups, salt restriction significantly raised serum total and LDL cholesterol, insulin, and uric acid concentrations. The largest increase in cholesterol occurred in reverse reactors, whose blood pressure rose in response to salt restriction. Plasma renin activity and aldosterone and noradrenaline concentrations rose in all groups during salt restriction, the largest increases again occurring in reverse reactors. Thus short-term sodium restriction has unfavorable effects on lipid and glucose metabolism in normotensive subjects, particularly those who derive no hemodynamic benefit from the intervention.

Weder and Egan found similar adverse effects of short-term salt restriction in 27 subjects including both hypertensive and normotensive individuals (*323*). Theirs was a randomized, placebo-controlled, double-blinded crossover comparison of 1-week periods of 20 and 208 mEq/day NaCl intake, with 2 weeks of ad libitum salt intake between phases. With salt restriction there was a trend ($p = .07$) toward increased total and LDL cholesterol. This probably resulted from plasma volume contraction, because hemoglobin, hematocrit, total protein, and albumin increased significantly. Together, these changes could increase whole-blood viscosity. Plasma norepinephrine, fasting plasma insulin, and the glucose/insulin ratio also increased significantly during salt restriction. These findings would recommend a cautious approach to salt restriction except for those for whom the benefits clearly outweigh the possible risks.

Another potential hazard of salt restriction was demonstrated in SHR and Wistar-Kyoto rats (*324*). On a low-salt diet, both strains were abnormally sensitive to blood loss and exhibited attenuated pressor responses to acute and chronic stress. Attenuation of the pressor response to stress was due primarily to decreased release of noradrenergic transmitter. Although compensatory responses were adequate to maintain homeostasis, the neurohumoral compensatory reserve was sharply curtailed.

As in healthy humans, it is difficult to induce a change in blood pressure in normotensive rats by manipulating dietary salt within a realistic range (*325*). Moreover, the response of different strains of laboratory rats to drastic changes of salt intake is extremely heterogeneous, and a paradoxical increase in blood pressure sometimes occurs during severe salt restriction. The causes for salt appetite and its general lack of relation to blood pressure were discussed.

A high-salt diet produced increases in systolic blood pressure, urinary protein excretion, and renal vascular lesions in SHR (*326*). Males were more salt-sensitive than females. An apparent relationship between systolic blood pressure and urinary protein excretion could not be assumed to be causal because the association disappeared when regression analyses were performed within dietary subgroups and because of the significant gender differences in protein excretion. The changes in blood pressure and protein excretion are most likely independent consequences of the high-salt diet.

Depending on the age and strain of rats, a high-salt diet can significantly increase left ventricular weight and this response is independent of cardiac volume or pressure overload (*327*). A high-salt diet caused left ventricular hypertrophy in young Wistar and Wistar-Kyoto rats but not in Dahl salt-resistant rats. The response in Wistar and Wistar-Kyoto strains was smaller in mature rats than in young ones.

The effect of long-term salt loading on blood pressure and aortic connective tissue components was studied in normotensive Wistar rats (*328*). Blood pressure of high-salt and control groups began to diverge by 90 days and after 180 days it was significantly elevated in NaCl-treated rats.

The only significant aortic connective tissue change after 360 days of massive salt ingestion was an increased concentration of sulfated glycosaminoglycans. The authors suggested that this increase, occurring in the late stage of hypertensive development, might contribute to the pathogenesis of atherosclerotic CVD.

The effects of salt are frequently considered to be effects of sodium, but the anion also plays a role. The effects of sodium chloride, sodium citrate, and placebo on pressor responses to graded norepinephrine and angiotensin II infusions were studied in salt-resistant and salt-sensitive normotensive subjects (*329*). Although the chloride significantly raised mean arterial blood pressure in salt-sensitive subjects, the citrate did not. However, the pressor response to norepinephrine and angiotensin II was greater with both salts than with placebo; it was also greater in salt-sensitive than in salt-resistant subjects. Thus, whereas the blood pressure increase was a response to sodium chloride, the pressor response was to sodium ion, and enhanced pressor responsiveness therefore cannot completely account for the NaCl-induced rise in blood pressure. A review of the literature also revealed the importance of the anion accompanying sodium, with regard to blood pressure (*330*). When hypertension was induced in Sprague-Dawley rats by infusion of angiotensin II, plasma norepinephrine increased with sodium chloride loading but not with sodium citrate (*331*). Maximum response to a ganglion blocker and increase in extracellular fluid volume were also greater with sodium chloride. Thus full expression of salt sensitivity in angiotensin II–induced hypertension depends on high intake of both sodium and chloride, and increased sympathetic nervous system activity may be involved.

OTHER

Allium *spp.*

Two papers briefly reviewed the health effects of garlic (*Allium sativum*), particularly with respect to the cardiovascular system (*332,333*). They pointed out common weaknesses in clinical studies, which make it difficult to interpret results, and discussed different types of garlic preparations. The first (*332*) concluded that the hypocholesterolemic effect of garlic is not yet firmly established in humans. The second (*333*) concluded that although evidence for garlic's ability to reduce cardiovascular risk factors is accumulating, proof is still incomplete. Some garlic preparations may be useful in treating hyperlipidemia and hypertension, but reductions in morbidity and mortality have not been demonstrated. In response to reference *333*, readers reported results of their studies using a dried garlic powder standardized to 1.3% alliin (*334*). In 7 out of 8 studies of more than 500 subjects, 0.6–0.9 g/day of garlic powder reduced plasma cholesterol and triglyceride concentrations by 5–20%. Animal experiments showed that this effect resulted from inhibition of hepatic HMG-CoA reductase and remodeling of plasma lipoproteins and cell membranes.

Extracts of garlic and wild garlic (*Allium ursinum*) and purified compounds from them were tested for their influence on cholesterol synthesis in a rat liver homogenate assay (*335*). Chloroform and acetone/chloroform extracts of both garlic and wild garlic inhibited cholesterol synthesis by 44–52% at a concentration of 166 µg/mL in this system. At 10^{-3} mol/L, ajoene, methylajoene, allicin, 2-vinyl-4*H*-1,3-dithiin, and diallyldisulfide inhibited cholesterol synthesis by 37–72%. The effect of the garlic extracts is thus due to the combined action of multiple sulfur-containing thiosulfinates, ajoenes, and dithiines.

Various garlic extracts and commercial garlic products were evaluated for their inhibition of collagen-stimulated in vitro platelet aggregation (*336*). A several-fold variation in activity among product brands was found, the best products being as active as fresh garlic clove homogenates. Which compounds were responsible for the activity depended on the nature of the preparation. Ajoene, found only in the oil macerates, had the highest specific activity of all the compounds tested but was present only in low concentrations. Based on quantity and specific activity, allicin and diallyl trisulfide were the most important garlic-derived sulfur compounds that inhibited platelet aggregation in this in vitro system; in vivo, diallyl trisulfide appears to be the most important.

Aqel et al. provided evidence that part of the hypotensive action of garlic juice stems from a direct relaxant effect on smooth muscle (*337*). They tested garlic juice using isolated segments of aorta, trachea, and intestines of rabbits and guinea pigs and isolated rabbit hearts. The juice inhibited norepinephrine-induced contraction of aortic rings in the presence and absence of calcium. It also inhibited acetylcholine- and histamine-induced contraction of tracheal smooth muscles, with and without calcium. Spontaneous movements of rabbit jejunum and guinea pig ileum were inhibited and the force of contraction in isolated hearts was reduced in a concentration-dependent manner.

Austrian investigators reported the dose-dependent inhibition of adenosine deaminase by an unidentified constituent of garlic and wild garlic, and hypothesized that the accumulation of adenosine provides a molecular basis for most of the clinical effects of *Allium* extracts (*338*). Although allicin is currently favored as the active principle of garlic, neither allicin nor any other putative active constituent (alliin, diallyl sulfide, diallyl disulfide, ajoene) had any important inhibitory effect on adenosine deaminase. A standard in vitro testing procedure was reported for this enzyme assay, which is suitable for quality assessment of raw or dried garlic and standardization of pharmaceutical products derived from garlic.

Herbs and spices

Five antiplatelet agents have been isolated from Chinese herbs (*339*). Apigenin from *Apium graveolens* and magnolol from *Magnolia officinalis* inhibit thromboxane synthesis. Osthole from *Angelica pubescens*, protopine from *Corydalis* tubers, and norathyriol from *Tripterospermum lanceolatum* inhibit phosphoinositide breakdown. All except apigenin markedly prolonged the tail bleeding time of mice in a dose-dependent manner 30 min after intraperitoneal injection. In endotoxin-induced disseminated intravascular coagulation in rats, 50–100 mg/kg of norathyriol prevented decreases in platelet counts and fibrinogen and the prolongation of plasma prothrombin time. At 100 mg/kg it also suppressed collagen- and ADP-induced ex vivo platelet aggregation in rat plasma. However, at doses up to 200 mg/kg none of the antiplatelet agents prevented acute thromboembolic death in mice.

During the first 5 days after irradiation, high doses of ^{60}Co (4.0–8.0 Gy) increase the rate of platelet aggregation in experimental animals (*340*). Radiation-protective effects of acetylsalicylic acid and Chinese drug plants were assessed in in vitro and in vivo tests. Aqueous extracts were made of five plants: *Carthamus tinctorius* L. flowers, *Sargentodoxae cuneata* (Oliv.) Rehd. and Wils. stems, *Paeonia lactiflora* (Pall.) and *Salvia miltiorrhiza* roots, and *Ligusticum chuanxiong* (Hort.) rhizomes. For in vitro tests, extracts were added to platelet-rich plasma from hearts of control and irradiated rabbits. For in vivo experiments, extracts were injected into mice daily for 4 days after irradiation and blood was drawn for testing 30 min after the last injection. In vitro, all extracts inhibited platelet aggregation by 23–53%. In vivo, the extracts and acetylsalicylic acid inhibited aggregation by 63–69% except for *S. miltiorrhiza*, which was slightly less active. Acetylsalicylic acid and all extracts except *C. tinctorius* increased the 30-day survival of irradiated mice by 20–50%. The survival time of animals that died was also increased.

Dietary curcumin (0.5%), capsaicin (15 mg%), ginger (50 mg%), and mustard (250 mg%) significantly increased the activity of hepatic cholesterol-7α-hydroxylase in rats (*341*). This is the rate-limiting enzyme in conversion of cholesterol to bile acids, an important pathway for eliminating cholesterol from the body. Black pepper (0.5%) and cumin (1.25%) had no effect on enzyme activity. The microsomal cholesterol content in serum and liver was significantly elevated in curcumin- and capsaicin-fed animals. Thus turmeric, red pepper, ginger, and mustard can enhance the conversion of cholesterol to bile acids. However, turmeric and red pepper simultaneously stimulate cholesterol synthesis, which may counterbalance their effect on bile acid synthesis and make their hypocholesterolemic action simply a result of interference with exogenous cholesterol absorption.

Protection of PUFAs against oxidative attack is necessary to realize their protective effects against CVD and other diseases. Several spice principles exhibited dose-related inhibition of ascorbate-initiated lipid peroxidation in preparations of rat liver microsomes (*342*). Curcumin (5–50 μM, from turmeric), eugenol (25–150 μM, from cloves) and capsaicin (25–150 μM, from red pepper) inhibited peroxidation by >90% at the highest concentration tested. Zingarone (from ginger) inhibited peroxidation at concentrations >150 μM, but linalool (coriander) and piperine (black pepper) had only a small effect at 500 μM. The protective effect of curcumin and eugenol was reversed by addition of high concentrations of Fe^{2+}.

Skim milk, orotic acid, and nucleotides

Skim milk has been reported to have hypolipidemic (*343,344*), hypotensive (*343*), and antiatherosclerotic (*345*) effects. In a study of free-living adults, 64 subjects maintained their typical diet supplemented with 1 quart per day of skim milk for 8 weeks, while 18 subjects who did not consume the supplemental milk served as controls for the known seasonal variation in lipid parameters (*343*). Supplemental milk consumption was associated with a significant (p = .037) reduction in serum triglycerides and a 6.6% decrease in serum cholesterol (p = .0004) in subjects whose baseline cholesterol level was >190 mg/dL. There was no significant change in these values in the low-cholesterol group. However, this group showed a sharp decrease in diastolic blood pressure, whereas the high-cholesterol group had a smaller decrease, compared with controls. These findings were discussed in terms of nutrients provided by the skim milk, for example, calcium and orotic acid. In studies with cholesterol-fed rabbits, animals fed skim milk powder had lower levels of plasma total cholesterol, triglycerides, phospholipids, LDL, and VLDL and higher HDL than controls (*344*). Lecithin:cholesterol acyltransferase activity was also lower in milk-fed animals. A second paper by these authors reported that skim milk feeding enhanced regression of cholesterol-induced atherosclerotic lesions in rabbits (*345*). Plasma cholesterol decreased faster during the regression period in milk-fed animals than in controls, and aortic cholesterol concentration decreased only in the milk-fed group. Aortic collagen, mucopolysaccharides, and calcium returned to normal during regression, whereas elastin continued to rise, in both milk-fed and control animals.

The effect of dietary nucleotides on the fatty acid composition of erythrocyte membrane phospholipids was studied in weanling rats, to establish this as an animal model for further biochemical investigations (*346*). Intake of nucleotides after weaning increased the degree of unsaturation of erythrocyte membranes, whereas phosphatidylcholine and sphingomyelin showed the opposite response and phosphatidylethanolamine did not change. Dietary nucleotides appear to affect the elongation of essential fatty acids similarly in weanling rats and newborn infants.

Alcohol

Norman Kaplan reviewed evidence for the benefits of moderate alcohol consumption (*347*). He cited consistent findings of J- or U-shaped curves showing moderate drinking to protect against coronary artery disease and ischemic stroke, and a threshold for hypertensive effects. He sees "bashing booze" as another example of the guilt-ridden trend to restrict all behaviors seen as deviant, in reaction to the excesses of the 1960s and 1970s.

The Caerphilly Prospective Heart Disease Study determined alcohol and SFA intake among 1600 men aged 49–66 years by a dietary questionnaire (*348*). Platelet aggregation induced by ADP and collagen was evaluated in a fasting blood sample. The odds ratio of a high response to aggregation was significantly reduced among drinkers (primary ADP, $p < .05$; secondary ADP, $p < .001$; collagen, $p < .02$). Significance was increased by adjusting for smoking and including only subjects with a high intake of SFAs or low intake of PUFAs. The responsiveness to thrombin was slightly increased at all levels of alcohol consumption. The authors concluded that part of alcohol's effect on CHD is mediated through a dose-dependent effect on specific platelet functions and modulated by the intake of dietary fat. The components of alcohol's

protective effect were further explored by Langer et al. (*349*). They studied a cohort of Japanese Hawaiian men who participated in the Honolulu Heart Program. In these subjects, roughly half of the protective effect of moderate alcohol consumption against CHD was attributed to an increase in HDL cholesterol. An additional 18% was related to decrease in LDL cholesterol, but this was counterbalanced by a 17% increase in risk due to increased systolic blood pressure. The remaining 50% of benefit may involve interference with thrombosis. These findings are consistent with findings in other populations and provide reasonable biological explanations for the beneficial effects of moderate alcohol consumption. However, another study of 37 nondrinkers, 147 moderate drinkers, 90 heavy drinkers, and 106 alcoholics found no favorable effect of moderate alcohol consumption on blood lipid profiles (*350*). The authors concluded that if moderate drinking protects against CHD it is not through a lipid mechanism.

Miscellaneous

The roots of the perennial shrub *Rosa rugosa* are traditionally used in Korea to treat diabetes mellitus (*351*). Experiments were performed to confirm the hypolipidemic effects of root extracts in rats. With a cholesterol-free diet, the extract slightly decreased total serum cholesterol; this was not seen when cholesterol was fed, suggesting an effect of the extract on endogenous cholesterol synthesis that was masked by dietary cholesterol. The extract had no effect on concentrations of total cholesterol in liver, although liver triglyceride content was reduced.

The hypocholesterolemic potential of *Cassia fistula*, a legume, was studied in hypercholesterolemic rats (*352*). Addition of *C. fistula* to the hypercholesterolemic diet reduced total cholesterol and lipids and increased phospholipids in blood, liver, spleen, kidney, and heart; total brain lipids were also reduced. Thus overall changes in lipid metabolism were beneficial. In addition, activities of SGOT, SGPT, and serum alkaline and acid phosphatases returned to near-normal values, as did levels of serum protein, albumin, globulin, free amino acids, uric acid, and creatinine. In comparable studies by the same research group, roots of licorice (*Glycyrrhiza glabra*), another traditional medicine, had similar effects on lipid distribution in hypercholesterolemic rats (*353*). Added to the hypercholesterolemic diet, licorice root improved liver and kidney function and lipid metabolism and also had a hypoglycemic effect. Licorice roots contain numerous bioactive saponins.

Pleurotus ostreatus, the common "oyster mushroom," showed hypocholesterolemic activity in genetically hypercholesterolemic rats (*354*). When added to a hypercholesterolemic diet it markedly decreased serum cholesterol levels, principally by reducing VLDL and LDL. The same research group showed that *P. ostreatus* could prevent the effects of chronic alcohol intake on serum and hepatic lipids in hamsters (*355*). After 8 weeks of drinking a 15% ethanol solution, serum cholesterol, triglycerides, and phospholipids were elevated and 40–60% of this was accounted for by increase in VLDL. Simultaneous feeding of the fungus reduced serum cholesterol to below levels in animals not given alcohol, and triglycerides and VLDL were 30% lower than in animals given alcohol; the alcohol-induced increase in hepatic cholesterol and triglycerides was also prevented.

A fraction from brewer's yeast inhibited in vitro cholesterol synthesis in cell-free and hepatocyte preparations from rat liver (*356*). Tests with several substrates indicated that the site of inhibition lay between acetyl-CoA and mevalonate. The effect was not due to chromium. One inhibitory substance in the yeast fraction was nicotinamide riboside.

Male Wistar rats were fed a hypercholesterolemic diet supplemented with the polyphenols quercetin, morin, or tannic acid (*357*). Tannic acid and morin effectively reduced plasma and liver lipids, whereas quercetin increased plasma LDL cholesterol after 10 weeks and had no effect on plasma total cholesterol or triglycerides or liver lipids. Tannic acid reduced hepatic lipase activity. There were no differences between groups in plasma alanine aminotransferase, alkaline phosphatase, or bilirubin. In studies with platelets from rabbits and humans (*358*), kaempferol, quercetin, fisetin, morin,

and myricetin inhibited aggregation to differing degrees, depending on the aggregation inducer. Myricetin most effectively inhibited ADP-induced platelet aggregation; kaempferol and morin were inactive. All compounds except myricetin completely inhibited aggregation in platelets challenged with arachidonic acid. Inhibition of aggregation was generally paralleled by inhibition of thromboxane B_2 synthesis. These and other results indicated that the major antiplatelet effect of the compounds tested was due to antagonism of thromboxane receptors and inhibition of thromboxane synthesis.

The maltodextrin fat substitute known as "Oatrim" has a favorable effect on serum lipid profiles (*359*). Not only can it replace a portion of dietary SFAs, but it also has intrinsic activity. Inglett and Grisamore reviewed its hypocholesterolemic effects and summarized its potential applications and commercial status.

It's not merely what and how much one eats, but how often, that determines cholesterol concentrations (*360*). A study of more than 2000 older adults found that age-adjusted total cholesterol concentrations for men and women reporting ≥4 meals per day averaged 0.23 mmol/L lower than for those who ate 1 or 2 meals per day. LDL concentrations were also lower in subjects who ate more frequently. The associations remained after adjustment for potential confounding factors. The authors concluded that an increase in meal frequency can have favorable effects with no other dietary modification.

Diet–gene interactions

Nutritional regulation of cholesterol synthesis and apoB kinetics were studied in normal subjects and subjects with familial hypercholesterolemia (*361*). Two dietary regimens were compared in a clinical research ward under isocaloric, metabolically steady-state conditions: the basal diet had a caloric distribution of 45% carbohydrate, 40% fat, and 15% protein; the test diet was Vivonex, 99% carbohydrate and 1% fat, administered through a nasogastric feeding tube. The major finding was that carbohydrate feeding reduced LDL cholesterol concentration and LDL apoB mass in subjects with familial hypercholesterolemia by increasing plasma clearance of LDL, whereas substantial catabolism of VLDL apoB took place in normal subjects.

Plasma lipid levels are also influenced by apoE phenotype. ApoE2 and apoE4 differ from "normal" apoE3 by a single amino acid substitution. Dallongeville et al. reported a metaanalysis of modulation of plasma triglyceride levels by apoE phenotype (*362*). Compared with apoE3/3 controls, E2/2 and E3/2 phenotypes have lower mean total cholesterol levels and E4/3 and E4/4 have higher; E4/2 values are slightly lower. Compared with apoE3/3, all phenotypes except E4/4 have higher triglyceride values. Differences for HDL cholesterol are not significant except for a slightly reduced level in E4/3. The authors conclude that in addition to the elevated cholesterol levels associated with the apoε4 allele, persons with the apoE4/3 phenotype may also be at increased risk for CVD by virtue of elevated plasma triglycerides and reduced HDL cholesterol.

A dietary study was conducted in subjects with different apoE and apoB genotypes (*363*). On both low- and high-cholesterol diets, apoε2/3 subjects had significantly lower LDL cholesterol levels than apoε3/3 subjects. However, there were no genotype-related differences in average lipid response to change from the low- to the high-cholesterol diet, indicating that these gene foci do not play an important role in the response of lipid levels to dietary cholesterol.

A study among ethnic groups differing in their risk of CHD showed that both genetic and environmental factors determine factor VII coagulant activity (*364*). Persons possessing the Gln_{353} allele of factor VII have factor VIIc levels significantly below average. In this study, however, Afro-Caribbeans had lower levels of factor VIIc than Europeans but did not differ in the frequency of Gln_{353}, suggesting that other factors, perhaps dietary fat, were involved in the low factor VIIc levels. Factor VIIc levels are generally positively correlated with plasma triglycerides; Gujarati Indians, who had the highest frequency of Gln_{353}, also had the highest level of triglycerides; their mean factor VIIc levels did not correspond to the high frequency of Gln_{353}. In the Gujaratis, triglycerides were correlated with the factor VII Arg_{353} allele but not with Gln_{353}. The

authors concluded that the effect of triglycerides on factor VIIc is genotype-specific and demonstrates a gene–environment interaction.

Large genetic variations in hepatic HMG-CoA reductase activity exist among various inbred mouse strains (*365*). C57BL/6 mice normally have levels of hepatic reductase mRNA 5 times higher than found in BALB/c mice, and this results in correspondingly greater hepatic reductase activity. However, diet interacts with genes to regulate expression of the HMG-CoA reductase gene. Cholesterol feeding had minimal effect on hepatic reductase activity and mRNA levels in BALB/c mice but reduced both measures more than 10-fold in C57BL/6 mice. The possible nature of the gene–diet interaction was discussed.

LITERATURE CITED

1. Herzberg, G.R. Dietary regulation of fatty acid and triglyceride metabolism. The 1990 Borden Award Lecture. *Can. J. Physiol. Pharmacol.* 69:1637–1647 (1991).

2. Shrapnel, W.S., G.D. Calvert, P.J. Nestel, and A.S. Truswell. Diet and coronary heart disease. *Med. J. Aust.* 156(Suppl.):S9–S16 (1992).

3. Ulbricht, T.L.V., and D.A.T. Southgate. Coronary heart disease: seven dietary factors. *Lancet* 338:985–992 (1991).

4. Sacks, F.M. The role of cereals, fats, and fibers in preventing coronary heart disease. *Cereal Foods World* 36:822–826 (1991).

5. Grundy, S.M. Multifactorial etiology of hypercholesterolemia: implications for prevention of coronary heart disease. George Lyman Duff Memorial Lecture. *Arterioscler. Thromb.* 11:1619–1635 (1991).

6. Slater, E.E., H.P. Dustan, R.H. Grimm, Jr., et al. Workshop: Metabolic and Nutritional Factors in Hypertension. Recommendations for treatment and prevention. *Hypertension* 18(Suppl. I):I-121–I-124 (1991).

7. Lindholm, L.H. Cardiovascular risk factors and their interactions in hypertensives. *J. Hypertens.* 9(Suppl. 3):S3–S6 (1991).

8. Roberts, D.C.K. Dietary factors in the fall in coronary heart disease mortality. *Prostaglandins Leukotrienes Essential Fatty Acids* 44:97–101 (1991).

9. Sigfusson, N., H. Sigvaldason, L. Steingrimsdotter, et al. Decline in ischaemic heart disease in Iceland and change in risk factor levels. *Br. Med. J.* 302:1371–1374 (1991).

10. Beevers, D.G., and J.S. Prince. Some recent advances in non-communicable diseases in the tropics. 1. Hypertension: an emerging problem in tropical countries. *Trans. Roy. Soc. Trop. Med. Hyg.* 85:324–326 (1991).

11. Stamler, J. Blood pressure and high blood pressure. Aspects of risk. *Hypertension* 18(Suppl. I):I-95–I-107 (1991).

12. Kaplan, N.M. Long-term effectiveness of nonpharmacological treatment of hypertension. *Hypertension* 18(Suppl. I):I-153–I-160 (1991).

13. Lloyd, J.K. Cholesterol: should we screen all children or change the diet of all children. *Acta Pædiatr. Scand.* Suppl. 373:66–72 (1991).

14. Ford, E.S., and R.S. Cooper. Risk factors for hypertension in a national cohort study. *Hypertension* 18:598–606 (1991).

15. Weizel, A. The cholesterol story. More questions than answers. *Atheroscler. Rev.* 23:273–280 (1991).

16. Sonnenberg, L.M., B.M. Posner, A.J. Belanger, et al. Dietary predictors of serum cholesterol in men: the Framingham cohort population. *J. Clin. Epidemiol.* 45:413–418 (1992).

17. Watts, G.F., B. Lewis, J.N.H. Brunt, et al. Effects on coronary artery disease of lipid-lowering diet, or diet plus cholestyramine, in the St Thomas' Atherosclerosis Regression Study (STARS). *Lancet* 339:563–569 (1992).

18. Sciarrone, S.E.G., L.J. Beilin, I.L. Rouse, and P.B. Rogers. A factorial study of salt restriction and a low-fat/high-fibre diet in hypertensive subjects. *J. Hypertens.* 10:287–298 (1992).

19. Fønnebø, V. Coronary risk factors in Norwegian Seventh-day Adventists: a study of 247 Seventh-day Adventists and matched controls. The Cardiovascular Disease Studies in Norway. *Am. J. Epidemiol.* 135:504–508 (1992).

20. Larsson, B., I. Johansson, G. Hellsten, et al. Blood lipids and diet in Swedish adolescents living in Norsjö, an area with high incidence of cardiovascular diseases and diabetes. *Acta Pædiatr. Scand.* 80:667–674 (1991).

21. Vartianen, E., H.J. Korhonen, P. Pietinen, et al. Fifteen-year trends in coronary risk factors in Finland, with special reference to North Karelia. *Int. J. Epidemiol.* 20:651–662 (1991).

22. Barker, M.E., S.I. McClean, J.J. Strain, and K.A. Thompson. Dietary behaviour and health in Northern Ireland: an exploration of biochemical and haematological associations. *J. Epidemiol. Commun. Health* 46:151–156 (1992).

23. Campos, H., W.C. Willet, R.M. Peterson, et al. Nutrient intake comparisons between Framingham and rural and urban Puriscal, Costa Rica. *Arterioscler. Thromb.* 11:1089–1099 (1991).

24. Aráuz, R.A. Monge, L. Muñoz, and M.T. Rojas. La dieta como factor de riesgo de la enfermedad cardiovascular en habitantes del area metropolitana, San Jose, Costa Rica. *Arch. Latinoam. Nutr.* 41:350–362 (1991).

25. Bacardi-Gascon, M., and A. Jimenez-Cruz. Diet and mortality from coronary heart diseases in Spain. *Ecol. Food Nutr.* 25:249–253 (1991).

26. Porrini, M., P. Simonetti, G. Testolin, et al. Relation between diet composition and coronary heart disease risk factors. *J. Epidemiol. Commun. Health* 45:148–151 (1991).

27. Singh, R.B., A.R. Sircar, R.G. Singh, et al. Dietary modulators of lipid metabolism in the Indian Diet–Heart Study (I.D.H.S.). *Int. J. Vit. Nutr. Res.* 62:73–82 (1992).

28. Singh, R.B., S.S. Rastogi, R. Verma, et al. An Indian experiment with nutritional modulation in acute myocardial infarction. *Am. J. Cardiol.* 69:879–885 (1992).

29. McMurry, M.P., M.T. Cerqueira, S.L. Connor, and W.E. Connor. Changes in lipid and lipoprotein levels and body weight in Tarahumara Indians after consumption of an affluent diet. *New Engl. J. Med.* 325:1704–1708 (1991).

30. Agheli, N., M. Cloarec, and B. Jacotot. Effect of dietary treatment on the lipid, lipoprotein and fatty acid compositions in type IV familial hypertriglyceridemia. *Ann. Nutr. Metab.* 35:261–273 (1991).

31. Garry, P.J., W.C. Hunt, K.M. Koehler, et al. Longitudinal study of dietary intakes and plasma lipids in healthy elderly men and women. *Am. J. Clin. Nutr.* 55:682–688 (1992).

32. Ullman, D., W.E. Connor, L.F. Hatcher, et al. Will a high-carbohydrate, low-fat diet lower plasma

lipids and lipoproteins without producing hypertriglyceridemia? *Arterioscler. Thromb.* 11:1059–1067 (1991).

33. Clevidence, B.A., J.T. Judd, A. Schatzkin, et al. Plasma lipid and lipoprotein concentrations of men consuming a low-fat, high-fiber diet. *Am. J. Clin. Nutr.* 55:689–694 (1992).

34. Barnard, R.J. Effects of life-style modification on serum lipids. *Arch. Intern. Med.* 151:1389–1394 (1991).

35. Grundy, S.M. Plasma lipid lowering in short-term life-style change. *Arch. Intern. Med.* 151:1275–1276 (1991).

36. Wood, P.D., M.L. Stefanick, P.T. Williams, and W.L. Haskell. The effects on plasma lipoproteins of a prudent weight-reducing diet, with or without exercise, in overweight men and women. *New Engl. J. Med.* 325:461–466 (1991).

37. Singh, R.B., S.S. Rastogi, R. Verma, et al. Randomised controlled trial of cardioprotective diet in patients with recent acute myocardial infarction: results of one year follow up. *Br. Med. J.* 304:1015–1019 (1992).

38. Fall, C.H.D., D.J.P. Barker, C. Osmond, et al. Relation of infant feeding to adult serum cholesterol concentration and death from ischaemic heart disease. *Br. Med. J.* 304:801–805 (1992).

39. Williams, J.K., M.S. Anthony, and T.B. Clarkson. Coronary heart disease in rhesus monkeys with diet-induced coronary artery atherosclerosis. *Arch. Pathol. Lab. Med.* 115:784–790 (1991).

40. Topping, D.L. Soluble fiber polysaccharides: effects on plasma cholesterol and colonic fermentation. *Nutr. Rev.* 49:195–203 (1991).

41. Shinnick, F.L., R. Mathews, and S. Ink. Serum cholesterol reduction by oats and other fiber sources. *Cereal Foods World* 36:815–821 (1991).

42. Challis, T. Oats and cholesterol. *Food Chem. Toxicol.* 29:651–653 (1991).

43. Leadbetter, J., M.J. Ball, and J.I. Mann. Effects of increasing quantities of oat bran in hypercholesterolemic people. *Am. J. Clin. Nutr.* 54:841–845 (1991).

44. Whyte, J.L., R. McArthur, D. Topping, and P. Nestel. Oat bran lowers plasma cholesterol levels in mildly hypercholesterolemic men. *J. Am. Diet. Assoc.* 92:446–449 (1992).

45. Bremer, J.M., R.S. Scott, and C.J. Lintott. Oat bran and cholesterol reduction: evidence against specific effect. *Aust. N.Z. J. Med.* 21:422–426 (1991).

46. Sacks, F.M., and J. Swain. The hypocholesterolemic effects of β-glucan. (Letter.) *JAMA* 266:1079 (1991).

47. Warshafsky, S. The hypocholesterolemic effects of β-glucan. (Letter.) *JAMA* 266:1079–1080 (1991).

48. Davidson, M.H., L.D. Dugan, J.H. Burns, et al. The hypocholesterolemic effects of β-glucan. (Reply.) *JAMA* 266:1079 (1991).

49. Spiller, G.A., J.W. Farquhar, J.E. Gates, and S.F. Nichols. Guar gum and plasma cholesterol. Effect of guar gum and an oat fiber source on plasma lipoproteins and cholesterol in hypercholesterolemic adults. *Arterioscler. Thromb.* 11:1204–1208 (1991).

50. Haskell, W.L., G.A. Spiller, C.D. Jensen, et al. Role of water-soluble dietary fiber in the management of elevated plasma cholesterol in healthy subjects. *Am. J. Cardiol.* 69:433–439 (1992).

51. Eliasson, K., K.R. Ryttig, B. Hylander, and S. Rössner. A dietary fibre supplement in the treatment of mild hypertension. A randomized, double-blind, placebo-controlled trial. *J. Hypertens.* 10:195–199 (1992).

52. Cara, L., M. Armand, P. Borel, et al. Long-term wheat germ intake beneficially affects plasma lipids and lipoproteins in hypercholesterolemic human subjects. *J. Nutr.* 122:317–326 (1992).

53. McIntosh, G.H., J. Whyte, R. McArthur, and P.J. Nestel. Barley and wheat foods: influence on plasma cholesterol concentrations in hypercholesterolemic men. *Am. J. Clin. Nutr.* 53:1205–1209 (1991).

54. Anderson, J.W., N.H. Gilinsky, D.A. Deakins, et al. Lipid responses of hypercholesterolemic men to oat-bran and wheat-bran intake. *Am. J. Clin. Nutr.* 54:678–683 (1991).

55. Kashtan, H., H.S. Stern, D.J.A. Jenkins, et al. Wheat-bran and oat-bran supplements' effects on blood lipids and lipoproteins. *Am. J. Clin. Nutr.* 55:976–980 (1992).

56. Anderson, J.W., S. Riddell-Lawrence, T.L. Floore, et al. Bakery products lower serum cholesterol concentrations in hypercholesterolemic men. *Am. J. Clin. Nutr.* 54:836–840 (1991).

57. Cara, L., C. Dubois, P. Borel, et al. Effects of oat bran, rice bran, wheat fiber, and wheat germ on

postprandial lipemia in healthy adults. *Am. J. Clin. Nutr.* 55:81–88 (1992).

58. Richter, W.O., B.G. Jacob, and P. Schwandt. Interaction between fibre and lovastatin. (Letter.) *Lancet* 338:706 (1991).

59. De Schrijver, R., D. Fremaut, and A. Verheyen. Cholesterol-lowering effects and utilization of protein, lipid, fiber and energy in rats fed unprocessed and baked oat bran. *J. Nutr.* 122:1318–1324 (1992).

60. Newman, R.K., C.F. Klopfenstein, C.W. Newman, et al. Comparison of the cholesterol-lowering properties of whole barley, oat bran, and wheat red dog in chicks and rats. *Cereal Chem.* 69:240–244 (1992).

61. Mongeau, R., R. Brassard, S. Malcolm, and B.G. Shah. Effect of dietary cereal brans on body weight and blood lipids in a long-term rat experiment. *Cereal Chem.* 68:448–453 (1991).

62. Kahlon, T.S., F.I. Chow, R.N. Sayre, and A.A. Betschart. Cholesterol-lowering in hamsters fed rice bran at various levels, defatted rice bran and rice bran oil. *J. Nutr.* 122:513–519 (1992).

63. Shimizu, H., M. Yamauchi, T. Kuramoto, et al. Effects of dietary konjac mannan on serum and liver cholesterol levels and biliary bile acid composition in hamsters. *J. Pharmacobio-Dyn.* 14:371–375 (1991).

64. Cara, L., P. Borel, M. Armand, et al. Effects of increasing levels of raw or defatted wheat germ on liver, feces and plasma lipids and lipoproteins in the rat. *Nutr. Res.* 11:907–916 (1991).

65. Koseki, M., H. Seki, M. Kazama, et al. Effects of pectin and lard on the production of short-chain fatty acids in the cecum, on the growth of colonic bacteria, and on the liver cholesterol level in rats. *Agric. Biol. Chem.* 55:1441–1448 (1991).

66. Arjmandi, B.H., J. Ahn, S. Nathani, and R.D. Reeves. Dietary soluble fiber and cholesterol affect serum cholesterol concentration, hepatic portal venous short-chain fatty acid concentrations and fecal sterol excretion in rats. *J. Nutr.* 122:246–253 (1992).

67. Mazur, A., E. Gueux, C. Felgines, et al. Effects of dietary fermentable fiber on fatty acid synthesis and triglyceride secretion in rats fed fructose-based diet: studies with sugar-beet fiber. *Proc. Soc. Exp. Biol. Med.* 199:345–350 (1992).

68. Mazur, A., C. Felgines, F. Nassir, et al. Apolipoprotein B gene expression in rat intestine. The effect of dietary fiber. *FEBS Lett.* 284:63–65 (1991).

69. Sanchez, A., and R.W. Hubbard. Plasma amino acids and the insulin/glucagon ratio as an explanation for the dietary protein modulation of atherosclerosis. *Med. Hypoth.* 36:27–32 (1991).

70. Maubois, J.L., J. Léonil, R. Trouvé, and S. Bouhallab. Les peptides du lait à activité physiologique. III. Peptides du lait à effet cardiovasculaire: activités antithrombotique et antihypertensive. *Lait* 71:249–255 (1991).

71. Miyoshi, S., T. Kaneko, Y. Yoshizawa, et al. Hypotensive activity of enzymatic α-zein hydrolysate. *Agric. Biol. Chem.* 55:1407–1408 (1991).

72. Turnbull, W.H., A.R. Leeds, and D.G. Edwards. Mycoprotein reduces blood lipids in free-living subjects. *Am. J. Clin. Nutr.* 55:415–419 (1992).

73. Bergeron, N., Y. Deshales, C. Lavigne, and H. Jacques. Interaction between dietary proteins and lipids in the regulation of serum and liver lipids in the rabbit. Effect of fish protein. *Lipids* 26:759–764 (1991).

74. Honda, J., M. Iwamoto, S. Shichijo, et al. BM-1, a platelet aggregation inhibitor from mackerel. (Letter.) *Lancet* 338:817 (1991).

75. Carroll, K.K. Review of clinical studies on cholesterol-lowering response to soy protein. *J. Am. Diet. Assoc.* 91:820–827 (1991).

76. Laurin, D., H. Jacques, S. Moorjani, et al. Effects of a soy-protein beverage on plasma lipoproteins in children with familial hypercholesterolemia. *Am. J. Clin. Nutr.* 54:98–103 (1991).

77. Beynen, A.C. Dietary protein and serum cholesterol. (Editorial.) *Nutrition* 8:110–111 (1992).

78. von Duvillard, S.P., A.F. Stucchi, A.H.M. Terpstra, and R.J. Nicolosi. The effect of dietary casein and soybean protein on plasma lipid levels in cebus monkeys fed cholesterol-free or cholesterol-enriched semipurified diets. *J. Nutr. Biochem.* 3:71–74 (1992).

79. Samman, S. The effect of Max Epa on low density lipoprotein metabolism: perspectives from an animal model. *Prostaglandins Leukotrienes Essential Fatty Acids* 43:83–85 (1991).

80. Baba, N., H. Radwan, and T. Van Italie. Effects of casein versus soyprotein diets on body composition and serum lipid levels in adult rats. *Nutr. Res.* 12:279–288 (1992).

81. Sjöblom, L., A. Eklund, L. Humble, et al. Plasma very low density lipoproteins from male rats fed casein or soybean protein diets: a comparison of fatty

acid composition and influence on prostanoid production. *J. Nutr.* 121:1705–1713 (1991).

82. Chiang, M.-T., and S. Kimura. Effect of dietary protein on the peroxidation of eicosapentaenoic acid in stroke-prone spontaneously hypertensive rats. *Int. J. Vit. Nutr. Res.* 61:239–243 (1991).

83. Terpstra, A.H.M., J.C. Holmes, and R.J. Nicolosi. The hypercholesterolemic effect of dietary soybean protein vs. casein in hamsters fed cholesterol-free or cholesterol-enriched semipurified diets. *J. Nutr.* 121:944–947 (1991).

84. Kromhout, D. Dietary fats: long-term implications for health. *Nutr. Rev.* 50(4):49–53 (1992).

85. Dolecek, T.A. Epidemiological evidence of relationships between dietary polyunsaturated fatty acids and mortality in the Multiple Risk Factor Intervention Trial. *Proc. Soc. Exp. Biol. Med.* 200:177–182 (1992).

86. Posner, B.M., J.L. Cobb, A.J. Belanger, et al. Dietary lipid predictors of coronary heart disease in men. The Framingham Study. *Arch. Intern. Med.* 151:1181–1187 (1991).

87. Kaplan, N.M. Lipid intervention trials in primary prevention: a critical review. *Clin. Exp. Hypertens. Theory Pract.* A14:109–118 (1992).

88. Reiser, R., and F.B. Shorland. Meat fats and fatty acids. In *Meat and Health*. A.M. Pearson and T.R. Dutson (eds.) *Adv. Meat Res.* 6:21–62 (1990).

89. Norum, K.R. Dietary fat and blood lipids. *Nutr. Rev.* 50:30–37 (1992).

90. Dietschy, J.M., L.A. Woollett, and D.K. Spady. Dietary fatty acids and the regulation of plasma low-density lipoprotein cholesterol levels. In *Atherosclerosis. Its Pathogenesis and the Role of Cholesterol.* P.C. Weber and A. Leaf (eds.). *Atheroscler. Rev.* 23:7–18 (1991).

91. Mazier, M.J.P., and P.J.H. Jones. Dietary fat quality and circulating cholesterol levels in humans: a review of actions and mechanisms. *Prog. Food Nutr. Sci.* 15:21–41 (1991).

92. Spiller, G.A. Health effects of Mediterranean diets and monounsaturated fats. *Cereal Foods World* 36:812–814 (1991).

93. Sacks, F.M., and W.W. Willett. More on chewing the fat: the good fat and the good cholesterol. *New Engl. J. Med.* 325:1740–1742 (1991).

94. Kritchevsky, D. Palm oil in lipid metabolism. *Nutr. Res.* 12(Suppl. 1):S31–S41 (1992).

95. Rukmini, C., and T.C. Raghuram. Nutritional and biochemical aspects of the hypolipidemic action of rice bran oil: a review. *J. Am. Coll. Nutr.* 10:593–601 (1991).

96. Nicolosi, R.J., L.M. Ausman, and D.M. Hegsted. Rice bran oil lowers serum total and low density lipoprotein cholesterol and apo B levels in nonhuman primates. *Atherosclerosis* 88:133–142 (1991).

97. Katan, M.B., and R.P Mensink. Isomeric fatty acids and serum lipoproteins. *Nutr. Rev.* 50(4):46–48 (1992).

98. Zock, P.L., and M.B. Katan. Hydrogenation alternatives: effects of *trans* fatty acids and stearic acid versus linoleic acid on serum lipids and lipoproteins in humans. *J. Lipid Res.* 33:399–410 (1992).

99. Nestel, P.J., M. Noakes, G.B. Belling, et al. Plasma cholesterol-lowering potential of edible-oil blends suitable for commercial use. *Am. J. Clin. Nutr.* 55:46–50 (1992).

100. Valsta, L.M., M. Jauhiainen, A. Aro, et al. Effects of a monounsaturated rapeseed oil and a polyunsaturated sunflower oil diet on lipoprotein levels in humans. *Arterioscler. Thromb.* 12:50–57 (1992).

101. Spiller, G.A., D.J.A. Jenkins, L.N. Cragen, et al. Effect of a diet high in monounsaturated fat from almonds on plasma cholesterol and lipoproteins. *J. Am. Coll. Nutr.* 11:126–130 (1992).

102. Mata, P., L.A. Alvarez-Sala, M.J. Rubio, et al. Effects of long-term monounsaturated- vs polyunsaturated-enriched diets on lipoproteins in healthy men and women. *Am. J. Clin. Nutr.* 55:846–850 (1992).

103. Wardlaw, G.M., J.T. Snook, M.-C. Lin, et al. Serum lipid and apolipoprotein concentrations in healthy men on diets enriched in either canola oil or safflower oil. *Am. J. Clin. Nutr.* 54:104–110 (1991).

104. Barr, S.L., R. Ramakrishnan, C. Johnson, et al. Reducing total dietary fat without reducing saturated fatty acids does not significantly lower total plasma cholesterol concentrations in normal males. *Am. J. Clin. Nutr.* 55:675–681 (1992).

105. Denke, M.A., and S.M. Grundy. Effects of fats high in stearic acid on lipid and lipoprotein concentrations in men. *Am. J. Clin. Nutr.* 54:1036–1040 (1991).

106. Bodenann, A., U. Ackermann-Liebrich, and U. Keller. Fleischkonsum und Serum-Cholesterinkonzentration. *Dtsch. Med. Wochenschr.* 116:1089–1094 (1991).

107. Heber, D., J.M. Ashley, M.E. Solares, et al. The effects of a palm-oil enriched diet on plasma lipids and lipoproteins in healthy young men. *Nutr. Res.* 12(Suppl. 1):S53–S59 (1992).

108. Garcia, P.A., K.B. Hanson, C. Kies, et al. Studies of women eating diets with different fatty acid composition. I. Plasma lipoproteins and steroid excretion. *J. Am. Coll. Nutr.* 10:315–321 (1991).

109. Cole, T.G., P.E. Bowen, D. Schmeisser, et al. Differential reduction of plasma cholesterol by the American Heart Association phase 3 diet in moderately hypercholesterolemic, premenopausal women with different body mass indexes. *Am. J. Clin. Nutr.* 55:385–394 (1992).

110. Prewitt, T.E., T.G. Unterman, R. Glick, et al. Insulin-like growth factor I and low-density-lipoprotein cholesterol in women during high- and low-fat feeding. *Am. J. Clin. Nutr.* 55:381–384 (1992).

111. Anonymous. Different effects of dietary saturated fatty acids on cholesterol metabolism in nonhuman primates. *Nutr. Rev.* 49:277–278 (1991).

112. Khosla, P., and K.C. Hayes. Comparison between the effects of dietary saturated (16:0), monounsaturated (18:1), and polyunsaturated (18:2) fatty acids on plasma lipoprotein metabolism in cebus and rhesus monkeys fed cholesterol-free diets. *Am. J. Clin. Nutr.* 55:51–62 (1992).

113. Hayes, K.C., and P. Khosla. Dietary fatty acid thresholds and cholesterolemia. *FASEB J.* 6:2600–2607 (1992).

114. Ney, D.M., H.-C. Lai, J.B. Lasekan, and M. Lefevre. Interrelationship of plasma triglycerides and HDL size and composition in rats fed different dietary saturated fats. *J. Nutr.* 121:1311–1322 (1991).

115. Chautan, M., M. Charbonnier, J. Léonardi, et al. Modulation of lipid chylomicron-synthesizing enzymes in rats by the dietary (n–6):(n–3) fatty acid ratio. *J. Nutr.* 121:1305–1310 (1991).

116. De Schrijver, R., D. Vermeulen, and E. Viaene. Lipid metabolism responses in rats fed beef tallow, native or randomized fish oil and native or randomized peanut oil. *J. Nutr.* 121:948–955 (1991).

117. Fernandez, M.L., E.C.K. Lin, and D.J. McNamara. Regulation of guinea pig plasma low density lipoprotein kinetics by dietary fat saturation. *J. Lipid Res.* 33:97–109 (1992).

118. Woollett, L.A., D.K. Spady, and J.M. Dietschy. Saturated and unsaturated fatty acids independently regulate low density lipoprotein receptor activity and production rate. *J. Lipid Res.* 33:77–88 (1992).

119. Woollett, L.A., D.K. Spady, and J.M. Dietschy. Regulatory effects of the saturated fatty acids 6:0 through 18:0 on hepatic low density lipoprotein receptor activity in the hamster. *J. Clin. Invest.* 89:1133–1141 (1992).

120. Teik, K.H., and D.T.S. Tan. Studies on the lipidemic property of dietary palm oil: comparison of the responses of serum, liver and heart lipids to dietary palm oil, palm oil triglycerides, coconut oil and olive oil. *Nutr. Res.* 12(Suppl. 1):S105–S115 (1992).

121. Hopkins, P.N. Effects of dietary cholesterol on serum cholesterol: a meta-analysis and review. *Am. J. Clin. Nutr.* 55:1060–1070 (1992).

122. McNamara, D.J. Relationship between blood and dietary cholesterol. In *Meat and Health.* A.M. Pearson and T.R. Dutson (eds.). *Adv. Meat Res.* 6:63–87 (1990).

123. Lehtimäki, T., T. Moilanen, T. Solakivi, et al. Cholesterol-rich diet induced changes in plasma lipids in relation to apolipoprotein E phenotype in healthy students. *Ann. Med.* 24:61–66 (1992).

124. Vorster, H.H., A.J.S. Benadé, H.C. Barnard, et al. Egg intake does not change plasma lipoprotein and coagulation profiles. *Am. J. Clin. Nutr.* 55:400–410 (1992).

125. Jones, M.P., and D.M. Heuman. Physiological responses to increased dietary cholesterol: the case of the egg man. *Hepatology* 14:1291–1293 (1991).

126. Ekstedt, B., E. Jönsson, and O. Johnson. Influence of dietary fat, cholesterol and energy on serum lipids at vigorous physical exercise. *Scand. J. Clin. Lab. Invest.* 51:437–442 (1991).

127. Otani, H., T. Kita, Y. Ueda, et al. Long-term effects of a cholesterol-free diet on serum cholesterol levels in Zen monks. *New Engl. J. Med.* 326:416 (1992).

128. Hennessy, L.K., J. Osada, J.M. Ordovas, et al. Effects of dietary fats and cholesterol on liver lipid content and hepatic apolipoprotein A-I, B, and E and LDL receptor mRNA levels in cebus monkeys. *J. Lipid Res.* 33:351–360 (1992).

129. Kushwaha, R.S., C.A. McMahan, G.E. Mott, et al. Influence of dietary lipids on hepatic mRNA levels of proteins regulating plasma lipoproteins in baboons with high and low levels of large high density lipoproteins. *J. Lipid Res.* 32:1929–1940 (1991).

130. Parks, J.S., and J.R. Crouse. Reduction of cholesterol absorption by dietary oleinate and fish oil in African green monkeys. *J. Lipid Res.* 33:559–568 (1992).

131. Gray, D.S., R.C. Sharma, H.P. Chin, and D.M. Kramsch. Body fat distribution affects responses to high fat cholesterol containing diet in male cynomolgus monkeys. (Letter.) *Atherosclerosis* 88:93–95 (1991).

132. Bhattacharyya, A.K., and J.P. Strong. Serum total bile acid concentration in rhesus monkeys: effects of feeding cholesterol and inhibiting cholesterol absorption and synthesis. *Ann. Nutr. Metab.* 36:55–60 (1992).

133. Laraki, L., X. Pelletier, and G. Debry. Effects of dietary cholesterol and phytosterol overload on Wistar rat plasma lipids. *Ann. Nutr. Metab.* 35:221–225 (1991).

134. Fungwe, T.V., L. Cagen, H.G. Wilcox, and M. Heimberg. Regulation of hepatic secretion of very low density lipoprotein by dietary cholesterol. *J. Lipid Res.* 33:179–191 (1992).

135. Manorama, R., and C. Rukmini. Serum lipids of rats fed crude and refined palm oil in high cholesterol and cholesterol free diets. *Nutr. Res.* 12(Suppl. 1):S93–S103 (1992).

136. Imaizumi, K., and M. Sugano. Effects of different saturated fats on various aspects of lipid metabolism in rats hypersensitive to dietary cholesterol. *Nutr. Res.* 12(Suppl. 1):S85–S91 (1992).

137. Surette, M.E., J. Whelan, G.-P. Lu, et al. Dependence on dietary cholesterol for $n-3$ polyunsaturated fatty acid–induced changes in plasma cholesterol in the Syrian hamster. *J. Lipid Res.* 33:263–271 (1992).

138. Burr, M.L. Fish food, fish oil and cardiovascular disease. *Clin. Exp. Hypertens. Theory Pract.* A14:181–192 (1992).

139. Wallingford, J.C., and E.A. Yetley. Development of the health claims regulations: the case of omega-3 fatty acids and heart disease. *Nutr. Rev.* 49:323–331 (1991).

140. Bønaa, K., K.S. Bjerve, and A. Nordøy. Habitual fish consumption, plasma phospholipid fatty acids, and serum lipids: the Tromsø Study. *Am. J. Clin. Nutr.* 55:1126–1134 (1992).

141. Gerhard, G.T., B.D. Patton, S.A. Lindquist, and R.C. Wander. Comparison of three species of dietary fish: effects on serum concentrations of low-density-lipoprotein cholesterol and apolipoprotein in normotri-glyceridemic subjects. *Am. J. Clin. Nutr.* 54:334–339 (1991).

142. Jacotot, B. The effect of polyunsaturated Ω-3 fatty acids on blood lipids and lipoprotein metabolism. In *Fish Oil and Blood-Vessel Wall Interactions.* Proceedings of the International Symposium, Granada, Spain, 23–25 Feb. 1990. P.M. Vanhoutte and Ph. Douste-Blazy (eds.). Paris, John Libbey Eurotext. Pp. 53–62 (1991).

143. Horrobin, D.F. Interactions between $n-3$ and $n-6$ essential fatty acids (EFAs) in the regulation of cardiovascular disorders and inflammation. *Prostaglandins Leukotrienes Essential Fatty Acids* 44:127–131 (1991).

144. Homma, Y., K. Ohshima, H. Yamaguchi, et al. Effects of eicosapentaenoic acid on plasma lipoprotein subfractions and activities of lecithin:cholesterol acyltransferase and lipid transfer protein. *Atherosclerosis* 91:145–153 (1991).

145. Beil, F.U., W. Terres, M. Orgass, and H. Greten. Dietary fish oil lowers lipoprotein(a) in primary hypertriglyceridemia. (Letter.) *Atherosclerosis* 90:95–97 (1991).

146. Dallongeville, J., L. Boulet, J. Davignon, and S. Lussier-Cacan. Fish oil supplementation reduces β-very low density lipoprotein in type III dysbetalipoproteinemia. *Arterioscler. Thromb.* 11:864–871 (1991).

147. Nenseter, M.S., A.C. Rustan, S. Lund-Katz, et al. Effect of dietary supplementation with $n-3$ polyunsaturated fatty acids on physical properties and metabolism of low density lipoprotein in humans. *Arterioscler. Thromb.* 12:369–379 (1992).

148. Ferretti, A., J.T. Judd, R. Ballard-Barbash, et al. Effect of fish oil supplementation on the excretion of the major metabolite of prostaglandin E in healthy male subjects. *Lipids* 26:500–503 (1991).

149. Fumeron, F., L. Brigant, V. Ollivier, et al. $n-3$ Polyunsaturated fatty acids raise low-density lipoproteins, high-density lipoprotein 2, and plasminogen-activator inhibitor in healthy young men. *Am. J. Clin. Nutr.* 54:118–122 (1991).

150. Franceschini, G., L. Calabresi, P. Maderna, et al. ω-3 fatty acids selectively raise high-density lipoprotein 2 levels in healthy volunteers. *Metabolism* 40:1283–1286 (1991).

151. Lindsey, S., A. Pronczuk, and K.C. Hayes. Low density lipoprotein from humans supplemented

with n–3 fatty acids depresses both LDL receptor activity and LDLr mRNA abundance in HepG2 cells. *J. Lipid Res.* 33:647–658 (1992).

152. Bellisola, G., S. Galassini, G. Moschini, et al. Selenium and glutathione peroxidase variations induced by polyunsaturated fatty acids oral supplementation in humans. *Clin. Chim. Acta* 205:75–85 (1992).

153. Kim, D.N., J. Schmee, C.S. Lee, et al. Reductions in serum thromboxane, prostacyclin, and leukotriene B_4 levels in swine fed a fish oil supplement to an atherogenic diet. *Exp. Mol. Pathol.* 55:1–12 (1991).

154. Lottenberg, A.M.P., H.C.F Oliveira, E.R. Nakandakare, and E.C.R. Quintão. Effect of dietary fish oil on the rate of very low density lipoprotein triacylglycerol formation and on the metabolism of chylomicrons. *Lipids* 27:326–330 (1992).

155. Smit, M.J., A.M. Temmerman, H. Wolters, et al. Dietary fish oil–induced changes in intrahepatic cholesterol transport and bile acid synthesis in rats. *J. Clin. Invest.* 88:943–951 (1991).

156. Boudreau, M.D., P.S. Chanmugam, S.B. Hart, et al. Lack of dose response by dietary n–3 fatty acids at a constant ratio of n–3 to n–6 fatty acids in suppressing eicosanoid biosynthesis from arachidonic acid. *Am. J. Clin. Nutr.* 54:111–117 (1991).

157. Parrish, C.C., D.A. Pathy, J.G. Parkes, and A. Angel. Dietary fish oils modify adipocyte structure and function. *J. Cell. Physiol.* 148:493–502 (1991).

158. Yanagita, T., N. Enomoto, and K. Yamamoto. Cholesterol-lowering effect of agemaki, a kind of shellfish, in mice. *J. Nutr. Sci. Vitaminol.* 37:313–318 (1991).

159. Schmidt, E.B., I.C. Klausen, S.D. Kristensen, et al. The effect of n–3 polyunsaturated fatty acids on Lp(a). *Clin. Chim. Acta* 198:271–289 (1991).

160. Brown, S.A., J. Morrisett, J.R. Patasch, et al. Influence of short term dietary cholesterol and fat on human plasma Lp[a] and LDL levels. *J. Lipid Res.* 32:1281–1289 (1991).

161. Luley, C., I. Lelieur, M. Hanisch, et al. Fish oil treatment and apolipoprotein(a). *Drug Res.* 42:77–80 (1992).

162. Hornstra, G., A.C. van Houwelingen, A.D.M. Kester, and K. Sundram. A palm oil–enriched diet lowers serum lipoprotein(a) in normocholesterolemic volunteers. (Letter.) *Atherosclerosis* 90:91–93 (1991).

163. Delplanque, B., J.L. Richard, and B. Jacotot. Influence of diet on the plasma levels and distribution of apoA-1-containing lipoprotein particles. *Prog. Lipid Res.* 30:159–170 (1991).

164. Stucchi, A.F., L.K. Hennessy, D.B. Vespa, et al. Effect of corn and coconut oil–containing diets with and without cholesterol on high density lipoprotein apoprotein A-I metabolism and hepatic apoprotein A-I mRNA levels in cebus monkeys. *Arterioscler. Thromb.* 11:1719–1729 (1991).

165. Srivastava, R.A.K., S. Jiao, J. Tang, et al. In vivo regulation of low-density lipoprotein receptor and apolipoprotein B gene expressions by dietary fat and cholesterol in inbred strains of mice. *Biochim. Biophys. Acta* 1086:29–43 (1991).

166. Srivastava, R.A.K., J. Tang, E.S. Krul, et al. Dietary fatty acids and dietary cholesterol differ in their effect on the in vivo regulation of apolipoprotein A-I and A-II gene expression in inbred strains of mice. *Biochim. Biophys. Acta* 1125:251–261 (1992).

167. Osada, J., A. Fernandez-Sanchez, J.L. Diaz-Morillo, et al. Hepatic expression of apolipoprotein A-I gene in rats is upregulated by monounsaturated fatty acid diet. *Biochem. Biophys. Res. Commun.* 180:162–168 (1991).

168. Harats, D., Y. Dabach, G. Hollander, et al. Fish oil ingestion in smokers and nonsmokers enhances peroxidation of plasma lipoproteins. *Atherosclerosis* 90:127–139 (1991).

169. Reaven, P., S. Parthasarathy, B.J. Grasse, et al. Feasibility of using an oleate-rich diet to reduce the susceptibility of low-density lipoprotein to oxidative modification in humans. *Am. J. Clin. Nutr.* 54:701–706 (1991).

170. Bonanome, A., A. Pagnan, S. Biffanti, et al. Effect of dietary monounsaturated and polyunsaturated fatty acids on the susceptibility of plasma low density lipoproteins to oxidative modification. *Arterioscler. Thromb.* 12:529–533 (1992).

171. Scaccini, C., M. Nardini, M. D'Aquino, et al. Effect of dietary oils on lipid peroxidation and on antioxidant parameters of rat plasma and lipoprotein fractions. *J. Lipid Res.* 33:627–633 (1992).

172. L'Abbé, M.R., K.D. Trick, and J.L. Beare-Rogers. Dietary (n–3) fatty acids affect rat heart, liver, and aorta protective enzyme activities and lipid peroxidation. *J. Nutr.* 121:1331–1340 (1991).

173. Stare, F.J. Nutrition research from respiration and vitamins to cholesterol and atherosclerosis. *Annu. Rev. Nutr.* 11:1–20 (1991).

174. Burr, M.L. *N*-3 and *N*-6 fatty acids, cholesterol, and coronary heart disease. In *Atherosclerosis. Its Pathogenesis and the Role of Cholesterol.* P.C. Weber and A. Leaf (eds.). *Atheroscler. Rev.* 23:251–258 (1991).

175. Israel, D.H., and R. Gorlin. Fish oils in the prevention of atherosclerosis. *J. Am. Coll. Cardiol.* 19:174–185 (1992).

176. Lorenz, R. Ω-3 fatty acids and risk of atherosclerosis. In *Fish Oil and Blood-Vessel Wall Interactions.* Proceedings of the International Symposium, Granada, Spain, 23–25 Feb. 1990. P.M. Vanhoutte and Ph. Douste-Blazy (eds.). Paris, John Libbey Eurotext. Pp. 133–139 (1991).

177. Mancini, M., and M. Parillo. Lipid intake and atherosclerosis. *Ann. Nutr. Metab.* 35(Suppl. 1):103–108 (1991).

178. Kumar, N., and O.P. Singhal. Atherosclerosis: are dairy products safe? *J. Soc. Dairy Technol.* 45(2):49–52(1992).

179. Rapp, J.H., W.E. Connor, D.S. Lin, and J.M. Porter. Dietary eicosapentaenoic acid and docosahexaenoic acid from fish oil. Their incorporation into advanced human atherosclerotic plaques. *Arterioscler. Thromb.* 11:903–911 (1991).

180. Seidelin, K.N., B. Myrup, and B. Fischer-Hansen. *n*-3 fatty acids in adipose tissue and coronary artery disease are inversely related. *Am. J. Clin. Nutr.* 55:1117–1119 (1992).

181. Maron, D.J., J.M. Fair, W.L. Haskell, et al. Saturated fat intake and insulin resistance in men with coronary artery disease. *Circulation* 84:2020–2027 (1991).

182. Rudel, L.L., J.K. Sawyer, and J.S. Parks. Dietary fat, lipoprotein structure, and atherosclerosis in primates. In *Atherosclerosis. Its Pathogenesis and the Role of Cholesterol.* P.C. Weber and A. Leaf (eds.). *Atheroscler. Rev.* 23:41–50 (1991).

183. Kritchevsky, D. Dietary fat and experimental atherosclerosis. *Int. J. Tissue Reactions* 13(2):59–65 (1991).

184. Greenberg, B. Effects of dietary fish oil in experimental models of atherosclerosis. In *Fish Oil and Blood-Vessel Wall Interactions.* Proceedings of the International Symposium, Granada, Spain, 23–25 Feb. 1990. P.M. Vanhoutte and Ph. Douste-Blazy (eds.). Paris, John Libbey Eurotext. Pp. 81–88 (1991).

185. Hodis, H.N., D.W. Crawford, and A. Sevanian. Cholesterol feeding increases plasma and aortic tissue cholesterol oxide levels in parallel: further evidence for the role of cholesterol oxidation in atherosclerosis. *Atherosclerosis* 89:117–126 (1991).

186. Kim, D.N., J. Schmee, C.S. Lee, et al. Comparison of effects of fish oil and corn oil supplements on hyperlipidemic diet induced atherogenesis in swine. *Atherosclerosis* 89:191–201 (1991).

187. Thomas, L.H. Ischaemic heart disease and consumption of hydrogenated marine oils in England and Wales. *J. Epidemiol. Commun. Health* 46:78–82 (1992).

188. Saynor, R., and T. Gillott. Long-term reduction in re-infarction rate, blood fibrinogen, and triglyceride and total cholesterol in patients taking Ω-3 fatty acids for ischaemic heart disease. In *Fish Oil and Blood-Vessel Wall Interactions.* Proceedings of the International Symposium, Granada, Spain, 23–25 Feb. 1990. P.M. Vanhoutte and Ph. Douste-Blazy (eds.). Paris, John Libbey Eurotext. Pp. 149–160 (1991).

189. Kaul, U., S. Sanghvi, V.K. Bahl, et al. Fish oil supplements for prevention of restenosis after coronary angioplasty. *Int. J. Cardiol.* 35:87–93 (1992).

190. Bairati, I., L. Roy, and F. Meyer. Double-blind, randomized, controlled trial of fish oil supplements in prevention of recurrence of stenosis after coronary angioplasty. *Circulation* 85:950–956 (1992).

191. Schuler, G., R. Hambrecht, G. Schlierf, et al. Myocardial perfusion and regression of coronary artery disease in patients on a regimen of intensive physical exercise and low fat diet. *J. Am. Coll. Cardiol.* 19:34–42 (1992).

192. Charnock, J.S., P.L. McLennan, K. Sundram, and M.Y. Abeywardena. Omega-3 PUFA's reduce the vulnerability of the rat heart to ischaemic arrhythmia in the presence of a high intake of saturated animal fat. *Nutr. Res.* 11:1025–1034 (1991).

193. Leprán, I., and L. Szekeres. Effect of dietary sunflower seed oil on the severity of reperfusion-induced arrhythmias in anesthetized rats. *J. Cardiovasc. Pharmacol.* 10:40–44 (1992).

194. Lehr, H.A., M.D. Menger, D. Nolte, and K. Messmer. Favorable effects of dietary fish oil on capillary perfusion homogeneity after ischemia and reperfusion. *Transplant. Proc.* 23:2356–2358 (1991).

195. Paulson, D.J., J.M. Smith, J. Zhao, and J. Bowman. Effects of dietary fish oil on myocardial ischemic/reperfusion injury of Wistar Kyoto and stroke-prone spontaneously hypertensive rats. *Metabolism* 41:533–539 (1992).

196. Papies, B., I. Schimke, V. Moritz, et al. Ischemic myocardial damage in spontaneously hypertensive rats (SHR) is enhanced after long-term feeding of an alpha-linolenic acid enriched diet. *Prostaglandins Leukotrienes Essential Fatty Acids* 43:111–117 (1991).

197. Lee, J.H., I. Ikeda, and M. Sugano. Dietary cholesterol influences on various lipid indices and eicosanoid production in rats fed dietary fat desirable for the protection of ischemic heart disease. *J. Nutr. Sci. Vitaminol.* 37:389–399 (1991).

198. Salonen, J.T. Dietary fats, antioxidants and blood pressure. *Ann. Med.* 23:295–298 (1991).

199. Kenny, D. The paradoxical effects of dietary fish oil on blood pressure. *Med. Hypoth.* 37:97–99 (1992).

200. Singer, P. α-Linolenic acid vs. long-chain *n*–3 fatty acids in hypertension and hyperlipidemia. *Nutrition* 8:133–135 (1992).

201. Oh, S.Y., J. Ryue, C.-H. Hsieh, and D.E. Bell. Eggs enriched in ω-3 fatty acids and alterations in lipid concentrations in plasma and lipoproteins and in blood pressure. *Am. J. Clin. Nutr.* 54:689–695 (1991).

202. Manatt, M.W., P.A. Garcia, C. Kies, and J. Dupont. Studies of women eating diets with different fatty acid composition. II. Urinary eicosanoids and sodium, and blood pressure. *J. Am. Coll. Nutr.* 10:322–326 (1991).

203. Radack, K., C. Deck, and G. Huster. The effects of low doses of *n*–3 fatty acid supplementation on blood pressure in hypertensive subjects. *Arch. Intern. Med.* 151:1173–1180 (1991).

204. Cobiac, L., P.J. Nestel, L.M.H. Wing, and P.R.C. Howe. Effects of dietary sodium restriction and fish oil supplements on blood pressure in the elderly. *Clin. Exp. Pharmacol. Physiol.* 18:265–268 (1991).

205. Cobiac, L., P.J. Nestel, L.M.H. Wing, and P.R.C. Howe. A low-sodium diet supplemented with fish oil lowers blood pressure in the elderly. *J. Hypertens.* 10:87–92 (1992).

206. Howe, P.R.C., Y.K. Lungershausen, P.F. Rogers, et al. Effects of dietary sodium and fish oil on blood pressure development in stroke-prone spontaneously hypertensive rats. *J. Hypertens.* 9:639–644 (1991).

207. Howe, P.R.C., P.F. Rogers, and Y. Lungershausen. Blood pressure reduction by fish oil in adult rats with established hypertension—dependence on sodium intake. *Prostaglandins Leukotrienes Essential Fatty Acids* 44:113–117 (1991).

208. Head, R.J., M.T. Mano, S. Bexis, et al. Dietary fish oil administration retards the development of hypertension and influences vascular neuroeffector function in the stroke prone spontaneously hypertensive rat (SHRSP). *Prostaglandins Leukotrienes Essential Fatty Acids* 44:119–122 (1991).

209. Shimamura, T., and A.C. Wilson. Influence of dietary fish oil on the aortic, myocardial, and renal lesions of SHR. *J. Nutr. Sci. Vitaminol.* 37:581–590 (1991).

210. Dierberger, B., M. Schäch, I. Anadere, et al. Effect of a diet rich in linseed oil on complex viscosity and blood pressure in spontaneously hypertensive rats (SHR). *Basic Res. Cardiol.* 86:561–566 (1991).

211. St. Louis, C., R.M.K.W. Lee, J. Rosenfeld, and A. Fargas-Babjak. Antihypertensive effect of γ-linolenic acid in spontaneously hypertensive rats. *Hypertension* 19(Suppl. II):II-111–II-115 (1992).

212. Mills, D.E., R.P. Ward, D. McCutcheon, et al. Attenuation of cyclosporine-induced hypertension by dietary fatty acids in the borderline hypertensive rat. *Transplantation* 53:649–654 (1992).

213. Renaud, S. Fatty acids (Ω-3), platelets and coronary disease. In *Fish Oil and Blood-Vessel Wall Interactions*. Proceedings of the International Symposium, Granada, Spain, 23–25 Feb. 1990. P.M. Vanhoutte and Ph. Douste-Blazy (eds.). Paris, John Libbey Eurotext. Pp. 141–147 (1991).

214. Bang, H.O. Coronary heart disease and Ω-3: epidemiological aspects. In *Fish Oil and Blood-Vessel Wall Interactions*. Proceedings of the International Symposium, Granada, Spain, 23–25 Feb. 1990. P.M. Vanhoutte and Ph. Douste-Blazy (eds.). Paris, John Libbey Eurotext. Pp. 109–116 (1991).

215. Lagarde, M., M. Groset, and M. Hajarine. Interaction between Ω-3 fatty acid and platelet phospholipids. In *Fish Oil and Blood-Vessel Wall Interactions*. Proceedings of the International Symposium, Granada, Spain, 23–25 Feb. 1990. P.M. Vanhoutte and Ph. Douste-Blazy (eds.). Paris, John Libbey Eurotext. Pp. 63–67 (1991).

216. Force, T., R. Milani, P. Hibberd, et al. Aspirin-induced decline in prostacyclin production in patients

with coronary artery disease is due to decreased endoperoxidase shift. Analysis of the effects of a combination of aspirin and *n*–3 fatty acids on the eicosanoid profile. *Circulation* 84:2286–2293 (1991).

217. Vane, J.R., and R.M. Botting. Heart disease, aspirin, and fish oil. (Editorial.) *Circulation* 84:2588–2590 (1991).

218. Akoh, C.C., and J.O. Hearnsberger. Effect of catfish and salmon diet on platelet phospholipid and blood clotting in healthy men. *J. Nutr. Biochem.* 2:329–333 (1991).

219. Wander, R.C., and B.D. Patton. Comparison of three species of fish consumed as part of a Western diet: effects on platelet fatty acids and function, hemostasis, and production of thromboxane. *Am. J. Clin. Nutr.* 54:326–333 (1991).

220. Ågren, J.J., H. Pekkarinen, H. Litmanen, and O. Hänninen. Fish diet and physical fitness in relation to membrane and serum lipids, prostanoid metabolism and platelet aggregation in female students. *Eur. J. Appl. Physiol.* 63:393–398 (1991).

221. Brown, A.J., and D.C.K. Roberts. Fish and fish oil intake: effect on haematological variables related to cardiovascular disease. *Thromb. Res.* 64:169–178 (1991).

222. Stroh, S., and I. Elmadfa. In-vitro-Untersuchungen zum Einfluß verschiedener Mischungsverhältnisse an ω-3- und ω-6-Fettsäuren auf die Thrombozytenaggregation und Thromboxansynthese in Humanthrombozyten. *Z. Ernährungswiss.* 30:192–200 (1991).

223. Malle, E., W. Sattler, E. Prenner, et al. Effects of dietary fish oil supplementation on platelet aggregability and platelet membrane fluidity in normolipemic subjects with and without high plasma Lp(a) concentrations. *Atherosclerosis* 88:193–200 (1991).

224. Vanderhoek, J.Y., N.W. Schoene, and P.-P.T. Pham. Inhibitory potencies of fish oil hydroxy fatty acids on cellular lipoxygenases and platelet aggregation. *Biochem. Pharmacol.* 42:959–962 (1991).

225. O'Keefe, S.F., M. Lagarde, A. Grandgirard, and J.L. Sebedio. *Trans n*–3 eicosapentaenoic and docosahexaenoic acid isomers exhibit different inhibitory effects on arachidonic acid metabolism in human platelets compared to the respective *cis* fatty acids. *J. Lipid Res.* 31:1241–1246 (1990).

226. Batres-Cerezo, R., J. Dupont, P.A. Garcia, et al. Studies of women eating diets with different fatty acid composition. III. Fatty acids and prostaglandin synthesis by platelets and cultured human endothelial cells. *J. Am. Coll. Nutr.* 10:327–339 (1991).

227. Beswick, A.D., A.M. Gehily, D.S. Sharp, et al. Long-term diet modification and platelet activity. *J. Intern. Med.* 229:511–515 (1991).

228. Kwon, J.-S., J.T. Snook, G.M. Wardlaw, and D.H. Hwang. Effects of diets high in saturated fatty acids, canola oil, or safflower oil on platelet function, thromboxane B_2 formation, and fatty acid composition of platelet phospholipids. *Am. J. Clin. Nutr.* 54:351–358 (1991).

229. Barre, D.E., and B.J. Holub. The effect of borage oil consumption on the composition of individual phospholipids in human platelets. *Lipids* 27:315–320 (1992).

230. Burri, B.J., R.M. Dougherty, D.S. Kelley, and J.M. Iacono. Platelet aggregation in humans is affected by replacement of dietary linoleic acid with oleic acid. *Am. J. Clin. Nutr.* 54:359–362 (1991).

231. Mutanen, M., R. Freese, L.M. Valsta, et al. Rapeseed oil and sunflower oil diets enhance platelet in vitro aggregation and thromboxane production in healthy men when compared with milk fat or habitual diets. *Thromb. Haemostasis* 67:352–356 (1992).

232. Bandyopadhyay, I., S. Saha, and J. Dutta. Effect of dietary fish oil on platelet aggregability: comparison between two oils with different eicosapentaenoic to arachidonic acid ratio. *Biochem. Int.* 25:919–928 (1991).

233. Heemskerk, J.W.M., M.A.H. Feijge, A. Kester, and G. Hornstra. Dietary fat modifies thromboxane A_2-induced stimulation of rat platelets. *Biochem. J.* 278:399–404 (1991).

234. Krumhardt, B., and J. Dupont. Rat platelet phospholipase A_2 activity and thromboxane synthesis are concomitantly affected by dietary linoleic acid. *J. Nutr. Biochem.* 2:443–448 (1991).

235. Brown, A.J., E. Pang, and D.C.K. Roberts. Persistent changes in the fatty acid composition of erythrocyte membranes after moderate intake of *n*–3 polyunsaturated fatty acids: study design implications. *Am. J. Clin. Nutr.* 54:668–673 (1991).

236. Ågren, J.J., and O.O. Hänninen. Effect of moderate freshwater fish diet on erythrocyte ghost phospholipid fatty acids. *Ann. Med.* 23:261–263 (1991).

237. Gibson, R.A., M.A. Neuman, S.L. Burnard, et al. The effect of dietary supplementation with eicosapentaenoic acid on the phospholipid and fatty acid composition of erythrocytes of marmoset. *Lipids* 27:169–176 (1992).

238. Semplicini, A., E. Casiglia, M. Marzola, et al. Effects of linoleic acid supplementation on blood pressure and kinetics of red cell sodium transport: the Piove di Sacco study. *J. Hypertens.* 9(Suppl. 6):S310–S311 (1991).

239. Vajreswari, A., and K. Narayanareddy. Effect of dietary fats on erythrocyte membrane lipid composition and membrane-bound enzyme activities. *Metabolism* 41:352–358 (1992).

240. Hagve, T.-A., Y. Johansen, and B. Christophersen. The effect of n–3 fatty acids on osmotic fragility of rat erythrocytes. *Biochim. Biophys. Acta* 1084:251–254 (1991).

241. Corbett, R., J.-F. Ménez, H.H. Floch, and B.E. Leonard. The effects of chronic ethanol administration on rat liver and erythrocyte lipid composition: modulatory role of evening primrose oil. *Alcohol Alcoholism* 26:459–464 (1991).

242. Sakai, K., and H. Okuyama. Effects of a high α-linolenate and high linoleate diet on hemolysis and lipid peroxidation of rat erythrocytes. *Chem. Pharm. Bull.* 39:1504–1506 (1991).

243. van den Berg, J.J.M., N.J. de Fouw, F.A. Kuypers, et al. Increased n–3 polyunsaturated fatty acid content of red blood cells from fish oil–fed rabbits increases in vitro lipid peroxidation, but decreases hemolysis. *Free Rad. Biol. Med.* 11:393–399 (1991).

244. Vanhoutte, P.M., and Ph. Douste-Blazy (eds.). *Fish Oil and Blood-Vessel Wall Interactions.* Proceedings of the International Symposium, Granada, Spain, 23–25 Feb. 1990. Paris, John Libbey Eurotext (1991).

245. Boulanger, C., V.B. Schini, H. Shimokawa, et al. Effect of chronic exposure to cod liver oil and Ω-3 unsaturated fatty acids on endothelium-dependent relaxations. In *Fish Oil and Blood-Vessel Wall Interactions.* Proceedings of the International Symposium, Granada, Spain, 23–25 Feb. 1990. P.M. Vanhoutte and Ph. Douste-Blazy (eds.). Paris, John Libbey Eurotext. Pp. 89–97 (1991).

246. Lehr, H.-A., C. Hübner, B. Finckh, et al. Dietary fish oil reduces leukocyte/endothelium interaction following systemic administration of oxidatively modified low density lipoprotein. *Circulation* 84:1725–1731 (1991).

247. Locher, R., A. Sachinidis, C. Brunner, and W. Vetter. Intracellular free calcium concentration and thromboxane A_2 formation of vascular smooth muscle cells are influenced by fish oil and n–3 eicosapentaenoic acid. *Scand. J. Clin. Lab. Invest.* 51:541–547 (1991).

248. Faraci, F.M., M.L. Armstrong, and D.D. Heistad. Dietary treatment of atherosclerosis abolishes hyperresponsiveness of retinal blood vessels to serotonin in monkeys. *Stroke* 22:1405–1408 (1991).

249. Ludwig, M., K.-O. Stumpe, A. Sauer, et al. Short-term high dietary cholesterol in early life induces persistent increases in arterial wall thickness and vascular reactivity to noradrenaline. *J. Hypertens.* 9(Suppl. 6):S136–S147 (1991).

250. Engler, M.M., J.W. Karanian, and N. Salem, Jr. Influence of dietary polyunsaturated fatty acids on aortic and platelet fatty acid composition in the rat. *Nutr. Res.* 11:753–763 (1991).

251. Engler, M.M., J.W. Karanian, and N. Salem, Jr. Ethanol inhalation and dietary n–6, n–3, and n–9 fatty acids in the rat: effect on platelet and aortic fatty acid composition. *Alcoholism Clin. Exp. Res.* 15:483–488 (1991).

252. Malis, C.D., A. Leaf, G.S. Varadarajan, et al. Effects of dietary ω-3 fatty acids on vascular contractility in preanoxic and postanoxic aortic rings. *Circulation* 84:1393–1401 (1991).

253. Edwards, I.J., A.K. Gebre, W.D. Wagner, and J.S. Parks. Reduced proteoglycan binding of low density lipoproteins from monkeys (*Macaca fascicularis*) fed a fish oil versus lard diet. *Arterioscler. Thromb.* 11:1778–1785 (1991).

254. Bruckner, G. Ω-3 fatty acids and microcirculation. In *Fish Oil and Blood-Vessel Wall Interactions.* Proceedings of the International Symposium, Granada, Spain, 23–25 Feb. 1990. P.M. Vanhoutte and Ph. Douste-Blazy (eds.). Paris, John Libbey Eurotext. Pp. 99–107 (1991).

255. Lehr, H.-A., C. Hübner, D. Nolte, et al. Dietary fish oil blocks the microcirculatory manifestations of ischemia–reperfusion injury in striated muscle in hamsters. *Proc. Natl. Acad. Sci. USA* 88:6726–6730 (1991).

256. Ellis, E.F., R.J. Police, L.Y. Dodson, et al. Effect of dietary n–3 fatty acids on cerebral microcirculation. *Am. J. Physiol.* 262:H1379–H1386 (1992).

257. Lee, A.G. Lipids and their effects on membrane proteins: evidence against a role for fluidity. *Prog. Lipid Res.* 30:323–348 (1991).

258. Vajreswari, A., and K. Narayanareddy. Effect of dietary fats on some membrane-bound enzyme activities, membrane lipid composition and fatty acid profiles of rat heart sarcolemma. *Lipids* 27:339–343 (1992).

259. McMurchie, E.J., S.L. Burnard, J.A. Rinaldi, et al. Cardiac membrane lipid composition and adenylate cyclase activity following dietary eicosapentaenoic acid supplementation in the marmoset monkey. *J. Nutr. Biochem.* 3:13–22 (1992).

260. Heinrich, J., U. Wahrburg, H. Martin, and G. Assmann. The effect of diets, rich in mono- or polyunsaturated fatty acids, on lipid metabolism and haemostasis. *Fibrinolysis* 4(Suppl. 2):76–78 (1990).

261. Müllertz, A., G. Hølmer, and J. Grøndahl-Hansen. Increased concentration of plasminogen activator inhibitor type-1 in plasma after intake of fish oil. *Fibrinolysis* 4(Suppl. 2):86–88 (1990).

262. Stewart-Phillips, J.L., J. Lough, and N.C. Phillips. The effect of a high-fat diet on murine macrophage activity. *Int. J. Immunopharmacol.* 13:325–332 (1991).

263. Steinberg, D. Antioxidants and atherosclerosis. A current assessment. (Editorial.) *Circulation* 84:1420–1424 (1991).

264. Duthie, G.G., C.T. Shortt, J.D. Robertson, et al. Plasma antioxidants, indices of lipid peroxidation and coronary heart disease risk factors in a Scottish population. *Nutr. Res.* 12(Suppl. 1):S61–S67 (1992).

265. Janero, D.R. Therapeutic potential of vitamin E in the pathogenesis of spontaneous atherosclerosis. *Free Rad. Biol. Med.* 11:129–144 (1991).

266. Pronczuk, A., Y. Kipervarg, and K.C. Hayes. Vegetarians have higher plasma alpha-tocopherol relative to cholesterol than do nonvegetarians. *J. Am. Coll. Nutr.* 11:50–55 (1992).

267. Wahlqvist, M.L., Z. Krivokuca-Bogetic, C.S. Lo, et al. Differential serum responses of tocopherols and tocotrienols during vitamin supplementation in hypercholesterolaemic individuals without change in coronary risk factors. *Nutr. Res.* 12(Suppl. 1):S181–S201 (1992).

268. Dieber-Rotheneder, M., H. Puhl, G. Waeg, et al. Effect of oral supplementation with D-α-tocopherol on the vitamin E content of human low density lipoproteins and resistance to oxidation. *J. Lipid Res.* 32:1325–1332 (1991).

269. Princen, H.M.G., G. van Poppel, C. Vogelezang, et al. Supplementation with vitamin E but not β-carotene in vivo protects low density lipoprotein from lipid peroxidation in vitro. Effect of cigarette smoking. *Arterioscler. Thromb.* 12:554–562 (1992).

270. DeMaio, S.J., S.B. King, III, N.J. Lembo, et al. Vitamin E supplementation, plasma lipids and incidence of restenosis after percutaneous transluminal coronary angioplasty (PTCA). *J. Am. Coll. Nutr.* 11:68–73 (1992).

271. Steiner, M. Influence of vitamin E on platelet function in humans. *J. Am. Coll. Nutr.* 10:466–473 (1991).

272. Verlangieri, A.J., and M.J. Bush. Effects of d-α-tocopherol supplementation on experimentally induced primate atherosclerosis. *J. Am. Coll. Nutr.* 11:131–138 (1992).

273. Kumar, C.T., V.K. Reddy, M. Prasad, et al. Dietary supplementation of vitamin E protects heart tissue from exercise-induced oxidant stress. *Mol. Cell. Biochem.* 111:109–115 (1992).

274. Simon, J.A. Vitamin C and cardiovascular disease: a review. *J. Am. Coll. Nutr.* 11:107–125 (1992).

275. McBride, J. Woes of a fruitless diet. *Agric. Res.* 40(5):13 (1992).

276. Jacques, P.F. Effects of vitamin C on high-density lipoprotein cholesterol and blood pressure. *J. Am. Coll. Nutr.* 11:139–144 (1992).

277. Hemilä, H. Vitamin C and lowering of blood pressure: need for intervention trials? (Letter.) *J. Hypertens.* 9:1076–1078 (1991).

278. Frei, B. Ascorbic acid protects lipids in human plasma and low-density lipoprotein against oxidative damage. *Am. J. Clin. Nutr.* 54:1113S–1118S (1991).

279. Chakrabarty, S., A. Nandi, C.K. Mukhopadhyay, and I.B. Chatterjee. Protective role of ascorbic acid against lipid peroxidation and myocardial injury. *Mol. Cell. Biochem.* 111:41–47 (1992).

280. Gerster, H. Potential role of beta-carotene in the prevention of cardiovascular disease. *Int. J. Vit. Nutr. Res.* 61:277–291 (1991).

281. Cabré, E., J.L. Periago, M.D. Mingorance, et al. Factors related to the plasma fatty acid profile in

healthy subjects, with special reference to antioxidant micronutrient status: a multivariate analysis. *Am. J. Clin. Nutr.* 55:831–837 (1992).

282. Smith, L.L. Another cholesterol hypothesis: cholesterol as antioxidant. *Free Rad. Biol. Med.* 11:47–61 (1991).

283. Kotchen, T.A., J.M. Kotchen, and M.A. Boegehold. Nutrition and hypertension prevention. *Hypertension* 18(Suppl. I):I-115–I-120 (1991).

284. Karppanen, H. Minerals and blood pressure. *Ann. Med.* 23:299–305 (1991).

285. Kesteloot, H. Relationship between dietary cations and blood pressure. *Ann. Nutr. Metab.* 35(Suppl. 1):109–118 (1991).

286. McCarron, D.A., and F.C. Luft. Heterogenität der Hypertonie: die unterschiedlichen Einflüsse der Elektrolytzufuhr. *Klin. Wochenschr.* 69(Suppl. XXV):97–102 (1991).

287. Marier, J.R. Dietary magnesium and drinking water: effects on human health status. In *Compendium on Magnesium and Its Role in Biology, Nutrition, and Physiology*. H. Sigel and A. Sigel (eds.). *Metal Ions in Biological Systems* 26:85–104 (1990).

288. Singh, R.B., S.S. Rastogi, U.V. Mani, et al. Does dietary magnesium modulate blood lipids? *Biol. Trace Elem. Res.* 30:59–64 (1991).

289. Hsieh, S.-T., H. Sano, K. Saito, et al. Magnesium supplementation prevents the development of alcohol-induced hypertension. *Hypertension* 19:175–182 (1992).

290. Siani, A., P. Strazzullo, A. Giacco, et al. Increasing the dietary potassium intake reduces the need for antihypertensive medication. *Ann. Intern. Med.* 115:753–759 (1991).

291. Overlack, A., H. Conrad, and K.O. Stumpe. The influence of oral potassium citrate/bicarbonate on blood pressure in essential hypertension during unrestricted salt intake. *Klin. Wochenschr.* 69(Suppl. XXV):79–83 (1991).

292. Mervaala, E.M.A., J.-J. Himberg, J. Laakso, et al. Beneficial effects of a potassium- and magnesium-enriched salt alternative. *Hypertension* 19:535–540 (1992).

293. Ganguli, M., and L. Tobian. In SHR rats, dietary potassium determines NaCl sensitivity in NaCl-induced rises of blood pressure. *Clin. Exp. Hypertens. Theory Pract.* A13:677–685 (1991).

294. McCarron, D.A. Epidemiological evidence and clinical trials of dietary calcium's effect on blood pressure. In *Calcium-Regulating Hormones. I. Role in Disease and Aging*. H. Morii (ed.). *Contrib. Nephrol.* 90:2–10 (1991).

295. McCarron, D.A., C.D. Morris, E. Young, et al. Dietary calcium and blood pressure: modifying factors in specific populations. *Am. J. Clin. Nutr.* 54:215S–219S (1991).

296. Saito, K., H. Sano, Y. Furata, et al. Calcium supplementation in salt-dependent hypertension. In *Calcium-Regulating Hormones. I. Role in Disease and Aging*. H. Morii (ed.). *Contrib. Nephrol.* 90:22–35 (1991).

297. Van der Vijver, L.P.L., M.A.E. van der Waal, K.G.C. Weterings, et al. Calcium intake and 28-year cardiovascular and coronary heart disease mortality in Dutch civil servants. *Int. J. Epidemiol.* 21:36–39 (1992).

298. Gillman, M.W., S.A. Oliveria, L.L. Moore, and R.C. Ellison. Inverse association of dietary calcium with systolic blood pressure in young children. *JAMA* 267:2340–2343 (1992).

299. Belizán, J.M., J. Villar, L. Gonzalez, et al. Calcium supplementation to prevent hypertensive disorders of pregnancy. *New Engl. J. Med.* 325:1399–1405 (1991).

300. Knight, K.B., and R.E. Keith. Calcium supplementation on normotensive and hypertensive pregnant women. *Am. J. Clin. Nutr.* 55:891–895 (1992).

301. Seely, S. Is calcium excess in Western diet a major cause of arterial disease? (Editorial.) *Int. J. Cardiol.* 33:191–198 (1991).

302. Peuler, J.D. Contrasting hemodynamic effects of high oral calcium in genetic models of salt-sensitive hypertension. *Clin. Exp. Hypertens. Theory Pract.* A13:709–717 (1991).

303. Hano, T., A. Baba, J. Takeda, et al. Antihypertensive effects of oral calcium supplementation in spontaneously hypertensive rats. In *Calcium-Regulating Hormones. I. Role in Disease and Aging*. H. Morii (ed.). *Contrib. Nephrol.* 90:36–41 (1991).

304. Oparil, S., Y.-F. Chen, H. Jin, et al. Dietary Ca^{2+} prevents NaCl-sensitive hypertension in spontaneously hypertensive rats via sympatholytic and renal effects. *Am. J. Clin. Nutr.* 54:227S–236S (1991).

305. Fujito, K., M. Yokomatsu, N. Ishiguro, et al. Effects of dietary calcium on erythrocyte sodium ion transport systems in spontaneously hypertensive rats.

In *Calcium-Regulating Hormones. I. Role in Disease and Aging.* H. Morii (ed.). *Contrib. Nephrol.* 90:54–58(1991).

306. Oshima, T., E.W. Young, K. Hermsmeyer, and D.A. McCarron. Modification of platelet and lymphocyte calcium handling and blood pressure by dietary sodium and calcium in genetically hypertensive rats. *J. Lab. Clin. Med.* 119:151–158 (1992).

307. Folkow, B. Critical review of studies on salt and hypertension. *Clin. Exp. Hypertens. Theory Pract.* A14:1–14 (1992).

308. Luft, F.C., and K.O. Stumpe (eds.) *Sodium Restriction as a Public Health Measure for the General Population.* International Symposium, Bonn, Oct. 5, 1990. *Klin. Wochenschr.* 69(Suppl. XXV) (1991).

309. Elliott, P. Sodium and blood pressure: a review of the evidence from controlled trials of sodium reduction and epidemiological studies. *Klin. Wochenschr.* 69(Suppl. XXV):3–10 (1991).

310. Hense, H.-W. Are the conclusions of INTERSALT applicable to the German population? *Klin. Wochenschr.* 69(Suppl. XXV):11–16 (1991);.

311. Cappuccio, F.P., N.D. Markandu, and G.A. MacGregor. Dietary salt intake and hypertension. *Klin. Wochenschr.* 69(Suppl. XXV):17–25 (1991).

312. Heagerty, A.M. Salt restriction, a sceptic's viewpoint. *Klin. Wochenschr.* 69(Suppl. XXV):26–29 (1991).

313. Watt, G.C.M. Does salt sensitivity exist? *Klin. Wochenschr.* 69(Suppl. XXV):30–35 (1991).

314. Skrabal, F., P. Kotanko, P. Wach, et al. Weitere Fortschritte bei der Salzsensitivitätshypothese beim Menschen. *Klin. Wochenschr.* 69(Suppl. XXV):36–40 (1991).

315. Blaustein, M.P., and J.M. Hamlyn. Pathogenesis of essential hypertension. A link between dietary salt and high blood pressure. *Hypertension* 18(Suppl. III):III-184–III-195 (1991).

316. Law, M.R., C.D. Frost, and N.J. Wald. Dietary salt and blood pressure. *J. Hypertens.* 9(Suppl. 6):S37–S41 (1991).

317. Swales, J.D. Dietary salt and blood pressure: the role of meta-analysis. *J. Hypertens.* 9(Suppl. 6):S42–S46 (1991).

318. Benetos, A., Y.-Y. Xiao, J.-L. Cuche, et al. Arterial effects of salt restriction in hypertensive patients. A 9-week, randomized, double-blind, crossover study. *J. Hypertens.* 10:355–360 (1992).

319. Feldman, R.D. A low-sodium diet corrects the defect in β-adrenergic response in older subjects. *Circulation* 85:612–618 (1992).

320. Turkkan, J.S., and D.S. Goldstein. Stress and sodium hypertension in baboons: neuroendocrine and pharmacotherapeutic assessments. *J. Hypertens.* 9:969–975 (1991).

321. Vasan, R.S., and J. Narula. Hypertension to normotension—? A case of 'summer-salt'. (Letter.) *Int. J. Cardiol.* 33:179–180 (1991).

322. Ruppert, M., J. Diehl, R. Kolloch, et al. Short-term dietary sodium restriction increases serum lipids and insulin in salt-sensitive and salt-resistant normotensive adults. *Klin. Wochenschr.* 69(Suppl. XXV):51–57 (1991).

323. Weder, A.B., and B.M. Egan. Potential deleterious impact of dietary salt restriction on cardiovascular risk factors. *Klin. Wochenschr.* 69(Suppl. XXV):45–50 (1991).

324. Ely, D.L., N.F. Paradise, and B. Folkow. Blood pressure and neurogenic adaptations to reduced dietary sodium in the SHR model of hypertension. *Klin. Wochenschr.* 69(Suppl. XXV):58–72 (1991).

325. Drüeke, T.B., and M. Muntzel. Heterogeneity of blood pressure responses to salt restriction and salt appetite in rats. *Klin. Wochenschr.* 69(Suppl. XXV):73–78 (1991).

326. Blizard, D.A., W.N. Peterson, S.S. Iskandar, et al. The effect of a high salt diet and gender on blood pressure, urinary protein excretion and renal pathology in SHR rats. *Clin. Exp. Hypertens. Theory Pract.* A13:687–697 (1991).

327. Yuan, B., and F.H.H. Leenen. Dietary sodium intake and left ventricular hypertrophy in normotensive rats. *Am. J. Physiol.* 261:H1397–H1401 (1991).

328. Takahashi, N., M. Iwama, M. Horiguichi, et al. Long-term exposure of Wistar rats to high dietary sodium chloride level. I. Changes in aortic connective tissue components. *Int. J. Vit. Nutr. Res.* 62:47–53 (1991).

329. Sharma, A.M., S. Schattenfroh, H.-M. Thiede, et al. Effects of sodium salts on pressor reactivity in salt-sensitive men. *Hypertension* 19:541–548 (1992).

330. Reusch, H.P., and F.C. Luft. Die Rolle des Chlorids in der Natrium-induzierten „salzsensitiven" Hypertonie. *Klin. Wochenschr.* 69(Suppl. XXV):90–96 (1991).

331. Sato, Y., E. Ogata, and T. Fujita. Role of chloride in angiotensin II-induced salt-sensitive hypertension. *Hypertension* 18:622–629 (1991).

332. Jacob, B.G., and P. Schwandt. Cholesterin-senkende Wirkung von Knoblauch? *Dtsch. Med. Wochenschr.* 117:397–398 (1992).

333. Mansell, P., and J.P.D. Reckless. Garlic. Effects on serum lipids, blood pressure, coagulation, platelet aggregation, and vasodilatation. *Br. Med. J.* 303:379–380 (1991).

334. Brosche, T., and D. Platt. (Letter.) Garlic. *Br. Med. J.* 303:785 (1991).

335. Sendl, A., M. Schliack, R. Löser, et al. Inhibition of cholesterol synthesis in vitro by extracts and isolated compounds prepared from garlic and wild garlic. *Atherosclerosis* 94:79–85 (1992).

336. Lawson, L.D., D.K. Ransom, and B.G. Hughes. Inhibition of whole blood platelet-aggregation by compounds in garlic clove extracts and commercial garlic products. *Thromb. Res.* 65:141–156 (1992).

337. Aqel, M.B., M.N. Gharaibah, and A.S. Salhab. Direct relaxant effects of garlic juice on smooth and cardiac muscles. *J. Ethnopharmacol.* 33:13–19 (1991).

338. Koch, H.P., W. Jäger, J. Hysek, and B. Körpert. Garlic and onion extracts. In vitro inhibition of adenosine deaminase. *Phytother. Res.* 5:50–52 (1992).

339. Teng, C.-M., F.-N. Ko, J.-P. Wang, et al. Antihaemostatic and antithrombotic effect of some antiplatelet agents isolated from Chinese herbs. *J. Pharm. Pharmacol.* 43:667–669 (1991).

340. Wang, H.-F., X. Li, Y.-M. Chen, et al. Radiation-protective and platelet aggregation inhibitory effects of five traditional Chinese drugs and acetylsalicylic acid following high-dose γ-irradiation. *J. Ethnopharmacol.* 34:215–219 (1991).

341. Srinivasan, K., and K. Sambaiah. The effect of spices on cholesterol 7α-hydroxylase activity and on serum and hepatic cholesterol levels in the rat. *Int. J. Vit. Nutr. Res.* 61:364–369 (1991).

342. Reddy, A.Ch.P., and B.R. Lokesh. Studies on spice principles as antioxidants in the inhibition of lipid peroxidation of rat liver microsomes. *Mol. Cell. Biochem.* 111:117–124 (1992).

343. Buonopane, G.J., A. Kilara, J.S. Smith, and R.D. McCarthy. Effect of skim milk supplementation on blood cholesterol concentration, blood pressure, and triglycerides in a free-living human population. *J. Am. Coll. Nutr.* 11:56–67 (1992).

344. Aggarwal, R.A.K., and V.K. Kansal. Influence of skim milk on plasma lipids, lipoproteins and lecithin: cholesterol acyltransferase activity in cholesterol fed rabbits. *Milchwissenschaft* 46:355–357 (1991).

345. Aggarwal, A.K., and V.K. Kansal. Regression of atherosclerosis in rabbit on skim milk diet. *Milchwissenschaft* 46:766–769 (1991).

346. Jiménez, J., J. Boza, Jr., M.D. Suárez, and A. Gil. Changes in fatty acid profiles of red blood cell membranes mediated by dietary nucleotides in weanling rats. *J. Pediatr. Gastroenterol. Nutr.* 14:293–299 (1992).

347. Kaplan, N. Bashing booze: the danger of losing the benefits of moderate alcohol consumption. *Am. Heart J.* 121:1854–1856 (1991).

348. Renaud, S.C., A.D. Beswick, A.M. Fehily, et al. Alcohol and platelet aggregation: the Caerphilly Prospective Heart Disease Study. *Am. J. Clin. Nutr.* 55:1012–1017 (1992).

349. Langer, R.D., M.H. Criqui, and D.M. Reed. Lipoproteins and blood pressure as biological pathways for effect of moderate alcohol consumption on coronary heart disease. *Circulation* 85:910–915 (1992).

350. Seppä, K., P. Sillanaukee, T. Pitkäjärvi, et al. Moderate and heavy alcohol consumption have no favorable effect on lipid values. *Arch. Intern. Med.* 152:297–300 (1992).

351. Lee, S.-Y., J.-D. Kim, Y.-H. Lee, et al. Influence of extract of *Rosa rugosa* roots on lipid levels in serum and liver of rats. *Life Sci.* 49:947–951 (1991).

352. El-Saadany, S.S., R.A. El-Massry, S.M. Labib, and M.Z. Sitohy. The biochemical role and hypocholesterolaemic potential of the legume *Cassia fistula* in hypercholesterolaemic rats. *Nahrung* 35:807–815 (1991).

353. Sitohy, M.Z., R.A. El-Massry, S.S. El-Saadany, and S.M. Labib. Metabolic effects of licorice roots (*Glycyrrhiza glabra*) on lipid distribution pattern, liver and renal functions of albino rats. *Nahrung* 35:799–806 (1991).

354. Bobek, P., E. Ginter, M. Jurcovicová, and L. Kuniak. Cholesterol-lowering effect of the mushroom *Pleurotus ostreatus* in hereditary hypercholesterolemic rats. *Ann. Nutr. Metab.* 35:191–195 (1991).

355. Bobek, P., E. Ginter, M. Jurcovicová, et al. Effect of oyster fungus (*Pleurotus ostreatus*) on serum

and liver lipids of Syrian hamsters with a chronic alcohol intake. *Physiol. Res.* 40:327–332 (1991).

356. Holdsworth, E.S., D.V. Kaufman, and E. Neville. A fraction derived from brewer's yeast inhibits cholesterol synthesis by rat liver preparations in vitro. *Br. J. Nutr.* 65:285–299 (1991).

357. Yugarani, T., B.K.H. Tan, and N.P. Das. Effects of polyphenolic natural products on the lipid profiles of rats fed high fat diets. *Lipids* 27:181–186 (1992).

358. Tzeng, S.-H., W.-C. Ko, F.-N. Ko, and C.-M. Teng. Inhibition of platelet aggregation by some flavonoids. *Thromb. Res.* 64:91–100 (1991).

359. Inglett, G.E., and S.B. Grisamore. Maltodextrin fat substitute lowers cholesterol. *Food Technol.* 45(6):104 (1991).

360. Edelstein, S.L., E.L. Barrett-Connor, D.L. Wingard, and B.A. Cohn. Increased meal frequency associated with decreased cholesterol concentrations; Rancho Bernardo, CA, 1984–1987. *Am. J. Clin. Nutr.* 55:664–669 (1992).

361. Stacpoole, P.W., K. von Bergmann, L.L. Kilgore, et al. Nutritional regulation of cholesterol synthesis and apolipoprotein B kinetics: studies in patients with familial hypercholesterolemia and normal subjects treated with a high carbohydrate, low fat diet. *J. Lipid Res.* 32:1837–1848 (1991).

362. Dallongeville, J., S. Lussier-Cacan, and J. Davignon. Modulation of plasma triglyceride levels by apoE phenotype: a meta-analysis. *J. Lipid Res.* 33:447–454 (1992).

363. Boerwinkle, E., S.A. Brown, K. Rohrbach, et al. Role of apolipoprotein E and B gene variation in determining response of lipid, lipoprotein, and apolipoprotein levels to increased dietary cholesterol. *Am. J. Hum. Genet.* 49:1145–1154 (1991).

364. Lane, A., J.K. Cruickshank, J. Mitchell, et al. Genetic and environmental determinants of factor VII coagulant activity in ethnic groups at differing risk of coronary heart disease. *Atherosclerosis* 94:43–50 (1992).

365. Hwa, J.J., S. Zollman, C.H. Warden, et al. Genetic and dietary interactions in the regulation of HMG-CoA reductase gene expression. *J. Lipid Res.* 33:711–725 (1992).

4

Other Effects of Diet

Inflammation and the immune response
Glucose metabolism, glucose tolerance, and
    diabetes
Endocrine system, metabolism, and reproduction
Kidney disease and function
Gastrointestinal tract
Stone diseases
Teeth and bones
Nervous system and behavior
Cataract
Drug metabolism and interactions
Growth, development, and aging

INFLAMMATION AND THE IMMUNE RESPONSE

Immunomodulation by dietary lipids

Chandra's presentation at a symposium on nutrition, immunomodulation, and AIDS provides background for this subject (*1*). He summarized animal studies and epidemiological observations showing how vitamins, minerals, and fats influence immune function. Chandra and Amorin reviewed the immunoregulatory actions of lipids, with emphasis on Chandra's studies in rodents (*2*). The following mechanisms of action have been suggested: modulation of eicosanoid synthesis, changes in composition and fluidity of cell membranes, altered number and density of surface receptors, changes in number and function of specific cell types, and altered production and action of cytokines. Deficiency of essential fatty acids reduces cell-mediated immune response, phagocyte function, and antibody production; but excess dietary fat also impairs these functions. In rodents, consumption of >16 energy percent (en%) fat suppresses cell-mediated immunity; fat restriction protects against disease and increases longevity in mice prone to develop autoimmune pathology. Thresholds that would produce comparable effects in humans have not been established. Maki and Newberne also reviewed the effect of type and quantity of dietary fat on the immune system, discussing what has been learned from models of systemic lupus erythematosus (*3*). They concluded that "overnutrition and obesity are not in our favor with respect to immunocompetence."

A study was conducted of seven healthy women living in a metabolic suite, to learn how the dietary fat and *n*–6 polyunsaturated fatty acid (PUFA) content affect immune status (*4*). During the first 20 days subjects were given a diet containing 5.2 en% *n*–6 PUFA and 41.1 en% total fat. During the next 40 days, three women ate a diet with 3.2 en% PUFA and 26.1 en% fat; the diet of the other four contained 9.1 en% *n*–6 PUFA and 31.1 en% fat. Subjects then crossed over to the other test diet for the last 40 days. Both reduced-fat diets caused significant increase in blastogenesis of peripheral blood

mononuclear cells cultured with phytohemagglutinin, concanavalin A, protein A, and pokeweed and in serum concentrations of C_3 and C_4 complement. However, no differences were seen between the high- and low-PUFA test diets. The authors concluded that a moderate increase in *n*–6 PUFA in the context of a moderate- to low-fat diet does not suppress the human immune system.

One way in which dietary fat influences the immune system is by modulating synthesis of inflammatory mediators. The *n*–6 PUFA arachidonic acid can be converted to leukotriene B_4, a potent inflammatory compound, by the action of 5-lipoxygenase. The *n*–6 PUFAs linoleic acid and dihomo-γ-linolenic acid (DGLA) also affect leukotriene B_4 synthesis (*5*). Neutrophils were isolated and purified from human blood and incubated with the calcium ionophore A23187 and fatty acid (0–100 µM), and lipoxygenase products were measured. Both linoleic acid and DGLA showed dose-related inhibition of leukotriene B_4 synthesis. This was associated with a dose-related increase in 15-lipoxygenase products, which themselves inhibited leukotriene B_4 synthesis. The authors concluded that diets rich in these *n*–6 fatty acids may have a therapeutic effect in inflammatory diseases in which leukotrienes have a pathogenic role. A study with neutrophils from human subjects given supplementary γ-linolenic acid (18:3*n*–6) showed a dose-dependent increase in DGLA (20:3*n*–6) in polymorphonuclear neutrophil phospholipids and a decreased capacity of calcium ionophore–activated cells to generate leukotriene B_4 (*6*).

Investigators studied the effect of excess dietary linoleate on leukotriene B_4-induced neutrophil responses in rats (*7*). Leukotriene B_4- and formyl-peptide-stimulated cells from rats fed 10 en% linoleic acid exhibited significantly greater luminol-augmented chemiluminescence than cells from control rats, indicating enhanced oxidative metabolism. There were no differences in response to concanavalin A. Leukotriene B_4 inhibited neutrophil aggregation in a dose-related way in the high-linoleate diet group but there were no differences between groups in chemotaxis. Thus linoleate supplementation is associated with a stimulus-specific modulation of neutrophil oxidative and aggregatory responses in a manner suggesting an effect on early receptor-linked or immediately post-receptor steps of stimulus–response coupling.

Because the expression of major histocompatibility antigens is necessary during an immune response, the possible influence of dietary fat on Ia antigen expression was investigated (*8*). Mice were fed diets enriched in one of four types of fatty acid: 18:2*n*–6, 18:1*n*–9, *n*–3, or saturated fatty acid (SFA). After stabilization on the experimental diets, some mice in each group were inoculated intraperitoneally with *Listeria monocytogenes*. In the peritoneum of noninfected mice, diet did not affect total cell yield or percentage of B cells, macrophages, or Ia$^+$ cells, but the *n*–3 group had a higher percentage of T cells. In infected mice, however, the *n*–3 group had the lowest percentage of T cells, macrophages, and Ia$^+$ cells in the peritoneum and the lowest density of Ia molecules on peritoneal exudate cells. Similarly, in the spleens of noninfected mice dietary fat did not affect the relationship between B cells and Ia expression, but it did influence Ia expression on B cells in infected mice. The data demonstrate that dietary fat influences murine peritoneal and splenic immune cell populations and Ia antigen expression, but the effects are not uniform for all immune tissues and cell types.

Metabolic changes in the thymus, spleen, and mesenteric lymph nodes were evaluated in rats fed *n*–3 PUFAs and control diets (*9*). Hexokinase activity was 4 times greater in the spleen and thymus, twice as great in the liver, and decreased by 35% in mesenteric lymph nodes of *n*–3-fed rats. Citrate synthase was decreased in spleen and lymph nodes and increased in thymus. Glucose-6-phospho-dehydrogenase activity was doubled in spleen and lymph nodes, slightly increased in thymus, and reduced by two-thirds in the liver. Glutathione peroxidase activity and total lipid peroxides increased in all tissues. These results show that dietary *n*–3 PUFAs cause important changes in lipid peroxidation and in enzymes of glycolysis, glutaminolysis, the pentose pathway, and the tricarboxylic acid cycle in immune tissues.

Another effect of dietary *n*–3 PUFAs is enhancement of tumor necrosis factor (TNF) production by murine resident peritoneal macrophages

(*10*). Mice were maintained for 5 weeks on 10 en% fat diets with different amounts of *n*–3 and *n*–6 PUFAs. Production of TNF, prostaglandin E$_2$, and 6-keto prostaglandin F$_{1\alpha}$ was monitored after in vitro stimulation of peritoneal macrophages with lipopolysaccharide. Macrophages from mice fed a high-*n*–3 diet produced 8 times as much TNF and half as much prostaglandin E$_2$ as cells from mice in other groups. However, the decrease in prostaglandin E$_2$ production could account for only part of the increase in TNF production in the high-*n*–3 group.

Because *n*–3 PUFAs and life-long energy restriction inhibit autoimmune disease in mice, Fernandes et al. tested these interventions in a murine model of AIDS (*11*). The effects of ad libitum and 40% energy-restricted diets, both with 5% corn oil, were compared with ad libitum diets containing 20% corn oil or fish oil. The energy-restricted and fish-oil diets significantly prolonged survival of mice injected with LpBM5 MuLV virus. Mice fed the protective diets showed smaller declines in interleukin-2 production and proliferative response to mitogens 4 weeks after injection of the virus. Mice in the fish-oil group had significantly lower levels of prostaglandin E$_2$; energy-restricted and fish-oil groups had lower levels of arachidonic acid in the spleen. Thus moderate energy restriction and dietary *n*–3 PUFAs modulated the production or response of lymphokines, including the immunosuppressive prostaglandin E$_2$, and delayed progression of the retroviral infection.

However, *n*–3 fatty acids may also decrease natural resistance to infection. Mice were fed diets rich in corn oil, hydrogenated coconut oil, or menhaden oil and then challenged with a virulent strain of *Salmonella typhimurium* (*12*). Mice fed fish oil had a sharply higher mortality rate than the other groups after a very low-dose *S. typhimurium* challenge. The authors could only speculate on the mechanism for this decreased resistance.

An immunosuppressive effect of dietary fish oil supplementation was also demonstrated in healthy men and confirmed by in vitro studies with eicosapentaenoic acid (EPA) (*13*). Subjects were injected with tetanus toxoid at the beginning of the trial; 4 received fish oil extract providing 2.4 g/day of EPA and 2 received olive oil placebo for 6 weeks.

Numerous immune variables were monitored throughout the intervention period and for 23 weeks of follow-up. Several showed no consistent change, but the mitogenic response to anti-CD3 and release of phytohemagglutinin- and pokeweed mitogen–stimulated interleukin-2 were reduced as a consequence of fish oil ingestion, and levels of serum immunoglobulins decreased in 3 of the 4 subjects receiving fish oil. Fish oil did not affect the systemic humoral response to the tetanus toxoid booster, although the specific in vitro response of peripheral blood lymphocytes to tetanus toxoid was compromised at week 3 in subjects who received fish oil. This might reflect a differential sensitivity of circulating B lymphocytes and bone marrow B lymphocytes to fish oil, or merely the necessity for a certain accumulation of EPA in lymphocyte membranes. All parameters modified by ingestion of fish oil were similarly altered by incubating normal lymphocytes with EPA in vitro.

To develop a biochemical explanation for the cardioprotective and immunomodulatory actions of n–3 PUFAs, Ferretti et al. compared the effects of a salmon diet and a reference diet on biosynthesis of prostaglandins E in 10 healthy men (*14*). Both diets contained 25 en% fat, but the n–6/n–3 ratio was 3.6 in the salmon diet and 19.5 in the reference diet. After stabilization on the reference diet 6 men were switched to the salmon diet for 40 days and 4 continued on the reference diet. The groups then switched diets for an additional 40 days. Prostaglandins E were measured as the major urinary metabolite. The salmon diet produced an average 24% decrease in urinary output of the metabolite, regardless of the order of the diets. A change of this magnitude in prostaglandin E synthesis would undoubtedly have clinically significant effects on cardiovascular and immune functions. The results of the change for the most part appear favorable, but other systems could be affected in ways as yet undetermined.

The effect of EPA on the inflammatory potential of neutrophils was evaluated by supplementing the diets of 12 young adults with 2.16 g/day of EPA or 12 g/day of olive oil for 4 weeks in a double-blind crossover study (*15*). Neutrophil function was assessed as luminol-enhanced chemiluminescence in response to platelet-activating factor and formyl-methionyl-leucyl-phenylalanine. An order effect was observed: neutrophil function was significantly reduced only in subjects who ingested EPA first. The authors concluded that dietary supplementation with EPA inhibits neutrophil responses to inflammatory mediators, but other fatty acids modify the effects of EPA.

Immunomodulation by nonlipid dietary components

VITAMIN E. A 2×3 factorial study examined the interactive effects of dietary fat and vitamin E on the immune system of the rat (*16*). Weanling female rats were fed diets containing corn oil or fish oil with 30, 300, or 900 mg/kg of vitamin E. With 30 mg/kg of vitamin E, the vitamin E content of splenocytes from rats fed fish oil was ~40% lower than that from the corn oil group. Fish-oil feeding consistently reduced prostaglandin E synthesis by 70–80%, regardless of vitamin E supplementation. Although rats fed fish oil with 900 mg/kg of vitamin E had the greatest antibody production against sheep red blood cells, this response was not correlated with changes in immune cell prostaglandin E production or α-tocopherol content. Other separate and interactive effects of fat and vitamin E were observed. The results challenge two widespread ideas: that vitamin E supplementation always leads to reduction in prostaglandin E production by immune tissues, and that fish-oil feeding has no measurable adverse effects on the immune system.

When healthy men ate a basal diet supplemented with fish oil, fish oil plus vitamin E, or placebo, the mitogenic responsiveness of peripheral blood mononuclear cells to concanavalin A was suppressed by fish oil alone but restored by addition of vitamin E (*17*). There was a highly significant positive relationship between plasma α-tocopherol concentration and responsiveness of T lymphocytes to concanavalin A.

CAROTENOIDS. A review by Bendich examined the many effects of carotenoids on immune function in normal animals and tumor-bearing animal models (*18*). Effects not related to vitamin A, such as direct inhibitory effects of carotenoids on malignant transformation, were of particular interest. Lymphocytes, macrophages, and natural killer cells are among the immune effector cells whose activities are affected by carotenoids. Synthesis and secretion of tumor cytotoxic factor(s) are enhanced. Evidence is also accumulating that carotenoids affect tumor cells directly, perhaps by their antioxidant activity, by depressing adenylate cyclase activity, or through generation of regulatory proteins.

A trial of β-carotene supplementation for 4 months in 11 patients infected with the HIV virus demonstrated modulation of certain immune markers (*19*). After 3 months of treatment the percentage of natural killer cells and activated lymphocytes were increased, but they subsequently declined. There were no treatment-related changes in total lymphocyte count or percentage of cells expressing CD11, CD8, or CD4 antigens.

In vitro studies of the effects of carotenoids on murine lymphocyte function and expression of cell-surface markers provided additional evidence that these actions are not related to provitamin A activity (*20*). Nor was it clear that the results could be explained merely by the oxygen-quenching capacity of the substances tested. In several assays using spleen cells, astaxanthin, which has no provitamin A activity, was either more active than β-carotene or showed activity while β-carotene was inactive.

ENERGY RESTRICTION. Although protein–energy malnutrition impairs immune function in humans, the individual effects of protein and energy deprivation have not been clarified. To show the effects of energy deprivation, 12 obese but otherwise healthy young adults were studied during 6 weeks on a commercial very-low-energy diet containing 93 g/day of protein (*21*). Significant decreases were observed in numbers of total leukocytes, neutrophils, lymphocytes, and monocytes beginning after the first or second week of the diet. Only lymphocyte counts returned to normal during the subsequent 1 or 2 weeks of refeeding. Except for a small decrease in CD4$^+$ cells, other mononuclear cells populations did not change. Phorbol ester–stimulated uptake of [^{3}H]thymidine decreased after 1 week; the response to concanavalin A, phytohemagglutinin, and pokeweed mitogen decreased after 6 weeks. Delayed-type hypersensitivity skin-test responses did not change. Decreases in circulating leukocyte counts and in vitro responses to mitogens with specificity for different cell subsets suggested that in some individuals, or with longer duration of energy deprivation, these responses could have clinical significance.

Although profound impairment of immune function has been observed in populations of developing countries, it was at first difficult to reproduce these observations consistently in laboratory animals (*22*). Paradoxically, nutritional restriction at times enhanced certain immune functions. It was then shown that undernutrition (40% energy restriction) without malnutrition regularly extended the lifespan of rodents while maintaining vigorous immunologic function and preventing many cancers and other immunologically based diseases of aging. A major influence of such undernutrition was the down-regulation of cellular proliferation and cell turnover in all of the rapidly replicating tissues studied. Expression of certain oncogenic retroviruses could also be inhibited in highly susceptible strains of mice.

MINERALS. A comprehensive review showed how dietary sodium, potassium, calcium, magnesium, and trace elements influence arachidonic acid metabolism and eicosanoid production (*23*; 253 references). Clinical disorders associated with changes in intake of these elements were discussed and pathways of arachidonate metabolism and the mode of action of eicosanoids were briefly reviewed. For most elements, no single process is involved but rather a series of complex interactions sometimes affecting levels of other elements. Other brief reviews considered the roles of selenium (*24*) and zinc (*25*) in the immune response.

LACTIC ACID BACTERIA. Several research groups have studied the influence of fermented milk foods on the immune response (*26–28*). In an 8-day trial, CD-1 mice were fed various fermented milks and the phagocytic activity of their pulmonary alveolar macrophages was determined during feeding and 7 days after the test feeding was stopped (*26*). Milks fermented by *Lactobacillus bulgaricus, Streptococcus cremoris, Streptococcus lactis,* or *Streptococcus thermophilus* did not stimulate phagocytic activity. Milks fermented by *Lactobacillus casei, Lactobacillus helveticus,* or *Bifidobacterium longum* enhanced phagocytic activity. None of the milks significantly affected the number of zymosan particles ingested by activated cells, indicating that the effect is restricted to resting cells. Possible mechanisms were discussed and the authors proposed that production of immunomodulatory peptides through bacterial-mediated proteolysis of milk proteins was responsible for the observed results. Other investigators studied the effect of natural and heated yogurt on specific and nonspecific immune defense mechanisms of mice (*27*). Both products increased phagocytic activity but neither affected lymphocytic activity. Natural yogurt protected against gastrointestinal infection after challenge with 10 LD_{50} of *S. typhimurium,* but not against challenge with 20 LD_{50} or with 10^7 cells of *Escherichia coli.* Heated yogurt was not protective. To test the prophylactic potential of yogurt containing *Lactobacillus acidophilus* against candidal vaginitis, women with recurrent *Candida* infection were assigned to eat no yogurt or to eat 8 oz/day of yogurt for 6-month periods in a crossover design (*28*). Vaginal and rectal colonization by lactobacilli and *Candida* and candidal vaginal infections were monitored. Daily yogurt ingestion decreased both candidal colonization and candidal infections.

OTHER. Some animal studies indicate that dietary nucleotides are necessary for maintenance of normal immune function (*29*). When healthy, term neonates were breast-fed or given SMA formula with or without 33 mg/L of nucleotides, there were no significant differences between groups in growth or incidence and severity of infections at 2 months. However, natural killer cell activity was significantly higher in breast-fed and nucleotide-supplemented groups when the infants were 2 months old, and production of interleukin-2 by stimulated mononuclear cells was greater in infants receiving nucleotide supplements than in the nonsupplemented SMA group. Natural killer cell activity declined in all groups when the infants were 4 months old, for

reasons that were not clear but could involve response to immunizing agents, dietary change, or maturation.

Peptides with opioid and immunomodulatory activity have been identified in the sequence of milk proteins, particularly caseins. Investigations of these peptides were recently reviewed (*30*). Their physiological significance is not clear. The in vivo expression of their activity depends on their release from the milk protein and on factors modulating their degradation, transport, and absorption. Among the bioactive peptides of milk are ones that influence macrophage, B-cell, and T-cell functions. Human breast milk contains immunoglobulins, enzymes, and growth factors that provide passive protection against infection. Other protein and peptide components have both suppressive and enhancing activity and may regulate development of the immune system by, for example, influencing induction of immune tolerance and prevention of hypersensitivities to food antigens. These substances have been found in sheep's and cow's milk as well as in human colostrum and late milk.

Incubation of the fungus *Mortierella alpina* with sesame oil increases the mycelial DGLA content but decreases production of arachidonic acid. In experiments with a cell-free fungal extract and rat liver microsomes, (+)sesamin specifically inhibited $\Delta 5$ desaturase activity at low concentrations (*31*). It did not inhibit $\Delta 6$, $\Delta 9$, or $\Delta 12$ desaturase activity. Sesamolin, sesaminol, and episesamin also specifically inhibited the $\Delta 5$ desaturase. This selective effect of sesame lignans on PUFA biosynthesis has implications for the arachidonic acid cascade and the immune response.

Effects of diet on specific immune responses and diseases

Zurier briefly summarized the involvement of essential fatty acids in inflammation, as eicosanoid precursors and as components of cell membranes (*32*). EPA has a small but reproducible dose-dependent antiinflammatory effect as adjunct therapy for rheumatoid arthritis, which may stem from a shift in the balance between cell-membrane 20-carbon fatty acids of the *n*–6 and *n*–3 series (*33*). These act competitively as eicosanoid precursors, and n–3 eicosanoids are less proinflammatory than n–6 eicosanoids. Cleland et al. measured the arachidonic acid and EPA content of neutrophil membranes from healthy men assigned to a high- or low-linoleate diet followed by the same diet supplemented with fish oil. In the initial phase, there was a significant difference between the high- and low-linoleate groups in the linoleic acid content of neutrophil phospholipids. Subsequent supplementation with fish oil increased the EPA in neutrophil phospholipids but the increase was greater in the low-linoleate group. This shows that dietary n–6 PUFAs inhibit the incorporation of EPA into neutrophil membranes and suggests that the antiinflammatory activity of EPA could be enhanced by limiting intake of linoleate.

ASTHMA. A year-long trial of fish oil supplements in patients with allergic asthma found a small improvement in forced expiratory volume after 9 months (*34*). This measure is not always correlated with the patient's subjective evaluation, and other studies may have failed to demonstrate an effect due to inappropriate dosage or inadequate treatment time.

Because high sodium intake reportedly increases bronchial reactivity in asthmatic men, the effects of low-, normal-, and high-sodium diets on peak expiratory flow were studied in 17 adults with mild asthma in an open randomized crossover trial (*35*). Mean 24-h urinary excretion of sodium (± SD) was 84 ± 32, 147 ± 45, and 201 ± 73 mmol for the three diets, respectively. Two-week periods of the low- and high-sodium diets had no effect on peak expiratory flow in these patients.

ATOPIC SKIN RESPONSES. The effect of dietary fish-oil supplementation on the antigen-induced cutaneous late-phase response was studied in 16 atopic subjects (*36*). At baseline, all subjects developed a late-phase response to intradermal allergen injection, with a mean area of induration at 6 h of 1840 ± 472 mm^2. Subjects were then randomized to receive fish oil (3.2 g/day of EPA and 2.2 g/day of docosahexaenoic acid [DHA]) or olive-oil placebo for 10 weeks. At the end of this period there were no

significant changes from baseline in the size of the immediate wheal-and-flare response or the extent of induration at 4 and 6 h. Nor were there any postdiet changes in the microscopic appearance of biopsy specimens from the lesions. The authors concluded that dietary fish oil does not inhibit the cutaneous late-phase response either clinically or histologically.

The rationale for treating atopic eczema with evening primrose oil and clinical results of such trials were reviewed by Kerscher and Korting (*37*). Evening primrose oil is rich in γ-linolenic acid. In humans, this compound is synthesized from linoleic acid by the action of $\Delta 6$ desaturase, an enzyme reported to be defective in persons who develop atopic eczema. Taken individually or subjected to metaanalysis, trials of evening primrose oil have demonstrated marked improvement in patients with atopic eczema. However, the long-term efficacy and safety of this treatment remain to be established.

LUPUS ERYTHEMATOSUS. A prospective double-blind crossover study assessed the effects of a low-fat diet supplemented with fish oil in patients with active systemic lupus erythematosus (*38*). The basal diet contained 20 en% fat, supplemented with 20 g of MaxEPA or 20 g of olive oil in the two 12-week test phases. The trial began with 2 weeks on the basal diet to test understanding and compliance, and there was an 8-week washout between test periods. Criteria for "ideal improvement," "useful improvement," no change, and deterioration were established for each subject. Fourteen of 17 patients achieved ideal or useful improvement while taking MaxEPA, whereas 13 of the 17 were static or worse while taking placebo. No important side effects occurred. This study demonstrates the potential for dietary treatment of systemic lupus erythematosus.

Autoantibodies from persons with systemic lupus erythematosus cross-react with the small nuclear ribonucleoprotein particles of many animals. Bullard-Dillard et al. investigated whether cross-reactivity also occurs between proteins of common dietary plants and anti-Sm autoantibodies from serum of lupus patients (*39*). They analyzed protein extracts from soybeans, corn, spinach, and carrots. At least one protein (M_r ~28,000) common to all the extracts was recognized by most of the anti-Sm sera tested. Affinity-purified antibody eluted from this plant protein specifically recognized the Sm proteins of a HeLa cell protein extract. Only autoimmune lupus sera with anti-Sm activity recognized the 28-kDa dietary plant protein. The authors suggested that studies in animals could elucidate the roles of dietary components in autoimmune disease.

Doctors in Japan reported the case history of a 16-year-old girl with systemic lupus erythematosus brought under control by change to a vegetarian diet (40). The patient's proteinuria, hypocomplementemia, and antinuclear and anti-DNA titers were difficult to control until, on the advice of her parents and without permission of her physicians, she tapered off steroids and started the vegetarian diet. Protein and caloric intake were much reduced with little reduction in fat. Between August 1985 and December 1986, antibody titers became normal, urinary excretion of protein decreased, and serum albumin rose; values of these parameters remained stable when the patient was last evaluated in March 1991.

RHEUMATOID ARTHRITIS. Das reviewed interactions between essential fatty acids, eicosanoids, cytokines, growth factors, and free radicals of relevance to designing therapeutic strategies for rheumatoid arthritis and other collagen vascular diseases (41). The pathobiology of rheumatoid arthritis and the role of T cells, cytokines, neutrophils, soluble-phase inflammatory mediators, and modulators of interleukin and TNF synthesis were summarized. The role of drugs such as cyclosporine, 1,25-dihydroxycholecalciferol, and pentoxyfylline was considered. Interactions between various factors and cell types were shown diagrammatically.

Because fish oil appears beneficial in treating rheumatoid arthritis and psoriasis, physicians in Switzerland asked whether fish can substitute for fish oil (42). They observed three parallel groups of rheumatology-clinic outpatients for 2 months: one group ate a normal diet without fish, one a normal diet including 700 g/week of fish, and one a normal diet without fish but with 7.5 g/day of fish oil.

Outcome measures were the lipid composition of platelet-rich plasma and serum cholesterol and triglycerides. The relative amounts of EPA and DHA increased significantly in the fish-diet and fish-oil groups, and triglyceride levels decreased slightly but significantly. Cholesterol did not change. The benefit from fish oil in patients with rheumatoid arthritis or psoriasis is thought to result from an increase in membrane n–3 PUFAs, but large numbers of fish-oil capsules are required. This study shows that similar effects may be achieved by eating several fish meals weekly, with no other change in eating habits.

The report of Kjeldsen-Kragh et al. on a controlled trial of fasting and a vegetarian diet as therapy in rheumatoid arthritis (43) generated active comment from readers (44–49). In the study, 27 rheumatoid arthritis patients in functional class II or III were assigned to a 4-week stay at a health farm, where they underwent a 7- to 10-day subtotal fast and were then put on individually adjusted gluten-free vegan diets for 3.5 months. During this phase and the one that followed any food that exacerbated symptoms was dropped from the diet. After the vegan diet a lactovegetarian diet was gradually introduced and maintained until the end of the 13-month study. Twenty-six controls stayed for 4 weeks at a convalescent home and ate an ordinary diet throughout the 13-month study. After 4 weeks at the health farm the diet group showed significant improvement as measured by number of tender joints, Ritchie's articular index, number of swollen joints, pain score, erythrocyte sedimentation rate, C-reactive protein, white blood cell count, and a health assessment questionnaire. Only pain score improved significantly in the controls. Even after a year, the diet group maintained an advantage in all measured indexes. In commenting on this report, Darlington and Ramsey summarized their corroboratory experience with dietary treatment of rheumatoid arthritis, adding some caveats and tentative explanations for the observed effects (44). Physicians at another clinic described their protocol for dietary treatment of rheumatoid arthritis patients (45). Still other physicians, however, reported that 20% of patients they surveyed had tried similar diet modifications on their own and given them up as ineffective (46).

French investigators tested a diet rich in raw fruits and vegetables with no cereals or dairy products, on the theory that this resembled the diet of our preagricultural ancestors, in whom rheumatoid arthritis was rare or absent (*47*). Of 46 adults in the study, 17 clearly improved and 19 were in complete remission for 1–5 years; the regimen was a failure in 10. Other readers suggested problematic aspects of the study design of Kjeldsen-Kragh et al., particularly noting differences in management of the two groups of patients (*48,49*). The authors clarified some points of misunderstanding in the last two letters (*50*).

One way in which dietary components trigger rheumatoid arthritis may involve a molecular mimicry mechanism similar to that postulated for the role of infectious agents in reactive arthritis (*51*). Serum antibodies from some (but not all) patients with rheumatoid arthritis recognized bovine albumin present in milk and serum. Residues 141–157 of the bovine albumin differ markedly from the corresponding fragment of human albumin but are highly homologous with human collagen type I, vitamin D–binding protein, and the complement component C1q. The immunogenicity of this fragment was confirmed by constructing a synthetic peptide with the same sequence and demonstrating specific reactivity for it in rheumatoid arthritis sera highly reactive toward bovine serum albumin. To a degree, immunogenicity was conformation-dependent: reactivity was higher with the intact native molecule than with the denatured molecule or the synthetic peptide.

GLUCOSE METABOLISM, GLUCOSE TOLERANCE, AND DIABETES

Direct and indirect actions of nutrients in regulating insulin secretion from pancreatic β cells were summarized in a brief review (*52*). The discussion included the Ca^{2+} cation and other second messengers, specific nutrients (glucose and other sugars, amino acids, free fatty acids and ketone bodies), and actions of neurotransmitters and gut hormones.

Dietary carbohydrate and fiber

To learn about specific metabolic effects of different diets, 22 lean adults and 23 obese adults were characterized by dietary history, anthropometric data, oral glucose tolerance, and insulin sensitivity (S_I) (*53*). S_I was inversely correlated with fat intake and directly correlated with fiber intake. There was no association between S_I and total energy, protein, or alcohol intake, or between S_I and the dietary polyunsaturated/saturated (P/S) fat ratio. There was a significant inverse association between basal glucose concentrations and fiber intake. The findings from this study support the conclusion that low-fiber, high-fat diets are associated with increased insulin resistance in healthy, free-living adults.

In a study of elderly subjects, body mass index and frequent intake of carbohydrates and pastries was positively associated with the incidence of glucose intolerance (*54*). Frequent intake of legumes was negatively associated with incidence of glucose intolerance. These relationships remained after controlling for age, gender, alcohol use, energy intake, prescribed diet, use of medications, and comorbidity. The authors concluded that energy balance and frequent eating of carbohydrate-rich foods are related to development of glucose intolerance in an elderly population.

A metabolic-ward study was conducted in 10 subjects with insulin-dependent diabetes mellitus (IDDM) (*55*). Subjects were stabilized on a control diet and then randomly assigned to 4 weeks of a high-carbohydrate, high-fiber diet or a low-carbohydrate, low-fiber diet. After a 6-week washout period they returned to the metabolic ward and were crossed over to the other diet for 4 weeks. Insulin requirements of the two diets were measured by artificial pancreas studies. Relative to the diet low in carbohydrate and fiber, the high-carbohydrate, high-fiber diet decreased basal insulin requirements, increased carbohydrate disposal per unit of insulin, and decreased total and HDL cholesterol. Glycemic control and other lipid fractions did not differ significantly between diets.

Wolever et al. reviewed the purpose, methodology, and clinical utility of the glycemic index (*56*). Within limits determined by the expected glycemic index difference and day-to-day variation of glycemic responses, it is possible to rank the glycemic potential of different meals in individual subjects. Although reducing fluctuations in blood glucose after meals has only a modest effect on overall control of blood glucose, it may benefit particular diabetic patients. More important, however, is the ability of diets with a low glycemic index to reduce blood lipids in hypertriglyceridemic subjects. Although high-carbohydrate diets are recommended for persons with diabetes and hyperlipidemia, the type of carbohydrate partially determines the metabolic response. Thus the glycemic index becomes a useful measure so that high-carbohydrate diets with the potential to increase blood glucose, insulin, and triglyceride concentrations can be avoided.

Various mechanisms have been proposed for the hypoglycemic effect of dietary fiber. When the relationship between the glycemic index and the total dietary fiber content of foods was analyzed, assuming a nonlinear regression curve for mechanistic reasons, the empirical equation obtained was $Y = 19.9 \, X^{-0.322}$ (57). Regression curves of the same type were obtained for soluble and insoluble dietary fiber. The correlations between observed glycemic index and glycemic indexes calculated from the regression curves for soluble and insoluble fiber were virtually identical (−.780 and −.781). However, at any given level, soluble dietary fiber gave a lower index than insoluble dietary fiber. This suggests that soluble fiber plays the more important role in the hypoglycemic effect of total dietary fiber. The authors proposed that when there is no published glycemic index for a food but its total dietary fiber content is known, an alternative glycemic index based on fiber be calculated from their regression equation.

In vivo and in vitro tests were conducted to study the mechanisms affecting the rate of digestion and absorption of starch in pasta (58). Healthy young adults ate test meals containing equivalent amounts of available carbohydrate as spaghetti, macaroni, spaghetti "porridge," bread made from spaghetti ingredients, and mashed potatoes. Blood glucose levels were monitored for 3 h and glycemic indexes were calculated from 90- or 120-min areas

under the glucose curves. The rate of starch hydrolysis was measured in vitro with foods in a form "as eaten." Results showed the importance of food structure in determining glycemic response. The more compact foods (spaghetti, macaroni) offered the enzymes limited access, resulting in lower glycemic indexes and lower peak blood glucose values. Differences between foods in the late-phase glucose response were also observed. In vivo and in vitro tests ranked the products similarly, and the authors recommended their new in vivo method for predicting glycemic response to various foods.

To settle arguments about whether the glycemic indexes for individual foods can predict the glycemic response to a mixed meal, investigators evaluated the short-term effects of exchangeable amounts of various carbohydrates on plasma glucose and insulin responses (59). Healthy subjects and subjects with non-insulin-dependent diabetes mellitus (NIDDM) were given five mixed meals of different ethnic origins. Each meal contained 50 g of carbohydrate, 15 g of protein, and 15 g of fat and was compared with a 50-g glucose load. The glycemic index and the insulin index did not rank the meals in the same order. The area under the glucose curve and the predicted glycemic index were highly correlated in both NIDDM and healthy subjects. The Polish meal of egg noodles, cheese, and raisins produced the greatest glycemic response; the Syrian meal of lentils and rice produced the smallest. However, the greatest insulinemic response was to the standard meal of white bread, cheese, milk, chocolate, and an orange. The authors concluded that the glycemic index is a valid measure, useful in diet planning, and that legume foods should be incorporated as carbohydrate sources in diets for subjects with NIDDM or impaired glucose tolerance.

To study the postprandial effects of meals with different amylose/amylopectin ratios, healthy men were given hot mixed meals containing 13 en% protein, 24 en% fat, 6 en% monosaccharides and disaccharides, and 57 en% polysaccharides (60). In one meal the amylose/amylopectin ratio was 0:100 and in the other, 45:55. Care was taken to achieve full gelatinization of starch granules, to rule out effects of "resistant starch." The amylose/amylopectin ratio had no important effect on postprandial triglycerides or breath hydrogen. High-amylose meals were reported as less palatable but more satiating. They produced smaller initial and late insulin responses and initial glucose response, but averaged over 6 h the glucose response was somewhat greater. The high-amylose meal also resulted in higher levels of free glycerol and free fatty acids after 6 h. The results showed that the amylose/amylopectin ratio has a significant influence on several postprandial responses and suggest that its manipulation could produce beneficial effects.

Finer reviewed "sweeteners and metabolic disorders" (*61*). Metabolism of nutritive sweeteners in the normal state and in diabetes mellitus, hyperlipidemia, glycogen storage diseases, disorders of fructose metabolism, and other metabolic diseases was discussed. Metabolism of aspartame by normal, phenylketonuric, and diabetic subjects was then reviewed. The author concluded that "normal" persons would derive little benefit from replacing sucrose with another nutritive or nonnutritive sweetener, but a variety of metabolic disorders determine the acceptability and safety of individual sweeteners for others. Another review (*62*) summarized evidence that increased sucrose consumption increases postprandial plasma glucose, insulin, and triglyceride concentrations and fasting total and VLDL triglyceride and cholesterol, and decreases HDL cholesterol concentration. Qualitatively similar changes have been reported in normal, hyperinsulinemic, and hypertriglyceridemic subjects and persons with NIDDM. The authors concluded that such changes should be viewed as the expected consequence of high-sucrose diets. Moreover, undesirable effects on carbohydrate and lipid metabolism have been demonstrated at sucrose levels typical of the diet of the average adult American. Because at present it is not possible to predict individual responses to this amount of dietary sucrose and individual responses may be of enormous clinical significance even when population-wide responses are modest, the authors advised limiting sucrose consumption and further modifying sucrose consumption on a case-by-case basis in accordance with metabolic status.

The nonobese diabetic mouse is a model in which the primary event in IDDM is autoimmunity against β cells (*63*). In this mouse, substituting sorbose for dietary sucrose resulted in lower body weight and lower blood glucose levels than in sucrose-fed controls. Urinary glucose secretion was also inhibited, but serum insulin levels were not affected. The authors suggested that dietary sorbose might similarly benefit diabetic patients.

To determine the metabolic effects of a high-fructose diet, healthy subjects were given two isocaloric test diets for 28-day periods in a crossover design (*64*). The diets were of similar composition, except that one contained 20% fructose and the other contained <3% fructose, with starch making up the difference. The most significant finding was that fasting serum total and LDL cholesterol were 9.0 and 11% higher, respectively, at the end of the fructose diet than at the end of the starch diet. This was primarily due to a decrease on the starch diet rather than to an increase with fructose, but this study could not show whether the change was due to the decreased fructose or increased starch content of the high-starch diet. There were no important differences in numerous other blood measurements, although lower values for peak plasma glucose on the first and last days of the fructose diet were on the threshold of statistical significance.

A review of trials of high-carbohydrate, high-fiber, reduced-fat diets for diabetics concluded that this regimen is beneficial and there is no reason to change it, except when large amounts of fiber are not tolerated (*65*). For some persons, partial replacement of fiber with complex carbohydrates of low glycemic index or with monounsaturated fatty acids (MUFAs) is acceptable. The modes of action of dietary fiber were discussed and long-term safety of high-fiber diets was considered. Riccardi and Rivellese stressed that discrepant results from studies of high-carbohydrate diets in diabetes can frequently be reconciled by taking dietary fiber into account (*66*). High-carbohydrate, high-fiber diets consistently improve glycemic control and reduce plasma cholesterol concentrations in diabetic subjects. Furthermore, such diets do not increase plasma insulin and triglyceride concentrations despite their increased carbohydrate content. However, some foods not particularly rich in dietary fiber also exert the beneficial effects of high-fiber foods. For example, a food's physical form influences its accessibility to digestive enzymes, determining its rate of digestion and absorption (see also reference *58*). These authors concluded that a diet low in cholesterol and saturated fat should be recommended to all diabetic patients, and the best way to achieve this is through a balanced increase in fiber-rich foods and unsaturated fat.

The glycemic and insulinemic effects of ingesting 7 g of soy or cellulose fiber before a normal breakfast were studied in 8 NIDDM patients (*67*). Glucose values were significantly lower for soy than for cellulose 30, 60, 90, and 120 min after fiber ingestion. Insulin curves were not significantly different. This demonstrated a positive influence of soy fiber, compared with cellulose fiber, in control of postprandial glycemia in NIDDM patients. Oat products also improve glucose metabolism and lower serum cholesterol in subjects with NIDDM, but this effect is generally attributed to water-soluble fiber (*68*). To test the effects of insoluble oat fiber, 8 lean men with NIDDM ate a conventional diabetes diet for 1 week, after which they were given a control diet with 30 g/day of insoluble oat fiber (incorporated into muffins) for 2 weeks in a hospital metabolic ward. On discharge they resumed their normal diet but continued to ingest 30 g/day of insoluble oat fiber (in muffins) for 10 weeks. The muffins were acceptable and produced no serious side effects. During the hospital phase of the study, fasting serum glucose decreased by 13%, LDL cholesterol by 8.9%, and apoB-100 by 17%; other serum lipid measures did not change significantly. However, the effects on glucose, LDL cholesterol, and apoB-100 were transient and levels returned to baseline during the subsequent ambulatory phase. More study of insoluble oat fiber was recommended.

Guar gum's effectiveness in reducing postprandial glucose and plasma insulin levels depends on its ability to increase the viscosity of digest in the small intestine (*69*). A study in nondiabetic young adults evaluated the postprandial effects of wheat breads containing guar gums having differing rheological properties (largely determined by molecular weight and particle size). Control bread was made from white wheat flour; in the test breads, this was replaced by guar gum samples at the level of 100 g/kg. Postprandial glucose response did not differ between breads. However, the insulin response to all guar breads was significantly lower than to the control, and the effect was apparently uninfluenced by large variations in molecular weight and particle size. Bread using guar gum of low molecular weight was judged most palatable.

Dietary lipids

The role of dietary fat as a risk factor for adult-onset NIDDM was assessed in a geographically based epidemiologic study (*70*). Information on current diet was obtained in 24-h diet recall interview, which preceded an oral glucose tolerance test. The resultant study population included 70 subjects with previously undiagnosed diabetes, 171 with impaired glucose intolerance, and 1076 normal controls. The adjusted odds ratios relating a 40-g/day increase in fat intake to NIDDM and impaired glucose tolerance were 1.51 and 1.62, respectively. These ratios increased to 3.03 and 2.67 when only diabetic subjects with fasting glucose >140 mg/dL and persons with impaired glucose tolerance confirmed at follow-up were included.

To test the hypothesis that the modern high-fat diet adversely affects carbohydrate metabolism regardless of genetic background, 12 nondiabetic Pima Indians and 12 nondiabetic Caucasians matched for age, sex, and obesity were studied on a metabolic ward (*71*). They were fed a traditional Pima diet and a modern diet, each for 2 weeks, in a randomized crossover design. Pimas and Caucasians responded similarly, except for larger changes in plasma lipids among the Pimas. Compared with the Pima diet (70% carbohydrate, 15% fat, 15% protein), the modern diet was associated with significantly decreased oral glucose tolerance and increased plasma cholesterol concentration. Reduced glucose tolerance was associated with reduced glucose-mediated glucose disposal, decreased acute insulin response to glucose, and decreased β-cell sensitivity to glucose. The authors concluded that diet composition affects the prevalence of NIDDM not only in Pima Indians, in whom it is the highest in the world, but also in Caucasians.

Yet another review of the effects of carbohydrate and fat intake on glucose and lipoprotein metabolism in persons with diabetes found interpretation difficult because changes due to differences in relative amounts of fat and carbohydrate, differences in the types of fat and carbohydrate, and differences in amount of dietary fiber and cholesterol were not always separated (*72*). The authors argued that the most characteristic defects in carbohydrate and lipoprotein metabolism are exacerbated by some low-fat, high-carbohydrate diets. Therefore simply replacing dietary fat (or more specifically, saturated fat) with carbohydrate is not necessarily the best way to reduce risk of coronary artery disease in diabetics. They suggested that diets containing usual amounts of fat, substituting unsaturated for saturated fats and greatly reducing cholesterol, offer the best overall metabolic control for persons with diabetes. In male New Zealand rabbits, however, ingestion of a high-fat (19%) diet with a P/S ratio of 2.7 produced elevated plasma triglyceride, phospholipid, and cholesterol concentrations, changed the distribution of cholesterol and phospholipids among lipoprotein fractions, and significantly diminished glucose tolerance and insulin secretion (*73*). Thus, compared to the 2% fat control diet, the high-fat diet evoked a diabetogenic condition.

To characterize the insulin resistance induced in rats by a high-fat diet, in vivo and in vitro tests were conducted in rats fed diets with 60 en% fat as lard and control chow diets with 12 en% fat (*74*). By oral glucose tolerance testing, the high-fat group exhibited hyperinsulinemia and insulin resistance. Levels of insulin binding to insulin receptors from muscle and liver were similar in the high-fat group and controls. However, in the high-fat group, in vitro autophosphorylation of purified insulin receptors on tyrosine residues was decreased in both liver and muscle; and in vivo tyrosine phosphorylation of insulin receptors and the endogenous substrate pp175 in response to insulin injection was decreased in the liver. No difference in phosphorylation of pp190 in muscle was observed. Levels of glucose transporters in crude membrane from muscle and liver were similar in the two groups. The authors concluded that insulin resistance in rats fed a high-fat diet is a postreceptor defect in muscle, although tyrosine phosphorylation of the insulin receptor and its endogenous substrate were decreased in the liver and this could have contributed to the altered metabolic state.

Dietary information was collected at baseline and 2-year follow-up to determine whether changes in dietary fat intake were related to changes in serum lipid levels in IDDM patients (*75*). Sex- and age-group-specific Spearman correlations between change in LDL cholesterol and change in dietary fat, saturated fat, and cholesterol intakes were significant for men 18–29 years old. Within this group, changes in percent saturated fat, percent fat, and Keys score were significantly and independently related to changes in LDL cholesterol.

A very brief review summarized the potential benefits of *n*–3 PUFAs in diabetes mellitus but warned of possible hazards as well (*76*). Although triglyceride levels are reduced after *n*–3 supplementation, glycemic balance is sometimes also degraded, particularly in NIDDM complicated by obesity. The mechanism of this is not understood. A more extensive review (152 references cited) highlighted the potentially antiatherogenic properties of marine lipids for diabetic subjects (*77*). In addition to their very low prevalence of coronary heart disease, Greenland Eskimos have a remarkably low incidence of diabetes. After discussing this and other epidemiologic observations and reviewing the nomenclature and biochemistry of fatty acids, the authors considered risk factors and metabolic disturbances that may account for the unusual proclivity of diabetic persons to develop atherosclerosis. They concluded that much lower doses of *n*–3 fatty acids than originally thought might reduce cardiovascular risk factors in diabetics without compromising glucose homeostasis. They recommended natural dietary sources of *n*–3 PUFAs (i.e., fish) for both IDDM and NIDDM patients, while taking a go-slow approach to fish oil supplementation.

A study conducted by the USDA, the National Cancer Institute, and Hoffmann–LaRoche described the effects of fish oil alone and in conjunction with vitamin E on hormones involved in carbohydrate and lipid metabolism (*78*). Forty healthy men were fed controlled diets providing 40 en% fat, with a minimum of *n*–3 fatty acids. During the first 10 weeks they took capsules supplying 15 g/day of mixed fat; during the second 10 weeks the capsules supplied 15 g/day of fish-oil concentrate; and during the final 8 weeks 200 mg/day of vitamin E was added to the fish oil. Fish-oil feeding significantly increased plasma concentrations of glucose and decreased triglycerides, cholesterol, insulin, growth hormone, somatomedin-C, and glucagon. Addition of vitamin E to the fish oil further reduced insulin and growth hormone and restored somatomedin-C to the level found with placebo fat. Vitamin E also sharply reduced concentration of dehydroepiandrosterone sulfate. The authors concluded that changes in plasma glucose and lipid levels caused by dietary fish oil could be explained by changes in hormones involved in carbohydrate and lipid metabolism.

Berdanier et al. studied the effects of life-long fish-oil feeding on male BHE/cdb rats, which are genetically programmed to develop NIDDM (*79*). Diets contained 1% corn oil plus an additional 1 or 9% corn oil, menhaden oil, or beef tallow. Although the high levels of menhaden oil and beef tallow retarded development of glucose intolerance and hyperlipemia, rats receiving the high level of menhaden oil had the shortest lifespan of all groups. Glomerulosclerosis appeared earliest and was most severe in this group, and rats with severe renal lesions also had mineralized foci in the aorta and heart. Rats fed the 2% fat diets differed little with respect to glucose tolerance and lipemia.

The ability of *n*–3 fatty acids to restore impaired glucose tolerance was evaluated in the fat-fed mouse model of NIDDM (*80*). Groups of animals were fed lab chow, lab chow plus 2.5 g/kg of SuperEPA, and diets containing 20 en% protein and 80 en% animal or vegetable fat alone or with 2.5 g/kg of SuperEPA. Fat-fed mice of both sexes became hyperglycemic and had impaired glucose tolerance, but the decay of plasma glucose during tolerance testing was significantly slower in groups fed animal fat. The only effect of SuperEPA supplementation was on males fed the animal fat diet. These mice gained less weight and had significantly less hyperglycemia and impairment of glucose tolerance than males fed animal fat without SuperEPA. In females but not males, animal fat diets raised

cholesterol levels significantly more than vegetable fat diets. The authors did not speculate on reasons for the sex-related differences in response. Obesity alone did not cause the impaired glucose tolerance because not all groups of fat-fed mice were obese. This model reflects many aspects of the metabolism that characterizes obese human NIDDM patients and may be useful in explaining the nongenetic part of the pathogenesis of NIDDM.

Nineteen middle-aged NIDDM patients were studied during three 2-month dietary periods (*81*). During the first and last phases they ate a low-fat, high-carbohydrate diet providing 10 en% PUFA, 10 en% SFA, and 5 en% MUFA. During the second phase total fat supplied 40 en% and MUFAs supplied 25 en%. There were no significant effects of diet on plasma glucose, total or HDL cholesterol, or triglycerides. These results indicate that a wider dietary choice can safely be made available to NIDDM patients.

In healthy adults, ingestion of 3.3 g of sodium propionate in bread containing 50 g of available carbohydrate acutely reduced the blood glucose response area by nearly half (*82*). One week of dietary supplementation with 9.9 g/day of sodium propionate in bread reduced the area under the blood glucose response curve by 38% and increased fecal bulk and bifidobacteria populations and ratio of anaerobes to aerobes. In in vitro tests, sodium propionate bread or mixture of sodium propionate with white bread inhibited the activity of salivary amylase. It therefore appears that propionate inhibits human amylolytic activity in addition to its reported effect on HMG CoA reductase activity. The results also suggest that ingestion of propionate bread increases the amount of undigested starch entering the colon, even though there was no substantial change in breath hydrogen (an index of carbohydrate malabsorption). Perhaps the presence of exogenous propionate in the colon inhibited bacterial hydrogen production. Methane production did increase when propionate bread was eaten.

Children with IDDM have altered essential fatty acid and prostaglandin metabolism, manifested by decreased levels of DGLA and arachidonic acid in serum total lipids, and increased plasma levels of prostaglandins E_2 and $F_{2\alpha}$ (*83*). A double-blind, placebo-controlled test was conducted in 11 children with IDDM to see if evening primrose oil, which is rich in γ-linolenic acid, could normalize these measures. Six children received 2 capsules/day of evening primrose oil for 4 months followed by 4 capsules/day for an additional 4 months. The lower dose did not alter prostaglandin levels, but with the higher dose DGLA levels increased significantly and prostaglandin E_2 decreased significantly. Biosynthetic pathways of prostaglandin biosynthesis and feedback between them were discussed.

The metabolism of medium-chain triglycerides differs markedly from metabolism of long-chain triglycerides (*84*). Both the intact medium-chain triglycerides and the hydrolyzed fatty acids are rapidly absorbed from the gut. They do not enter the lymphatics and peripheral circulation as chylomicrons but are transported directly to the liver, where they are readily metabolized. In a 5-day crossover design, the metabolic effects of a 40% fat diet containing 77.5% of fat calories as medium-chain triglycerides and an isocaloric diet containing long-chain triglycerides were compared. Seven subjects with NIDDM showed improved glycemic control during medium-chain triglyceride feeding, as measured by preprandial glucose excursion. The amount of glucose needed to maintain euglycemia during intravenous insulin infusion was increased not only in diabetics but also in hypertriglyceridemic subjects and, to a lesser extent, normal controls. Medium-chain triglycerides increased the rate of insulin-mediated glucose disposal but did not alter basal glucose metabolism or insulin-mediated suppression of hepatic glucose output. Fasting serum β-hydroxybutyrate levels increased in normal controls but not in diabetics. The authors concluded that medium-chain triglycerides increase insulin-mediated glucose metabolism in NIDDM patients by increasing insulin-mediated glucose disposal, and thus may be a useful adjunct to conventional therapy for NIDDM.

Other dietary and lifestyle factors

Life expectancy of diabetics is reduced more by pathologic changes in the vascular system than by acute complications of insulin deficiency. Rösen et al. reviewed evidence for the role of oxidative stress in development of the vascular complications of diabetes (*85*). They first considered whether the observed effects stem from a true increase in oxidative stress or from a decreased capacity to compensate for it. Impaired regeneration of free-radical scavengers due to decreased availability of NADPH may be involved. Another explanation invokes the formation of advanced glycosylation end products, in which increased levels of blood sugar facilitate nonenzymatic addition of sugars to the free amino groups of proteins, with subsequent rearrangement to yield stable ketoamines. Whatever the mechanism, preliminary data indicate that treatment with antioxidants (vitamin E, vitamin C, glutathione) can retard or prevent development of the vascular complications of diabetes. The ability of vitamin E to inhibit protein glycosylation in vivo was evaluated in patients with IDDM (*86*). Matched groups of 10 subjects each received 0, 600, or 1200 mg/day of vitamin E for 2 months. Fasting plasma glucose, mean daily plasma glucose, fasting labile hemoglobin A_1, and glycosylated proteins were measured at baseline and after 1 and 2 months of treatment. Hyperglycemic clamp studies were also performed. Glycemic indexes did not change during the study, but there were significant, dose-related reductions in fasting labile hemoglobin A_1, stable hemoglobin A_1, and glycosylated proteins in groups receiving vitamin E. Thus protein glycosylation can be reduced in diabetic subjects with no accompanying change in plasma glucose.

A prospective cohort study of >84,000 women in the USA assessed dietary risk factors for clinical NIDDM (*87*). During the 6-year follow-up 702 new cases were identified. After controlling for body mass index, previous weight change, and alcohol intake, no associations were found between risk of NIDDM and intake of total energy, protein, sucrose, carbohydrate, or fiber. Significant inverse associations were found for intake of vegetable fat, potassium, calcium, and magnesium. These associations were attenuated in obese women. A separate study showed that magnesium supplements can improve glucose handling in the elderly (*88*). Although plasma concentrations and urinary loss of magnesium were similar in young and old nonobese adults, concentrations of magnesium in the erythrocytes were significantly lower in older subjects. Four weeks of supplementation with 4.5 g/day of magnesium significantly increased erythrocyte magnesium concentration and improved insulin response and action. The increase in erythrocyte magnesium was inversely correlated with erythrocyte membrane microviscosity.

Proteins, particularly cow's milk proteins, are important dietary triggers of the autoimmune process leading to IDDM in genetically predisposed individuals (89). Studies in the spontaneously diabetic BB rat showed that eliminating intact cow's milk proteins from the diet during the weaning period (13–23 days) significantly reduced the incidence of IDDM even when the animals were later exposed to these proteins; withdrawal of cow's milk proteins from diets of animals exposed during weaning did not protect them from developing IDDM. Among both humans and rats, newly identified diabetics exhibit higher levels of antibodies to cow's milk proteins (β-lactoglobulin and bovine serum albumin) than normal controls. Moreover, antibodies to bovine serum albumin cross-reacted with a pancreatic β-cell membrane protein of M_r 69,000, which is thought to be induced by interferon. These observations and results of additional molecular studies led the authors to hypothesize that bovine milk proteins share antigenic epitopes with host-cell proteins and through molecular mimicry can trigger an autoimmune response in genetically predisposed individuals, resulting in clinical expression of IDDM. The rat experiments further suggest that there is a specific window of sensitivity during infancy. This hypothesis is testable and could lead to prevention of IDDM in some children. An epidemiologic study compared the age-standardized incidence rates of childhood IDDM with consumption of cow's milk (90). Diabetes registries and data on fluid cow's milk consumption from Finland, Sweden, Norway, Great Britain, Denmark, the USA, New Zealand, the Netherlands, Canada, France, Israel, and Japan were used. The data fit a linear regression model, with $r = .96$ and 94% of the geographic variation in incidence of IDDM explained by differences in milk consumption. A matched case–control study investigated

the role of early infant feeding in development of IDDM in Blacks and Whites (91). Among Whites but not Blacks, diabetics were less likely than controls to have been breast-fed. Duration of partial and exclusive breast feeding did not differ between diabetics and controls in either Blacks or Whites. In Blacks, however, the first exposure to breast-milk substitutes occurred at an earlier age in diabetic subjects than in controls. This relationship was true for all breast-milk substitutes, whether or not they contained cow's milk protein. The authors pointed out that a recent trend toward increased breast feeding has not been accompanied by a reduced incidence of IDDM, as would be expected if breast feeding alone were protective. However, this study does implicate early infant diet in development of childhood IDDM.

Swanston-Flatt et al. reviewed traditional medicines and foods used to treat diabetes before the introduction of insulin in 1922 (92). A list of 40 traditional dietary adjuncts used to treat diabetes in the U.K. includes many ordinary foods and spices such as chili pepper, ginger, tarragon, thyme, cabbage, garlic, onion, pea, turnip, mushrooms, apple, lemon, lime, blackberry, and sweet corn. Data showing effects of various adjuncts on glucose and insulin levels, food and fluid intake, and body weight in normal and diabetic rats were presented; in general, changes were seen only after induction of diabetes by streptozotocin. Guayusa, mushroom, burdock, nettle, agrimony, lucerne, coriander, eucalyptus, and juniper all improved glucose or insulin levels or both. The authors cautioned that "natural" is not synonymous with "safe" and many of these traditional remedies are toxic if consumed in large quantities. Rhizomes of the Indonesian vegetable and medicinal plant *Curcuma xanthorrhiza* Roxb. ameliorated the diabetic symptoms of growth retardation, hyperphagia, polydipsia, and elevated serum glucose and triglycerides in streptozotocin-induced diabetic rats (93). It also improved the ratio of arachidonate to linoleate in liver phospholipids and modified the amount and composition of fecal bile acids. These investigations have not been extended to models of NIDDM.

The short-term effects of red wine drunk with meals were assessed in 5 men with IDDM and 10 with NIDDM (*94*). On two consecutive days the men ate identical meals, accompanied in random order by two glasses of water or two glasses of red wine. Insulin requirement was determined by an artificial pancreas for the IDDM patients, and glucose tolerance was evaluated from the postprandial glycemic level in NIDDM patients. There were no significant differences between meals in terms of insulin requirement. There was a smaller rise in blood glucose in NIDDM patients after the meal with wine; insulin levels were comparable, although the peak was reached later after wine. The authors concluded that moderate consumption of red wine with meals has no adverse effect on glycemic control in diabetics. The wine contains tannins and phytates that might explain its action.

After reviewing the literature, O'Dea analyzed data from 28 reports on "lifestyle diseases" of Australian Aborigines (*95*). An additional 27 reports on obesity, NIDDM, insulin resistance, and related subjects were used to help interpret the data on Aborigines. The review discussed the transition of the Aborigines from the hunter–gatherer lifestyle to a westernized lifestyle, which revealed their unusual vulnerability to NIDDM. The author concluded that insulin resistance, which was advantageous for survival in the traditional lifestyle, is the underlying metabolic characteristic that predisposes this people to obesity, NIDDM, and coronary heart disease when they adopt the Western lifestyle and diet.

A study of insulin-resistant subjects, subjects with NIDDM, and normal controls evaluated the effects of an intensive 3-week program of diet and exercise on hyperinsulinemia and associated risk factors for atherosclerosis (*96*). All participants underwent a physical examination and treadmill test, on which individualized walking programs were based. Their diet followed the Pritikin Eating Plan, which prescribes <10 en% fat, 10–15 en% protein, and 75–80% en% carbohydrate. All groups had significant decreases in all risk factors, but the changes were greatest in the NIDDM patients. Seventeen of the 29 insulin-resistant subjects achieved normal fasting insulin levels.

NIDDM has been suggested to be a manifestation of a "thrifty genotype" that aids fuel conservation (*97*). To test this hypothesis, NIDDM and normal subjects were studied after 6 days on a 700-calorie diet and 6 days on a 2800-calorie diet. With 2800 calories per day diabetics had a higher median basal plasma glucose level than controls, but with the energy-restricted diet there was no difference. The two groups had similar plasma insulin levels, but these were 2–3 times higher on the high-calorie diet. Postprandial insulin levels also increased to a similar extent in the two groups. On both diets, NIDDM subjects had an impaired first-phase insulin response to an intravenous glucose load. NIDDM and control groups experienced similar weight loss and similar increase in plasma ketone bodies on the energy-restricted diet. The authors saw no evidence of a "thrifty" response in the NIDDM group and suggested that a potentially harmful genetic defect persisted during evolution not because it conferred an advantage but because under the prevailing conditions it did not confer a disadvantage.

ENDOCRINE SYSTEM, METABOLISM, AND REPRODUCTION

A study of endocrine and metabolic effects of long-term food restriction in rats found that such restriction preserves the integrity of many metabolic functions (*98*). From the age of 6 weeks until they were 28 weeks old, male Fischer rats were fed 60% of the food consumed by ad libitum–fed controls, plus a vitamin supplement. "Young" controls were analyzed when they were 3 months old; "old" controls, after 28 weeks. Old diet-restricted animals showed no significant age-related change in serum levels of luteinizing hormone, testosterone, or T_4, whereas these values were decreased in old controls. Serum triglycerides were reduced in diet-restricted animals but elevated in old controls, relative to young controls. Serum cholesterol was significantly elevated in both groups of old rats, but more so in rats fed ad libitum.

Insulin-like growth factor-I (IGF-I) and -II peptides are structurally related to insulin and their secretion is nutritionally regulated (*99*). These growth factors and their binding proteins are major links between nutrient intake and cellular anabolic responses. The review by Clemmons and Underwood summarized the autocrine, paracrine, and endocrine actions of IGF; nutritional control of IGF-I synthesis, secretion, and plasma concentrations; nutritional regulation of IGF-binding protein concentrations; and control of IGF action by binding proteins. Nutrient restriction apparently produces resistance to IGF-I and growth hormone by mechanisms that are manifest at multiple points in the IGF biosynthetic pathway.

In addition to peptides with opioid and immunostimulating activities (30), milk also contains peptides with growth-factor activity (100). Nabet et al. reviewed the modes of transmission and principal mechanisms of action of growth factors, citing the most important growth factors in various tissues and biological fluids (100). They summarized the biochemical composition of two whey fractions and their growth-promoting activity in cell culture. Among the bioactive constituents of milk are ACTH, progesterone, α-fetoprotein, gastrin, histamine, insulin, thyroid-stimulating hormone, luteinizing hormone, and prolactin.

Another review considered the effects of dietary estrogens on a variety of reproductive processes and biochemical events (101). A phenolic ring enables numerous substances to bind to the estrogen receptor, frequently conferring on them activity as estrogen agonists or antagonists. Isoflavonoids are such "phytoestrogens"; they are defensive compounds whose synthesis is largely controlled by environmental circumstances and whose concentrations in food can therefore be highly variable. Biochemical actions of phytoestrogens may be receptor- or membrane-linked; they can affect ion transport, enzyme secretion, and numerous enzyme activities. Because endogenous steroidal and catecholamine estrogens also play a role in many of these processes, it is likely that many activities of plant flavonoids are attributable to their estrogen-like structures. Thus dietary phytoestrogens provide a background against which endogenous estrogen acts.

The estrogenic action of the phytoestrogen coumestrol was examined in immature female rats fed concentrations of coumestrol that might occur in a normal human diet (102). Coumestrol competitively inhibited binding of estrogen to the estrogen receptor and exerted a cumulative dose-dependent uterotrophic effect. Isoflavonoids in lab chow had similar effects, compared with a control semipurified diet. Because rats lack the sex hormone–binding globulin found in primates the implications of these findings for humans are not entirely clear. They suggest, however, that the dietary phytoestrogen coumestrol is a potent estrogen that must be considered in estimates of the total lifetime estrogenic load to which humans are exposed. The same research group reported that dietary coumestrol has agonistic effects on estrogen-dependent processes in immature female rats (103). After 4 days of treatment, induction of progestin receptors was observed in the uterus, pituitary, and hypothalamus–preoptic area. Vaginal opening was accelerated and occurred at a lower body weight; prolonged treatment led to irregularity in vaginal cycles, suggesting that coumestrol induced permanent changes in reproductive function.

An interesting commentary concerned dietary phytoestrogens and the menopause in Japan (104). It has been observed that Japanese women have a much lower frequency of hot flushes than Canadian women. When urinary excretion of phytoestrogens was determined in Japanese subjects living in the Kyoto area, levels of genistein, daidzein, and equol 100–1000 times higher than levels of endogenous estrogens were found. These compounds bind to estrogen receptors and act as weak estrogens. The authors suggested that the estrogenic effects of dietary phytoestrogens might be particularly noticeable in the background of low endogenous estrogen in postmenopausal women, perhaps explaining why women whose diets contain large quantities of phytoestrogens have a lower frequency of hot flushes and other menopausal symptoms.

The effects of dietary components on physical and hormonal sexual maturation were examined in pubertal girls (105). Results of multivariate analysis indicated that fiber was the most important factor; breast development was slower and hormonal concentrations lower in girls who consumed less dietary fiber. The authors suggested that this effect is mediated by the hypothalamus–pituitary–gonad system.

A reader hypothesized that the observed effects were due to mild zinc deficiency resulting from the phytate content of the diet (*106*); this was the explanation for delayed puberty in an Iranian village (J.A. Halsted et al., *Am. J. Med.* 53:277, 1972). In their response the authors discussed problems in extrapolating conclusions of the earlier study to their results (*107*). They could not rule out a role for zinc in their study but suggested it was unlikely because of the normal growth and greater prepubertal height of the girls with slower pubertal development.

A cohort of 213 girls (aged 10 years ± 9 months) was followed for 4 years, until 82% of the 194 parents who responded reported that their daughter had had her first menstrual period (*108*). Analysis of dietary information and other measures showed that the relative risk of menarche before the age of 12.5 years was 2.0 for the tallest girls compared with the shortest, and 2.1 for the fattest girls compared with the leanest. Menarcheal age was not associated with intake of energy or energy-adjusted intake of protein, fat, or carbohydrate. The results support the idea that nutritional factors influence age at menarche mainly through their effects on accumulation of adipose tissue.

A double-blind crossover trial was conducted in 33 women with premenstrual syndrome, to determine the effects of calcium supplementation on perimenstrual symptoms (*109*). By factor analysis four factors (negative affect, water retention, food, and pain) accounted for 67% of the total variance in scale scores. Calcium supplementation significantly reduced negative affect, water retention, and pain during the luteal phase and pain during the menstrual phase.

The effect of dietary fat on length of the follicular phase of the menstrual cycle was evaluated in a controlled-diet setting (*110*). Thirty healthy subjects were randomized to diets containing low (0.3) or high (1.0) P/S ratios. After a free-living baseline period of one menstrual cycle, subjects were placed on a high-fat (40 en%) diet for four cycles and then on a low-fat (20 en%) diet for four cycles, maintaining the designated P/S ratio. Both low-fat diets significantly increased the length of the follicular phase. There was also a trend toward an increased length of the follicular phase with the diets having a P/S ratio of 0.3, but the number of subjects was too small to draw definite conclusions about this.

Lean white fish was substituted for other sources of animal protein in diets of postmenopausal women at high risk of coronary heart disease to investigate effects on plasma lipoproteins and endogenous sex hormones (*111*). Both test diets provided 19% protein, 52% carbohydrate, and 29% lipids, with a P/M/S ratio of 1.1:1:1. Animal protein was supplied as either fish or a combination of beef, pork, egg, and milk. The fish diet caused significantly higher levels of plasma total, HDL, and HDL$_3$ cholesterol and LDL-apoB, showing it to have no beneficial effect on these variables in postmenopausal women. It also significantly increased levels of sex hormone–binding globulin. Because the P/M/S ratio was the same in both diets, leaving the nature of the animal protein as the major difference, the authors concluded that fish protein prevents the reduction of plasma cholesterol by PUFAs. It is also plausible that sex hormone–binding globulin modulated the cholesterol and lipoprotein response to fish protein.

A case–control study assessed the relationship between calcium intake in the first 20 weeks of pregnancy and risk of preeclampsia and gestational hypertension (*112*). Subjects were 172 women with preeclampsia, 251 with gestational hypertension, and 505 controls who delivered their first baby in Quebec City or Montreal in 1984–1986. Dietary calcium was not associated with preeclampsia. For gestational hypertension, however, the adjusted odds ratio decreased progressively from 1.0 in the lowest quartile of calcium consumption to 0.60 in the highest. Other studies conducted in Guatemala and Argentina and at the Johns Hopkins Hospital, Baltimore, evaluated the role of calcium in pregnancy-induced hypertension and low birth-weight (*113*). The authors concluded that by lowering blood pressure during pregnancy, calcium supplementation may also influence the incidence of preeclampsia or the gestational age at which it develops. In addition, calcium's effect on smooth muscle relaxation could decrease the incidence of prematurity. These results may be mediated by calcium's influence on circulating parathyroid hormone and renin concentrations, which modulate intracellular transport of ionized calcium; the same mechanism may be responsible for reducing uterine activity.

Community diet-related differences in blood pressure during pregnancy were assessed in Inuit women from seven communities in the Keewatin region of the Northwest Territories (*114*). Women from the three communities with the highest consumption of fish and marine mammals had significantly lower mean diastolic blood pressure values during the last 6 hours of pregnancy. This relationship was independent of other factors. These women were also less likely to have been hypertensive during pregnancy than women from the four communities where less marine food was consumed. Data from harvest of marine mammals and fish by Inuit hunters from the various communities and from diet surveys were substantiated by levels of EPA in cord serum.

A paper by Secher and Olsen (reference *86* in chapter 4, *Food Safety 1991*) on fish oil and preeclampsia drew comment by several readers (*115–117*). Baker and Pipkin pointed out that platelet angiotensin II binding sites and angiotensin II pressor sensitivity are both increased in patients with preeclampsia. One suggested explanation for this is that there is an inherited or acquired defect in platelet membranes of women with preeclampsia, for which fish oil might compensate. This is a testable hypothesis. However, Pipkin further pointed out possible hazards of fish-oil supplementation during pregnancy (*116*), and other readers stressed that all fish-oil and *n*–3 PUFA preparations are not equivalent and that in the long run low-dose aspirin might provide the same benefits as fish oil during pregnancy and be better accepted (*117*). Secher et al. responded to the concerns of these correspondents (*118*).

The high birth weights and long duration of pregnancy in the Faroe Islands led Olsen et al. to hypothesize that high intake of marine *n*–3 PUFAs prolongs gestation by shifting the balance of production of prostaglandins involved in parturition (*119*). In a randomized controlled trial they compared the effects of a fish-oil supplement, an olive-oil supplement, and no supplement on length of gestation and weight and length of the newborn. Subjects were 533 healthy Danish women in the 30th week of pregnancy. Average duration of gestation, birth weight, and birth length were greatest in the fish-oil group and least in the olive-oil group, the differences in gestation reflecting a shift in the entire distribution. After adjustment for length of gestation, differences in average birth weight and length were not significant. Diet surveys revealed that duration of gestation also increased with increasing fish consumption, regardless of the supplement tested. Because fish-oil supplementation in late pregnancy seemed to delay delivery without affecting fetal growth or impairing parturition, the authors postulated that the supplement was acting on processes leading to initiation of parturition.

To determine whether diet can modify the embryotoxic effects of diabetes, female rats were made diabetic by streptozotocin injection 2 weeks before mating (*120*). Groups of pregnant rats were then maintained on a standard diet, a purified high-protein diet, and a purified diet with normal protein content. Control nondiabetic pregnant rats were fed the standard diet. Rats fed the normal-protein diet showed a higher rate of embryo resorption, lower fetal weight, and higher frequency of major malformations than the other groups. This experiment could not distinguish between a protective effect of a high-protein diet and a harmful effect of a high-carbohydrate diet.

KIDNEY DISEASE AND FUNCTION

Ahmed reviewed evidence associating diet with chronic renal disease and demonstrating that dietary manipulation can slow the loss of residual renal function (*121*). When ingested over long periods of time, excess dietary protein can increase normal blood flow and glomerular filtration rate. According to one theory, this predisposes healthy individuals to progressive glomerular sclerosis and deterioration of renal function, which in turn may accelerate development of the sclerosis. Restricting dietary protein, phosphorus, or both generally retards the loss of renal function in patients with chronic renal insufficiency. Lipids are also implicated in this process.

Donadio reviewed the potential of *n*–3 PUFAs in treating immune renal disease (*122*). He discussed the sources, nomenclature, and biological activities of *n*–3 and *n*–6 PUFAs. Studies in experimental models of glomerular injury and clinical trials of fish oil supplementation in patients with renal disorders were then summarized. Among the reported benefits of fish oil are prevention or amelioration of proteinuria; prolonged survival; improvement in blood rheology, platelet aggregation, and lipid parameters; and perhaps diminution of cyclosporine-induced nephrotoxicity and inhibition of inflammatory and atherogenic mechanisms in lupus nephritis. In another review, Holub et al. discussed animal studies and clinical trials of *n*–3 PUFAs for modification of renal disorders (*123*). These studies indicate that fish oil acts by modifying the fatty acid composition of membrane phospholipids in platelets, the glomerulus, and inflammatory cells. This results in changes in arachidonic acid metabolism, with decreased production of thromboxane A_2, leukotriene B_4, and platelet-activating factor, which have been implicated in various renal pathophysiologies.

A study in rats revealed how dietary fish oil interferes with renal arachidonic acid metabolism (*124*). One group of male weanling rats was fed an ad libitum diet enriched in fish oil; pair-matched controls were fed the same basic diet with safflower oil substituted for fish oil, each rat being given the amount eaten the day before by the experimental animal paired with him. Fish oil had antidiuretic and antinatriuretic effects that correlated with reduced renal cortical endogenous prostaglandin E_2. It altered the renal ratio of prostacyclin to thromboxane A_2 in favor of vasodilation. After 6 months of fish-oil feeding, rats showed increased proteinuria and decreased glomerular filtration rate and estimated renal plasma flow. The possible role of lipid peroxidation and free radical formation in these deleterious effects was discussed. After uninephrectomy, fish-oil feeding augmented the compensatory increase in glomerular filtration rate by the remaining kidney. In a study of the effects of dietary fat on glomerular hemodynamics, groups of young male rats were fed diets containing 20% fat as coconut oil, sunflower oil, or fish oil (*125*). Micropuncture studies were performed after 4–6 weeks of feeding. Rats fed fish oil exhibited increased single-nephron glomerular filtration rates and single-nephron plasma flow. These changes were not associated with altered glomerular capillary hydraulic pressure or glomerular ultrafiltration coefficient. The increased single-nephron plasma flow resulted from a 37% decrease in efferent arteriolar resistance. These hemodynamic actions may partly explain fish oil's effects on the course of experimental and clinical renal disease.

A 12-week trial of daily fish-oil supplementation (1.8 g of EPA and 1.2 g of DHA) was conducted in nondiabetic patients with chronic renal insufficiency (*126*). Measurements of renal function were made at baseline, at the end of fish-oil supplementation, and again 12 weeks later. Glomerular filtration rate and effective renal plasma flow did not change during the study. Erythrocyte viscosity improved significantly. There were increases in HDL and HDL_2 cholesterol and decreases in VLDL cholesterol and triglycerides; total and LDL cholesterol tended to increase. Values of most plasma lipid parameters had returned to baseline 12 weeks after fish-oil supplementation was stopped. Thus daily ingestion of fish oil had a favorable effect on erythrocyte deformability but had both positive and negative effects on the lipid profile; whether the favorable effects outweigh the unfavorable has not been established.

The effect of dietary proteins and lipids was studied in 24 patients with primary membranous glomerulopathy whose proteinuria was in the nephrotic range (*127*). The test diets were a normal mixed-protein diet containing <30 en% fat and <200 mg of cholesterol, and a low-protein vegetarian diet supplemented with essential amino acids, containing <30 en% fat and essentially no cholesterol, with carbohydrate making up for the reduction in protein. Both diets contained 10 en% linoleic acid, but the low-protein diet had a higher P/S ratio. After at least 1 month on the normoprotein diet, subjects ate the normoprotein and low-protein diets for periods of 3 months in a randomized crossover design. Protein restriction had no effect on glomerular filtration rate, urinary protein loss, and serum albumin concentration. Serum total and LDL cholesterol and proteinuria were significantly lower than baseline levels after both diet periods, probably as a result of reducing dietary fat intake.

Nephrotic patients with persistent proteinuria also have various lipid abnormalities that may promote atherosclerosis and more rapid progression of renal disease (*128*). The effects of a low-fat, high-fiber, vegetarian soy-based diet on hyperlipidemia were evaluated in 20 untreated subjects with chronic glomerular diseases, stable severe proteinuria, and hyperlipidemia. During the 8-week test-diet period there were significant decreases in total, LDL, and HDL cholesterol, apoA, and apoB, but serum triglyceride concentrations did not change. Urinary protein excretion and creatinine clearance decreased significantly. Values of all variables except creatinine clearance had returned to near-baseline levels 8 weeks after the subjects resumed their usual diets. A study of steroid-resistant nephrotic patients with normal serum creatinine levels evaluated a vegan diet supplemented with essential amino acids and keto analogues (*129*). Free and albumin-bound serum fatty acids were measured after patients had eaten a free mixed-protein diet and after they had eaten the supplemented vegan diet for an average of 1 month. The following significant changes were observed after the test-diet period: decreased proteinuria, serum cholesterol, and serum free palmitic acid, and increased free serum linoleic acid. There were also nonsignificant increases in all albumin-bound fatty acids (C18:2, C18:1, C18, and C16) whether expressed as nmol/mL of serum or as nmol/nmol of albumin.

A central feature of glomerulosclerosis is the pathological accumulation of extracellular matrix in diseased glomeruli, and transforming growth factor β1 has widespread regulatory effects on extracellular matrix. The effects of dietary protein restriction were studied in a rat model of glomerulonephritis (*130*). Feeding of a low-protein diet rapidly reduced the elevated expression of transforming growth factor β1 and its mRNA that ordinarily occur after induction of glomerulonephritis in this model. These rats did not develop excess glomerular extracellular matrix and had less proteinuria than controls.

Selenium deficiency is the putative cause of Balkan endemic nephropathy. Data on selenium deficiency in Yugoslavia were reviewed, with reference to selenium content of rocks, soils, stream sediments, cereal crops, and human serum, tissues, and scalp hair (*131*).

GASTROINTESTINAL TRACT

Dietary influences on the gastric mucosa and ulcer disease

Marotta and Floch reviewed the association between diet and gastric and duodenal ulcer disease, and discussed the dietary treatment of ulcers (*132*). The remarkable historical shifts in diet therapy may result from the lack of evidence that diet plays any major role in either healing or relapse. The authors concluded that there is now little role for dietary therapy and no need to place patients with gastric ulcer disease on restrictive diets, although it is prudent to avoid spices that cause discomfort, coffee (not necessarily caffeine in general), and alcohol. The putative beneficial effects of a high-fiber diet may stem not from the fiber but from an unidentified protective factor in such diets; alternatively, there may be no direct benefit of high-fiber diets but rather a detrimental effect of low-fiber diets.

While results of diet therapy for ulcer disease are equivocal, epidemiologic studies continue to show a relationship between diet and incidence of gastric and duodenal ulcers. A prospective study of Hawaiian men of Japanese ancestry born between 1900 and 1919 identified 280 incident cases of gastric ulcer and 149 of duodenal ulcer after 149,291 person-years of observation (*133*). Risk of both forms of ulcer was directly related to pack-years of cigarette smoking, but there was no association with alcohol intake. Risk of gastric ulcer was positively associated with use of table salt or soy sauce; there was no association with other Oriental foods, milk, or fruit. Risk of duodenal ulcer was inversely associated with consumption of a Western-style diet around 1940 and with eating two or more servings of bread per day.

An experiment in rats showed that intragastric administration of as little as 10 µL of fish oil 30 min before intragastric administration of ethanol significantly reduced the lesion score (*134*). When administered daily for 2 weeks with the last dose given 48 h before the ethanol, only the highest dose of fish oil (1000 µL) was protective.

Because eicosanoids mediate defensive and inflammatory processes in the gut mucosa and dietary fatty acids are precursors in eicosanoid biosynthesis, the effects of dietary fat on mucosal eicosanoid biosynthesis and development of duodenal ulcers were studied in rats (*135*). A low-fat rodent diet was supplemented with 8% by weight of sunflower or cod liver oil and fed to groups of rats for 4 weeks. Plasma fatty acid profiles changed as expected. Production of prostaglandin E_2, 6-keto-prostaglandin $F_{1\alpha}$, thromboxane B_2, and leukotriene B_4 were sharply reduced in the cod liver oil group; prostaglandin E_3 and leukotriene B_5 were undetectable in the sunflower oil group. In rats with duodenal damage induced by cysteamine, the cod liver oil diet palliated the progression of chronic ulcerative lesions and shortened the course of the disease. This effect was associated with reduction in luminal release of thromboxane and leukotriene B_4 during the chronic stage of the inflammatory lesions.

The effects of ellagic acid on gastric H^+,K^+-ATPase activity were studied in mucosal preparations from hog stomach, and effects on acid secretion and gastric ulcers were studied using a stress-ulcer model in rats (*136*). Ellagic acid inhibited gastric H^+,K^+-ATPase activity by 50% at 2.1×10^{-6} M; this inhibition was competitive with respect to ATP and noncompetitive with respect to K^+. In rats, gastric lesions were induced by water immersion and restraint. Intraperitoneal administration of ellagic acid at doses >5 mg/kg significantly reduced acid secretion and the occurrence of gastric lesions. The authors postulated that this was due to inhibition of H^+,K^+-ATPase activity.

In another rat study, feeding diets with 9–10% menhaden oil reduced sucrase activity and production of prostaglandin E_2 and leukotriene B_4 in the small-intestinal mucosa and appeared to stimulate

mucosal regeneration after methotrexate-induced injury (*137*).

Intestinal effects of dietary fiber

Eastwood and Morris summarized observations on the function of dietary fiber along the gastrointestinal tract, attempting to extend these principles to other dietary constituents (*138*). They reviewed structure–function relationships of dietary fiber with respect to hydration, cell wall structures, and physiological properties. Transport of nutrients and digesta viscosity in the foregut were discussed. Equations describing the role of dietary fiber in small-intestinal function were presented. Other sections covered effects on steroid metabolism, cecal fermentation, and fecal parameters. By attempting to classify dietary fiber in a more physical manner, recognizing the diverse actions of different fibers at various sites, the authors hoped to provide a model to explain and predict the physiological action of polymers in general.

MacDonald et al. found that different dietary fibers had different effects on insulin receptors in the rat intestinal mucosa (*139*). Relative to a fiber-free diet, corn bran increased insulin binding in the duodenum by 30% and in the ileum by 50%, but decreased it by 44% in the jejunum. Guar gum increased binding in the colon by 73% but decreased binding in the jejunum by 40%. Wheat and oat brans increased binding 50% in the small intestine. Receptor autophosphorylation was 30% greater with fiber-free or wheat bran diets than with cellulose or oat bran. The authors postulated that these changes in receptor binding and activity are related to the altered rates of cell proliferation reported by others in response to dietary fiber.

A feeding study in pigs showed that 6% guar gum, compared with cellulose or a fiber-free diet, reduced glucose absorption and production of insulin, gastric inhibitory polypeptide, and insulin-like growth factor-1 but did not change the hepatic insulin and gastric inhibitory polypeptide extraction coefficients (*140*). Ingestion of guar gum roughly doubled the hepatic extraction coefficient of gut-produced insulin-like growth factor and decreased pancreatic glucagon secretion.

To test the physiological and metabolic effects of *Plantago ovata* seeds and husks in rats, a fiber-free elemental diet was supplemented with 100 or 200 g/kg of *P. ovata* seeds or husks or wheat bran (*141*). At the higher concentration, all supplements significantly increased fecal wet and dry weight but the husks were most effective. The *Plantago* supplements increased intestinal length and weight, but wheat bran had little or no effect. *Plantago* preparations also tended to have greater effects on fecal bacterial mass, total acetate in cecal contents and feces, fecal bile acid excretion, and β-glucuronidase activity. The three dietary fibers inhibited mucosal digestive enzyme activities to different degrees, or enhanced enzyme activity in the ileum.

Two feeding studies in pigs documented gastrointestinal effects of various wheat and oat fractions (*142,143*). The wheat products tested were refined flour, aleurone, pericarp and testa, and bran; rolled oats and oat bran were also tested. The first study documented differences in the digestibility and bulking properties of the various fractions (*142*). The second documented effects on microbial activity and production of short-chain fatty acids in the gastrointestinal tract (*143*). Together, they showed that the gastrointestinal effects of various types of cereal dietary fiber are highly correlated with the chemical and structural composition of the cell wall materials. The authors believe that these observations in pigs are also valid for humans.

To see whether guar and psyllium are fermented by human fecal bacteria in vivo as they are in vitro, a control polysaccharide-free diet and the same diet supplemented with 20 g of guar or psyllium were fed to normal young adults (*144*). Breath hydrogen and methane and serum acetate concentrations were measured. Ingestion of guar produced a nonsignificant increase in breath hydrogen and a significant increase in breath methane; there were significant differences in serum acetate concentrations in the order guar > psyllium > control. The authors concluded that guar is fermented in the human colon but their data do not permit conclusions about psyllium. In assessing the effects of increased colonic fermentation on serum lipids, the same research group unexpectedly found that supplementation of metabolic diets with lactulose, while apparently increasing intestinal fermentation, also significantly increased fasting serum total and LDL cholesterol and apoB levels (*145*). The authors concluded that certain rapidly fermented substrates may raise rather than lower serum lipids, perhaps by increasing the amount of acetate absorbed from the colon. For fermentation to contribute to the hypolipidemic effect of fiber, sufficient propionate must be produced to offset the effects of increasing the amount of acetate available as a precursor for lipid synthesis. This is a property of certain viscous fibers such as purified gums and pectins.

Intestinal effects of dietary fat

A randomized, double-blind, placebo-controlled crossover trial evaluated the effects of fish-oil supplementation in patients with active ulcerative colitis (*146*). Rectal dialysate levels of leukotriene B_4 decreased from 71.0 pg/mL at baseline to 27.7 pg/mL after 4 months of supplementation with 3.24 g/day of EPA and 2.16 g/day of DHA. Significant histological improvement was seen and significant weight gain occurred. Seven patients who were receiving concurrent treatment with prednisone were able to halve their average dose during fish-oil supplementation. No significant changes occurred during the placebo period. Although the gains were modest and did not justify recommending fish oil as sole therapy for acute ulcerative colitis, the authors suggested consideration of fish-oil supplements for patients who require long-term continuous steroid treatment to control symptoms. In another clinical trial, patients with active ulcerative colitis or Crohn's disease were randomized to receive capsules of MaxEPA or olive oil for 12 weeks while eating their customary diet (*147*). With fish oil, concentrations of EPA and DHA were significantly increased in colonic mucosal lipids, while arachidonic acid levels fell progressively throughout the study. Fish oil suppressed mucosal prostaglandin E_2, thromboxane B_2, and 6-keto-prostaglandin $F_{1\alpha}$. These changes would be expected to benefit inflammatory bowel disease. Olive oil supplementation significantly increased oleic acid in colonic mucosa while decreasing stearic acid and DHA; eicosanoid synthesis was not affected.

A high-fat, low-fiber Western-type diet was a significant risk factor for torsion of the colon in vervet monkeys (African green monkeys, *Cercopithecus aethiops*) (*148*). Other risk factors were male sex, older age, and a solitary and relatively sedentary existence in a confined space. The longer mesentery and larger abdomen in the adult male probably increases his risk of torsion.

STONE DISEASES

According to a review of the role of environmental factors in the development of idiopathic renal calcium stones, there is little doubt that dietary factors (particularly hypernutrition) are involved but specific cause–effect relationships elude identification and proof (*149*). Although "eating too much" is considered a risk factor, studies of eating habits in Germany show that most men consume too many calories, too much fat and protein, and too little carbohydrate; there is not necessarily a difference between men who develop stones and men who do not. The reviewer also felt that current interest in renal stones emphasizes oxalate at the expense of other dietary substances involved in stone formation. Among the dietary factors implicated are liquid intake and total and relative amounts of calcium, magnesium, sodium, phosphorus, and perhaps other minerals including anions. The role of vitamin D was also discussed, but more with reference to exposure to sunlight than to dietary sources. Lipids bind calcium in the intestine and can thus influence calcium and oxalate absorption; they are found in the matrix of urinary stones; and phosphatidylethanolamine has been considered a precursor of oxalate, which induces lipid peroxidation, which, in turn, is enhanced during stone formation in rats. Ingestion of fish oil has reduced urinary calcium and oxalate in patients with recurrent calcium urolithiasis. Mechanisms have also been suggested for the involvement of excessive protein intake in stone formation. Although numerous pathways of carbohydrate metabolism lead to oxalate production, the influence of fiber and complex carbohydrates has not been thoroughly studied. High alcohol

consumption may be a risk factor because it is frequently associated with hyperuricosuria, hyperphosphaturia, and hypercalciuria. The authors concluded that much needs to be done to understand how the Western diet interacts with hormones and metabolism to affect renal function, renal tissue minerals and oxalate, and the composition of urine.

Hughes and Norman reviewed the literature on diet and calcium stones with the goal of developing dietary guidelines for reducing the risk of recurrent stone formation (*150*). They recommended moderating intake of calcium, oxalate, protein, sodium, and alcohol and increasing intake of dietary fiber and water. Research is needed to document the long-term effects of dietary modification on urinary risk factors and rates of recurrence of calcium stones. Responding to this review, a reader suggested that dietary oxalate–bashing may obscure the fact that an increasing incidence of renal stones has been accompanied since the turn of the century by a decreasing consumption of foods rich in oxalates (*151*). What has increased in parallel with incidence of stones is intake of fat, sodium, and animal protein. Also, although Hughes and Norman considered vegetarian diets problematic because they can lead to increased excretion of oxalate, the reader pointed out that despite their higher oxalate intake, vegetarians have a lower-than-expected incidence of urinary stone disease.

The hypothesis that a shift in eicosanoid metabolism toward the $n-3$ pathway protects against development of kidney stones was tested by feeding EPA in a rat model of nephrocalcinosis (*152*). Two groups of rats were given injections of calcium gluconate to induce stone formation. Rats in one of these groups were fed MaxEPA before and during the period of calcium gluconate injections; a control group received saline injections. Nephrocalcinosis was readily induced in the positive controls but was prevented by fish-oil treatment. Urinary calcium excretion was significantly reduced in the treated animals. Treatment of 12 recurrent, hypercalciuric, hyperoxaluric stone-formers with MaxEPA for 8 weeks also reduced hypercalciuria and hyperoxaluria in these animals.

To measure the extent to which different dietary fibers can reduce renal calcium excretion, 15 healthy women were given a standardized calcium-rich diet with no bran and the same diet supplemented with 36 g of rice, soy, or wheat bran (*153*). Each diet was eaten for 5 days. All bran diets tended to decrease renal calcium excretion and increase renal oxalic acid excretion, but rice bran was most effective ($p < .01$). The relative supersaturation of urine with calcium oxalate increased on all diets but the increase failed to reach statistical significance. The greatest increase in relative supersaturation, ~21%, occurred with wheat bran, which failed to alter renal calcium excretion significantly; the authors therefore concluded that oxalic acid excretion has a greater influence than calcium on this measure.

As is the case for renal stones, dietary risk factors for development of gallstones are not clearly established. A prospective analysis of 4730 women hospitalized with gallstone disease examined the role of dietary factors, dieting, and fasting period (*154*). After an average of 10 years of follow-up, 216 incident cases of gallstone disease were confirmed. Risk was positively associated with dieting and length of the overnight fasting period. High fiber intake was slightly protective. The effect of fat and total energy were age-dependent.

Two studies evaluated the effects of dietary fat on biliary lipids and cholesterol gallstone formation in African green monkeys, a useful animal model for this disease (*155,156*). Diets for the first study contained 0.34 g of cholesterol per 100 g of food with 42% of energy as lard or safflower oil (*155*). Groups of females were fed these diets throughout pregnancy and lactation. At weaning their sons were placed on the same diet until they were killed at 16 (prepubertal), 32 (peripubertal), or 60 (young adult) months of age. The type of dietary fat had no influence on composition of biliary lipids but had the anticipated effect on plasma lipids. Cholesterol gallstones were found in 2 of 23 of the young-adult animals, one from each diet group; no stones were found in younger monkeys. Gallbladder bile from 32-month-old monkeys had significantly more cholesterol and a higher cholesterol saturation index than bile from older or younger monkeys. The authors concluded that these peripubertal increases were not clinically significant in terms of gallstone formation. In the second study, adult males were fed

diets containing cholesterol and 42 en% fat (*156*). In one group, half of the fat was derived from lard and in the other, from menhaden oil. After 2.5–3 years 67% of animals fed the lard diet had cholesterol gallstones, compared with only 22% of the animals fed fish oil. The cholesterol saturation index was also higher in the lard-fed group. No difference in bile acid profiles was found. Fish-oil feeding led to higher levels of *n*–3 fatty acids in biliary phospholipids, and in liver perfusion studies these animals had a higher biliary lipid secretion rate. The authors concluded that the enhanced biliary phospholipid secretion, probably favored by enrichment of biliary phospholipids with relatively less hydrophobic *n*–3 fatty acids, produced a less lithogenic gallbladder bile.

TEETH AND BONES

Effects of diet on dental health

A review of sweeteners and dental health summarized the concept of dental caries as a multifactorial disease involving susceptible teeth, a cariogenic substrate, and cariogenic microorganisms (*157*). Clinical, animal, and bacteriologic studies of the cariogenicity of nutritive and nonnutritive sweeteners were then discussed.

Different populations of our Stone-Age ancestors also suffered from various degrees of dental caries that may have been diet-related (*158*). The $^{13}C/^{12}C$ ratio of bone collagen provides information about the relative importance of classes of foods in the diet. Depending on their photosynthetic pathway, land plants incorporate different proportions of carbon-12 and carbon-13 from the atmosphere. Temperate grasses and most shrubs and trees use the Calvin, or C_3, pathway, whereas tropical grasses use the C_4 system; marine organisms have a $^{13}C/^{12}C$ ratio similar to that of C_4 plants. Where there were no C_4 grasses, isotopic analysis of bones of hunter–gatherers reveals the proportions of marine and terrestrial foods eaten. Stable carbon isotope measurements and incidences of dental caries were presented for prehistoric human skeletons from different regions of Cape Province, South Africa. Isotope measurements showed that marine foods varied in importance through time, across space, and by sex. The incidence of caries was lowest among coastal skeletons in the southwestern Cape, intermediate at a noncoastal site in the southwest, and highest at a site in the southern Cape. In coastal skeletons, individuals who ate large amounts of seafood had a lower incidence of caries than persons who ate a more mixed marine and terrestrial diet. The high incidence of caries in the southern site may have resulted from low levels of fluoride in the groundwater.

A Finnish study of risk factors in dental erosion found considerable risk associated with eating citrus fruits oftener than twice a day, drinking soft drinks daily, or ingesting apple vinegar or sports beverages at least once weekly (*159*).

Two papers from Japan reported anticaries effects of green tea (*160,161*). An extract of polyphenolic compounds from *Camellia sinensis* inhibited attachment of a *Streptococcus mutans* strain to saliva-coated hydroxyapatite discs, inhibited formation of water-insoluble glucan from sucrose by a crude preparation of glucosyltransferase from *S. mutans*, and when added to drinking water, decreased the caries scores in specific pathogen–free rats infected with *S. mutans* and fed a cariogenic diet (*160*). A second study reported the effects of tea polyphenols on fissure caries induced by indigenous cariogenic bacteria in conventional rats (*161*). Groups of male rats were given 0.1–0.5% tea polyphenols in their diet or drinking water for 40 days. By both routes of administration, tea polyphenols significantly reduced the number of total fissure caries lesions, enamel lesions, lesions reaching the dentinoenamel junction, and advanced dentin lesions. Rats eating a cariogenic diet with 0.1% tea polyphenols had ~40% fewer total fissure caries lesions than controls. No toxic effects were observed.

Effects of diet on bone health and development of osteoporosis

Burckhardt and Heaney edited a volume of papers from the first symposium entirely devoted to nutritional aspects of osteoporosis (*162*). The major topics at the symposium were nutrition and the development of peak bone mass, nutrition and maintenance of bone health, and nutritional strategies for preventing and treating osteoporosis. Nutrition primarily affects bone mass, which is only one factor in bone fragility and osteoporosis. It is very important, however: a difference as small as 5% in bone mass can mean a 40% difference in risk of fracture. Nor is bone health a single-nutrient issue. Anderson and Hendersen discussed dietary factors that limit or modify development of peak bone mass (*163*). Besides calcium these include protein, calories, phosphorus, vitamin D, and several micronutrients. Cumming reviewed a selection of papers on the relationship between calcium intake and bone mass in women (*164*). Of 33 bone sites evaluated in 16 intervention studies, only 4 sites underwent greater bone loss in the calcium-supplemented group than in controls, and 3 of these were vertebral. There was a trend toward increasing benefit of calcium with age. The majority of 29 cross-sectional studies showed a small positive relationship between bone mass and dietary calcium intake; this was most consistent for premenopausal women. Studies in perimenopausal women or groups with a very wide age range generally produced inconsistent or inconclusive results, perhaps through failure to account for menopausal age. However, the 11 longitudinal studies of calcium intake and bone mass in women produced the most confusing and inconsistent results of all. From case–control and cohort studies of fracture risk, Cumming could not state the role of calcium. The strongest conclusion of the review was that calcium supplements reduce the rate of bone loss in postmenopausal women. Another review in this symposium volume concluded that calcium intake is important in determining bone mass early and late in life, but in the perimenopausal period the large effects of menopause tend to overwhelm any effects of calcium (*165*).

A population-based study of perimenopausal women in Switzerland identified several risk factors and protective factors (*166*). It found that only 16% of Swiss women aged 45–54 had an "adequate" intake of calcium, and 22% were at risk of osteoporosis based on inadequate calcium intake.

Moreover, a calcium-poor diet was positively associated with other unhealthy habits such as physical inactivity, smoking, and frequent alcohol consumption.

A 10-year longitudinal study in the Netherlands beginning with a group of healthy perimenopausal women eating their habitual diets evaluated the role of dietary calcium in the natural history of osteoporosis (167). Radial cortical bone mineral content was measured annually, at which time food consumption was estimated by the cross-check dietary history method. After 8 years, bone mineral content of the lumbar spine and right femoral neck were measured in a subgroup of women selected on the basis of low (<800 mg/day) and high (>1350 mg/day) calcium intake and rate of cortical bone loss (<0.5 and >2.5%/year). Cortical bone mass decreased during the first 6–7 years after menopause at an average rate of 1.6%/year, regardless of the amount of calcium in the diet. Nor did calcium intake have a differential effect on cortical and trabecular bone mass in this study. Higher body mass index, however, appeared protective for postmenopausal cortical (but not trabecular) bone. The authors suggested that this was due to generation of estrogens from adipose tissue in amounts sufficient to protect cortical bone, or perhaps to mechanical loading of the skeleton.

A review by Charles et al. emphasized that obligatory losses of calcium through skin, intestine, and urine are significant and relationships between dietary calcium and obligatory loss are complex (168). It is not presently known to what extent minimal obligatory calcium loss at different ages in males and females is related to intrinsic loss of skeletal calcium or to a lack of calcium preservation in kidney, skin, and intestine. At least three mechanisms of bone loss operate in adult life, and the effects of dietary calcium on these individual processes are not known. Before recommendations for calcium intake can be made with confidence it is necessary to know if and how dietary calcium and calcium supplements influence bone metabolism. However, some changes in the calcium nutrition and metabolism of the elderly have been described (169). Calcium intake tends to decrease with age, and the availability of dietary calcium may be further reduced in persons adhering to widely recommended high-fiber diets. In addition, the small intestine's fractional calcium absorption and ability to adapt to low calcium intake are thought to decrease with age. Postmenopausal women with low calcium intakes can reduce bone loss by increasing their dietary calcium; the threshold of calcium to lessen spinal bone loss appears higher than that for the radius and femoral neck. Optimal intake of calcium for the very old needs further study.

Eaton and Nelson discussed human calcium requirements and calcium nutrition from an evolutionary perspective (170). We evolved in a high-calcium nutritional environment. The earliest primates were insectivorous, and the calcium content of insects is relatively high. Later primates ate a more mixed diet, still including insects and other invertebrates but adding fruits, leaves, and a few small vertebrates. If their plant foods were similar to foods of contemporary nonhuman primates, they were excellent sources of calcium. The need of present-day apes and monkeys to consume a great deal of low-energy plant food ensures a high calcium intake; the same situation probably prevailed for human ancestors. The last period when the collective human gene pool interacted with bioenvironmental circumstances typical of those in which it evolved was the Late Paleolithic, ~20,000–35,000 years ago. The advent of plant agriculture began to upset the balance between calcium and phosphorus in plant foods: most uncultivated plants provide more calcium than phosphorus, but grains have 10 times more phosphorus than calcium. Assuming exercise and dietary patterns of the Stone Age to be "natural," calcium intake was roughly twice that of contemporary humans and levels of physical exertion were certainly greater. Modifying the modern diet to more closely approximate that for which we are genetically programmed could have an important positive impact on health.

Weaver discussed the relationship between osteoporosis and the bioavailability of calcium (171). She reviewed studies of calcium intake and bone mass and age- and hormone-related aspects of calcium absorption. Isotopic tracer techniques permit labeling of individual foods to evaluate calcium absorption. These studies show that calcium is absorbed from most plant foods as efficiently as from dairy products, unless they have unusually high concentrations of oxalic or phytic acid. However, few plant foods contain calcium in sufficient concentrations or can be tolerated in sufficient quantities to replace dairy products for most people. Bioavailability was also the theme of a review by Charles (*172*). Again, the value of isotopic tracer studies to measure the availability of calcium from specific sources was stressed. In deciding whether increased calcium intake is advisable, it is important to consider the calcium absorptive status of the subject, the source and nature of the added calcium (e.g., milk or a supplement), when and how the calcium (if a supplement) is dispensed, the subject's compliance, and how the regimen is to be evaluated.

The reduction in bone mass that leads to osteoporosis is partly genetically determined and partly determined during growth, as well as in later life (*173*). Significant correlations for bone mass were found between mothers and daughters and between fathers and daughters, but the largest and most highly significant correlations were between a daughter's value and the mean value for her parents. Insofar as risk factors for osteoporosis are determined early in life, osteoporosis may be considered a pediatric disease. The author reviewed calcium intake and calcium balance at different parts of the life cycle, concluding that the very highest requirements for calcium are during infancy and adolescence, followed by childhood and young adulthood. A calcium balance study in adolescent girls was particularly interesting: it revealed that urinary calcium excretion was not related to calcium intake as it is in adults, suggesting that urinary excretion by the girls represented obligatory loss and they were retaining dietary calcium at a high rate. In view of these findings, a study of dietary calcium and the bone mineral status of healthy white children and adolescents was disturbing (*174*). Most children aged 2–11 years met the recommended calcium intake of 800 mg/day for that age group, but only 15% of 11- to 16-year-olds met their recommended intake of 1200 mg/day. Dietary calcium intake was significantly correlated with bone mineral status.

Serum determinations of calcium, phosphate, magnesium, alkaline phosphatase, parathyroid hormone, 25-hydroxyvitamin D, and 1,25-dihydroxyvitamin D were in the normal range and were not correlated with bone mineral status. A multiple regression model of vertebral bone mineral density in healthy white girls 8–18 years old showed that 81% of the variance was described by maturational age, chronological age, and calcium intake (*175*). All three were significant predictors of vertebral bone mineral density. Thus again it appears that calcium nutrition during adolescence influences peak bone mass.

An interesting study of osteoporosis and calcium intake compared these variables with the incidence of hip fracture in Japan and the USA (*176*). Bone mass and calcium intake were lower in Japanese women than in their white U.S. counterparts. Paradoxically, although the prevalence of osteoporosis was comparable in the two nations, the incidence of hip fracture appeared to be much less in Japan. Assuming that the difference in hip fracture incidence is real, the authors speculated that bone quality factors other than density protect against fracture or, alternatively, that elements of the Japanese lifestyle might strengthen the pelvic muscles and provide skill and agility to prevent falls.

Four papers by Heaney discussed the role of nutrition in preventing and treating osteoporosis (*177–180*). Inadequate calcium intake may contribute to low bone mass and ultimately to osteoporotic fractures by limiting the attainment of maximum genetically programmed skeletal mass during growth, or by aggravating bone loss in later life (*177*). Ample calcium intake throughout life will prevent both of these consequences, but no amount of calcium supplementation can compensate for bone loss due to inactivity, hormone deficiency, alcohol abuse, smoking, or any other factor: "The only disorder [calcium] can be expected to alleviate is calcium deficiency." To the extent that calcium deficiency is prevalent in Western society, however, it contributes to the osteoporotic fracture burden. The annual costs of hip fracture to Western nations are extremely high and are certain to rise as the proportion of the very old in the population rises (*178*). Nutrition is involved in several aspects of this problem: calcium, in its relationship to bone density—but also general nutritional status, as it affects musculature and fat protecting the hip, aspects of bone quality other than density, and recovery from hip fracture. Protein nutrition may be particularly important in the elderly. The impact of calcium intake on bone health must be considered in the broad context of osteoporotic fracture (*179*). Only to the extent that calcium deficiency contributes to bone fragility will a high calcium intake protect against such fracture. Thus in the USA, where more than half of women have an inadequate calcium intake, an important part of the osteoporotic fracture burden is calcium-related and preventable by increasing calcium intake; in other countries where calcium nutrition is generally adequate (e.g., Denmark and the Netherlands), a population-wide program to increase calcium intake would provide less benefit. Because primary prevention of osteoporosis involves achieving the full genetic potential for bone mass, adequate lifelong calcium intake is important (*180*). Calcium utilization and requirements throughout the life cycle were reviewed. Secondary prevention, such as calcium supplements, exercise, and hormone replacement, protects whatever bone mass exists in adulthood.

In his review of the literature on calcium, calcium metabolism, and skeletal health in women, Kanis attempted to show why others have drawn opposite conclusions from the same data—some arguing that all mixed diets contain sufficient calcium, others claiming that most of the world's population is calcium-deficient (*181*). He described bone remodelling in women and how it responds in osteoporosis or to a change in calcium nutrition. He discussed reasons why some epidemiologic studies find an association between lifetime intake of calcium and bone density or fracture risk, while others find no such association. Many studies, for example, fail to account for energy intake and energy expenditure (i.e., exercise). He criticized the calculation of dietary requirements from calcium balance studies showing a relationship between external calcium balance and dietary calcium intake, saying the correlation is an artefact arising from the appearance of calcium intake on both sides of the equation. His discussion of skeletal metabolism after

menopause showed that postmenopausal women are able to adapt to increments in dietary intake and there is probably a place for calcium supplementation in this group. However, he argued that only an association, not a causal relationship, has been demonstrated between calcium intake and osteoporotic fracture rate.

A study in healthy postmenopausal women with no history of calcium supplementation found a mean calcium consumption of 606 ± 302 mg/day, based on a food-frequency questionnaire (*182*). Subjects who consumed less than the population mean had significantly lower vertebral bone mineral density than subjects with intakes above the mean. Univariate regression analyses revealed that bone mineral density was significantly correlated with calcium intake and body weight. These data are consistent with the hypothesis that calcium intake is a determinant of skeletal health in postmenopausal women.

Calcium balance studies in 85 women with postmenopausal crush-fracture osteoporosis found that overall calcium balance correlated significantly with energy content ($r = .31$), protein ($r = .22$), calcium ($r = .28$), phosphate ($r = .27$), and coffee ($r = -.21$) when ^{47}Ca kinetic data were analyzed by a modified expanding calcium pool model (*183*). However, with a multiple backward linear regression model, only calcium and coffee intake had significant effects. Coffee consumption greater than 1000 mL/day induced an extra calcium loss of 1.6 mmol of calcium per day; consumption of 1 or 2 cups had little impact.

A critical review of a report by Dawson-Hughes et al. (chapter 4, reference *158*, *Food Safety 1991*) against the background of information on calcium intake and metabolism in postmenopausal women drew several conclusions (*184*). First, since rates of bone loss at clinically important sites (spine and hip) are low in postmenopausal women with normal bone mass, studies of postmenopausal women with low bone mass would probably be more fruitful and clinically relevant. Because individual variation in bone loss is high, it is necessary to make multiple measurements of bone changes over long periods in large groups of subjects to evaluate any intervention. Calcium supplementation is of no use in preventing bone loss during the perimenopausal period, but women 6 years or more past menopause can benefit from calcium supplementation if their habitual intake is very low. In these women, calcium carbonate prevented significant bone loss from the femoral neck and radius, but not from the spine; calcium citrate malate protected all three sites. The possible advantage of calcium citrate malate over calcium carbonate needs further study. Finally, additional strategies may be necessary for long-term arrest of bone loss in most postmenopausal women. Dawson-Hughes also reviewed controlled clinical trials of calcium supplementation and bone loss, discussing requisite features of an appropriate trial (*185*). Like others, she concluded that the responsiveness of postmenopausal women to calcium supplementation depends on menopausal age. Although some studies found that bone loss from the radius could be attenuated by very high doses of calcium during the perimenopausal period, no amount of calcium influenced the rate of vertebral bone loss at this time. Again, late-postmenopausal women can benefit from calcium supplements if their habitual intake of calcium is very low. Bone loss from the hip needs more study. At any site, fracture risk depends on many indexes; but total mineral content is a good predictor and can be measured reproducibly.

In contrast, one 2-year controlled trial of very high-dose calcium supplementation (1000 and 2000 mg/day) in perimenopausal women did find a reduction in vertebral bone loss (*186*). The supplement was administered as effervescent tablets containing calcium lactogluconate and calcium carbonate. Twenty-two of the 295 women who entered the trial dropped out because of gastrointestinal side effects. The mean lumbar bone loss in controls after 2 years was 8.5%, compared with 1.3% in the 1000 mg/day group and 0.7% in the 2000 mg/day group. The decrease in lumbar bone loss was significant in the first year but not the second and there was no effect on metacarpal cortical bone loss. Subjects taking supplements also had significantly decreased serum alkaline phosphatase, osteocalcin, and 1,25-dihydroxyvitamin D and a decreased urinary hydroxyproline/creatinine ratio after one year, but the decrease in osteocalcin was

no longer significant after two years. Long-term effects of calcium supplementation on lumbar bone loss need further study.

A 2-year study in perimenopausal women with low forearm bone density compared the effects of exercise, exercise plus calcium supplementation, and exercise plus hormone replacement on bone loss from three forearm sites (*187*). An untreated group of women with normal bone density served as controls. Significant bone loss in the distal forearm occurred in the control and exercise groups (2.7 and 2.6% per year, respectively). In the exercise plus calcium group the rate of bone loss was 0.5%/year; and bone density increased 7.5% per year in the group treated with exercise and hormone replacement. Although exercise plus hormone replacement was more effective than exercise plus calcium, it was associated with a relatively high rate of side effects such as breast tenderness and vaginal bleeding.

Toss emphasized the importance of considering how a wide range of lifestyle factors influence bone mass at various sites (*188*). Specifically mentioned were exercise, dieting, body mass index, tobacco smoking, alcohol consumption, caffeine consumption, exposure to sunlight, and dietary protein, phosphate, vitamin D, and fiber. Interaction of these variables with sex and age should also receive attention.

A cross-cultural epidemiologic survey of the association between dietary animal protein and hip fracture asked whether the metabolic acid–osteoporosis hypothesis could help explain the observed variation in fracture incidence among women older than 50 years (*189*). Catabolism of protein, particularly animal protein, is the source of most metabolically produced acid, and metabolic acidosis can lead to bone buffering with bone dissolution. Regression analysis of hip fracture data in women from 34 studies in 16 countries revealed a strong positive relationship with dietary animal protein. The association could not be explained by either calcium or total caloric intake. Because there is a plausible biological basis for the animal protein–hip fracture association, the authors believe that further study of the metabolic acid hypothesis is warranted.

A study of 27 ovolactovegetarian and 37 nonvegetarian women 28–45 years old concluded that their differences in dietary practices had no important effects on their bone biology or reproductive history (*190*). There were no significant differences in urinary calcium excretion or spinal bone density between groups. In both groups, caffeine intake was positively associated with urinary calcium excretion but not with bone density.

Risk factors for osteoporosis have been more thoroughly studied in Caucasian women than in Asians. Because the two groups differ considerably in dietary habits, lifestyle, and gene pools, a study of the effect of diet and lifestyle on bone mass was conducted in female Japanese college students (*191*). Forearm bone mineral density was significantly correlated with habitual physical activity and with calcium intake since infancy; the effects of exercise and calcium intake on the ratio of bone density to bone width were additive. Intakes of protein and total energy were also positively correlated with bone density, whereas dieting and skipping meals were associated with reduced bone density. A history of breast-feeding was positively associated with bone density, perhaps because of the poor nutritional quality of formulas used in Japan at the time or to some effect of breast-feeding on subsequent eating behavior. Smoking, alcohol drinking, and sun exposure did not contribute to the variability in bone density in this study. Possible explanations for this are that the subjects were too young to be affected by these factors and that these factors do not affect peak bone mass.

In growing rats, a high-fat, high-sucrose diet had adverse effects on structural and mechanical properties of the vertebrae (*192*). Although there were no differences in body mass between the experimental group and controls, rats fed the high-fat, high-sucrose diet for 10–12 weeks showed significantly smaller cross-sectional areas, lengths, and volumes of the L_6 vertebra. Adverse effects on mechanical properties were measured as reduced initial maximum load, energy at initial maximum load, and strain energy density at initial maximum load. The authors concluded that in immature rats the experimental diet impaired vertebral strength, morphology, and mechanical integrity.

NERVOUS SYSTEM AND BEHAVIOR

Connor (*193*) and Connor et al. (*194*) discussed dietary n–3 fatty acids in terms of their effects on plasma lipids and lipoproteins and their role as essential fatty acids for the brain and retina. n–3 fatty acid deficiency has recently been characterized in rhesus monkeys. Its clinical features are much more subtle than those of n–6 fatty acid deficiency. When female monkeys were fed a semipurified diet throughout pregnancy with safflower oil as the only fat source and their infants were weaned on the same diet, the infants' growth was normal, fatty liver did not develop, and there were no skin or fur symptoms even after long-term depletion. However, vision was impaired, the electroretinogram was abnormal, and water intake was excessive. Plasma and tissues had reduced levels of $18:3n$–3 and $22:6n$–3, and increased levels of $22:4n$–6 and $22:5n$–6. DHA, which is uniquely prominent in phospholipid membranes of the retina, brain, and spermatozoa, was reduced by 50% in the retina and 75% in the cerebral cortex in neonates; the deficit was even greater when the animals were 22 months old. The reduction in DHA was compensated by an increase in n–6 fatty acids, particularly 22:5, so that the polyunsaturation of the phospholipid membranes was approximately maintained. Although fish-oil feeding rapidly normalized the fatty acid profile, there was no improvement in electroretinogram abnormalities even after 9 months of repletion. The polydipsia may be related to altered brain biochemistry but did not appear to be mediated by renal disease, osmotic regulation, or abnormalities of the posterior pituitary hormones.

Another review of the role of α-linolenic acid and long-chain n–3 PUFAs in neonatal brain development summarized studies in rodents and monkeys (*195*). Changes in brain fatty acid profiles in response to dietary manipulations were discussed. In both rats and monkeys, n–3 PUFA deficiency is associated with changes in the electroretinogram and visual acuity. Most studies of cognitive function have used rodents. Although various degrees of learning impairment have been described, these studies are fraught with methodologic and interpretational problems. Behavioral responses to n–3 feeding or deficiency were summarized in a table. The author concluded that within limits the developing brain can regulate its concentration of 22:6n-3 in response to dietary deficiency or excess of 18:3n-3 or the long-chain derivatives. Although there is ample evidence for specific effects of n–3 PUFAs on retinal function, putative effects on cognitive function in rodents can still be considered equivocal.

Studies of n–3 PUFAs as pharmacologically active substances abound but there are few studies of their role as essential nutrients. Bjerve et al. reviewed clinical observations of their own group and others (*196*). Reported cases of n–3 deficiency in humans are limited to two children and eight adults. In adults, deficiency was associated with inflammatory changes in skin and hair follicles. The children had neurologic symptoms, retarded growth, and skin changes, which responded favorably when dietary n–3 PUFAs were increased. Bjerve et al. found concentrations of n–3 PUFAs in plasma total phospholipids to be a reliable index of dietary intake. Attempts to estimate dietary requirements for n–3 PUFAs suggested that the minimum level to prevent deficiency is 260–290 mg/day of 18:3n–3 or 100–200 mg/day of long-chain n–3; the optimal intake was calculated to be 860–900 mg/day of 18:3n–3 or 350–400 mg/day of long-chain n–3. Determining n–3 requirements is most critical for preterm infants because the major part of fetal accretion of these fatty acids takes place during the last 8 weeks of gestation and preterm very-low-birth-weight infants have small tissue reserves of n–3 fatty acids. The authors summarized their studies of preterm infants and emphasized the need to determine optimum levels of n–3 PUFAs for infant formulas and formulas for feeding malnourished and critically ill patients.

Two studies in rats documented responses of brain fatty acid profiles to dietary fat. Weanling rats were fed semipurified diets containing 40 en% fat, in which the dietary 18:2n–6/18:3n–3 ratio varied incrementally by factors of ~4 from 1.8 to 165 while amounts of other fatty acids were held constant (*197*). The experimental diets rapidly and specifically altered the proportions of n–6 and n–3 22-carbon fatty acids in several membrane fractions of the brain: dietary 18:2n–6/18:3n–3 ratio and membrane n–6/n–3 ratio were strongly correlated, although the magnitude of the response to a particular dietary ratio varied among the individual fatty acids. An important observation was that the diet-induced accumulation of specific fatty acids continued throughout the 12-week experiment, even after rapid neural growth had stopped. A two-generation study evaluated the response of fatty acid profiles in brain and heart phospholipid subclasses to n–3 PUFAs of marine and vegetable origin (*198*). Female rats were fed experimental diets from weaning until they were 18 weeks old; offspring of these animals ate the same diet as their mother until the age of 18 weeks. The experimental diets had the same amounts of n–3 and n–6 fatty acids (n–3/n–6 = 0.8), but only the marine-oil diet provided long-chain n–3 PUFAs. In heart phosphatidylethanolamine, the highest levels of long-chain n–3 fatty acids were attained in the marine-oil group and there were no marked differences between the two generations, whereas in the linseed-oil group there was a considerable increase in 22:6n–3 from the first to the second generation, reflecting the mammal's limited ability to desaturate and elongate 18:3n–3 fatty acids. In brain phosphatidylethanolamine and phosphatidylserine, fatty acid profiles of the two generations were similar, but again, marine oil was more effective than linseed oil at increasing long-chain n–3 and decreasing long-chain n–6 fatty acids.

A study in neonatal piglets evaluated the effect of dietary linoleic and α-linolenic acids on the DHA and saturated fatty acid content of liver and brain (*199*). All combinations of low (16%) and high (30 or 35%) 18:2n–6 with 1 and 4% 18:3n–3 were tested, with coconut oil making up the remainder of the fat; n–6/n–3 ratios ranged from 4 to 30. There was a significant inverse relationship between dietary 18:3n–3 and hepatic phospholipid palmitic acid (16:0), but no influence of dietary 18:2n–6. In brain, 4% 18:3n–3 combined with 16% 18:2n–6 also reduced deposition of 16:0. MUFAs in brain and liver were significantly decreased by high formula levels of either n–3 or n–6. DHA in hepatic phospholipids and total brain lipids was significantly higher when formula contained 4% 18:3n–3. The authors concluded that influences of essential fatty acids on the nonessential fatty acids that also modulate the properties of structural membranes should be considered in establishing dietary requirements for essential fatty acid. Another study in neonatal piglets compared the effectiveness of dietary α-linolenic acid, fish oil, and sow's milk as sources of membrane DHA (22:6n–3) in the retina and synaptic plasma membrane (*200*). It found that 18:3n–3 supplied in formula was about one-quarter as effective as long-chain n–3 fatty acids as a source of membrane DHA. At the higher level tested, formula 18:3n–3 supported deposition of DHA comparable to that from natural milk. Fish oil also supported tissue levels of DHA comparable to those from natural milk, but decreased the level of 22:4n–6, suggesting interference with n–6 metabolism.

Chronic administration of ethanol affects fatty acid profiles and metabolism in numerous tissues. Two studies in rats demonstrated that γ-linolenic acid counteracts the effects in brain. Male Wistar rats were fed a nutritionally balanced liquid diet containing ethanol with or without 10% evening primrose oil for 21 days (*201*). Controls were pair-fed isocaloric sucrose and the amount of rat chow eaten by the experimental rat the previous day. Ethanol alone significantly reduced the percentage of arachidonic acid and increased the linoleate/arachidonate ratio in phosphatidylinositol in cortical synaptosomal fractions; concomitant administration of evening primrose oil reversed the effect of ethanol. Behavioral effects of ethanol and their modification by evening primrose oil were evaluated in a model of fetal alcohol syndrome (*202*). Rats were given ethanol with or without evening primrose oil throughout pregnancy, nursing, and weaning. Controls received the basal diet with or without evening primrose oil. The offspring were tested at about 60 days of age for locomotor activity and behavior in the Morris maze. Ethanol alone significantly suppressed daytime activity in males and females; evening primrose oil prevented this effect. Evening primrose oil significantly enhanced learning in the Morris maze, whether or not alcohol was administered. The ability of γ-linolenic acid to

attenuate the neurotoxic effects of chronic ethanol consumption may have practical implications.

To evaluate the peroxidizability of brain lipids after long-term ingestion of oils with different oxidative stability, male mice were fed diets containing perilla oil, lard, or rapeseed oil for 15 months (*203*). All diets contained 5 mg of α-tocopherol acetate per 100 g. Brain lipids were then extracted and their fatty acid composition, tocopherol content, and levels of thiobarbituric acid–reactive substances determined. Dietary fat influenced brain fatty acid composition as expected. α-Tocopherol content was significantly elevated in the perilla oil group. Despite its high oxidizability, perilla oil had little effect on the lipid peroxidation status of brain homogenates as measured by thiobarbituric acid and the rate of oxygen absorption induced by a free-radical initiator. The authors attributed this to the increased level of α-tocopherol in the brains of these mice. They concluded that dietary α-linolenic acid does not increase the susceptibility of brain lipids to free radical–initiated peroxidation when α-tocopherol supply is adequate, and that the influence of dietary oil on the peroxidizability of brain lipids is more complex than would be predicted from simple consideration of the oxidizability of the oil.

A study in neonatal mice showed that the fatty acid composition of brain and liver are influenced postnatally by the mother's fat intake (*204*). This is at least partly regulated at the mRNA level. When pups were nursed by mothers fed a fat-free or 5% coconut-oil diet, peak levels of mRNA for proteolipid protein and myelin basic protein were lower than in pups whose mothers were fed corn oil. Brain levels of mRNA for stearoyl CoA desaturase (which affects the rate of myelin synthesis) and LDL receptor were also altered by neonatal fat intake. This response was tissue-specific: when nursing mothers were fed fat-free diets, mRNA for stearoyl CoA desaturase was decreased in their pups' brains but elevated in liver; mRNA for LDL receptor was decreased in brain but unaffected in liver. The divergent responses of developing brain and liver to dietary fatty acids represent metabolic adaptations at the tissue level and could not be predicted from fatty acid profile data alone.

In his 1989 Borden Award lecture, Young reviewed the effects of tryptophan, folic acid, and carbohydrate meals on brain serotonin synthesis, mood, and behavior (*205*). When normal men ingested tryptophan-deficient mixtures of amino acids to deplete their brain tryptophan and serotonin, significant lowering of mood occurred as measured by the depression scale scores of the Multiple Affect Adjective Checklist. The mood-lowering effect was relatively resistant to environmental manipulation. In a similar test of patients recovered from depression, tryptophan depletion caused a full depressive relapse. Low tryptophan is also associated with increased aggressive responding in humans and other animals and can block the analgesic effect of morphine in humans. It is not involved in any simple way with carbohydrate craving. In addition, folic acid deficiency lowered brain serotonin and mood. Although carbohydrate meals can have clear effects on human mood and behavior, a brain serotonin mechanism is considered unlikely; other known mechanisms could easily mediate these effects. In rats, serotonin synthesis and catabolism in the fetal brain is controlled by the mother's intake of tryptophan (*206*). Oral administration of tryptophan to pregnant rats during the second half of gestation produced increases of tryptophan in fetal tissues that had not yet peaked at a dose of 1000 mg/kg. Concentrations in the brain were 300% higher than in the carcass and 600% higher than in the placenta. Changes in brain tryptophan induced parallel changes in serotonin and 5-HIAA but did not affect tyrosine, dopamine, or norepinephrine.

Muldoon et al. tested the hypothesis that the reported association between cholesterol reduction and destructive or aggressive behavior reflects changes in serotonergic activity in the central nervous system (CNS) (*207*). They studied adult male cynomolgus monkeys that had been eating a high-fat, high-cholesterol diet or a low-fat, low-cholesterol diet for at least 5 months. CNS serotonergic activity was measured as the prolactin response to fenfluramine challenge. Mean total plasma cholesterol concentration was 420 mg/dL in the high-fat group and 154 mg/dL in the low-fat group. Median baseline prolactin concentrations did not differ between groups. However, distributions of the prolactin response to fenfluramine challenge differed significantly, the lowest prolactin concentrations aggregating among animals fed the low-fat diet. Although confirmatory behavioral and neurochemical data were not obtained and the time course of the response was not characterized, these observations were consistent with the hypothesis. Possible mechanisms were discussed, but the study did not support any one over another.

The effect of selenium supplementation on mood in a population that might have subclinical selenium deficiency was assessed in a double-blind crossover study (*208*). Subjects took low-selenium or high-selenium yeast-based tablets daily for 5 weeks in random order, with a 6-month washout period between. Dietary intake of selenium was estimated from responses to a food frequency questionnaire, and all subjects completed the Profile of Moods States before, midway through, and after each 5-week trial. The change in mood while taking the active tablet was inversely correlated with the amount of dietary selenium; the lower the dietary selenium, the more reports of anxiety, depression, and fatigue decreased after selenium therapy. The implications of these findings for populations whose food supply contains low levels of selenium were discussed.

In rats, manipulation of dietary macronutrients alters the density of D2 dopamine receptors in the brain (*209*). Groups of young adult males were pair-fed with isocaloric diets containing 8% protein and 80% carbohydrate, 20% protein and 68% carbohydrate, or 52% protein and 36% carbohydrate for 36 weeks. The low-protein group had a decrease in density of D2 dopamine receptors in the striatum (28%) and mesolimbic (36%) regions, with no change in receptor affinity. Although the changes were statistically significant, their physiological importance is not known. They may, however, explain some of the behavioral changes induced by long-term protein deficiency. Dietary protein's effect on dopaminergic systems was also implicated in a neuroelectrical study of rats (*210*). Beginning when they were weanlings, rats were fed 50% or 24% casein diets ad lib for 36–40 weeks. Then were then anesthetized with α-chloralose and urethane and EEG recordings of evoked and event-related potentials were made, using an alerting stimulus–imperative stimulus conditioning paradigm. The high-protein diet caused an increase in central arousal mechanisms, as measured by cortical negativity response. This specifically involved increased excitability of the motor cortex and was not associated with a disorder of information processing in the cerebral cortex as measured by brainstem auditory-evoked responses and somatosensory-evoked potentials. Although the study showed that motor but not sensory cortical potentials are amplified by a high-protein diet and are consistent with the idea that high dietary protein stimulates dopaminergic activity, the authors stressed the limits their paradigm places on interpretation of the results.

Lemongrass tea made from leaves of *Cymbopogon citratus* (DC) Stapf. is a popular folk remedy for various nervous and gastrointestinal disturbances (*211*). In rats, oral administration of an infusion of fresh lemongrass leaves produced dose-dependent analgesia for the hyperalgesia induced by carrageenin or prostaglandin E_2, but not by dibutyryl cAMP. This indicated a peripheral rather than central site of action. The major analgesic component of the infusion was identified as the terpene myrcene. Myrcene's peripheral analgesic action was confirmed by additional testing using a commercial preparation of the compound. Myrcene-type compounds may represent a new class of peripheral analgesics with a profile of action different from that of aspirin-like drugs.

Animal experimentation has shown that weanlings prefer the diet ingested by their nursing mother and are more likely to accept novel foods if they experienced a wide range of flavors during suckling. Mennella and Beauchamp evaluated the effects of garlic on the sensory qualities of human milk and the infant's nursing behavior (*212*). Women who participated in the study ate a bland diet before the test days, when they were given garlic capsules or placebo. Evaluation of milk samples by a sensory panel showed that garlic ingestion increased the intensity of the milk's odor and that the effect peaked 2 hours after ingestion. Infants spent more time attached to the breast, sucked more, and tended to ingest more milk when the milk smelled like garlic. The authors postulated not only that maternal diet affects the sensory qualities of milk, potentially influencing later food preferences of the child, but that the effect extends to the in utero situation, where the fetus swallows and is bathed in amniotic fluid whose sensory qualities reflect maternal diet. They recommended further investigation of the extent to which prenatal and neonatal sensory experiences influence the human infant's willingness to accept novel foods at weaning and subsequently.

Although foods high in refined sugar are claimed to exacerbate hyperactivity and increase aggressive behavior, controlled studies have not confirmed an effect on hyperactivity, have yielded equivocal results regarding inattention, and have generally not investigated aggressive behavior (*213*). Wender and Solanto assessed cognitive attention and aggressive behavior in response to a sugar challenge in a randomized crossover design. Children between 5.5 and 7.5 years old who met DSM-III criteria for attention deficit disorder with hyperactivity as well as other criteria for oppositional disorder and hyperkinesis were paired with controls matched for age, sex, socioeconomic status, and IQ. They were tested immediately after ingestion of a flavored beverage containing 35 g of sucrose, 175 mg of saccharin, or 175 mg of aspartame. These challenges were given with a high-carbohydrate breakfast. Although children with attention deficit disorder with hyperactivity were significantly more aggressive than controls, neither sugar nor placebo altered the aggressive behavior of either group. However, sugar increased inattention, measured by a continuous-performance task, in the group with attention deficit disorder. The authors suggested that this might represent a response to the combination of sugar challenge and high-carbohydrate meal and further studies would be needed to determine its clinical significance.

A behavioral study evaluated the effects of dietary fat and cholesterol on adult male cynomolgus monkeys living in social groups (*214*). For 22 months, monkeys were fed a "luxury" high-fat, high-cholesterol diet or a "prudent" diet containing 30 en% fat and 0.05 mg of cholesterol per kilocalorie of diet. Monkeys eating the luxury diet had higher total serum cholesterol and lower HDL cholesterol than those eating the prudent diet. The occurrence of 21 behaviors commonly exhibited by this species in captivity was monitored. Monkeys eating the prudent diet initiated significantly more contact aggression (slap/grab/push, grapple, or bite) than their luxury-fed counterparts. No other agonistic or affiliative behaviors differed between groups. Differences in contact aggression appeared during the first 3 months in dominant animals but were not apparent until later in submissive animals. Many questions could not be answered by this study—for example, whether the luxury diet suppressed aggressivity or the prudent diet enhanced it. However, the results are consistent with the idea that low serum cholesterol is associated with increased aggressive or antisocial behavior.

Horrobin reviewed the evidence for a relationship between schizophrenia and metabolism of essential fatty acids and eicosanoids (*215*). Direct and indirect evidence points to an impairment of prostaglandin E_1 metabolism in schizophrenia. Biochemical comparisons of schizophrenic and normal subjects in 6 countries have demonstrated reduced levels of linoleic acid and elevated levels of 22-carbon *n*–6 and *n*–3 essential fatty acids in plasma or brain phospholipids of schizophrenics. Moreover, clinical trials of γ-linolenic and dihomo-γ-linolenic acids, prostaglandin E_1 precursors, have shown modest therapeutic benefits. In view of the lack of progress using drugs based on the "dopamine concept" of schizophrenia and the known interactions between the essential fatty acid–eicosanoid and dopamine systems, Horrobin argued that it is time for thorough evaluation of the link between schizophrenia and the essential fatty acid–eicosanoid system. In the same issue of *Prostaglandins Leukotrienes and Essential Fatty Acids* Vaddadi reviewed the rationale for and results of using γ-linolenic acid to treat schizophrenia and tardive dyskinesia (*216*). According to one hypothesis, the elevated dopamine/prostaglandin E_1 ratio commonly observed in schizophrenics could be normalized either by reducing dopamine hyperfunctioning or by increasing prostaglandin E_1 levels. Limited success with the first approach prompted studies of the second. Treatment with phenoxymethyl penicillin, a drug that stimulates production of prostaglandin E_1, has had antipsychotic

effects alone and in conjunction with γ-linolenic acid. Modest beneficial effects from administration of prostaglandin E_1, α-linolenic acid, or dihimo-γ-linolenic acid have also been reported. In patients with either schizophrenia or tardive dyskinesia, the best results are associated with treatment combining essential fatty acids with supplements containing micronutrients involved in converting them to prostaglandins.

A case–control study of lifestyle and dietary factors in idiopathic Parkinson's disease was undertaken in Germany to generate new hypotheses regarding importance of factors in early life and the rural environment (*217*). Parkinson's disease was significantly associated with living in a village and harvesting mushrooms during childhood. There were no differences between patients and controls in childhood water supply, fishing in fresh or salt water, or eating self-harvested fish. Patients had a greater preference for almonds and plums; there was no difference between patients and controls in intake of mushrooms, peanuts, oil-dressed salad, fish, animal offal, or foods known to harbor heavy metals and pesticides. Perhaps the major findings of this study were that patients with Parkinson's disease are no exception to the rule that dietary habits frequently change during life, and that the putative role of dietary vitamin E in the development and course of Parkinson's disease is more complex than previously thought. However, other investigators reported an international comparison that showed striking positive correlations between age-adjusted Parkinson's disease mortality rates and per capita consumption of total protein ($r = .58$, $p < .02$) and meat ($r = .64$, $p < .01$) (*218*). Of 24 countries, New Zealand had the fourth highest Parkinson's disease mortality and the highest per capita consumption of protein; Mexico and Japan were lowest on both measures. The associations remained after adjustment for estimated annual income, which is a rough index of access to advanced medical care. These findings were put forward to generate new hypotheses relating to the role of diet in the etiology of Parkinson's disease.

Possible links between diet and multiple sclerosis have also been considered (*219*). The geographic pattern of multiple sclerosis in the Near

East and Mediterranean countries offers opportunities to test dietary hypotheses. Prevalence is relatively high in southern Europe, Israel, and Cyprus, and low in Libya, Tunisia, Saudi Arabia, and among native Kuwaitis. There is a particularly remarkable difference in prevalence between Malta (4/100,000) and Sicily (30–60/100,000). Consumption of 16 nutrients and 76 commodities from the FAO list were compared with prevalence of multiple sclerosis in 10 countries of the Mediterranean–Near East region; those that showed a significant association were further tested in a world-wide sample of 21 countries and in 6 northern/central vs. 5 southern European countries. Per capita consumption of these items in Italy and Malta were also noted. Nine items were associated with multiple sclerosis in the first three tests: animal protein, total fat, calcium, riboflavin, pork, total meat, margarine, coffee, beer, and smoke preservation of foods. Of these, only margarine, coffee, and smoke preservation agreed with the multiple sclerosis gradient between Italy and Malta. Plausible epidemiologic and biological arguments can be made for the association between smoked and cured meat and multiple sclerosis, but it would be justifiable to test all nine variables in case–control studies.

van Meer advanced the hypothesis that development of poliomyelitis is related to consumption of refined sugar (*220*). He cited some anomalies in the history of polio—cases in which large gatherings took place during epidemics yet no increase in dissemination of the disease occurred. He related polio epidemics to statistics on sugar production and consumption and documented a higher incidence of polio in a given geographic area in subpopulations who ate refined sugar than in subpopulations who ate less refined or brown sugar. He correlated polio epidemics to a shift from brown to white sugar, as in Jamaica after World War II. There is also evidence associating elevated blood sugar levels with increased susceptibility to polio. Intriguingly, polio epidemics have been associated with campaigns to eradicate insects with DDT, whose pharmacological action in humans is to increase levels of blood sugar. His contention was that it takes more than the poliovirus and a nonimmune person to produce a case of polio.

CATARACT

A review of risk factors for cataract development mentioned lack of specific nutrients (*221*). Certain metabolic disorders, e.g., diabetes, are also risk factors and nutritional factors may underlie these disorders. Another review discussed "sugar cataracts" in evaluating risk factors in human cataractogenesis, noting that the polyol metabolic pathway is important only in the pathogenesis of juvenile diabetic cataracts (*222*). Therapeutic use of retinoids has been implicated in cases of cataracts and other eye problems.

Taylor et al. reviewed the role of reduced proteolytic capacity in cataract formation and discussed evidence that the functions of antioxidants and proteases are related (*223*). They demonstrated that the proteolytic capabilities of the lens are compromised by aging and exposure to light and oxygen; cumulative damage results in lens opacity. Antioxidants are protective in vivo and in vitro, and antioxidant status can be enhanced by dietary means in humans and experimental animals. In rodents, caloric restriction also retards cataract formation but the mechanism is not associated with levels of plasma ascorbate. An estimated one-half of cataract surgeries would be unnecessary if cataract development could be delayed by 10 years. Another review discussed free radical–related pathogenesis of senile cataract and possibilities for prevention and palliation by antioxidants, including dietary antioxidants (*224*). Glutathione metabolism and the role of blood chemical and biochemical parameters were emphasized.

It has been suggested that the initial action of selenite in the selenite model of cataractogenesis in rodents is as an oxidant (*225*). Intraperitoneal injection of sodium selenite into 10-day-old rat pups produced cataracts in >95% of controls within 5 days; daily administration of vitamin C beginning in 8-day-old pups reduced incidence of cataracts to ~15%. Lenses of selenite-treated pups had sharply reduced levels of ATP, reduced glutathione, and soluble proteins and increased levels of malondialdehyde; pups treated with vitamin C and selenite had near-normal levels of these substances. These observations are consistent with the hypothesis that selenite cataract is due to oxidative stress in the lens and that vitamin C is anticataractogenic.

Associations between cataract prevalence and diet were determined in a 50% random sample of Beaver Dam (Wisconsin) Eye Study participants (*226*). The type and severity of lens opacities was determined by grading of photographs and dietary information was based on a food frequency questionnaire. Dietary intake of linoleic acid, vitamin E, niacin, zinc, and lutein was negatively associated with cataract risk, but intake of vitamin E or zinc supplements was not associated with cortical cataract risk. The severity of nuclear sclerosis was negatively associated with intake of several dietary carotenoids. Total vitamin A and vitamin C intake from diet and supplements also reduced risk for nuclear sclerosis.

DRUG METABOLISM AND INTERACTIONS

The effects of macronutrients, micronutrients, several nonnutritive dietary chemicals, and ethanol on cytochromes P450 and xenobiotic metabolism were reviewed in the context of the multiplicity and substrate specificity of these enzymes (*227*). Although the actions of several dietary chemicals on individual P450 isozymes have been established, the actions of macronutrients and most micronutrients are largely unknown. By having dissimilar effects on various P450 forms, a nutrient may have diverse effects on drug metabolism. Thus chronic ethanol consumption increases the rate of metabolic clearance of some drugs (meprobamate, pentobarbital, aminopyrine, tolbutamide, propranolol, rifampicin, testosterone), whereas acute consumption impairs metabolism of many drugs, including some in the former list. In general, nutritional deficiencies decrease rates of xenobiotic metabolism; thiamin and mild riboflavin deficiency, however, enhance it. P450IIE1 was used to illustrate the dietary modulation of P450 enzymes and the effect of this on chemical toxicity and carcinogenicity. Most studies are done using hepatic microsome

preparations from rodents. Although these can reveal the basic principles of how a dietary factor affects drug metabolism, specific results do not necessarily apply to other tissues or species. Another, more comprehensive, review considered the effects of dietary nutrients and restriction on P450 enzymes and the mixed function oxidase system in terms of species differences, malnutrition, variability in drug metabolism, aging, and dietary influences on the metabolism of P450 substrates other than drugs (*228*).

A study in rats examined the effects of type of dietary fat and the fat/carbohydrate ratio on hepatic microsomal P450IIE1 activity (*229*). In low- (0.5%) and high-fat (35%) diets the type of fat made no difference, whereas with 5 or 20% fat, corn oil and fish oil produced higher P450IIE activity than saturated or monounsaturated fats. A high ratio of dietary fat to carbohydrate increased levels of P450IIE1 and total P450 enzymes. The authors concluded that the constitutive P450 enzyme level is regulated by the type of dietary fat and the fat/carbohydrate ratio.

The effects of a single dose of garlic oil (500 mg/kg) and 5 daily doses (each 50 mg/kg) on hepatic phase I and II biotransformation enzymes were studied in rats (*230*). The single dose significantly depressed cytochrome P450, aminopyrine N-demethylase, and aniline hydroxylase activity without affecting microsomal protein content, cytochrome b_5, NADPH–cytochrome c reductase, benzphetamine N-demethylase, or cytosolic glutathione S-transferase. Analysis of serum enzymes revealed no evidence of hepatic toxicity. In contrast, daily administration significantly increased hepatic cytochrome P450, aminopyrine N-demethylase, and benzphetamine N-demethylase activities without affecting the other parameters. These results suggest a dose-related effect of garlic oil on the hepatic drug-metabolizing enzyme system.

In rats, eating a diet containing 2.5% cooked brussels sprouts for only 2 days significantly induced small-intestinal P4502B1 and hepatic P4501A2 (*231*). Additional dose-dependent effects were seen when larger amounts (up to 20%) were fed for up to 28 days. Some activities were enhanced, whereas others were diminished. The authors suggested that these metabolic alterations are responsible for the decreased cancer risk in rodents and humans attributed to cruciferous vegetables.

A feeding study in rats determined the dose–response curves for effects of dietary flavonoids on activity of drug-metabolizing enzymes (*232*). Flavone, flavanone (which differs from flavone by the absence of one double bond in the pyrone ring), and tangeretin (a polymethoxylated flavone) were added to purified diets at levels of 20–2000 ppm. The threshold for activity of flavone and flavanone depended on the enzyme in question. No level of tangeretin tested affected monooxygenase activities, although the 2000-ppm dose induced ethoxyresorufin deethylase and UDP-glucuronyl transferase. The authors emphasized that these levels of flavonoids are likely to occur in normal human diets and that the effects of low, even subthreshold, doses of multiple compounds are likely to be additive. These findings support the hypothesis that the anticarcinogenicity of flavonoids is related to their effects on drug-metabolizing enzymes.

A long-term study was conducted in rats to determine the effects of a high-salt diet on hepatic drug-metabolizing and glutathione-related enzyme systems (*233*). No changes were observed for 180 days. However, feeding 8% salt for 360 days resulted in decreased cytochrome P450 content and increased glutathione peroxidase activity, accompanied by reduced capacity of hepatic tissue to activate benzo[*a*]pyrene in bacterial mutagenesis assays. Thus, although it appeared unlikely that a long-term high-salt diet is involved in the carcinogenic effects of benzo[*a*]pyrene, such a diet could diminish the ability to detoxify xenobiotic compounds and thereby favor various pathological processes.

Manipulations of the macronutrient composition of the diet can markedly alter oxidative drug metabolism in humans (*234*). Eight healthy adults were fed a 44% protein, 35% carbohydrate diet for 14 days; then, after a 3-day washout period, they were given an isocaloric 10% protein, 70% carbohydrate diet for 14 days. On days 11 and 13 of each dietary period they were given acetaminophen and oxazepam, respectively. These drugs are metabolized primarily by conjugation. Change from the high-protein, low-carbohydrate diet to the low-protein, high-carbohydrate produced a 14% increase in urinary recovery of acetaminophen glucuronide and a 32% increase in oxazepam glucuronide. These increases were at the expense of other metabolic pathways, as there were no significant changes in the metabolic clearance rates of the drugs.

GROWTH, DEVELOPMENT, AND AGING

Influence of dietary fat on development and aging

EFFECTS OF MATERNAL DIET ON FATTY ACID COMPOSITION OF BREAST MILK AND FETAL AND NEONATAL TISSUES. The essential fatty acid status of Inuit and Dutch neonates was compared by analyzing phospholipids from venous cord plasma and umbilical cord tissue (*235*). Total SFAs and MUFAs were significantly higher and PUFAs significantly lower in Inuits. Reduced amounts of the longer-chain and highly unsaturated fatty acids, both *n*–3 and *n*–6, accounted for most of the difference in PUFA content; in contrast, amounts of linoleic and dihomo-γ-linolenic acids were significantly higher in the Inuit neonates. The lower *n*–3 status in Inuit neonates in the context of a higher maternal dietary supply points to genetic differences between the Inuits and Dutch in the handling of these substances. In particular, evidence suggests a lesser expression of Δ5-desaturase in Inuit neonates. The authors postulated that the Inuit fetus will be very susceptible to developing severe *n*–3 deficiency if Inuit women adopt the Western diet.

The fatty acid composition of samples of breast milk from Nigerian and Japanese women was determined by gas chromatography (*236*). Cultural dietary differences were reflected: milk of Nigerian women contained more SFAs, arachidonic acid, and eicosatrienoic and docosatetraenoic acids, whereas milk of Japanese women contained more MUFAs and *n*–3 PUFAs. A Canadian study evaluated the effect of an Efamol supplement on the total fat and essential fatty acid composition of human milk after prolonged lactation (*237*). Thirty-six women completed 8 months of breast feeding after starting the study; 18 received Efamol and 18 received placebo. Total fat and essential fatty acid contents of the milk decreased during the study in the placebo group but rose in the Efamol group. A remarkably high proportion of the supplemental fatty acids could be accounted for by their appearance in the milk. These results show that milk composition can readily be manipulated by changing the maternal diet and may be of particular importance in neonatal nutrition when prolonged breast feeding is desirable.

The effect of *trans* fatty acids in a mother's diet on the composition of her milk has been of some concern because *trans* fatty acids can influence essential fatty acid metabolism (*238*). In studies of pigs, the effects of dietary *trans* fatty acids from hydrogenated oils on milk composition were evaluated in colostrum and 21 days postpartum. Feeding *trans*-containing fats led to secretion of *trans* fatty acids in the milk; levels in colostrum and milk were similar. Feeding up to ~29% of *trans* fats had no consistent effect on the level of polyenoic fatty acids but did reduce the level of SFAs and increase the level of *cis* + *trans* monoenoic fatty acids. Increasing dietary linoleic acid did not affect secretion of *trans* fatty acids but did raise the linoleic acid level in the milk. The authors concluded that the effects of dietary *trans* fatty acids on the fat content and fatty acid composition of sow's colostrum and milk were minor to moderate.

To determine the effects on progeny of long-term feeding of diets containing different types and amounts of fat to the mother, female rats were fed one of four experimental diets from weaning (*239*). The low-fat diet contained 4.5% fat, half corn oil and half beef tallow. Three high-fat diets contained 30% tallow and 2% corn oil, 16% tallow and 16% corn oil, or 2% tallow and 30% corn oil. Offspring of these rats were killed at birth or weaning for evaluation of growth and fatty acid composition. Newborns of mothers fed the high-PUFA diet weighed less than the other newborns, but the difference was no longer apparent in weanlings. The carcass composition of neonates and body weight of weanlings were unaffected by maternal diet, although weanlings from dams fed the high-fat diets contained a higher percentage of carcass lipids. Fatty acid composition varied with diet as expected.

Studies in mice evaluated effects of the n–3/n–6 ratio in the mother's diet on her offspring. Beginning at mating, females were fed one of 6 diets containing similar amounts of total PUFAs but with n–3/n–6 ratios ranging from 0 to 4 (*240*). Distribution of fatty acids in the phosphatidylcholine and phosphatidylethanolamine fractions of heart, kidney, and liver was measured in 12-day-old sucklings. As the dietary n–3/n–6 ratio increased to ~0.5, tissue levels of 20:5n–3, 22:5n–3, and 22:6n–3 increased and 18:2n–6 and 20:4n–6 decreased. The two phospholipid subclasses responded similarly but there were differences between tissues. A higher n–3/n–6 ratio in tissue than in milk indicated that the pups preferentially incorporated n–3 over n–6 into their tissues. This effect was restricted to preformed long-chain n–3 PUFAs, which bypassed the rate-limiting Δ6 desaturation step: when the 18:3n–6 Δ6 desaturation product of 18:2n–6 was given in the maternal diet, incorporation of n–3 fatty acids was suppressed. In similar experiments, brains of 12-day-old pups were analyzed (*241*). Increasing n–3/n–6 ratios were associated with slightly smaller brains relative to body weight. The predominant n–3 and n–6 fatty acids in milk were 20:5n–3 and 18:2n–6, whereas in brain they were 22:6n–3 and 20:4n–6. The n–3/n–6 ratio of milk lipids showed a strong linear relationship with diet, but the relationship with brain phosphatidylcholine and phosphatidylethanolamine was quadratic, maximum responses occurring at dietary ratios of 0.25–0.5.

NEONATAL DIET. Innis comprehensively reviewed essential fatty acids in growth and development (*242*; contains 566 references). She discussed the biochemistry and metabolism of essential fatty acids and their role in development of the CNS and other organs, clinical studies of dietary n–3 and n–6 fatty acids in term and premature infants, and approaches to determining fatty acid requirements in growth and development. She also edited the proceedings of a symposium on lipids in infant nutrition (*243*). Sessions at this symposium addressed geographic variations in the fatty acid composition of human milk, dietary influences on lipoproteins during infancy, lipid nutrition and energy balance in very premature infants, and the role of and requirements for long-chain fatty acids in infancy.

Questions still remain about the optimal fatty acid mix for infant formulas; neonatal piglets are a useful model with which to resolve these issues. From birth to 15 days of age, piglets were fed sow's milk or formulas containing various mixtures of n–3 and n–6 fatty acids (*244*). Although all formulas contained similar quantities of 18:2n–6 fatty acids, increasing dietary n–3 had significant effects on tissue fatty acid composition, and brain showed important differences from liver and plasma. This study did not confirm reports that fish oil increases 20:5n–3 and decreases 20:4n–6 in brain; however, there was a dose-related decrease in 24:4n–6 and increase in 20:5n–3 in liver, which showed no evidence of reaching a maximum over the concentration range of dietary long-chain PUFAs studied. In view of this the authors urged further study of the effects of formula composition on tissue levels of these important eicosanoid precursors, and caution in use of fish oils low in n–6 long-chain PUFAs for infant formulas.

AGING. Nestel reviewed the issues related to dietary fat recommendations for the elderly (*245*). They include changing food preferences and eating habits in older persons, problems in maintaining proper weight, the relationship of dietary fat to the major chronic diseases afflicting the elderly, and other nutritional considerations.

One process that decreases in aging rats is the Δ6-desaturation of linoleic and α-linolenic acids (*246*). A way to circumvent this would be to provide the 6-desaturated metabolite, γ-linolenic acid, directly. The 6-desaturation of linoleic and α-linolenic acids in liver microsomes of young and old rats was studied in animals fed a basal diet with soybean oil or a diet supplemented with evening primrose oil, which is rich in γ-linolenic acid. Liver microsome preparations from young rats showed no diet-related difference in Δ6-desaturase activity on either substrate, indicating that when this activity is at or near its peak, variations in diet do not influence it. In microsomes from old animals, however, desaturase activity was significantly greater in animals fed the evening primrose oil diet. The fatty acid compositions of the microsomes corresponded to findings related to desaturase activity. Other dietary effects on the microviscosity and fatty acid composition of microsomal membranes were discussed.

Influence of diet restriction on aging

IMMUNE RESPONSE. Because of the reported effects of diet restriction on age-related decline of the immune system in various rodent models, these effects were evaluated in CFY Sprague-Dawley rats (*247*). From weaning, male rats were fed ad libitum or given an amount of food that maintained body weight at ~50% that of the pair-matched ad libitum-fed control. Diet-restricted animals yielded smaller lymphoid organs and numbers of lymphocytes than their fully fed controls. There were phenotypic differences and large differences in the mitogen responses of individual animals within a dietary group. However, the authors found no evidence that dietary restriction improved B- or T-cell responses in spleen, Peyer's patches, brachial/axillary lymph nodes, or mesenteric nodes in either 12- or 20-month-old rats. Nor were they able to demonstrate an age-related decline in lymphocyte performance, suggesting that results of such testing are strain-dependent. Nevertheless, compared with control serum, serum from diet-restricted rats enhanced T-cell mitogen responses, suggesting that serum factors can modify the intrinsic ability of lymphocytes to proliferate in response to mitogens.

In perhaps the first demonstration that diet restriction can enhance immunity to an actual infectious agent, Effros et al. studied a long-lived F1 hybrid mouse strain (*248*). At weaning, females were randomly assigned to one of two isonutrient diets, differing only in total calories (as carbohydrate). "Controls" were mildly calorie-restricted; "restricted" mice were severely calorie-restricted. Antigen-specific recall was measured as the proliferation of memory spleen cells after a second exposure to the influenza virus. Old controls had a very low response, whereas responses of young controls and old restricted mice were similar. Antibody production in old restricted animals was between that in old and young controls. T cells from old diet-restricted mice consistently showed a greater proliferative response than control T cells; in some cases their response was comparable to that from young controls. Diet restriction also reduced the age-related decline in antigen presentation. These improvements apparently reflect the activity of more than one mechanism at several levels.

DNA REPAIR. Hepatic DNA polymerases from C57BL/6 mice undergo an age-related decline in specific activity and fidelity, which can be attenuated by diet restriction (*249,250*). Testing was done in diet-restricted and control mice 6, 16, and 26 months old; differences in survival rates between the two groups began to be apparent at ~26 months. Polymerase preparations from diet-restricted mice showed a smaller age-related decline in specific activity and copied synthetic DNA templates with greater fidelity than enzymes from controls. Treatment of the enzymes with inositol-1,4-bisphosphate consistently improved the fidelity of polymerase α in both diet groups at all ages, but had no effect on polymerase β. The authors suggested that interaction of DNA polymerases with phosphoinositide hydrolysis products increases the enzymes' specific activity and fidelity, and these interactions could be an important mechanism moderating the age-related decrease in function of DNA polymerases. A second paper reported that UV-initiated unscheduled DNA synthesis was significantly higher in hepatocytes from weanlings and 18-month-old calorie-restricted mice than in hepatocytes from 18-month-old controls (*250*). These results suggest that calorie restriction could ameliorate the age-related deterioration of cellular mechanisms involved in reducing the rate at which mutations accumulate, potentially delaying the age of onset of mutation-associated diseases.

OTHER EFFECTS OF DIET RESTRICTION. Age-related lesions were evaluated as biomarkers in a study of effects of diet restriction in mice (*251*). All lesions observed in all organs of 1134 mice of 4 genotypes were described. Half of the mice were

diet-restricted and half were controls fed ad libitum; insofar as possible, mice representing each combination of sex, strain, and diet group were killed for study after 12, 18, 24, and 30 months. Diet restriction significantly reduced the occurrence of total lesions, total tumors, and total lymphoid nodules of various organs in mice of the same age, sex, and genotype; all of these markers generally increased with age in both diet groups. The authors concluded that total tumors, total lymphoid nodules, total lesions, and absence of lesions are all markers independent of lifespan that reflect the diminished rate of aging induced by diet restriction.

Two seldom-considered effects of diet restriction in rodents are reduction of average body temperature and decreased membrane microviscosity (*252*). Diet restriction was accomplished by feeding female rats every other day. This regimen reduced their mean body temperature by ~1°C, although the temperature pattern of these animals was more complex than the simple circadian rhythm exhibited by controls fed ad libitum. Membranes from splenic lymphocytes, hepatocytes, and cerebellum of such diet-restricted animals showed reduced microviscosity compared with membranes from controls, even taking into account the 1°C in vivo temperature difference. Implications of these observations were discussed.

Diet restriction decreased age-related hypertrophy of astrocytes in the mouse hippocampus and dentate gyrus (*253*). In the frontal and parietal cortex of calorie-restricted mice astroglia were significantly smaller than those of controls at 6 months but not at older ages, suggesting that calorie restriction delayed neocortical astrocyte development. The authors discussed the significance of these observations, arguing that they indicate more than a simple delay of aging in the brain. In rats, food restriction affects age-related morphometric parameters of cerebellar synapses (*254*). Six-month-old rats have a greater number and surface density of synapses than 27- to 28-month-old rats fed ad libitum; food restriction prevents the decrease in number and decreases the reduction in surface density of synaptic contacts. This may explain the improved motor coordination and performance observed in old diet-restricted animals.

Other effects of diet on development and aging

Meydani reviewed the biochemical changes leading to age-associated changes in the immune response, particularly as influenced by dietary antioxidants and prooxidants (255). Splenocytes from old mice and peripheral blood mononuclear cells from older adults produced significantly more prostaglandin E_2 and their plasma contained higher levels of thiobarbituric acid–reactive substances than were found in their younger counterparts. In both aged mice and older human subjects, vitamin E supplementation reduced prostaglandin E_2 synthesis while increasing interleukin-2 production, mitogenic response to concanavalin A, and the delayed hypersensitivity skin test reaction. In humans, vitamin E also reduced levels of thiobarbituric acid–reactive substances. In old mice, glutathione supplementation improved the mitogenic response and delayed hypersensitivity skin test reaction. In contrast, when older women were given prooxidant EPA and DHA supplements, their production of cytokines and the mitogenic response to phytohemagglutinin decreased and production of thiobarbituric acid–reactive substances increased. The beneficial effects of antioxidants and the detrimental effects of prooxidants are consistent with the hypothesis that changes in free radical reactions and lipid peroxidation with aging contribute to the age-related decline of the immune response.

In the evolution of inquiries on nature vs. nurture into inquiries on nature interacting with nurture, the importance and complexity of nutrition's role have become recognized. Blizard discussed the "nature of nurture" in the etiology of hypertension, in terms of genetic models and the influence of the maternal environment—with emphasis on diet (256). Many physiological systems that undergo rapid change during the preweaning period (such as the sympathetic nervous system and the renin–angiotensin system) may mediate the influence of the maternal environment; the mother's behavior and genetic constitution can influence development of these systems; and nutritional factors are involved at all levels in these phenomena. Any physiological mechanism proposed as a link between a mother's behavior and the physiology of her adult offspring must recognize the role of nutrition.

A 10-year study of Pregnavite Forte F confirmed the efficacy of folic acid supplementation for at-risk women in reducing the incidence of fetuses with neural tube defects (257). It emphasized the importance of beginning the vitamin supplement at least 4 weeks before conception, and repeating it during every pregnancy. Review of intervention trials and observational studies prompted the U.S. FDA to recommend that all women in the USA who are capable of becoming pregnant should consume 0.4 mg/day of folic acid for the purpose of reducing their risk of having a pregnancy affected by spina bifida or other neural tube defect (258). Except under a physician's supervision, intakes ≥ 1 mg/day were not advised. Four intervention studies, summarized in tabular form, found that high-dose folic acid supplementation reduced the risk of pregnancies affected by neural tube defects by 60–100% in women who had had prior affected pregnancies. Three case–control studies and a prospective cohort study found risk reductions of 60, 75, 0, and 72% in high-risk women for various levels and durations of folate supplementation. The average dietary consumption of folic acid by women in the USA is ~0.2 mg/day. Three strategies for reaching the recommended level would be to improve dietary habits, fortify the food supply, or use supplements. From a public health perspective, the most promising approach has not been selected. However, women who select foods consistent with the U.S. Dietary Pyramid are likely to consume diets containing ≥ 0.4 mg/day. It is expected that adequate folate intake will avert up to 50% or more of neural tube defects.

In Wistar rats, the type and amount of dietary protein influence lifespan and metabolism (259). Groups of 23-month-old females were placed on diets containing 19% protein, three-quarters of which was of animal origin, or 8.8% protein exclusively of vegetable origin. Analysis of hepatic free amino acids revealed higher contents of glycine + alanine and tyrosine and a much lower phenylalanine/tyrosine ratio in the low-protein group. Levels of valine and leucine were higher in the high-protein group, but isoleucine levels were not affected by diet. Levels of dopamine in the medial hypothalamus and of serotonin in the lateral hypothalamus were significantly lower in the low-protein group; the median lifespan of these animals was 24% longer. These observations indicate that dietary protein can modify metabolic activity and lifespan and that CNS regulation may be involved.

The relatively long gestation and high birth weight of babies born to Faroe Islanders have been attributed to the marine-based diet of the mothers. However, this view was challenged by a study comparing gestational period and birth weight of infants born to residents of the Orkney Islands and the Scottish mainland (*260*). Residents of Orkney eat 30% more fish than residents of Aberdeen; their babies are larger and gestation is slightly longer. However, there were other differences between the two groups that could cause the difference in birth weight. Factors most strongly related to birth weight were the mother's height, weight, and smoking habits; smoking could also explain the slightly shorter gestation in Aberdeen. A small but significant proportion of the variation in birth weight was explained by the mother's residing in Orkney; this may be related to a number of genetic or environmental factors, only some of which are dietary.

The role of nutritional factors in development of glucose intolerance in normoglycemic subjects is not clearly understood. A 3-year study was conducted in 175 normoglycemic elderly adults who were evaluated initially by a glucose tolerance test and dietary history and followed up by annual glucose tolerance testing and physical examination (*261*). About 60% of the subjects reported eating fish, with an average consumption of 24.2 g/day. Among fish-eaters, the incidence of glucose intolerance was significantly lower than among those who did not eat fish. The inverse association persisted after accounting for age, sex, and possible confounding baseline characteristics. This suggests that in an elderly population, habitual consumption of small amounts of fish may protect against development of impaired glucose tolerance and diabetes mellitus.

Calcium deficiency is considered common in humans and it is aggravated in aging; parathyroid hormone mobilizes calcium from bone to restore serum calcium depleted during calcium deficiency

(*262*). Fujita reviewed the interrelationships among calcium, the parathyroids, and aging. He emphasized that disturbances in calcium gradients and pools are inevitably associated with cell dysfunction, damage, and death as well as with aging. Calcium bioavailability and the effects of calcium supplementation on hypertension and diabetes mellitus were briefly reviewed.

Until 1984, dietary intake of selenium in Finland was relatively low (*263*). At that time, a decision was made to add sodium selenate to multinutrient fertilizers used in agriculture, with the objective of raising the selenium concentration in cereals tenfold. By 1990 the average daily intake of adult Finns had increased from 20–50 µg to 0.11 mg and the selenium content of breast milk had more than doubled. The authors estimated that the current selenium intake of infants in Finland is ~11 µg/day, which falls at the low end of the U.S. National Research Council recommendations. However, there were no overt signs of selenium deficiency in infants before selenium fertilization began. Effects of recent agricultural changes on selenium intake and concentrations in human milk are being monitored. An investigator in Australia has suggested a link between poor maternal selenium status during pregnancy or low selenium content in milk and sudden infant death syndrome (SIDS) (*264*). Both Tasmania and South Island, New Zealand, have selenium-deficient soils and high rates of SIDS. There are other associations between poor selenium status and cardiac and musculoskeletal abnormalities, including sudden cardiac death in children and pregnant young women. Increased risk of SIDS in formula-fed infants may be related to the low selenium content of some infant formulas. The author postulated a mechanism for the protective role of selenium, concluding that although a few authors argue that selenium is unlikely to have anything to do with SIDS, the problem is too serious for this possibility to go uninvestigated. Correspondence on the SIDS–selenium connection emphasized that SIDS is probably not a single entity (*265*). For example, the sudden death seen in calves and lambs, in Keshan disease, and in acute cardiomyopathy may be responsive to selenium treatment. The epidemiology of Keshan disease and its association with selenium-deficient soils and inadequate supply of selenium in breast milk was summarized. The author posed questions relating to the role of antioxidant systems in protecting the endothelium, the vulnerability of an infant's antioxidant status, and the role of endothelial dysfunction in SIDS. A commentary on this letter presented additional intriguing epidemiologic evidence for an association of selenium status and antioxidant systems generally with SIDS (*266*). Appropriate animal models are available for study of this subject.

LITERATURE CITED

1. Chandra, R.K. Nutrition and immunoregulation. Significance for host resistance to tumors and infectious diseases in humans and rodents. *J. Nutr.* 122:754–757 (1992).

2. Chandra, R.K., and S.A.D. Amorin. Lipids and immunoregulation. *Nutr. Res.* 12(Suppl. 1):S137–S145 (1992).

3. Maki, P.A., and P.M. Newberne. Dietary lipids and immune function. *J. Nutr.* 122:610–614 (1992).

4. Kelley, D.S., R.M. Dougherty, L.B. Branch, et al. Concentration of dietary *n–6* polyunsaturated fatty acids and the human immune status. *Clin. Immunol. Immunopathol.* 62:240–244 (1992).

5. Iversen, L., K. Fogh, G. Bojesen, and K. Kragballe. Linoleic acid and dihomogammalinolenic acid inhibit leukotriene B_4 formation and stimulate the formation of their 15-lipoxygenase products by human neutrophils in vitro. Evidence of formation of antiinflammatory compounds. *Agents Actions* 33:286–291 (1991).

6. Ziboh, V.A., and M.P. Fletcher. Dose–response effects of dietary γ-linolenic acid–enriched oils on human polymorphonuclear-neutrophil biosynthesis of leukotriene B_4. *Am. J. Clin. Nutr.* 55:39–45 (1992).

7. Gyllenhammar, H., J. Palmblad, and B. Ringertz. Effects of an essential fatty acid–supplemented diet on leukotriene B_4-induced rat neutrophil functions. *Scand. J. Clin. Lab. Invest.* 51:525–532 (1991).

8. Huang, S.-C., M.L. Misfeldt, and K.L. Fritsche. Dietary fat influences Ia antigen expression and immune cell populations in the murine peritoneum and spleen. *J. Nutr.* 122:1219–1231 (1992).

9. Guimarães, A.R.P., and R. Curi. Metabolic changes induced by W-3 polyunsaturated fatty acid rich–diet (W-3 PUFA) on the thymus, spleen and mesenteric lymph nodes of adult rats. *Biochem. Int.* 25:689–695 (1991).

10. Hardardottir, I., and J.E. Kinsella. Tumor necrosis factor production by murine resident peritoneal macrophages is enhanced by dietary *n–3* polyunsaturated fatty acids. *Biochim. Biophys. Acta* 1095:187–195 (1991).

11. Fernandes, G., V. Tomar, N. Mohan, and J.T. Venkatraman. Potential of diet therapy on murine AIDS. *J. Nutr.* 122:716–722 (1992).

12. Chang, H.R., A.G. Dulloo, I.R. Vladoianu, et al. Fish oil decreases natural resistance of mice to infection with *Salmonella typhimurium*. *Metabolism* 41:1–2 (1992).

13. Virella, G., K. Fourspring, B. Hyman, et al. Immunosuppressive effects of fish oil in normal human volunteers: correlation with the in vitro effects of eicosapentanoic [sic] acid on human lymphocytes. *Clin. Immunol. Immunopathol.* 61:161–176 (1991).

14. Ferretti, A., G.J. Nelson, and P.C. Schmidt. Salmon-rich diet inhibits arachidonate cyclooxygenation in healthy men. *J. Nutr. Biochem.* 2:547–552 (1991).

15. Thompson, P.J., N.L.A. Misso, M. Passarelli, and M.J. Phillips. The effect of eicosapentaenoic acid consumption on human neutrophil chemiluminescence. *Lipids* 26:1223–1226 (1991).

16. Fritsche, K.L., N.A. Cassity, and S.-C. Huang. Dietary (*n–3*) fatty acid and vitamin E interactions in rats: effects on vitamin E status, immune cell prostaglandin E production and primary antibody response. *J. Nutr.* 122:1009–1018 (1992).

17. Kramer, T.R., N. Schoene, L.W. Douglass, et al. Increased vitamin E intake restores fish-oil–induced suppressed blastogenesis of mitogen-stimulated T lymphocytes. *Am. J. Clin. Nutr.* 54:896–902 (1991).

18. Bendich, A. β-Carotene and the immune response. *Proc. Nutr. Soc.* 50:263–274 (1991).

19. Garewal, H.S., N.M. Ampel, R.R. Watson, et al. A preliminary trial of beta-carotene in subjects infected with the human immunodeficiency virus. *J. Nutr.* 122:728–732 (1992).

20. Jyonouchi, H., R.J. Hill, Y. Tomita, and R.A. Good. Studies of immunomodulating actions of carote-

noids. I. Effects of β-carotene and astaxanthin on murine lymphocyte functions and cell surface marker expression in in vitro culture system. *Nutr. Cancer* 16:93–105 (1991).

21. Field, C.J., R. Gougeon, and E.B. Marliss. Changes in circulating leukocytes and mitogen responses during very-low-energy all-protein reducing diets. *Am. J. Clin. Nutr.* 54:123–129 (1991).

22. Good, R.A., and E. Lorenz. Nutrition and cellular immunity. *Int. J. Immunopharmacol.* 14:361–366 (1992).

23. Peplow, P.V. Modification to dietary intake of sodium, potassium, calcium, magnesium and trace elements can influence arachidonic acid metabolism and eicosanoid production. *Prostaglandins Leukotrienes Essential Fatty Acids* 45:1–19 (1992).

24. Turner, R.J., and J.M. Finch. Selenium and the immune response. *Proc. Nutr. Soc.* 50:275–285 (1991).

25. Woodward, B. Zinc, a pharmacologically potent essential nutrient: focus on immunity. *Can. Med. Assoc. J.* 145:1469 (1991).

26. Moineau, S., and J. Goulet. Effect of feeding fermented milks on the pulmonary macrophage activity in mice. *Milchwissenschaft* 46:551–554 (1991).

27. Perdigon, G., S. Alvarez, M.E. Nader de Macias, et al. Behaviour of natural and heated yogurt in the immune system and preventive capacity on enteric infections. *Milchwissenschaft* 46:410–416 (1991).

28. Hilton, E., H.D. Isenberg, P. Alperstein, et al. Ingestion of yogurt containing *Lactobacillus acidophilus* as prophylaxis for candidal vaginitis. *Ann. Intern. Med.* 116:353–357 (1992).

29. Carver, J.D., B. Pimentel, W.I. Cox, and L.A. Barness. Dietary nucleotide effects upon immune function in infants. *Pediatrics* 88:359–363 (1991).

30. Coste, M., and D. Tomé. Milk peptides with physiological activities. II. Opioid and immunostimulating peptides derived from milk proteins. *Lait* 71:241–247 (1991).

31. Shimizu, S., K. Akimoto, Y. Shinmen, et al. Sesamin is a potent and specific inhibitor of Δ5 desaturase in polyunsaturated fatty acid biosynthesis. *Lipids* 26:512–516 (1991).

32. Zurier, B. Essential fatty acids and inflammation. *Ann. Rheum. Dis.* 50:745–746 (1991).

33. Cleland, L.G., M.J. James, M.A. Neumann, et al. Linoleate inhibits EPA incorporation from dietary fish-oil supplements in human subjects. *Am. J. Clin. Nutr.* 55:395–399 (1992).

34. Dry, J., and D. Vincent. Effect of a fish oil diet on asthma: results of a 1-year double-blind study. *Int. Arch. Allergy Appl. Immunol.* 95:156–157 (1991).

35. Lieberman, D., and D. Heimer. Effect of dietary sodium on the severity of bronchial asthma. *Thorax* 47:360–362 (1992).

36. Thien, F.C.K., B.A. Atkinson, A. Khan, et al. Effect of dietary fish oil supplementation on the antigen-induced late-phase response in the skin. *J. Allergy Clin. Immunol.* 89:829–835 (1992).

37. Kerscher, M.J., and H.C. Korting. Treatment of atopic eczema with evening primrose oil: rationale and clinical results. *Clin. Invest.* 70:167–171 (1992).

38. Walton, A.J.E., M.L. Snaith, M. Locniskar, et al. Dietary fish oil and the severity of symptoms in patients with systemic lupus erythematosus. *Ann. Rheum. Dis.* 50:463–466 (1991).

39. Bullard-Dillard, R., J. Chen, S. Pelsue, et al. Anti-Sm autoantibodies of systemic lupus erythematosus cross react with dietary plant proteins. *Immunol. Invest.* 21:193–202 (1992).

40. Shigemasa, C., T. Tanaka, and H. Mashiba. Effect of vegetarian diet on systemic lupus erythematosus. (Letter.) *Lancet* 339:1177 (1992).

41. Das, U.N. Interaction(s) between essential fatty acids, eicosanoids, cytokines, growth factors and free radicals: relevance to new therapeutic strategies in rheumatoid arthritis and other collagen vascular diseases. *Prostaglandins Leukotrienes Essential Fatty Acids* 44:201–210 (1991).

42. Fahrer, H., F. Hoeflin, B.H. Lauterburg, et al. Diet and fatty acids: can fish substitute for fish oil? *Clin. Exp. Rheumatol.* 9:403–406 (1991).

43. Kjeldsen-Kragh, J., M. Haugen, C.F. Borchgrevink, et al. Controlled trial of fasting and one-year vegetarian diet in rheumatoid arthritis. *Lancet* 338:899–902 (1991).

44. Darlington, L.G., and N.W. Ramsey. Diets for rheumatoid arthritis. (Letter.) *Lancet* 338:1209 (1991).

45. Maberly, D.J., and H.M. Anthony. Diets for rheumatoid arthritis. (Letter.) *Lancet* 338:1210 (1991).

46. Helliwell, P.S., and A. Rewilak. Diets for rheumatoid arthritis. (Letter.) *Lancet* 338:1209–1210 (1991).

47. Seignalet, J. Diet, fasting, and rheumatoid arthritis. (Letter.) *Lancet* 339:68–69 (1992).

48. Abuzakouk, M., and C. O'Farrelly. Diet, fasting, and rheumatoid arthritis. (Letter.) *Lancet* 339:68 (1992).

49. Pananyi, G.S. Diet, fasting, and rheumatoid arthritis. (Letter.) *Lancet* 339:69 (1992).

50. Kjeldsen-Kragh, J., M. Haugen, and Ø. Fførre. Diet therapy in rheumatoid arthritis. (Reply.) *Lancet* 339:250 (1992).

51. Pérez-Maceda, B., J.P. López-Bote, C. Langa, and C. Bernabeu. Antibodies to dietary antigens in rheumatoid arthritis—possible molecular mimicry mechanism. *Clin. Chim. Acta* 203:153–165 (1991).

52. Flatt, P.R., C.R. Barnett, O. Shibier, and S.K. Swanston-Flatt. Direct and indirect actions of nutrients in the regulation of insulin secretion from the pancreatic β cells. *Proc. Nutr. Soc.* 50:559–566 (1991).

53. Lovejoy, J., and M. DiGirolamo. Habitual dietary intake and insulin sensitivity in lean and obese adults. *Am. J. Clin. Nutr.* 55:1174–1179 (1992).

54. Feskens, E.J.M., C.H. Bowles, and D. Kromhout. Carbohydrate intake and body mass index in relation to the risk of glucose intolerance in an elderly population. *Am. J. Clin. Nutr.* 54:136–140 (1991).

55. Anderson, J.W., J.A. Zeigler, D.A. Deakins, et al. Metabolic effects of high-carbohydrate, high-fiber diets for insulin-dependent diabetic individuals. *Am. J. Clin. Nutr.* 54:936–943 (1991).

56. Wolever, T.M.S., D.J.A. Jenkins, A.L. Jenkins, and R.G. Josse. The glycemic index: methodology and clinical implications. *Am. J. Clin. Nutr.* 54:846–854 (1991).

57. Nishimune, T., T. Yakushiji, T. Sumimoto, et al. Glycemic response and fiber content of some foods. *Am. J. Clin. Nutr.* 54:414–419 (1991).

58. Granfeldt, Y., and I. Björck. Glycemic response to starch in pasta: a study of mechanisms of limited enzyme availability. *J. Cereal Sci.* 14:47–61 (1991).

59. Indar-Brown, K., C. Norenberg, and Z. Madar. Glycemic and insulinemic responses after ingestion of ethnic foods by NIDDM and healthy subjects. *Am. J. Clin. Nutr.* 55:89–85 (1992).

60. van Amelsvoort, J.M.M., and J.A. Weststrate. Amylose-amylopectin ratio in a meal affects postprandial variables in male volunteers. *Am. J. Clin. Nutr.* 55:712–718 (1992).

61. Finer, N. Sweeteners and metabolic disorders. In *Handbook of Sweeteners*. S. Marie and J.R. Piggott (eds.). London, Blackie and Son Ltd. Pp. 225–247 (1991).

62. Hollenbeck, C.B., and A.M. Coulston. The effects of increased sucrose consumption on carbohydrate and lipoprotein metabolism in individuals with insulin resistance. In *Sugars in Nutrition*. M. Gracey, N. Kretchmer, and E. Rossi (eds.). *Nestlé Nutrition Workshop Series* 25:169–178 (1991).

63. Furuse, M., C. Kimura, H. Takahashi, and J.-I. Okumura. Prevention of the incidence of diabetes by dietary sorbose in nonobese diabetic mice. *J. Nutr.* 121:1135–1138 (1991).

64. Swanson, J.E., D.C. Laine, W. Thomas, and J.P. Bantle. Metabolic effects of dietary fructose in healthy subjects. *Am. J. Clin. Nutr.* 55:851–856 (1992).

65. Anderson, J.W., and A.O Akanji. Dietary fiber—an overview. *Diabetes Care* 14:1126–1131 (1991).

66. Riccardi, G., and A.A. Rivellese. Effects of dietary fiber and carbohydrate on glucose and lipoprotein metabolism in diabetic patients. *Diabetes Care* 14:1115–1125 (1991).

67. Librenti, M.C., M. Cocchi, E. Orsi, et al. Effect of soya and cellulose fibers on postprandial glycemic response in type II diabetic patients. *Diabetes Care* 15:111–113 (1992).

68. Anderson, J.W., C.C. Hamilton, J.L. Horn, et al. Metabolic effects of insoluble oat fiber on lean men with type II diabetes. *Cereal Chem.* 68:291–294 (1991).

69. Ellis, P.R., F.M. Dawoud, and E.R. Morris. Blood glucose, plasma insulin and sensory responses to guar-containing wheat breads: effects of molecular weight and particle size of guar gum. *Br. J. Nutr.* 66:363–379 (1991).

70. Marshall, J.A., R.F. Hamman, and J. Baxter. High-fat, low-carbohydrate diet and the etiology of non-insulin-dependent diabetes mellitus: the San Luis Valley Diabetes Study. *Am. J. Epidemiol.* 134:590–603 (1991).

71. Swinburn, B.A., V.L. Boyce, R.N. Bergman, et al. Deterioration in carbohydrate metabolism and lipoprotein changes induced by modern, high fat diet in Pima Indians and Caucasians. *J. Clin. Endocrinol. Metab.* 73:156–165 (1991).

72. Hollenbeck, C.B., and A.M. Coulston. Effects of dietary carbohydrate and fat intake on glucose and

lipoprotein metabolism in individuals with diabetes mellitus. *Diabetes Care* 14:774–785 (1991).

73. Mlekusch, W., A.M. Taupe, K. Vrecko, et al. Effect of a high fat diet on plasma lipids, lipoprotein lipase, lecithin:cholesterol acyltransferase, and insulin function in adult rabbits. *J. Nutr. Biochem.* 2:616–622 (1991).

74. Okamoto, M., M. Okamoto, S. Kono, et al. Effects of a high-fat diet on insulin receptor kinase and the glucose transporter in rats. *J. Nutr. Biochem.* 3:241–250 (1992).

75. Stuhldreher, W., and T. Orchard. Impact of dietary change on serum lipid levels in insulin-dependent diabetes mellitus: the epidemiology of diabetes complications adult population. (Abstract.) *Am. J. Epidemiol.* 134:741 (1991).

76. Berthezene, F. Ω-3 fatty acid and diabetes mellitus. In *Fish Oil and Blood-Vessel Wall Interactions.* P.M. Vanhoutte and Ph. Douste-Blazy (eds.). Paris, John Libbey Eurotext. Pp. 129–131 (1991).

77. Malasanos, T.H., and P.W. Stacpoole. Biological effects of ω-3 fatty acids in diabetes mellitus. *Diabetes Care* 14:1160–1179 (1991).

78. Bhathena, S.J., E. Berlin, J.T. Judd, et al. Effects of ω3 fatty acids and vitamin E on hormones involved in carbohydrate and lipid metabolism in men. *Am. J. Clin. Nutr.* 54:684–688 (1991).

79. Berdanier, C.D., B. Johnson, D.K. Hartle, and W. Crowell. Life span is shortened in BHE/cdb rats fed a diet containing 9% menhaden oil and 1% corn oil. *J. Nutr.* 122:1309–1317 (1992).

80. Islin, H., K. Capito, S.E. Hansen, et al. Ability of omega-3 fatty acids to restore the impaired glucose tolerance in a mouse model for type-2 diabetes. Different effects in male and female mice. *Acta Physiol. Scand.* 143:153–160 (1991).

81. Bonanome, A., A. Visonà, L. Lusiani, et al. Carbohydrate and lipid metabolism in patients with non-insulin-dependent diabetes mellitus: effects of a low-fat, high-carbohydrate diet vs a diet high in monounsaturated fatty acids. *Am. J. Clin. Nutr.* 54:586–590 (1991).

82. Todesco, T., A.V. Rao, O. Bosello, and D.J.A. Jenkins. Propionate lowers blood glucose and alters lipid metabolism in healthy subjects. *Am. J. Clin. Nutr.* 54:860–865 (1991).

83. Arisaka, M., O. Arisaka, and Y. Yamashiro. Fatty acid and prostaglandin metabolism in children with diabetes mellitus. II.—The effect of evening primrose oil supplementation on serum fatty acid and plasma prostaglandin levels. *Prostaglandins Leukotrienes Essential Fatty Acids* 43:197–201 (1991).

84. Eckel, R.H., A.S. Hanson, A.Y. Chen, et al. Dietary substitution of medium-chain triglycerides improves insulin-mediated glucose metabolism in NIDDM subjects. *Diabetes* 41:641–647 (1992).

85. Rösen, P., R. Oestreich, and D. Tschöpe. Vitamin E and diabetes. *Fat Sci. Technol.* 93:425–431 (1991).

86. Ceriello, A., D. Giugliano, A. Quatraro, et al. Vitamin E reduction of protein glycosylation in diabetes. New prospect for prevention of diabetic complications? *Diabetes Care* 14:68–72 (1991).

87. Colditz, G.A., J.E. Manson, M.J. Stampfer, et al. Diet and risk of clinical diabetes in women. *Am. J. Clin. Nutr.* 55:1018–1023 (1992).

88. Paolisso, G., S. Sgambato, A. Gambardella, et al. Daily magnesium supplements improve glucose handling in elderly subjects. *Am. J. Clin. Nutr.* 55:1161–1167 (1992).

89. Martin, J.M., B. Trink, D. Daneman, et al. Milk proteins in the etiology of insulin-dependent diabetes mellitus (IDDM). *Ann. Med.* 23:447–452 (1991).

90. Dahl-Jørgensen, K., G. Joner, and K.F. Hanssen. Relationship between cows' milk consumption and incidence of IDDM in childhood. *Diabetes Care* 14:1081–1083 (1991).

91. Kostraba, J.N., J.S. Dorman, R.E. LaPorte, et al. Early infant diet and risk of IDDM in Blacks and Whites. *Diabetes Care* 15:626–631 (1992).

92. Swanston-Flatt, S.K., P.R. Flatt, C. Day, and C.J. Bailey. Traditional dietary adjuncts for the treatment of diabetes mellitus. *Proc. Nutr. Soc.* 50:641–651 (1991).

93. Yasni, S., K. Imaizumi, and M. Sugano. Effects of an Indonesian medicinal plant, *Curcuma xanthorrhiza* Roxb., on the levels of serum glucose and triglyceride, fatty acid desaturation, and bile acid excretion in streptozotocin-induced diabetic rats. *Agric. Biol. Chem.* 55:3005–3010 (1991).

94. Gin, H., P. Morlat, J.M. Ragnaud, and J. Aubertin. Short-term effect of red wine (consumed during meals) on insulin requirement and glucose tolerance in diabetic patients. *Diabetes Care* 15:546–548 (1992).

95. O'Dea, K. Westernisation, insulin resistance and diabetes in Australian Aborigines. *Med. J. Aust.* 155:258–264 (1991).

96. Barnard, R.J., E.J. Ugianskis, D.A. Martin, and S.B. Inkeles. Role of diet and exercise in the management of hyperinsulinemia and associated atherosclerotic risk factors. *Am. J. Cardiol.* 69:440–444 (1992).

97. Levy, J.C., G.M. Ward, B.A. Naylor, et al. Masking of diabetic phenotype on a low-energy diet despite persistence of impaired insulin response. *Metabolism* 40:1009–1015 (1991).

98. Stokkan, K-A., R.J. Reiter, M.K. Vaughan, et al. Endocrine and metabolic effects of life-long food restriction in rats. *Acta Endocrinol. (Copenh.)* 125:93–100 (1991).

99. Clemmons, D.R., and L.E. Underwood. Nutritional regulation of IGF-I and IGF binding proteins. *Annu. Rev. Nutr.* 11:393–412 (1991).

100. Nabet, P., F. Belleville-Nabet, and G. Linden. Les peptides du lait à activités physiologiques. I. Facteurs de croissance dans le lait et le lactosérum. *Lait* 71:225–239 (1991).

101. Whitten, P.L., and F. Naftolin. Dietary estrogens: a biologically active background for estrogen action. In *The New Biology of Steroid Hormones*. R.B. Hochberg and F. Naftolin (eds.). New York, Raven Press. *Serono Symp. Publ.* 74:155–167 (1991).

102. Whitten, P.L., E. Russell, and F. Naftolin. Effects of a normal, human-concentration, phytoestrogen diet on rat uterine growth. *Steroids* 57:98–106 (1992).

103. Whitten, P.L., and F. Naftolin. Effect of a phytoestrogen diet on estrogen-dependent reproductive processes in immature female rats. *Steroids* 57:56–61 (1992).

104. Adlercreutz, H., E. Hämäläinen, S. Gorbach, and B. Goldin. Dietary phyto-oestrogens and the menopause in Japan. (Letter.) *Lancet* 339:1233 (1992).

105. de Ridder, C.M., J.H.H. Thijssen, P. Van't Veer, et al. Dietary habits, sexual maturation, and plasma hormones in pubertal girls: a longitudinal study. *Am. J. Clin. Nutr.* 54:805–813 (1991).

106. Sandstead, H.H. Growth, sexual maturation, and dietary fiber in pubertal girls. (Letter.) *Am. J. Clin. Nutr.* 55:1186 (1992).

107. de Ridder, C.M., J.H.H. Thijssen, and P. Van't Veer. Growth, sexual maturation, and dietary fiber in pubertal girls. (Reply.) *Am. J. Clin. Nutr.* 55:1186–1187 (1992).

108. Maclure, M., L.B. Travis, W. Willett, and B. MacMahon. A prospective cohort study of nutrient intake and age at menarche. *Am. J. Clin. Nutr.* 54:649–656 (1991).

109. Alvir, J.M.J., and S. Thys-Jacobs. Premenstrual and menstrual symptom clusters and response to calcium treatment. *Psychopharmacol. Bull.* 27:145–148 (1991).

110. Reichman, M.E., J.T. Judd, P.R. Taylor, et al. Effect of dietary fat on length of the follicular phase of the menstrual cycle in a controlled diet setting. *J. Clin. Endocrinol. Metab.* 74:1171–1175 (1992).

111. Jacques, H., L. Noreau, and S. Moorjani. Effects on plasma lipoproteins and endogenous sex hormones of substituting lean white fish for other animal-protein sources in diets of postmenopausal women. *Am. J. Clin. Nutr.* 55:896–901 (1992).

112. Marcoux, S., J. Brisson, and J. Fabia. Calcium intake from dairy products and supplements and the risks of preeclampsia and gestational hypertension. *Am. J. Epidemiol.* 133:1266–1272 (1991).

113. Repke, J.T., and J. Villar. Pregnancy-induced hypertension and low birth weight: the role of calcium. *Am. J. Clin. Nutr.* 54:237S–241S (1991).

114. Popeski, D., L.R. Ebbeling, P.B. Brown, et al. Blood pressure during pregnancy in Canadian Inuit: community differences related to diet. *Can. Med. Assoc. J.* 145:445–454 (1991).

115. Baker, P., and F.B. Pipkin. Fish-oil and pre-eclampsia. (Letter.) *Br. J. Obstet. Gynaecol.* 98:499–500 (1991).

116. Pipkin, F.B. Fish-oil and pre-eclampsia. (Letter.) *Br. J. Obstet. Gynaecol.* 98:737 (1991).

117. McCormack, M.J., and G. Constantine. Fish-oil and pre-eclampsia. (Letter.) *Br. J. Obstet. Gynaecol.* 98:737–738 (1991).

118. Secher, N.J., S.F. Olsen, and J.D. Sørensen. Fish-oil and pre-eclampsia. (Letter.) *Br. J. Obstet. Gynaecol.* 98:738–740 (1991).

119. Olsen, S., J.D. Sørensen, N.J. Secher, et al. Randomised controlled trial of effect of fish-oil supplementation on pregnancy duration. *Lancet* 339:1003–1007 (1992).

120. Giavini, E., M.L. Broccia, M. Prati, and G.D. Roversi. Diet composition modifies embryotoxic effects induced by experimental diabetes in rats. *Biol. Neonate* 59:278–286 (1991).

121. Ahmed, F.E. Effect of diet on progression of chronic renal disease. *J. Am. Diet. Assoc.* 91:1266–1270 (1991).

122. Donadio, J.V., Jr. Omega-3 polyunsaturated fatty acids: a potential new treatment of immune renal disease. *Mayo Clin. Proc.* 66:1018–1028 (1991).

123. Holub, B.J., D.J. Philbeck, A. Parbtani, and W.F. Clark. Dietary lipid modification of renal disorders and ether phospholipid metabolism. *Biochem. Cell Biol.* 69:485–489 (1991).

124. Logan, J.L., U.F. Michael, and B. Benson. Dietary fish oil interferes with renal arachidonic acid metabolism in rats: correlations with renal physiology. *Metabolism* 41:382–389 (1992).

125. Schmitz, P.G., M.P. O'Donnell, B.L. Kasiske, and W.F. Keane. Glomerular hemodynamic effects of dietary polyunsaturated fatty acid supplementation. *J. Lab. Clin. Med.* 118:129–135 (1991).

126. Schaap, G.H., H.J.G. Bilo, J.R. Beukhof, et al. The effect of short-term omega-3 polyunsaturated fatty acid supplementation in patients with chronic renal insufficiency. *Curr. Ther. Res.* 49:1061–1070 (1991).

127. D'Amico, G., G. Remuzzi, G. Maschio, et al. Effect of dietary proteins and lipids in patients with membranous nephropathy and nephrotic syndrome. *Clin. Nephrol.* 35:237–242 (1991).

128. D'Amico, G., M.G. Gentile, G. Manna, et al. Effect of vegetarian soy diet on hyperlipidaemia in nephrotic syndrome. *Lancet* 339:1131–1134 (1992).

129. Cupisti, A., G.M. Ghiggeri, E. Morelli, and G. Barsotti. Fatty acids serum levels in nephrotic patients on a pure vegetarian diet. (Letter.) *Nephron* 60:376–377 (1992).

130. Okuda, S., T. Nakamura, T. Yamamoto, et al. Dietary protein restriction rapidly reduces transforming growth factor $\beta 1$ expression in experimental glomerulonephritis. *Proc. Natl. Acad. Sci. USA* 88:9765–9769 (1991).

131. Maksimovic, Z.J. Selenium deficiency and Balkan endemic nephropathy. *Kidney Int.* 40(Suppl. 34):S-12–S-14 (1991).

132. Mavotta, R.B., and M.H. Floch. Diet and nutrition in ulcer disease. *Med. Clin. North Am.* 75:967–979 (1991).

133. Kato, I., A.M.Y. Nomura, G.N. Stemmermann, and P.-H. Chyou. *Am. J. Epidemiol.* 135:521–530 (1992).

134. Leung, F.W. Fish oil protection against ethanol-induced gastric mucosal injury in rats. (Letter.) *Digest. Dis. Sci.* 37:636–637 (1992).

135. Lugea, A., S. Videla, J. Vilaseca, and F. Guarner. Antiulcerogenic and antiinflammatory actions of fatty acids on the gastrointestinal tract. *Prostaglandins Leukotrienes Essential Fatty Acids* 43:135–140 (1991).

136. Murakami, S., Y. Isobe, H. Kijima, et al. Inhibition of gastric H^+, K^+-ATPase and acid secretion by ellagic acid. *Planta Med.* 57:305–308 (1991).

137. Vanderhoof, U.A., D.J. Blackwood, H. Mohammadpour, and J.H.Y. Park. Effect of dietary menhaden oil on normal growth and development and on ameliorating mucosal injury in rats. *Am. J. Clin. Nutr.* 54:346–350 (1991).

138. Eastwood, M.A., and E.R. Morris. Physical properties of dietary fiber that influence physiological function: a model for polymers along the gastrointestinal tract. *Am. J. Clin. Nutr.* 55:436–442 (1992).

139. MacDonald, R.S., L. Steel-Goodwin, and R.J. Smith. Influence of dietary fiber on insulin receptors in rat intestinal mucosa. *Ann. Nutr. Metab.* 35:328–338 (1991).

140. Nunes, C.S., and K. Malmlöf. Glucose absorption, hormonal release and hepatic metabolism after guar gum ingestion. *Reprod. Nutr. Dev.* 32:11–20 (1992).

141. Leng-Peschlow, E. *Plantago ovata* seeds as dietary fibre supplement: physiological and metabolic effects in rats. *Br. J. Nutr.* 66:331–349 (1991).

142. Bach Knudsen, K.E., and I. Hansen. Gastrointestinal implications in pigs of wheat and oat fractions. 1. Digestibility and bulking properties of polysaccharides and other major constituents. *Br. J. Nutr.* 65:217–232 (1991).

143. Bach Knudsen, K.E., B. Borg Jensen, J.O. Andersen, and I. Hansen. Gastrointestinal implications in pigs of wheat and oat fractions. 2. Microbial activity in the gastrointestinal tract. *Br. J. Nutr.* 65:233–248 (1991).

144. Wolever, T.M.S., P. ter Wal, P. Spadafora, and P. Robb. Guar, but not psyllium, increases breath methane and serum acetate concentrations in human subjects. *Am. J. Clin. Nutr.* 55:719–722 (1992).

145. Jenkins, D.J.A., T.M.S. Wolever, A. Jenkins, et al. Specific types of colonic fermentation may raise low-density-lipoprotein-cholesterol concentrations. *Am. J. Clin. Nutr.* 54:141–147 (1991).

146.   Stenson, W.F., D. Cort, J. Rodgers, et al. Dietary supplementation with fish oil in ulcerative colitis. *Ann. Intern. Med.* 116:609–614 (1992).

147.   Hillier, K., R. Jewell, L. Dorrell, and C.L. Smith. Incorporation of fatty acids from fish oil and olive oil into colonic mucosal lipids and effects upon eicosanoid synthesis in inflammatory bowel disease. *Gut* 32:1151–1155 (1991).

148.   Fincham, J.E., J.V. Seier, and C.J. Lombard. Torsion of the colon in vervet monkeys: association with an atherogenic Western-type of diet. *J. Med. Primatol.* 21:44–46 (1992).

149.   Schwille, P.O., and U. Herrmann. Environmental factors in the pathophysiology of recurrent idiopathic calcium urolithiasis (RCU), with emphasis on nutrition. *Urol. Res.* 20:72–83 (1992).

150.   Hughes, J., and R.W. Norman. Diet and calcium stones. *Can. Med. Assoc. J.* 146:137–143 (1992).

151.   Fromberg, M. Diet and calcium stones. (Letter.) *Can. Med. Assoc. J.* 146:1894 (1992).

152.   Buck, A.C., R.Ll. Davies, and T. Harrison. The protective role of eicosapentaenoic acid (EPA) in the pathogenesis of nephrolithiasis. *J. Urol.* 146:188–194 (1991).

153.   Jahnen, A., H. Heynck, B. Gertz, et al. Dietary fibre: the effectiveness of a high bran intake in reducing renal calcium excretion. *Urol. Res.* 20:3–6 (1992).

154.   Sichieri, R., J.E. Everhart, and H. Roth. A prospective study of hospitalization with gallstone disease among women: role of dietary factors, fasting period, and dieting. *Am. J. Public Health* 81:880–884 (1991).

155.   Scobey, M.W., M.S. Wolfe, and L.L. Rudel. Age- and dietary fat-related effects on biliary lipids and cholesterol gallstone formation in African green monkeys. *J. Nutr.* 122:917–923 (1992).

156.   Scobey, M.W., F.L. Johnson, J.S. Parks, and L.L. Rudel. Dietary fish oil effects on biliary lipid secretion and cholesterol gallstone formation in the African green monkey. *Hepatology* 14:679–684 (1991).

157.   Wennerholm, K., C.-G. Emilson, and D. Birkhed. Sweeteners and dental health. In *Handbook of Sweeteners.* S. Marie and J.R. Piggott (eds.). Glasgow, Blackie and Son Ltd. Pp. 205–224 (1991).

158.   Sealy, J.C., M.K. Patrick, A.G. Morris, and D. Alder. Diet and dental caries among later Stone Age inhabitants of the Cape Province, South Africa. *Am. J. Phys. Anthropol.* 88:123–134 (1992).

159.   Järvinen, V.K., L.L. Rytömaa, and O.P. Heinonen. Risk factors in dental erosion. *J. Dent. Res.* 70:942–947 (1991).

160.   Otake, S., M. Makimura, T. Kuroki, et al. Anticaries effects of polyphenolic compounds from Japanese green tea. *Caries Res.* 25:438–443 (1991).

161.   Sakanaka, S., N. Shimura, M. Aizawa, et al. Preventive effect of green tea polyphenols against dental caries in conventional rats. *Biosci. Biotech. Biochem.* 56:592–594 (1992).

162.   Burckhardt, P., and R.P. Heaney (eds). *Nutritional Aspects of Osteoporosis.* New York, Raven Press. *Serono Symp. Publ.* 85 (1991).

163.   Anderson, J.J.B., and R.C. Henderson. Dietary factors in the development of peak bone mass. In Burckhardt, P., and R.P. Heaney (eds). *Nutritional Aspects of Osteoporosis.* New York, Raven Press. *Serono Symp. Publ.* 85:3–20 (1991).

164.   Cumming, R.G. Epidemiology of calcium intake and bone health. In Burckhardt, P., and R.P. Heaney (eds). *Nutritional Aspects of Osteoporosis.* New York, Raven Press. *Serono Symp. Publ.* 85:159–173 (1991).

165.   Abraham, R., J. Pearson, and J. Reeve. Calcium intake: important in early menopause? In Burckhardt, P., and R.P. Heaney (eds). *Nutritional Aspects of Osteoporosis.* New York, Raven Press. *Serono Symp. Publ.* 85:191–203 (1991).

166.   Gass, R., and F. Gutzwiller. Nutritional risk factors for osteoporosis; a population based study of perimenopausal women in Switzerland. In Burckhardt, P., and R.P. Heaney (eds). *Nutritional Aspects of Osteoporosis.* New York, Raven Press. *Serono Symp. Publ.* 85:181–190 (1991).

167.   van Beresteijn, E.C.H., P.R. Dekker, H.J. van der Heiden-Winkeldermaat, et al. The habitual calcium intake from milk products and its significance for bone health; a 10-year longitudinal study. In Burckhardt, P., and R.P. Heaney (eds). *Nutritional Aspects of Osteoporosis.* New York, Raven Press. *Serono Symp. Publ.* 85:205–212 (1991).

168.   Charles, P., E.F. Eriksen, C. Hasling, et al. Nutrition and the obligatory calcium losses. In Burckhardt, P., and R.P. Heaney (eds). *Nutritional Aspects of Osteoporosis.* New York, Raven Press. *Serono Symp. Publ.* 85:263–277 (1991).

169. Dawson-Hughes, B. Effects of calcium intake on calcium retention and bone density in postmenopausal women. In Burckhardt, P., and R.P. Heaney (eds). *Nutritional Aspects of Osteoporosis.* New York, Raven Press. *Serono Symp. Publ.* 85:331–345 (1991).

170. Eaton, S.B., and D.A. Nelson. Calcium in evolutionary perspective. *Am. J. Clin. Nutr.* 54:281S–287S (1991).

171. Weaver, C.M. Calcium bioavailability and its relation to osteoporosis. *Proc. Soc. Exp. Biol. Med.* 200:157–160 (1992).

172. Charles, P. Calcium absorption and calcium bioavailability. *J. Intern. Med.* 231:161–168 (1992).

173. Matkovic, V. Osteoporosis as a pediatric disease: role of calcium and heredity. *J. Rheumatol.* 19(Suppl. 33):54–59 (1992).

174. Chen, G.M. Dietary calcium and bone mineral status of children and adolescents. *Am. J. Dis. Child.* 145:631–634 (1991).

175. Sentipal, J.M., G.M. Wardlaw, J. Mahan, and V. Matkovic. Influence of calcium intake and growth indexes on vertebral bone mineral density in young females. *Am. J. Clin. Nutr.* 54:425–428 (1991).

176. Fujita, T., and M. Fukase. Comparison of osteoporosis and calcium intake between Japan and the United States. *Proc. Soc. Exp. Biol. Med.* 200:149–152 (1992).

177. Heaney, R.P. Calcium in the prevention and treatment of osteoporosis. *J. Intern. Med.* 231:169–180 (1992).

178. Heaney, R.P. Hip fracture: a nutritional perspective. *Proc. Soc. Exp. Biol. Med.* 200:153–156 (1992).

179. Heaney, R.P. Effect of calcium on skeletal development, bone loss, and risk of fractures. *Am. J. Med.* 91(Suppl. 5B):23S–28S (1991).

180. Heaney, R.P. Lifelong calcium intake and prevention of bone fragility in the aged. *Calcif. Tissue Int.* 49(Suppl.):S42–S45 (1991).

181. Kanis, J.A. Calcium requirements for optimal skeletal health in women. *Calcif. Tissue Int.* 49(Suppl.):S33–S41 (1991).

182. Andon, M.B., K.T. Smith, M. Bracker, et al. Spinal bone density and calcium intake in healthy postmenopausal women. *Am. J. Clin. Nutr.* 54:927–929 (1991).

183. Hasling, C., K. Søndergaard, P. Charles, and L. Mosekilde. Calcium metabolism in postmenopausal osteoporotic women is determined by dietary calcium and coffee intake. *J. Nutr.* 122:1119–1126 (1992).

184. Anonymous. Calcium supplementation and bone loss in postmenopausal women. *Nutr. Rev.* 49:184–187 (1991).

185. Dawson-Hughes, B. Calcium supplementation and bone loss: a review of controlled clinical trials. *Am. J. Clin. Nutr.* 54:274S–280S (1991).

186. Elders, P.J., J.C. Netelenbos, P. Lips, et al. Calcium supplementation reduces vertebral bone loss in perimenopausal women: a controlled trial in 248 women between 46 and 55 years of age. *J. Clin. Endocrinol. Metab.* 73:533–540 (1991).

187. Prince, R.L., M. Smith, I.M. Dick, et al. Prevention of postmenopausal osteoporosis. *New Engl. J. Med.* 325:1189–1195 (1991).

188. Toss, G. Effect of calcium intake vs. other lifestyle factors on bone mass. *J. Intern. Med.* 231:181–186 (1992).

189. Abelow, B.J., T.R. Holford, and K.L. Insogna. Cross-cultural association between dietary animal protein and hip fracture: a hypothesis. *Calcif. Tissue Int.* 50:14–18 (1992).

190. Lloyd, T., J.M. Schaeffer, M.A. Walker, and L.M. Demers. Urinary hormonal concentrations and spinal bone densities of premenopausal vegetarian and nonvegetarian women. *Am. J. Clin. Nutr.* 54:1005–1010 (1991).

191. Hirota, T., M. Nara, M. Ohguri, et al. Effect of diet and lifestyle on bone mass in Asian young women. *Am. J. Clin. Nutr.* 55:1168–1173 (1992).

192. Salem, G.J., R.F. Zernicke, and R.J. Barnard. Diet-related changes in mechanical properties of rat vertebrae. *Am. J. Physiol.* 262:R318–R321 (1992).

193. Connor, W.E. *N*-3 fatty acids: effects on the plasma lipids and lipoproteins and on neural development. *Atheroscler. Rev.* 23:191–220 (1991).

194. Connor, W.E., M. Neuringer, and S. Reisbick. Essential fatty acids: the importance of *n*–3 fatty acids in the retina and brain. *Nutr. Rev.* 50:21–29 (1992).

195. Wainwright, P.E. α-Linolenic acid, long-chain *n*–3 fatty acids, and neonatal brain development. *Nutrition* 7:443–446 (1991).

196. Bjerve, K.S., L. Thoresen, K. Bønaa, et al. Clinical studies with α-linolenic acid and long-chain *n*–3 fatty acids. *Nutrition* 8:130–132 (1992).

197. Dyer, J.R., and C.E. Greenwood. Neural 22-carbon fatty acids in the weanling rat respond rapidly and specifically to a range of dietary linoleic to α-linolenic fatty acid ratios. *J. Neurochem.* 56:1921–1931 (1991).

198. Alsted, A.-L., and C.-E. Høy. Fatty acid profiles of brain phospholipid subclasses of rats fed *n*–3 polyunsaturated fatty acids of marine or vegetable origin. A two generation study. *Biochim. Biophys. Acta* 1125:237–244 (1992).

199. Arbuckle, L.D., F.M. Rioux, M.J. MacKinnon, and S.M. Innis. Formula α-linolenic (18:3(*n*–3)) and linoleic (18:2(*n*–6)) acid influence neonatal piglet liver and brain saturated fatty acids, as well as docosahexaenoic acid (22:6(*n*–3)). *Biochim. Biophys. Acta* 1125:262–267 (1992).

200. Arbuckle, L.D., and S.M. Innis. Docosahexaenoic acid in developing brain and retina of piglets fed high or low α-linolenate formula with and without fish oil. *Lipids* 27:89–93 (1992).

201. Corbett, R., F. Berthou, B.E. Leonard, and J.-F. Ménez. The effects of chronic administration of ethanol on synaptosomal fatty acid composition: modulation by oil enriched with gamma-linolenic acid. *Alcohol Alcoholism* 27:11–14 (1992).

202. Duffy, O., J.-F. Ménez, and B.E. Leonard. Effects of an oil enriched in gamma linolenic acid on locomotor activity and behaviour in the Morris Maze, following in utero ethanol exposure in rats. *Drug Alcohol Dependence* 30:65–70 (1992).

203. Terao, J., A. Nagao, H. Suzuki, and M. Yamazaki. Effect of dietary fats (perilla oil, lard, rapeseed oil) on peroxidizability of mouse brain lipids. *J. Agric. Food Chem.* 39:1477–1481 (1991).

204. DeWille, J.W., and S.J. Farmer. Postnatal dietary fat influences mRNAs involved in myelination. *Dev. Neurosci.* 14:61–68 (1992).

205. Young, S.N. Some effects of dietary components (amino acids, carbohydrate, folic acid) on brain serotonin synthesis, mood, and behavior. *Can. J. Physiol. Pharmacol.* 69:893–903 (1991).

206. Arevalo, R., D. Afonso, R. Castro, and M. Rodriguez. Fetal brain serotonin synthesis and catabolism is under control by mother intake of tryptophan. *Life Sci.* 49:53–66 (1991).

207. Muldoon, M.F., J.R. Kaplan, S.B. Manuck, and J.J. Mann. Effects of a low-fat diet on brain serotonergic responsivity in cynomolgus monkeys. *Biol. Psychiatry* 31:739–742 (1992).

208. Benton, D., and R. Cook. The impact of selenium supplementation on mood. *Biol. Psychiatry* 29:1092–1098 (1991).

209. Hamdi, A., E.S. Onaivi, and C. Prasad. A low protein–high carbohydrate diet decreases D2 dopamine receptor density in rat brain. *Life Sci.* 50:1529–1534 (1992).

210. Brock, J.W., and C. Prasad. Motor, but not sensory, cortical potentials are amplified by high-protein diet. *Physiol. Behav.* 50:887–893 (1991).

211. Lorenzetti, B.B., G.E.P. Souza, S.J. Sarti, et al. Myrcene mimics the peripheral analgesic activity of lemongrass tea. *J. Ethnopharmacol.* 34:43–48 (1991).

212. Mennella, J.A., and G.K. Beauchamp. Maternal diet alters the sensory qualities of human milk and the nursling's behavior. *Pediatrics* 88:737–744 (1991).

213. Wender, E.H., and M.V. Solanto. Effects of sugar on aggressive and inattentive behavior in children with attention deficit disorder with hyperactivity and normal children. *Pediatrics* 88:960–966 (1991).

214. Kaplan, J.R., S.B. Manuck, and C. Shively. The effects of fat and cholesterol on social behavior in monkeys. *Psychosom. Med.* 53:634–642 (1991).

215. Horrobin, D.F. The relationship between schizophrenia and essential fatty acid and eicosanoid metabolism. *Prostaglandins Leukotrienes Essential Fatty Acids* 46:71–77 (1992).

216. Vaddadi, K.S. Use of gamma-linolenic acid in the treatment of schizophrenia and tardive dyskinesia. *Prostaglandins Leukotrienes Essential Fatty Acids* 46:67–70 (1992).

217. Vieregge, P., C. v. Maravic, and H.-J. Friedrich. Life-style and dietary factors early and late in Parkinson's disease. *Can. J. Neurol. Sci.* 19:170–173 (1992).

218. Coughlin, S.S., J.H. Pincus, and P. Karstaedt. An international comparison of dietary protein consumption and mortality from Parkinson's disease. *J. Neurol.* 239:236–237 (1992).

219. Lauer, K. The food pattern in geographical relation to the risk of multiple sclerosis in the Mediterranean and Near east region. (Letter.) *J. Epidemiol. Commun. Health* 45:251–252 (1991).

220. van Meer, F. Poliomyelitis: the role of diet in the development of the disease. *Med. Hypoth.* 37:171–178 (1992).

221. Müller-Breitenkamp, U., and O. Hockwin. Risk factors in cataract development: a review. In *Distribution of Cataracts in the Population and Influencing Factors*. K. Sasaki and O. Hockwin (eds.). *Dev. Ophthalmol.* 21:60–65 (1991).

222. Lerman, S. Evaluation of risk factors in human cataractogenesis. In *Distribution of Cataracts in the Population and Influencing Factors*. K. Sasaki and O. Hockwin (eds.). *Dev. Ophthalmol.* 21:120–128 (1991).

223. Taylor, A., J. Jahngen-Hodge, L.L. Huang, and P. Jacques. Aging in the eye lens: roles for proteolysis and nutrition in formation of cataract. *Age* 14:65–71 (1991).

224. Ferrer, J.V., J. Sastre, F.V. Pallardó, et al. Senile cataract: a review on free radical related pathogenesis and antioxidant prevention. *Arch. Gerontol. Geriatr.* 13:51–59 (1991).

225. Devamanoharan, P.S., M. Henein, S. Morris, et al. Prevention of selenite cataract by vitamin C. *Exp. Eye Res.* 52:563–568 (1991).

226. Mares-Perlman, J.A., B.E.K. Klein, R. Klein, et al. Relation between cataract and nutrient intake from diet and supplements. (Abstract.) *Am. J. Epidemiol.* 134:758 (1991).

227. Yang, C.S., J.F. Brady, and J.-Y. Hong. Dietary effects on cytochromes P450, xenobiotic metabolism, and toxicity. *FASEB J.* 6:737–744 (1992).

228. Anderson, K.E., and A. Kappas. Dietary regulation of cytochrome P450. *Annu. Rev. Nutr.* 11:141–167 (1991).

229. Yoo, J.-S. H., S.M. Ning, C.B. Pantuck, et al. Regulation of hepatic microsomal cytochrome P450IIE1 level by dietary lipids and carbohydrates in rats. *J. Nutr.* 121:959–965 (1991).

230. Dalvi, R.R. Alterations in hepatic phase I and phase II biotransformation enzymes by garlic oil in rats. *Toxicol. Lett.* 60:299–305 (1992).

231. Wortelboer, H.M., C.A. de Kruif, A.A.J. van Iersel, et al. Effects of cooked brussels sprouts on cytochrome P-450 profile and phase II enzymes in liver and small intestinal mucosa of the rat. *Food Chem. Toxicol.* 30:17–27 (1992).

232. Siess, M.-H., A.M. Le Bon, and M. Suschetet. Dietary modification of drug-metabolizing enzyme activities: dose–response effect of flavonoids. *J. Toxicol. Environ. Health* 35:141–152 (1992).

233. Horiguchi, M., M. Iwama, N. Takahashi, et al. Long-term exposure of Wistar rats to high dietary sodium chloride level. II. Changes in hepatic drug-metabolizing and glutathione-related enzyme systems. *Int. J. Vit. Nutr. Res.* 62:54–59 (1992).

234. Pantuck, E.J., C.B. Pantuck, A. Kappas, et al. Effects of protein and carbohydrate content of diet on drug conjugation. *Clin. Pharmacol. Ther.* 50:254–258 (1991).

235. Hornstra, G., M.D.M. Al, J.M. Gerrard, and M.M.G. Simonis. Essential fatty acid status of neonates born to Inuit mothers: comparison with Caucasian neonates and effect of diet. *Prostaglandins Leukotrienes Essential Fatty Acids* 45:125–130 (1992).

236. Ogunleye, A., A.T. Fakoya, S. Niizeki, et al. Fatty acid composition of breast milk from Nigerian and Japanese women. *J. Nutr. Sci. Vitaminol.* 37:435–442 (1991).

237. Cant, A., J. Shay, and D.F. Horrobin. The effect of maternal supplementation with linoleic and γ-linolenic acids on the fat composition and content of human milk: a placebo-controlled trial. *J. Nutr. Sci. Vitaminol.* 37:573–579 (1991).

238. Pettersen, J., and J. Opstvedt. *Trans* fatty acids. 4. Effects on fatty acid composition of colostrum and milk. *Lipids* 26:711–717 (1991).

239. Hausman, D.B., H.M. McCloskey, and R.J. Martin. Maternal dietary fat type influences the growth and fatty acid composition of newborn and weanling rats. *J. Nutr.* 121:1917–1923 (1991).

240. Huang, Y.-S., P.E. Wainwright, P.R. Redden, et al. Effect of maternal dietary fats with variable *n–3/n–6* ratios on tissue fatty acid composition in suckling mice. *Lipids* 27:104–110 (1992).

241. Wainwright, P.E., Y.S. Huang, B. Bulman-Fleming, et al. The effects of dietary *n–3/n–6* ratio on brain development in the mouse: a dose response study with long-chain *n–3* fatty acids. *Lipids* 27:98–103 (1992).

242. Innis, S.M. Essential fatty acids in growth and development. *Prog. Lipid Res.* 30:39–103 (1991).

243. Innis, S.M. (ed.). *Lipids in Infant Nutrition*. Proceedings of a symposium, 29–30 August 1991. *J. Pediatr.* 120(4 Part 2, Suppl.) (1992).

244. Arbuckle, L.D., F.M. Rioux, M.J. MacKinnon, et al. Response of (*n*–3) and (*n*–6) fatty acids in piglet brain, liver and plasma to increasing, but low, fish oil

supplementation of formula. *J. Nutr.* 121:1536–1547 (1991).

245. Nestel, P.J. Dietary fat for the elderly: what are the issues? In *Nutrition of the Elderly.* H. Munro and G. Schlierf (eds.). New York, Vevey/Raven Press, Ltd. *Nestlé Nutrition Workshop Series* 29:119–127 (1992).

246. Biagi, P.L., A. Bordoni, S. Hrelia, et al. γ-Linolenic acid dietary supplementation can reverse the aging influence on rat liver microsome Δ^6-desaturase activity. *Biochim. Biophys. Acta* 1083:187–192 (1991).

247. Riley-Roberts, M.-L., R.J. Turner, P.M. Evans, and B.J. Merry. Lymphoproliferative responses in diet-restricted and aging Sprague-Dawley rats. *Exp. Gerontol.* 27:201–209 (1992).

248. Effros, R.B., R.L. Walford, R. Weindruch, and C. Mitcheltree. Influences of dietary restriction on immunity to influenza in aged mice. *J. Gerontol.:Biol. Sci.* 46:B142–B147 (1991).

249. Srivastava, V.K., R.D. Tilley, R.W. Hart, and D.L. Busbee. Effect of dietary restriction on the fidelity of DNA polymerases in aging mice. *Exp. Gerontol.* 26:453–466 (1991).

250. Srivastava, V.K., and D.L. Busbee. Decreased fidelity of DNA polymerases and decreased DNA excision repair in aging mice: effects of caloric restriction. *Biochem. Biophys. Res. Commun.* 182:712–721 (1992).

251. Bronson, R.T., and R.D. Lipman. Reduction in rate of occurrence of age related lesions in dietary restricted laboratory mice. *Growth Dev. Aging* 55:169–184 (1991).

252. Pieri, C., M. Falasca, F. Moroni, et al. Diet restriction, body temperature and physicochemical properties of cell membranes. *Arch. Gerontol. Geriatr.* 12:179–185 (1991).

253. Castiglioni, A.J., Jr., M.E. Legare, D.L. Busbee, and E. Tiffany-Castiglioni. Morphological changes in astrocytes of aging mice fed normal or caloric restricted diets. *Age* 14:102–106 (1991).

254. Pieri, C., F. Marcheselli, M. Falasca, et al. Food restriction in female Wistar rats, IV. Morphometric parameters of cerebellar synapses. *Arch. Gerontol. Geriatr.* 13:161–166 (1991).

255. Meydani, S.N. Dietary modulation of the immune response in the aged. *Age* 14:108–115 (1991).

256. Blizard, A. Genetic models in brain and behavior research, part IV. Nature/nurture and the nature of nurture in the etiology of hypertension. *Experientia* 48:311–314 (1992).

257. Holmes-Siedle, M., R.H. Lindenbaum, and A. Galliard. Recurrence of neural tube defect in a group of at risk women: a 10 year study of Pregnavite Forte F. *J. Med. Genet.* 29:134–135 (1992).

258. Centers for Disease Control. Recommendations for the use of folic acid to reduce the number of cases of spina bifida and other neural tube defects. *Morbid. Mortal. Weekly Rep.* 41(RR-14):1–7 (1992).

259. Medovar, B.Ja., K.J. Petzke, T.G. Semesko, et al. Zur Wirkung unterschiedlicher Proteindiäten auf Lebensdauer und ausgewählte biochemische Parameter von alten Ratten. *Nahrung* 35:961–967 (1991).

260. Harper, V., R. MacInnes, D. Campbell, and M. Hall. Increased birth weight in northerly islands: is fish consumption a red herring? *Br. Med. J.* 303:166 (1991).

261. Feskens, E.J.M., C.H. Bowles, and D. Kromhout. Inverse association between fish intake and risk of glucose intolerance in normoglycemic elderly men and women. *Diabetes Care* 14:935–941 (1991).

262. Fujita, T. Calcium, parathyroids and aging. In *Calcium-Regulating Hormones. I. Role in Disease and Aging.* H. Morii (ed.). Basel, Karger. *Contrib. Nephrol.* 90:206–211 (1991).

263. Kantola, M., and T. Vartiainen. Selenium content of breast milk in Finland after fertilization of soil with selenium. *J. Trace Elem. Electrolytes Health Dis.* 5:283–284 (1991).

264. McGlashan, N.D. Low selenium status and cot deaths. *Med. Hypoth.* 35:311–314 (1991).

265. FitzHerbert, J.C. SIDS and selenium. (Letter.) *Med. J. Aust.* 156:220 (1992).

266. Jeffery, H. SIDS and selenium. (Comment.) *Med. J. Aust.* 156:220–221 (1991).

5

Measurement and Bioavailability of Food Components

Analysis of food components
Sources of constituents
Bioavailability of food components
Modifying the composition of foods

ANALYSIS OF FOOD COMPONENTS

Antioxidants

Kochhar and Rossell summarized the types and uses of antioxidants in food systems and then discussed a broad range of methods for their detection, measurement, and evaluation (*1*; 352 references cited). Austrian workers discussed and compared HPLC and capillary gas chromatography (GC) methods for quantitative analysis of tocopherols in plant oils (*2*). For GC it was first necessary to saponify the oil sample. Tocopherols were then extracted quantitatively with cyclohexane. Results by HPLC and GC were highly correlated ($r = .9994$). Measurements for 95% of the samples assayed by the two methods agreed within ±16.7 µg/g. Other investigators described a reversed-phase HPLC method for simultaneous measurement of retinol, tocopherols, α- and β-carotene, lycopene, and β-cryptoxanthin in human plasma (*3*). The determination involves sequential use of two detectors with programmable wavelength, a spectrophotometer to detect carotenoids in the visible spectrum, and a fluorometer to measure retinol and the tocopherols.

Dietary fiber

A collaborative study to validate a method for determining the soluble and insoluble dietary fiber components of foods was reported (*4*). The method is a modification of that adopted as final action by the AOAC for determining total dietary fiber. Twenty-two foods and food products were tested by providing each of 39 collaborators with 7 test samples and a standard in a staggered design for duplicate blind analysis. The relative standard deviations overall and for specific test samples were presented and the high variability associated with some samples was discussed. The method for insoluble dietary fiber was adopted first action by AOAC International but the method for soluble dietary fiber requires further study.

A nonenzymatic gravimetric method was described for determining total dietary fiber in fruits and vegetables that contain little starch and are frequently eaten raw (*5*). The authors demonstrated that in foods such as these a hydrolysis step is unnecessary: extraction with hexane and dilute alcohol yielded residues of comparable weight to those obtained after enzyme treatment. For the 10 fruits and vegetables tested, results agreed well with those from the American Association of Cereal Chemists (AACC) and the AOAC procedures for total dietary fiber.

A collaborative AOAC–AACC study of methods for determining soluble, insoluble, and total dietary fiber was conducted in 11 laboratories to evaluate a modified enzymatic–gravimetric procedure (*6*). The modification involved minor modification of older AOAC methods, to reduce analysis time and improve precision. Phosphate buffer was replaced by MES-TRIS, one pH adjustment step was eliminated, and reaction and filtration volumes were reduced. Twenty samples of cereal and grain products, fruits, and vegetables were sent to the participating laboratories for duplicate blind analysis. The total dietary fiber values calculated by summing values for soluble and insoluble dietary fiber agreed closely. Mean values determined by the modified and unmodified methods were in extremely close agreement but the modification substantially improved precision. The modification has been adopted first action by AOAC International.

Gravimetric and chemical methods for determining dietary fiber in cereal products were reviewed (*7*). Published values for soluble, insoluble, and total fiber content of oat groats, bran, and hulls were presented and discussed. When specific information about chemical components is not required, the quicker gravimetric methods yield acceptable results.

Fatty acids

The fatty acid composition of fish-oil capsules from various sources world-wide was determined by GC (*8*). Ratios of eicosapentaenoic acid (EPA) to docosahexaenoic acid (DHA) were determined and several samples of fish were also analyzed. Twenty-three samples represented fish oils or fish-oil concentrates; 3 were ethyl esters of fish oil fatty acids.

Most fish-oil capsules contained ~30% *n*–3 fatty acids with an EPA/DHA ratio of ~3:2. Capsules containing fatty acid ethyl esters had ~50% *n*–3 fatty acids, with an EPA/DHA ratio of ~3:2. No admixture with other edible oils was detected.

Thiosulfinates

Reversed-phase HPLC was used to separate and quantitate all alkyl and alkenyl thiosulfinates, including configurational isomers, in homogenates of garlic cloves (*9*). The variability of bulbs from different domestic and foreign sources and the variability between bulbs or cloves from the same source was documented, and changes during storage were demonstrated. The authors proposed a method for standardizing the determination of allicin from garlic, discussing it in terms of other published procedures. The same research group reported the quantitation of sulfides and dialk(en)yl thiosulfinates in commercial garlic products by HPLC (*10*). Thiosulfinates were released only from garlic cloves and garlic powders, whereas vinyldithiins and ajoenes were found only in products containing garlic macerated in vegetable oil, and the diallyl, methyl allyl, and dimethyl sulfide series occurred only in products containing the oil of steam-distilled garlic. The total content of sulfur compounds depended on the type of product. Garlic powders in particular were extremely variable, but the general variability (up to 33-fold for steam-distilled garlic oils) shows the importance of analysis before garlic products are used in situations where their content of sulfur compounds is important.

SOURCES OF CONSTITUENTS

Lipids

TRANS FATTY ACIDS. A reassessment of the availability of *trans* fatty acids in the U.S. diet compared published estimates for 1984 with new estimates for 1989 (*11*). Availability from total food service fats and oils was unchanged. The 1989 value for industrial fats and oils was somewhat higher, partly because more complete data were available. In contrast, the per capita availability of *trans* fatty acids from household salad and cooking oils, household shortenings, and all margarines and spreads decreased between 1984 and 1989. The reassessed value for total *trans* fatty acids was 8.1 g/day per person, similar to the 1984 estimate of 7.6 g/day per person. The total may increase because of the recent switch by many establishments from tallow to partially hydrogenated vegetable oils for use in frying. Estimates were based on several sources of data on market size and share of various major and minor products and product brands and on *trans* fatty acid data provided by industry. Estimates for food service fats and oils were adjusted for wastage.

The fatty acid compositions of rapeseed and soybean oils marketed in France were determined by gas liquid chromatography (*12*). Total *trans*-18:3 fatty acids accounted for up to 3% of total fatty acids in the samples tested. This represents a 30% isomerization rate. The two main geometrical isomers of linolenic acid always had the *cis,cis,trans* (~48%) and *trans,cis,cis* (~41%) configurations, regardless of the degree of isomerization. About 6.5% of the *cis,trans,cis* isomer was found. The only di-*trans* isomer abundant enough to be quantitated was the *trans,cis,trans* (~5%). Mono-*trans* isomers of linoleic acid were also present, but at levels 13–14 times lower than linolenic acid isomers.

Geometrical and positional isomers of linoleic acid in a partially hydrogenated Canadian canola oil–based margarine were separated by gas liquid chromatography (*13*). *cis*-9,*trans*-13-Octadecadienoic acid was identified as the major isomer by partial hydrazine reduction and mass spectral studies. Other quantitatively important isomers were *cis*-9,*trans*-12; *trans*-9,*cis*-12; and *cis*-9,*cis*-15. These were also the major isomers found in other hard and soft vegetable-oil margarines in the Canadian retail market. A variety of minor isomers were identified as well. Amounts of the *trans*-9,*trans*-12 isomer were generally 0.5% of the total fatty acids. This research group has also reported a more complete fatty acid analysis of 50 brands of margarine sold in Canada (*14*). Total *trans* fatty acids in hard margarines ranged from 26 to 50%, and in soft margarines, from 0 to 38%. A high concentration of *trans* fatty acids was found in margarines based on canola or soybean oil.

FISH-OIL LIPIDS. Several factors affect the fat, cholesterol, and *n*–3 fatty acid content of "sardines" harvested off the coast of Maine (*15*). Fat content ranged from 5% in juvenile Atlantic herring (*Clupea harengus harengus*) sampled in June and October to 11% in maturing herring sampled before the spawning season in July. Canning liquids—vegetable oil, fish oil, or cookout liquid—influenced the fat content of the finished product. Comparing across four catch dates, fluctuations in fat content were greater than ±20% from the mean for similarly processed samples. Cookout liquid appeared to be the best canning solution, as it enhanced the amounts of EPA and DHA in the product while contributing minimally to the cholesterol content. The authors concluded that because of the large differences within even a single catch of sardines, compliance with labeling requirements would be difficult unless extensive sampling for nutritional analysis was conducted. Wide variation was also found in the cholesterol content of South African fish oils (*16*). In 118 samples it ranged from 0.37 to 1.96%. The cholesterol levels of anchovy oils peaked during winter (July and August) and fell by roughly two-thirds to their lowest values in March and April. The cholesterol content was inversely related to the oil yield of the fish. Cholesterol was confirmed as the major sterol in anchovy (*Engraulis capensis*) and red-eye (*Etrumeus whiteheadii*) oils.

The highly unsaturated *n*–3 fatty acids in muscle of wild and farmed eels (*Anguilla anguilla*) from northern Italy were measured (*17*). Farmed eels were richer in DHA and EPA than wild animals, and addition of cod liver oil to their diet augmented accumulation of these fatty acids without affecting the total lipid content. The authors proposed two indexes of the nutritional quality of fish for populations at high risk of chronic degenerative disease: fish lipid quality, calculated as (EPA + DHA)/total lipids, and atherogenic index, calculated as the fatty acid ratio (14:0 + 16:0)/(20:5*n*–3 + 22:6*n*–3).

High concentrations of *n*–3 fatty acids are synthesized by most groups of algae and provide the dietary source of these substances for fish. It is growth rate that determines an alga's economic potential for biomass or fatty acid production. Growth and EPA production were evaluated in 26 cultures from collections in the USA, U.K., and Canada and 10 strains isolated from fresh-water reservoirs in Thailand (*18*). The most EPA was produced by strains of *Chlorella minutissima* and *Phaeodactylum tricornutum*; the latter also produced very high biomass in culture, making its total yield of EPA greater than that of any other strain. The best EPA producers had low contents of DHA and arachidonic acid, which simplifies EPA recovery. No isolate from Thailand produced EPA or DHA. Palmitic, oleic, linoleic, and linolenic acid were the major fatty acids in Thai strains.

OTHER. Eighteen native Australian plants were evaluated as potential oilseed crops: two species of *Lasiopetalum*, two of *Thomasia*, and *Rulingia platycalyx*, all of the family Sterculiaceae; *Mukia maderaspatama*, a member of the Cucurbitaceae; and 12 species of *Dodonaea*, from the Sapindaceae (*19*). The major fatty acids in all of these were linoleic (43–76%), oleic (10–23%), and palmitic (8–15%). Sterculiaceae seed oils generally contain significant amounts of cyclopropene and its dihydro derivatives, but these were not found in *Lasiopetalum* or *Thomasia*. Some cucurbit seed oils contain conjugated unsaturated fatty acids, but oil from *M. maderaspatama* did not. These variations within families highlight the need for analysis of any species considered for economic exploitation.

Chung discussed the analysis, nature, and content of cereal grain lipids (*20*). The review included tocol derivatives, carotenoids, and sterols. The lipid content of whole grains and various grain fractions was discussed.

The concentration of conjugated linoleic acid (CLA) was determined in cheese processed under various conditions (*21*). Overall, the concentration was in the range of 3.2–8.9 mg per gram of fat. Processing cheddar cheese at 80 or 90°C under atmospheric conditions increased CLA content; processing under nitrogen and 70 or 85°C had no effect. There was a dose-related increase in CLA formation as the concentration of whey protein concentrate and its low-molecular-weight fraction was increased from 0 to 6%.

Fiber and carbohydrate

Marlett reported the content and composition of dietary fiber in 117 common foods (*22*). She tested 23 fruits, 33 vegetables, 41 grain products, 7 legumes, 4 nuts, and 9 miscellaneous foods. Within each group the fiber concentration was fairly constant, although composition was heterogeneous. Values for soluble fiber were lower than generally reported because of the analytic methods used. Cellulose accounted for about half the total fiber in legumes, but for only one-third or less in the other groups. Hemicelluloses comprised about half the total fiber in grains, 25–35% in other groups. Pectin varied widely. The author suggested that these food groups can be used to rank intake of dietary fiber into low, medium, and high categories.

The carbohydrate composition of cereal grains was discussed by Becker and Hanners (*23*). They considered various fractions of wheat, corn, rice, oats, barley, sorghum, millet, rye, *Triticale* spp., wild rice, and amaranth.

Vitamins and antioxidants

A study of the vitamin C content of major food sources for this vitamin revealed extremely large sample variability (*24*). For some foods the mean value varied by a factor of 2. Even foods collected from the same market or geographic region sometimes varied considerably. The relative amounts of ascorbic acid and dehydroascorbic acid also showed a wide range of values. Although these findings complicate estimates of vitamin C intake when only a few foods provide the major source, in practice, a diverse diet should compensate for the day-to-day variability in vitamin C content of particular foods.

In contrast to the variability in vitamin C content, mean values for α- and β-carotene and vitamin A in foods are relatively stable (*25*). Evaluation of a variety of fruits and vegetables from markets in Cairo and Alexandria found no significant differences between locations or times of analysis. Vitamin A activity and other values determined

in this study agreed well with published values in the USDA *Handbook No. 8.*

The active constituents of green tea were analyzed by high-performance thin-layer chromatography (*26*). The content of polyphenols tended to increase from spring to autumn, whereas caffeine remained stable. Total polyphenols ranged from 9.36 to 12.91%, and caffeine varied between 1.82 and 2.94. Although green tea components have antitumor, antimutagenic, and antioxidant activity, the authors concluded from their analyses that Chinese people would have to at least double the amount of tea they drink in order to benefit from its therapeutic effects.

In Finland, results of supplementing all multinutrient agricultural fertilizers with selenium, beginning in 1984, are now being measured as increased selenium levels in Finnish foods (*27,28*). In all cases, selenium levels in domestic agricultural products increased (*27*). Food groups evaluated were cereals, fruits and vegetables, meat and meat products, dairy products and eggs, and ready-to-eat foods. Selenium intake of the general population now probably meets the recommendations. Only diets with a very exceptional composition provide <0.05 mg or >0.2 mg per 10 MJ. Based on these results of the fertilization program, the Finnish Ministry of Agriculture switched to a uniform level of selenium supplementation in 1990 (*28*). Previously, a higher amount of selenium had been applied to grain fields; now grain is fertilized at the same rate as other crops. Changes in the selenium content of whole milk, cheese, and eggs from 1975–1977 to 1989 were shown. Most of the increase occurred in the first two years after selenium fertilization started.

BIOAVAILABILITY OF FOOD COMPONENTS

Minerals

Turnlund reviewed methods for using stable isotopes to study the bioavailability of dietary minerals (*29*). The usual absorption of minerals ranges from <1% to >90%, depending on the mineral in question, its chemical form, and other nutritive and non-nutritive components of the diet. By using stable isotope tracers as labels, the minerals in a particular food or meal can be distinguished from minerals from other sources and their metabolic fate followed. Multiple isotopes of the same element and multiple elements can be studied simultaneously. The design and conduct of studies in human subjects was discussed and results of such studies, particularly for iron, copper, and zinc, were summarized. As Fairweather-Tait pointed out, because many trace elements are so poorly and variably absorbed by the body, knowledge of their intake is of little use in evaluating whether the supply is adequate (30). Methods of assessing bioavailability include chemical balance studies, use of radioisotopes and stable isotopes, measuring rate of repletion or plasma appearance, and in vitro techniques. Factors involved in the bioavailability of specific minerals were summarized.

Just as other nutrient and nonnutrient components of food influence mineral utilization, so do methods of food processing and preparation (31). For example, fermentation affects the bioavailability of zinc and iron in beer, wine, yogurt, and African tribal foods. Differences in the conditions of heat treatments such as time, temperature, moisture, and degree of browning may influence the availability of iron. Effects of Maillard browning were discussed in some detail; the author has not noted the adverse effects of browning on availability of zinc and iron reported by others. How mineral availability is affected by curing and cooking meat, seed germination (sprouts), processing of soy products, food packaging and storage, food additives, and milling of grain was covered briefly.

The influence of various dietary components on manganese absorption were evaluated in adult subjects who consumed test meals labeled with ^{52}Mn or ^{54}Mn (32). The meals were infant diets (human milk and a cow's-milk formula) and wheat bread. Manganese absorption was not correlated with either whole-blood manganese status or indexes of iron status. Addition of calcium to human milk significantly decreased manganese absorption. Phytate, phosphate, or ascorbic acid added to infant formula and iron added to wheat bread had no effect on manganese absorption. At least in these foods, manganese absorption in humans is not significantly affected by dietary factors considered likely to have an effect. These findings do not agree with results from some animal studies.

CALCIUM. To determine how fiber constituents other than phytate modify mineral balance, young adults ate test diets for three 22-day periods in a 3×3 crossover design (33). The diets were a normal basal diet, basal diet supplemented with 15 g of low-phytate barley fiber, and a modified high-fiber diet containing less protein; they contained similar amounts of calcium, magnesium, zinc, and iron. Apparent balances were calculated as intake minus urinary and fecal excretion except for iron, whose absorption was measured as intake minus fecal excretion. The mean balances on the three diets were 0.2, 1.9, and –0.8 mmol calcium; 0.3, –0.2, and –0.5 mmol magnesium; 3.0, –4.6, and –18.4 µmol zinc; and 16.1, 5.4, and –23.2 µmol iron absorption. These values are small compared with the mineral content of the diet, and the authors concluded that as much as 25 g/day of the fiber would have no adverse effects on mineral retention provided the diet contained adequate utilizable trace elements.

The bioavailability of calcium from a calcium supplement and calcium-fortified food products was evaluated by calcium balance studies in young adults (34). Controlled experimental diets were provided for 7-day periods in a randomized block design. The largest positive calcium balance was achieved with fortified orange juice. The difference was significant when fortified orange juice was compared with self-selected diet or fortified milk or cheese, and nonsignificant compared with calcium carbonate tablet or fortified soda. Whether the food vehicle or the form of calcium used for fortification was responsible for the differences in bioavailability was not determined. However, based on assays of alkaline phosphatase, the author believes that the form (Ca_3PO_4) explained the lower calcium balance observed when the fortified cheese product was provided.

The bioavailability of calcium and zinc in infant formulas based on protein hydrolysates was measured in infant rhesus monkeys (35). Infants were fed diets radiolabeled with ^{47}Ca and ^{65}Zn, and whole-body radioactivity was measured immediately after dosing and 7 days later. The bioavailability of calcium was greater in formulas based on casein or whey protein hydrolysates than in the two soy/collagen hydrolysate formulas. When the different calcium contents of the formulas were considered, retention from 4 of the 5 milk protein hydrolysates remained higher than from the soy/collagen products, although the differences were not great. The bioavailability of zinc was also greater in the milk products, but total zinc retention was similar with the soy/collagen products because of their higher zinc content.

Serna-Saldivar et al. confirmed earlier findings that lime treatment during preparation of tortillas increases their calcium content and that this calcium is highly bioavailable (*36*). Femurs of rats fed tortillas had better properties (e.g., greater density, mineral content, and breaking strength) than femurs of rats fed raw grains. Tortillas made from quality protein maize produced better results than tortillas made from regular corn or sorghum. Rats fed quality protein maize products had the highest levels of serum albumin, probably reflecting the higher quality of the dietary protein. Hypocalcemia was related to low serum albumin levels. Results of another feeding study in rats showed that addition of Bengal gram to wheat chapatis significantly improved calcium absorption and retention (*37*). The authors concluded that no risk of protein-induced hypercalciuria is incurred when cereals are supplemented with legumes.

Metabolic studies were conducted in men to study the effect of oat bran on calcium absorption and on calcium, phosphorus, magnesium, and zinc balance (*38*). Subjects ate controlled diets during a 40-day baseline control period and a 32-day experimental phase, in which four oat-bran muffins constituted part of the daily diet. Consumption of oat bran led to a significant increase in urinary phosphorus excretion and decreases in urinary calcium excretion. Intestinal absorption of calcium, determined with ^{47}Ca, did not change, whereas endogenous fecal calcium increased slightly but significantly. Overall, the daily intake of four oat-bran muffins, which doubled the dietary fiber intake, did not change calcium, magnesium, and zinc balances and improved nitrogen and phosphorus balances.

IRON. Comparative studies in human subjects and rats demonstrated that rodents are not a valid model for quantitative assessment of dietary factors in human iron nutrition (*39*). Using identical methodology and test meals for both species, absorption studies were conducted to measure the effects of ascorbic acid and meat (enhancers) and tea, bran, and soy protein (inhibitors) on absorption of nonheme iron. Meat and tea had a marked effect in humans but not in rats, and rats' response to ascorbic acid, soy protein, and bran was far smaller.

Preliminary assessment of new varieties of grain amaranth suggested that amaranth cereal is an ideal vehicle for fortification with NaFeEDTA, ferrous fumarate, or $FeSO_4$ (*40*). However, iron absorption from the unfortified cereal appeared to be low. These studies were performed in rats and must be confirmed in humans.

Sandberg reviewed the effects of food processing on phytate hydrolysis and the availability of iron and zinc in cereal and vegetable foods (*41*). She showed how understanding of phytate hydrolysis and the formation of promoting factors makes it possible to nutritionally optimize food processing. By manipulating parameters of soaking, malting, and fermentation and addition of phytase, phytate content can be decreased and the bioavailability of iron and zinc increased.

Considerable variation in density of bioavailable iron exists in typical Central African meals (*42*). By combining measurement of exchangeability of nonheme iron and use of the extrinsic tag method, it was possible to evaluate the absorption of nonheme iron from meals contaminated with environmental iron, as African meals frequently are. Three meals labeled with ^{59}Fe and ^{55}Fe, with cereals, roots, and plantain forming the major staple foods, were prepared under realistic conditions and fed to healthy men. Less than half of the exogenous (contaminating) iron exchanged with the organic radioiron tracer; this iron did not enter the nonheme iron pool from which iron is thought to be absorbed. Iron absorption from the meals (1.4–5.1%) was much lower than absorption from typical European meals. Greatest absorption was from the plantain-based meal. Iron deficiency in Africa was discussed.

Jackson and Lee reviewed the conflicting reports on the effect of dairy products on iron availability (43). Possible sources of disagreement are methodologic differences, test species, the chemical form of dietary iron, and overall composition of the test meal. Studies in human subjects demonstrate the superiority of human milk to cow's milk in terms of bioavailability of iron, although the basis for this has not been explained. Human milk contains less casein, phosphate, and calcium, components which may inhibit iron absorption. However, the authors see little danger that dairy products will have significant adverse effects on iron absorption against the background of a complex meal. Similar conclusions were reached in an Agricultural Research Service study (44). Milk drunk with a mixed meal neither enhanced nor suppressed iron absorption. Studies of iron absorption from human and cow's milk found that the milk's calcium content could account for at least 70% of the difference in bioavailability of iron (45). When $CaCl_2$ was added to human milk to equalize the calcium content of the milks, iron absorption was roughly halved in healthy young adults. No evidence for an enhancer of iron absorption was found in human milk. Implications of these results for the mineral composition of infant formulas were discussed.

The effect of manganese and zinc on iron absorption was studied in adult volunteers (46). Because of the large individual variability in iron absorption, the experiments were designed so that subjects served as their own controls. $FeSO_4$ was radiolabeled with ^{55}Fe or ^{59}Fe, according to whether it was administered alone or in conjunction with manganese or zinc. The minerals were provided either in a solution or in a hamburger meal. Blood was drawn 2 weeks after the last dose to determine the $^{55}Fe/^{59}Fe$ ratio. Total retention of ^{59}Fe was measured by whole-body counting; retention of ^{55}Fe was calculated from the isotopic ratio. Addition of 7.5 or 15 mg of manganese to 3 mg of iron in solution reduced iron absorption by 21 and 34%, respectively; 15 mg of manganese given in the

hamburger meal reduced iron absorption by 40%. Fractional iron absorption was strongly dose-dependent, indicating direct competitive inhibition by manganese. Addition of 15 or 45 mg of zinc also interfered significantly with absorption of 3 mg of iron when given as a water solution, but not when given in the hamburger meal. The authors postulated that when dietary ligands are present there is no interaction between iron and zinc. They emphasized that these results apply only to nonheme dietary iron, but can be considered representative for interactions between nonheme iron and the major portion of dietary zinc and manganese.

Other

The effects of postharvest storage, processing, and chemical interactions on the bioavailability of ascorbic acid, thiamin, vitamin A, carotenoids, and minerals were reviewed (47). These nutrients were chosen as representative of those whose reactivity makes them vulnerable to losses. The authors discussed specific reactions of concern and ways to prevent or compensate for losses.

The plasma response to β-carotene has been reported to be smaller after ingestion of carotene-rich foods than after equivalent doses of β-carotene supplements. The hypothesis that pectin reduces the plasma β-carotene response was tested in healthy young women (48). In a crossover design, subjects were given controlled meals with and without 12 g of citrus pectin. Immediately after each meal, a capsule containing 25 mg of β-carotene was administered. Plasma samples were obtained 0, 8, 30, 48, and 192 h after the meals for quantitation of β-carotene by HPLC. At the 30-h time point, mean plasma carotene levels were significantly lower after the pectin meal than after the meal without pectin. They were also lower after 48 and 192 h, but the differences between meals were not significant due to the wide variation in individual plasma levels and responsiveness. The mean *increase* in plasma β-carotene concentrations in response to the pectin meal was less than half the increase in the absence of pectin at 30, 48, and 192 h. The clear implication of this is that data based on purified supplements may not be directly translatable into food recommendations based on β-carotene content because of effects of other dietary components.

The bioavailability of starch in several wheat-based bread products was studied in terms of the glucose and insulin responses of healthy subjects and the rate and extent of in vitro starch digestion (*49*). Evaluated were three white wheat bread products varying in crust/crumb ratio, three products with a high soluble-fiber content, and two coarse-wheat breads. Although there were no substantial differences in starch hydrolysis related to properties of the starch itself, significant differences were related to food structure in the digestion studies. Metabolic responses were greatest to the white-bread products and least to the coarse bread with intact kernels and the high-fiber bread with oat bran.

MODIFYING THE COMPOSITION OF FOODS

Meats

A volume in the *Advances in Applied Biotechnology* series was devoted to technologies and strategies for reducing the fat and cholesterol content of foods (*50*). Major sections dealt with meat production and processing, processed foods, processing and formulation of dairy products, and eggs and egg substitutes. Of particular relevance was a chapter on altering the fat composition of meat by dietary modification (*51*). Partial replacement of palmitic acid with stearic or oleic acid would be desirable because neither of the latter two substances raises serum cholesterol in humans. Feeding growing pigs a high-oleate diet sharply increases the oleate content of their muscle and adipose tissue while reducing palmitate and other saturated fatty acids. Similar achievement in modifying beef fat has been elusive because rumen microorganisms hydrogenate unsaturated fatty acids. To circumvent ruminal biohydrogenation, cattle have been fed fatty acids in various forms. Limited success has been attained by feeding high-oleate sunflower seed, which increases stearate and decreases palmitate. Differences in fat metabolism among breeds of cattle need further study.

Several studies of dietary manipulation of fatty acid composition in pigs were reported (*52–54*). Morgan et al. fed pigs four experimental diets, all based on barley, soybean meal, and fish meal (*52*). Diet 1 contained 50 g/kg of tallow. The other diets contained 50 g/kg of soybean oil, either unsupplemented (diet 2) or supplemented with 7.5 g/kg of γ-linolenic acid (diet 3) or 9.5 g/kg of the product EPAnoil (providing EPA and DHA) (diet 4). High levels of linoleic and linolenic acid were found in fat samples from pigs fed diets 2–4. This resulted in a ratio of polyunsaturated fatty acids (PUFAs) to saturated fatty acids (SFAs) of ~1.0, compared with a ratio of 0.3–0.7 for tallow-fed pigs (depending on the sampling site). γ-Linolenic acid supplementation did not consistently increase arachidonic acid production, but EPAnoil significantly increased levels of EPA and DHA in body lipids. Feeding experiments in Germany tested a range of 18:2 + 18:3 fatty acids from 10.9 to 26.3 g per kilogram of feed (*53*). Dietary fat had a highly statistically significant effect on composition of backfat. Increases in linoleic and linolenic acid were at the expense of oleic, stearic, and palmitic acid. The authors concluded that the relative polyenic acid content of pig fat can be accurately predetermined by the composition of the feed and animals can be tailored to specific market requirements. In another study, pigs were fed a control diet or a test diet containing 2, 4, or 6% fish oil for 4 weeks before slaughter (*54*). EPA and DHA began to increase in the fish-oil groups within the first week; rates of increase were greater during the first two weeks than during the final two weeks. Increases in EPA and DHA were dose-related and came primarily at the expense of oleic and linoleic acid.

Fatty acid composition of poultry meat is also influenced by diet. In a study of broiler chickens, the fatty acid composition of white and dark meat reflected the fatty acid profile of the full-fat seeds or reconstituted meal and oil in the diet (*55*). Feeding full-fat flax seeds or reconstituted flax oil and meal increased the deposition of α-linolenic acid, EPA, and 18:3*n*–3 fatty acid; the oil-plus-meal combination enhanced 18:2*n*–6 content more than the corresponding full-fat seed, and replacing oil with animal tallow in the mixtures decreased the level of 18:2n–6. Heat pretreatment of the seeds or reconstituted mixtures had no important effect on the results. Preliminary experiments in ducklings demonstrated a clear potential to manipulate and improve the fatty acid profile by diet (56). Birds given linseed oil or MaxEPA supplements from the age of 22 days until slaughter at 44 days had increased carcass levels of n–3 PUFAs.

Dairy products

Ney reviewed the basis for the dietary recommendations of the National Cholesterol Education Program, the effects of dietary milk fat on blood cholesterol level, and the rationale and feasibility of strategies for modifying the lipid composition of milk (57). Milk fat has an unusual fatty acid profile. About 10% of the fatty acids contain fewer than 12 carbon atoms, and stearic and oleic acid comprise ~35%; these fatty acids are not considered hypercholesterolemic. Supercritical fluid extraction, steam stripping, molecular conversion, and fractionation technologies are available for reducing the already relatively low cholesterol content of milk fat. Various diets for dairy cows are also being evaluated. For example, heat treatment of soybeans protects the PUFAs from complete microbial hydrogenation in the rumen. However, partial hydrogenation produces *trans* isomers and the health effects of *trans* fatty acids in milk are not known. Thus the technology to modify the composition of milk fat exists, and economic considerations will determine the methods used for various applications.

Attempts were made to increase the content of α-linolenic acid and its elongation products in milk by adding flax seed to the diet of dairy cows (58). Only 1% of dietary 18:3n–3 was transferred to milk fat. However, roughly half of the 18:3 fatty acid was transferred to the milk when linseed oil was infused directly into the abomasum. Δ6-Desaturase activity is low in the cow, and DHA was not detected in the milk. The authors concluded that bovine lipid metabolism allows high transfer rates of n–3 fatty acids from linseed oil into milk fat if ruminal biohydrogenation is prevented. Another study in dairy cows produced somewhat different results (59). It found that feeding supplemental unprotected PUFAs as sunflower or safflower seeds significantly lowered the concentrations of short- and medium-chain fatty acids and increased the concentrations of long-chain unsaturated fatty acids in milk fat and butter.

Eggs

Progress in modifying the lipid profile of egg yolk was discussed by Hargis and Van Elswyk (60). Fatty acid composition is readily modified by diet. Increasing the level of dietary unsaturated fats increases the degree of unsaturation in the egg yolk, and depending on the oil fed, increases linoleic acid at the expense of oleic acid. The level of SFAs is less manipulatable but can be increased by feeding ≥10% saturated fat. Enrichment of yolk with n–3 PUFAs can be accomplished but the acceptability, stability, and benefits of such eggs require evaluation. In contrast, the cholesterol content of egg yolk is refractory to dietary modification (61). Normal dietary manipulation of fat and fiber, drugs, and selective breeding have produced only modest reductions, and the author believes that current technology is unlikely to allow changes of practical significance. After reviewing the lack of success, he asked whether the cholesterol content of eggs *should* be changed, in view of the minor influence of dietary cholesterol on blood cholesterol levels in most normal humans.

After preliminary observations that the n–3 PUFA content of eggs from range-fed chickens in Greece was at least 8-fold higher than that of conventional eggs in U.S. supermarkets, Simopoulos and Salem investigated the effect of diet on yolk fatty acid composition (62). They were particularly interested in evaluating egg yolk as a source of PUFAs for infants. Comparison of the lipid profiles of Greek eggs, conventional U.S. eggs, and two types of n–3-enriched eggs (from hens fed fish meal or flax seed) indicated that the fatty acid composition of Greek eggs can be approximated by dietary manipulation. Furthermore, such eggs could provide much of the n–3 requirement of preterm and older infants.

Jiang and Sim fed PUFA-enriched chicken eggs to rats and examined the effects on fatty acid composition and cholesterol levels in plasma and tissue (*63*). Consumption of *n*–3-enriched yolks significantly reduced plasma and liver total cholesterol. Hepatic total lipids and phospholipids were enriched in linolenic acid, EPA, and DHA, with concomitant reduction of arachidonic acid in the phospholipid fraction. Consumption of eggs enriched in *n*–6 PUFAs (chiefly linoleic acid) caused a comparable reduction in plasma cholesterol, but significantly elevated hepatic cholesterol. The results demonstrate that alterations in egg yolk composition achieved by manipulating diets of laying hens can favorably affect lipid parameters in animals that eat these eggs.

Plant products

Hildebrand reviewed the potential of genetic engineering to improve food quality by manipulation of fatty acid metabolism in plants (*64*). He discussed genes for desaturases and lipoxygenases and biotechnological possibilities for their use as adjuncts to breeding programs. A review by Somerville considered prospects for genetically modifying the composition of edible oils from higher plants (*65*). Techniques for introducing new genes into agronomic plants are well established, and in theory it is possible to genetically engineer higher plants to produce fats and oils with predetermined fatty acid composition. Somerville addressed biological and technical constraints of this approach. Triglycerol biosynthesis in developing seeds was reviewed and examples of specific applications of genetic engineering (reducing palmitic acid content, producing medium-chain triglycerides, and regulating unsaturation and triglyceride composition) were discussed. As an example of the improvement in oil quality achievable by genetic modification, Wong and Swanson reviewed the story of canola oil (*66*). Beginning with conventional breeding programs in the early 1960s and progressing through microspore mutagenesis techniques, erucic acid content was drastically reduced and oleic acid increased. Today's canola oil has the lowest SFA level of any high-oleate vegetable oil.

Marine macroalgae are potential alternatives to fish oil as a source of *n*–3 PUFAs (*67*). Twelve species of Chlorophyta, Phaeophyta, and Rhodophyta from the Arabian Gulf were surveyed. Phaeophyta and Rhodophyta generally were richer than Chlorophyta in eicosatetraenoic acid and EPA and poorer in linolenic acid. In most species, incubation at 5°C decreased the relative amount of palmitic acid, but only in the Phaeophyta and Rhodophyta did the concentration of 20:4 and 20:5 increase at the lower temperature. These PUFAs occurred at high levels in monogalactosyldiacylglycerols and digalactosyldiacylglycerols. Corresponding galactosyldiacylglycerols in the Chlorophyta were rich in 18:3 and 16:3 fatty acids. The authors concluded that Phaeophyta and Rhodophyta, even from hot regions, are potential sources for C_{20} PUFAs and can be further enriched in these compounds by low-temperature incubation for a few days.

Literature Cited

1. Kochhar, S.P., and J.B. Rossell. Detection, estimation, and evaluation of antioxidants in food systems. In *Food Antioxidants*. B.J.F. Hudson (ed.). New York, Elsevier Applied Science. Pp. 19–64 (1990).

2. Ulberth, F., H. Reich, and W. Kneifel. Zur Analytik von Tocopherolen—ein Methodenvergleich zwischen HPLC und GC. *Fat Sci. Technol.* 94:51–54 (1992).

3. Hess, D., H.E. Keller, B. Oberlin, et al. Simultaneous determination of retinol, tocopherols, carotenes and lycopene in plasma by means of high-performance liquid chromatography on reversed phase. *Int. J. Vit. Nutr. Res.* 61:232–238 (1991).

4. Prosky, L., N.-G. Asp, T.F. Schweizer, et al. Determination of insoluble and soluble dietary fiber in foods and food products: collaborative study. *J. AOAC Int.* 75:360–367 (1992).

5. Li, B.W., and M.S. Cardozo. Nonenzymatic-gravimetric determination of total dietary fiber in fruits and vegetables. *J. AOAC Int.* 75:372–374 (1992).

6. Lee, S.C., L. Prosky, and J.W. De Vries. Determination of total, soluble, and insoluble dietary fiber in foods—enzymatic–gravimetric method, MES-TRIS buffer: collaborative study. *J. AOAC Int.* 75:395–416 (1992).

7. Vollendorf, N.W., and J.A. Marlett. Dietary fiber methodology and composition of oat groats, bran, and hulls. *Cereal Foods World* 36:565–570 (1991).

8. Sagredos, A.N. Fettsäuren-Zusammensetzung von Fischölkapseln. *Fat Sci. Technol.* 93:184–191 (1991).

9. Lawson, L.D., S.G. Wood, and B.G. Hughes. HPLC analysis of allicin and other thiosulfinates in garlic clove homogenates. *Planta Med.* 57:263–270 (1991).

10. Lawson, L.D., Z.-Y.J. Wang, and B.G. Hughes. Identification and HPLC quantitation of the sulfides and dialk(en)yl thiosulfinates in commercial garlic products. *Planta Med.* 57:363–370 (1991).

11. Hunter, J.E., and T.H. Applewhite. Reassessment of *trans* fatty acid availability in the US diet. *Am. J. Clin. Nutr.* 54:363–369 (1991).

12. Wolff, R.L. *trans*-Polyunsaturated fatty acids in French edible rapeseed and soybean oils. *J. Am. Oil Chem. Soc.* 69:106–110 (1992).

13. Ratnayake, W.M.N., and G. Pelletier. Positional and geometrical isomers of linoleic acid in partially hydrogenated oils. *J. Am. Oil Chem. Soc.* 69:95–105 (1992).

14. Ratnayake, W.M.N., R. Hollywood, and E. O'Grady. Fatty acids in Canadian margarines. *Can. Inst. Sci. Technol. J.* 24:81–86 (1991).

15. Krzynowek, J., D.S. Uljua, L.J. Panunzio, and R.S. Maney. Factors affecting fat, cholesterol, and omega-3 fatty acids in Maine sardines. *J. Food Sci.* 57:63–65,111 (1992).

16. de Koning, A.J., and T. Mol. The cholesterol content of South African fish oil and its seasonal variation. *Fat Sci. Technol.* 94:60–63 (1992).

17. Abrami, G., F. Natiello, P. Bronzi, et al. A comparison of highly unsaturated fatty acid levels in wild and farmed eels (*Anguilla anguilla*). *Comp. Biochem. Physiol.* 101B:79–81 (1992).

18. Yongmanitchai, W., and O.P. Ward. Screening of algae for potential alternative sources of eicosapentaenoic acid. *Phytochemistry* 30:2963–2967 (1991).

19. Rao, K.S., G.P. Jones, D.E. Rivett, and D.J. Tucker. Fatty acid composition of newer seed oils. *Fat Sci. Technol.* 94:37–38 (1992).

20. Chung, O.K. Cereal lipids. In *Handbook of Cereal Science and Technology*. K.J. Lorenz and K. Kulp (eds.). New York, Marcel Dekker, Inc. *Food Sci. Technol.* 41:497–508 (1991).

21. Shantha, N.C., E.A. Decker, and Z. Ustunol. Conjugated linoleic acid concentration in processed cheese. *J. Am. Oil Chem. Soc.* 69:425–428 (1992).

22. Marlett, J.A. Content and composition of dietary fiber in 117 frequently consumed foods. *J. Am. Diet. Assoc.* 92:175–186 (1992).

23. Becker, R., and G.D. Hanners. Carbohydrate composition of cereal grains. In *Handbook of Cereal Science and Technology*. K.J. Lorenz and K. Kulp (eds.). New York, Marcel Dekker, Inc. *Food Sci. Technol.* 41:469–496 (1991).

24. Vanderslice, J.T., and D.J. Higgs. Vitamin C content of foods: sample variability. *Am. J. Clin. Nutr.* 54:1323S–1327S (1991).

25. Abdel-Kader, Z.M. Determination of carotenoids in foods by high-performance liquid chromatography. *Nahrung* 35:689–693 (1991).

26. Min, Z., and X. Peigen. Quantitative analysis of the active constituents in green tea. *Phytother. Res.* 5:239–240 (1991).

27. Eurola, M.H., P.I. Ekholm, M.E. Ylinen, et al. Selenium in Finnish foods after beginning the use of selenate-supplemented fertilisers. *J. Sci. Food Agric.* 56:57–70 (1991).

28. Ekholm, P., M. Ylinen, M. Eurola, et al. Effects of general soil fertilization with sodium selenate in Finland on the selenium content of milk, cheese and eggs. *Milchwissenschaft* 46:547–550 (1991).

29. Turnland, J.R. Bioavailability of dietary minerals to humans: the stable isotope approach. *Crit. Rev. Food Sci. Nutr.* 30:387–396 (1991).

30. Fairweather-Tait, S.J. Bioavailability of trace elements. *Food Chem.* 43:213–217 (1992).

31. Johnson, P.E. Effect of food processing and preparation on mineral utilization. In *Nutritional and Toxicological Consequences of Food Processing*. M. Friedman (ed.). New York, Plenum Press. *Adv. Exp. Med. Biol.* 289:483–498 (1991).

32. Davidson, L., Å. Cederblad, B. Lönnerdal, and B. Sandström. The effect of individual dietary components on manganese absorption in humans. *Am. J. Clin. Nutr.* 54:1065–1070 (1991).

33. Wisker, E., R. Nagel, T.K. Tanudjaja, and W. Feldheim. Calcium, magnesium, zinc, and iron balances in young women: effects of a low-phytate barley-fiber concentrate. *Am. J. Clin. Nutr.* 54:553–559 (1991).

34. Kohls, K. Calcium bioavailability from calcium fortified food products. *J. Nutr. Sci. Vitaminol.* 37:319–328 (1991).

35. Rudloff, S., and B. Lönnerdal. Calcium and zinc retention from protein hydrolysate formulas in suckling rhesus monkeys. *Am. J. Dis. Child.* 146:588–591 (1992).

36. Serna-Saldivar, S.O., L.W. Rooney, and L.W. Greene. Effects of lime treatment on the bioavailability of calcium in diets of tortillas and beans: bone and plasma composition in rats. *Cereal Chem.* 69:78–81 (1992).

37. Gupta, S., and B.L. Kawatra. Effect of cereal–legume *chapati* diets on absorption and retention of calcium. *Plant Foods Hum. Nutr.* 42:165–173 (1992).

38. Spencer, H., C. Norris, J. Derler, and D. Osis. Effect of oat bran muffins on calcium absorption and calcium, phosphorus, magnesium and zinc balance in men. *J. Nutr.* 121:1976–1983 (1991).

39. Reddy, M.B., and J.D. Cook. Assessment of dietary determinants of nonheme-iron absorption in humans and rats. *Am. J. Clin. Nutr.* 54:723–728 (1991).

40. Ologunde, M.O., R.L. Shepard, O.A. Afolabi, and O.L. Oke. Bioavailability to rats of iron from fortified grain amaranth flour. *Int. J. Food Sci. Technol.* 26:493–500 (1991).

41. Sandberg, A.-S. The effect of food processing on phytate hydrolysis and availability of iron and zinc. In *Nutritional and Toxicological Consequences of Food Processing.* M. Friedman (ed.). New York, Plenum Press. *Adv. Exp. Med. Biol.* 289:499–508 (1991).

42. Galan, P., F. Cherouvrier, L. Mashako, et al. Iron bioavailability from African meals with rice, cassava, or plantain forming the staple food. *J. Clin. Biochem. Nutr.* 10:217–224 (1991).

43. Jackson, L.S. The effect of dairy products on iron availability. *Crit. Rev. Food Sci. Nutr.* 31:259–270 (1992).

44. Wood, M. Milk doesn't block cereal's iron. *Agric. Res.* 39(8):26 (1991).

45. Hallberg, L., L. Rossander-Hultén, M. Brune, and A. Gleerup. Bioavailability in man of iron in human milk and cow's milk in relation to their calcium contents. *Pediatr. Res.* 31:524–527 (1992).

46. Rossander-Hultén, M. Brune, B. Sandström, et al. Competitive inhibition of iron absorption by manganese and zinc in humans. *Am. J. Clin. Nutr.* 54:152–156 (1991).

47. Clydesdale, F.M., C.-T. Ho, C.Y. Lee, et al. The effects of postharvest treatment and chemical interactions on the bioavailability of ascorbic acid, thiamin, vitamin A, carotenoids, and minerals. *Crit. Rev. Food Sci. Nutr.* 30:599–638 (1991).

48. Rock, C.L., and M.E. Swendseid. Plasma β-carotene response in humans after meals supplemented with dietary pectin. *Am. J. Clin. Nutr.* 55:96–99 (1992).

49. Holm, J., and I. Björk. Bioavailability of starch in various wheat-based bread products: evaluation of metabolic responses in healthy subjects and rate and extent of in vitro starch digestion. *Am. J. Clin. Nutr.* 55:420–429 (1992).

50. Haberstroh, C., and C.E. Morris (eds.). *Fat and Cholesterol Reduced Foods: Technologies and Strategies.* The Woodlands, TX, Portfolio Pub. Co. *Adv. Appl. Biotechnol.* 12 (1991).

51. Smith, S.B. Dietary modification for altering fat composition of meat. In *Fat and Cholesterol Reduced Foods: Technologies and Strategies.* C. Haberstroh and C.E. Morris (eds.). The Woodlands, TX, Portfolio Pub. Co. *Adv. Appl. Biotechnol.* 12:75–97 (1991).

52. Morgan, C.A., R.C. Noble, M. Cocchi, and R. McCartney. Manipulation of the fatty acid composition of pig meat lipids by dietary means. *J. Sci. Food Agric.* 58:357–368 (1992).

53. Fischer, K., P. Freudenreich, K.H. Hoppenbrock, and W. Sommer. Einfluß produktionstechnischer Bedingungen auf das Fettsäurenmuster im Rückenspeck von Mastschweinen. *Fleischwirtschaft* 72:200–205 (1992).

54. Irie, M., and M. Sakimoto. Fat characteristics of pigs fed fish oil containing eicosapentaenoic and docosahexaenoic acids. *J. Anim. Sci.* 70:470–477 (1992).

55. Ajuyah, A.O., K.H. Lee, R.T. Hardin, and J.S. Sim. Influence of dietary full-fat seeds and oils on total lipid, cholesterol and fatty acid composition of broiler meats. *Can. J. Anim. Sci.* 71:1011–1019 (1991).

56. Farrell, D.J. Manipulation of growth, carcass composition and fatty acid content of meat-type ducks using short-term feed restriction and dietary additions. *J. Anim. Physiol. Anim. Nutr.* 65:146–153 (1991).

57. Ney, D.M. Potential for enhancing the nutritional properties of milk fat. *J. Dairy Sci.* 74:4002–4012 (1991).

58. Hagemeister, H., D. Precht, M. Franzen, and C.A. Barth. α-Linolenic acid transfer into milk fat and its elongation by cows. *Fat Sci. Technol.* 93:387–391 (1991).

59. Stegeman, G.A., R.J. Baer, D.J. Schingoethe, and D.P. Casper. Composition and flavor of milk and butter from cows fed unsaturated dietary fat and receiving bovine somatotropin. *J. Dairy Sci.* 75:962–970 (1992).

60. Hargis, P.S., and M.E. Van Elswyk. Modifying yolk fatty acid composition to improve the health quality of shell eggs. In *Fat and Cholesterol Reduced Foods: Technologies and Strategies.* C. Haberstroh and C.E. Morris (eds.). The Woodlands, TX, Portfolio Pub. Co. *Adv. Appl. Biotechnol.* 12:249–260 (1991).

61. Naber, E.C. Cholesterol content of eggs: can and should it be changed? In *Fat and Cholesterol Reduced Foods: Technologies and Strategies.* C. Haberstroh and C.E. Morris (eds.). The Woodlands, TX, Portfolio Pub. Co. *Adv. Appl. Biotechnol.* 12:261–276 (1991).

62. Simopoulos, A.P., and N. Salem, Jr. Egg yolk as a source of long-chain polyunsaturated fatty acids in infant feeding. *Am. J. Clin. Nutr.* 55:411–414 (1992).

63. Jiang, Z., and J.S. Sim. Effects of dietary *n*–3 fatty acid–enriched chicken eggs on plasma and tissue cholesterol and fatty acid composition of rats. *Lipids* 27:279–284 (1992).

64. Hildebrand, D.F. Altering fatty acid metabolism in plants. *Food Technol.* 46(4):71–74 (1992).

65. Somerville, C.R. Prospects for genetic modification of the composition of edible oils from higher plants. *Food Biotechnol.* 5:217–228 (1991).

66. Wong, R.S.-C., and E. Swanson. Genetic modification of canola oil: high oleic acid canola. In *Fat and Cholesterol Reduced Foods: Technologies and Strategies.* C. Haberstroh and C.E. Morris (eds.). The Woodlands, TX, Portfolio Pub. Co. *Adv. Appl. Biotechnol.* 12:153–164 (1991).

67. Al-Hasan, R.H., F.M. Hantash, and S.S. Radwan. Enriching marine macroalgae with eicosatetraenoic (arachidonic) and eicosapentaenoic acids by chilling. *Appl. Microbiol. Biotechnol.* 35:530–535 (1991).

Part II: Safety of Food Components

6

Assessment of Food Safety

General and acute toxicity
Mutagenicity and carcinogenicity
Reproductive and developmental toxicity
Neurological toxicity and behavioral effects
Immunotoxicity

GENERAL AND ACUTE TOXICITY

Papers from a 1990 symposium on "Food Safety Assessment" were recently published (*1*). Among the topics discussed and reviewed were risk assessment, including several computer models; laboratory testing of ingredients; evaluation guidelines; assessing microbial safety; impacts of diet; and evaluations of irradiated foods, antioxidants, color additives, olestra, nitroso compounds, urethane, and potato glycoalkaloids.

Many reports from a 1990 symposium on "Nutritional and Toxicological Consequences of Food Processing" were also concerned with various aspects of food safety assessment (*2*). Both deleterious substances, such as heterocyclic amines in cooked meats, tin, lipid peroxides, and food allergens, as well as protective substances, such as anticarcinogenic fatty acids, were discussed. Emphasis was on chemicals in foods which may be created or altered during food processing.

Various aspects of the economics of food safety were covered in another volume (*3*). Consumer demands for food and food safety were discussed as were applications of risk assessment methodology to food safety. Economic impacts of foodborne disease were described and consumer perceptions of several food safety issues (pesticide residues, fat consumption) were considered.

Two recent reviews were devoted to the topic of government regulation of food safety in the USA. Various federal agencies and the important federal laws relevant to ensuring a safe food supply were described in one paper (*4*). The other review (*5*) summarized the roles of federal, state, and local governments in protecting consumers against food hazards. Some historical background was given and the interplay of science and societal considerations in shaping food safety policies was discussed.

Reports from a 1990 symposium on "Trends in Biological Dosimetry" considered numerous methods for the detection of toxic effects (*6*). These included analyses of structure–activity relationships, detection of DNA and protein adducts and genotoxic effects. Biomonitoring of human populations was discussed along with data on human exposures to lead, dioxin, and nitrosamines.

Toxicological studies in animals have yielded a wealth of information but the relevance of all this data to humans is not certain. Guidelines for the extrapolation of safety data from animals to humans were included in a recent edition of *Guide to Clinical Trials* (*7*). Topics discussed included types of toxicological studies, predicting adverse human effects from results of these studies, and issues and controversies related to extrapolation of data, such as doses to use, clinical vs. toxicological endpoints, threshold effects, species specificities, whether pathologists should read tissue slides blind or unblind, and paradoxical effects observed.

Statistical methods for analyzing results of short-term genotoxic tests were reviewed with an eye to promoting further research into biostatistical issues and methods of analysis (*8*). Methods for analyzing data from the Ames *Salmonella*/microsome assay are the best developed and were discussed for their applicability to other short-term tests. Appropriate methods for the design and analysis of various in vivo and in vitro short-term tests were described and recommended.

Traditional measures of acute toxicity, such as the classical LD_{50} test, have been criticized for ethical and scientific reasons. Both the fixed-dose procedure and the up-and-down method require the use of fewer animals and were found to be acceptable alternatives to the classical test in assays for acute oral toxicity with 10 compounds (*9*). In the fixed-dose procedure, 10 rats were dosed at one of 4 dose levels selected on the basis of a sighting study which involved 3–4 animals. Rats were observed for 14 days after treatment. Depending on the outcome of the first dose group, a second dose group was used. The compounds were rated as very toxic, toxic, harmful, or unclassified according to EC criteria. In the up-and-down method, female rats were dosed one at a time, starting the first animal at the best estimate of the LD_{50}. If this animal was alive after 24 h, the next animal was given a dose 1.3 times higher than the first; if the first animal died, the next animal was given a dose 1.3 times lower. This dosing routine was continued until 4 animals had been treated after reversal of the initial outcome.

Useful data on signs of toxicity and gross autopsy findings were also obtained from these assays.

Primary cultures of human hepatocytes were compared with cultured rat hepatocytes, mouse non-hepatic 3T3 cells, and mouse LD_{50} tests for their accuracy in predicting human toxicity of 10 chemicals (10). Cells were exposed to the chemicals for 24 h and then assayed by the MTT test which detects mitochondrial enzyme activity. Results from these experiments were compared with information on human acute lethal dosages. All the chemicals except one had roughly similar effects on the 3 cell culture systems but, overall, the data indicated that human acute toxicity was most accurately predicted by the human hepatocyte culture.

MUTAGENICITY AND CARCINOGENICITY

Physiochemical properties and structure–activity relationships

Proceedings of a 1990 international workshop on QSAR (quantitative structure–activity relationships) in environmental toxicology were recently published (11). QSAR techniques and molecular descriptors were presented and their relationship to biological processes such as biokinetics, bioaccumulation, toxicity, and mechanism of action, were discussed. Reports from 10 research groups considered the applications of QSAR methods in practice.

In a QSAR investigation of the role of hydrophobicity in regulating mutagenicity in the Ames test, 88 aromatic and heteroaromatic amines were tested with *S. typhimurium* TA98 with S9 activation, 67 amines were activated and tested with strain TA100 (12), and 117 aromatic and heteroaromatic nitro compounds (13) were tested without activation in strain TA100. Hydrophobicity of the compounds was found to play a major role in determining mutagenicity while electronic effects were less important. Hydrophobic and electronic effects had a similar influence on mutagenicity by the amines in TA98 and in TA100 suggesting that these molecular properties were important during the activation

process. The number of aromatic rings in the amines was important in determining mutagenicity in strain TA98 only. Certain other structural features should be investigated but the QSARs derived here appear to be reasonable and self-consistent.

The CASE Program (Computer-Automated Structure Evaluation), an expert system that automatically selects relevant descriptors for structure–activity relationships, was used to analyze the binding of 136 polycyclic aromatic hydrocarbons (PAHs), substituted dibenzo-*p*-dioxins, dibenzo-furans, and biphenyls whose binding affinities were measured by sucrose density gradients and of 87 PAH, nitro-PAH, halo-PAH, and *N*-heterocyclic compounds whose binding affinities were measured by electrofocusing (14). Certain molecular structures relevant for binding to the intracellular TCDD or Ah receptor were identified by CASE: for halogenated aromatic hydrocarbons, fragments containing lateral halogens and a longitudinal hydrogen appeared important whereas the fragments of PAH and heterocyclic compounds which were important contained the classical "bay" region. It may be that two different recognition sites are involved in Ah receptor binding.

Data from a number of assays of mutagenicity, cytogenotoxicity, carcinogenicity, sensory irritation, male rat-specific $\alpha2\mu$-nephrotoxicity, and maximum tolerated dose were used as learning sets in CASE analyses and then, using this information, a large, randomly chosen population of chemicals (N≥1300) was analyzed for potential toxicity (15). The compounds were then sorted out by their responses to specific tests and the overlap among the tests was determined. The data demonstrate that none of the currently used short-term tests are highly predictive of rodent carcinogenicity but that they reflect a spectrum of partially overlapping mechanisms. Since there are significant non-overlapping domains among the tests, it is possible to identify batteries of complementary tests for subclasses of chemicals. Results from these test batteries should provide more reliable information on potential carcinogenicity.

Efforts are being made to predict the carcinogenicity of 44 chemicals currently being screened for rodent carcinogenicity by the U.S. National

Toxicology Program. Two recent analyses have investigated the importance of electrophilic reactivity of these compounds. Electrophilic reactivity was estimated by a formula which assigned a numerical value to various elements and electrophilic groups in the molecules. This analysis predicted that 11 compounds were probable carcinogens and another 15 were possible mutagens (*16*). Experimental determination of the rate constant of electron attachment in cyclohexane for 31 of the 44 chemicals indicated that 16 of the compounds would be carcinogenic (*17*). Similar results were obtained from the experimental and the calculated predictions of carcinogenicity.

Of 58 epoxides tested, 16 failed to induce sister chromatid exchanges in Chinese hamster V79 cells (*18*). Comparison of activity as related to structure indicated that mono-substituted epoxides had the highest genotoxic potency. While the results obtained with V79 cells generally agreed with those obtained with the Ames test, some differences were observed which may be due to differences in cellular uptake of the chemicals or in detoxification reactions.

Microbial test systems

The influence of different metabolic activation system (rat liver S9 preparations) concentrations on the dose–response exhibited by promutagens in the *Salmonella* spiral and plate assays was studied using a factorial experimental design (*19*). Mutagens were tested at 13 concentrations using 10 different S9 concentrations (0.1–4.0 mg protein/plate for standard plate assays and 0.25–4.9 mg-equivalents in the spiral assay). Results from these experiments demonstrated that even small differences in S9 concentrations can affect the measured mutagenic potency and that S9–compound interactions cannot be generalized through the use of interaction studies. Furthermore, spiral assay data and plate assay data for promutagens are not directly comparable unless the S9 concentrations for all chemical doses are also comparable.

An alternative metabolic activation system for promutagens in the Ames assay utilizes extracts of mammalian cells expressing P450 cDNAs.

Activation of several food-related promutagens (aflatoxin B_1, PhIP, MeIQ, Trp-P-1) by cell extracts expressing P450IA2 cDNA was dramatically increased when the preincubation method rather than the plate incorporation method was used (*20*). Preincubation also significantly increased revertant yield when low concentrations of S9 mix were used as the activating system.

In a series of experiments in two laboratories with 10 mutagens (*21*) and with 10 promutagens (*22*) an attempt has been made to identify selected chemicals which could be used as reference materials to calibrate the *Salmonella* assay so as to provide more quantitative estimates of mutagenic potency. Ten doses of each chemical were tested using *S. typhimurium* strain TA100, with 1.1 mg protein (S9)/plate used to activate the promutagens in the plate incorporation procedure. Low variability of results was observed with most of the test compounds, indicating that they could be used for bioassay controls and potentially as reference standards in comparative bioassays. When used as reference standards, an appropriate dose range must be used and care must be given to the number and spacing of doses if highly reproducible slope values are to be generated.

Results of *Salmonella* mutagenicity tests of 311 coded chemicals with and without preincubation with an S9 from Aroclor-induced rats or hamsters were reported (*23*). Three laboratories were involved in testing and 8 strains of *S. typhimurium* were used. A chemical was designated nonmutagenic only if it tested negative in strains TA98, TA100, TA1535, and TA97 and/or TA1537 with and without activation. Of the compounds tested, 120 were mutagenic, 172 were nonmutagenic, and 19 were questionable with either borderline results or giving different results in different laboratories.

Since different strains of *S. typhimurium* are sensitive to different types of mutagens, experiments were conducted with 103 direct mutagens and 7 tester strains to define the best associations for screening new compounds (*24*). Use of strains TA100 and TA1538 detected 86% of the mutagens while 97% and 99% of the mutagens were detected by combinations of 4 strains (TA100, TA102, TA1537, TA1538) and of 5 strains (TA97, TA102, TA1535,

TA1537, TA1538), respectively. Detection of 100% of the mutagens required the use of 6 strains.

The Microscreen assay, which utilizes *E. coli* WP2s(λ), was developed as a means of testing very small samples. A total of 133 compounds, including 111 which had been tested in the *Salmonella* assay and 66 which had also been tested in rodent bioassays, were tested with the Microscreen (*25*). Concordance between the two microbial assays was 71% and was about 70% between the rodent carcinogenicity assays and the Microscreen. The Microscreen assay was able to detect halogenated compounds better than the *Salmonella* assay and should prove useful in detecting mutagens, particularly when sample size is limiting.

Genotoxicity tests using Drosophila

Effects of chemical and physical agents on recombination events in germ line cells of male and female *Drosophila melanogaster* were reviewed (*26*). Since meiotic recombination does not normally occur in male germ line cells, chemically induced male recombination may form a basis for a fast, one-generation screening assay. Of 25 agents tested in male germ cells, 24 of them, including alkylating, intercalating and cross-linking agents, direct-acting compounds and those requiring metabolic activation, did induce male recombination.

Ten known carcinogens (including safrole and benz(α)pyrene) were tested using the *zeste-white* somatic mutation assay with *D. melanogaster* (*27*). All the tested compounds produced significant increases in the eye spot frequency, indicating that this test is highly sensitive to these compounds. This assay should be further tested using carcinogens with different modes of action.

Methods employing cultured mammalian cells in vitro

GENOTOXICITY ASSAYS. Fragments of human thyroid tissue obtained during the course of prescribed surgery were cultured and examined for their suitability as reliable models for genotoxicity studies (*28*). Positive dose-related increases in DNA fragmentation were observed after these cell cultures were exposed for 1 h to 4 different direct-acting alkylating agents. However, no increase in DNA damage occurred when the cells were exposed to 2 procarcinogens. The level of mixed function oxidase activity in these thyroid cells is apparently too low to activate the procarcinogens.

Proceedings of a workshop on "Micronuclei as an Index of Cytogenetic Damage" at the 1991 annual meeting of the Environmental Mutagen Society were recently summarized (*29*). Information concerning the production of micronuclei, what protocols are now accepted or proposed internationally, recent results obtained, and new methods and protocols likely to be forthcoming was reported. In addition, a single protocol was proposed which would satisfy the requirements of 6 regulatory authorities in Canada, the European Economic Community, the Organization for Economic Co-operation and Development, Japan, and the USA.

Many in vitro genotoxicity assays are considered poor predictors of rodent carcinogencity because of their low specificity, which results in a high false-positive rate. Ten compounds, reported to be noncarcinogenic in the literature, were tested concurrently in the Chinese hamster ovary cell/hypoxanthine–guanine phosphoribosyl transferase (CHO/HGPRT) mutation assay and the CHO micronucleus assay to determine their use in predicting rodent carcinogenicity (*30*). Four compounds gave negative results in both assays, with and without metabolic activation. One compound, dichlorvos, tested positive in both assays and has recently been shown to induce tumors in rodents. All 5 of the other compounds were positive in the micronucleus assay, and only 1 of them was equivocally positive in the mutation assay. These results indicate that the CHO/HGPRT assay provides more relevant results when screening chemicals for potential carcinogenicity.

Primary cultures of mouse epidermal keratinocytes were exposed to various concentrations of 4 polycyclic aromatic hydrocarbons (PAHs) to investigate the relationship between DNA adduct formation and the induction of unscheduled DNA synthesis (UDS) (*31*). Within the linear dose–response range (0.005–0.25 µg/mL) for each chemical, a good correlation was observed between the level of UDS detected and the amount of DNA adducts present. However, measurement of DNA adducts proved to be a more sensitive indicator of genotoxicity. Adducts could be detected at PAH concentrations of 0.005 and 0.01 µg/mL while UDS could not be detected below concentrations of 0.01 µg/mL. Thus, the UDS assay would be more useful for rapid screening for relatively strong genotoxic agents.

ACTIVATION OF PROMUTAGENS AND PROCARCINOGENS. Since many cultured cells are unable to metabolically activate promutagens and procarcinogens, this activation is often achieved by addition of a rat hepatic microsomal preparation (S9 mix). However, the S9 mix is cytotoxic and this extracellular activation may not be as effective as that occurring intracellularly. Therefore, several other methods to metabolically activate these compounds have been proposed. Two research groups have developed protocols using metabolically competent liver cell cultures as both the activating system and the target for DNA damage. In experiments with an established human hepatoma cell line (Hep G2), dose-dependent increases in frequencies of micronuclei and sister chromatid exchanges (SCEs) were observed after treatments with all 5 indirectly acting procarcinogens tested [safrole, cyclophosphamide (CP), dimethyl nitrosamine, hexamethylphosphoramide, and benzo[*a*]pyrene (B[a]P)] and with 2 directly acting carcinogens (methyl methanesulfonate and mitomycin C) but not with the non-carcinogen, pyrene (*32*). Mutations at the HGPRT locus in a continuous Chinese hamster epithelial liver cell culture were increased by exposure to the procarcinogens CP, B[a]P, aflatoxin B_1 (AFB_1), and 7,12-dimethylbenz[a]anthracene and by exposure to 2 direct-acting carcinogens (*33*). Several parameters were examined to establish optimal assay conditions, and activities of various enzymes involved in metabolism of promutagens were measured. These assay systems are promising alternatives to the rodent liver S9 homogenate in short-term tests.

Another alternative to rodent liver S9 activation is the use of microcarrier-attached rat hepatocytes (*34*). Primary cultures of these hepatocytes grown on collagen-coated dextran microcarriers retained their initial level of ethoxycoumarin deethylase activity for 24 h and 25% of the initial activity was present for up to 48 h. When these microcarrier-attached hepatocytes were cocultured with BALB/c 3T3 cells cytotoxicity of CP was expressed in a time- and concentration-dependent manner. Without the hepatocytes, CP was not cytotoxic. This assay system may also be useful in studying indirectly acting carcinogens and mutagens.

Two new Chinese hamster cell lines genetically engineered to metabolic competence by the introduction of cytochrome P450 genes have been assessed for their ability to detect procarcinogens. Chinese hamster cells (CHL, originally derived from the lung of a newborn hamster) containing a monkey cytochrome P-450IA1 DNA were 25 times as sensitive to the cytotoxic effects of AFB_1 than the parental CHL cells (*35*). This hypersensitivity was almost completely abolished by a specific inhibitor of P-450IA. AFB_1 also induced mutations at the HGPRT locus in the new cell line but not in the parental CHL line.

Three Chinese hamster V79 cell lines genetically engineered to contain one of 3 rat liver cytochrome P450 genes were evaluated for the detection of procarcinogens in the micronucleus assay (*36*). Increased frequencies of micronuclei were observed in strain SD1 (containing P450b or CYP2B1) exposed to CP, in strain XEM2 (containing P450c or CYP1A1) exposed to B[a]P, in strain XEMd-MZ (containing CYP1A2 or P450d) exposed to 2-aminoanthracene, and in all strains exposed to sterigmatocystin. These strains may be useful not only for the detection of procarcinogens but also for investigating mechanisms of bioactivation and genotoxicity.

DETECTION OF TUMOR PROMOTERS. In most cultured cells containing the Epstein-Barr virus (EBV), the virus remains latent but it can be induced by a number of compounds which activate protein kinase C and which are also known tumor promoters. In the Burkitt lymphoma line Raji, the viral genome has been deleted such that only an abortive lytic cycle can be induced. A genetically engineered strain of Raji containing a reporter gene, chloramphenicol–acetyltransferase (CAT), under the control of an EBV early promoter, has been evaluated as an in vitro test system for tumor promoters (*37*). CAT activity is low in untreated cells but high after treatment with various EBV inducers, such as phorbol esters, sodium butyrate, and iododeoxyuridine. This cell line may provide a simple, quantitative, and reproducible test system for tumor promoters which activate protein kinases C.

Short-term in vivo tests

During recent years, an enormous amount of data has accumulated concerning the genotoxic effects of a number of chemicals in a variety of short-term in vivo tests. A recent issue of *Mutation Research* was devoted to a description and discussion of a method to compare and combine short-term genotoxicity test data (*38*). This method combines the major parameters of testing (dose, metabolic activation, sign of response) into a single score which could be pooled by test, by class of tests (e.g., prokaryotic gene mutation) and by family of classes (e.g., in vitro tests) hierarchically into a composite score for a chemical. This system should be able to deal with redundant, incomplete, and conflicting results and provide a weight-of-evidence analysis for the tested chemicals.

Analysis of results from in vivo sister chromatid exchange (SCE) assays using different methods of data transformation was described and evaluated (*39*). When two different data sets were analyzed using (1) no transformation (SCE count/cell); (2) natural logarithm of (1 + SCE count/cell); (3) square root of (0.5 + SCE count/cell); (4) one-fourth power of (SCE count/cell averaged for each animal); and (5) median SCE count/cell, none of the transformations appeared to offer any advantage in the assessment of whether a test agent induces SCE in a dose-related manner. A method for determining, subject to budgetary constraints, the desired number of animals/dose group and cells scored/animal was also proposed.

Three commercially available cooking oils (olive, peanut, and sunflower seed) which are commonly used as vehicles in toxicological tests were found to induce a cytotoxic effect on mouse bone marrow (*40*). Mice were given single i.p. injections of 4 mL oil/kg body weight and then femoral bone marrow samples were examined 30–72 h later. Although none of the oils appeared to alter the frequency of micronucleated polychromatic erythrocytes (PCEs), all 3 oils significantly reduced the PCE/red blood cell ratio at 30 h. This cytotoxic effect may affect results obtained with in vivo micronucleus tests.

A special issue of *Mutation Research* (*41*) reviewed various aspects of a new method for the micronucleus test using rodent peripheral blood reticulocytes with acridine orange supravital staining. These reports from the Collaborative Study Group for the Micronucleus Test demonstrated a dose-dependent increase in micronucleated peripheral reticulocytes in response to 23 test chemicals. Most chemicals gave the greatest response at 48 h post-dosing. Since this assay generates reproducible and reliable data it provides an attractive alternative to the conventional bone marrow assay.

Since aneuploid and polyploid cells are observed in 75% of spontaneous abortions and in 2% of live-born children, a need exists for a convenient, reliable screening assay for aneuploidic agents. Testicular material from male mice given i.p. injections of one of ten known or suspect spindle poisons was examined 6, 14, and 22 h after dosing to determine induction of hyperploidy by chromosome counting and to determine effects on testicular cell proliferation (*42*). Seven of the chemicals increased the frequencies of hyperploid secondary spermatocytes and also induced meiotic delay in primary and/or secondary spermatocytes. It appeared that meiotic delay was indicative of aneuploidy induction and could serve as a prescreen for aneuploidic agents.

To determine possible biochemical parameters which could be early signs of carcinogenicity in rodents, female rats were gavaged with 2 dose levels of 111 chemicals (including 49 known carcinogens) (*43*). The animals were sacrificed 21 h later and were examined for hepatic DNA damage, hepatic ornithine decarboxylase activity, serum alanine aminotransferase activity, and hepatic cytochrome P-450 content. The 4 biochemical assays were complementary to each other. Taken together, results from these assays had a much greater concordance with results from rodent carcinogenicity tests than other short-term in vitro and in vivo assays.

These biochemical tests may be a useful component in complementary batteries of tests for predicting rodent carcinogenicity.

Two transgenic mouse strains containing *lac* genes from *E. coli* have been constructed and used for the in vivo detection of mutations. Muta™Mouse has approximately 40 copies of the *lacZ* gene incorporated via lambda phage into a single site on both chromosomes of a homologous pair in each cell (*44*). These genes were microinjected into fertilized hybrid eggs (BALB/c × DBA/z) which were then implanted into female mice to be carried to term. A second transgenic mouse strain has been constructed to contain approximately 30 copies per chromosome of a lambda shuttle vector containing the *lacI* gene in cells of C57BL/6 mice (*45*). Both types of transgenic mice were exposed to a variety of chemicals, and 3–7 days later body tissues were collected and analyzed. DNA was extracted from the tissues and the shuttle vector containing the *lac* genes was recovered by addition of lambda packaging extract. These phages were allowed to infect *E. coli* cells and, following an overnight incubation, phage containing mutant *lacI* or *lacZ* genes produce clear plaques while phage with non-mutant genes produce blue plaques on indicator plates containing Xgal. These mice have been used successfully to detect mutations in a variety of tissues. This assay system should allow extrapolation of in vitro data on genotoxicity of chemicals to whole animals.

Medium-term tests in rodents

Early indicators of non-genotoxic carcinogenesis were reviewed in a series of papers in an issue of *Mutation Research* (*46*). Non-genotoxic carcinogens may produce specific, identifiable effects in animals exposed for periods as short as 90 days. These effects are all associated with cell replication and include cell necrosis, organ enlargement, biochemical changes, and hormonal disturbances. Such changes in rodent kidney, bladder, liver, pancreas, stomach, skin, and thyroid tissues were described and the validity of considering these early changes as indicators of non-genotoxic carcinogenesis was discussed.

In a rapid production model for pancreatic carcinogenesis in hamsters, diethylnitrosamine (DEN) was shown to be a weak initiator of pancreatic carcinogenesis (*47*). This model was developed to incorporate the principle of selection based on resistance to cytotoxicity, originally demonstrated for liver carcinogenesis in rats. Hamsters were dosed with DEN or another known initiator, *N*-nitrosobis-(2-oxopropyl)amine (BOP), and then subjected to 3 cycles of augmentation: 4 days on a choline-deficient diet supplemented with toxic DL-ethionine, followed by a basal diet containing L-methionine and a dose of BOP. Animals were sacrificed and examined 10 weeks after the beginning of the experiment. BOP followed by augmentation resulted in 100% incidence of total pancreatic lesions and 89.5% of carcinomas. Corresponding incidences were 65% and 15% for DEN followed by augmentation, and 21% and 0% for augmentation alone. This assay may be useful in identifying etiological factors involved in human pancreatic cancer development.

Two similar medium-term assays requiring 20–24 weeks to complete have been developed to assess the tumor-promoting potential of various chemicals in rats. In the first assay, three potent carcinogens, DEN, *N*-methyl-*N*-nitrosourea (MNU), and *N*-bis(2-hydroxypropyl)nitrosamine (DHPN), were sequentially administered during a 4-week period to rats to initiate tumors in a variety of organs (*48*). Of 14 chemicals administered during the subsequent 16 weeks, 11 were found to modify the incidence of at least one type of neoplastic lesion and 7 targeted more than two organs. Results for these compounds as compared to results from previous long-term carcinogenicity assays indicated that this medium-term multiple-organ bioassay was a reliable measure of tumor-promoting activity.

Following 4 weeks of injections of MNU, the incidences of preneoplastic and neoplastic lesions induced by 6 known carcinogens were enhanced in their target organs (*49*). Apparently prior treatment with MNU sensitized the tissues to the effects of the carcinogens, allowing detection of their effects after only 20 weeks. This system could be used as a whole-body medium-term screening assay for detecting environmental carcinogens.

Long-term bioassays for carcinogenesis

Thousands of long-term carcinogenicity experiments have been conducted during the past 30 years. To aid researchers in pinpointing relevant data, two recent analyses of large databases have organized experimental results according to 34 or 35 target organs or systems affected by the test chemicals. Both analyses report that the liver is the most frequent target organ, with lungs, mammary glands, stomach, kidney, and hematopoietic system often affected. One analysis utilized the Carcinogenic Potency Database which included results of 3969 experiments testing the effects of 533 chemicals (50). Most of the experiments have used rats or mice and overall results indicate that 76% of rat carcinogens are positive in mice and 71% of mouse carcinogens are positive in rats. Data from the Technical Reports Series of the National Cancer Institute and the National Toxicology Program were analyzed in the second study (51). This database includes information on 379 chemicals tested in 1394 experiments. These toxicology studies were typically carried out using both sexes of two species of rodents (usually the Fischer 344 rat and the B6C3F1 mouse strains) with an exposure time of about two years. These analyses may aid in risk assessment and in designing further experiments.

Prior to the appearance of full-fledged colon cancer in laboratory rats, altered crypts, called aberrant crypt foci (ACF), can be observed in colon mucosal sections. In a study to determine whether these ACF are preneoplastic lesions, colon mucosal samples from rats given a single carcinogenic dose of 1,2-dimethylhydrazine-HCl were examined at intervals of 2 to 57 weeks post-dosing (52). ACF were present at all time intervals in treated rats and were also present when adenocarcinomas were observed. The number of ACF with 4 or more crypts and those exhibiting a higher grade of nuclear atypia increased significantly at or beyond 19 weeks. These features of ACF strongly support the hypothesis that ACF are precursor lesions of colon cancer.

Two diets, widely used in toxicological studies, were compared with respect to their influence on spontaneous neoplasia and neoplastic responses to 2-acetylaminofluorene (2-AAF) (53). Mice were fed either a purified diet (AIN-76A) or a non-purified natural ingredient diet (NIH-07) for up to 2 years. Various doses of 2-AAF were added to the diets of males (0–60 ppm) and females (0–150 ppm). In most cases AIN-fed animals attained higher maximum body weights and died earlier than their NIH-fed counterparts. Consumption of the AIN-76A diet was also associated with a higher spontaneous frequency of liver neoplasia and a higher frequency of 2-AAF-induced bladder neoplasia in males and a higher frequency of 2-AAF-induced liver tumors in females. This study demonstrates the importance of diet selection in carcinogenicity studies and suggests that dietary effects may be related to effects on body weight.

Since all chemicals are toxic at some dose and this dose may vastly exceed likely human exposure, the maximum tolerated dose (MTD) regime for carcinogenicity testing may not be valid (54). The safer the chemical, the higher the MTD, but the higher the MTD, the more likely it is that various biochemical and physiological distortions will occur and result in toxicity-induced cancer. The authors suggest that a minimally toxic dose, the highest subtoxic dose that can be tolerated by the animals over a long period of time without demonstrable toxicity or histopathology, is more appropriate for carcinogenicity bioassays.

About half the substances tested at their MTD are found to induce cancer, and this may be a direct effect of their stimulatory effect on cell proliferation when given in such high concentrations. Pariza (55) proposed that this chemically induced mitogenesis be considered an undesirable toxic effect and that MTD be redefined as the highest dose that may be fed without inducing mitogenesis. Since MTDs determined in this way are likely to be lower than those determined by current procedures, a safety factor could be employed to provide an added level of protection. For example, the acceptable daily intake of a substance that does not induce cancer at its MTD would be set at 1% of that MTD.

Indices of human exposure to carcinogens

Biomonitoring of humans to detect exposure to environmental and occupational carcinogens provides more relevant information than environmental monitoring because it takes into account individual differences in absorption, metabolism and repair. A number of sensitive techniques not requiring radiolabelled carcinogens were developed recently for the detection of carcinogen–DNA adducts and have been reviewed recently (56). These techniques include immunologic methods with polyclonal and monoclonal antisera, [^{32}P]post-labeling of modified nucleotides, fluorescence spectroscopy, and GC/MS. Advantages and disadvantages of the different techniques were discussed. Levels of detection of the adducts are generally at the femto or atto mole level (i.e., 1 adduct/10^8 or 10^{10} nucleotides). While some techniques are more sensitive or specific than other methods, cost is also a concern in choosing a method for epidemiological studies.

Fluorescence line-narrowing spectroscopy is a highly sensitive and selective analytical technique for the detection and characterization of DNA adducts in organisms exposed to PAHs. Liver DNA from fish exposed to benzo[a]pyrene (100 mg BP/kg fish) was found, by this method, to contain a major DNA adduct derived from syn-benzo[a]pyrene diol-epoxide. This method has a detection limit of about 1 adduct/10^8 normal basepairs for 100 µg DNA (57).

Many human cancers contain mutations in the *p53* tumor suppressor gene, and those detected in lung and liver cancers are primarily G:C to T:A transversions. Since such transversions are known to be induced by BP and aflatoxin B_1, a study was done using DNA polymerase fingerprint analysis to identify *p53* nucleotides affected by these carcinogens (58). Of 14 nucleotide residues known to be mutated in lung cancers, 13 were targets of BP. Similarly, aflatoxin B_1 caused G:C to A:T transversions at a known mutational hot spot in liver cancers. These data indicate that most of the mutations identified in lung and liver cancers occur in nucleotides selectively targeted by two major carcinogens etiologically associated with these tumors.

Micronucleus frequencies were determined in lymphocytes of capillary blood from 250 healthy persons aged 6–88 years to test the method and obtain a normal range of values (59). In the younger age groups, 6–20 and 21–45, the micronucleus frequency ranged from 0–1% with averages of 0.14 and 0.09, respectively. Older age groups had significantly higher mean micronucleus frequencies, 0.24–0.25. The percentage of persons with micronuclei in their lymphocytes was also significantly higher in the older age groups (30.6%) than in the younger groups (16.5%). No significant differences in micronucleus frequencies were observed between males and females of similar age. This appears to be a convenient and sensitive method for monitoring humans for exposure to environmental mutagens and carcinogens.

Three in vitro lymphocyte proliferation assays using cells from rats were evaluated for their ability to detect exposure to toxins (60). At the lowest concentrations tested, 8 toxic compounds induced changes in at least one assay. Splenocytes from rats exposed in vivo to chromate or cadmium responded differently when the cells were assayed in vitro with added chromate or cadmium. Thus, it may be possible to use these assays to detect exposure to a variety of toxicants.

To determine the normal range of variability in chromosomal aberrations (CA), sister chromatid exchanges (SCE) and mitogen-induced blastogenesis in cultured peripheral lymphocytes from humans, 8 blood samples were obtained from each of 48 healthy volunteers (24 male, 24 female) over a two-year period (61). Neither sex, age, nor lifestyle factors (smoking, alcohol and caffeine intake, etc.) appeared to affect the results on the 3 tests but there was a significant effect of both year and season of sampling for all 3 endpoints. The frequency of SCEs was lower during summer and autumn while that of CAs was nearly always lower during autumn and winter. These results highlight one of the difficulties in human monitoring and emphasize the need for concurrent sampling of control and exposed populations.

Another difficulty in monitoring human populations lies in individual variations in susceptibility to induced chromosomal damage. In assays for induction of SCEs by diepoxybutane (DEB) in lymphocytes from 55 healthy women, those from 11 women were significantly more sensitive to DEB (62). Baseline SCE frequencies were also significantly higher in these individuals. Given the relatively high population frequency of this sensitivity to DEB, it is likely that individual variations could distort conclusions about the induction of SCEs by environmental toxins unless such DEB sensitivity is taken into account.

Risk assessment

In a recent review, Pariza (*63*) traced the evolution of risk assessment as applied to food safety. Sources of uncertainty related to the many assumptions made in estimating risks were considered and the difficulties in interpretation of risk assessments were discussed.

Interpretation of the vast amount of data from various genotoxicity and carcinogenicity experiments engenders much debate with many new ideas and variations of older ones. A series of articles in *Environmental Health Perspectives* was devoted to "Databases of Genotoxicity and Carcinogenicity and Their Usefulness for Hazard Evaluation" (*64*). Another series in *Environmental Carcinogenesis Reviews* considered risk assessment from a scientific approach as well as from governmental and industrial viewpoints as part of a special issue devoted to an "Approach to a Consensus for the Basis of Regulation of Environmental Chemicals" (*65*).

Human biomonitoring data (concentrations in adipose tissue), pharmacodynamic and pharmacokinetic parameters in humans and animals, and selected dose-response data from animal carcinogenicity studies were utilized in a cancer risk assessment for chlordane and heptachlor (*66*). Conversion factors based on body surface area were used to extrapolate animal data to humans. Conservative estimates from the Global 82 linearized multistage mathematical model yielded unit cancer risks of 1.8×10^{-4} for heptachlor and 1.4×10^{-4} for chlordane via all potential routes of human exposure. U.S. EPA estimates of risk, based on estimated exposure doses from ambient air and drinking water without regard to pharmacokinetics, were 3-fold higher for chlordane and 8-fold higher for heptachlor. The authors argue that risk assessments which incorporate all the scientifically valid and biologically relevant data available will be more reliable and enable us to best protect public health.

Epidemiological studies have been useful in identifying some human carcinogens and may also be useful in indicating substances which are noncarcinogenic to humans if enough information on exposure and adequate followup periods are considered. Important aspects of a data collection and analysis for epidemiological studies were reviewed and discussed with an eye to improving their value in quantitative risk assessments (*67*). Attempts should be made to more accurately determine exposure since the use of "ever/never" exposure and of "duration" of exposure without consideration of intensity of exposure may give misleading results. Models for data analysis need to be revised to be more applicable to epidemiological studies so as to incorporate factors such as variability in dose rate over time and a diminishing of relative risk within a few decades after exposure.

To a large extent, regulatory agencies base their decisions on carcinogenic risks to humans on results of rodent carcinogenicity studies. But controversy continues as to the predictive value of these assays. A recent review (*68*) emphasized the qualitative and quantitative comparisons of data from high-dose experiments with mice and rats and between rodents and humans. These authors concluded that the carcinogenic potencies of chemicals in rats and mice correlate well and that, for chemicals for which good data on human exposure are available, the upper limits on potencies in humans are consistent with rodent potencies. Using data from carcinogenic studies with 22 chemicals, these same authors made a quantitative comparison between rodent and human carcinogenic potencies (*69*). For 18 chemicals the human evidence is consistent with predictions based on the rodent bioassays, and for 2 chemicals it was inconsistent. For the remaining 2 chemicals there was insufficient data to make a useful comparison between rodents and humans.

Mammalian cell mutagenicity assays were evaluated for their role in genotoxicity testing of industrial chemicals with an emphasis on the widely used CHO/HGPRT assay and the mouse lymphoma L5178Y tk+/- mutation assay (*70*). The CHO/HGPRT assay is apparently a highly specific assay but might be less sensitive to some types of mutagens while the mouse lymphoma assay appeared to be sensitive but might have a lower specificity due to experimental artifacts such as pH change and osmolality changes. Industrial and regulatory perspectives on such testing were discussed.

Results of 4 genotoxicity assays [Ames test, mouse lymphoma L5178Y mutation assay, chromosomal aberrations (CA) in CHO cells, and sister chromatid exchange (SCE) in CHO cells] in 4 different databases were compared (71). Factor analysis was used to model different pieces of information and permitted a quantitative scale which measured similarities and dissimilarities among assay performances. The Ames test and the CA test performed similarly while the SCE assay and the mouse lymphoma assay were similar in performance to each other.

Data from the Gene-Tox database and the RTECS database (Registry of Toxic Effects of Chemical Substances) were compared and evaluated for their ability to predict carcinogenic potency (72). Several models were used to estimate carcinogenic potency but there were no statistically significant differences between predictions of the different models and no statistically significant difference between the abilities of the two databases to predict carcinogenicity. Databases focusing primarily on mutagenicity appear inadequate in predicting a multistage process like carcinogenesis.

Guidelines for mutagenicity testing as revised by the Office of Toxic Substances and the Office of Pesticide Programs include 3 tests in the initial tier: the Salmonella assay, an in vitro mammalian gene mutation assay and an in vivo cytogenetics assay which may be either an assay for CA or micronuclei in bone marrow (73). If these tests indicate a mutagenicity concern, further tests should be conducted. Recommendations for protocol in the initial testing and for further testing as indicated were discussed.

A recent paper outlined the administrative arrangements for conducting risk assessments and the requirements for ascertaining whether a substances is "toxic" with respect to human health according to the Canadian Environmental Protection Act (74). To date, a health risk assessment of 2 priority compounds, polychlorinated dibenzodioxins and polychlorinated dibenzofurans, has been completed with both groups of compounds considered "toxic" on the basis of their effects in rodent assays and their levels in the environment.

Genotoxicity testing and data interpretation as applied in the Netherlands in the context of regulation of chemicals were discussed in a recent paper (75). Several aspects of short-term genotoxicity tests were considered including the following: their ability to predict carcinogenicity; the limited database on the performance of short-term in vivo assays; the relevance of devising separate strategies to test for carcinogenicity and for germ-cell mutagenicity; and the use of short-term tests to distinguish between genotoxic and non-genotoxic carcinogens. Examples were given of the use of these tests in the toxicological evaluation of chemicals in the Netherlands.

Different governments and agencies differ in their approaches to cancer risk assessment. While some governments (many in Europe) evaluate each chemical on a case-by-case basis and may not have standardized risk assessment procedures for regulatory decisions, other (such as the USA) consider all animal carcinogens to be presumptive human carcinogens regardless of available knowledge on mechanisms of carcinogenicity. The Netherlands does consider mechanisms of carcinogenicity in its regulatory decisions (76). An international expert panel has been convened to discuss these different approaches and attempt to reach some international consensus.

REPRODUCTIVE AND DEVELOPMENTAL TOXICITY

The protocol for Reproductive Assessment by Continuous Breeding (RACB), originally designed for use with mice has been modified for use with rats (77). During the second phase of RACB, mice were continually bred for a 14-week period, producing 5 litters of pups. There was some question as to whether rats would be able to produce 5 litters in rapid succession, but the Sprague-Dawley rats used here did so. The standard RACB design was modified slightly for the rats to allow greater time for gestation and delivery but otherwise the RACB protocol for rats was the same as that for mice so that comparable data could be obtained.

Behavioral tests are a required component of developmental toxicity studies submitted to some regulatory agencies. To aid in determining an optimal test battery for such effects, 12 pharmaceutical agents were tested in 2 or more of 28 Segment I, II, and/or III studies with Sprague-Dawley rats (*78*). Behavioral effects, as determined by lowest-observable-effect levels, occurred in each study design, and no one design appeared more likely to produce a behavioral effect than any other. A study design proposed by an international group of scientists appears to be optimal for testing behavioral effects. This study design includes the exposure periods of Segment II and III studies with specialized behavioral safety designs conducted, as needed, to identify dose–response relationships, critical periods, and the full manifestation of effects.

The frog embryo teratogenesis assay:*Xenopus* (FETAX) was evaluated for its ability to assess mixtures of toxicants (*79*). Nine combinations of developmental toxicants were tested at concentrations known to induce malformations. Concentration addition was observed for 3 combinations in which both chemicals were believed to act by the same teratogenic mechanism. Response additive joint action was observed for the other 6 combinations in which the chemicals had different modes of action. These results indicate that FETAX should be useful for mixture toxicity hazard assessment.

In order to evaluate *Drosophila* as a screening system for developmental toxicants, 32 chemicals were tested at 14 concentrations and all statistically significant defects were noted (*80*). From these data, two structural defects, a bent humeral bristle and a notch in the wing blade, were chosen as markers in a new bioassay procedure. These two defects showed a consistent dose–response in flies treated with a variety of toxicants, were not elicited by most presumed non-developmental toxicants, and were rare spontaneous occurrences. Using these two defects as criteria, 10 of 13 known developmental toxicants and 4 of 5 non-developmental toxicants were correctly identified. This assay may be

useful in screening chemicals for their potential developmental toxicity.

Responses of rat and chick limb bud micromass cultures to 8 chemicals of diverse structure, potency and mechanism were compared (*81*). Two endpoints were used: extractable alcian blue stain as a measure of differentiation to chondrocytes and extractable neutral red stain as an index of proliferation. Rat and chick responses to 3 of the chemicals were indistinguishable and were similar for the other chemicals. However, it was not possible to draw conclusions about the predictability of micromass cultures because none of the parameters proposed to define a positive result in this assay was completely satisfactory.

A modified submerged culture system was developed to study responses of embryonic palatal tissue from rats, mice, and humans to 5 teratogens (*82*). The tissues were cultured in serum-free medium in disposable flasks on a rocker platform with the culture medium changed daily. This assay system could distinguish between various mechanisms of clefting as produced by the different compounds. However, the tissues showed an increased responsiveness to some chemicals in the presence of serum, suggesting that an unknown factor in serum may be required for full activity.

A Dirichlet–trinomial distribution for modelling data from reproductive and developmental studies was presented (*83*). With current statistical methods, the effects of a treatment on the number of deaths and the effect on the number of malformations are analyzed separately. But this method allows for simultaneous analysis of multiple endpoints. Using a real data set on effects of hydroxyurea, this analysis procedure was compared with an analysis based on the beta-binomial model.

Statistical methods for analyzing developmental toxicity data were described and reviewed (*84*). The methods included distribution-free, nonparametric analyses and several models involving parametric distributions such as the beta-binomial density. For quantitative analyses, the litter should be considered as the experimental unit.

Although specific developmental and reproductive toxicity tests may be important in testing drugs and pesticides, it has been suggested that a simple acute toxicity test may be just as useful in predicting reproductive and developmental toxicity for other chemicals (*85*). A comparison of available acute toxicity information on a number of compounds, identified as potential human reproductive or developmental toxicants, with their respective likely human threshold doses indicated that most toxicants were a potential threat to humans only if exposure approached levels that were lethal to rats or mice. However, the human embryo is highly sensitive to some compounds, such as thalidomide, which exhibit a low toxicity in routine developmental toxicity tests.

NEUROTOXICITY AND BEHAVIORAL EFFECTS

Various approaches to determine neurotoxic effects were reviewed and discussed in a recent book edited by Tilson and Mitchell (*86*). Parameters such as morphological effects on cultured cells, neuronal proteins and brain neurochemistry, evoked potentials, motor function, sensory dysfunction, cognition, and developmental effects may be assessed to detect neurotoxicity. Risk assessment and detection of neurotoxicity in humans were also discussed.

Proceedings of the third meeting of the International Neurotoxicity Association held in 1991 in Italy were published in a 1992 issue of *Neurotoxicology* (*87*). Symposium topics included neurotoxicity in humans, developmental neurotoxicity, in vitro neurotoxicity tests, and neurobehavioral toxicity.

Role of toxicants in neurological disorders was the overall theme of papers presented at the 8th International Neurotoxicology Conference in 1990 and recently published in *Neurotoxicology* (*88*). Some neurotoxins may exert effects after a long latency and may be involved in central nervous system degeneration, cancer, and Parkinson's disease. The use of various animal models and in vitro and tissue culture methods in elucidating disease etiology was described and discussed.

Papers presented at a symposium on "Screening for Neurotoxicity" at the 1990 annual meeting of the American College of Toxicology reviewed several screening methods for assessing neurotoxicity (*89*). Use of these tests in evaluating regulated food chemicals and drugs was discussed.

Sagittal slices of rat brain were found to be a sensitive in vitro model for the toxic effects of acrylamide (*90*). Incubation of these brain slices under oxygen in artificial cerebrospinal fluid with acrylamide resulted in a dose- and time-dependent inhibition of several lysosomal enzymes and glyceraldehyde 3-phosphate dehydrogenase. Inhibition of lysosomal enzymes was also observed in vivo in the brain of rats dosed with acrylamide. This in vitro method may be useful in studying the mechanism of toxicity of a variety of neurotoxicants.

As a potential in vitro model for neurotoxicity, a method was developed for the culture of chick brain cells (embryonic day 7) in monolayer and in reaggregate cultures (*91*). Differentiation of nerve and glial cells was monitored with monoclonal antibodies against neurofilament protein (NF) and glial fibrillary acidic protein (GFAP). The expression of NF could be used as a sensitive cytotoxicity endpoint while GFAP expression could serve as an endpoint for monitoring differentiation.

A good deal of data are available in the literature describing the effects of lesions, in different areas of the brain, on behavior. Using such information on the effects of brain lesions in monkeys on reversal learning and delayed spatial learning, it was possible to suggest possible loci for neurotoxic effects of lead and PCBs (*92*). Symptoms produced by these toxins closely resembled the reported effects of lesions in the frontal cortex. Such correlations may be useful in identifying further tests which could aid in understanding the mechanism of neurotoxic effects of different neurotoxins. Although motor activity is an important measure of neurotoxicity, the effects of chemicals on motor activity may be influenced by other variables in the laboratory environment and apparatus. Therefore, an interlaboratory comparison of motor activity experiments in 6 laboratories was conducted to determine whether similar toxic effects were detected in laboratories using different experimental protocols and apparatus (*93*). Analyses indicated that there was a relatively restricted range of within-laboratory variability and reliability in control values and that these ranges were comparable for the different laboratories. In nearly every case, all laboratories were capable of detecting qualitatively similar changes in motor activity following acute exposure to a variety of chemicals.

The Neurobehavioral Evaluation System (NES) is a widely used battery of tests including perceptual–motor, memory, learning, attention, and reaction time tests. To examine the reliability of 11 tests and a mood rating scale contained in NES, these tests were administered to 66 subjects on two testing days separated by at least 7 days (*94*). Results indicated that all but the learning–memory test are satisfactory for comparing group performance in laboratory studies. For the assessment of complex perceptual–motor performance both the symbol–digit substitution and pattern comparison tests are reliable, while for assessment of response speed and attention, the CPT and switching attention tests were the most reliable. Since the number of subjects was not large and all were young, well-educated males, the authors urge some caution in interpreting these results.

IMMUNOTOXICITY

In a recent book various topics related to clinical immunotoxicology were reviewed and discussed (*95*). These included basic principles of immunotoxicology (including methods for assessment of toxicity), models of immunotoxic mechanisms, and environmental and occupational immunotoxins, including dioxin, organophosphorus compounds, and some metals.

Some xenobiotic compounds are potent suppressors of the in vitro primary humoral response of murine splenocytes. Experiments with human tonsillar lymphocytes indicate that they may also be used in evaluating the direct immunotoxic potential of some antibiotics (*96*). Both human and murine lymphocytes responded similarly to acetoxydimethylnitrosamine and to acrolein as seen by the dose-dependent inhibition of pokeweed mitogen–induced cell proliferation and Ig(M+A+G) response

caused by similar concentrations of the toxins. Dioxin did not exert these effects on either splenocyte type but did have some other toxic effects on murine, but not human, splenocytes.

A screening battery of assays to detect immunotoxicity has been used during the past 10 years to investigate 51 selected compounds. Data from these studies has been analyzed to determine the ability of each test and of test combinations to detect immunotoxic compounds (*97*). Results indicated that only 2 or 3 immune tests are sufficient to predict immunotoxicity in rodents. The tests most highly correlated with immunotoxicity were the splenic antibody plaque forming cell response (78%) and cell surface marker analysis (83%). Potential immunotoxic compounds were also likely to be rodent carcinogens but no relationship was observed between immunotoxicity and mutagenicity in in vitro genotoxicity tests.

LITERATURE CITED

1. Finley, J.W., S.F. Robinson, and D.J. Armstrong. *Food Safety Assessment.* Washington, D.C., American Chemical Society. *ACS Symp. Ser.* 484 (1992).

2. Friedman, M. *Nutritional and Toxicological Consequences of Food Processing.* New York, Plenum Pub. Corp. *Adv. Exp. Med. Biol.* 289 (1991).

3. Caswell, J.A. *Economics of Food Safety.* New York, Elsevier Sci. Pub. Co., Inc. (1991).

4. Labuza, T.P., and W. Baisier. The role of the federal government in food safety. *Crit. Rev. Food Sci. Nutr.* 31:165–176 (1992).

5. Thonney, P.F., and C.A. Bisogni. Government regulation of food safety: interaction of scientific and societal forces. *Food Technol.* 46(1):73–80 (1992).

6. Gledhill, B.L., and F. Mauro. *New Horizons in Biological Dosimetry.* New York, Wiley–Liss (1991).

7. Spilker, B. Extrapolation of safety (i.e., toxicological) data from animals to humans. In *Guide to Clinical Trials.* New York, Raven Press, Chap. 88, pp. 675–683 (1991).

8. Edler, L. Statistical methods for short-term tests in genetic toxicology: the first fifteen years. *Mutat. Res.* 277:11–33 (1992).

9. Yam, J., P.J. Reer, and R.D. Bruce. Comparison of the up-and-down method and the fixed-dose procedure for acute oral toxicity testing. *Food Chem. Toxicol.* 29:259–263 (1991).

10. Jover, R., X. Ponsoda, J.V. Castell, and M.J. Gómez-Lechón. Evaluation of the cytotoxicity of ten chemicals on human cultured hepatocytes: predictability of human toxicity and comparison with rodent cell culture systems. *Toxicol. in vitro* 6:47–52 (1992).

11. Multiple authors. *QSAR in Environmental Toxicology.* Proceedings of the Fourth International Workshop, Veldhoven, Netherlands, 16–20 September 1990. *Sci. Total Environ.* Vol. 109 and 110 (1991).

12. Debnath, A.K., G. Debnath, A.J. Shusterman, and C. Hansch. A QSAR investigation of the role of hydrophobicity in regulating mutagenicity in the Ames test: 1. Mutagenicity of aromatic and heteroaromatic amines in *Salmonella typhimurium* TA98 and TA100. *Environ. Molec. Mutagen.* 19:37–52 (1992).

13. Debnath, A.K., R.L. Lopez de Compadre, A.J. Shusterman, and C. Hansch. Quantitative structure–activity relationship investigation of the role of hydrophobicity in regulating mutagenicity in the Ames test: 2. Mutagenicity of aromatic and heteroaromatic nitro compounds in *Salmonella typhimurium* TA100. *Environ. Molec. Mutagen.* 19:53–70 (1992).

14. Rannug, U., M. Sjögren, A. Rannug, et al. Use of artificial intelligence in structure–affinity correlations of 2,3,7,8-tetrachlorodibenzo-*p*-dioxin (TCDD) receptor ligands. *Carcinogenesis* 12:2007–2015 (1991).

15. Rosenkranz, H.S., Y.P. Zhang, and G. Klopman. Implications of newly recognized relationships between mutagenicity, genotoxicity and carcinogenicity of molecules. *Mutat. Res.* 250:25–33 (1991).

16. Benigni, R. QSAR prediction of rodent carcinogenicity for a set of chemicals currently bioassayed by the US National Toxicology Program. *Mutagenesis* 6:423–425 (1991).

17. Bakale, G., and R.D. McCreary. Prospective k_e screening of potential carcinogens being tested in rodent bioassays by the US National Toxicology Program. *Mutagenesis* 7:91–94 (1992).

18. von der Hude, W., S. Carstensen, and G. Obe. Structure–activity relationships of epoxides: induction of sister-chromatid exchanges in Chinese hamster V79 cells. *Mutat. Res.* 249:55–70 (1991).

19. Claxton, L.D., V.S. Houk, J.C. Allison, and J. Creason. Evaluating the relationship of metabolic activation system concentrations and chemical dose concentrations for the Salmonella spiral and plate assays. *Mutat. Res.* 253:127–136 (1991).

20. Trottier, Y., W.I. Waithe, and A. Anderson. The detection of promutagen activation by extracts of cells expressing cytochrome P450IA2 cDNA: preincubation dramatically increases revertant yield in the Ames test. *Mutat. Res.* 281:39–45 (1992).

21. Claxton, L.D., V.S. Houk, L.G. Monteith, et al. Assessing the use of known mutagens to calibrate the *Salmonella typhimurium* mutagenicity assay: I. Without exogenous activation. *Mutat. Res.* 253:137–147 (1991).

22. Claxton, L.D., V.S. Houk, J.R. Warner, et al. Assessing the use of known mutagens to calibrate the *Salmonella typhimurium* mutagenicity assay: II. With exogenous activation. *Mutat. Res.* 253:149–159 (1991).

23. Zeiger, E., B. Anderson, S. Haworth, et al. Salmonella mutagenicity tests: V. Results from the testing of 311 chemicals. *Environ. Molec. Mutagen.* 19(Suppl. 21):2–14 (1992).

24. Bonneau, D., V. Thybaud, C. Melcion, et al. Optimum associations of tester strains for maximum detection of mutagenic compounds in the Ames test. *Mutat. Res.* 252:269–279 (1991).

25. Rossman, T.G., M. Molina, L. Meyer, et al. Performance of 133 compounds in the lambda prophage induction endpoint of the Microscreen assay and a comparison with *S. typhimurium* mutagenicity and rodent carcinogenicity assays. *Mutat. Res.* 260:349–367 (1991).

26. Würgler, F.E. Effects of chemical and physical agents on recombination events in cells of the germ line of male and female *Drosophila melanogaster. Mutat. Res.* 250:275–290 (1991).

27. Batiste-Alentorn, M., N. Xamena, A. Creus, and R. Marcos. Genotoxicity studies with the unstable *zeste-white* (UZ) system of *Drosophila melanogaster*: results with ten carcinogenic compounds. *Environ. Molec. Mutagen.* 18:120–125 (1991).

28. Mattioli, F., L. Robbiano, F.P. Mattioli, and G. Brambilla. Use of human thyroid cell primary cultures for genotoxicity studies. *Toxicol. in vitro* 6:149–153 (1992).

29. Heddle, J.A., M.C. Cimino, M. Hayashi, et al. Micronuclei as an index of cytogenetic damage: past,

present, and future. *Environ. Molec. Mutagen.* 18:277–291 (1991).

30. Oshiro, Y., C.E. Piper, P.S. Balwierz, and S.G. Soelter. Chinese hamster ovary cell assays for mutation and chromosome damage: data from noncarcinogens. *J. Appl. Toxicol.* 11:167–177 (1991).

31. Gill, R.D., B.E. Butterworth, A.N. Nettikumara, and J. DiGiovanni. Relationship between DNA adduct formation and unscheduled DNA synthesis (UDS) in cultured mouse epidermal keratinocytes. *Environ. Molec. Mutagen.* 18:200–206 (1991).

32. Natarajan, A.T., and F. Darroudi. Use of human hepatoma cells for *in vitro* metabolic activation of chemical mutagens/carcinogens. *Mutagenesis* 6:399–403 (1991).

33. Turchi, G., A. Nardone, and F. Palitti. Application of an epithelial liver cell line, metabolically competent, for mutation studies of promutagens. *Mutat. Res.* 271:79–88 (1992).

34. Voss, J.-U., and H. Seibert. Microcarrier-attached rat hepatocytes as a xenobiotic-metabolizing system in cocultures. *Cell Biol. Toxicol.* 7:387–399 (1991).

35. Sawada, M., R. Kitamura, and T. Kamataki. Stable expression of monkey cytochrome P-450IA1 cDNA in Chinese hamster CHL cells and its application for detection of mutagenicity of aflatoxin B_1. *Mutat. Res.* 265:23–29 (1992).

36. Ellard, S., Y. Mohammed, S. Dogra, et al. The use of genetically engineered V79 Chinese hamster cultures expressing rat liver *CYP1A1, 1A2* and *2B1* cDNAs in micronucleus assays. *Mutagenesis* 6:461–470 (1991).

37. Polack, A., G. Laux, M. Hergenhahn, et al. Short-term assays for detection of conditional cancerogens I. Construction of DR-CAT Raji cells and some of their characteristics as tester cells. *Int. J. Cancer* 50:611–616 (1992).

38. International Commission for Protection against Environmental Mutagens and Carcinogens (ICPEMC). *A Method for Combining and Comparing Short-term Genotoxicity Test Data. Mutat. Res.* 266:1-60 (1992).

39. Murphy, S.A., R.R. Tice, M.G. Smith, and B.H. Margolin. Contributions to the design and statistical analysis of in vivo SCE experiments. *Mutat. Res.* 271:39–48 (1992).

40. Simula, A.P., and B.G. Priestly. Influence of vegetable oil vehicles on bone-marrow proliferation in the mouse micronucleus test. *Mutat. Res.* 261:83–84 (1991).

41. Organizing Committee of CSGMT/JEMS-MMS. *Micronucleus Test with Rodent Peripheral Blood Reticulocytes by Acridine Orange Supravital Staining. Mutat. Res.* 278:81–208 (1992).

42. Miller, B.M., and I.-D. Adler. Aneuploidy induction in mouse spermatocytes. *Mutagenesis* 7:69–76 (1992).

43. Kitchin, K.T., J.L. Brown, and A.P. Kulkarni. Predictive assay for rodent carcinogenicity using in vivo biochemical parameters: operational characteristics and complementarity. *Mutat. Res.* 266:253–272 (1992).

44. Myhr, B.C. Validation studies with Muta™Mouse: A transgenic mouse model for detecting mutations in vivo. *Environ. Molec. Mutagen.* 18:308–315 (1991).

45. Kohler, S.W., G.S. Provost, A. Fieck, et al. Analysis of spontaneous and induced mutations in transgenic mice using a lambda ZAP/*lacI* shuttle vector. *Environ. Molec. Mutagen.* 18:316–321 (1991).

46. Multiple authors. *Early Indicators of Nongenotoxic Carcinogenesis.* Proceedings of the Joint ECTOC/IPCS Workshop. Brussels, 1990. *Mutat. Res.* 248:211–374 (1991).

47. Amanuma, T., K. Mizumoto, M. Tsutsumi, et al. Initiating activity of diethylnitrosamine in a rapid production model for pancreatic carcinomas in Syrian hamsters. *Jpn. J. Cancer Res.* 82:632–637 (1991).

48. Fukushima, S., A. Kagiwara, M. Hirose, et al. Modifying effects of various chemicals on preneoplastic and neoplastic lesion development in a wide-spectrum organ carcinogenesis model using F344 rats. *Jpn. J. Cancer Res.* 82:642–649 (1991).

49. Uwagawa, S., H. Tsuda, T. Inoue, et al. Enhancing potential of 5 different carcinogens on multiorgan tumorigenesis after initial treatment with N-methyl-N-nitrosourea in rats. *Jpn. J. Cancer Res.* 82:1397–1405 (1991).

50. Gold, L.S., T.H. Slone, N.B. Manley, and L. Berstein. Target organs in chronic bioassays of 533 chemical carcinogens. *Environ. Health Perspect.* 93:233–246 (1991).

51. Huff, J., J. Cirvello, J. Haseman, and J. Bucher. Chemicals associated with site-specific neoplasia in 1394 long-term carcinogenesis experiments in

laboratory rodents. *Environ. Health Perspect.* 93:247–270 (1991).

52. McLellan, E.A., A. Medline, and R.P. Bird. Sequential analyses of the growth and morphological characteristics of aberrant crypt foci: putative preneoplastic lesions. *Cancer Res.* 51:5270–5274 (1991).

53. Fullerton, F.R., D.L. Greenman, and T.J. Bucci. Effects of diet type on incidence of spontaneous and 2-acetylaminofluorene-induced liver and bladder tumors in BALB/c mice fed AIN-76A diet versus NIH-07 diet. *Fund. Appl. Toxicol.* 18:193–199 (1992).

54. Carr, C.J., and A.C. Kolbye, Jr. A critique of the use of the maximum tolerated dose in bioassays to assess cancer risks from chemicals. *Reg. Toxicol. Pharmacol.* 14:78–87 (1991).

55. Pariza, M.W. A new approach to evaluating carcinogenic risk. *Proc. Natl. Acad. Sci. USA* 89:860–861 (1992).

56. Santella, R.M. DNA adducts in humans as biomarkers of exposure to environmental and occupational carcinogens. *Environ. Carcinogen. Ecotoxicol. Rev.* C9:57–81 (1991).

57. Jankowiak, R., P. Lu, G.J. Small, et al. Fluorescence line-narrowing spectrometry: a versatile tool for the study of chemically initiated carcinogenesis. *J. Pharm. Biomed. Anal.* 8:113–121 (1990).

58. Puisieux, A., S. Lim, J. Groopman, and M. Ozturk. Selective targeting of *p53* gene mutational hotspots in human cancers by etiologically defined carcinogens. *Cancer Res.* 51:6185–6189 (1991).

59. Xue, K.-X., G.-J. Ma, S. Wang, and P. Zhou. The in vivo micronucleus test in human capillary blood lymphocytes: methodological studies and effect of ageing. *Mutat. Res.* 278:259–264 (1992).

60. Snyder, C.A., and C.D. Valle. Lymphocyte proliferation assays as potential biomarkers for toxicant exposures. *J. Toxicol. Environ. Health* 34:127–139 (1991).

61. Anderson, D., A.J. Francis, P. Godbert, et al. Chromosome aberrations (CA), sister-chromatid exchanges (SCE) and mitogen-induced blastogenesis in cultured peripheral lymphocytes from 48 control individuals sampled 8 times over 2 years. *Mutat. Res.* 250:467–476 (1991).

62. Wiencke, J.K., M.R. Wrensch, R. Miike, and N.L. Petrakis. Individual susceptibility to induced chromosome damage and its implications for detecting genotoxic exposures in human populations. *Cancer Res.* 51:5266–5269 (1991).

63. Pariza, M.W. Risk assessment. *Crit. Rev. Food Sci. Nutr.* 31:205–209 (1992).

64. Multiple authors. Databases of genotoxicity and carcinogenicity and their usefulness for hazard evaluation. *Environ. Health Perspect.* 96:3-112 (1991).

65. Arcos, J., M. Argus, and Y. Woo, eds. *Approach to a Consensus for the Basis of Regulation of Environmental Chemicals. J. Environ. Sci. Health* C8(2) (1990–91).

66. Adeshina, F., and E.L. Todd. Application of biological data in cancer risk estimations of chlordane and heptachlor. *Reg. Toxicol. Pharmacol.* 14:59–77 (1991).

67. Shore, R.E., V. Iyer, B. Altshuler, and B.S. Pasternack. Use of human data in quantitative risk assessment of carcinogens: Impact on epidemiologic practice and the regulatory process. *Reg. Toxicol. Pharmacol.* 15:180–221 (1992).

68. Goodman, G., and R. Wilson. Predicting the carcinogenicity of chemicals in humans from rodent bioassay data. *Environ. Health Perspect.* 94:195–218 (1991).

69. Goodman, G., and R. Wilson. Quantitative prediction of human cancer risk from rodent carcinogenic potencies: A closer look at the epidemiological evidence for some chemicals not definitively carcinogenic in humans. *Reg. Toxicol. Pharmacol.* 14:118–146 (1991).

70. Li, A.P., C.S. Aaron, A.E. Auletta, et al. An evaluation of the roles of mammalian cell mutation assays in the testing of chemical genotoxicity. *Reg. Toxicol. Pharmacol.* 14:24–40 (1991).

71. Benigni, R., and A. Guiliani. Simultaneous evaluation of genotoxicity data from different sources: a multivariate statistical approach. *Mutat. Res.* 266:71–76 (1992).

72. Travis, C.C., L.A. Wang, and J.M. Morris. Comparison of the Gene-Tox and RTECS data bases as predictors of carcinogenic potency. *Mutat. Res.* 279:261–268 (1992).

73. Dearfield, K.L., A.E. Auletta, M.C. Cimino, and M.M. Moore. Considerations in the U.S. Environmental Protection Agency's testing approach for mutagenicity. *Mutat. Res.* 258:259–283 (1991).

74. Armstrong, V.C., and R.C. Newhook. Assessing the health risks of priority substances under the

Canadian Environmental Protection Act. *Reg. Toxicol. Pharmacol.* 15:111–121 (1992).

75. Kramers, P.G.N., A.G.A.C. Knaap, C.A. van der Heijden, et al. Role of genotoxicity assays in the regulation of chemicals in The Netherlands: considerations and experiences. *Mutagenesis* 6:487–493 (1991).

76. Whysner, J., and G.M. Williams. International cancer risk assessment: the impact of biologic mechanisms. *Reg. Toxicol. Pharmacol.* 15:41–50 (1992).

77. Gulati, D.K., E. Hope, J. Teague, and R.E. Chapin. Reproductive toxicity assessment by continuous breeding in Sprague-Dawley rats: a comparison of two study designs. *Fund. Appl. Toxicol.* 17:270–279 (1991).

78. Lochry, E.A., and M.S. Christian. Behavioral evaluations in reproductive safety assessments. *J. Am. Coll. Toxicol.* 10:585–591 (1991).

79. Dawson, D.A., and T.S. Wilke. Evaluation of the frog embryo teratogenesis assay:*Xenopus* (FETAX) as a model system for mixture toxicity hazard assessment. *Environ. Toxicol. Chem.* 10:941–948 (1991).

80. Lynch, D.W., R.L. Schuler, R.D. Hood, and D.G. Davis. Evaluation of *Drosophila* for screening developmental toxicants: Test results with eighteen chemicals and presentation of a new *Drosophila* bioassay. *Teratogen. Carcinogen. Mutagen.* 11:147–173 (1991).

81. Brown, N.A., and R. Wiger. Comparison of rat and chick limb bud micromass cultures for developmental toxicity screening. *Toxicol. in vitro* 6:101–107 (1992).

82. Abbott, B.D., and A.R. Buckalew. Embryonic palatal responses to teratogens in serum-free organ culture. *Teratology* 45:369–382 (1992).

83. Chen, J.J., R.L. Kodell, R.B. Howe, and D.W. Gaylor. Analysis of trinomial responses from reproductive and developmental toxicity experiments. *Biometrics* 47:1049–1058 (1991).

84. Piergorsch, W.W., and J.K. Haseman. Statistical methods for analyzing developmental toxicity data. *Teratogen. Carcinogen. Mutagen.* 11:115–133 (1991).

85. Marks, T.A. A retrospective appraisal of the ability of animal tests to predict reproductive and developmental toxicity in humans. *J. Am. Coll. Toxicol.* 10:569–584 (1991).

86. Tilson, H.A., and C.L. Mitchell, eds. *Neurotoxicology.* New York, Raven Press (1992).

87. Multiple authors. Proceedings of the Third Meeting of the International Neurotoxicity Association. *Neurotoxicology* 13(1) (1992).

88. Multiple authors. *Role of Toxicants in Neurological Disorders.* Proceedings of the Eighth International Neurotoxicology Conference, Little Rock, Arkansas, October 1–4, 1990. *Neurotoxicology* 12(3) (1991).

89. Multiple authors. Symposium Proceedings: Screening for Neurotoxicity II—The Eleventh Annual Meeting of the American College of Toxicology, 30 October 1990, Orlando, FL. *J. Am. Coll. Toxicol.* 10(6):661–732 (1991).

90. Ravindranath, V., and K. S. Pai. The use of rat brain slices as an *in vitro* model for mechanistic evaluation of neurotoxicity-studies with acrylamide. *Neurotoxicology* 12:225–234 (1991).

91. Wyle-Gyurech, G.G., and C.A. Reinhardt. Differentiation of embryonic chick brain cells in monolayer and reaggregate cultures: a potential model *in vitro* for neurotoxicity. *Toxicol. in vitro* 5:419–425 (1991).

92. Levin, E.D., S.L. Schantz, and R.E. Bowman. Use of the lesion model for examining toxicant effects on cognitive behavior. *Neurotoxicol. Teratol.* 14:131–141 (1992).

93. Crofton, K.M., J.L. Howard, V.C. Moser, et al. Interlaboratory comparison of motor activity experiments: implications for neurotoxicological assessments. *Neurotoxicol. Teratol.* 13:599–609 (1991).

94. Arcia, E., and D.A. Otto. Reliability of selected tests from the neurobehavioral evaluation system. *Neurotoxicol. Teratol.* 14:103–110 (1992).

95. Newcombe, D.S., N.R. Rose, and J.C. Blom, eds. *Clinical Immunotoxicology.* New York, Raven Press (1992).

96. Wood, S.C., J.G. Karras, and M.P. Holsapple. Integration of the human lymphocyte into immunotoxicological investigations. *Fund. Appl. Toxicol.* 18:450–459 (1992).

97. Luster, M.I., C. Portier, D.G. Pait, et al. Risk assessment in immunotoxicology. I. Sensitivity and predictability of immune tests. *Fund. Appl. Toxicol.* 18:200–210 (1992).

Intentional (Direct) Additives

Preservatives
Nitrate, nitrite, and N-nitroso compounds
Food preservation by irradiation
Antioxidants
Sweeteners
Flavors and flavor enhancers
Food colors
Vitamins
Stabilizers, thickeners, and conditioners
Fat substitutes
Other additives

One method used to assess whether there is a significant possibility that consumers will be exposed to excessive amounts of food additives is the Danish Budget Method: if the daily amount of food and drink consumed contains no more of the additive than its ADI (acceptable daily intake), then consumers should be protected from overexposure to the additive. In a recent paper the potential applications, the versatility, and some inherent limitations of the Budget Method were discussed (1). Basic assumptions underlying the method were reassessed and additional correction factors were considered. Using calculations on intense sweeteners as an example, the usefulness of the Budget Method in distinguishing between additives which are unlikely to be consumed in excess from those which deserve closer scrutiny was illustrated. Finally, appropriate and inappropriate uses of the Budget Method were described.

PRESERVATIVES

Sulfiting agents

An estimated 5–10% of asthmatics have adverse reactions to sulfites, with steroid-dependent asthmatics being at greater risk for acute asthma attacks following sulfite ingestion. A recent review described such reactions and discussed estimates of prevalence, methods for accurate diagnosis of sulfite sensitivity, and proposed mechanisms to account for such reactions (2). As yet no one single mechanism has been identified to account for sulfite reactions, and even sulfite-sensitive individuals do not react to the ingestion of all sulfited foods equivalently.

Allergic sheep were used to investigate possible mechanisms of metabisulfite(MBS)-induced bronchoconstriction (3). Lung resistance was found to increase significantly in a dose-dependent manner when the sheep inhaled aerosols containing 25, 50, and 100 mg MBS/mL. Pretreatment with an anticholinergic reagent (ipratropium bromide), an antiasthma drug (nedocromil), or the bradykinin B_2-receptor antagonist, NPC-567,

blocked the MBS-induced bronchoconstriction. However, the histamine H_1-receptor antagonist, chlorpheniramine, did not prevent this reaction to MBS. Thus, it appears that in allergic sheep, inhalation of MBS stimulates bradykinin B_2-receptors with subsequent activation of cholinergic mechanisms leading to bronchoconstriction.

Although sulfiting agents are not permitted in meat and meat derivatives in the USA, Spain and other European countries do allow the use of sulfites in the manufacture of fresh sausages. An improved method of extraction of free and total sulfites from sausage, involving the use of a sodium phosphate buffer, pH 10, containing 1 mL glycerol/L, has been used to obtain recoveries averaging 86.4% (range 77–97%) (4). Following extraction, samples were analyzed by HPLC with electrochemical detection. In reproducibility assays, coefficients of variation of 3.3 and 5% were obtained for free and total sulfites, respectively. Analyses of 48 samples of fresh sausage using this technique revealed that 62% had total sulfite levels >450 µg SO_2/g, the level permitted by Spanish law.

Total sulfite in commercially available thixotropic materials based on methylcellulose and hydroxypropylmethylcellulose was determined by ion exclusion chromatography with electrochemical detection (5). Sulfite was extracted by dissolving the materials in 5% sodium sulfate, and then bound sulfite was released by adjusting the pH to 11.0. Samples were applied to an Aminex HPX-87H ion exclusion column and sulfite was detected by oxidation at a platinum electrode maintained at 600 mV. Mean sulfite recovery from samples spiked at 10–50 ppm was 91%. Aldehydes did not interfere with the analyses at concentrations <100-fold excess.

An enzyme electrode using the enzyme sulfite oxidase immobilized onto pig intestine was developed for the determination of sulfite in foods and feeds (6). Glutaraldehyde bovine serum albumin was used to immobilize the enzyme. Various parameters such as temperature, pH, and buffer composition were optimized and sulfite was quantitated by monitoring amperometrically the production of hydrogen peroxide. A linear response was obtained in the range of 5.2×10^{-6} to 1.0×10^{-3} M.

This assay was sensitive and gave reproducible results and will be further evaluated in analyses of foods and feeds.

Two automated methods have been described for the determination of sulfur dioxide in wine. In one method the characteristic UV absorption bands of sulfur dioxide were measured by gas-phase molecular absorption spectrometry (*7*). Sulfur dioxide was released from white wine samples by reaction with NaOH and then its absorbance was determined as it passed into a flow-through absorption cell in an atomic absorption spectrometer. This method has a detection limit of 0.2 µg/mL and the calibration graph was linear up to 120 µg/mL. Samples could be analyzed at the rate of 20/hour.

In another approach with the same sample output rate, sulfur dioxide in wine was determined by flow injection analysis and gas diffusion (*8*). Wine samples were hydrolyzed to release bound sulfite and then a gas-permeable membrane was used for a preliminary separation to allow analyses of any color of wine. Sulfur dioxide was reacted with *p*-aminoazobenzene and formaldehyde in an acid medium and the products were monitored colorimetrically. Determination limits were 2 ppm for total sulfur dioxide and 0.2 ppm for free sulfur dioxide.

Organic acids

A 19-year-old Belgian female reportedly experienced a severe anaphylactic reaction following ingestion of beef, chipped potatoes, and mustard sauce (*9*). About 1 week previously she had generalized itching after eating cheese. The principal food preservative in both the cheese and the mustard was sodium benzoate. During several weeks on a diet without this preservative, she remained symptom-free. An oral challenge with 20 mg sodium benzoate induced localized urticaria and generalized itching. A thorough physical examination revealed that the patient had an unsuspected acute left maxillary sinusitis. Following treatment with antibiotics and local therapy, a second oral challenge indicated a higher tolerance to sodium benzoate than before (only localized itching after ingestion of 120 mg).

Since traces of benzene, possibly arising from added benzoate, have been detected in some drinks, 97 samples of various fruits, juices, and drinks were surveyed for traces of benzene (*10*). Headspace sampling with analysis by GC/MS enabled detection with confirmation of benzene levels as low as 0.03 µg/kg. With selected ion monitoring the detection limit was 0.02 µg/kg. Benzene was detected at levels ranging from 0.018 in a fruit juice to 3.83 µg/kg in a soft drink labeled to contain benzoate. Benzene at 1.81 µg/kg was present in a cranberry drink with no declared benzoate. Average benzene levels in juices and in soft drinks labeled to contain benzoate (0.672 and 0.793 µg/kg, respectively) were about 12 times higher than levels in similar products without added benzoate. Non-carbonated drinks with and without benzoate contained averages of 0.395 and 0.116 µg/kg, respectively. Since all of these concentrations were much lower than the Canadian and EPA guideline of 5 µg/kg, they are not considered to pose a health hazard.

Four food additives (benzoic, sorbic, propionic and caprylic acids) were successfully determined by ion-paired capillary electrophoresis with on-column UV detection at 190 nm (*11*). The concentration of tetrabutyl ammonium hydrogen sulfate was optimized to ensure the best migration of the solutes. Detection limits were 200 pg for propionic and caprylic acids, 100 pg for sorbic acid, and 20 pg for benzoic acid. This method was applied to the determination of benzoic acid in oyster sauce.

Simultaneous determination of sorbic, dehydroacetic, and benzoic acids was achieved by GC/MS utilizing chemical ionization (*12*). Samples of commercially available cheese, jam, juice, and cuttlefish were treated with NaCl solution and then sulfuric acid. Preservatives were extracted with ether and then injected into the system. Minimum detectable amounts of the 3 compounds were 200–500 pg. The chemical ionization mass fragmentographic method was about 10-fold more sensitive than the electron impact method. Neither the solvent peak nor other contaminants interfered with determination of these preservatives.

Sorbic acid and potassium sorbate tested negative in a variety of in vivo and in vitro genotoxicity assays (*13*). Oral administration of sorbic acid to mice at doses up to 5 g/kg body weight failed to induce sister chromatid exchanges or micronuclei in bone marrow cells. This compound also did not induce unscheduled DNA synthesis in cultured human A549 cells. Potassium sorbate did not cause significant effects in the alkaline elution assay with DNA either in vivo with rats or in vitro. In contrast to these two compounds, sodium sorbate was very sensitive to oxidative degradation and the main product of this degradation was mutagenic in the Ames test.

In a short-term assay (7 days), administration of diets containing 4% propionic or butyric acid to rats, mice, and hamsters resulted in damage and cellular proliferation in the epithelium of the forestomach of all 3 species (*14*). Rats appeared to be the most sensitive species and butyric acid was the more potent compound. It is suggested that long-term feeding of these compounds may cause a cycle of continued damage and repair eventually resulting in tumor formation.

Three reports of a petroleum-like aroma or an obnoxious odor in chikuwa (a kind of Japanese fish paste) led to an investigation of the preparation and handling of this product (*15*). The unusual odor was identified by GC as styrene but no styrene was detected in the packaging material for the chikuwa. The food was found to be contaminated with a yeast, *Pichia carsonii*, at a level of 5.4×10^6 cfu/g, and this same yeast was an environmental contaminant in the food processing plant. This yeast proved to be capable of producing styrene from cinnamic acid, which was an antimicrobial ingredient of the fish paste.

NITRATE, NITRITE, AND *N*-NITROSO COMPOUNDS

Nitrate and nitrite in foods

Nitrite and nitrate levels were measured by a colorimetric method and by a specific ion electrode method, respectively, in commercially processed and home processed spinach and beets (*16*). Nitrate and nitrite levels in home frozen spinach were lower but not significantly different from those in comparable commercially frozen products. However, nitrate levels in home canned beets were significantly higher than those in commercially canned products. During the home canning process, the cooking water for beets was then used for the canning liquid, and this water most likely had a high concentration of nitrate released from the beets during cooking. During commercial canning, fresh water is used for the canning liquid. Commercially produced pickled and Harvard beets had significantly lower nitrate/nitrite levels than other processed beets, presumably due to the diluting effects of added sugar.

An HPLC method and an enzymatic method were compared for the determination of nitrate in a variety of fruits, vegetables, and wines (*17*). With nitrate levels in the range of 5–80 mg/L, results from both assays were comparable and reproducible. At concentrations below 5 mg/L, the enzymatic method gave more reliable results.

Compared to an HPLC method, the cadmium reduction–Griess method (Cd–Griess) was found to consistently underestimate the concentration of nitrate in fresh and cured meats (*18*). Analyses of 5 samples of fresh and 3 samples of cured meats by HPLC revealed nitrate levels of 6.2–26.7 nmol/g and 124–3018 nmol/g, respectively. Corresponding values obtained by Cd–Griess were 0–17.2 nmol/g and 9.4–941 nmol/g, respectively. Recovery of nitrate added to chicken breast was 80.1% for HPLC and 31.1% for Cd–Griess.

Effects of storage temperature, initial sodium nitrite levels, and smoking on the levels of nitrite in herring and trout were measured during storage up to 28 days (*19*). Fish fillets were treated for 15 min with sodium nitrite solutions of 5–20% and then stored at −30°C or at +7°C. Nitrite levels were found to decrease slightly in frozen samples but decreased significantly during storage at refrigeration temperatures. The reduction depended on the salt concentration of the brine, the pretreatment of the sample, and the freshness of the fish. Smoking reduced nitrite levels by half while storage at +4°C further decreased nitrite concentrations.

There has been some concern that high nitrate levels in drinking water will lead to high nitrate levels in milk from cows consuming this water. During a 10-month period in France, nitrate levels were monitored in drinking water from 4 sources and in associated cow's milk (*20*). Average nitrate levels in the water sources were 9.3, 30.8, 64.3 and 135.2 mg/L and corresponding levels in milk were 1.19, 1.32, 1.31, and 1.64 mg/L. Thus, nitrate levels in milk remained low despite very high levels in some water sources.

Several photometric analytical methods for the determination of nitrate in milk were discussed and an automated method using a flow stream analyzer, ADM 300, was proposed as a convenient and reliable method (*21*). High nitrate concentrations (3.2 and 5.6 mg/L) were detected in the milk of two cows 2 h after dosing with 5 or 10 g sodium nitrate/kg live weight. This excess nitrate was rapidly cleared from the animals and by 24 h milk nitrate levels had decreased to normal levels (about 1 mg/L).

Results of an inter-laboratory study on the precision of the xylenol method for the determination of nitrate in milk products were presented (*22*). Samples tested were milk powder (12 mg nitrate/kg), whey powder (106 mg/kg), and freeze-dried cheese (8 mg/kg and 92 mg/kg). Repeatability varied from 2 to 9 mg/kg and reproducibility varied from 4 to 23 mg/kg.

Biological effects of nitrate and nitrite

To assess the genotoxic risk to humans of consumption of nitrate-contaminated drinking water, peripheral lymphocytes of 78 Dutch women exposed to different nitrate levels in drinking water were examined (*23*). The women were grouped according to low (0.13 mg nitrate/L drinking water), medium (32 mg/L), and high (average of 133.5 mg/L) exposure and were also questioned about any other dietary or medicinal sources of nitrate, cigarette smoking, and alcohol consumption. Women in the high-exposure group excreted more urinary nitrogen but there was no significant difference among the groups in the frequencies of sister chromatid exchanges in peripheral lymphocytes. Only cigarette smoking was associated with a small but significant increase in chromosomal damage.

Effects of subchronic poisoning with potassium nitrate and sodium nitrite on the intestinal absorption of D-xylose were studied in rats given daily doses of 5 or 10 mg sodium nitrite/kg body weight or 50 or 100 mg potassium nitrate/kg (*24*). Exposure to nitrite, but not to nitrate, reduced the absorption of xylose and decreased the activity of Na^+/K^+-ATPase and of alkaline phosphatase. Lactic acid levels in the nitrite-treated rats were higher than in controls.

Endogenous nitrosation

Fecal concentrations of apparent total *N*-nitroso compounds (ATNC) in 14 subjects consuming their normal free-choice diet ranged from 40 to 590 mg (N-NO)/kg feces (*25*). Wide variations in fecal and urinary ATNC were also observed in a single individual monitored over a 2-month period: a 5-fold range in fecal and a 13-fold range in urinary ATNC concentrations. Dietary nitrate was shown to have an effect on fecal ATNC levels. After 8 days on a low nitrate diet, fecal ATNC levels in 8 volunteers averaged 82 mg (N-NO)/kg (range of non-detectable to 143 mg/kg) while after 3 days on a high nitrate diet, fecal ATNC levels averaged 307 mg/kg (range of 73 to 714 mg/kg). These results suggest that dietary nitrate levels are an important factor influencing endogenous nitrosation and fecal ATNC concentrations.

In a study designed to determine whether differences in endogenous nitrosating ability were related to gastric cancer incidence, nitrosation in 80 healthy volunteers from regions of high and low incidence of gastric cancer in Italy was assessed using the *N*-nitrosoproline (NPRO) test (*26*). Background levels of urinary nitrate and NPRO were higher in subjects from the high incidence area but only the NPRO levels were significantly greater. Urinary levels of nitrate and NPRO (in 12-h samples) were measured after an oral dose of 500 mg L-proline and compared to background levels. Urinary excretion of NPRO approximately doubled after the proline loading dose in both groups, indicating that their nitrosating abilities were similar. Thus, geographic variation in gastric cancer incidence did not correlate with differences in nitrosating ability.

Cholangiocarcinoma, one of the most common cancers in northeast Thailand, is associated epidemiologically with infestations of the liver fluke, *Opisthorchis viverrini*, and with higher levels of urinary nitrosamines. In an investigation of the relationship between these two possible risk factors, 99 healthy volunteers from regions of high, moderate, and low incidence of cholangiocarcinoma were examined for infestation with this fluke and for endogenous nitrosating ability (*27*). None of the subjects in the low incidence areas carried this parasite while 29–85% of those in the 3 moderate and high incidence areas studied were infested. Endogenous nitrosating ability, as determined by the NPRO test with and without ascorbic acid, was found to be significantly higher in parasitized individuals than in non-parasitized individuals in the high incidence area. These results suggest that the parasitic infection induces some physiological change which enhances endogenous nitrosation, thereby increasing the cancer risk. Low levels of preformed nitrosamines were also detected in some fermented fish and pork food items frequently consumed in northeast Thailand.

A significant increase in urinary NPRO was observed in 16 subjects following consumption of a meal containing about 172 mg nitrate and 2.4 g proline compared to a meal containing no added proline (*28*). In a second study, inclusion of an additional mg of ascorbic acid in the proline–nitrate diet significantly decreased urinary NPRO levels in 13 of 19 subjects tested. Considerable interindividual variation was observed in nitrosating ability, and this was associated with variations in conversion of meal nitrate to salivary nitrite.

Ascorbic acid also appeared to inhibit gastric nitrosation in individuals given doses of 200 mg sodium nitrate followed by 1 g ascorbic acid (*29*). Just prior to and 1, 2, and 4 hours following dosing with nitrate, with or without ascorbic acid, samples of gastric juice were collected and analyzed for *N*-nitroso compounds. While a great deal of individual variation was observed, statistical analysis revealed that global mean concentrations of gastric *N*-nitroso compounds were significantly reduced after ingestion of ascorbic acid.

One possible explanation for individual variation in nitrosating ability is a variation in numbers of salivary nitrate-reducing organisms. To investigate this variable, endogenous nitrosation was measured in 16 volunteers before and after treatment with an oral antiseptic (*30*). The antiseptic caused a 94% reduction in salivary nitrate-reducing bacteria resulting in a decline from 17% to 4% in the amount of salivary nitrate which was converted to nitrite in vivo. This, in turn, was correlated with 62 and 74% decreases in the excretion of NPRO and *N*-nitrosothiazolidine-4-carboxylic acid. These data indicate that interindividual variation in oral nitrate–reducing capacities may account for some of the variability in nitrosamino acid excretion.

Endogenous nitrosation may also occur in the urinary bladder of individuals with chronic urinary infections. Analyses of samples of saliva, gastric juice, blood, feces, and urine from 40 controls revealed that levels of nitrate and of 4 nitrosatable amines were highest in urine. Average excretion of nitrite and of 4 nitrosamines was significantly higher in 30 spine-injured paraplegics and in 12 patients with bladder augmentations (both groups with chronic bladder infections) as compared to controls without bladder infections (*31*).

In vitro experiments under simulated gastric conditions were conducted to determine the potential for endogenous nitrosation of compounds in Chinese salted fish (*32*) and of Nigerian vegetables and spices (*33*). Samples of food were incubated for 1 h at 37°C with simulated gastric juice and nitrite. *N*-nitrosodimethylamine (NDMA) was the only volatile nitrosamine detected from the salted fish digestion and was the major nitrosamine from the Nigerian foods. *N*-nitrosopiperidine was detected in one digested Nigerian food, ugwu. Ascorbic acid significantly decreased nitrosamine formation in the salted fish but did not decrease the mutagenicity of the digested fish. There was insufficient NDMA formed during the digestion to account for the observed mutagenicity. This indicates that some other non-nitroso mutagen is present.

Nitrite treatment of 16 tryptophan-related compounds (known to be metabolites of tryptophan in humans) was found to introduce a hydroxy group into the indole or benzene ring and this converted them to mutagenic compounds (*34*). None of the compounds was mutagenic before nitrite treatment but 11 were mutagenic, without activation, to *Salmonella typhimurium* after incubation for 1 hour with nitrite.

Incubation of the fried food mutagens IQ, MeIQ, Glu-P-1, and Trp-P-1 with nitrite at pH 3 for 1 h resulted in the conversion of Glu-P-1 and Trp-P-1 to weak or non-mutagenic compounds and of IQ and MeIQ to extremely strong, direct acting mutagens in the Ames test (*35*). The nitrosation products of MeIQ were resolved by TLC into 7 bands, four of which were highly mutagenic. These compounds may have physiological significance in gastrointestinal tumorigenesis.

Occurrence of N-*nitroso compounds and their formation in foods*

Literature, published prior to July 1991, concerning the occurrence and formation of nonvolatile *N*-nitrosamines in foods and beverages has been reviewed (*36*). Of the total apparent *N*-nitrosamines in food, less than 10% have been identified and 12–21% are nonvolatile *N*-nitrosamines. *N*-nitrosoproline (NPRO) and *N*-nitrosothiazolidine-4-carboxylic acid (NTCA) are the two non-volatile *N*-nitrosamines most commonly identified in the diet.

Apparent total *N*-nitroso compounds (ATNC) in 25 smoked and unsmoked fried bacon samples were found to average 2700 µg (N-NO)/kg [range of 430–6800 µg (N-NO)/kg] (*37*). ATNC in smoked samples were, on the average, higher than in the unsmoked samples but the difference was not significant. Protein-bound NPRO was the most abundant nitroso compound in unsmoked bacon, averaging 260 µg/kg and accounting for 4% of the ATNC. In smoked bacon, average levels of NPRO, NTCA, *N*-nitrosothiazolidine (NTHZ), and 2-(hydroxymethyl)-3-nitrosothiazolidine-4-carboxylic acid (NHMTCA) were 305, 660, 340, and 180 µg/kg, respectively. Only about 16% of the ATNC could be identified as known *N*-nitrosamines.

Since a high gastric cancer mortality in some regions of China has been associated with consumption of certain salted, fermented fish products, such as fish sauce, *N*-nitroso compounds and genotoxins were determined in 49 fish sauce samples collected from villages in this high-risk area (*38*). Before nitrosation (incubation for 1 h at 37°C with sodium nitrite), total nitroso compounds ranged from 0.2 to 16 µmoles/L. After nitrosation at pH 2 and pH 7, nitrosamine levels rose by up to 4800- and 100-fold, respectively. Commonly occurring volatile nitrosamines were not detected in any samples. NPRO and nitrososarcosine constituted up to 1% and 0.7%, respectively, of the total nitroso compounds. Prior to nitrosation none of the fish sauce samples were genotoxic in the SOS chromotest while after nitrosation all were weakly genotoxic.

Using GC with thermal energy analysis, 31.5% of 38 alcoholic drinks and 215 food samples tested in West Germany in 1989–1990 had detectable levels of volatile *N*-nitrosamines (*39*). Using this data and data from the German Nutritional Report of 1988, average daily intakes of 0.011 µg NPYR and 0.015 µg *N*-nitrosopiperidine (NPIP) were calculated. Intakes of NDMA were estimated to be 0.28 and 0.17 µg/day for men and women, respectively. This difference in NDMA ingestion is due to different dietary practices including the greater consumption of beer by males (619.4 g/day vs 185 g/day for females).

Of 258 food samples and 53 beverages collected in eastern France, 89% contained detectable levels of NDMA (*40*). Highest concentrations, up to 16 µg/kg, were found in stone fruit spirits. Smoked fish, smoked meat and nitrite-cured meat also contained appreciable amounts of this nitrosamine. NDMA in beer averaged 0.28 µg/L, lower than in the past, due to improvements in brewing.

Effects of processing conditions on NPRO and *N*-nitrososarcosine (NSAR) levels in Estonian meats, fish, and cheese were investigated (*41*). NPRO levels in processed meats ranged from 5 to 353 µg/kg but were not detectable in raw materials. Nitrosamines were formed during salting and smoking, while frying of ham and sausage further enhanced NPRO levels. Smoked cheeses and fish also consistently had higher nitrosamine levels (131 and 16 µg/kg, respectively) than unsmoked samples.

A variety of meats, fish, and alcoholic beverages were obtained from markets in Lagos, Nigeria, and tested for the presence of nitrosamines (*42*). Most of the samples had detectable levels of nitrosamines, with the highest levels found in grilled, spiced meat (0.8–0.9 mg nitrosamine as nitrosodiethanolamine/kg) and in the spiced meat before grilling (0.9–1.6 mg/kg). The coating spice was believed to contain peanut powder, pepper, vegetable oil and a salt mixture.

Since marine fish contain nitrosable compounds in their flesh, the question arises as to whether frankfurters made of pork and minced fish or surimi have greater concentrations of nitrosamines than occur in all-meat frankfurters. In experiments with frankfuters made with all meat, with 15% fish, and with 50% fish, NDMA levels were found to vary with cooking method. Highest levels were found in samples fried, grilled, or broiled, and lowest levels in uncooked and boiled samples (*43*). Both raw and cooked samples made with fish had higher NDMA levels: raw all-meat frankfurters, no detectable NDMA; with 15% surimi, 0.5 ppb NDMA; with 50% surimi, 0.8 ppb. For broiled frankfurters the NDMA levels were 0.2, 1.5, and 4.0 ppb, respectively. However, NTHZ and NTCA levels were not significantly greater in fish-containing frankfurters compared to all-meat frankfurters (*44*).

Concentrations of NHMTCA in 30 samples of smoked meats and bacon were determined by a newly developed procedure based on derivatization of NHMTCA with diazomethane and analysis by HPLC with thermal energy analysis (*45*). Seventeen of the meat products contained 10–540 ppb NHMTCA. Addition of NHMTCA to raw bacon followed by frying resulted in decarboxylation of the nitrosamine to yield NHMTHZ. NHMTHZ was detected only in fried bacon.

Faba beans and members of the Brassica family of vegetables (broccoli, cabbage, turnips, etc.) contain indole compounds which may be converted to nitrosamines by reaction with nitrite. Nitrosation of 4-chloro-methoxyindole (from faba beans) and of indole-3-acetonitrile (from brassicas) produced compounds which were mutagenic to *Salmonella typhimurium* TA100, were potent inducers of sister chromatid exchanges in Chinese hamster V79 cells,

and significantly inhibited gap junctional intercellular communication (*46*). Tests with 8 indole compounds derived from indole glucosinolate revealed that all became mutagenic to *S. typhimurium* TA98 and TA100 and to *E. coli* WP2 uvrA/pKM101 after treatment with nitrite at pH 3 (*47*). Activation of the nitrosated compounds by an S9 mix was not necessary for mutagenicity and, in fact, S9 mix decreased the mutagenicity of some compounds.

A yellow substance (YS), identified as a β-carboline compound, has been isolated from soy sauce by HPLC and shown to be weakly mutagenic to *S. typhimurium* TA100 without S9 mix (*48*). Treatment with nitrite at pH 3.2 increased mutagenicity 7.5 times. YS was present in regular fermented soy sauce at a concentration of 2 µg/mL and in some other types of soy sauce at concentrations of 0.38–0.79 µg/mL. Heating at 120°C for 20 minutes doubled the mutagenicity in all 3 types of soy sauce.

Biological effects of N-nitroso compounds

Attempts to explain the preponderance of diabetic Icelandic males who were born in October have focused on foods eaten by their parents approximately 9 months previously and, specifically, on the smoked cured mutton which is a favorite food around Christmas time (*49*). Experiments with CD 1 mice demonstrated that male progeny of parents where either the mother or both parents had been fed this mutton developed diabetes. Further assays using various fractions of mutton revealed that water-extracted meat samples were not diabetogenic while the water extract of smoked cured meat, smoked cured fat and meat with added NTCA all exerted diabetogenic effects on male progeny. Diabetogenic effects could be observed even in the third litter after consumption of the tainted meat ceased. It appears that some nitrosamine(s) may be an etiological factor in the development of diabetes.

A supplementary issue of *Cancer Research* consisted of a full report of the British Industrial Biological Research Association's large carcinogenesis bioassays investigating the effects of *N*-nitrosodiethylamine (NDEA), NDMA, NPYR, and NPIP (*50*). A total of 4080 rats were exposed to drinking water containing NDEA or NDMA in various concentrations to elucidate dose–effect responses for liver and esophageal cancer. At low doses of the nitrosamines, a linear relationship was observed between dose and tumor incidence such that, at a dose of 1 ppm NDEA or NDMA about 25% of the rats developed a liver neoplasm and at 0.1 ppm about 2.5% developed neoplasms. There was no indication of a "threshold." At low dose levels NDEA appeared to be about twice as potent as NDMA. Effects of NPIP and NPYR were tested on 584 rats with dose–response relationships observed for NPYR and liver tumors and for NPIP and tumors of the liver and upper gastrointestinal tract similar to those observed for NDEA and NDMA, except that NPYR and NPIP were less potent. Carcinogenic effects of NDEA on female mice and female hamsters and on older rats were also studied. A detailed statistical analysis of all the data is included.

Data from several experiments on diethylnitrosamine(DEN)-induced hepatocarcinogenesis in rodents was analyzed within the framework of a two mutation carcinogenesis model (*51*). Results indicated that the probability of initiation was proportional to the number of O^4-ethyldeoxythymidine DNA adducts resulting from DEN exposure, indicating that these adducts represent promutagenic lesions. Experimental data indicate that DEN can act as both an initiator and a promoter although the mechanism for promotion is not clear.

Excretion and distribution of two ^{14}C-labeled MTCAs (β-carboline compounds isolated from soy sauce) and the nitrosated forms of these compounds were investigated in orally dosed rats (*52*). Most of the two labeled MTCAs were eliminated in feces within 24 h while the nitrite-treated MTCAs were mainly excreted in the urine. When the nitrosated compounds were administered, some radioactivity was detected in the liver and kidney as well as in the gastrointestinal tract, but with the untreated MTCAs, radioactivity was detectable only in the gastrointestinal tract and in the feces. In vitro experiments have shown that nitrosation converts the MTCAs into direct-acting mutagens.

Pancreatic ductular adenocarcinoma has a poorly understood etiology in humans but can be induced in Syrian golden hamsters by β-substituted nitrosamines. Activation of these nitrosamines in hamsters has been reviewed (*53*). Experimental studies have demonstrated that pancreatic tissue is more efficient than hepatocytes in generating mutagens from these nitrosamines and these activated compounds can alkylate DNA. However, the roles of hepatic metabolism and detoxification reactions have not yet been clarified.

Many nitrosamines are known to be activated by cytochrome P-450 enzymes but some organs in which nitrosamine-induced cancers occur are not rich in these enzymes. In vitro experiments with *N*-nitrosomethylaniline (which causes tumors in lungs of mice and in the esophagus of rats) have demonstrated that it can be oxidized by peroxidase in the presence of hydrogen peroxide to produce carcinogens which bind covalently to DNA and tRNA (*54*). Since some lung cells are rich in peroxidases, they may be particularly susceptible to effects of this carcinogen.

Organ specificity of carcinogens may be partly a result of organ-specific activation. Specificity may also be affected by hepatic metabolism of the nitrosamine. Metabolism of NDEA and *N*-nitrosomethyl-*n*-pentylamine (NMPentA) was investigated in rats in vivo and in livers of rats pretreated with 3-methylcholanthrene, phenobarbital, or arochlor, all of which are potent inducers of P450 enzymes (*55*). About half of the radioactivity from the labeled nitrosamine doses was eliminated by exhalation while 15.6–27% was excreted in urine. Glucuronides were formed by hepatocytes in vitro, with the extent of glucuronidation determined by the lipophilicity of the nitrosamine. Although glucuronidation is generally considered a detoxification reaction, glucuronides could be transported to other organs where a glucuronidase could liberate the ultimate carcinogen.

Detection and assay of N-*nitroso compounds*

Simultaneous determination of two nonvolatile *N*-nitroso compounds, 2-(hydroxymethyl)-*N*-nitrosothiazolidine-4-carboxylic acid (HMNTCA) and 2-(hydroxymethyl)-*N*-nitrosothiazolidine (HMNTHZ), in smoked meats and cheese has been achieved by use of HPLC with a thermal energy analyzer (*56*).

Samples were extracted with methanol or acetonitrile, defatted with isooctane, cleaned up on an acidic alumina sample preparation cartridge, derivatized, and then injected into the HPLC apparatus. Confirmation was carried out by gas–liquid chromatographic–mass spectrometric analysis. Recoveries of these two compounds added to various products at concentrations of 10–20 and 50–200 ppb averaged 94% and 79%, respectively. Several parts of the procedure were discussed to point out steps which are critical to success.

Volatile *N*-nitrosamines in hams processed with elastic rubber netting probably originate from amine precursors in the rubber and nitrite used in curing. Solid phase extraction of the nitrosamines was found to yield more accurate results than mineral oil distillation or low-temperature vacuum distillation in the determination of these nitrosamines by gas chromatography with chemiluminescent detection (*57*). A meat sample was thoroughly mixed with anhydrous sodium sulfate and Celite, packed into a column, and extracted directly with dichloromethane. The extract was then passed through a separate silica gel column before GC analysis. Analysis of a sample spiked with 2,6-dimethylmorpholine demonstrated that artifactual nitrosamines were formed during extraction by the two distillation methods but no artifacts were noted with the solid-phase extraction method.

A second check sample survey for the determination of *N*-nitrosamines in beer and malt was organized by the International Agency for Research on Cancer with results submitted by 16 laboratories from Canada, Europe, and the USA (*58*). Each laboratory received two beer samples, one containing 0.5 µg/L *N*-nitrosodimethylamine (NDMA) and the other containing 4 µg NDMA/L and 30 µg *N*-nitrosoproline (NPRO)/L and two naturally contaminated malts and standard solutions containing NDMA, NPRO, and *N*-nitrosopyrrolidine (NPYR) with instructions to use a method of their own choice. Compared to results from a previous, similar check study, there was a distinct improvement in the analysis of NDMA, with fewer outliers and a better distribution of results. However, little improvement was noted for the analysis of the other two compounds.

FOOD PRESERVATION BY IRRADIATION

Toxicological studies

Irradiated sugar solutions are mutagenic to *Salmonella* tester strain TA100 and one of the main products of γ-radiolysis of D-glucose and D-fructose, glucasone, has been implicated as a mutagenic agent. Glucasone has also been found to be cytotoxic to Chinese hamster V79 cells in the presence of cupric ions (*59*). Hydrogen peroxide was detected in solutions of glucasone and cupric ions, and further experiments demonstrated that catalase effectively inhibited the cytotoxic effects of glucasone. Since this compound may be present in irradiated foods containing sugars, further experiments are underway to determine whether its presence in foods presents a health risk.

Radiation-induced buildup of lipid hydroperoxides in whole egg powder and in egg yolk powder was monitored as a function of dose, dose rate, and the presence of oxygen (*60*). Anaerobic conditions severely limited formation of hydroperoxides. An induction dose of 2.5 kGy was observed in air in both powders, independent of the dose rate. The accumulation of hydroperoxides was inversely proportional to the dose rate. Therefore, to avoid extensive degradation, egg powders should be irradiated at the highest available dose rate by a dose not exceeding 2.5 kGy. At this dose any contaminating *Salmonella* populations would be reduced by a factor of 1000 and organoleptic changes would not be a concern.

Toxic effects of a 10% solution of irradiated cocoa were examined in the wing spot assay in *Drosophila melanogaster* (*61*). Irradiated cocoa appeared to cause a significantly greater number of small wing spots but not of large single spots or twin spots as compared to controls exposed to unirradiated cocoa or to no cocoa. However, media containing 10% cocoa, whether or not irradiated, killed about 80% of the *Drosophila* larvae. This makes it difficult to interpret the mutagenicity data in terms of potential human health hazards.

Available information on the effects of γ-irradiation on pesticides in solution or in foods was recently reviewed (*62*). Generally, pesticide degradation is greater in irradiated aqueous solutions than in aliphatic solvents or in foods. Some degradation products have been identified in organic solvents but very few analyses have been performed with irradiated foods. Some addition products between molecules of solvent and pesticides have been observed. The toxicological significance of pesticide degradation products is very difficult to assess, particularly since pesticide levels in foods are usually very low.

Most food irradiation plants are radioisotope plants based on ^{60}Co but some electron beam irradiation facilities have recently been commissioned. Induction of radioactivity was measured in samples of chicken, prawns, cheeses, and spices irradiated on the electron linear accelerator HELIOS at 20 MeV and at 10 MeV (the regulatory maximum energy permitted) (*63*). No measurable radioactivity was induced at 10 MeV. To assess effects of a possible malfunction of an electron beam irradiation facility, samples were irradiated to the regulatory limit of 10 kGy at 20 MeV. One day after irradiation, cheeses contained 0.0068 Bq/g and the other samples 0.0135 Bq/g of radioactivity. These levels are about 5–10-fold lower than radioactivity naturally found in low-sodium salts and in pepper and turmeric because of their potassium contents.

Detection of irradiated foods

In an evaluation of electron spin resonance (ESR) as a method for identifying irradiated foods, 21 European laboratories participated in analyses of samples of beef and trout bones, sardine scales, pistachio nut shells, dried grapes and papaya, and poultry bones (*64*). No difficulties were encountered in identifying irradiated meat bones and dried fruit. Results were not as good with fish, although the success rate improved with increasing doses of radiation. Analysis of pistachio nuts proved very difficult because irradiation produced very small changes in spectral shape.

Free radicals produced in chicken bone by ^{137}Cs γ-rays were measured by ESR and used to quantitatively estimate the radiation dose (*65–67*). Additive re-irradiation of the bone gave a reproducible dose–response function which could be used to estimate the initial dose. Analysis of the data by linear regression analysis and by exponential fitting analysis revealed that the latter gave a better estimate of the initial absorbed radiation dose.

ESR has also been used to detect irradiated whiting (fish) and scampi (Norway lobster). Fins, scales, and vertebrae of whiting irradiated at 1–10 kGy were analyzed for free radical concentrations (*68*). All 3 sample types could be used to qualitatively detect irradiation; analyses of vertebrae gave the best quantitative estimates of radiation dose. Signals from irradiated, freeze-dried, ground vertebrae did not change significantly after fish were stored for 21 days at 3°C. A linear response with increasing irradiation dose was observed in analyses of the cuticle of scampi (*69*). Freeze drying of the cuticle resulted in a larger signal, and peak height was found to be a reliable method of quantification. After 14 days' storage at –20°C or at +5°C, ESR signals declined 8% and 27%, respectively.

A variety of irradiated foods has been examined in an investigation of the application of ESR for control of irradiated foods (*70*). As in previous studies identification of irradiated poultry and fish bones was straightforward. ESR was also useful in detection of irradiated pears which had a stronger signal than unirradiated fruits and of irradiated dates and mushrooms which gave a multicomponent signal. Some spices (white mustard, paprika, and chili) produced no ESR signal before irradiation but did afterwards. The radiation-induced ESR signal in black pepper was highly sensitive to moisture. Preliminary experiments with irradiated stones of cherries, plums, lemons, apple pips, raspberries, cranberries, red currants, blackcurrants, gooseberries, and tomatoes demonstrated the induction of short-lived ESR signals of no practical use for the control of food irradiation.

Irradiation of lipids causes formation of compounds not normally present in foods, and these may be possible biomarkers for detection of irradiation. Following irradiation of chicken, C_{n-1} and C_{n-2} alkanes and alkenes (n being the carbon number of the parent fatty acid) are formed and can be detected by separation of the hydrocarbons using florasil chromatography followed by GC analysis using a flame ionization detector (*71*). Irradiation of cholesterol produces two compounds, 6-keto-cholestanol and 7-ketocholestanol, that are not now known to be present in foods (*72*). These compounds may be detected by GC/MS and, if they are found in irradiated meat and poultry and absent in unirradiated foods, they may also be useful markers.

Phenylalanine, a constituent of most food proteins, is converted to o-, m-, or p-tyrosine by irradiation. Since o-tyrosine is not normally found in food, it has been proposed as a marker for irradiated meats. Analyses of 18 chicken breast samples revealed a mean background level of o-tyrosine of 0.18 ppm (*73*). The radiation dose–response curve was found to be linear within the range of 1–10 kGy with a slope of 0.127 ppm. Postirradiation storage at 4 or 8°C until spoilage did not significantly affect levels of o-tyrosine.

During irradiation of foods some of the thymine present in DNA may be converted to thymine glycol. A fluorimetric assay for thymine glycol was investigated as a possible method for detecting irradiated foods (*74*). However, analyses of irradiated chicken meat and of DNA from irradiated chicken meat proved unsuitable for this purpose due to interference by one of the reagents, o-aminobenzaldehyde.

ANTIOXIDANTS

Effects of ascorbic acid and curcumin on quercetin-induced DNA damage, lipid peroxidation, and protein degradation were investigated in rat liver nuclei under aerobic conditions in the presence of equimolar concentrations of iron or copper (*75*). In the presence of either metal, both antioxidants were found to enhance DNA damage and lipid peroxidation but only ascorbic acid increased protein degradation. These results demonstrate that although curcumin and ascorbic acid can exert antioxidant and anticarcinogenic effects, they also have pro-oxidant properties.

Variations in amperometric methods for the determination of ascorbic acid and sulfite were investigated to optimize accuracy and reduce the effects of contaminants (*76*). Samples of beer containing these two antioxidants were first subjected to ion exclusion chromatography. Analysis with a pulsed amperometric detector using a single applied voltage to the platinum working electrode was unsuccessful apparently due to contamination of the relatively small surface area of the platinum electrode. Satisfactory results were obtained with a standard amperometric cell (whose electrode has a much larger surface area) but remarkably superior results were obtained when this cell was operated in a pulsed mode and cleaning cycles were continually applied during the analysis. Recoveries of the antioxidants from spiked beers averaged 95–118%, indicating that the method is free of interference.

An HPLC method utilizing a reversed-phase C18 column and gradient elution with water/acetonitrile/methanol/isopropanol was used to analyze oils for the presence of 9 commonly used, synthetic phenolic antioxidants (*77*). Oil samples were diluted with isopropanol/hexane and then applied to the column. Antioxidants were detected by UV light. This method was also appropriate for the simultaneous determination of triglycerides and tocopherols and thus may allow study of the inhibition effects of the antioxidants.

Ascorbic acid

In addition to its promoting effects for rat bladder tumors, it has been suggested that ascorbic acid, which is metabolized to oxalate, may have a role in the development of calcium oxalate lithogenesis. To test this hypothesis, 15 patients with unilateral nephrostomy tubes after extracorporeal shock wave lithotripsy were orally dosed with 0 (control), 100, 500, 1000, or 2000 mg ascorbic acid on days 2 and 3 postoperatively (*78*). Successive 6-h specimens were collected before and after dosing from both kidneys from all patients. A statistically significant increase in urinary oxalate was observed in all patients dosed with ≥500 mg ascorbic acid. This represented an increase in oxalate excretion of

6–13 mg/day/1000 mg ascorbic acid supplement, an amount which would increase the risk of urolithiasis.

A method for the direct and simultaneous determination of ascorbic acid and isoascorbic acid (erythorbic acid) in food products by paired-ion reverse-phase HPLC has been developed (*79*). Food samples, preserved with metaphosphoric acid, were homogenized and injected into the system, and the antioxidants were separated using a mobile phase containing metaphosphoric acid, sodium acetate, and tetrabutylammonium hydrogen sulfate, pH 5.4. Detection of the compounds was achieved by amperometry using a glassy carbon electrode and Ag/AgCl reference electrode. Detection limit was 0.5 ng antioxidant. Analysis of 12 samples of ground beef suspected of being adulterated with erythorbic acid revealed that 8 contained detectable levels of ascorbic or erythorbic acids. Apparently these antioxidants are used by some retailers to maintain the fresh appearance of ground beef.

Ascorbic acid is one of several additives which may be present in soft drinks, and its determination may be complicated by the presence of these other additives as well as by various colored compounds in the drinks. Therefore, a method utilizing 2nd and 3rd order derivative spectrophotometric data was developed for the determination of ascorbic acid in soft drinks (*80*). A blank solution was prepared using the soft drink, and ascorbic acid levels were determined by standard addition. Concentrations of 0.5–0.7 µg/mL could be determined without interference from other additives and coloring matter.

Butylated hydroxyanisole (BHA)

In a recent review, the physical and chemical characteristics of BHA were summarized and its metabolism in animals and humans was described (*81*). Evidence from toxicological studies indicates that BHA is not genotoxic but does induce carcinogenesis in the forestomach of rodents. The mechanism of carcinogenicity is unknown but some evidence implicates reactive oxygen species, in particular, hydroxyl radicals.

One hypothesis suggests that the tumorigenicity of BHA results from the induction of an inflammatory response with subsequent cell proliferation. However, in rats fed a diet containing 1.5% BHA for 2 weeks, BHA was found to inhibit both prostaglandin and hydroxy fatty acid release from linoleic and arachidonic acids in the forestomach, glandular stomach and colon/rectum (*82*). Therefore, it seems unlikely that inflammatory action is directly responsible for the enhancement of cell proliferation by BHA.

Experiments demonstrating the carcinogenic effects of BHA generally use high doses of this compound, thus raising the possibility that contaminants in commercial BHA preparations contribute to the tumorigenic effects. Commercial BHA consists primarily of 3-BHA (about 93.8%), with about 5% 2-BHA and 5 related phenolic compounds comprising the remaining 1.2%. In recent experiments, the carcinogenicity of purified 3-BHA (>99.6% by HPLC) and 3 of the minor phenolic contaminants was assessed in Syrian golden hamsters fed diets containing 1% of these compounds (*83*). After 24 weeks the animals were sacrificed and their forestomachs examined histopathologically. Both 3-BHA and one of the other compounds, 2,5-di-tert-butyl hydroquinone, induced severe hyperplasia and papillomas while the other compounds induced only a mild hyperplasia in a few animals.

Butylated hydroxytoluene (BHT)

Depending on the concentrations used, BHT may have a protective effect by inhibiting the toxicity of many chemicals or it may, itself, exhibit a concentration-dependent toxicity. In experiments using the red blood cell fragility assay, BHT at concentrations <60 nmol/mg protected against osmotic fragility while higher concentrations enhanced fragility (*84*). Protective effects correlated with decreased membrane fluidity as measured by fluorescence polarization while enhanced fragility was associated with increased fluidity. In rat hepatocyte suspensions, BHT at high concentrations also increased membrane fluidity, resulting in enzyme leakage from mitochondrial membranes. It appears that membrane fluidity changes are at least in part responsible for some of the cytotoxic and chemoprotective effects of BHT.

Dietary BHT (100, 300, 1000, 3000, and 6000 ppm) modulates the carcinogenic effects of 2-acetylaminofluorene (AAF) (*85*). Rats were fed diets containing 50 ppm AAF and BHT for up to 76 weeks with some animals from each group sacrificed at 12, 24, 36, and 48 weeks. At the highest concentration BHT caused an increase in the incidence and multiplicity of bladder neoplasms and at 3000 ppm it increased nodular hyperplasia of the bladder. However, BHT inhibited the induction of liver altered foci by AAF in a dose-dependent manner and reduced the incidence of hepatocellular carcinomas and the multiplicity of liver neoplasms. Numbers of neoplasms/animal were reduced to about 60% and 28% of the numbers induced by AAF alone, by BHT concentrations of 100 and 300 ppm and of 1000–6000 ppm, respectively.

Dietary BHT concentrations of 0.4 and 0.8% significantly inhibited the formation of 7,12-dimethylbenz[*a*]anthracene(DMBA)–DNA adducts in the mammary gland of female rats (*86*). Examination of the levels of specific adducts formed revealed that the formation of the adduct of the antidiastereomer of DMBA and deoxyguanosine was preferentially inhibited. This inhibition of adduct formation may explain the protective effect of BHT on the initiation of DMBA-induced mammary carcinogenesis.

Since BHT has been reported to cause hemorrhage in rats, mice and guinea pigs were fed diets containing 0–5% BHT for up to 30 days and examined for hemorrhagic effects (*87*). No guinea pigs and only 4 mice housed in wire-bottom cages developed lung hemorrhages. Prothrombin time was reduced in most groups of treated mice but only in guinea pigs dosed with 1% dietary BHT. A dose-related toxic nephrosis occurred in mice fed 1.35–5.0% BHT in the diet. The nephrotoxic ED_{50} was 2.3 g/kg body weight/day in a one-month study.

Mutagenicity of some fried food mutagens and of 3,3'-dichlorobenzidine (DCB) to *Salmonella typhimurium* TA98 was enhanced by BHT (*88,89*). While BHA and *n*-propyl gallate inhibited the mutagenicity of IQ, MeIQ, and MeIQx, BHT at high concentrations (>50 μg/plate) significantly enhanced the mutagenicity of IQ and MeIQ. All of these experiments utilized an S9 activation system. At concentrations of 4 and 20 μM, BHT enhanced the mutagenicity of DCB by 32 and 21%, respectively, and the covalent binding of DCB to DNA by 76 and 328%, respectively. BHT altered the profile of metabolites produced from DCB by an S9 mix by causing the formation of one entirely new metabolite, increasing the relative amount of another metabolite, and decreasing the amounts of 3 metabolites.

Kojic acid

Kojic acid, an antibacterial metabolite produced by some species of *Penicillium* and *Aspergillus*, is used as a food additive to prevent enzymatic browning due to polyphenol oxidase. Results of recent in vitro genotoxicity assays demonstrated that this compound is mutagenic to *S. typhimurium* TA98 and TA100, with and without S9 activation, using both plate incorporation and preincubation methods (*90*). Furthermore, kojic acid was found to induce dose-related increases in sister chromatid exchanges and chromosomal aberrations in Chinese hamster ovary cells.

Ethoxyquin

Groups of male and female F344 rats were fed a diet containing 0.5% ethoxyquin for 4 weeks to 18 months to investigate the development of nephrotoxicity (*91*). Male rats proved to be much more susceptible, developing an interstitial degeneration of the papillary tip by 4 weeks and a complete form of papillary necrosis by 24 weeks. In females these papillary changes developed later and they never progressed beyond the interstitial phase. Proximal tubule hyperplasia was observed in treated males at later sampling times but there was no evidence that ethoxyquin directly induced preneoplastic lesions.

Ethoxyquin is an antioxidant used to retard the decomposition of some pigments and has proved useful in protecting the natural red color of paprika. A new procedure for the determination of ethoxyquin in paprika, eliminating the necessity of removing other colored substances, has been developed (*92*). Samples were extracted with ethyl acetate and then analyzed by reverse-phase HPLC using gradient elution (acetonitrile:water) and UV detection at 270 nm. Results were linear in the range of 2–50 µg/mL. Greater sensitivity (detection limit of 0.2 µg/mL) could be achieved with fluorimetric detection with excitation at 311 nm and emission at 444 nm. Ethoxyquin levels in 13 commercial samples ranged from undetectable to 235 µg/g.

SWEETENERS

Aspartame

During the years 1986–1990, the FDA's Adverse Reaction Monitoring System received 251 reports of epileptic seizures associated with aspartame intake (*93*). Of these, 124 were classified as Group D (highly unlikely that the reported symptoms were associated with ingestion of aspartame) and 41 were classified as Group A (symptoms recurred each time a product containing aspartame was consumed). The other 86 cases were assigned to intermediate groups with some indications that aspartame, or the foods it was present in, might be associated with the seizures. Since these data are from a passive surveillance system, further double-blind controlled scientific studies should be conducted to elucidate the association between aspartame and seizures.

In a double-blind study on two consecutive days, 10 children with newly diagnosed but untreated generalized absence seizures were challenged with 40 mg aspartame/kg on one day and a sucrose-sweetened drink on the other day (*94*). Following aspartame, the total duration of spike-wave discharge per hour was significantly increased for the group as a whole. Spike wave bursts/hour were increased in 7 patients and mean length of spike bursts was longer in 8 patients after aspartame ingestion as compared to sucrose ingestion. Thus, aspartame appears to exacerbate the amount of EEG spike in some children with absence seizures.

Following advertisements for persons with hypersensitivity reactions to aspartame, 61 subjects were screened (*95*). Twenty of the subjects with suggestive symptoms were willing to participate in a single-blind challenge and, of these, only 3 had a positive response. In further, double-blind challenges all 3 tested negative. In this geographic area (Washington, D.C. area), it proved difficult to recruit patients with a true aspartame allergy.

Since some anecdotal evidence has associated aspartame with some symptoms of central nervous dysfunction, 13 pilots were tested in a double-blind study of aspartame effects using the SPARTANS cognitive test battery of aviation-relevant information-processing tasks (*96*). Subjects were tested during 5 sessions: pretest and posttest controls and 3 randomly ordered test periods following ingestion of 50 mg aspartame/kg body weight, a placebo, or ethyl alcohol as a positive control. Although alcohol affected both psychomotor and spatial abilities, there were no detectable decrements associated with aspartame ingestion.

The clearance of plasma phenylalanine (Phe) and the availability to the brain of Phe, tyrosine (Tyr), and tryptophan (Trp) was investigated in 6 healthy males gives 0.56 g Phe in the form of 1.0 g aspartame or 12.2 g bovine albumin (*97*). Following an overnight fast, subjects consumed one of the test doses or water, and venous blood samples were collected and analyzed during the next 4 hours. Results demonstrated a marked and persistent increase in the availability of Phe to the brain following ingestion of aspartame but not following protein intake. Phe was cleared from the plasma faster after consumption of protein compared with aspartame.

Both humans and experimental animals rapidly metabolize aspartame in the gastrointestinal tract to Phe, aspartic acid and methanol. Pharmacokinetic studies with rats and mice given doses of up to 2000 mg aspartame/kg revealed that maximal plasma Phe and Tyr concentrations occurred within 1 hour after dosing and returned to baseline within 4–8 hours regardless of the size of the dose (*98*). Comparisons of the plasma levels of these amino acids in rodents with data previously obtained from human volunteers indicated that rodents require a 2–6 times higher dose of aspartame than humans to produce similar increases in plasma phenylalanine/large neutral amino acid ratios.

In aqueous solutions aspartame slowly decomposes to yield methanol, two different isomers of L-aspartyl-L-phenylalanine (α- and β-Asp-Phe), and cyclo-Asp-Phe. Depending on their pH and storage conditions, aspartame-containing beverages may contain varying quantities of these products. Absorption and metabolism of these 3 peptide decomposition products at concentrations of 0.5–40 mmol/L, were investigated in studies with rat jejunal segments (99). Phe and α-Asp-Phe were rapidly absorbed from the jejunum by carrier-assisted uptake while β-Asp-Phe and cyclo-Asp-Phe slowly diffused from the lumen. Homogenates of rat liver and intestinal mucosa catalyzed the hydrolysis of α- but not of β- or cyclo-Asp-Phe. Rat cecal contents and homogenates of *E. coli* cultures hydrolyzed both α- and β- but not cyclo-Asp-Phe.

Three fruit preparations used in making flavored yogurt and containing 2130–2280 ppm aspartame were analyzed for decomposition products during storage for 6 months at 3 different temperatures (100). Initial pH of the fruit preparations was 3.6–4.0 and no changes occurred during storage. After 6 months storage at 4.4, 21.1, and 32.2 °C, approximately 85%, 60%, and 25%, respectively, of the initial aspartame could be recovered.

An improved HPLC method was developed for the determination of aspartame and its degradation product, diketopiperazine (cyclo-Asp-Phe), in various cacao powder, emulsifier and thickening agents containing dessert powders (101). This procedure was used to determine stability of aspartame when various dessert powders were mixed with boiling water and allowed to cool for 80 minutes. No degradation was detected in gelatin-based desserts (pH 3), whereas in products containing milk or cacao (pH 6), degradation of aspartame was estimated at 20–35%.

Saccharin

A previous short-term study demonstrating an increased agglutinability of bladder epithelial cells in response to concanavalin A in analbuminemic rats fed a saccharin-containing diet suggested that these rats might be useful in screening for bladder carcinogens. However, in a long-term study, no bladder carcinomas were observed in either normal or analbuminemic rats fed a diet containing 5% sodium saccharin for 80 weeks (102).

High levels of dietary sodium saccharin increase proliferation of urothelial cells and lead to the formation of silicate-containing precipitate and microcrystals in the urine of male rats. In experiments with rats fed 7.5% sodium saccharin, no increase in total urinary silicon was observed as compared to controls (103). However, saccharin was bound to male rat urinary proteins and it was suggested that these complexes served as a nidus for the formation of silicate-containing precipitate and crystals. These crystals are apparently cytotoxic to bladder epithelium resulting in regenerative hyperplasia.

Fructose

Fructose, which naturally occurs in honey and fruits, has become a more common dietary component since high fructose corn syrups are now used to sweeten many beverages and processed foods. In a recent review, metabolic and nutritional aspects of fructose were discussed and the evidence for adverse effects of fructose was evaluated (104). Some data indicate that dietary fructose causes elevated serum triglycerides, exacerbates the severity of symptoms of copper deficiency, and induces hyperuricemia. This review concludes that normal dietary levels of fructose would not have adverse effects for most people but there may be subgroups, such as those with gout and some diabetics with hypertriglyceridemia, which may experience harmful effects from fructose ingestion.

To determine whether the effects of dietary fructose on various aspects of glucose metabolism can affect tumor growth and development, control and thymoma-implanted mice were fed diets containing 16.5% glucose or fructose (105). Control mice fed fructose had higher blood glucose, insulin, and triglyceride levels than glucose-fed controls. Tumors were detected earlier and tumor size (23 days after implantation) was greater in fructose-fed animals. These results suggest that the hyper-insulinemic effect of fructose may enhance the growth of some types of tumors.

Other sweeteners

Neohesperidin dihydrochalcone (NHDC), an intensely sweet derivative of a flavanone glycoside present in citrus fruit, has been proposed as a nonnutritive sweetener for soft drinks and other products. In a subchronic oral toxicity test rats were fed diets containing 0, 0.2, 1.0, and 5% NHDC for 13 weeks (*106*). No treatment-related ophthalmic, hematological, or histopathological effects were observed at any dose. In the highest dose group, a marked cecal enlargement was noted early in the study and plasma urea concentrations and urinary pH were decreased. These changes appear to be adaptive responses and not clear manifestations of toxicity. The intermediate dose, providing about 750 mg NHDC/kg body weight was considered the no-effect level.

A recent review of a book detailing toxicity studies of acesulfame-K concluded that data from extensive testing of this sweetener indicated that it would be a safe additive (*107*) Acute toxicity studies demonstrated an oral LD_{50} of 7431 mg/kg body weight. Results from numerous studies on genotoxicity, teratogenicity, and carcinogenicity were negative. The only caution mentioned by the reviewer was that many of these experiments were done by the research department of the producer and vendor of acesulfame-K. However, there was no reason to suspect that the experimental results were not credible.

FLAVORS AND FLAVOR ENHANCERS

Two recent reviews described the evolution of the process of safety evaluation of flavoring substances by the Expert Panel of the Flavor and Extract Manufacturer's Association during the past 30 years (*108,109*). The procedures used and criteria employed for GRAS (generally recognized as safe)

determinations were discussed. The evaluations are an ongoing process as new information becomes available and proposals are made for substances to be used in greater concentrations or in a wider variety of foods.

Monosodium glutamate (MSG)

Papers from a recent ILSI Symposium summarized available data on "The Scientific Facts about MSG" (*110*). Sensitivity to MSG, glutamate and brain function, and the kinetics of glutamate in relation to its neurotoxicity were some of the topics considered. Sensitivity to MSG is not rare but it varies in intensity and is nearly always associated with sensitivity to other substances such as salicylates or amines.

A special issue of *Physiology and Behavior* was devoted to papers from the Second International Symposium on Umami (*111*). MSG and 5'-ribonucleotides are known to be the principal umami substances. Symposium papers were mainly concerned with the nature of umami as a flavor and its use in foods but several papers described interactions between MSG and the nervous system.

In a collaborative study involving 11 laboratories, an enzymatic method for the determination of free glutamic acid in meat products and dried soups was evaluated (*112*). Glutamate dehydrogenase oxidatively deaminates L-glutamic acid, producing NADH and oxoglutarate. When the NADH reacts with an indicator, it forms a compound detectable at 492 nm. A total of 14 samples (7 each of sausage and of dried cauliflower soup) with glutamate contents varying between 0.4 and 16 g/kg were assayed. Reproducibility standard deviations, which reflect variation between laboratories, were 12–16% for sausage (0.4–1.3 g glutamate/kg) and 4.6% for the dried soup (7–16 g glutamate/kg).

Other flavoring compounds

Mutagenicity of smoke condensates from 6 types of wood used for flavoring and preserving food in Nigeria was evaluated using the Ames test (*113*). All the smoke condensates induced dose-dependent increases in mutations but their potency varied between 0.04 and 0.9 revertants/µg condensate in *S. typhimurium* TA100. Concentrations of individual polycyclic aromatic hydrocarbons (PAH) also varied among the different smoke condensates. Generally, those with higher concentrations of PAHs exerted greater mutagenic effects. However, mutagenicity assays using PAHs in the concentrations present in the smoke condensates indicated that the PAHs alone cannot account for the mutagenicity of the condensates.

Benzophenone is occasionally used as a flavoring in non-alcoholic drinks, frozen dairy products, baked goods, and puddings in concentrations ranging from 0.57 to 3.27 ppm. Estimates of the daily intake of this flavoring in the USA range from 0.32 µg to 0.33 mg per person. In a safety evaluation of this compound, rats were given dietary doses of 20 mg benzophenone/kg body weight/day for 90 days or 100 or 500 mg/kg/day for 28 days (*114*). Some treatment-related effects were seen in the mid- and high-dose animals, although not all effects were observed in both sexes at both dose levels. These effects included hepatocellular enlargement, decreases in erythrocyte count, hemoglobin, and hematocrit, and an increase in total bilirubin. The no-effect-level was demonstrated at 20 mg/kg/day, which would be equivalent to an intake of 1200 mg/day for a 60-kg human.

Long-term carcinogenicity studies demonstrated that *d*-limonene induces kidney tumors in male but not in female F344 rats and not in either sex of mice. A metabolite of *d*-limonene binds to a urinary protein, α_{2u}-globulin, specific to male rats. In male rats gavaged for 14 consecutive days with 300 mg *d*-limonene/kg/day, no significant changes were noted in serum α_{2u}-globulin but urinary levels of the kidney form of this protein were increased, implying disruption or exfoliation of kidney proximal tubule cells (*115*). In a 32-week initiation–promotion study, male F344 rats treated with *N*-ethyl-*N*-hydroxyethylnitrosamine for 2 weeks followed by 30 weeks of promotion with *d*-limonene showed an increase in cell proliferation in the proximal tubules and an increase in renal adenomas and atypical hyperplasias (*116*). However, no increases in cell proliferation or tumors or preneoplastic lesions were observed in similarly treated males of the α_{2u}-globulin-deficient rat strain, NCI-Black Reiter. These

studies indicate that this male rat specific urinary protein is necessary for the cytotoxic and carcinogenic effects of *d*-limonene. Humans are therefore most likely not susceptible to carcinogenic effects of *d*-limonene.

Myrcene, a major constituent of oil of bay and hop and also present in the herb lemon grass, was evaluated, in concentrations up to 1000 µg/mL, for its genotoxic effects on mammalian cells in vitro (*117*). Negative results were obtained with tests for chromosomal aberrations and sister chromatid exchanges in human lymphocytes and for mutations at the hprt-locus in hamster V79 cells. All tests were done with and without activation by an S9 mix. There were no indications of induced cytotoxicity. However, myrcene did appear to reduce the toxic and mutagenic effects of cyclophosphamide in V79 cells and may therefore have antimutagenic properties.

FOOD COLORS

Effects of the color additive Caramel Color III (ammonia caramel, AC) on the immune system of rats were investigated in a 4-week study in which rats were fed diets containing 2–3 ppm or 11–12 ppm pyridoxine and provided with drinking water containing 4% AC (*118*). Compared to controls (no AC), rats dosed with AC on the low pyridoxine diet had reduced levels of B and T lymphocytes with reduced cell numbers in spleen, popliteal lymph nodes, and blood. Decreased numbers of ED2[+] macrophages were present in the thymic cortex. All these effects were either less pronounced or absent in rats on the high pyridoxine diet, suggesting that the effects of AC may be mediated through some effect on a pyridoxine-dependent process.

Two long-term studies (104 and 109 weeks) were conducted to determine toxic and/or carcinogenic effects of dietary allura red (FD&C Red No. 40) in two strains of mice (*119*). Diets containing 0, 0.37, 1.39, or 5.19% allura red were fed to dams throughout mating, gestation, and lactation and then to their offspring at the same concentrations they were exposed to in utero. No treatment-related adverse effects were observed, so that 5.19% was the no-observable-adverse-effect level. This corresponds to approximately 7300 and 8300 mg allura red/kg/day for male and female mice, respectively.

Carcinogenicity of cochineal, a red coloring used in foods and other products, was evaluated in B6C3F$_1$ mice (*120*). Mice were fed diets containing 0, 3, or 6% cochineal for two years. By the end of the study, mice of all groups developed various tumors but there was no significant difference in tumor incidence between the different dietary groups. This lack of carcinogenicity is consistent with results of short-term in vitro assays of this compound.

Some reproductive, developmental, and behavioral parameters in mice were apparently affected by dietary amaranth (a red color additive) (*121*). Parent mice were fed 0, 0.03, 0.09, or 0.27% dietary amaranth from 4 weeks prior to mating through gestation and lactation. Pups were continued on their respective parental diet during 8 weeks of observation. No major toxic effects were observed in the pups but there were significant reductions in olfactory orientation in both sexes and in direction of swimming on postnatal day 4 in male pups. Survival index of the 0.27% amaranth group was reduced on postnatal day 21 as compared to controls.

Mutagenicity of metanil yellow and orange II, two azo dyes commonly used as food colors, was assessed in a diploid human lymphoblast cell line, AHH-1, which is competent for xenobiotic metabolism (*122*). Both compounds induced significant numbers of mutations at the HPRT locus in AHH-1 cells during a long-term (20 days), low-dose (30 nM orange II or 50 nM metanil yellow) study. Concentrations required to double the spontaneous mutation rate were 22 nM for metanil yellow and 12 nM for orange II.

Since chronic feeding of metanil yellow and orange II have been reported to cause alterations in liver weight and, in some cases, hepatic lesions, experiments were conducted to determine whether these compounds can induce hepatic lipid peroxidation (*123*). Rats were given ip injections of 80 mg metanil yellow/kg body weight, 80 mg orange II/kg, or a mixture of 40 mg of each color/kg for 3 consecutive days and then sacrificed 1 day after the last dose. When administered alone, both compounds induced significant increases in NADPH-dependent enzymatic lipid peroxidation in nuclear, mitochondrial, and microsomal membranes. Relatively lower levels of lipid peroxidation were caused by orange II. Results with the mixture of the two compounds demonstrated an additive or synergistic effect.

In clastogenicity assays with rats and mice, FD&C Yellow No. 6, a widely used colorant, induced no significant increases in bone marrow micronucleated polychromatic erythrocytes in either species following gavage with a single dose of 500, 1000, or 2000 mg/kg of the food color (*124*). A structurally related azo dye, Solvent Yellow 14, which is not approved for use in foods, did exert clastogenic effects in rats but not in mice.

Green S, a food color approved in India and some other countries, was found to induce sister chromatid exchanges (SCEs) and chromosomal aberrations (CAs) in mice (*125*). The minimum effective doses (injections) which induced SCEs and CAs were 50 and 200 mg Green S/kg body weight, respectively.

A thin-layer chromatographic/liquid secondary ion mass spectrometric method was developed to rapidly separate and identify the 11 food dyes that are permitted in Japan (*126*). Glycerol and magic bullet were found to ensure good stability and reproducibility of the mass spectra. For the reversed phase TLC, two solvent systems were used: one for the separation of xanthene dyes containing methanol, methyl ethyl ketone, and sodium sulfate and another for the other dyes containing methanol, acetonitrile, and sodium sulfate. Thioglycerol was used to concentrate diffused spots on the plate. This method provided satisfactory mass spectra for all the food dyes except indigo carmine.

A method utilizing capillary isotachophoresis has been applied to the determination of synthetic food colorants (*127*). Food dyes were extracted with methanol–ammonia solution (powdered samples), with n-amylalcohol (liquid samples), or by adsorption on powdered or granulated polyamides followed by extraction with methanol–ammonia. First, the food dyes in samples were determined qualitatively by paper chromatography and this was followed by analytical evaluations of isotachopherograms from columns using an electrolyte system with HCl as the leading electrolyte, acetic acid as the terminating electrolyte, pH 3.5, and β-alanine as the counter ion. Fifteen food samples, including pudding mixes, powdered beverages, and hard candies, were analyzed using this method.

Amaranth and indigo carmine have been determined at the ppb level by voltammetric analysis using silver-based mercury film electrodes (*128*). The two food dyes were detected at different reduction potentials: –0.11 V for indigo carmine and –0.24 V for amaranth. Thus they could be determined separately without interfering with each other. Response of both colorants was linear in a concentration range of 0–100 ng/mL.

VITAMINS

Vitamin A

A congenital abnormality in the eye was reported in an infant whose mother had consumed excessive amounts of vitamin A during pregnancy (*129*). Examination of the "enlarged left eye" revealed an hourglass-shaped cornea and iris with a reduplicated lens. During pregnancy, the mother had taken a multivitamin tablet almost daily and had eaten 3 meals containing liver a week during the first trimester. Considering these and other usual dietary sources of vitamin A, it was estimated that she took an average daily dose of 25,000 IU vitamin A during the first trimester. Recommended dietary intake of vitamin A should not exceed 10,000 IU/day because teratogenic effects have been reported at doses as low as 20,000 IU.

In response to such reports, the Department of Health in Great Britain has recommended that women not take vitamin A supplements and not consume liver during pregnancy (*130*). Standard reference books give the vitamin A levels in ox and chicken liver as 16,500 and 9,300 μg/100 g,

respectively. But recent tests indicate that ox liver contains 27,000–29,580 μg/100 g and that chicken liver contains 13,210–37,000 μg/100 g. The recommended daily intake of vitamin A is 750 μg, rising to 1200 μg for nursing mothers.

Data from a Hungarian study designed to investigate the protective effects of periconceptional multivitamin supplementation on the occurrence of neural tube defects indicated that daily vitamin supplements containing 6000 IU of vitamin A taken from 1 month before gestation to the 12th week of pregnancy did not exert teratogenic effects (*131*). Comparison of the 1203 and 1510 births in the vitamin-exposed and non-exposed groups, respectively, revealed no excess of congenital abnormalities usually associated with high intakes of vitamin A among the infants of mothers taking supplements.

Niacin

Five outbreaks of facial flushing accompanied by a feeling of warmth and pruritis involving about 150 people occurred in Israel among people who had consumed frozen ground beef or processed veal steaks (*132*). Analysis of available meat samples were negative for histamines but revealed the presence of 0.3–1.5 g niacin/kg meat. Samples of meat taken directly from one supplier of the implicated meat contained 2.4–6.0 g niacin/kg meat. Naturally occurring levels of niacin in skeletal muscle meat range up to 0.07 g/kg and recommended daily intakes range from 6–19 mg. Although niacin is an illegal meat additive in Israel, it is sometimes used as a color enhancer. Niacin is heat stable and therefore not destroyed by cooking.

Vitamin D

An unusual series of 8 cases of hypervitaminosis D was described from Massachusetts (*133*). None of the patients reported taking cod liver oil, fish oil, vitamin D supplements, or health food supplements but all had elevated serum 25-hydroxyvitamin D concentrations (mean = 731 nmol/L; normal range 22–200 nmol/L). Six patients had elevated serum levels of vitamin D_3 and 7 had hypercalcemia.

All stated that they drank milk (118–710 mL/day) from the same local dairy. Analyses of vitamin D-fortified milk from the dairy revealed concentrations of vitamin D_3 ranging from undetectable to 245,840 IU/L. According to federal regulations, fortified milk should contain 400 IU of vitamin D/quart. It appeared that vitamin D was added to the milk sporadically and sometimes in excess.

Vitamin E

Palm vitee, a vitamin E-containing extract of palm oil, contains approximately 20% α-tocopherol and 80% tocotrienols. In acute toxicity tests, mice and rats were fed daily doses of 250, 500, 1000, or 2500 mg palm vitee/kg body weight/day for 30 days (*134*). Although treated mice gained significantly more weight during the experiment and some sluggish motor activity was observed, no treatment-related physical or behavioral abnormalities were noted. Some minor and inconsistent fluctuations in mean arterial pressure and heart rate occurred in anesthetized cats injected with 2–20 mg palm vitee/kg. These doses of palm vitee are approximately 60–600 times higher than the normal daily vitamin E dosage in humans.

STABILIZERS, THICKENERS, AND CONDITIONERS

Carrageenan

Since oxygen free radicals are known to be involved in a wide variety of inflammatory conditions, the role of these radicals in carrageenan-induced intestinal injury was investigated (*135*). On day 1 a group of rats was sensitized by giving them an injection of lambda degraded carrageenan and adjuvant. Then on day 8, all rats were given carrageenan in drinking water and some groups also received one of 3 drugs, allopurinol, superoxide dismutase–polyethylene glycol, or dimethyl sulfoxide, until day 38. All 3 oxyradical scavengers significantly attenuated intestinal injury as measured by 4 indices of inflammation. These results indicate that oxyradicals are also involved in carrageenan-induced intestinal injury.

A simple, rapid colorimetric method using Alcian blue reagent was developed for the determination of carrageenan in jellies and salad dressings (*136*). This reagent was added to a neutralized, aqueous defatted (if necessary) sample and the resulting carrageenan–Alcian blue complex was collected, dissolved in monoethanolamine and determined colorimetrically at 615 nm. Detection limit for the method was 0.05%, and recoveries from jellies and salad dressings averaged 93.3% and 91.9%, respectively. Results were similar to those obtained by a capillary GC method.

High titer antisera to κ-carrageenan produced in rabbits and guinea pigs, along with rabbit serum as a capture antibody and guinea pig serum as a detector antibody, were used in a sandwich ELISA to detect κ-carrageenan in foods (*137*). Assay results were linear in a range of 16–256 nm/mL, and recoveries of κ-carrageenan added to jellies and puddings averaged 88–94%. Minimal sample preparation was required and the antisera showed no cross-reactivity to 6 other thickeners tested.

Potassium bromate

Acute oral toxicity of potassium bromate, used as a food additive mainly for the treatment of wheat flour, was investigated in experiments with rats given doses of 85, 159, 325 and 602 mg/kg (*138*). None of the animals died within 72 h after the lowest dose while only 20% survived a dose of 159 mg/kg. LD_{50} value in rats was estimated to be 157 mg/kg. About 95% of the potassium bromate was absorbed from the stomach within 30 min of dosing and about 13% was excreted in the urine within 24 h. Trace amounts of methemoglobin were detected in blood of animals and significant hemochromatosis was observed in the kidney, spleen and liver.

Primary cultures of rat kidney and liver cells and homogenates of kidney, liver, heart, and brain of rats were exposed to potassium bromate to investigate the formation of potentially toxic active oxygen species (*139*). Hydroxyl radicals were generated in kidney cells and homogenates but not in liver and only to a limited extent in brain and heart. This reaction was effectively inhibited by singlet oxygen scavengers. Singlet oxygen production was confirmed by chemiluminescence. These active oxygen species are most likely involved in the toxic and carcinogenic effects of potassium bromate.

Potassium bromate was also found to induce micronuclei in peripheral blood reticulocytes of male mice in the same manner as in polychromatic erythrocytes of bone marrow (140). Mice were injected with 18.8–212 mg potassium bromate/kg and blood cells were collected 24–96 h later and stained with acridine orange to detect micronuclei.

Brominated vegetable oils

Brominated vegetable oils (BVO) have been used to adjust the density of citrus flavoring oils in soft drinks, but toxicological studies have indicated that BVO are a cumulative health hazard. A simple, precise colorimetric method for the detection of BVO in soft drinks has been developed (141). BVO were extracted with ether and the organic bromides changed to inorganic form by the addition of a small amount of zinc dust. Lead dioxide was added to liberate bromine, which was detected by a color change in fluorescein-impregnated filter paper. Concentrations as low as 10 ppm can be detected.

Chlorinated bleaching adducts in flour-containing foods

During routine residue analyses using a procedure designed to detect chlorinated herbicides, bakery products and other flour-containing food items were found to contain a series of unusual halogenated compounds (142). These compounds were present in bleached but not in unbleached flours. GC/MS with chemical ionization revealed the presence of more than 8 chlorinated derivatives of indigenous fatty acids. The most prominent residue was that of 9,10-dichloro-12-octadecanoic acid which was commonly found in some cakes at levels higher than 20 ppm. Toxicological significance of these compounds has not yet been determined.

Tragacanth gum

Tragacanth gum is a complex polysaccharide widely used in cosmetic, pharmaceutical, and food products. In an oral toxicity study this gum was fed to mice for 13 weeks at dietary levels of 0.625, 1.25, 2.5, and 5.0% (143). No treatment-related effects were noted in clinical signs, body or organ weights, urinalysis or hematology tests. Single or small numbers of tiny nodules (squamous cell hyperplasia) were observed in the forestomach of some treated males. Further studies of mice dosed for 48 weeks with 5% gum failed to demonstrate a consistent effect of the gum on hyperplasia or DNA synthesis in forestomach epithelium. Thus, the oral toxicity of tragacanth gum in mice was concluded to be negligible.

FAT SUBSTITUTES

Following intravenous administration of olestra to rats and monkeys, there was no evidence of its metabolism, and 74% of the dose to monkeys was recovered from the liver after 48 h while 58–96% of the dose to rats was found in the liver at 24 h (144). However, when fed in the diet (8% to monkeys and 9% to rats) for 24–29 months, no olestra was detected in monkey liver as determined by TLC (limit of determination, 34 µg/g) and none was detected in liver samples from 47 of 50 rats analyzed by HPLC (determination limit 1.6 µg/g). Very low concentrations of olestra were found in the other 3 rats (2–4 µg/g). These results are similar to previous results and indicate that very little, if any, olestra is absorbed from the gastrointestinal tract.

During two 2-year studies, olestra was fed to rats at dietary levels of 0, 0.99, 4.76, and 9.09% to determine any toxic effects (145). No evidence of adverse effects was detected by data on growth and feed consumption, ophthalmoscopic examinations, organ weights, serum chemistry, hematology, urinalysis, or histopathological evaluations. Relative to controls, there was a higher incidence of basophilic liver foci in olestra-fed females but these were not associated with liver tumors, alterations in liver function, or increases in liver weight.

A 20-month study with beagle dogs fed olestra at 0, 5, or 10% of the diet likewise demonstrated a lack of toxic and carcinogenic effects of this fat substitute (*146*). No olestra-related effects were seen on growth, hematology, serum biochemistry, or histopathology.

OTHER ADDITIVES

Ethylenediaminetetraacetic acid (EDTA)

Na_2EDTA, a widely used chelating agent in foods, was tested for its ability to induce bone marrow micronuclei, dominant lethal mutations, and sperm-head abnormalities in mice (*147*). Oral doses of 5–15 mg EDTA/kg body weight/day for 5 consecutive days failed to induce obvious signs of toxicity or alterations in sperm counts or the incidences of sperm-head abnormalities or post-implantation embryonic deaths. However, acute doses of EDTA (5–20 mg/kg) did induce a dose-dependent increase in micronucleated polychromatic erythrocytes at 24 h.

A reversed-phase ion-pair HPLC method for the determination of EDTA in the liquid of canned mushrooms was developed (*148*). Cupric chloride was added to filtered samples prior to injection into the HPLC system. The Cu^{++}–EDTA complex was separated using a water–methanol mobile phase containing tetrabutylammonium as the counter ion and detected by UV at 300 nm. Determination limit was 10 mg EDTA/L and a linear response was obtained between 7 and 178 mg EDTA/L. Recoveries of added EDTA averaged 101–106%.

Purified cellulose

Safety of industrially purified cellulose was recently reviewed and updated based on literature published since the 1972 GRAS declaration (*149*). Since molecular chlorine is used to remove lignan in the purification process, trace amounts of organochlorine residuals may be present in the purified

cellulose. However, the available literature indicates that chronic ingestion of purified cellulose during the entire lifespan of rats and mice does not result in any increase in neoplasia, spontaneous disease, or adverse reproductive or developmental effects. Neither does purified cellulose appear to promote carcinogenesis or alter the absorption or metabolism of other dietary components.

Alkaline cellulase

Alkaline cellulase is isolated from submerged cultures of the fungus *Humicola insolens* and is used as a processing aid in brewing and baking. In a series of studies to evaluate the safety of this enzyme, there was no evidence that the enzyme caused reproductive toxicity or mutations (*150*). General toxicity was low, with a no-adverse-effect level in rats of 420 mg enzyme TOS/kg. Mild effects were noted when the skin and eye were exposed to this enzyme. Since humans would most likely be exposed to a maximum of 0.1 mg enzyme TOS/kg/day by ingestion of beer and bread, alkaline cellulose can be regarded as safe for the consumer. Evidence also indicates that *H. insolens* can be regarded as non-toxigenic and non-pathogenic.

Calcium lactate

Long term toxicity/carcinogenicity studies of calcium lactate in rats gave negative results (*151*). Calcium lactate, widely used as a calcium supplement in a variety of foods, was added to drinking water of rats at levels of 0, 2.5, or 5% during a two-year study. No significant dose-related increases were observed in tumor incidences or in any toxic lesions.

LITERATURE CITED

1. Bär, A., and G. Würtzen. Assessing the use of additives in food: a reappraisal of the Danish budget method. *Lebensm. Wiss. Technol.* 23:193–202 (1990).

2. Bush, R.K., E. Zoratti, and S.L. Taylor. Diagnosis of sulfite and aspirin sensitivity. *Clin. Rev. Allergy* 8:159–179 (1991).

3. Mansour, E., A. Ahmed, A. Cortes, et al. Mechanisms of metabisulfite-induced bronchoconstriction: evidence for bradykinin B_2-receptor stimulation. *J. Appl. Physiol.* 72:1831–1837 (1992).

4. Paíno-Campa, G., M.J. Peña-Egido, and C. García-Moreno. Liquid chromatographic determination of free and total sulphites in fresh sausages. *J. Sci. Food Agric.* 56:85–93 (1991).

5. Reim, R.E. Total sulfite in cellulosics by ion exclusion chromatography with electrochemical detection. *J. Food Sci.* 56:1087–1090,1094 (1991).

6. Nabirahni, M.A., and R.R. Vaid. Development and application of an immobilized enzyme electrode for the determination of sulfite in foods and feeds. *Anal. Lett.* 24:551–565 (1991).

7. Arowolo, T.A., and M.S. Cresser. Automated determination of sulphite by gas-phase molecular absorption spectrometry. *Analyst* 116:1135–1139 (1991).

8. Bartroli, J., M. Escalada, C.J. Jorquera, and J. Alonso. Determination of total and free sulfur dioxide in wine by flow injection analysis and gas-diffusion using *p*-aminoazobenzene as the colorimetric reagent. *Anal. Chem.* 63:2532–2535 (1991).

9. Michils, A., G. Vandermoten. J. Duchateau, and J.-C. Yernault. Anaphylaxis with sodium benzoate. *Lancet* 337:1424–1425 (1991).

10. Page, B.D., H.B.S. Conacher, D. Weber, and G. Lacroix. A survey of benzene in fruits and retail fruit juices, fruit drinks, and soft drinks. *J. AOAC Int.* 75:334–340 (1992).

11. Ng, C.L., H.K. Lee, and S.F.Y. Li. Analysis of food additives by ion-pairing electrokinetic chromatography. *J. Chromatogr. Sci.* 30:167–170 (1992).

12. Kakemoto, M. Simultaneous determination of sorbic acid, dehydroacetic acid and benzoic acid by gas chromatography–mass spectrometry. *J. Chromatogr.* 594:253–257 (1992).

13. Jung, R., C. Cojocel, W. Müller, et al. Evaluation of the genotoxic potential of sorbic acid and potassium sorbate. *Food Chem. Toxicol.* 30:1–7 (1992).

14. Harrison, P.T.C., P. Grasso, and V. Badescu. Early changes in the forestomach of rats, mice and hamsters exposed to dietary propionic and butyric acid. *Food Chem. Toxicol.* 29:367–371 (1991).

15. Shimada, K., E. Kimura, Y. Yasui, et al. Styrene formation by the decomposition by *Pichia carsonii* of *trans*-cinnamic acid added to a ground fish product. *Appl. Environ. Microbiol.* 58:1577–1582 (1992).

16. Bednar, C.M., C. Kies, and M. Carlson. Nitrate-nitrite levels in commercially processed and home processed beets and spinach. *Plant Foods Hum. Nutr.* 41:261–268 (1991).

17. Gromes, R., D. Glaser, B. Sattig, and B. Schnellbacher. Bestimmung des nitratgehaltes in lebensmitteln mit HPLC und einem neuen enzymatischen test. *Dtsch. Lebensm.-Rundsch.* 87:346–350 (1991).

18. Sanderson, J.E., J.R. Consaul, and K. Lee. Nitrate analysis in meats; comparison of two methods. *J. Food Sci.* 56:1123–1124 (1991).

19. Karl, H. Bestimmung des nitritgehaltes in räucherfischen und anderen fischprodukten. *Dtsch. Lebensm.-Rundsch.* 88:41–45 (1992).

20. Kammerer, M., L. Pinault, and H. Pouliquen. Teneur en nitrate du lait. Relation avec sa concentration dans l'eau d'abreuvement. *Ann. Rech. Vét.* 23:131–138 (1992).

21. Geissler, C., O. Steinhöfel, and M. Ulbrich. Zum nitratgehalt in der milch. *Arch. Anim. Nutr., Berlin* 41:649–656 (1991).

22. Feier, U., and P.-H. Goetsch. Inter-laboratory studies on precision characteristics of analytical methods. II. Determination of nitrate content in milk and milk products—xylenol method. *Milchwissenschaft* 46:170,172 (1991).

23. Kleinjans, J.C.S., H.J. Albering, A. Marx, et al. Nitrate contamination of drinking water: evaluation of genotoxic risk in human populations. *Environ. Health Perspect.* 94:189–193 (1991).

24. Grudzinski, I., and A. Szymanski. The effect of subchronic poisoning with potassium nitrate and sodium nitrite on the processes of intestinal absorption of D-xylose in rats. *Arch. Environ. Contam. Toxicol.* 21:447–452 (1991).

25. Rowland, I.R., T. Granli, O.C. Bøckman, et al. Endogenous *N*-nitrosation in man assessed by measurement of apparent total *N*-nitroso compounds in faeces. *Carcinogenesis* 12:1395–1401 (1991).

26. Knight, T., R. Pirastu, D. Palli, et al. Nitrate and *N*-nitrosoproline excretion in two Italian regions with contrasting rates of gastric cancer: the role of nitrate and other factors in endogenous nitrosation. *Int. J. Cancer* 50:736–739 (1992).

27. Srivatanakul, P., H. Ohshima, M. Khlat, et al. *Opisthorchis viverrini* infestation and endogenous nitrosamines as risk factors for cholangiocarcinoma in Thailand. *Int. J. Cancer* 48:821–825 (1991).

28. Knight, T.M., D. Forman, H. Ohshima, and H. Bartsch. Endogenous nitrosation of L-proline by dietary-derived nitrate. *Nutr. Cancer* 15:195–203 (1991).

29. Kyrtopoulos, S.A., B. Pignatelli, G. Karkanias, et al. Studies in gastric carcinogenesis. V. The effects of ascorbic acid on *N*-nitroso compound formation in human gastric juice *in vivo* and *in vitro*. *Carcinogenesis* 12:1371–1376 (1991).

30. Shapiro, K.B., J.H. Hotchkiss, and D.A. Roe. Quantitative relationship between oral nitrate-reducing activity and the endogenous formation of *N*-nitrosoamino acids in humans. *Food Chem. Toxicol.* 29:751–755 (1991).

31. Tricker, A.R., B. Pfundstein, T. Kälble, and R. Preussmann. Secondary amine precursors to nitrosamines in human saliva, gastric juice, blood, urine and faeces. *Carcinogenesis* 13:563–568 (1992).

32. Weng, Y.-M., J.H. Hotchkiss, and J.G. Babish. *N*-Nitrosamine and mutagenicity formation in Chinese salted fish after digestion. *Food Addit. Contam.* 9:29–37 (1992).

33. Atawodi, S.E., E.N. Maduagwu, R. Preussmann, and B. Spiegelhalder. Potential of endogenous formation of volatile nitrosamines from Nigerian vegetables and spices. *Cancer Lett.* 57:219–222 (1991).

34. Hashizume, T., H. Santo, H. Tsujisawa, et al. Mutagenic activities of tryptophan metabolites before and after nitrite treatment. *Food Chem. Toxicol.* 29:839–844 (1991).

35. Lin, J.-K., J.T. Cheng, and S.Y. Lin-Shiau. Enhancement of the mutagenicity of IQ and MeIQ by nitrite in the Salmonella system. *Mutat. Res.* 278:277–287 (1992).

36. Tricker, A.R., and S.J. Kubacki. Review of the occurrence and formation of non-volatile *N*-nitroso compounds in foods. *Food Addit. Contam.* 9:39–69 (1992).

37. Massey, R.C., P.E. Key, R.A. Jones, and G.L. Logan. Volatile, non-volatile and total *N*-nitroso compounds in bacon. *Food Addit. Contam.* 8:585–598 (1991).

38. Chen, C.S., B. Pignatelli, C. Malaveille, et al. Levels of direct-acting mutagens, total *N*-nitroso compounds in nitrosated fermented fish products, consumed in a high-risk area for gastric cancer in southern China. *Mutat. Res.* 265:211–221 (1992).

39. Tricker, A.R., B. Pfundstein, E. Theobald, et al. Mean daily intake of volatile *N*-nitrosamines from foods and beverages in West Germany in 1989–1990. *Food Chem. Toxicol.* 29:729–732 (1991).

40. Mavelle, T., B. Bouchikhi, and G. Debry. The occurrence of volatile *N*-nitrosamines in French foodstuffs. *Food Chem.* 42:321–338 (1991).

41. Hamburg, A., and A. Hamburg. N-Nitrosoproline and N-nitrososarcosine in Estonian foodstuffs. *J. Food Safety* 12:149–159 (1992).

42. Coker, H.A.B., A.E. Thomas, and A. Akintonwa. Determination of the total level of nitrosamines in select consumer products in Lagos area of Nigeria. *Bull. Environ. Contam. Toxicol.* 47:706–710 (1991).

43. Fiddler, W., J.W. Pensabene, R.A. Gates, et al. N-Nitrosodimethylamine formation in cooked frankfurters containing Alaska pollock (*Theragra chalcogramma*) mince and surimi. *J. Food Sci.* 57:569–571,595 (1992).

44. Pensabene, J.W., W. Fiddler, R.A. Gates, et al. N-Nitrosothiazolidine and its 4-carboxylic acid in frankfurters containing Alaska pollock. *J. Food Sci.* 56:1108–1110 (1991).

45. Sen, N.P., P.A. Baddoo, S.W. Seaman, and D. Weber. 2-(Hydroxymethyl)-*N*-nitrosothiazolidine-4-carboxylic acid in smoked meats and bacon and conversion to 2-(hydroxymethyl)-*N*-nitrosothiazolidine during high-heat cooking. *J. Food Sci.* 56:913–915 (1991).

46. Tiedink, H.G.M., L.H.J. de Haan, W.M.F. Jongen, and J.H. Koeman. *In-vitro* testing and the carcinogenic potential of several nitrosated indole compounds. *Cell Biol. Toxicol.* 7:371–386 (1991).

47. Sasagawa, C., and T. Matsushima. Mutagen formation on nitrite treatment of indole compounds derived from indole-glucosinolate. *Mutat. Res.* 250:169–174 (1991).

48. Oshita, I., H. Kanamori, M. Mizuta, and I. Sakamoto. A mutagenic β-carboline derivative in soy sauce. *Shokuhim Eiseigaku Zasshi* 32:272–277 (1991).

49. Stowers, J.M., and S.B.W. Ewen. Possible dietary factors in the induction of diabetes and its inheritance in man, with studies in mice. *Proc. Nutr. Soc.* 50:287–298 (1991).

50. Multiple authors. Full report of the British Industrial Biological Research Association carcinogenesis bioassays (with an invited article discussing these assays). *Cancer Res.* 51:6409–6491 (1991).

51. Travis, C.C., T.W. McClain, and P.D. Birkner. Diethylnitrsoamine-induced hepatocarcinogenesis in rats: a theoretical study. *Toxicol. Appl. Pharmacol.* 109:289–304 (1991).

52. Nagahara, A., and S. Kumagai. Excretion and distribution of nitrite-treated or untreated 1-methyl-1,2,3,4-tetrahydro-β-carboline-3-carboxylic acid in rats. *Food Chem. Toxicol.* 29:243–247 (1991).

53. Lawson, T., D. Nagel, and D. Rogers. The activation of β-substituted nitrosamines that are carcinogenic to the pancreas. *Int. J. Pancreatol.* 20:9–21 (1991).

54. Stiborová, M., E. Frei, H. H. Schmeiser, et al. Peroxidase oxidizes *N*-nitrosomethylaniline to ultimate carcinogen(s) binding to DNA and transfer RNA in vitro. *Cancer Lett.* 63:53–59 (1992).

55. Wiench, K., E. Frei, P. Schroth, and M. Wiessler. 1-C-Glucuronidation of *N*-nitrosodiethylamine and *N*-nitrosomethyl-*n*-pentylamine *in vivo* and in primary hepatocytes from rats pretreated with inducers. *Carcinogenesis* 13:867–872 (1992).

56. Sen, N.P., P.A. Baddoo, S.W. Seaman, and D. Weber. Simultaneous determination of 2-(hydroxymethyl)-*N*-nitrosothiazolidine-4-carboxylic acid and 2-(hydroxymethyl)-*N*-nitrosothiazolidine in smoked meats and cheese. *J. Agric. Food Chem.* 40:221–226 (1992).

57. Pensabene, J.W., W. Fiddler, and R.A. Gates. Solid-phase extraction method for volatile *N*-nitrosamines in hams processed with elastic rubber netting. *J. AOAC Int.* 75:438–442 (1992).

58. Castegnaro, M. International *N*-nitroso compounds check sample programme: report on the performance in the second study dedicated to their determination in beer and malt. *Food Addit. Contam.* 8:577–584 (1991).

59. Nakayama, T., K. Terazawa, and S. Kawakishi. Cytotoxicity of glucosone in the presence of cupric ion. *J. Agric. Food Chem.* 40:830–833 (1992).

60. Katusin-Razem, B., B. Mihaljevic, and D. Razem. Radiation-induced oxidative chemical changes in dehydrated egg products. *J. Agric. Food Chem.* 40:662–668 (1992).

61. Zimmering, S., O. Olvera, M.P. Cruces, et al. Irradiated cocoa tested in the wing spot assay in *Drosophila melanogaster. Mutat. Res.* 281:169–171 (1992).

62. Lépine, F.L. Effects of ionizing radiation on pesticides in a food irradiation perspective: a bibliographic review. *J. Agric. Food Chem.* 39:2112–2118 (1991).

63. Findlay, D.J.S., T.V. Parsons, and M.R. Sene. Experimental electron beam irradiation of food and the induction of radioactivity. *Appl. Radiat. Isot.* 43:567–575 (1992).

64. Raffi, J., M.H. Stevenson, M. Kent, et al. European intercomparison on electron spin resonance identification of irradiated foodstuffs. *Int. J. Food Sci. Technol.* 27:111–124 (1992).

65. Desrosiers, M.F., G.L. Wilson, C.R. Hunter, and D.R. Hutton. Estimation of the absorbed dose in radiation-processed food--1. Test of the EPR response function by a linear regression analysis. *Appl. Radiat. Isot.* 42:613–616 (1991).

66. Desrosiers, M.F. Estimation of the absorbed dose in radiation-processed food--2. Test of the EPR response function by an exponential fitting analysis. *Appl. Radiat. Isot.* 42:617–619 (1991).

67. Desrosiers, M.F. Electron spin resonance for monitoring radiation-processed meats containing bone. *J. Food Sci.* 56:1104–1105 (1991).

68. Stewart, E.M., M.H. Stevenson, and R. Gray. Use of ESR spectroscopy for the detection of irradiated whiting (*Merlangius merlangus*). *J. Sci. Food Agric.* 55:653–660 (1991).

69. Stewart, E.M., M.H. Stevenson, and R. Gray. Detection of irradiation in scampi tails—effects of sample preparation, irradiation dose and storage on ESR response in the cuticle. *Int. J. Food Sci. Technol.* 27:125–132 (1992).

70. Stachowicz, W., G. Strzelczak-Burlinska, J. Michalik, et al. Application of electron paramagnetic resonance (EPR) spectroscopy for control of irradiated food. *J. Sci. Food Agric.* 58:407–415 (1992).

71. Ammon, J., G. Mildau, W. Ruge, and H. Delincée. Nachweis einer bestrahlung von hühnerfleisch durch gaschromatographische messung von radiolyseprodukten aus der fettfraktion. *Dtsch. Lebensm.-Rundsch.* 88:35–37 (1992).

72. Maerker, G., and K.C. Jones. Gamma-irradia-

tion of individual cholesterol oxidation products. *J. Am. Oil Chem. Soc.* 69:451–455 (1992).

73. Chuaqui-Offermanns, N., and T. McDougall. Background levels and radiation dose yield of o-tyrosine in chicken meat. *J. Food Protect.* 54:935–938 (1991).

74. Ewing, D.D., and T.M. Stepanik. Ineffectiveness of a fluorometric method for identifying irradiated food based on thymine glycol. *J. Food Sci.* 57:660–663 (1992).

75. Sahu, S.C., and M.C. Washington. Effect of ascorbic acid and curcumin on quercetin-induced nuclear DNA damage, lipid peroxidation and protein degradation. *Cancer Lett.* 63:237–241 (1992).

76. Wagner, H.P., and M.J. McGarrity. The use of pulsed amperometry combined with ion-exclusion chromatography for the simultaneous analysis of ascorbic acid and sulfite. *J. Chromatogr.* 546:119–124 (1991).

77. Andrikopoulos, N.K., H. Brueschweiler, H. Felber, and C. Taeschler. HPLC analysis of phenolic antioxidants, tocopherols and triglycerides. *J. Am. Oil Chem. Soc.* 68:359–364 (1991).

78. Urivetzky, M., D. Kessaris, and A.D. Smith. Ascorbic acid overdosing: a risk factor for calcium oxalate nephrolithiasis. *J. Urol.* 147:1215–1218 (1992).

79. Behrens, W.A., and R. Madere. Quantitative analysis of ascorbic acid and isoascorbic acid in foods by high-performance liquid chromatography with electrochemical detection. *J. Liq. Chromatogr.* 15:753–765 (1992).

80. García Montelongo, F., M.J. Sánchez, J.C. García Castro, and A. Hardisson. 2nd and 3rd Order derivative spectrophotometric determination of ascorbic acid in soft drinks. *Anal. Lett.* 24:1875–1883 (1991).

81. Verhagen, H., P.A.E.L. Schilderman, and J.C.S. Kleinjans. Butylated hydroxyanisole in perspective. *Chem.-Biol. Interact.* 80:109–134 (1991).

82. Schilderman, P.A.E.L., W. Engels, J.J.M. Wenders, et al. Effects of butylated hydroxyanisole on arachidonic acid and linoleic acid metabolism in relation to gastrointestinal cell proliferation in the rat. *Carcinogenesis* 13:585–591 (1992).

83. Lam, L.K.T., and P. Garg. Tumorigenicity of di-tert-butyl-substituted hydroquinone and hydroxyanisoles in the forestomach of Syrian golden hamsters. *Carcinogenesis* 12:1341–1344 (1991).

84. Shertzer, H.G., G.L. Bannenberg, M. Rundgren, and P. Moldéus. Relationship of membrane fluidity, chemoprotection, and the intrinsic toxicity of butylated hydroxytoluene. *Biochem. Pharmacol.* 42:1587–1593 (1991).

85. Williams, G.M., T. Tanaka, H. Maruyama, et al. Modulation by butylated hydroxytoluene of liver and bladder carcinogenesis induced by chronic low-level exposure to 2-acetylaminofluorene. *Cancer Res.* 51:6224–6230 (1991).

86. Singletary, K.W., and J.M. Nelshoppen. Selective *in vivo* inhibition of rat mammary 7,12-dimethylbenz[*a*]anthracene–DNA adduct formation by dietary butylated hydroxytoluene. *Carcinogenesis* 12:1967–1969 (1991).

87. Takahashi, O. Haemorrhages due to defective blood coagulation do not occur in mice and guinea-pigs fed butylated hydroxytoluene, but nephrotoxicity is found in mice. *Food Chem. Toxicol.* 30:89–97 (1992).

88. Chen, C., A.M. Pearson, and J.I. Gray. Effects of synthetic antioxidants (BHA, BHT and PG) on the mutagenicity of IQ-like compounds. *Food Chem.* 43:177–183 (1992).

89. Ghosal, A., and M.M. Iba. Enhancement by butylated hydroxytoluene of the in vitro activation of 3,3'-dichlorobenzidine. *Mutat. Res.* 278:31–41 (1992).

90. Wei, C.I., T.S. Huang, S.Y. Fernando, and K.T. Chung. Mutagenicity studies of kojic acid. *Toxicol. Lett.* 59:213–220 (1991).

91. Hard, G.C., and G.E. Neal. Sequential study of the chronic nephrotoxicity induced by dietary administration of ethoxyquin in Fischer 344 rats. *Fund. Appl. Toxicol.* 18:278–287 (1992).

92. Viñas, P., M. Hernández Córdoba, and C. Sánchez-Pedreño. Determination of ethoxyquin in paprika by high-performance liquid chromatography. *Food Chem.* 42:241–251 (1991).

93. Tollefson, L., and R.J. Barnard. An analysis of FDA passive surveillance reports of seizures associated with consumption of aspartame. *J. Am. Diet. Assoc.* 92:598–601 (1992).

94. Camfield, P.R., C.S. Camfield, J.M. Dooley, et al. Aspartame exacerbates EEG spike-wave discharge in children with generalized absence epilepsy: A double-blind controlled study. *Neurology* 42:1000–1003 (1992).

95. Garriga, M.M., C. Berkebile, and D.D. Metcalfe. A combined single-blind, double-blind, placebo-controlled study to determine the reproducibility of hyper-

sensitivity reactions to aspartame. *J. Allergy Clin. Immunol.* 87:821–827 (1991).

96. Stokes, A.F., A. Belger, M.T. Banich, and H. Taylor. Effects of acute aspartame and acute alcohol ingestion upon the cognitive performance of pilots. *Aviat. Space Environ. Med.* 62:648–653 (1991).

97. Møller, S.E. Effect of aspartame and protein, administered in phenylalanine-equivalent doses, on plasma neutral amino acids, aspartate, insulin and glucose in man. *Pharmacol. Toxicol.* 68:408–412 (1991).

98. Hjelle, J.J., R.E. Dudley, M.P. Marietta, et al. Plasma concentrations and pharmacokinetics of phenylalanine in rats and mice administered aspartame. *Pharmacology* 44:48–60 (1992).

99. Lipton, W.E., Y.-N. Li, M.K. Younoszai, and L.D. Stegink. Intestinal absorption of aspartame decomposition products in adult rats. *Metabolism* 40:1337–1345 (1991).

100. Fellows, J.W., S.W. Chang, and W.H. Shazer. Stability of aspartame in fruit preparations used in yogurt. *J. Food Sci.* 56:689–691 (1991).

101. Große-Wächter, S., and U. Dirks. Bestimmung von aspartam und seinem cyclisierungsprodukt diketopiperazin in desserterzeugnissen mittels HPLC. *Z. Lebensm. Unters. Forsch.* 193:344–346 (1991).

102. Homma, Y., Y. Kondo, T. Kakizoe, et al. Lack of bladder carcinogenicity of dietary sodium saccharin in analbuminaemic rats, which are highly susceptible to *N*-nitroso-*n*-butyl-(4-hydroxybutyl)amine. *Food Chem. Toxicol.* 29:373–376 (1991).

103. Cohen, S.M., M. Cano, R.A. Earl, et al. A proposed role for silicates and protein in the proliferative effects of saccharin on the male rat urothelium. *Carcinogenesis* 12:1551–1555 (1991).

104. Henry, R.R., P.A. Crapo, and A.W. Thorburn. Current issues in fructose metabolism. *Annu. Rev. Nutr.* 11:21–39 (1991).

105. Yam, D., A. Fink, I. Nir, and P. Budowski. Insulin–tumor interrelationships in Thymoma bearing mice. Effects of dietary glucose and fructose. *Br. J. Cancer* 64:1043–1046 (1991).

106. Lina, B.A.R., H.C. Dreef-van der Meulen, and D.C. Leegwater. Subchronic (13-week) oral toxicity of neohesperidin dihydrochalcone in rats. *Food Chem. Toxicol.* 28:507–513 (1990).

107. Jones, J.M. Everything you wanted to know about the safety of acesulfame-K... *Cereal Foods World* 37:329–330 (1992).

108. Woods, I.A., and J. Doull. GRAS evaluation of flavoring substances by the expert panel of FEMA. *Reg. Toxicol. Pharmacol.* 14:48–58 (1991).

109. Oser, B.L., and R.A. Ford. FEMA expert panel: 30 years of safety evaluation for the flavor industry. *Food Technol.* 45(11):84–88,93–94,97 (1992).

110. Multiple authors. ILSI MSG Symposium. The scientific facts about MSG. *Food Aust.* 43(7):S3–S17 (1991).

111. Multiple authors. Umami—Proceedings of the Second International Symposium on Umami. *Physiol. Behav.* 49(5) (1991).

112. Hattula, M.T., and H.C. Wallin. Enzymatic determination of free glutamic acid in dried soups and in minced sausages: NMKL collaborative study. *J. Assoc. Off. Anal. Chem.* 74:921–925 (1991).

113. Asita, A.O., M. Matsui, T. Nohmi, et al. Mutagenicity of wood smoke condensates in the Salmonella/microsome assay. *Mutat. Res.* 264:7–14 (1991).

114. Burdock, G.A., D.H. Pence, and R.A. Ford. Safety evaluation of benzophenone. *Food Chem. Toxicol.* 29:741–750 (1991).

115. Saito, K., S. Uwagawa, H. Kaneko, and A. Yoshitake. Behavior of α_{2u}-globulin accumulating in kidneys of male rats treated with *d*-limonene: kidney-type α_{2u}-globulin in the urine as a marker of *d*-limonene nephropathy. *Toxicology* 79:173–183 (1991).

116. Dietrich, D.R., and J.A. Swenberg. The presence of α_{2u}-globulin is necessary for d-limonene promotion of male rat kidney tumors. *Cancer Res.* 51:3512–3521 (1991).

117. Kauderer, B., H. Zamith, F.J.R. Paumgartten, and G. Speit. Evaluation of the mutagenicity of β-myrcene in mammalian cells in vitro. *Environ. Molec. Mutagen.* 18:28–34 (1991).

118. Houben, G.F., H. van den Berg, M.H.M. Kuijpers, et al. Effect of the color additive caramel color III and 2-acetyl-4(5)-tetrahydroxybutylimidazole (THI) on the immune system of rats. *Toxicol. Appl. Pharmacol.* 113:43–54 (1992).

119. Borzelleca, J.F., J.W. Olson, and F.E. Reno. Lifetime toxicity/carcinogenicity studies of FD & C Red No. 40 (allura red) in mice. *Food Chem. Toxicol.* 29:313–319 (1991).

120. Mori, H., H. Iwata, T. Tanaka, et al. Carcinogenicity study of cochineal in B6C3F$_1$ mice. *Food Chem. Toxicol.* 29:585–588 (1991).

121. Tanaka, T. Effects of amaranth on F$_1$ generation mice. *Toxicol. Lett.* 60:315–324 (1992).

122. Rastogi, P.B., W.G. Thilly, and L. Shirnamé-Moré. Long-term low-dose mutation studies in human cells: metanil yellow and orange II. *Mutat. Res.* 249:265–273 (1991).

123. Ramachandani, S., M. Das, and S.K. Khanna. Lipid peroxidation of ultrastructural components of rat liver induced by metanil yellow and orange II: comparison with blend. *Toxicol. Indust. Health* 8:63–75 (1992).

124. Westmoreland, C., and D.G. Gatehouse. The differential clastogenicity of Solvent Yellow 14 and FD & C Yellow No. 6 *in vivo* in the rodent micronucleus test (observations on species and tissue specificity). *Carcinogenesis* 12:1403–1407 (1991).

125. Giri, A.K., S.S. Sivan, K.A. Khan, and N. Sethi. Sister chromatid exchange and chromosome aberrations in mice after in vivo exposure of Green S– a food colorant. *Environ. Molec. Mutagen.* 19:223–226 (1992).

126. Harada, K.-i., K. Masuda, M. Suzuki, and H. Oka. Separation and identification of food dyes by thin-layer chromatography/liquid secondary ion mass spectrometry. *Biol. Mass Spectrom.* 20:522–528 (1991).

127. Karovicová, J., J. Polonský, A. Prībela, and P. Simko. Isotachophoresis of some synthetic colorants in foods. *J. Chromatogr.* 545:413–419 (1991).

128. Mo, S., J. Na, H. Mo, and L. Chen. Voltammetric determination of indigo carmine and amaranth on a silver-based mercury film electrode. *Anal. Lett.* 25:899–909 (1992).

129. Evans, K., and M.U. Hickey-Dwyer. Cleft anterior segment with maternal hypervitaminosis A. *Br. J. Opthalmol.* 75:691–692 (1991).

130. Anonymous. Pregnant women advised to avoid eating liver. *Vet. Rec.* 127:414 (1990).

131. Dudas, I., and A.E. Czeizel. Use of 6,000 IU vitamin A during early pregnancy without teratogenic effect. (Letter.) *Teratology* 45:335-336 (1992).

132. Gross, E.M., Y. Roth, V. Uzieli, et al. Multiple outbreaks of niacin (nicotinic acid) intoxication due to addition of meat "enhancer" to products by two different meat processors. *J. Food Protect.* 55:116–119 (1992).

133. Jacobus, C.H., M.F. Holick, Q. Shao, et al. Hypervitaminosis D associated with drinking milk. *New Engl. J. Med.* 326:1173–1177 (1992).

134. Oo, S.L., P. Chang, and K.E. Chan. Toxicological and pharmacological studies on palm vitee. *Nutr. Res.* 12(Suppl. 1):S217–S222 (1992).

135. Moyana, T., and J-M. A. Lalonde. Carrageenan-induced intestinal injury: possible role of oxygen free radicals. *Ann. Clin. Lab. Sci.* 21:258–263 (1991).

136. Yabe, Y., T. Ninomiya, T. Tatsuno, and T. Okada. Simple colorimetric determination of carrageenan in jellies and salad dressings. *J. Assoc. Off. Anal. Chem.* 74:1019–1022 (1991).

137. Arakawa, S., H. Ishihara, O. Nishio, and S. Isomura. A sandwich enzyme-linked immunosorbent assay for κ-carrageenan determination. *J. Sci. Food Agric.* 57:135–140 (1991).

138. Kawana, K., T. Nakaoka, Y. Horiguchi, et al. Toxicological study of potassium bromate. I. Absorption, metabolism and excretion of potassium bromate after oral administration in rats. *Eisei Kagaku* 37:258–265 (1991).

139. Sai, K., S. Uchiyama, Y. Ohno, et al. Generation of active oxygen species *in vitro* by the interaction of potassium bromate with rat kidney cell. *Carcinogenesis* 13:333–339 (1992).

140. Awogi, T., K. Murata, M. Uejima, et al. Induction of micronucleated reticulocytes by potassium bromate and potassium chromate in CD-1 male mice. *Mutat. Res.* 278:181–185 (1992).

141. Krishna Murthy, M.N., S. Rajalakshmi, J.A. Satyabodha, and K.V. Nagaraja. A qualitative colorimetric test for brominated vegetable oil in soft drinks. *J. Assoc. Off. Anal. Chem.* 74:698–699 (1991).

142. Heikes, D.L. Mass spectral identification and gas chromatographic determination of chlorinated bleaching adducts in flour-containing food items. *J. Agric. Food Chem.* 40:489–491 (1992).

143. Hagiwara, A., H. Tanaka, D. Tiwawech, et al. Oral toxicity study of tragacanth gum in B6C3F1 mice: development of squamous-cell hyperplasia in the forestomach and its reversibility. *J. Toxicol. Environ. Health* 34:207–218 (1991).

144. Wood, F.E., B.R. DeMark, E.J. Hollenbach, et al. Analysis of liver tissue for olestra following long-term feeding to rats and monkeys. *Food Chem. Toxicol.* 29:231–236 (1991).

145. Wood, F.E., W.J. Tierney, A.L. Knezevich, et al. Chronic toxicity and carcinogenicity studies of olestra in Fischer 344 rats. *Food Chem. Toxicol.* 29:223–230 (1991).

146. Miller, K.W., F.E. Wood, S.B. Stuard, and C.L. Alden. A 20-month olestra feeding study in dogs. *Food Chem. Toxicol.* 29:427–435 (1991).

147. Muralidhara, and K. Narasimhamurthy. Assessment of *in vivo* mutagenic potency of ethylenediaminetetraacetic acid in albino mice. *Food Chem. Toxicol.* 29:845–849 (1991).

148. de Jong, J., A. van Polanen, and J.J.M. Driessen. Determination of ethylenediaminetetraacetic acid and its salts in canned mushrooms by reversed-phased ion-pair liquid chromatography. *J. Chromatogr.* 553:243–248 (1991).

149. Anderson, R.L., J.W. Owens, and C.W. Timms. The toxicity of purified cellulose in studies with laboratory animals. *Cancer Lett.* 63:83–92 (1992).

150. Greenough, R.J., and D.J. Everett. Safety evaluation of alkaline cellulase. *Food Chem. Toxicol.* 29:781–785 (1991).

151. Maekawa, A., Y. Matsushima, H. Onodera, et al. Long-term toxicity/carcinogenicity study of calcium lactate in F344 rats. *Food Chem. Toxicol.* 29:589–594 (1991).

8

Indirect Additives, Residues, and Contaminants

Antimicrobial drugs
Other veterinary drugs
Pesticides
Packaging materials
Polynuclear aromatic hydrocarbons (PAHs)
Polyhalogenated aromatic hydrocarbons
Other organic residues
Heavy metals (general)
Aluminum
Arsenic
Cadmium
Fluoride
Lead
Mercury
Selenium
Tin
Vanadium
Other inorganic residues and contaminants
Radionuclides

A variety of residues and contaminants in milk and milk products were reviewed in a recent monograph (*1*). These include: veterinary drugs and pharmacologically active compounds; pesticides; heavy metals and other trace elements; nitrate, nitrite, and nitrosamines; mycotoxins; polychlorinated biphenyls (PCBs); polychlorinated dibenzo-*p*-dioxins and dibenzofurans; and detergents and disinfectants. Sources of contamination, methods for analysis, and residue levels found in foods and their significance were discussed.

Governmental programs for monitoring and evaluating residues of pesticides and of drugs in meat were described in a volume devoted to the topic of meat and health (*2*). Ongoing programs monitor meat and poultry for violative residues and categorize them according to hazard. Periodically, FDA, FSIS, and EPA are also involved in the investigation and control of isolated contamination incidents.

It has been suggested that the millions of tons of newspapers generated annually in the USA be shredded and used as bedding for cattle. To determine whether this practice would introduce contaminants such as heavy metals or hydrocarbons into the meat of cattle, the concentrations of 16 hydrocarbons and of cadmium, copper, lead, and mercury were determined in blood and liver of 8 cattle bedded on shredded newspapers and compared with those in 8 cattle bedded on sawdust (*3*). Average length of the feeding period was 140 days. Neither mercury nor any of the hydrocarbons were detected in liver or blood of any animal or in samples of sawdust and newspapers used for bedding. Copper was present in both sawdust and newspapers at concentrations of 3.31 and 17.2 mg/kg, respectively. Newsprint also contained 0.68 mg Cd/kg and 2.1 mg Pb/kg. The newspaper used in this experiment had been sorted to remove magazines and colored materials and this undoubtedly decreased heavy metal concentrations. The only heavy metal detected in the cattle was copper, found at levels of 0.69 and 0.72 mg/L in blood and of 28.7 and 38.8 mg/kg in meat of cattle on newspaper and sawdust, respectively. This is well below the toxic level of 250–800 mg Cu/kg in cattle liver.

Heavy metals, pesticides, PCBs, polycyclic aromatic hydrocarbons (PAHs), and dioxins are the main residue concerns in seafoods. A recent review provided an overview of these toxicants, pointing out contamination sources and estimated seafood-related consumption of the various metals and organic compounds (*4*). Generally these compounds are not considered a significant problem in commercially harvested seafood but may be a problem with sport-caught fish and shellfish, particularly in certain regions. For example, analyses of fish caught in lakes and the river near Frankfort, Germany, showed that 44% were contaminated with toxaphene and 93% with pentachlorophenol (*5*). In about 50% of these cases, the toxin levels were close to the tolerance levels.

Information on dietary intake of chemical contaminants from 39 countries participating in the Global Environmental Monitoring System established by the UN has been compared with toxicologically acceptable intake levels (*6*). Average dietary intakes of lead exceed or approach provisional tolerable weekly intake (PTWI) in Cuba, Italy, and Thailand, while average intakes of cadmium exceed the PWTI only in Thailand. Drinking water, beverages, cereals, vegetables, and fruit have been identified as sources of Pb, and cereals and root and tuber vegetables are the main sources of cadmium. The contribution of fish to the total intake of mercury varied, according to different dietary habits, from 20% in some European countries to 85% in Finland and the USA. Generally, dietary intakes of mercury and of organochlorine and organophosphorus pesticides did not exceed acceptable daily intakes.

A variety of raw foods collected from different regions in India were found to be significantly contaminated with several chlorinated pesticides (*7*). Meat and dairy products were the prime sources of human dietary exposure. Butter samples contained average levels of 2800, 1400, 42, and 740 ng/g wet weight of ΣHCH (hexachlorocyclohexane), ΣDDT, aldrin, and dieldrin, respectively. Levels of these pesticides in meat and animal fat averaged 480, 100, 2.4, and 8.3 ng/g, respectively. Estimated dietary intakes of aldrin and dieldrin exceeded the acceptable daily intakes recommended by FAO/WHO. Residues of PCBs, HCB, and heptachlor in foods and estimated intakes were relatively low.

Heptachlor and HCB residue levels were also low in food samples from Bangkok (*8*). PCBs were detected in all food samples but at low concentrations. Highest levels of ΣHCH (59 ng/g) and aldrin (57 ng/g) were detected in butter, of ΣDDT (100 ng/g) in chicken fat, and of dieldrin (130 ng/g) in pork fat. Contamination with aldrin and dieldrin are of greatest concern because these are of greater toxicity to humans.

Mass spectrometric methods used for identification and confirmation of trace level residues of contaminants in foods were evaluated with respect to criteria desirable in a regulatory sample case (*9*). At concentrations in the low parts-per-million to parts-per-trillion range, various data manipulations or alternate choices of approaching the analytical problem of confirmation must be used to ensure an acceptable result.

An electrochemical enzyme immunoassay procedure for the detection of low concentrations of toxic substances in solution has been developed (*10*). The biosensor has two major elements: an electrical conducting layer having immobilized enzyme, polyclonal or monoclonal antibodies, and other necessary reagents, and the electronic components used in the signal readout. These provide an amperometric immunoassay based on coupling the immunoreaction to the enzyme electrode response by using a soluble, electrochemically active indicator. The method should have broad applicability in detecting trace amounts of toxins in small volumes.

A mixture of hydrocarbons and organochlorine compounds has been successfully separated by sorption chromatography on a two-step microcolumn of silica and aluminum oxide and determined by GC using a dual-detector system (flame ionization detection–electron capture detection) (*11*). The mixture was first applied to the silica oxide column and aliphatic hydrocarbons and chlorinated hydrocarbons were eluted with *n*-hexane. Then aromatic compounds with 1–2 rings, polynuclear hydrocarbons with 3–4 rings and polynuclear hydrocarbons with 5–6 rings were eluted from the aluminum oxide column with *n*-hexane-methylene chloride in

proportions of 9:1, 7:3, and 2:8, respectively. Finally, heterocyclic compounds with O, S, and N atoms were recovered with acetone–methanol (2:1). Chlorinated compounds, including PCBs and various pesticides and herbicides, were present in different fractions according to their chemical characteristics.

ANTIMICROBIAL DRUGS

Two recent WHO publications evaluating the toxicological significance of certain veterinary drug residues in human foods have been reviewed (*12,13*). The reports include general discussions of topics such as the application of safety factors to no-observed-effect levels and withdrawal times as well as toxicity data from the literature on a number of specific drugs and recommendations for Acceptable Daily Intakes and Maximum Residue Limits. Safety concerns include possible allergic reactions, effects on the mammalian nervous system, and the potential induction of drug-resistant coliforms in the human intestine.

Papers from a symposium on "Biological Models to Determine the Safety of Bound Residues in the Tissues of Food-Producing Animals" were published in *Drug Metabolism Reviews* (*14*). Various in vitro and in vivo assay systems were described along with approaches to interpreting results in order to assess possible risks to humans.

Of 337 milk samples obtained from shops in Europe and analyzed for antibiotic residues by the microbial receptor assay (Charm test II) and by 4 different microbial inhibitor assays, about 1.5% were found to contain detectable antibiotics (*15*). Penicillin, chloramphenicol, and gentamicin were detected in 7, 1, and 2 samples, respectively. Results for tests for sulfonamides could not be interpreted with certainty.

Neomycin was the most commonly found antibiotic in tissues from 967 bob veal calves which had tested positive in the calf antibiotic and sulfonamide test (CAST) (*16*). Specimens of muscle, liver and kidney were analyzed for penicillins, tetracyclines, streptomycin, chloramphenicol, neomycin, gentamicin, tylosin, and sulfonamides, with positive results in 81, 59, 86, 0, 425, 53, 8, and 86 calves, respectively. Unidentified microbial inhibitors were present in 291 calves. Neomycin concentrations in kidney specimens ranged from 0.25 to >100 ppm.

An HPLC method for the simultaneous determination of olaquindox, morantel, furazolidone, nitrofurazone, and carbadox residues in swine muscle was developed (*17*). Drugs were extracted with acetonitrile, cleaned up on an alumina column, and then separated on an Inertsil C8 column with a mobile phase of acetonitrile–water–acetic acid (3:97:1). All the drugs could be detected at 340 nm. Detection limit for each drug was 0.03 ppm and recoveries from spiked samples averaged 75%.

β-*Lactam antibiotics*

An allergic reaction possibly resulting from consumption of contaminated chicken occurred in a 21-year-old female who had been vacationing in Tenerife (*18*). Shortly after an evening meal she developed severe pruritis and a generalized rash, followed by swelling in her limbs and difficulty in swallowing. She had previously experienced similar symptoms after receiving penicillin. A local Spanish medical practitioner informed her that in Tenerife chicken may contain penicillin. (Sometimes antibiotics are used in washing carcasses.) It was not possible to test this chicken for drug residues. Although there have been a few well-documented cases of allergic reactions occurring in sensitized individuals consuming milk containing penicillin residues, it is considered unlikely that penicillin-tainted foods present a great risk (*19*). Residues, when present, are generally in very low concentrations and the oral route is known to be much less sensitizing, with low epitope density complexes formed in vivo. However, the occasional cases which occur illustrate the need to carefully control and monitor antibiotic residues in foods.

A modified procedure for the *Bacillus stearothermophilus* disk assay has been successfully used to determine ampicillin residues as low as 0.025 µg/g in muscle tissue of channel catfish and striped bass (*20*). Recoveries of ampicillin from spiked muscle ranged from 99 to 104%. This assay was used to monitor the elimination of an intravascular dose of ampicillin and demonstrated that the half-life of ampicillin in the muscle was 3.6 hours.

A capillary GC method has been developed for the determination of 7 penicillin residues in bovine muscle, liver, kidney, adipose tissue and milk (*21*). Samples were extracted with acetonitrile under slightly acidic conditions and cleaned up by liquid–liquid partitioning steps and anion exchange chromatography. The penicillin residues were methylated with diazomethane and then analyzed by GC with a programmed temperature vaporization, separated on a methyl silicone fused silica column with nitrogen-specific thermionic detection. Limits for detection in all tissues were well below 3 µg/kg and recoveries ranged between 65–80% for milk and 50–70% in bovine tissues.

A previously described HPLC procedure has been modified for the confirmation of penicillin residues in animal tissues, with detection limits of 5 ng/g (*22*). Samples were first mixed with acetonitrile and then cleaned up by partitioning prior to isocratic analysis with 0.01 M phosphate buffer–acetonitrile. Penicillins were detected at 210 nm. This method was sensitive and relatively simple, with recoveries >90% in most cases.

Liquid chromatographic methods have also been described for the determination of penicillin residues in milk. A method utilizing an automated cleanup procedure and isocratic chromatography with 0.01 M phosphate buffer–acetonitrile detected as little as 1 ng penicillin/mL, with recoveries of 87–97% from spiked samples (*23*). An ion pairing LC method which can determine 4 commonly used penicillins at the 3–4 ppb level in milk utilized tetrabutylammonium hydrogen sulfate to form ion pairs which were then separated on an LC column using an aqueous acetonitrile mobile phase (*24*). Overall recoveries were >82.9%. A third LC method involved ultrafiltration of milk diluted with methanol, acetonitrile, and water and then separation by ion-paired chromatography (*25*). Penicillins were detected using ultraviolet photodiode array detection

(UV–PDA) and confirmed by thermospray LC–MS. Limits of detection for 3 penicillins were 50–100 ppb for LC with UV–PDA and 100–200 ppb for thermospray LC–MS detection.

Sulfonamides

Disposition and elimination of sulfadimethoxine (SDMX) in the skin of broiler chickens was investigated in chickens given drinking water containing 1000 ppm SDMX for 5 days (*26*). Although SDMX disappeared rapidly from liver, kidney, muscles, and fat (below detectable levels in 3–5 days), it was still present at levels >0.1 µg/g in skin after 10 days. A waterproof bandage applied to the skin of some broilers did not affect SDMX residue levels, indicating that external contamination was not responsible for the high level in the skin. SDMX appeared to be distributed evenly throughout the entire skin area.

No decrease in a sulfonamide concentration of 5 µg/g was observed in luncheon meat during the different stages of processing and storage (4°C up to 27 days) (*27*). On the other hand, raw fermented sausages, which have a lower pH and a reduced water-holding capacity in their proteins, retain <40% of their initial level of sulfamethazine (SMZ) after 10 days of ripening. However, these results should be evaluated cautiously because the breakdown products of SMZ may retain their toxicity.

Enzyme immunoassays can provide a simple and reliable means of detecting antibiotic residues. Five commercial immunochemical test kits for SMZ in milk with detectabilities of 1–10 ppb were evaluated and compared with analyses by HPLC with electrochemical detection and by high performance thin-layer chromatography (HPTLC) (*28*). When used as directed all the test kits reliably detected SMZ in raw and processed milk at <10 ppb. Another two ELISAs, utilizing polyclonal antibodies raised to SMZ and to sulfanilamide (SNA) were developed and found to successfully detect 10 ppb SMZ and 100 ppb SNA in milk (*29*). The specificity of both assays was excellent, with little cross-reactivity. However, with an increasing number of different sulfonamide compounds being used in food animals, it would be efficient to have an immunoassay

which could detect a number of different sulfonamide compounds. Use of a sulfathiazole derivative chemically linked to a protein so that its aromatic amino group was exposed allowed isolation of antibodies which reacted with more than one sulfonamide (*30*). One set of these antibodies when used in an indirect competitive ELISA could detect 9 structurally different sulfonamides at concentrations of <2 nM/assay.

Two HPLC systems for the detection of SMZ in milk have been described. In one procedure, chloroform was used to extract the antibiotic from milk, and this extract was then cleaned up on a cyclobond I column prior to HPLC (*31*). Use of a methanol/ammonium acetate buffer eluted SMZ which was then determined by UV absorbance. Recoveries ranged from 83–88%, with a detection limit of 5 ppb. The second method utilized a C-18 cartridge for cleanup followed by HPLC with a mobile phase consisting of a sodium acetate buffer and acetonitrile (*32*). Recoveries from spiked samples averaged 74%, with a detection limit of 10 µg/kg. A survey of 215 European milk samples revealed that none contained this antibiotic.

A simple procedure has been developed for the determination of 13 sulfonamides by HPTLC and 11 sulfonamides by HPLC in milk, meat, and eggs (*33*). Samples were extracted with dichloromethane and defatted using a silica cartridge. Sulfonamides were eluted with phosphate buffer, extracted with ethyl acetate, and the resulting solution was divided into two portions for analysis by HPLC with a diode array or UV detector at 266 nm and by HPTLC on silica plates. Detection limits were 2 and 10 µg/kg for HPLC and HPTLC, respectively. Of 105 samples of Swiss pork and 98 samples of pork from other European countries, 83 and 50, respectively, contained sulfonamides, with 23 and 7, respectively, containing SMZ residues above the legal limit of 100 µg/kg. No sulfonamide residues were detected in 50 samples of fresh, powdered, or condensed milk or in 20 samples of fresh, powdered, or frozen eggs.

A quantitative HPTLC method for the detection of sulfonamides in animal tissue and in milk has been developed (*34*). Samples were first extracted with ethyl acetate and then cleaned up by solid phase extraction (meat) or matrix solid phase dispersion (milk). A three-multiple development chromatographic system was used for the separation, and derivatization with fluorescamine allowed detection of as little as 0.32 ng/spot. This method could distinguish 5 different sulfonamides when they were present in meat extracts.

Several modifications to HPLC methods for analysis of sulfonamides in meats have been proposed. Pre-column derivatization with fluorescamine allowed detection of 0.01 ng sulfaquinoxaline/g and 0.005 ng/g of 7 other sulfa drugs with an average recovery of 92.6% from fortified samples (35). No laborious cleanup steps were required and the method performed well in field trials testing 37 samples of meats. Small meat samples of only 1 g could be analyzed in a method based on solid-phase dispersion (36). Muscle tissue was blended with coated silica and packed into a syringe barrel. The sample was defatted with hexane and then the sulfonamides were eluted with dichloromethane and analyzed by HPLC with UV diode array detection. Detection limit was 0.01 ppm. Ion spray mass spectrometry analyses with 21 sulfonamide drugs demonstrated that all of them gave positive ion mass spectra with abundant protonated molecules and no fragmentation (37). This type of MS analysis in conjunction with HPLC provided a reliable and sensitive means for detection and identification of sulfonamide residues in salmon tissue.

Capillary zone electrophoresis at pH 7.0 was able to separate different sulfonamides from mixtures dissolved in pork extract (38). At this pH, 14 of 16 drugs tested can be determined and 12 of them can be identified by using the effective mobilities. Only a very simple pretreatment of meat was required before analysis. Limit of detection for the method varied from 2–9 ppm for a pressure injection of 10 s. This method may be applicable to assays for a variety of veterinary drugs in meat extracts.

Tetracyclines

Oxytetracycline (OTC) is used to control a bacterial disease in lobsters held in captivity for commercial sale. Recent experiments have shown that the Delvotest P procedure, a simple, sensitive test currently used to detect antibiotic residues in milk, can be used to detect OTC residues in lobster hemolymph at concentrations as low as 0.03 µg/mL (39). Assays of 18 lobster hemolymph samples using this technique and the more time-consuming zone-diffusion test demonstrated that both methods were able to detect the 14 positive samples.

HPLC methods using a solid-phase extraction protocol have been modified for determination of tetracyclines in bovine and porcine muscle in high sample loads with smaller final sample volumes (40) and in chinook salmon (41). Meat samples, spiked with OTC, tetracycline or chlortetracycline were extracted with Water Environmental Sep-Pak cartridges and then analyzed by HPLC using a mobile phase of phosphate, citrate, acetonitrile with tetamethylammonium chloride and EDTA. The antibiotics were detected at levels as low as 10 ng/g using diode ray detection. OTC in fish was extracted with a Sephadex G-25 column, chromatographed with a mobile phase of methanol–phosphate buffer (pH 2.25), and detected by UV at 365 nm. Detection limit was 0.05 ppm with an average recovery of 74.4% for spiked samples. OTC levels in muscles of salmon fed a medicated feed were found to exhibit a half-life of 5.4 days.

Analyses for OTC in whole blood or serum by HPLC utilizing a Hisep shielded hydrophobic phase column with a mobile phase of methanol/oxalic acid (42) or a polystyrene enrichment column with a mobile phase of acetonitrile/phosphoric acid/ heptanesulfonic acid (43) are capable of detecting antibiotic concentrations as low as 50 ng/mL. Both procedures allow direct injection of samples, and one has been fully automated (43).

Routine surveillance of hog carcasses for antibiotic residues using a bioassay and TLC revealed the presence of an unknown substance which behaved like tetracycline (44). This same substance was also found in an implicated swine feed premix. Further analyses by HPLC, reversed-phase TLC, and MS isolated and identified the substance as lumichrome, a photodegradation product of riboflavin, a vitamin commonly added to swine feed. Improper storage of feed may have caused degradation of riboflavin in the feed.

Analyses of 68 milk samples with 3 microbial antibiotic assays gave equivocal results: 45 were positive in the Arla microtest, 40 were positive in the Valio T101 test, and all were negative in the Delvotest SP (*45*). Only one of these samples was positive for tetracyclines when assayed by LC and immunoassay. These contradictory results were explained by further experiments which demonstrated that lipolysis of milk fat, resulting in free fatty acids, can cause false-positive results in the microbial non-agar assays and also interfere in the confirmation by the Charm test II.

Confirmation of OTC, tetracycline, and chlortetracycline residues in bovine milk at levels of 100 ng/mL has been achieved with a method using particle beam LC/MS (*46*). Milk samples were filtered and cleaned up on a C-18 cartridge which retains the tetracyclines. After elution from this column, the antibiotics were separated on a Novapak C-18 column with methanol/oxalic acid/acetonitrile as the mobile phase. The compounds were identified by negative chemical ionization with selective ion monitoring.

OTC is used to treat bacterial diseases in bee colonies and, if not properly used, may be present in honey (*47*) and pollen pellets (*48*) from treated hives. Two days after administration of OTC, honey in combs near the feeder may contain as much as 90.8 ppm OTC. OTC degrades rapidly in the next two weeks and then more gradually until it is undetectable after 6–8 weeks. Little OTC was present in royal jelly except immediately after antibiotic administration. However, OTC is transferred to pollen pellets when treated bees cement pollen grains together to form pellets. Once contaminated, the pellets contain detectable OTC for 4 years.

Chloramphenicol

Confirmation and quantification of chloramphenicol (CAP) residues in eggs and in cow's urine and muscle has been achieved by a method based on gas chromatography/negative ion chemical ionization mass spectrometry (*49*). [$^{37}Cl_2$]Chloramphenicol was used as an internal standard. Selective ion monitoring enabled the determination of CAP at levels of 3 µg/L in urine with a coefficient of variation of 8%. Limit of detection of the method was 0.1 ppb for urine, muscle, and eggs.

An analytical strategy utilizing different analytical principles was devised for the regulatory control of CAP residues in meat (*50*). A simple immunochemical card test with a limit of detection of about 2 µg/kg was used for direct screening in meat. A collaborative test, involving 13 Dutch laboratories and 554 samples, indicated that at CAP concentrations >8 µg/kg, no false negatives were found. CAP concentrations in positive samples were quantitated by a liquid chromatographic method with a limit of detection of about 1 µg/kg. Identity of CAP can be confirmed by using diode array ultraviolet detection (at concentrations exceeding 10 µg/kg) or by GC/MS in the electron impact mode. Preliminary experiments indicate that this analytical procedure is also appropriate for control of CAP residues in milk.

Quinoline antibiotics

Residues of flumequine (FQ), a relatively new antibacterial drug, in muscles and eggs of treated laying hens were monitored to determine rate of clearance (*51,52*). Following a single oral or intramuscular dose, FQ was detectable in serum, muscles, and egg yolk for 24–36 h, 24–36 h, and 6 days, respectively, after dosing. A similar retention pattern was observed when hens were given 5 successive daily doses of FQ. Highest tissue levels detected were 1.26–1.30 µg/g in muscle (at 3 h), 3.55–4.20 µg/g in egg white (1 day after dosing), and 0.18–0.38 µg/g in egg yolk (5 days after dosing).

FQ is cleared much more slowly from fish muscles. Pharmacokinetic studies with European eels given a single i.m. injection of FQ demonstrated that they absorb and eliminate this drug slowly, with half-lives of 33 and 255 hours for these processes (*53*). Salmon dosed with FQ, oxolinic acid (OX), enrofloxacin (ER), and sarafloxacin retained these antibiotics for prolonged periods in skin and bones (> 6 months) (*54*). OX and ER residues were detectable in muscle tissue 60 days after dosing. These extended periods of drug retention indicate that withdrawal periods in fish should be longer than the 5 days recommended for pigs and dairy cows. However, when rainbow trout were treated with OX orally (in medicated feed) they eliminated the drug within 10–15 days after treatment (*55*). The maximum muscle tissue level of OX measured was 2.9 µg/g at about 7 days.

A method using a simplified sample preparation of salmon tissue and fluorometric detection was developed for determination of OX residues by liquid chromatography (*56*). Tissue samples were mixed with sodium sulfate and then extracted with ethyl acetate. Following liquid partitioning, extracts were chromatographed with acetonitrile/methanol/oxalic acid with fluorescence detection at 327 nm excitation and 369 nm emission. Recoveries ranged from 71–83% in spiked samples. Using different sensitivity settings calibration curves were linear from 10–2000 ppb. Data from an interlaboratory evaluation of this method demonstrated good reproducibility relative standard deviations of 11.5–18.3%, with mean recoveries ranging from 77.2–84.5% (*57*). This method has been recommended for regulatory purposes in Canada.

OX and OX-related metabolites were successfully determined in channel catfish muscle by use of matrix solid-phase dispersion isolation and liquid chromatography (*58*). Mean percent recovery was 83% and limit of detection was 0.05 µg/g. Using this method, OX was detected in muscle and 4 OX-related metabolites were detected in bile of treated fish. The extraction method used here proved to be simpler and more effective than others which have been described.

Simple and rapid methods for extraction and analysis of residues of FQ, OX, ER, and sarafloxacin (SF) with detection limits of 5 ng/g (OX and ER) and 10 ng/g (FQ and SF) have been developed (*59,60*). Samples of fish tissues were extracted with acetonitrile and ammonia and then defatted with organic solvents prior to HPLC. Approximately 30 samples per day could be processed using this method and, in addition, large quantities of chemicals are not required.

An ion trap detector, in combination with capillary GC and chemical ionization conditions, proved sensitive enough to determine carbadox-

related residues (as the methyl ester of quinoxaline-2-carboxylic acid) at 3 µg/kg or higher in pork liver (*61*). Use of an internal standard allowed correction for losses during sample preparation. Recoveries from spiked samples ranged from 101 to 110%.

Nitrofuran antibiotics

Although nitrofurans have mutagenic and carcinogenic properties, they are still used to prevent and treat gastrointestinal infections in some farm animals. Tissues from veal calves orally dosed with furaltadone and furazolidone 3–4 hours before slaughter were examined for drug residues (*62*). Both drugs were rapidly degraded in liver, kidney, and muscle tissue after slaughter, with no parent nitrofurans detectable in edible tissues after 24 h. Thus, these tissues cannot be used for residue monitoring purposes. Little information is so far available on the nature and toxicity of degradation products of these drugs.

In vitro and in vivo assays with pigs and pig hepatocytes indicate that furazolidone is metabolized to a compound bound to proteins (*63*). A newly developed method demonstrated that at least 70% of the bound residues still contained the 3-amino-2-oxazolidinone (AOZ) side chain of furazolidone. Even after a withdrawal period of 14 days, liver samples of piglets orally treated with this drug contained 14% releasable AOZ, equivalent to 0.3 µg furazolidone/g tissue.

Matrix solid-phase dispersion was used to isolate furazolidone from poultry muscle, with an average percentage recovery of 99.8% (*64*). The chicken muscle was blended with octadecylsilyl-derivatized silica and used to prepare a column. Hexane was used to remove lipids and then dichloromethane eluted furazolidone which was quantified by HPLC utilizing UV detection. Minimal detectable limit was 156 pg/column.

Residues of nitrofurazone were determined by liquid chromatography in liver, breast, and thigh tissues from 42-day-old chickens which had been fed a diet containing 0.0055% nitrofurazone from hatching (*65*). Drug residue levels were always much higher in liver than in skeletal muscle tissue but quite a bit of variation was observed between individual birds and between tissue samples ground before analysis and unground tissues.

Other antibiotics

A method has been developed for the confirmation and quantification of dimetridazole and ipronidazole and their alcohol metabolites in turkey tissues by HPLC separation followed by thermospray tandem mass spectrometry (66). Control and fortified (2 and 10 ppb) turkey tissues were analyzed with no evidence of interference from the control tissues. Another metabolite of dimetridazole has been isolated from porcine plasma and identified as an *N*-demethylation product (67). This metabolite was present at lower levels than the alcohol metabolite in tissues of treated animals but neither metabolite was detectable 49 h after withdrawal.

Two sensitive methods have been developed for the detection of the antibiotic fumagallin in honey (68). A reversed-phase HPLC system method with a detection limit of 100 ppb was useful in identifying decomposition products of fumagallin. An indirect ELISA method was capable of detecting 20 ppb fumagallin in honey and could also detect neofumagallin, a major product of light decomposition. At these detection limits, neither fumagallin nor its metabolites were detected in 16 honey samples, including 4 samples from a beekeeper who regularly used fumagallin.

Since lincomycin cannot be distinguished from other antibiotics by microbiological tests, an HPLC procedure was developed for the determination of this antibiotic in milk and tissues (69). An automated HPLC system was used for cleanup, and then samples were loaded on a reversed-phase C-18 column and lincomycin was eluted with an acetonitrile gradient. Mean recoveries were 89–99% with detection limits of 20 (muscle and milk) and 50 (liver and kidney) ppb.

Tissue distribution and depletion of virginiamycin and its two components, M and S, were measured in rainbow trout (70). These compounds were fed to trout for 15 days, and some fish were sacrificed for analysis on days 3, 6, 11, and 16. Fish were also examined 2 and 5 days after the end of dosing. There was no evidence of accumulation of the antibiotic or its components in any tissues of the fish. At 2 days postdosing <10 ng of virginiamycin per g muscle was detected.

OTHER VETERINARY DRUGS

Anthelminthics

An HPLC/fluorescence detection method for detection of ivermectin in swine tissues was found to give average recoveries of 85% in analyses of kidney, liver, fat, and muscle specimens spiked at 6–150 ppb (71). Limits of detection and quantitation were 1 and 5 ppb, respectively. Ivermectin levels in swine dosed orally or by subcutaneous injection were highest in fat and liver, with an overall rapid depletion in all tissues. Suggested withdrawal time for swine orally dosed for 1 week in feed was 5 days and for swine dosed by injection, 18 days.

Levamisole and thiabendazole were assayed in meat with recoveries varying from 63 to 75% by an HPLC method with detection by a photodiode array detector at 240 nm for levamisole and at 300 nm for thiabendazole (72). Detection limits for the two compounds in meat were 25 and 5 µg/kg, respectively. A collisional spectroscopy procedure has been developed for simultaneous detection of these two drugs and three other related benzimidazole anthelminthics in sheep milk (73). The method involves injection of crude milk extracts and selection and collision of the most abundant ionic species obtained under electron impact ionization. Limits of detection ranged from 0.6 to 2.8 ppb and more than 5 samples per hour could be processed. Sheep given single oral therapeutic doses of the drugs excreted detectable drug residues in milk during the following 72 h.

Matrix solid-phase dispersion, using octadecylsilyl-derivatized silica column packing material, followed by liquid chromatography with UV detection achieved an overall recovery of 93% of the anthelminthic chlorsulon from milk samples spiked at 50–200 ppm (74). Compared to classical isolation techniques, this method was shorter with fewer steps and consumed smaller quantities of solvents.

Hormones and hormone-like agents

Papers from the 1990 International Meeting on Anabolics in France included a number of reports on toxicological effects of the anabolics used in food animals, primarily veal calves (75). The regulatory status of these drugs in the USA and in several European countries was discussed.

A multiresidue HPLC method has been developed for the determination of anabolic steroids in animal tissue (76). Samples were first extracted with methanol and then with two solid-phase extraction systems (Carbopack B and Amberlite CG-400 I) to separate the neutral from the acidic anabolics. Extracts were analyzed by HPLC with UV, electrochemical, and fluorimetric detection. Various analytical parameters were optimized and recoveries were found to be >83.6%.

A highly sensitive GC–negative-ion chemical ionization MS method has been developed for the determination of 19-nortestosterone, testosterone, and trenbolone (77). Hormones were extracted from meat and urine samples using an immunoaffinity column and then derivatized with carboxymethoxylamine and pentafluorobenzyl bromide. After further silylation these derivatives were detectable by GC–MS at levels of 0.06 ppb for trenbolone and 0.02 ppb for the other compounds.

β-AGONISTS. Clenbuterol, a β-agonist used illegally in Europe in cattle because of its anabolizing effects, has been responsible for several outbreaks of food poisoning recently. In France, 22 persons complained of tremor, headaches, tachycardia, and dizziness 1–3 hours after consuming veal liver (78). Analyses of the implicated liver revealed clenbuterol residues at concentrations of 0.375–0.50 µg/g. All patients recovered uneventfully. Three outbreaks of clenbuterol poisoning involving a total of 426 cases occurred in Spain between 1989–1992 (79). The affected persons had consumed cow's liver and in one outbreak the source was traced to a cooked dish including accidentally contaminated cinnamon.

Pharmacokinetics and residues of clenbuterol were monitored by enzyme immunoassay in tissues of veal calves given twice-daily doses of 5 µg/kg for 3 weeks (80). Tissue samples were examined from calves after 0, 3.5, and 14 days of withdrawal. Clenbuterol levels were always highest in the eye: 118 ng/g (0 days) and 15.1 ng/g (at 14 days). Average drug levels in liver and skeletal muscle were 46 and 4.5 ng/g, respectively, at 0 days and 0.6 and <0.08 ng/g after 14 days' withdrawal. Most tissues had acceptable residue levels after 2 weeks of withdrawal.

An enzyme immunoassay for the detection of clenbuterol in tissues of treated calves has been developed and found to have a limit of detection of 0.15 and 0.3 ppb in urine and liver, respectively (81). In calves treated orally with 2 µg clenbuterol/kg/day for 15 days, all tissues examined contained <0.3 µg/kg of the drug after 7 days' withdrawal, and only the liver had detectable levels of the drug (0.8 µg/kg) after 3 days' withdrawal.

Other toxins

Following a case of suspected intentional poisoning of beverages from industrial production in Italy, a method was developed for the rapid determination of coumatetralyl, an anticoagulant rodenticide, in cola- and orange-type soft drinks (82). Samples were cleaned up on a diatomaceous earth cartridge, with further clean-up by silica gel chromatography required for orange-type soft drinks. Reversed-phase HPLC with diode-array detection could determine as little as 10 µg coumatetralyl/kg in beverages. Recovery of this toxin from spiked samples was >80%.

PESTICIDES

Toxicological effects and safety assessment

In a review of 63 outbreaks of toxicity caused by alimentary exposure to pesticides, various factors causing or leading up to these epidemics were analyzed with a view to preventing such outbreaks in the future (*83*). Four mechanisms of contamination were identified: (a) Contamination during transport or storage. Sixteen such episodes were described, 10 of which were caused by parathion. Typical cases involved powders such as sugar and flour which were transported or stored with the pesticide or in a place previously contaminated by the pesticide. (b) Ingestion of seed dressed for sowing. Of the 10 episodes reported, 8 were due to organic mercury fungicides, including one in which a pig fed the dressed seed was the vehicle for poisoning. Such outbreaks may occur during times of food shortage, when treated seed were distributed after farmers had already sown their own grain, when local people were unable to read the warning label on bags of seed, or when people mistakenly believed that washing the dye off the treated seeds also removed the poison. (c) Use of pesticides in food preparation because of their organoleptic similarity to foods. Flour, sugar, and salt are the foodstuffs most commonly confused with pesticides of similar appearance. In the 22 episodes investigated, doses ingested were usually high, rapidly inducing gastrointestinal symptoms. (d) Presence of pesticides in water or food owing to misuse near harvesting time, misuse of containers, contamination of groundwater, and use of excessively high doses in agriculture. Fifteen episodes were described in this category, with the largest involving 1042 cases in the USA who ingested watermelon contaminated with aldicarb. A number of preventive measures were suggested to reduce the incidence of such epidemics.

In an investigation to determine possible health effects of chronic low-level ingestion of organophosphate and carbamate pesticides (which inhibit acetylcholinesterase activity), plasma cholinesterase activity was compared at baseline in January and in August in 331 schoolteachers in Denmark (*84*). A wide inter-individual variation in cholinesterase activity was observed. Although overall plasma cholinesterase activity measured in August did not differ significantly, in the highest exposure group (those who consumed exclusively commercial, sprayed fruits and vegetables) an average decrease of 2% in plasma cholinesterase activity was noted during the spraying season. No decrease occurred in groups with less exposure.

An increased mortality due to pancreatic cancer was associated with exposure to DDT and related compounds in a cohort of 5886 chemical workers (*85*). Twenty-eight cases and 112 matched controls were compared for work exposure to chemicals and lifestyle factors. Exposure to DDT was associated with a relative risk of 4.8 for pancreatic cancer, with workers having the longest exposure (average of 47 months) having a greater risk (7.4). Smoking was identified as an independent risk factor but controlling for smoking and other possible confounders did not appreciably alter the calculated risks.

Clastogenic effects of pesticide exposure were observed in 26 pesticide applicators in India (*86*). All the applicators were nonsmokers and did not consume alcohol, and most reported ill health effects such as severe giddiness and nervous disorders. The frequency of total chromosomal aberrations in peripheral lymphocytes was significantly higher in these applicators than in 26 controls without such exposure to pesticides.

Potential toxicologic effects of bound pesticide residues were reviewed (*87*). Although these residues may escape detection by conventional analytical methods, recent studies have demonstrated that even lignin-bound pesticide residues may be bioavailable to animals and humans consuming treated plants and may have toxicological significance. Better analytical methods and more data are required for a more reliable assessment of the possible risks of these bound residues. The pattern of excretion of [^{14}C]-pirimiphos-methyl (a post-harvest insecticide) in rats fed wheat-bound residues of this pesticide indicated that the bound residues are bioavailable (*88*). Rats fed diets containing 1.17 and 7.5 ppm of the bound insecticide for 3–5 months had a statistically significant decrease in lymphocytes and monocytes and an increase in serum alkaline phosphatase activity. At the higher dose there was also a significant decrease in pseudocholinesterase activity.

The fourth annual report summarizing results from the FDA's residue monitoring program from October 1989 to September 1990 has been published (*89*). During this time 19,962 foreign and domestically produced food samples (19,146 surveillance and 816 compliance samples) were analyzed. Of the surveillance samples, 60% of domestic and 64% of foreign samples had no detectable residues while a total of 2.8% had violative levels of residues. The estimated dietary intakes of pesticides were generally well below the standards established by FAO/WHO and by EPA.

More than 40 compounds are applied postharvest on fruits and vegetables to extend their lives and preserve quality (*90*). Those used most commonly include 8 fungicides, 2 fumigants, and an antiscald compound. Persistence and distribution of residues of these compounds in the edible portions of fresh fruits and vegetables have been reviewed. So far, studies on residual behavior have been reported for only a few compounds and on a limited number of foods but the available data are presented and discussed here.

Roles played by governmental agencies, the agrochemical industry, pesticide users and applicators, and food manufacturing and retail industries in controlling pesticide residues to ensure food safety were reviewed (*91*). Although pesticide use has resulted in environmental problems and occupational risks, the author concluded that there was no direct evidence that pesticide residues in foods contribute significantly to chronic disease.

Because the procedures used for establishing pesticide tolerances are complicated and do not involve data on health effects, these tolerances cannot really be considered as safety standards. However, these tolerances are commonly perceived as safety standards and may be used as a basis for food safety legislation. The tolerances do serve a useful function as enforcement tools and may discourage pesticide misuse (*92*).

Multiresidue methods

A computer program has been developed to calculate optimal conditions for reversed-phase liquid chromatography column switching in pesticide residue analysis (*93*). Based on experimentally determined relations between retention and mobile phase composition, the program calculates the displacement of analytes and sample interferences. This simulation procedure was evaluated for the simultaneous determination of procymidone and iprodione in fennel. The program accurately predicted retention times and peak volumes of the two pesticides and of a major interfering compound in fennel under stepwise gradient conditions.

Many multiresidue systems designed to detect a variety of pesticide residues in foods use gas chromatography for determination. Extraction of these residues and procedures for their cleanup vary with different food types. Activated Florasil and ethyl acetate cleanup generally result in recoveries of >80% for a great variety of pesticides, including carbamate, organochlorine, organophosphate, synthetic pyrethroid, triazine, urea, and other pesticides, in fruits and vegetables (*94–96*). Extraction by matrix solid-phase dispersion utilizes octadecylsilyl derivatized silica reverse-phase material mixed with the sample and fashioned into a column (*97*). Pesticides are then eluted from the column with acetonitrile and directly analyzed by GC with electron capture detection. In analyses of catfish muscle for 9 chlorinated pesticides, recoveries of 82–96% were achieved.

A new extraction procedure involving a nontoxic, nonflammable, and inexpensive solvent medium is the supercritical fluid extraction system. Samples are mixed with diatomaceous earth (which disperses the sample and adsorbs water) and then extracted with supercritical fluid carbon dioxide. Samples ranging from 95% water to pure lipophilic oils can be extracted efficiently this way. When combined with gas chromatography, analyte recoveries in excess of 85% have been achieved for over 30 types of pesticides at incurred levels ranging from 0.005–2 ppm in carrots, lettuce, peanut butter, hamburger, butter fat and potatoes (*98*). Supercritical fluid extraction has also been combined with (a) an enzyme immunoassay to detect the presence of alachlor in fortified lard and liver and (b) a cholinesterase assay to detect carbofuran (a cholinesterase inhibitor) in frankfurters (*99*).

Approximately 10% of pesticides contain fluorine and, in Canada, 5 fluorinated chemicals are registered for use. A method has been devised for the determination of these pesticides in foods at the low parts-per-billion level utilizing fluorine nuclear magnetic resonance spectroscopy (*100*). The level of sensitivity achieved permitted the direct analysis of fluorine-containing compounds in liquid food products such as vegetable oil and wine. Detection limits varied from 0.008 to 0.028 mg/kg, depending on the number of fluorine atoms in the compounds. Factors influencing sensitivity of this method were analyzed and discussed.

A gas chromatographic method with ion trap detection has been developed for the determination of 17 pesticides, 12 of which are not generally included in other multimethods (*101*). Samples of fruits and vegetables were homogenized, extracted with acetone, and cleaned up by gel permeation chromatography. Analyses for 4 other pesticides using this method were unsuccessful.

Using a rapid multiresidue screening procedure for 110 pesticides, a total of 5628 produce samples were extracted, analyzed and evaluated within 6.5 hours of receipt (*102*). The method involves homogenization of a produce sample with acetonitrile, followed by solvent concentration and exchange, and then GC for organochlorine and organophosphorus pesticides and LC for carbamate pesticides. Because of the rapid turnaround required, sample cleanup steps were abbreviated. However, this resulted in deposition of contaminating substances in the gas chromatograph injector and on the capillary precolumn, necessitating a rigorous schedule of preventive maintenance every 3 days. Confirmation of residues was accomplished by GC/MS.

A GC method with flame photometric detection, designed to quantitate organophosphorus pesticides in fatty as well as nonfatty foods, successfully detected 28 pesticides (*103*). Foods were divided into 4 groups depending on the type of extraction required (acetone or acetone/water) and cleanup procedures (active carbon-Celite, disposable minicolumns of Kieselguhr-type material, or disposable minicolumns of bonded-phase silica). Detection limits for the different pesticides ranged from 0.07 ng to 1.31 ng. Recoveries from spiked samples of apples, whole milk, olive oil, pasta, and eggs averaged 81–89%. This method would be suitable for a total diet study.

A total of 31 organochlorine pesticides can be routinely detected by simultaneous injection of samples into two dissimilar capillary columns with an electron capture detector attached to one column and an electrolytic conductivity detector to the other (*104*). Quantitation limits ranged from 0.05 to 1.5 ng for different compounds. Both fatty and nonfatty foods can be analyzed by using appropriate extraction methods.

A variety of pesticides can also be determined by gas chromatography/microwave induced plasma/ atomic emission detection (GC/MIP/AED) in fruits and vegetables (*105*). With a few exceptions, recoveries of organochlorine and organophosphorus pesticides averaged 91.7–109.3% and 73.2%, respectively. Recoveries of carbamate pesticides were inconsistent quantitatively. This assay system proved easy to use and simple to maintain. In a comparison of several detection methods for pesticide residues separated by GC, AED was found to have a much better selectivity than electron capture detection, electrolytic conductivity detection, nitrogen–phosphorus detection, and flame photometric detection for determination of organochlorine, organophosphorus, and organofluorine pesticides in 12 types of fruits and vegetables (*106*).

Fumigants

Methyl bromide is a widely used fumigant used to control termites and to destroy pests in soils, warehouses, mills, and other places where food is stored. Following oral administration of 8.3 µmol ^{14}C-labelled methyl bromide to rats, radioactivity was detected in liver, lungs, stomach, and forestomach (*107*). Highest levels of labelled, methylated guanine residues in DNA were observed in the gastrointestinal tract. These results demonstrate that methyl bromide is a potentially genotoxic compound.

Methyl bromide residues have been detected in foods exposed to fumigation. Significantly higher bromide levels, about 54 mg/kg, were present in tomato fruits grown in fumigated greenhouses as compared to controls in unfumigated greenhouses (*108*). Experiments involving fumigation of foods packaged in a variety of plastic, glass, metal, and cardboard containers revealed that some packaging materials provided an effective barrier to the fumigants methyl bromide and sulfuryl fluoride (*109*). No fumigant residues were detected in vacuum-packed foods in metal or glass, in factory-sealed PETE containers of oil or peanut butter, or in bologna in Barex packaging. However, the fumigants were able to penetrate porous packaging (cardboard), HDPE tubs and polyurethane-bagged foods by polymer permeation, and glass and plastic containers which had been opened and reclosed—by diffusion through air channels in closures. Highest fumigant levels detected were in margarine in an HDPE tub (151 ppm methyl bromide) and in peanut butter in a reclosed PETE jar (106 ppm). Even though these foods were fumigated at maximum exposure rates with minimum commodity aeration, residues of both fumigants were less than expected.

An automated, closed-system GC method was developed for the determination of methyl bromide residues in nuts (*110*). Samples were blended with sodium sulfate in a sealed container, warmed to 26°C, and then the headspace gas was automatically sampled and analyzed by GC. The method was simple, sensitive, and reproducible. Of 1132 samples of 11 types of nuts, methyl bromide was detected in only three: 0.03 ppm in pistachios, and 0.017 ppm and 0.014 ppm in two samples of processed walnuts. These low levels were expected since most of the nuts had been heat treated.

Another fumigant, 1,2-dibromoethane (EDB), is a mutagen and, after activation by glutathione S-transferase, is a potent carcinogen in rodents. Since fetuses of several laboratory rodents do not have this activating enzyme, experiments were carried out with human fetal liver to determine whether it was capable of activating EDB (*111*). Glutathione S-transferase was found to be very active in this tissue and metabolized EDB with high efficiency. These data suggested that the human fetus may be at greater risk from EDB toxicity than the adult.

Fungicides

Dithiocarbamates and ethylenethiourea (ETU). Chronic toxicity and carcinogenicity of ETU, a metabolite of ethylenebisdithiocarbamate (EBDC), was investigated in rats and mice orally dosed with this chemical (a) during the perinatal period (up to 8 weeks of age) only, (b) as an adult only (for 2 years starting at 8 weeks), and (c) during both perinatal and adult periods (*112*). Dietary exposure levels during the perinatal period were 9–90 ppm (rats) and 33–330 ppm (mice) and during the adult period were 25–250 ppm (rats) and 100–1000 ppm (mice). ETU did not induce tumors in rodents in group (a) but induced similar levels of thyroid tumors in both rats and mice in groups (b) and (c). ETU also had carcinogenic effects on the liver and pituitary gland of mice. Effects of nabam (an EBDC fungicide) and ETU on kidney function and morphology were examined in rats provided with drinking water containing 0–200 mg/L nabam or 0–300 mg/L ETU for 28 days (*113*). Neither compound appeared to affect kidney function although ETU was excreted in the urine after exposure to both compounds. High doses of ETU did induce some ultrastructural alterations in epithelial cells of renal proximal tubuli.

A reduction of 2.5- to 4-fold in residues of EBDC on leafy greens was achieved by washing in water for 3 minutes (*114*). However, levels were still relatively high, ranging from 4.62 to 9.54 ppm. Washing in a strong detergent further decreased residue concentrations to 1.15–2.23 ppm. Spinach retained more EBDC than the other greens regardless of treatment.

An HPLC procedure, involving a single extraction step with methanol, was developed for the determination of ETU in peels of potatoes, tomatoes, and apples (*115*). The foods were sprayed with mancozeb (EBDC) and then samples were analyzed after 0, 2, 4, and 7 days at 20°C. Detection limit was 0.1 ppm and recoveries ranged from 80 to 97%. Levels of ETU were observed to decline slowly on all the foods, with a half-life of about 6 days. Mancozeb disappeared much more slowly from field-sprayed apricots (*116*). Only about 10% was lost during the first 3 weeks after application. Variable amounts, ranging from 35 to 70%, of mancozeb were washed from the fruit by dipping in water.

A commercial particle beam liquid chromatography/mass spectrometry method, with a detection limit of 5 ppb, has also been used to detect ETU in crops (*117*). Residues were extracted from lettuce, applesauce, banana pulp, and papaya pulp containing as little as 5 ng ETU, and then the mass spectra obtained were matched with the NBS library reference EI spectrum. Isotopically labelled ETU was used as an internal standard. Recoveries of ETU from spiked samples were usually 80–90%.

BENZIMIDAZOLE FUNGICIDES. To determine the effects of microwave- and oven-baking on residues of thiabendazole in potatoes, peelings and flesh of treated potatoes were analyzed by reverse-phase HPLC with fluorescence and UV detection (*118*). Thiabendazole was present primarily in the peels of raw potatoes (mean of 12.2 mg/kg) with trace amounts (0.09 mg/kg) in the flesh. Residue levels were not significantly different after cooking by either method and there was no evidence that residues migrated from the peel into the flesh during cooking.

Thiabendazole residues in potatoes have also been successfully analyzed by HPTLC (*119*). Samples were homogenized and extracted with dichloromethane prior to spotting on a TLC plate. In comparison with HPLC, the HPTLC method was less sensitive but it could detect residues of about 0.4 mg/kg (about 0.1 the maximal permissible residue). Two sprout inhibitors, chlorpropham and propham, were also detected on these TLC plates.

Reversed-phase HPLC procedures with fluorescence detection have been described for determination of thiabendazole in citrus fruits (*120*) and of carbendazim in blueberries (*121*). Using acetonitrile/phosphate buffer as the mobile phase, 0.05 mg/kg thiabendazole could be quantified. The mobile phase for carbendazim determination was acetonitrile/methanol/water/monoethanolamine, and a detection limit of 15 ng/g was achieved.

A polyclonal enzyme immunoassay was developed to detect MBC, the degradation product of the fungicide benomyl on blueberries (*122*). The entire analysis took about 25 minutes since no cleanup step was required. Detection limit was 18 ppb and none of 40 field samples analyzed was found to contain residues approaching the tolerance of 15 ppm.

OTHER FUNGICIDES. An interlaboratory evaluation of the determination of captan, folpet, and captafol in tomatoes, cucumbers and apples using a wide-bore capillary column GC with electron capture detection has been conducted (*123*). The food samples were spiked with 3 levels of each fungicide and recoveries ranged from 86.2% to 115.4%. Interlaboratory coefficients of variation ranged from 2.8–9.7% for tomatoes and cucumbers and from 1.5 to 22.1% for apples.

Aliette, a fungicide used on pineapples and citrus fruits, has been evaluated for its carcinogenic potential using a consensus peer review process and EPA's guidelines for risk assessment (*124*). Based on carcinogenicity studies in rodents, in which male rats exposed to high doses of aliette developed bladder tumors, this fungicide has been categorized group C—a possible human carcinogen. However, this compound was not carcinogenic in female rats or in mice of either sex. Aliette tested negative in a variety of short-term genotoxicity assays. Its mechanism for carcinogenicity in male rats is unknown.

Herbicides and growth regulators

Paraquat and Diquat, herbicides registered in the USA for a variety of applications, are known to be toxic to humans. An ion-pairing LC method using a silica analytical column, sodium chloride as the ion pairing reagent and acetonitrile as the organic modifier has been developed for the determination of these herbicides in high-moisture food crops (*125*). The two herbicides were quantified by diode array UV absorbance at their wavelengths of maximum absorbance. Average recoveries from spiked samples of potatoes, corn, turnips, and asparagus ranged from 79.3 to 104.8%. Sensitivity of the method was about 0.01 ppm.

Metabolic residues of metolachlor, an herbicide chemically related to alachlor, a suspected carcinogen, were determined in tomatoes using GC/MS with a detection limit of 11–12 µg/kg (*126*). Tomato samples were hydrolyzed by acid and the metolachlor metabolites were derivatized prior to analysis. Recoveries of 87–96% were achieved for tomatoes fortified with 50–200 µg/kg metolachlor.

Proposals have been made for the preharvest use of glyphosate on some cereals, oilseeds, and pulses. Therefore, an LC method with postcolumn fluorescence detection has been developed for the determination of this herbicide in various cereals and beans (*127*). Samples were extracted with chloroform/water and then cleaned up on cation and anion exchange columns. Limits of detection of glyphosate ranged from 0.07 to 0.14 ppm in different crops, and average recoveries were 90.9–98.1%.

Dinoseb is an herbicide used on raspberries in Canada but not registered for this purpose in the USA. An HPLC method was capable of detecting as little as 0.025 ppm dinoseb in raspberries with average recoveries of 78.6–85.5% in spiked samples (*128*). Analyses of raspberries from 7 farms using dinoseb revealed no detectable residues on the berries.

Apples from trees of 5 varieties which had been sprayed with daminozide (Alar 85) for 1 year or for 21 years were assayed to determine residue levels of this growth regulator (*129*). "Top Red" apples, from trees sprayed for only one year at rates of 2.2–9.0 kg/ha, had no detectable daminozide residues when tested two or three years after cessation of spraying. "Golden Delicious," "Starking," "Rome," and "Red King" apples from trees which had long-term exposure to alar (2.2–4.5 kg/ha) still contained low levels (<1 ppm) of alar one year after spraying stopped. "Rome" and "Golden Delicious" had higher average residue levels (0.81–0.92 ppm) than the other varieties (0.05–0.2 ppm).

When treated with nitrite at pH 3 both daminozide and its breakdown product, unsymmetrical dimethylhydrazine (UDMH), were nitrosated to form *N*-nitrosodimethylamine (NDMA) (*130*). Under conditions of nitrite excess, yields of NDMA were 74.5% from daminozide and 48.2% from UDMH. Since NDMA is carcinogenic and this nitrosation reaction could occur in the gastrointestinal tract, caution should be exercised in the use of daminozide on crops intended for human consumption.

Use of a standard GC/MS method for determination of daminozide residues in high protein foods such as peanuts and peanut butter results in co-elution of some interfering substance(s) with daminozide. To eliminate this problem, following hydrolysis of daminozide to UDMH and distillation of the UDMH, glacial acetic acid was added to correct the pH to 5–6 (*131*). This step reduced interference and permitted minimum detection and determination limits of 0.005 ppm and 0.02 ppm, respectively, in high protein samples such as peanuts.

Maleic hydrazide, a growth regulator used on onions and potatoes, is known to have some toxic effects. A simple method for determination of this compound in foods, utilizing solid-phase extraction cartridges for clean up and then anion exchange HPLC with UV detection, has been developed (*132*). For samples spiked with 1.5–15 mg/kg, recoveries averaged 81–107%.

Insecticides

Residues of aldicarb in peeled potato tubers were found to decrease only slightly after cooking in boiling water and in the microwave (*133*). Aldicarb was applied to potato fields at rates of 1, 3 (adequate for pest control), 5, 10, and 25 kg/ha, and potatoes were sampled biweekly from 7 to 20 weeks later. Initial levels of aldicarb were very high (0.35–16.12 mg/kg at different application rates) but decreased during growth so that at maturity (20 weeks) residues were 0.03–1.94 mg/kg. However, neither cooking method completely destroyed aldicarb. For aldicarb concentrations of 0.21–0.45 mg/kg before cooking (from potatoes exposed to 3 and 5 kg/ha), cooking destroyed or washed out 30–38% of the residues.

Competitive ELISAs have been developed for the determination of 3 major organophosphate pesticides, fenitrothion (FN), chlorpyrifos-methyl (CPM), and pirimiphos-methyl (PIRM) (*134*). Each assay was specific for a single compound with no significant cross-reaction with the other pesticides and only limited reactions with major metabolites of the pesticides. Pesticides were extracted from grain and milling fractions with methanol. As little as 0.08 ppm FN, 0.2 ppm CPM, and 0.03 ppm PIRM could be detected in whole wheat grains. Results obtained with the ELISAs correlated well with results from GC analyses. An HPLC assay for PIRM demonstrated that residue levels on lettuce exceeded maximum residue limits (1 mg/kg) immediately after application but dropped significantly one to two weeks after application (*135*).

A rapid and sensitive HPLC method has been developed for the determination of abamectin and its delta 8,9-isomer in tomatoes (*136*). Samples were simultaneously homogenized and extracted with acetonitrile/water/hexane and then cleaned up on an aminopropyl solid-phase extraction cartridge. The pesticides were derivatized with trifluoroacetic anhydride/1-methylimidazole and then quantified by HPLC with fluorescence detection. The quantitation limit was 5 ppb, with recoveries of abamectin averaging 95%.

GC with fluorescence spectrometry was used to determine residues of carbaryl and its hydrolysis product, 1-naphthol, in apples and strawberries (*137*). The two compounds were separated by liquid chromatography prior to derivatizing with trimethyl anilinium hydroxide and GC analysis. Limit of detection was 0.14 ppm and recoveries of 72–77% were achieved with fruit samples spiked with carbaryl at 5.5 ppm.

A rapid HPLC procedure was used to study persistence of the acaricide fenbutatin oxide in peaches and nectarines (*138*). Detection limit of the method was 0.05 ppm and recoveries of 90.6–101.3% were achieved. Fruit trees were sprayed at the recommended rate and twice this rate and then fruits were collected and examined at weekly intervals. In both field and greenhouse experiments, residue concentrations decreased during 29 days after spraying but at the same time the fruits were growing. The apparent decrease in residue levels was mainly a dilution effect caused by the increased size of the fruits.

Bioavailability and characterization of bound residues of radiolabelled fenvalerate applied at 100 ppm to wheat were measured during the following 6 months (*139*). Residues were classified as surface (washed off with acetone/water), extractable (extracted with methanol for 24 h), and bound (not extractable). At 1–5 months of storage, concentrations of fenvalerate in each of these fractions were about 15%, 80%, and 6%, respectively. Supercritical fluid extraction liberated about 96% of the radio-

activity in the bound residues, of which 75% was identified as fenvalerate. When these bound residues were fed to rats, about 60% was eliminated in the feces and the remainder in the urine within 90 h. Approximately one-third of the excreted radioactivity was intact fenvalerate. These experiments demonstrate that the bound residues are bioavailable and should be evaluated toxicologically.

Fate and distribution of [^{14}C]-fenvalerate were monitored in cows and chickens fed dietary levels of 0.11–79 ppm and 9–160 ppm, respectively, of the pesticide (*140*). Fenvalerate was found to distribute rapidly as the unchanged molecule in the milk cream, egg yolk, body fat, and muscle tissue during consumption of contaminated feed. However, these residues dissipated rapidly when the animals were returned to untreated feed. Residue levels in various animal products were below the allowable daily intake even under the worst-case dietary exposure scenario.

Lactating dairy cows fed grain contaminated with the insecticide deltamethrin (2 or 10 mg/kg feed) for 28 days accumulated the pesticide primarily in fat with little or none detected in liver or muscle tissue (*141*). Residue levels in milk ranged up to 0.018 and 0.053 μg/g in cows given the higher and lower doses of deltamethrin. These residues dissipated rapidly when cows were returned to uncontaminated feed.

Various methods have been developed for the extraction of organochlorine pesticides from fatty samples. A single-step partition between *n*-hexane and acetonitrile on disposable cartridges of Kieselguhr type material followed by Florasil cleanup and solid-matrix sulfuric acid treatment recovered 72–104% of 18 organochlorine pesticides spiked into olive oil (*142*). A supercritical fluid cleanup procedure utilizing a mobile phase of carbon dioxide or methanol/carbon dioxide on an alumina or a silica column recovered 93–111% of 6 organochlorines from lard and chicken fat (*143*). Eleven organochlorines were extracted from milk, with an efficiency of 90–110%, by a one-step solvent extraction with ethyl acetate–acetone–methanol by ultrasonication (*144*). Extracts were further cleaned up on silica cartridges and then assayed by capillary GLC with electron capture detection.

PACKAGING MATERIALS

A wide variety of volatile compounds which may be present in different packaging materials was reviewed with some discussion of methods for detection (*145*). Such compounds include solvents, residual monomers of plastics, acetaldehyde, nitrosamines (from rubber netting), PCBs from paperboard, and many others. These compounds may leach into foods depending on the type of food and the storage conditions but most have been detected in foods in such minute quantities that they are probably toxicologically insignificant.

Toxicological studies

Butyl benzyl phthalate (BBP), a plasticizer used in food containers and wrapping materials, can migrate into food. Developmental toxicity of BBP was assayed in pregnant Wistar rats fed diets containing 2% BBP during various stages of pregnancy (*146,147*). Food consumption and body weight gain decreased in treated rats, so effects in treated rats were compared to those in pair-fed controls. Complete resorption of all implanted embryos occurred in all females given BBP on days 0–11 or 0–20 of pregnancy. Post-implantation loss was increased (as compared to controls) in females fed BBP on days 0–7 and 7–16 but not in females dosed on days 16–20 and 11–20 of pregnancy. Cleft palate was the most common teratogenic effect noted in the offspring, affecting 54% and 95% of pups whose mothers were fed BBP on days 11–20 and 7–16, respectively. Fusion of sternebrae occurred in 16.4% and 52% of pups in the same dose groups, respectively.

Cellulose acetate, a polymer used as a food packaging material, is generally recognized as safe although it has been occasionally associated with cases of dermatitis. To assess the potential for adverse effects from oral ingestion of this compound, rats were fed dietary levels of 0, 500, 2500, and 5000 mg cellulose acetate/kg body weight for 94–96 days (*148*). These doses correspond to 7.2–10.0% of the diet. No adverse treatment-related effects were observed in hematology, clinical chemistry, ophthalmology, food consumption, gross pathology, or histopathology at the end of the experiment.

Since workers in polyvinyl chloride (PVC) production plants in the 1970s were observed to have an increased incidence of angiosarcomas in the liver, there has been some concern that residual vinyl chloride monomer (VCM) in PVC-packaged foods may migrate into foods and be ingested. A lifetime (149 week) oral carcinogenicity study with rats investigated the effects of ingestion of PVC powder with a high VCM content (*149*). Actual exposures to VCM were 0, 0.014, 0.13, and 1.3 mg VCM/kg body weight/day. In the highest dose group, a variety of hepatic lesions, including neoplastic nodules, hepatocellular carcinomas, and angiosarcomas were observed. Only basophilic foci of hepatocellular alteration were observed in females (not males) of the lower dose groups. There was no evidence of tumors or pathological changes in other organs in any group. It was concluded that 0.13 mg VCM/kg/day is the no-observed-effect level with respect to induction of tumors in rats.

Melamine, used to produce a wide variety of tableware, can be released from these products into some food-simulating solvents and beverages, particularly at high temperatures and under acidic conditions. Intestinal distribution and absorption of melamine were examined in male rats fed diets containing 1% melamine for 1 week (*150*). Melamine concentrations in contents of the gastrointestinal tract were as follows: stomach, 3040 ppm; upper part of small intestine, 487 ppm; lower part of small intestine, 158 ppm; large intestine, 283 ppm. Concentrations in blood and urine averaged 22.6 and 5050 ppm, respectively. Melamine was not absorbed from the stomach but was absorbed exponentially from the small intestine and excreted in the urine.

Packaging components in foods, their migration and determination

Effects of long-term use of melamine tableware on the release of melamine monomers and formaldehyde was measured in cups used in a cafeteria during 4 years and in new cups given a repetitive heat treatment with 4% acetic acid at 95°C for 30 min (*151*). In a standard migration test using water at 60°C for 30 min, neither new cups nor those used for 3 and 4 years released formaldehyde above the detection limit of 0.1 ppm. In the same test, new cups, 3-year-old and 4-year-old cups released 0.03, 0.02, and 0.01 ppm melamine. Cups treated with acetic acid for 20 cycles (estimated to correspond to about 13.4 years of use) released 0.2 ppm formaldehyde and 0.12 ppm melamine in the migration test with water.

Because of the problem of leaching of di-(2-ethylhexyl) phthalate (DEHP) from DEHP-plasticized milk tubing into milk the use of such tubing has been banned in Denmark. About 6 months after the ban, milk samples from 1 German and 14 Danish dairies were analyzed for DEHP residues using a GC procedure with a detection limit of 0.05–0.2 mg/L (*152*). Only 2 samples had detectable levels of DEHP at concentrations of 0.05–0.14 mg/L. Such low levels probably do not constitute a health risk since the tolerable daily intake, according to the EEC Scientific Committee for Food, is 25 µg/kg body weight.

A polymeric plasticizer, poly(butylene adipate), has been used as a replacement for di(2-ethylhexyl) adipate (DEHA) in cling films to reduce levels of plasticizer migration. Seven individual oligomers have been identified from these new cling films, and their migration into olive oil was measured (*153*). Low-molecular-weight species, constituting 24% of the parent plasticizer, were found to account for more than 90% of plasticizer migration. After exposure of the oil to the film for 12 h at 23°C, a total of 390 mg total polymeric plasticizer was detected in the olive oil.

Sisal bags, primarily used for storing and transporting coffee and cocoa beans, are treated with a batching oil during manufacture. In a recent study, the potential for this oil, primarily a mixture of mineral oil products, to contaminate stored foods was investigated (*154*). Concentrations of total hydrocarbons and of aromatics from used bags ranged from 0.3–39 g/kg of bag and from <0.1–2.7 g/kg, respectively. GC analyses of the oils from the bags (originating in at least 5 countries) revealed a wide variation in composition of the oils. Residues detected in foods were typically 10–100 mg/kg, with most of the contamination probably involving molecules of <25 carbon atoms.

In a broad study of a variety of food packaging materials, important food contamination by hydrocarbons was noted for sisal bags, cardboard boxes, and wax-coated paper/cardboard (*155*). Paraffins from the packing materials were isolated by liquid chromatography and characterized by GC. Shells of cocoa beans near the fabric of sisal bags contained 1380 mg oil components/kg while those from the center of the bag had only 210 mg/kg contamination. Paraffins, which constitute 26% of waxed paper, migrate readily into salami in contact with the paper, reaching a concentration of 900 mg wax/kg meat. This migration process is strongly temperature-dependent. Little contamination was observed in cheese coated with paraffin. Pralines, individually wrapped in aluminum foil (with a very thin layer of paper glued to the foil by a wax) were found to be contaminated with 30–100 mg wax/kg.

Mineral hydrocarbons are used as flow promoters at levels up to 7–8% by weight in rigid polystyrene containers, such as cups for hot and cold beverages. In migration experiments, these hydrocarbons were detected in cold beverages (beer, apple juice, cola) at concentrations <0.1 mg/kg and in hot beverages (coffee, hot chocolate, tea, chicken soup) at levels <0.5 mg/kg (*156*). Cold drinks were analyzed after 16 h at room temperature while hot drinks remained in the cups for 1 h at 100°C.

GC/MS using selected ion monitoring was used to determine residual α-methyl styrene (α-MSt) in styrene-based polymers and to measure its migration into 4 food simulants (*157*). This procedure allowed quantitation of α-MSt at levels of 10 and 0.1 µg/g in the polymer and in the simulants, respectively. No migration of α-MSt was observed from food-grade polystyrene and styrene–acrylonitrile sheets into the 4 food simulants, nor from food-grade acrylonitrile–butadiene–styrene (ABS) into water, 4% acetic acid, or 20% ethanol. Low levels of α-MSt did migrate from ABS into *n*-heptane, resulting in concentrations of 0.08–0.15 µg/g heptane.

Some components of plastic packaging materials may migrate into foods during microwave cooking. To determine whether this is strictly a thermal effect or whether the microwave energy itself influences migration, five plastics, representing the most common materials used in microwave applications, were tested (*158*). In one set of experiments, empty containers were microwaved and then compared to untreated containers in migration testing into olive oil. In other experiments, migration into iso-octane during microwaving of these containers was compared to migration from identical containers, which had received equivalent thermal treatment, into the same solvent. Migration of plasticizers, oligomers, antioxidants, and volatile components were monitored and no difference was observed between microwave-treated plastics and those which had received an equivalent heat treatment.

Experiments using the food simulant miglyol, a fractionated coconut oil, and a commercial meat- and vegetable-filled pastry designed for microwave susceptor cooking demonstrated that measurable amounts of the diglycidyl ether of Bisphenol A (DGEBA) migrate through the poly(ethylene terephthalate) (PET) film into both the food and the oil during microwaving (*159*). DGEBA is an acrylic/epoxy adhesive used in susceptor packaging. Average concentrations of 1.33 and 8.59 µg/g DGEBA were determined in the food and the oil, respectively.

A reverse-phase LC column with fluorescence detection has been developed for the determination of DGEBA in water, 15% ethanol, and 3% acetic acid (*160*). Detection limit for the method was 0.1 µg/L with recoveries of nearly 100% from spiked samples. Relative precision at 200 µg/L was 3.4%.

POLYNUCLEAR AROMATIC HYDROCARBONS (PAHS)

Sources of dietary exposure to PAHs

A survey of cooked foods and herbs and spices obtained at markets in South India was conducted to determine levels of PAHs (*161*). Chrysene was detected in nearly all the pyrolysed samples, with highest levels measured in salted, sun-dried, oil-fried ribbon fish (18.57 µg/g). High levels of dibenzanthracene were detected in a decoction of a pyrolyzed mixture of cumin seeds, mint leaves, and cardamom (31.15 µg/g), salted and fried chillies (27,48 µg/g), and fried whitebait fish (12.34 µg/g). Benzo(*a*)pyrene (BP) concentrations were highest in the aforementioned ribbon fish (60.17 µg/g), whitebait fish (5.73 µg/g), and the cumin seed mixture (6.4 µg/g) and in seer fish (10.29 µg/g). Such high levels of PAHs in prepared foods may be related to the very high incidence of stomach cancer in South India.

Carrots were grown in control soils and in soils amended at 3 sludge application rates (15, 55, 180 t/ha) to determine their uptake of 15 PAH compounds (*162*). The applied sludge contained 17.2 mg PAH/kg. Cores of carrots grown in sludge-amended soil contained slightly higher PAH levels (3.6–4.2 µg/kg fresh weight) than those in control soils (1.9 µg/kg) but the difference was not significant. Carrot peels from the treated soils, however, did contain elevated PAH concentrations: 12.0–17.5 µg/kg compared to 7.6 µg/kg in control carrots. Such low levels probably do not pose a risk to human health.

Crustaceans and shellfish from polluted waters may accumulate high levels of PAHs. Blue crabs from a highly contaminated urban estuary in Virginia were found to contain PAH concentrations as high as 11 mg/kg dry weight in hepatopancreas and 3.1 mg/kg in muscle (*163*). Other organochlorines were detected in lower amounts. After 48 hours of exposure to PAHs in waste crankcase oil, "Cherrystone" clams were monitored for depuration of accumulated PAHs (*164*). Although there was quite a bit of variability in tissue levels of PAHs, there was no evidence of decreasing PAH concentrations in clams tested during 45 days following exposure.

Approximately 80% of the total dietary intake of PAHs is estimated to come from the cereals and the oils/fats food groups. To determine which individual food items are major contributors to PAH intake, a range of retail products from these food groups was analyzed for 11 PAH compounds (*165*). PAH levels were low in fish and animal-derived oils (e.g. butter, 0.06 µg BP/kg) but higher and more variable in vegetable oils (average of 1.29 µg BP/kg). Margarine was the major dietary source of PAHs in this group, accounting for about 70% of the PAH intake, although individual samples of the same brand of margarine varied by as much as a factor of 20 in PAH content. BP levels were low (<0.1 µg/kg) in white flour and bread but higher in bakery goods containing higher levels of edible oils. Refining of crude oils was found to significantly reduce PAH levels in oils.

Biological effects of PAHs

A multimedia transport model was used to evaluate environmental partitioning of BP and to identify the major sources of human exposure (*166*). Results demonstrated that BP partitions mainly into soil (82%) and that the food chain is the predominant route of human exposure. Inhalation and drinking of contaminated water are only minor sources of BP. The long-term average daily intake of BP in the USA is estimated to be 2.2 µg, with the food chain accounting for about 97% of this. Since there is an increased lifetime risk of 3.5×10^{-4} associated with exposure to background levels of BP, ingestion of food items contaminated with BP may pose a serious health risk.

To determine levels of excretion of the pyrene metabolite 1-hydroxypyrene (1-OHPY), 5 human volunteers consumed one meal with grilled hamburgers containing 22,450 ng BP/kg, and their urine samples following this meal were analyzed (*167*). 1-OHPY levels in these samples were 4–12 times higher than in a period when the volunteers consumed low BP levels (12–78 ng/kg). The high urinary levels of 1-OHPY were comparable to those measured in cases of occupational exposure to PAHs. Although dietary PAH concentrations can be reduced by avoiding certain foods and food preparation methods, it is difficult to completely eliminate them.

Effects of PAHs on human chorionic gonadotrophin (HCG) secretion by first trimester placental explants in vitro has been investigated (*168*). In both static and dynamic cultures, BP and 3-methylcholanthrene at 50 µM stimulated HCG production. This increased secretion of HCG continued after withdrawal of the PAH compounds. The in vivo effects of this alteration in hormone levels are unknown at this time.

Formation of BP–DNA adducts in human monocytes and lymphocytes was compared in in vitro experiments (*169*). Following incubation with BP, DNA adducts were found in monocytes but only occurred in lymphocytes after stimulation with phytohemagglutinin. Incubation of both cell types with the activated epoxide form of BP led to a similar pattern of DNA adducts. It appears that unstimulated lymphocytes are unable to activate promutagens like BP.

POLYHALOGENATED AROMATIC HYDROCARBONS

In a recent article, sources, environmental distribution, and risk assessment studies of polychlorinated dibenzo-*p*-dioxins (PCDDs), polychlorinated dibenzofurans (PCDFs), and polychlorinated biphenyls (PCBs) were reviewed (*170*). PCBs were manufactured for industrial purposes while PCDDs and PCDFs were unintentional by-products of a number of reactions. All these compounds are now widespread in the environment, including many foods. Although concentrations are usually low (except in cases of industrial accidents and environmental incidents) toxicity of some congeners is very high. Toxic equivalency factors (TEFs) have been calculated for different congeners of these compounds, and the use of TEFs in risk assessments for exposure to PCBs, PCDFs, and PCDDs was discussed.

Proceedings of the Tenth International Symposium on Chlorinated Dioxins and Related Compounds, held in Germany in 1990, were published in two issues of *Chemosphere* (*171,172*). Among the topics covered were analytical methods; formation and destruction of PCBs, PCDDs, and PCDFs; presence of these compounds in foods and paper products; toxicology; and risk assessment.

Analyses of human adipose tissue samples for 54 toxic substances (pesticides, PCBs, PCDDs, and

PCDFs, and volatiles) by the National Human Adipose Tissue Survey has been sorted by U.S. census divisions (*173*). Based on these data, it appears that persons living in the South Atlantic, East South Central, West South Central, and East North Central regions were exposed to greater amounts of toxic substances. Further investigations should try to pinpoint the sources of contamination in these areas.

Tissue samples (liver, adipose tissue, kidneys, testes, and prostate glands) were collected during autopsy of 8 males in western Oregon and analyzed for residues of pentachlorophenol (PCP), non-chloro-2-phenoxyphenol (NCPP), and some other chlorinated contaminants (*174*). Electron capture GC was used to quantitate the residues, and electron capture negative ion MS was used to confirm their identity. All tissues tested for PCP were positive, with concentrations ranging from 0.007 ppm in subcutaneous fat to 4.14 ppm in testes. Highest levels of NCPP were also found in testes (0.59 ppm). Other chlorinated compounds detected in fat included PCDDs and DDE.

Fat samples from 168 corpses in Zaragoza, Spain, were analyzed for residues of DDE, hexachlorobenzene (HCB), and β-hexachlorocyclohexane (β-HCH) (*175*). Concentrations of DDE (0.09–12.0 ppm) and β-HCH (0.01–3.39 ppm) were intermediate among those reported for other countries. However, the average residue level of HCB (2.95 ppm) was much higher than that reported in other countries. The origin of this high level of contamination is unknown.

Serum PCB and DDT levels in groups of 115 Great Lakes fish eaters and of 95 non-fish-eating controls were determined in 1989 and compared to levels previously measured in these individuals in 1982 (*176*). Substantial and significant decreases in mean serum DDT levels occurred in both groups during this time period but only a slight decrease in PCB levels was noted. There was no association between individual changes in serum levels of these compounds and self-reported changes in consumption of Great Lakes fish.

The use of blood samples for the estimation of body burden of organochlorine compounds has been evaluated in two studies. Analyses of paired serum/adipose tissue samples from 12 healthy volunteers in Finland revealed a positive correlation for DDT when concentrations were calculated on a fat-weight basis and for PCB and HCB when the calculations were based on wet weight (*177*). The association between blood cells and adipose tissue was weaker and no correlation between residues found in liver and adipose tissue was observed in samples from 23 autopsy cases. Positive relationships for residue concentrations of HCB, β-HCH, oxychlordane, and DDE in adipose tissue and blood were also observed in samples from 25 patients in Canada (*178*). However, no good relationship was observed for residues of a number of other chlorinated compounds.

Residues of several organochlorine chemicals in skin lipids were analyzed and compared to residues in adipose tissue samples of 23 subjects in Japan (*179*). Skin lipids were collected by wiping the face with cotton and cleaned up by gel permeation chromatography and sulfuric acid prior to GC analysis. Correlation coefficients for skin lipid/adipose tissue concentrations of DDE, β-HCH, and oxychlordane were 0.93, 0.92, and 0.68, respectively. Skin lipids of monkeys (*Macaca fascicularis*) were also analyzed for organochlorine residues and compared to residues in adipose tissue and blood (*180*). A mixture of β-HCH, DDT, and *trans*-lindane was injected subcutaneously into monkeys 5 times at weekly intervals. Chemical residues were determined 4–9 weeks after the last injection. Correlation coefficients for residue levels in blood and adipose tissue ranged from 0.83 to 0.94 and for skin lipids and adipose tissue were generally in the range of 0.72–0.83. Analysis of skin lipids may be another useful non-invasive approach for the estimation of body burdens of some organochlorine contaminants.

Elevated levels of PCBs, DDTs, HCHs, and aldrin and dieldrin were detected in animal fat, butter, meat, and seafood samples collected in different parts of Vietnam (*181*). Estimated average daily intakes of the 4 groups of residues were 3.7, 19, 6.3, and 0.55 µg/person, respectively. Fish, shellfish, and crustaceans were the primary source of DDTs, while cereals and vegetables were the primary sources of PCBs and HCHs. Significant residues of aldrin and dieldrin were detected in peanut oil, animal fat, and caviar.

Ten commercially available coffee filter papers (4 unbleached, 3 chlorine-bleached, and 2 peroxide-bleached, and 1 bleached, chlorine-free sample) were analyzed to determine residues of semi-volatile organics, dibenzofurans, and dioxins (*182*). PCDDs were not detected in any papers, while a single dioxin isomer was detected in one unbleached paper. A brominated compound was detected in an unbleached paper and a chlorine-bleached paper and tributyl phosphate, a plasticizer, was found in one oxygen-bleached paper. There was no direct relationship between bleaching methods and presence of halogenated residues in the filter papers.

Polychlorinated biphenyls (PCBs)

Bioaccumulation, metabolism, and toxicity of PCBs were recently reviewed (*183*). PCBs in the environment and their accumulation in the food chain were briefly discussed. In vivo and in vitro metabolism of PCBs by various enzymes in different organisms was summarized, and data on toxic and potentially carcinogenic effects were reported. Another paper reviewed the problem of PCBs in the environment from the point of view of an analytical chemist (*184*). Sources of contamination, fate in the environment, toxic properties, and limitations and purposes of analytical methods are complex and interrelated problems which should be considered. Further research should be directed to methods for congener-specific analysis.

PCB EXPOSURE AND HEALTH EFFECTS IN HUMANS. Results from studies of 3 cohorts exposed to PCB-contaminated fish from the Great Lakes Basin— the Michigan Sports Fisherman Cohort, the Michigan Maternal/Infant Cohort, and the Wisconsin Maternal/Infant Cohort—were summarized and compared with each other and with data from other geographic areas (*185*). A comprehensive evaluation of data on 7 major categories of exposure sequelae as related to consumption of contaminated fish affirmed the relationship between PCB exposure and (a) transplacental passage of PCB molecules and (b) alterations in health status during the neonatal period and early infancy. The relationship between other effects (maternal health, composite activity, and memory scale deficits) and PCB exposure was judged to be indeterminate.

Data from a North Carolina cohort, originally containing 859 newborns, also indicated that exposure to relatively high PCB levels in utero can affect early postnatal development but does not appear to have long-lasting effects (*186*). The mothers of these children did not have occupational or other special exposure to PCBs. Although some motor abnormalities and psychomotor delay had been observed in the first 2 years in the infants with the highest 5% exposure to PCBs, no significant differences were noted in scores on the McCarthy Scales of Children's Abilities at 3, 4, or 5 years or in 506 school report cards evaluated in later years.

In a pilot study, fat samples from 20 women with breast cancer and from 20 women with benign breast disease were analyzed for PCBs and several chlorinated pesticides (*187*). Significantly higher levels of PCBs, DDT, and DDE were found in fat from the women with cancer. Although the sample size was small and it was not possible to control for all other established risk factors, the results suggest that environmental contaminants may play a role in the development of breast cancer.

Peripheral lymphocytes from 32 workers occupationally exposed to PCBs and from 40 controls were subjected to cytogenetic analysis (*188*). A significantly higher incidence of aberrant cells and sister chromatid exchanges was observed in workers who had been exposed to PCBs for >10 years. Plasma PCB levels in workers exposed to PCBs for 11–15 years and for 16–25 years were 487 and 420 μg PCB/L, respectively, while the controls averaged 1.5–3 μg/L. However, another study of workers exposed to Aroclors 1254, 1242, and 1016 (*189*) found no significant associations between lipid PCB levels and clinical indicators of hepatotoxicity, hypertension, or pulmonary impairment. Neither was there evidence of chloracne or increased cancer mortality.

Coplanar PCBs, which are approximate stereoisomers of dioxin, have been found to be the most toxic PCB congeners. Levels of three coplanar congeners, #77, #126, and #169, were determined in 62 human adipose tissue samples from autopsies in 5 Ontario cities (*190*). Congener #77 was below the detection limit (20 pg/g) in most samples. Mean values for congener #126 were 235 and 370 pg/g and for congener #169 were 46 and 94 pg/g in males and females, respectively. These levels were comparable to some data from Japan but higher than some other results from North America. Mean coplanar PCB levels in milk from 96 mothers in Quebec were 8.07, 80.46, and 32.71 pg/g for congeners #77, #126, and #169, respectively (191). In this population, these PCB levels present a greater risk to infants than dioxins and dibenzofurans.

Mono-ortho and di-ortho coplanar PCBs in 100 samples of mother's milk in Germany averaged 44 (congener #118), 168 (#138), 27 (#156), and 25 (#170) µg/kg (192). These levels represent approximately 3 times the toxicity of dioxins and dibenzofurans in these milk samples.

A rapid and relatively simple LC method utilizing a porous graphitic column has been developed for the isolation of mono-ortho- and non-ortho-substituted PCBs from human milk (193). These PCBs could be determined at the parts-per-trillion level, and recoveries from spiked samples ranged from 90 to 104%.

BIOLOGICAL EFFECTS AND TOXICITY OF PCBs. Developmental/reproductive toxicity tests of PCBs in laboratory animals have been reviewed with respect to species sensitivity, sensitivity of the endpoints scored, biological plausibility, study quality and relevance to humans (194). Various measures of postnatal growth, development, and function were affected at the lowest doses studied. Lowest-observable-adverse-effect levels for rodents and for non-human primates were determined to be 0.25 and 0.08 mg/kg/day, respectively. No no-adverse-effect level was detected.

To determine alterations in the blood lipids and hepatic enzymes of pups being nursed by PCB-treated mothers, females rats were gavaged with 50 mg/kg of a PCB mixture every two days from postnatal days 2–20 (195,196). Tissue residues were highest at postnatal day 21 with mean levels of 60.31, 4.46, and 701.9 µg/g present in liver, brain, and fat, respectively, of female rats. These concentrations decreased steadily with time, as the animals grew and some PCBs were eliminated, so that at

postnatal day 300 residues in the same tissues were 0.22, 0.08, and 20.5 µg/g. Markedly increased hepatic triacylglycerol levels seen at day 21 decreased to normal levels by day 40 in females. Differences in DNA, RNA, and protein contents of the liver also returned to control levels within 60 days. However, some differences in hepatic drug-metabolizing enzymes persisted through postnatal day 180.

Recent epidemiological data suggest that prenatal exposure to PCBs has a greater effect than postnatal exposure on neuropsychological disorders. Results from cross-fostering studies with rats lead to similar conclusions (197). Female rats were fed diets containing 0 or 30 mg PCB/kg, and after the birth of their pups, half of the pups were nursed by females on the alternate diet. Levels of PCBs in the brains of offspring of treated females averaged 0.21 mg/kg at birth. After 22 days of nursing, pups of treated dams, who were nursed by untreated dams, had <0.07 mg PCBs/kg in the brain while the pups nursed by treated dams had brain levels of 0.3–0.36 mg/kg. Results from two behavioral assays, active avoidance learning and visual discrimination learning, demonstrated that prenatally exposed rats, even though their brain levels of PCBs were lower when tested, performed worse than those with only a postnatal exposure to PCBs.

Ten-day-old male mice given a single oral dose of 0.41 or 41 mg 3,3',4,4'-tetrachlorobiphenyl (TCB) displayed significantly different spontaneous motor behavior from controls when tested at 4 months (198). In addition, mice receiving the highest dose of TCB had a minor, but significant, increase in the density of muscarinic cholinergic receptors in the hippocampus. This alteration in the neonatal mouse brain may lead to permanent physiological and behavioral changes in the adult.

A homogeneous cell line, PC12, was used to investigate the relative potency of 43 PCB congeners as neurotoxicants (199). Congeners with ortho-, or ortho-,para-chlorine substitutions were found to cause the greatest decrease in cell dopamine levels. Increasing congener chlorination did not correlate with a decrease in potency. Similar effects were observed in non-human primate brains. Additional in vitro experiments indicated that the PCBs inhibited tyrosine hydroxylase activity, thereby decreasing dopamine levels (*200*). Thus, planar, dioxin-like congeners, which appear to be the most hepatotoxic and immunotoxic, do not appear to be neurotoxic.

Promoting activity of various PCB congeners in rat liver carcinogenesis has been compared to effects of these congeners on a variety of enzymatic changes in this organ (*201*). Female rats were initiated with diethylnitrosamine and then treated once a week with 15 or 150 μmol PCB/kg body weight for 8 weeks. Three congeners (2,2',4,5'- and 3,3',4,4'-tetrachlorobiphenyls and 2,3,4,4',5-pentachlorobiphenyl) exerted promoting effects, increasing the volumetric fraction of enzyme-altered foci in the liver. Induction of liver growth and of microsomal cytochrome P450 content in the liver correlated well with promoting activity and may be used to predict promoting activity in short-term assays.

Many suspected and established tumor promoters inhibit intercellular communication. Inhibition of cell–cell communication by different congeners of PCBs was investigated by the scrape loading/dye transfer assay and microinjection technique (*202*). Results indicated that substitution in the ortho position from the carbon bridge was essential for the ability to inhibit intercellular communication and that an increase in the number of ortho substituents enhanced potency. TCDD-like PCBs, with a planar conformation, did not inhibit dye transfer between cells.

Expression of 5 out of 10 protooncogenes examined was enhanced in livers of rats fed diets containing 0.05% of a mixture of PCBs (*203*). This altered expression was transcriptionally regulated and was more pronounced in rats treated with PCBs beginning at weaning than in adult rats. Correlations between altered protooncogene expression and tumor promoting activity have yet to be demonstrated.

After 55 months of exposure to 0, 5, 20, 40, or 80 μg dietary PCB/kg body weight/day, non-specific immune parameters were examined in rhesus monkeys (*204*). All treated groups had significantly higher serum hemolytic complement activity as compared to controls. Significant dose-related increases were observed in natural killer cell activity, thymosin alpha-1 levels, and interferon levels. Thus,

long-term exposure to PCBs appears to modulate several immune parameters.

Thyroid status of pups whose mothers consumed 50 ppm PBB or 250 ppm PCB during pregnancy and lactation was depressed, with a greater effect on T4 than on T3 (*205*). PBB caused minimal effects on the function of the hypothalamus–pituitary–adrenal axis but PCB caused decreased corticosterone levels before and after stimulation of axis function.

Recent data suggests that an Ah-mediated production of PCB metabolites may be responsible for alterations in thyroid hormone levels and vitamin A metabolism (*206*). Results from a variety of studies both in vitro and in vivo have been summarized and discussed with respect to the mechanisms of toxicity of PCBs. It appears that toxic symptoms caused by PCBs are partly induced by parent compounds and partly by metabolites, particularly the hydroxy metabolites generated from relatively planar PCB congeners.

PCBs IN FOODS AND FOOD-PRODUCING ANIMALS. Samples of fresh fruits and vegetables, fish, eggs, cereals, meat, and dairy products were collected from an area in Yugoslavia near an electro-industrial plant using PCBs and were analyzed to determine the extent of contamination (*207*). Although there was some variation in residue levels, some fish and egg samples had PCB levels which exceeded the tolerances set by the FDA. It was estimated that leafy vegetables and unpeeled fruits contributed about 3 times as much as foods of animal origin to the intake of PCBs. Total intake of dietary PCBs was estimated to be 6.2 mg/year/person in 1988 (3 years after the plant ceased operations).

A total of 46 samples of fresh fish and 101 samples of canned fish from the central Adriatic were analyzed for PCB residues (*208*). Mean PCB concentrations were 0.194 mg/kg in canned fish (primarily sardines) and 0.059 and 0.287 mg/kg in fresh fish from control and polluted areas, respectively. Canned cod liver from Poland was found to be contaminated with 1.2–2.6 μg/g of total PCBs with concentrations of 10 toxic coplanar PCBs ranging from 360 to 690 ng/g (*209*). Since PCB levels in some cans exceed the tolerance limit, this food is a potential health hazard. Coplanar PCBs were also detected in 30 samples of fish (striped bass) and 6 mussel samples from marine and estuarine waters of New York and in one composite sample of freshwater mussels from the same state (*210*). Concentrations of total coplanar PCBs in fish ranged from 0.1 to 2.02 µg/g wet weight, in marine mussels ranged from 7.5 to 18.0 ng/g dry weight, and in freshwater mussels averaged 112.9 ng/g dry weight. A recently developed method which combined sulfuric acid cleanup, carbon chromatography, and high resolution GC was used to determine levels of the PCB congeners.

Residues of PCBs were determined in milk fat, ear wax, and hair of cattle to determine their suitability for screening for carcass residues of PCBs (*211*). Samples were collected from 46 cattle from farms known to be contaminated with PCBs. When levels of the PCB congeners 138, 153, and 180 did not exceed 0.06, 0.05, and 0.03 mg/kg, respectively, in milk fat or 0.03, 0.03, and 0.02 mg/kg in ear wax, then maximum total PCB residues in meat and fat did not exceed statutory maximum PCB limits.

Experiments to determine the uptake of PCBs from soil by barley and tomato plants demonstrated that these plants lack an active transport system for these compounds (*212*). However, the plants readily trapped airborne PCBs volatilized from the soil, and concentrations as high as 19 ppb were detected in leaves of plants grown on soil containing 1 g of a mixture of Aroclors/50 g soil.

Polychlorinated dibenzo-p-dioxins (PCDDs) and polychlorinated dibenzufurans (PCDFs)

OCCURRENCE AND EFFECTS OF PCDDs AND PCDFs IN HUMANS. In a recent review (*213*), the available data on cancer risk to humans exposed to 2,3,7,8-tetrachlorodibenzo-*p*-dioxin (TCDD) was evaluated. Of 10 case–control studies of the relationship between exposure to phenoxys/chlorophenols (which may be contaminated with TCDD) and the incidence of malignant lymphomas, two reported a statistically significant association with non-Hodgkin's lymphoma but did not indicate whether subjects were exposed specifically to TCDD. One other study reported a statistically significant association with phenoxys containing TCDD. Of 15 case–control studies of soft-tissue sarcomas, less than half found a statistically significant relationship with TCDD exposure. Results of cohort studies of workers with occupational exposure to TCDD have provided little additional evidence of an increased risk for these types of cancer.

Some other epidemiological studies supported the hypothesis that TCDD is a human carcinogen. Followup mortality data on a cohort of 1583 chemical plant workers in Germany indicated an excess of deaths from cancer among the most highly exposed workers as compared to national mortality statistics for West Germany and to mortality in a cohort of male gas workers (*214*). A hospital-based case–control study of testicular cancer indicated an approximately two-fold increase in risk for this cancer among veterans who served in Vietnam (*215*). A historical cohort study of mortality in an international register of 18,910 production workers or sprayers (from 10 countries) exposed to TCDD revealed no excess in all-cause mortality, for all neoplasms, for the most common epithelial cancers, or for lymphomas (*216*). Increased risks were observed for soft-tissue sarcomas and for cancers of the testicle, thyroid, other endocrine glands, and nose and nasal cavity. However, because of the small number of cases, these results are difficult to interpret.

However, other investigations of persons exposed to TCDD report no long-term effects on health. A case–control study of 281 workers in a chemical plant, occupationally exposed to TCDD, and of 260 unexposed controls found no evidence of an elevated risk for clinical hepatic or gastrointestinal disease (*217*). Of 19,637 young people (aged 1–19 years) living in an area near Seveso, Italy, which was contaminated with TCDD after an explosion in a chemical plant in 1976, no excess mortality due to all causes was observed as compared to a control population of nearly 100,000 living in surrounding districts (*218*). None of 186 children who contracted chloracne, a reversible marker for TCDD intoxication, have died. Followup study of this exposed population continues.

Epidemiological studies on persons in Missouri who were exposed to TCDD from contaminated oil used to control dust have so far revealed no adverse effects on immune function (*219*). Further study of this exposed population also continues.

TCDD levels measured in the fat of breast milk of 14 Dutch mothers ranged from 5.35 to 17.0 ng/kg (*220*). Considering the concentrations and toxicities of 17 different furan and dioxin congeners, toxic equivalents in this milk ranged from 29.85 to 92.88 ng/kg. Four babies of these mothers had bleeding problems and their mothers' milk was found to have significantly higher levels of TCDD compared to the milk from the other 10 mothers. This supports the theory that TCDD alters vitamin K metabolism, thereby affecting blood coagulation.

Since animal studies have indicated that dioxin influences thyroid hormone status, thyroxine (T4), thyroid-binding globulin (TBG), and thyrotropin (TSH) levels were measured in 38 healthy term, breast-fed infants (*221*). At 11 weeks, mean TSH levels, mean T4 values and the T4/TBG ratio were all significantly higher in infants with a high exposure to dioxin [29.2–62.7 ng toxic equivalents (TEQ)/kg] in breast milk than in infants with a low exposure (8.7–28 ng TEQ/kg).

Two PCDD mixtures containing defined amounts of certain congeners were added to human hepatoma cell cultures to test their ability to induce P4501A1 enzymes (*222*). Compared to results previously obtained with rat hepatocytes and rat hepatoma cells, PCDDs were much less potent in the human cells, requiring 8- to 19-fold higher PCDD concentrations to induce the same level of P450 enzyme activity. Enzyme induction appeared to be largely due to the additive effects of the 2,3,7,8-substituted constituents. Induction of an enzyme associated with cytochrome P4501A1 in a human colon adenocarcinoma cell line was also found to require much higher levels of PCDD than mouse hepatoma cells (*223*). Characterization of the Ah receptor in these mouse and human cells revealed that the human Ah receptor had a much lower affinity for PCDD than the mouse receptor. These experiments support other observations indicating that humans are less sensitive than rodents to the effects of dioxin.

TOXICOLOGICAL EFFECTS IN ANIMALS. Nearly all estimates of risk to humans from exposure to TCDD have been based on extrapolations from a two-year chronic toxicity and oncogenicity study of TCDD's effects in rats reported by Kociba et al. in 1978. However, since histopathological criteria for proliferative lesions in rat liver have changed significantly since 1978, a reevaluation of the liver slides from this experiment has recently been conducted by an independent panel of pathologists (*224*). Using current National Toxicology Program criteria, female rats were judged to have about two-thirds fewer tumors than originally reported and the no-observed-effect level for hepatocellular carcinomas was 0.01 µg/kg/day rather than 0.001 µg/kg/day. These estimates indicate that carcinogenic risk to humans from exposure to TCDD is at least 16- fold lower than the previous estimates.

Data relating to the importance of the Ah (aryl hydrocarbon) receptor in mediating toxicity of TCDD in humans and experimental animals have been reviewed (*225*). TCDD apparently enters cells by passive diffusion and then binds to the Ah receptor. Several mammalian species are known to possess these receptors, although they differ in physicochemical properties. Such differences may partially explain the different degrees of toxicity of TCDD to different species. Despite extensive research efforts we still do not completely understand the mechanisms of TCDD toxicity, but this review summarizes and discusses the information obtained from many toxicity studies in animals.

Five different TCDD-responsive cDNA clones have been isolated from a human keratinocyte cell line and examined to elucidate the effects of TCDD at the molecular level (*226*). One clone was found to encode plasminogen activator inhibitor-2, a factor that influences growth and differentiation by regulating proteolysis of the extracellular matrix. Another clone encoded cytokine interleukin-1β, which functions in the regulation of cell proliferation and differentiation and in inflammation and immune responses. A third clone encoded genes for cytochrome P4501A1 (CYP1A1). Thus, TCDD, like other tumor-promoting agents, alters the expression of growth-regulatory genes.

Effects of dioxin on Ah receptor-dependent changes in protein–DNA interactions at the CYP1A1 transcriptional promoter were investigated in intact mouse hepatoma cells (227). Dioxin induced a change in promoter accessibility probably by altering chromatin structure. In uninduced cells, the promoter is inaccessible to its binding proteins.

Data on the changes in immunocompetence induced by TCDD have also been reviewed. One review considers recent information on possible mechanisms of immunotoxicity including the roles of the Ah receptor, calcium, phosphorylation, and hormones (228). Another review, by the same authors (229), focuses on recently published studies in animals investigating the effects of TCDD on innate immunity, host resistance, and lymphocyte homing and development and studies of immune function in exposed human populations.

Immunotoxic effects of TCDD have been shown to include alterations of T-cell function. An injection of 50 µg TCDD/kg body weight in male mice 4 days prior to challenge with ovalbumin significantly suppressed antigen-specific T-cell proliferation and interleukin-2 production in response to the ovalbumin (230). Experiments with mice gavaged with 5 µg TCDD/kg demonstrated that TCDD reduced the activity of carrier-induced T-helper cells (231). In vitro cultures of spleen cells from sheep red blood cell-primed, TCDD-treated mice produced fewer plaque-forming cells than cells from primed, vehicle-treated controls.

Natural killer cell activity was increased at 28 days in mice given an injection of 5 µg TCDD/kg followed by 3 weekly injections of 1.42 µg TCDD/kg (232). This dose of TCDD caused thymic atrophy and histological signs of liver damage and lipid accumulation. The increased activity of natural killer cells, observed in both the spleen and the blood, may be part of a general compensatory activation of the body's defenses caused by disturbances in the function of other parts of the immune system.

Different strains of mice vary in their Ah-mediated responses to an acute dose of TCDD, with DBA/2 mice being a low-responder strain. However, recent experiments with this strain of mice demonstrated that a subchronic oral dose of TCDD (0.3, 1.0, or 3.0 µg/kg for 14 days) enhances the suppression of humoral immunity by approximately 10-fold when compared to mice receiving the same total amount of TCDD as a single, acute dose (233). These results are important to consider when attempting to assess risk to humans from ingestion of chronic low doses of TCDD.

Antiestrogenic effects of TCDD were recently reviewed (234). In female rats TCDD inhibits a number of estradiol-induced effects, including uterine weight increase, estrogen and progesterone receptor levels, epidermal growth factor receptor binding, and c-fos protooncogene mRNA levels. TCDD also exerts antiestrogenic effects on human breast cancer cells in culture inhibiting the 17β-estradiol-induced proliferation of these cells. Doses of 1.0–30.0 µg TCDD/kg did not alter serum estradiol levels in mice but did induce a dose-dependent decrease in hepatic and uterine estrogen receptor proteins as determined by an enzyme immunoassay and equilibrium binding assays (235).

In male rats, TCDD (100 µg/kg, orally) decreased testosterone synthesis (236). This inhibition does not appear to be due to a defect in the luteinizing hormone (LH) receptor but TCDD does inhibit the LH-stimulated mobilization of cholesterol to cytochrome $P450_{scc}$. This steroidogenic inhibition occurred within one day of dosing.

Male offspring of females treated with 0.064, 0.16, 0.4, or 1.0 µg TCDD/kg on day 15 of pregnancy were monitored for effects on androgenic status (237), sexual behavior (238), and spermatogenesis and reproductive capability (239). Signs of overt toxicity, a slight decrease in live births and reduced body weight gain, were observed at only the two highest doses. Doses as low as 0.16 µg/kg produced statistically significant decreases in the ano-genital distance, delays in testicular descent, and decreases in copulatory rates. Statistically significant decreases in daily sperm production were observed at the lowest maternal dose tested although the morphology and mobility of the sperm appeared to be unaffected. Despite these effects on male reproductive characteristics, when these rats were mated with untreated females, little, if any, effect on male fertility was seen and the survival and growth of offspring were unaffected.

OCCURRENCE IN FOODS. Fourteen samples of fish, representing 5 species, from the Rhine and Neckar rivers in Germany were analyzed for residues of PCDDs and PCDFs (*240*). Concentrations of these compounds in the fillets ranged from 0.25 to 2.75 ng FHO–TEQ (toxicity equivalents)/kg on a fresh weight basis. The daily intake of PCDDs and PCDFs by an average fish consumer was estimated to be 0.07–0.72 pg FHO–TEQ/kg body weight. This would be less than the limit of 1 pg/kg recommended by the German Federal Health Office.

An H-4-II E Bioassay was evaluated as a screening method for detecting residues of PCDDs, PCDFs, and related compounds in fish and other environmental samples (*241*). Results from analyses of contaminated herring using this bioassay and a chemical assay of TCDD equivalents were nearly identical. Certain coplanar polychlorinated biphenyls, polychlorinated naphthalenes, and a mixture of polybrominated diphenyl ethers were also active as enzyme inducers in this assay.

Since chlorinated diphenyl ethers (CDPEs) can potentially interfere with determinations of PCDDs and PCDFs, a procedure was devised to remove CDPEs from fish samples prior to analysis for PCDDs by GC/MS (*242*). Fish samples were extracted with methylene chloride and sodium sulfate and then separated by gel permeation chromatography. Then CDPEs were completely removed by cleanup on a microalumina column and a carbon fiber column. CDPE levels in carp and northern pike from Lake Ontario ranged from 768–14,005 ng/g while the corresponding PCDF levels were 58–254 pg/g.

Trace amounts of PCDDs and PCDFs formed during the bleaching of paper with chlorine are present in paper used for food packaging. This has stimulated a number of investigations into possible contamination of milk stored in bleached paper cartons. A method utilizing multiple column cleanup steps and high resolution GC and quadropole mass spectrometry detected levels of 0.02–0.07 ppt TCDD and 0.12–0.71 ppt TCDF in cartoned whole milk from U.S. dairies in 1989 (*243*). Milk was sampled immediately after the cartons were filled and sealed. No TCDD or TCDF was found in bulk milk before packaging.

Bleached paperboard used for milk cartons, which was manufactured in Canada prior to mid-1989, was found to contain 1.4–55 ng TCDD toxic equivalents (TEQ)/kg paperboard while that produced later contained <1 ng/kg (the detection limit) (*244*). Between 3 and 25% of the TEQ in the old cartons was transferred into milk, with whole and 2% milk accumulating about double the concentration found in skim milk.

Swedish milk samples analyzed prior to packaging were found to contain low levels of contamination with PCDDs and PCDFs (*245*). This contamination was greater in samples from southern Sweden (0.6–0.7 pg TCDFs/g milk fat) than in samples from the north (0.4 pg/g). This difference is believed to result from long-range transport of particulate matter from central Europe. Laboratory experiments indicated that migration of PCDFs into milk from old bleached cartons increased with the length of storage.

A highly automated clean-up procedure utilizing Gilson *x-y-z* robots for injection, fraction collection, and solid-phase extraction has been developed for the determination of PCDDs and PCDFs in milk at the sub-ppt range (*246*). This method includes gel permeation chromatography, alumina clean-up and porous graphitized carbon chromatography, followed by analysis by GC with high resolution MS. Samples were efficiently cleaned up and the high degree of automation allowed the analysis of 6 milk samples per day along with 2 quality control samples and a blank.

All samples of striped bass, crabs, and lobsters collected in Newark Bay and the New York Bight were found to be contaminated by TCDD and a series of other hazardous 2,3,7,8-substituted congeners and some less hazardous PCDD and PCDF congeners (*247*). The highest TCDD concentration was found in crab hepatopancreas (>6000 ppt wet tissue weight). However, the meat of this crab contained only 100 ppt TCDD. In general, many congeners were detected in the crustacea while 2,3,7,8-substituted compounds were the only forms found in fish. An unknown compound, possibly a tetrachlorodibenzothiophene, was a dominant peak in most of the crustacean samples.

Other polyhalogenated aromatic compounds

POLYBROMINATED BIPHENYLS (PBBs). A group of 51 rural Michigan residents exposed to PBBs in 1973–1974 were examined to determine hexabromobiphenyl (HBB) levels and cytochrome P-450I activity (*248*). Thirty-six of the subjects still had detectable levels of HBB in their sera with a median concentration of 12 ppb and a maximum concentration of 860 ppb. Median HBB half-life was calculated to be 12 years. Compared to a control group of urban non-smokers who were not exposed to PBBs, the group of PBB-exposed residents had, on the average, elevated cytochrome P-450I activity as evidenced by the caffeine breath test and the caffeine urinary metabolite ratio. Test results from the exposed group were similar to those obtained from urban smokers.

POLYCHLORINATED DIPHENYL ETHERS (PCDEs). PCDEs are formed as by-products in the synthesis of chlorinated phenols and have been detected in a variety of environmental samples, including fish, crustaceans, and avian eggs. The chemistry, metabolism, uptake and excretion, and toxic effects of these compounds have been reviewed (*249*). PCDEs are potent immunotoxins in mice, and data suggest that they contribute significantly to the toxicity of mixtures of halogenated aromatics.

TETRACHLOROBENZYLTOLUENES (TCBTs). Ugilec 141, a mixture of TCBTs, has been used in place of PCBs for some applications in Germany. Toxic effects of these compounds were evaluated in mice and compared with effects of a commercial PCB mixture and of PCB-77 (3,3',4,4'-tetrachlorobiphenyl) (*250*). Ah-responsive and Ah-non-responsive mice were injected with 50 or 200 mg/kg body weight of the test compounds and sacrificed 7 days later for examination of liver, thyroid glands, and blood. Similar toxicological changes, both qualitative and quantitative, were induced in the mice by all three compounds. It appears that Ugilec poses environmental and health risks which are similar to PCBs and it would not, therefore, be a good substitute for PCBs.

HEXACHLOROBENZENE (HCB). HCB is a ubiquitous environmental contaminant with a variety of toxic effects, including dysfunction in the female reproductive system. Dose-related histopathological effects were observed in the surface epithelium of the ovary of cynomolgus monkeys dosed orally for 90 days with 0.1, 1.0, and 10 mg HCB/kg body weight/day (*251*). Examination of the ovaries of the treated monkeys revealed alterations in cell shape and large numbers of lysosomes in the cytoplasm. Affected cells in the highest dose group were in an advanced stage of degeneration. These effects may be related to altered hormonal levels.

A battery of behavioral tests was used to assess developmental neurotoxicity of HCB in rats (*252*). Two weeks prior to mating, female rats were gavaged with 10 or 100 mg HCB/kg body weight. Although HCB did not affect weight gain by the pups or the dams, HCB did significantly and adversely affect results on a number of behavioral tests in the pups. These results demonstrated that behavioral tests were a more sensitive indicator than physical measurements of developmental toxicity of HCB in rats.

In both humans and rats, HCB induces a hepatic porphyria characterized by increased hepatic accumulation and urinary excretion of uroporphyrin. An experimental model was developed to study HCB-induced porphyria in rats (*253*). Rats were gavaged with different daily doses of HCB to attain cumulative doses of 200–1500 mg HCB/kg body weight, and urinary porphyrin levels were measured. The approximate minimally effective cumulative dose was 400 mg/kg regardless of the daily dose. The porphyria, once induced, persisted for 500–600 days. A similar long-term porphyria has been observed in some humans exposed to high levels of HCB.

Subchronic, nephrotoxic effects of HCB were investigated in rats orally dosed with 50 or 100 mg HCB/kg, 5 days a week for 50 or 15 days, respectively (*254*). Analyses of urine of treated rats revealed no evidence of renal dysfunction. However, histological examination of male rat kidneys demonstrated degenerative and regenerative cellular foci and accumulation of α2u-globulin in kidney cells. This male rat–specific nephropathy could explain the higher incidence of kidney tumors in male as compared to female rats.

OTHER ORGANIC RESIDUES

Toxic oil syndrome

Toxic oil syndrome, which affected about 20,000 people in Spain in 1981 and resulted in >300 deaths, was caused by ingestion of denatured rapeseed oil containing aniline, which had been intentionally added since the oil was not intended for human consumption. Early symptoms of intoxication included urticaria, dyspnea and intense eosinophilia in peripheral blood. Four years after the outbreak, 436 subjects were reassessed to determine the persistence of respiratory symptoms (255). Of these subjects, 89.4% still suffered dyspnea and/or cough, 66.3% had neurological disorders, 39.2% had osteoarticular symptoms, and about 20% had hepatic involvement and sclerodermatous changes.

Information on the epidemiology, clinical features, and etiology of toxic oil syndrome (TOS) were summarized and reviewed in the *Journal of the American College of Cardiology* as background to a series of articles on cardiovascular manifestations of toxic oil syndrome and related diseases (256). Although individual symptoms of TOS had been observed in other diseases, the combination of symptoms and their progression in TOS at first appeared to be unique. However, clinical manifestations of eosinophilia myalgia syndrome (EMS), occurring in epidemic form in the USA in 1989, were strikingly similar to those of intermediate and chronic stages of TOS. In addition, the major damage to coronary arteries and the conduction system and neural structures in the heart which was observed in careful postmortems of 11 toxic oil victims resembled those described in cases of EMS (257). To test the hypothesis that altered tryptophan metabolism occurred during the acute phase of both syndromes, the tryptophan metabolites L-kynurenine and quinolinic acid, and neopterin, a marker of interferon-gamma (IFN-γ) were determined in blood obtained during the acute phase of each syndrome (258). All 3 compounds were significantly elevated in patients with TOS and EMS as compared to healthy control subjects. These data suggest that the rate-limiting enzyme of the kynurenine pathway of L-tryptophan metabolism was activated in both syndromes by cytokines including IFN-γ, and that products of tryptophan metabolism may have played a role in the pathogenesis of both TOS and EMS.

Although fatty acid anilides have been isolated, identified and implicated as the toxic agents responsible for TOS, it is not clear whether these anilides themselves or some secondary products were the actual etiological agents. Experiments with oleic acid anilide, heated oleic acid anilide, linoleic acid anilide, and heated linoleic acid anilide demonstrated that these compounds exerted a variety of effects on liver enzymes and immunological functions in rats (259,260). Rats were gavaged on alternate days for 2 weeks with 250 mg/kg of one of those compounds and then were sacrificed and examined 1, 7, and 28 days after the last dose. Results supported the hypothesis that fatty acid anilides played a role in the etiology of TOS.

Manufacturing processes at 2 French rapeseed oil companies, which had been identified as the ones exporting the denatured rapeseed oil implicated in TOS, were investigated (261). The oil exported to Spain was part of a batch, the rest of which was sold for human consumption in France—apparently without any adverse health effects. Prior to export, aniline equivalent to 2% of the weight of the oil was added to most of the Spanish oil. Since this denatured oil was not intended for human consumption, inspected trucks were not used for shipment to Spain, and so it is possible that contamination of the Spanish oil occurred in the tank trucks used for shipping.

Chloroform

A method has been developed for the simultaneous determination of residual chlorine and volatile chlorinated organic compounds (VCOC) in vegetables treated with sodium hypochlorite (262). Samples were incubated in phosphate buffer with KCN for 30 min and then the headspace gas was analyzed by GC with electrochemical detection. Analysis of 66 commercially available vegetables (in Japan) using this method revealed that four (1 cabbage, 3 soybean sprouts) contained chlorinated compounds, with residual chlorine ranging from 0.14–3.7 µg/g and chloroform ranging from 15–241 ng/g.

Tetrachloroethylene (perchloroethylene, PCE)

PCE residues, found in olive oil in the late 1980s, were found to result from use of this compound as a solvent in the determination of the oil content of olives. A rapid screening method for detection of PCE residues by headspace capillary GC was capable of quantifying residue levels as low as 0.001 mg/kg. Analyses of 98 different olive oil samples revealed that none had residue levels >0.1 mg/kg (European Commission guideline concentration) and 81 had PCE residues <0.01 mg/kg (263).

1,3-Dichloro-2-propanol (1,3-DCP-OH)

1,3-DCP-OH, which has been detected in some foods such as soy sauce, soup spices and instant soups, is known to have mutagenic and carcinogenic properties. Recent investigations into the genotoxic mechanism of this compound revealed that it can be converted into epichlorohydrin in buffer solutions (264). This derivative is responsible for the genotoxic effects of 1,3-DCP-OH in the SOS Chromotest. An S9 activation system was not necessary for epichlorohydrin formation.

Cyclohexylamine (CHA)

CHA is a corrosion inhibitor commonly added to steam generation systems. A sensitive method using the rubidium nitrogen detector was developed for the determination of CHA residues on vegetables blanched with primary steam generated from systems using CHA (265). Snap beans and green peppers blanched in this way were found to contain CHA residues of 3.63 and 0.73 ppm, respectively. Although a number of toxic effects have been attributed to CHA, for the following reasons CHA residues on blanched vegetables

will probably not present a health hazard: (a) Most food processors use secondary steam, generated from tap water, to blanch vegetables. (b) Washing of vegetables prior to cooking and the cooking process itself would probably remove some CHA residues if they were present. The authors note that there are a number of other commonly used steam additives which could potentially contaminate foods or be inhaled by workers exposed to primary steam.

Cyanide

Following an incident of cyanide contamination of grapes in 1989, an ion chromatographic method was developed for the determination of cyanide contamination of fruit (266). Results using this analysis were in good agreement with those from a colorimetric cyanide test kit at cyanide concentrations of 45–300 ppm. Detectable levels of cyanide in spiked fruit samples were found to decrease on standing such that the test kit could detect cyanide contamination for only 3 days after contamination. The HPLC method, however, could still detect residues after 2–3 weeks. Toxicity studies in rats demonstrated that the apparent decrease in cyanide concentration with time was correlated with a decrease in toxicity (267). These changes were dependant on the pH of the fruit juice or homogenate: Generally, when the natural pH of the fruit was >4, cyanide content and toxicity sharply decreased with time while for fruits with a natural pH <4 only slight decreases in toxicity and cyanide concentration were observed.

Formaldehyde

Formaldehyde may be present in fruits and vegetables naturally on the order of parts per million. Formaldehyde (FA) and hexamethylenetetramine (HMT), which slowly decomposes to FA under acidic conditions, are antimicrobial additives used during the production of certain cheeses. Biochemical aspects, acute and short-term toxicity studies, assays for reproductive and developmental toxicity, and long-term carcinogenicity studies following oral administration of FA and HMT have been reviewed (*268*). Chronic oral administration of FA causes cytotoxic effects on the stomach mucosa, but even at doses as high as 100 mg/kg body weight/day it does not induce tumors. Three different studies in rats have demonstrated a no-observed-effect level of 10–20 mg/kg/day for chronic oral administration.

Formaldehyde is also added to ruminant feed to protect dietary proteins from ruminal digestion. To determine whether this dietary formaldehyde is carried over into milk, dairy goats were fed a diet containing soybean oil–meal either untreated or treated with 0.3% formaldehyde to provide daily intakes of 0, 0.63. or 1.26 mg formaldehyde (*269*). The different diets had no effect on milk production but mean formaldehyde levels in milk correlated directly with dietary intake: 0.033, 0.083, and 0.153 mg/kg, respectively.

Diesel contaminants and other hydrocarbons

Recent oil spills and the problems associated with storing fish next to diesel fuel on boats raise the possibility of contamination of fish with petroleum products. A semiquantitative capillary column GC method has been developed for the determination of diesel fuel contamination in canned seafood (*270*). The diesel contaminants are extracted from the fish by steam distillation and then from the condensate with *n*-hexane. Recoveries from seafood samples spiked at 40–400 ppt ranged from 72 to 102%. Diesel fuel grades 1, 2, and 5 can be distinguished by this procedure.

Fish exposed to oil spills may take up and extensively metabolize some aromatic hydrocarbons. Recently, a relatively rapid, semiquantitative method combining enzymatic hydrolysis, methylene chloride extraction, and hexane/potassium hydroxide partitioning with HPLC fluorescence analysis was developed to estimate polar fluorescent aromatic compounds (FAC; e.g. aromatic hydrocarbon metabolites) in fish tissues (*271*). Concentrations of polar FACs in muscles of rock sole exposed to Prudhoe Bay crude oil were linearly proportional to dose. Concentrations of polar FACs were about 15-fold higher in liver than in muscle tissue of contaminated fish.

A survey of a variety of foods from Switzerland revealed that many were contaminated with mineral oil products used as lubricating oils/greases or as release agents (*272*). Hydrocarbons were isolated from food extracts on a silica gel column and then analyzed by coupled LC–GC. Paraffins, used as a release agent by bakeries, were detected in the bottom crust of wholemeal bread at a concentration of 330 mg/kg. A mineral oil product detected in a hard bonbon candy was found to correspond to that in a lubricant grease recommended for use in the food industry. Of 24 bonbons and caramels tested, 8 contained such oils at concentrations between 50 and 1300 mg/kg (as well as up to 2300 mg/kg hydrocarbons on the surface, originating from the wax paper packaging). Many chocolate samples were contaminated with various mineral oil products, one of which appeared to be a vaseline. The toxicological significance of these contaminants remains to be determined.

HEAVY METALS (GENERAL)

Monographs, proceedings, round tables, and discussions of the "Seventh International Symposium on Trace Elements in Man and Animals" have been published (*273*). Metabolic effects, toxicity, environmental sources and methods for analysis were described and discussed for a wide variety of metals and halides.

Metals in foods and food-producing animals

In a Canadian comprehensive total diet study, lead and cadmium levels were determined in 105 different food composites prepared in the summer of 1985 and in another 105 prepared in late autumn, 1985 (*274*). Mean Cd level was 13.7 ng/g (range of <0.07–297 ng/g), and the estimated dietary ingestion by adults averaged 14.5 g/day. Only shellfish and potato chips contained Cd concentrations which consistently exceeded 100 ng/g. Mean Pb level was 29.9 ng/g (range of 1.42–407 ng/g), and the estimated dietary ingestion by adults averaged 36.4 g/day. Raisins and several canned foods (beans, tomatoes, citrus fruits, applesauce, peaches, plums and cherries) had relatively high lead levels. Some samples were apparently contaminated in-house with lead, and the necessity for careful procedures for contamination control was discussed.

Essential and toxic minerals were assayed in Swedish market-basket diets collected in 1987 (*275*). Sixty food items were purchased from three shops in 4 major cities. Estimated intakes of essential minerals were generally close to recommended levels, and estimated daily intakes of mercury (1.8 µg), lead (17 µg), and cadmium (12 µg) were low compared to provisional tolerable intakes set by FAO/WHO.

In 1983 in England, approximately 88% of canned foods were in soldered cans, but by 1987 only about 17% of the cans in use were soldered. Monitoring of lead concentrations in canned foods during this period revealed a decline in lead levels in the canned foods (*276*). During spring 1987, only 1 can (sardines in a soldered can) contained a concentration of lead above the statutory limit of 1 mg/kg. Average tin levels in >98% of canned foods were well below 200 mg/kg, with only 3 cans (asparagus, 1984; tomato soup and spaghetti, 1985) exceeding 250 mg/kg. Both asparagus and tomato products are known to be corrosive to tin.

Cadmium and lead levels in raw, blanched, and canned peas from Spain were determined using atomic absorption spectrometry (*277*). Both lead and cadmium levels decreased during blanching, but then lead levels for all pea sizes increased during canning (welded cans) to a final concentration of 0.084–0.180 mg/kg. Cadmium levels in smaller peas increased more during canning than in larger peas. Mean levels of Cd (0.01 µg/g) and Pb (0.092 µg/g) would provide an estimated daily intake of 0.1 µg Cd and 1.1 µg Pb.

Plants may also acquire heavy metal contaminants from the soil they grow in. Residues of oil bottom ash and fly ash from oil-fired electric power plants are usually high in elements such as vanadium, nickel, aluminum, and molybdenum. To test whether such elements would be taken up by crops growing on soil contaminated with this ash, swiss chard (*Beta vulgaris*) was grown in soil containing 2% bottom ash or 1% fly ash (*278*). Significantly higher levels of all 4 minerals were found in plants grown on the ash-amended soil as compared to plants grown on the same soil without ash.

Soybeans and cowpeas grown on 3 different types of Alabama acid mine spoils were found to accumulate significantly elevated levels of Mn, Pb, Zn, and Ni (*279*). Some other legumes tested were unable to grow on these mine spoils even though they had been amended to contain recommended levels of N, P, K, Ca, and Mg prior to plant growth. Acidity (pH) of the spoils ranged from 3.9 to 4.9. Old silver mine dump materials, many containing high levels of Cd, Zn, and Pb, contaminate garden soils in Aspen, Colorado. Leafy vegetables, like lettuce, were found to accumulate the highest levels of the metals, up to 45 mg Pb/kg, 11.9 mg Cd/kg, and 444 mg Zn/kg (*280*).

Consumption of crayfish (*Procambarus clarkii*) has increased and they are now raised in ponds in Louisiana for commercial distribution. Because they are detritus feeders and are known to accumulate metals from the environment, wild and pond-raised crayfish from Louisiana were examined for mineral residues (*281*). Higher levels of most of the 22 elements were detected in the hepatopancreas (fat) as compared to the tail muscle. However higher concentrations of Cd were present in the tail (1.17 mg/kg) than in the fat (0.34 mg/kg). Mercury and lead levels were below or just slightly above the detection limits of 2.0 and 5.0 mg/kg, respectively. Arsenic averaged 4 mg/kg and vanadium concentrations ranged from 0.32 to 0.84 mg/kg. No significant differences were detected between wild and pond-raised crayfish.

Surveys of cadmium and lead levels in cattle (*282*) and sheep (*283*) in Germany revealed significant levels of contamination in internal organs of animals grown near former mineral mining areas and smelters. Cd concentrations in liver and kidneys of cattle from contaminated areas averaged 0.28 and 1.29 mg/kg fresh weight, respectively, while corresponding values in sheep were 0.29 and 0.547 mg/kg. Lead levels in cattle averaged 0.53 (liver) and 0.69 (kidneys) mg/kg and in sheep were 0.369 (liver) and 0.349 (kidneys) mg/kg. Average contaminant levels exceeded the guidelines for both metals in both organs of cattle and for Cd in sheep kidneys. Meat samples of both cattle and sheep contained much lower levels of contamination.

During a routine monitoring program of slaughter animals in Canada, residues of As, Cd, Cu, Hg, Pb, Se, and Zn were determined in liver and kidney tissues of cattle, swine, poultry, horses, calves, and sheep (*284*). Highest levels of As were found in avian and porcine samples, with averages of 0.36 and 0.26 µg/g, respectively, in liver. Cd and Hg levels were highest in horses, with averages of 27.7 µg Cd/g and 0.18 µg Hg/g in kidneys. Copper, at concentrations >150 µg/g, was present predominantly in livers from calves and sheep. Lead was detected in all species but concentrations >2 µg/g were found in only 3 kidney samples, 2 from cattle and 1 from a horse. Relatively high Zn levels were detected in livers of horses (67.3 µg/g), pigs (65.6 µg/g), and calves (70.2 µg/g). Overall, Cd residues appear to be of the most concern.

During 1987–1989, yeast produced as a nutritional supplement in Czechoslovakia (VITEX) was analyzed for heavy metal contaminants (*285*). Levels of Cd, Hg, and Pb were in the ranges of 0.3–5.12, 0.008–0.187, and 0.21–3.01 mg/kg, respectively. Five of the samples exceeded the government standards for Hg and 94 exceeded the standards for Cd. Spent sulfite liquor from a wood-pulp mill, used as a growth medium for the yeast, was identified as the main source for the cadmium and possibly the mercury contamination. The highest mercury level, however, was detected in a sample of KOH.

To ensure the safety of shellfish exports from Chile, an analytical quality control procedure was developed to detect contamination with Cd, Cu, and Hg (*286*). Three different analytical techniques (differential pulse anodic stripping voltammetry, neutron activation analysis, and atomic absorption spectrometry) were used. Standard certified reference materials were also analyzed to assure accurate determinations. Results obtained in analyses of molluscs from 3 different locations using all 3 methods were similar. Cd levels in the viscera of these molluscs were found to be an order of magnitude higher than those in non-visceral tissue.

A method for the determination of arsenic and selenium in foods by continuous hydride generation–atomic absorption spectrometry has been developed (*287*). No carrier gas was required for the transport of hydrides to the atomizer because enough hydrogen was generated during the reaction of the acid analyte solution and the reductant to effectively transport the hydrides. Detection limits for As and Se in foods were 3 and 5 ng/g, respectively. Recoveries of Se and As from spiked food samples (spinach, tuna in oil, corn, fish sticks, infant cereal) were 93–108%.

Occurrence and effects of heavy metals in humans

A U.N.-sponsored international pilot monitoring study on exposure to Pb and Cd has been set up in Beijing, Yokohama, Stockholm, and Zagreb (*288*). Exposure to these metals via air, food, and beverages was determined for 12–17 non-smoking women at each site during 7 consecutive days. Airborne particulates, duplicate diets, feces, and blood were collected and analyzed. Results obtained indicated that the diet was the main source of exposure to Cd and Pb in all groups except for Pb exposure in the Zagreb subjects. For many subjects there was great day-to-day variation in dietary intake of Pb and Cd, indicating that certain occasionally consumed foods were major sources of these metals.

The suitability of ear wax as a biological monitoring medium for metals was investigated in two volunteers (*289*). Samples were analyzed for 38 elements by inductively coupled plasma atomic emission spectroscopy. As, Pb, and Cd were detected in the wax at concentrations of 150–220, 13–14, and 0.67–1.6 µg/g dry weight, respectively. Clearly, further testing is required to determine whether metal concentrations in wax are directly related to exposure levels and to metal concentrations in internal organs. Some previous studies demonstrated that certain pesticides can also be detected in ear wax.

Although some analyses of bones of ancient humans demonstrate that these people had up to a 500-fold lower body burden of lead as compared to contemporary humans, other studies indicate that the difference in lead levels is much less. Recent meticulous analyses of bone samples of 14 North

American Pecos Indians living around A.D. 1400 revealed that both Cd and Pb concentrations in these bones were approximately 50-fold lower than in contemporary humans (*290*). Skeletal concentrations of zinc and silver, however, do not appear to have increased in modern humans.

Carcinogenic properties of 13 metals and their compounds have been reviewed with reference to data from epidemiological studies and short-term and long-term bioassays (*291*). Certain elements, including As, Pb, and Cd were considered comprehensively while others, including Se, Mn, and Zn, were discussed briefly.

A recent volume in *Methods in Enzymology* was devoted to metallothionein (*292*). This protein can bind 7–10 g atoms of metal/mol and may function in the absorption and tissue uptake of metals and their transport, storage, and detoxification. Papers in this volume discuss the toxicological and nutritional significance of metallothionein and methods for its induction, isolation, characterization, and quantification.

ALUMINUM

Absorption and distribution of aluminum

Mechanisms of gastrointestinal absorption and renal excretion of aluminum have recently been reviewed (*293*). Normal daily intake of aluminum for adults varies between 9 and 14 mg. However, persons ingesting aluminum-containing drugs may consume much higher levels. Gastrointestinal absorption of aluminum is facilitated by citrate and 1,12-dihydroxyvitamin D and is inhibited by calcium, fluoride, tannin, and silicic acid. The primary route for excretion of absorbed aluminum is through the kidneys, with only a minor fraction excreted by the bile.

In studies with rats fed 1 mg Al/g diet, citrate was found to increase retention of aluminum in bones, although this effect was not linearly correlated with dietary levels of citrate (*294*). An increase in calcium intake from 67 to 250 μmol/g diet reduced aluminum concentrations in bone. Rats

injected with aluminum were found to retain 20-fold more Al in bones and 100-fold more Al in kidney and liver than rats fed aluminum. Thus Al absorption in healthy animals is very low.

Ingestion of 900 mg aluminum hydroxide with 2 mg ascorbic acid by 13 healthy volunteers resulted in significantly higher urinary excretion of Al than occurred following ingestion of aluminum hydroxide alone (*295*). This 3–4-fold higher excretion of Al probably reflects enhanced gastrointestinal absorption of Al in the presence of ascorbic acid.

Biological effects and toxicity of aluminum

In July 1988, 20 tons of aluminum sulfate were discharged into treated reservoir water in Scotland. This resulted in major contamination of the water supply, and local residents and vacationers reported various degrees of acute, but generally transient, illness. Advisory groups convened in 1989 and 1990 concluded that although persistent toxic effects were possible, they were unlikely because the exposure was transient. To date there has been no evidence of an increased incidence of symptoms or illness attributable to the exposure to Al. A developmental followup study of children who were in utero during the incident and continued surveillance of the health of this community were recommended (*296*).

Experimental animal models of chronic motor neuron degeneration (for example, Western Pacific forms of amyotrophic lateral sclerosis, ALS) developed in rabbits and nonhuman primates were summarized and results were discussed (*297,298*). ALS-like motor neuron pathology can be induced in cynomolgus monkeys by administration of a low-calcium diet for 4 years, with or without supplemental Al, and in rabbits by intracisternal injections of aluminum chloride for prolonged periods. Such models suggest that exposure to environmental Al may also cause neuronal degeneration in humans.

Two ALS cases from the Kii peninsula of Japan were found to have extraordinarily high Al levels, low Mg concentrations, and high Ca/Mg ratios in central nervous system tissues as compared to controls who died from non-neurological causes (*299*). Soils and drinking water in high incidence areas of ALS are known to contain high levels of aluminum and low levels of Ca and Mg. These data indicate that a dysfunction in calcium and magnesium metabolism may result in Al deposition in nervous tissue.

Both genetic and environmental factors appear to be important in the development of Alzheimer's disease (AD). Four independent lines of evidence indicating that Al is an important risk factor for AD have been summarized and discussed (*300*). These include the following types of studies: (a) effects of prolonged exposure to trace amounts of Al; (b) Al accumulation in AD-affected brain tissue; (c) epidemiological studies correlating Al levels in drinking water and AD; and (d) treatments with trivalent metal ion–binding agents which have been shown to slow the progression of AD.

One epidemiological study in Ontario, involving 2344 patients with a diagnosis of AD or presenile dementia and 2232 patients with non-psychiatric diagnoses, found that the relative risk of AD increased with increasing concentrations of Al in drinking water, with a relative risk of 1.46 associated with Al concentrations ≥ 0.2 mg/L (*301*). Another epidemiological study in Ontario involving a cohort of 782 males (now 76 years old) also demonstrated increased mental impairment in subjects consuming drinking water high in Al (*302*). In addition, the data showed a strong association between water fluoride concentrations and dementia: men drinking water high in Al and low in F are about 3 times more likely to have some form of mental impairment than those living in areas where drinking water is high in F and low in Al.

On the other hand, an epidemiological study in Switzerland in which 800 persons (81–85 years old) were given an mnestic test revealed no differences in mnestic and naming skills between residents from areas with high (98 µg/L) or low (4 µg/L) aluminum concentrations in drinking water (*303*). Since this mnestic test is known to discriminate between healthy and demented octagenarians, and approximately 73% of dementias in this area are cases of AD, it appears that aluminum in drinking water is unrelated to this disease.

Aluminum has paradoxical effects on the skeletal system: on one hand, it can be toxic to human bone metabolism (vitamin D-resistant osteomalacia and diminished bone remodeling activity) while on the other, it can exert both mitogenic and antiproliferative effects in animals and in cell cultures. Data regarding these toxic and trophic osseus effects were reviewed and possible explanations were offered for these differing effects (*304*).

Some patients with chronic renal failure develop renal osteodystrophy with substantial deposition of aluminum in bone and diminished bone cell activity and bone formation. Recent data on the pathophysiology of aluminum-related bone disease was summarized, including consideration of the role of aluminum in inhibiting mineralization, interactions between aluminum and bone cells, and the role of aluminum in the pathogenesis of renal osteodystrophy (*305*).

Effects of aluminum on the stromal cells of rat bone marrow were investigated using a combination of in vivo exposure and in vitro culture of bone marrow cells (*306*). Aluminum was found to decrease macrophage count, erythrocyte count, and the hemoglobin level in peripheral blood while it also stimulated the number of fibroblasts.

Occurrence and detection of aluminum in foods

Aluminum levels were determined in a number of individual foods obtained in Swedish markets and in 24-h duplicate diets collected from women living in the Stockholm area (*307*). Most foods contained very little aluminum, with the highest levels detected in soy-based infant formula powder (14 mg Al/kg), casein-based infant formula powder (6–7 mg/kg), barley (1.6 mg/kg), tea (1.3 mg/kg), prawns (1.3 mg/kg), and rye flour (1.1 mg/kg). Beverages in aluminum cans had Al levels similar to those in glass bottles. Duplicate diets supplied an average of 13 mg Al. The major source of Al in these diets was a chocolate mint cake made with sodium aluminum phosphate in the baking soda. Tea and aluminum utensils were estimated to supply approximately 4 and 2 mg Al/day, respectively.

Recent interest in mechanisms of aluminum toxicity have prompted some concern regarding aluminum concentrations in infant formulae and milk powders. Analyses of 3 soy-based and 7 cow's milk–based infant formulae in England in 1990 revealed average Al concentrations of 3.9 and 0.4 mg/kg, respectively (*308*). These levels were, on average, 37–45% lower than concentrations measured in the same brands purchased between 1985–1987. For comparison, Al levels in retail soya milk (7 samples), 14 samples of retail cow's milk, and 8 samples of breast milk were 5–285 µg/L, 4–33 µg/L, and 3–79 µg/L, respectively. Analyses of 44 brands of milk powder in Singapore by inductively coupled argon plasma–optical emission spectrometry demonstrated average Al concentrations of 0.74, 6.1, and 1.1 mg/kg in cow's milk–based infant formulae, soybean-based infant formulae, and cow's milk–based milk powders, respectively (*309*).

Aluminum levels determined in several commercially available brands of pure orange juice averaged 5.9 µmol/L in 8 samples described as fresh and 6.9 µmol/L in 9 samples of reconstituted pure juice (*310*). Aluminum concentration in tap water was <0.5 µmol/L at the time of the study.

To investigate the possibility that aluminum beverage cans contribute to dietary Al intake, 106 samples of beverages in aluminum and glass containers were assayed to determine Al levels (*311*). Non-cola soft drinks in aluminum cans contained approximately 6 times as much Al (33.4 µmol/L) than similar drinks in glass bottles. Al in canned cola drinks averaged 24.4 µmol/L—about 3-fold higher than that in corresponding bottled drinks. No significant difference was detected in Al level in canned vs. bottled beer. In general, higher Al levels were correlated with lower pH.

Under simulated cooking conditions, fluoride was found to enhance the leaching of Al from metallic Al utensils, even at neutral pH (*312*). After boiling for 0.5 h, 0.05, 0.47, and 4.03 µg Al/g was leached from utensils when fluoride concentrations were 0, 1, and 10 µg/g, respectively.

In an evaluation of the quality of aluminum determination in food-type matrices by a variety of methods, 24 laboratories analyzed two blind powders and two duplicate diets, one of which was spiked with 15.87 mg Al/kg (*313*). Overall performance was very disappointing, with wide variations in aluminum concentrations reported for the same samples. Eleven of the laboratories had one or more major problems with their aluminum determinations. Best results were obtained from laboratories using wet-pressurized digestion in combination with electrothermal atomic absorption spectrometry. Laboratories using dry-ashing for sample decomposition obtained unreliable results.

ARSENIC

An acute, massive epidemic of arsenic poisoning involving 718 persons occurred in Argentina in 1987 following contamination of meat with an acaricide, sodium arsenite (*314*). Vandals broke into a butcher shop at night and poured the solution over the meat. The butcher, not realizing the meat had been poisoned, sold it. Meat samples were not available for analysis but urine samples from 307 subjects were analyzed and found to contain <3.6 to >1000 µg As/dL. A greater incidence and severity of symptoms was correlated with higher urinary arsenic levels, with increased diarrhea, vomiting and systemic symptoms occurring at >75 µg/dL. Prompt treatment prevented fatalities and none of the cases reported symptoms related to the poisoning 1 year after the episode.

Ingestion of inorganic arsenic is known to cause skin cancer but whether it also causes internal cancers is still a matter of controversy. Epidemiological data related to this question have recently been reviewed (*315*). At various times populations have been exposed to high arsenic levels in medicines, in wine substitutes and in drinking water which was either naturally or artificially contaminated. The most informative studies are from Taiwan and Japan and strongly suggest that high arsenic intake can cause cancers in the bladder, kidney, lung, and liver. Another reviewer, in discussing data available on the risk of arsenic ingestion concluded that a daily intake of 400 µg/day is safe (*316*). Arsenic appears to be an indirect carcinogen. Ingestion of elevated levels of arsenic results in arsenical hyperpigmentation of the skin, which is readily detectable and predictive of cancer risk in most cases. These skin lesions can aid in monitoring potentially carcinogenic arsenic exposures.

Between 1971 and 1987, 25,648 people living in southeastern Hungary and using well water contaminated with arsenic were surveyed to determine health effects (*317*). Data from this group were compared with that from another group of 20,836 people living in similar conditions (life style, occupation, socio-economic status) except that their drinking water was low in arsenic. Many cases of arsenical hyperkeratosis and hyperpigmentation were observed in the contaminated area but no serious vascular disorders nor excess incidence or mortality from cancer were noted. A high proportion of spontaneous abortions and stillbirths occurred in the contaminated area and this difference was statistically significant.

Rodents exposed to arsenic in drinking water develop porphyrinuria. However, a pilot study of 21 individuals in Mexico exposed to arsenic in drinking water (0.39 mg/L) revealed no increase in urinary porphyrins when compared to 19 controls exposed to 0.012 mg As/L (*318*). In another study involving 11 people from this same area of high As exposure and 13 controls no significant differences were observed between the groups in percentages of chromosomal aberrations and frequencies of sister chromatid exchanges in peripheral lymphocytes (*319*). However, the average generation time of lymphocytes was significantly longer in the As-exposed subjects.

A total of 225 samples including 79 species of edible mushrooms, most of which were collected in France, Germany, the Netherlands, and Switzerland, were analyzed for arsenic (*320*). Most cultivated mushrooms (*Agaricus bisporus*, shiitake, and oyster mushrooms) and wild-growing dried mushrooms of commerce (boletus, morels, and chanterelles) had low As concentrations (0.2–0.5 mg/kg dry weight). Several other species sold at Swiss markets, including wild species of *Agaricus*, had higher As levels, sometimes exceeding 10 mg/kg. Highest As levels occurred in *Laccaria amethystina*

(up to 250 mg/kg). However, most of the arsenic in this species is present as methylated arsinic acids of low toxicity. Considerable variation was observed in As levels in some individuals of the same species originating in different areas.

Although concentrations of 10 μM sodium arsenite exerted both cytotoxic and neoplastic transforming effects on BALB/3T3 cells, arsenobetaine, the main form of arsenic in certain seafoods, failed to induce either effect at concentrations as high as 500 μM (*321*). About 95% of the arsenobetaine taken up by the cells was present in the cytosol and no intracellular degradation of this compound was detected. These results support the view that arsenobetaine ingested with marine foodstuffs presents little health risk.

A method for the determination of arsenic by microwave acid dissolution in a closed Teflon bomb followed by hydride generation atomic absorption spectrometry has been developed (*322*). Analytical detection limit was 0.146 μg/L with recoveries of 96.3–100% from spiked samples. Analyses of the muscles of 32 fish species commonly caught off the coast of Spain indicated low arsenic levels (0.396–45.7 μg/g).

A simple HPLC method has been developed for the determination of arsonium compounds (arsenobetaine, arsenocholine and tetramethylarsonium cations) in seafood and human urine (*323*). Samples were extracted with methanol, cleanup with an anion exchange and liquid partitioning and then separated on a cyanopropyl bonded-phase column. Analytes were detected on-line by thermochemical hydride generation–atomic absorption spectrometry. For spiking levels of 0.1–2.8 μg/g sample, recoveries were >83%.

CADMIUM

Toxicology and methods for analysis of cadmium have been extensively reviewed (*324*). Topics considered were persistence and speciation of Cd in the environment; bioaccumulation of Cd and intake by humans; monitoring procedures; regulatory standards; and procedures for quantification. While a variety of analytical methods are available for Cd determination, sample preparation remains the most troublesome step in analyses for Cd.

Cadmium in foods and the environment

A nationwide survey including 30,311 families in 17 Spanish administrative areas recorded the types and amounts of food used during a 7-day period by these families (*325*). These data were correlated with data from different research laboratories on heavy metal contamination in Spanish foods. Analyses indicated that intakes of arsenic, mercury, and lead were below acceptable daily intake (ADI) levels but intake of cadmium exceeded the ADI in some regions of the country. Foods identified as having relatively high Cd concentrations were: squid (0.67 mg/kg); turnip leaves (0.6 mg/kg); mussels (0.49 mg/kg); sardines (0.34 mg/kg); kidney (0.28 mg/kg); grouper (0.25 mg/kg); and tuna (0.23 mg/kg).

Since leafy vegetables generally accumulate more Cd from soil than other types of vegetables, bioavailability of Cd to lettuce has been investigated by several research groups. Soil pH was found to significantly affect Cd uptake by lettuce and cabbage from sludge-treated soil under field conditions (*326*). Liming of soil to maintain an average pH of 7.0, as compared to the original average pH of 6.5, reduced average Cd levels in lettuce from 13.8 to 4.4 µg/g and in cabbage from 5.8 to 4.4 µg/g. Uptake of Cd and its translocation were found to vary in 4 lettuce varieties known to concentrate different amounts of Cd (*327*). The highest Cd line had the highest uptake rate and translocated the greatest percentage of its uptake to the shoot. The lowest Cd lines had an intermediate uptake rate and translocated the lowest percentage of Cd to the shoot. However, no difference in Cd uptake was observed in another study utilizing 16 lettuce varieties tested in soil and in 8 varieties tested in water culture (*328*).

Analyses of 17 rice samples collected at intervals between 1820 and 1987 in Japan revealed relatively low Cd levels in samples from 1820–1890 (0.0175–0.057 µg/g) followed by a rapid increase in Cd levels during 1912–1925, when use of mineral fertilizers began, to a high of 0.173 µg/g in the most recent samples (*329*). Some batches of phosphorite fertilizer were shown to have Cd levels as high as 77 ppm. The use of these fertilizers over time has enriched the soil with Cd and produced higher Cd levels in rice.

Analysis of samples of oyster mushrooms (*Pleurotus ostreatus*) obtained from a mushroom farm and retail stores in Czechoslovakia for mineral content demonstrated that lead and mercury levels were below the regulatory limits (*330*). However, 40% of the samples exceeded the permissible level of cadmium (0.5 mg/kg dry weight).

Goats and forage plants at several locations (near to and removed from Pb, Zn sulfide mines) in Greece were analyzed for Cd contamination (*331*). Average Cd levels in the plants (grass and *Trifolium*) and in livers and kidneys of goats from the areas near the mines had approximately twice the concentration of Cd as compared to those from areas distant from the mines. Mean Cd levels were 3.51 mg/kg in kidney and 1.53 mg/kg in liver of animals on the contaminated sites.

Cd levels were monitored in various tissues and milk of dairy cows fed for up to 554 days on a normal, control feed or feed supplemented with 1 or 5 ppm Cd (*332*). Cd concentrations in milk from the high Cd group did not differ significantly from controls. At 554 days Cd levels in muscle tissue did not differ significantly among the groups, although the high Cd group had accumulated significantly more Cd in kidneys (132.17 µg/g) and liver (14.41 µg/g) than controls (2.95 and 0.48 µg/g, respectively). Low levels (<2.6 µg/g) of Cd also accumulated in adrenal glands, ovaries, spleen, and uteri of the high-dose cows at 554 days.

Rock phosphate, which may contain as much as 99 ppm Cd, may be fed to pigs as a mineral supplement. To determine whether this practice would result in dangerous levels of Cd in kidneys of pigs, kidneys from 315 culled sows (the oldest age group of slaughtered pigs) were analyzed for Cd concentrations (*333*). Mean Cd concentration was 0.6 mg/kg, with only 3 kidneys exceeding the maximum permissible concentration (MPC, 2.5 mg/kg) and another 5 containing concentrations between 75 and 100% of the MPC. All 8 of these pigs were ≥4 years of age (well beyond the usual age for culling) and none had been given rock phosphate as a supplement. Pigs fed dietary Cd (0.44, 0.89, 2.21 or 4.43 mg/kg as cadmium chloride or 0.6 or 1.2 mg/kg as rock phosphate) during growth from 8 to 90 kg were found to accumulate Cd only in liver and kidney (*334*). Organ levels of Cd were directly related to dietary concentrations, with maximum concentrations of 2.01 and 12.25 mg/kg detected in liver and kidney, respectively.

Occurrence and effects of cadmium in humans

Epidemiological and physiological studies continue among some populations in Japan with high exposures to cadmium resulting from industrial and mining pollution of water sources and farm fields. Examination of mortality data for 256 and 275 residents of Sasu, Nagasaki Prefecture, a Cd-polluted area, revealed that Cd-induced renal tubular dysfunction led to excess mortality. In the one study (*335*), urinary β_2-microglobulin was independently and significantly related to mortality in men but not in women. Further study (*336*) demonstrated that serum β_2-microglobulin as well as total urinary protein were significantly related to mortality in both sexes, independent of age.

To investigate effects of Cd on collagen metabolism, serum and urinary hydroxyproline levels were determined in a total of 68 Japanese women (60–93 years old): 12 women with itai-itai disease (nephropathy and osteomalacia); 13 women classified as itai-itai observation patients (nephropathy only); 19 osteoporosis patients; and 24 patients with unrelated diseases (controls) (*337*). Urinary β_2-microglobulin levels and free hydroxyproline levels were significantly higher in the two Cd-exposed groups, indicating that Cd caused some disorder of collagen and/or amino acid metabolism.

Since Cd is known to cause kidney damage and 1,25-dihydroxyvitamin D [1,25(OH)$_2$D] is produced in the proximal tubules of the kidney by hydroxylation of 25-hydroxyvitamin D [25(OH)D], serum levels of 25(OH)D and 1,25(OH)$_2$D were measured in 7 women living in a Cd-polluted area in Toyama, Japan (*338*). Although all the women had severe renal tubular dysfunction, serum levels of 1,25(OH)$_2$D were within the normal range for 6 subjects. Serum 1,25(OH)$_2$D levels were significantly correlated with creatinine clearance.

Belgium, the principal Cd producer in Europe, also has areas with high cadmium pollution. Although Cd levels in blood and urine of 1283 people living in 2 high-exposure areas were significantly elevated as compared to 803 persons in 2 low-exposure areas, there were no significant differences in the prevalence of hypertension and other cardiovascular diseases between the two populations (*339*). However, Cd exposure did appear to affect calcium metabolism in these study populations (*340*). When data were adjusted for significant covariates, a significant and positive correlation was found between urinary Cd levels and serum alkaline phosphatase activity in both sexes and a significant, negative correlation was observed between urinary Cd and serum total calcium levels in men.

A subset of the Belgian study population consisting of 230 rural subjects was studied to determine the relationship between soil Cd levels and urinary Cd levels (*341*). Soil in the polluted area contained 7.4 ppm Cd and had a pH of 6.5 while corresponding values for the non-polluted area were 1.2 ppm Cd, pH 6.0. When data were adjusted for age, urinary Cd levels correlated significantly with soil Cd levels. These rural populations consume locally grown vegetables, some of which probably accumulate Cd, and in this way Cd is transferred from the soil to humans.

In a study of 166 Caucasian men in Paris, the distribution of hair Cd levels was skewed and was significantly correlated with smoking status (*342*). Hair Cd concentrations averaged 0.21, 0.78, and 0.67 µg/g for non-smokers, ex-smokers, and current smokers, respectively. Hair Cd levels were also significantly and inversely correlated with Na$^+$–K$^+$ pump activity in current smokers. Such a correlation had previously been observed in in vitro studies.

Heavy metal fallout from smelters in the USSR has caused significant pollution in northern Finland. Among these pollutants is cadmium which is deposited on lichen, the principal food of reindeer.

Blood Cd levels were measured in 230 male reindeer herders in northern Finland and were found to be twice as high in men who ate reindeer meat at least twice a week compared to men who ate it less often (*343*). A geographical gradient was observed in blood Cd levels, increasing from southwest to northeast with highest levels closest to the smelters.

Effects of cadmium in experimental animals and cell cultures

A recent issue of *Toxicology* was devoted to a review of effects of chronic cadmium exposure in animal models (*344*). Effects at the cellular level and at the organ level were considered along with a discussion of the contribution of cell biological and histochemical studies to risk assessments for human health.

Metallothionein (MT) gene expression was determined in lymphocytes of rats exposed to 1–100 ppm cadmium chloride in drinking water to assess the feasibility of using this induced gene expression as a means for screening human populations at risk (*345*). After 6- and 13-week exposure to 100 ppm Cd, MT gene expression in lymphocytes was enhanced 2- and 3-fold, respectively. Cd concentrations in kidneys of these rats were 19.6 (6 weeks) and 32.7 (13 weeks) μg/g. Thus, this assay could detect Cd exposure well below the point of nephrotoxicity (200 ppm Cd in kidney). Since humans absorb 3–6 times more Cd from the gastrointestinal tract than rodents, this assay should be able to detect lower levels of oral exposure in humans.

Although most oral toxicity studies of cadmium have used cadmium chloride, this is not likely to be the form in which cadmium occurs in the diet. In both animals and plants Cd is bound to a metallothionein-like protein. In experiments with rats fed diets containing 30 ppm Cd-MT or 30 ppm $CdCl_2$, a relatively higher accumulation of Cd in kidneys was observed after 4 weeks in the Cd-MT group (*346*). However, since hepatic Cd levels were lower in this group, indirect renal accumulation of Cd by redistribution from the liver might be lower for Cd-MT-fed rats. In a short-term test using radio-labelled Cd, pretreatment of rats with Zn (which induces metallothionein) caused a reduction in uptake of Cd into the liver and an increase in the kidney (*347*). These experiments indicate that intestinal MT enhances the absorption of Cd and its translocation to the kidney.

Dietary calcium also affects MT levels and Cd absorption. Rats fed a low Ca diet (0.1% Ca) with 100 mg Cd/L in drinking water for 8 weeks accumulated significantly higher Cd levels in liver and kidney and had higher MT levels in plasma, liver, and kidney compared to rats fed a normal diet (0.8% Ca) supplemented with the same amount of Cd (*348*). All diets were isocaloric. Low Ca diets were also found to enhance deposition of Cd in various regions of the brain, the spinal cord, and the femur (*349*).

In experiments testing the effects of other metals (Ca, Mg, Mn, Cu, Fe, Zn, and Se) on oral toxicity of Cd in rats, only iron, specifically as Fe^{2+}, appeared to have a significant effect (*350*). Supplements containing extra iron significantly decreased (by up to 80%) Cd accumulation in liver and kidneys. Addition of ascorbic acid to the iron supplement enhanced iron absorption but nullified the protective effect of iron.

Chronic exposure of male rats to drinking water containing 10 mg Cd/L for 52 weeks resulted in pathological testicular alterations as well as liver and kidney damage (*351*). Fertility tests of treated rats revealed that only 61% were able to sire young when mated with untreated females.

FLUORIDE

A risk assessment perspective on water fluoridation reviewed toxicological data and estimates of exposure for the general population (*352*). From optimally fluoridated water (0.7–1.2 mg/L), the daily maximum fluoride intake for adults has been estimated as 0.034 mg/kg. Dietary sources of fluoride may provide another 0.2–3.4 mg F/day for adults. Altogether, then, a typical adult would consume approximately 0.042 mg/kg/day while rats, which developed osteosarcomas during long-term carcinogenicity studies, were exposed to fluoride levels of 5.2 and 8.6 mg/kg. Therefore, the currently available data suggests that the practice of water fluoridation is not detrimental to health.

Survival and weight gain of rats and mice were not affected by 2 years of exposure to drinking water containing 11, 49, or 79 ppm fluoride during long-term assays by the National Toxicology Program (*353*). Some dose-related dental effects (tooth mottling) were observed in the treated rats and mice, and female rats given the highest dose had an increased incidence of osteosclerosis. No fluoride-related neoplasms were observed in mice and female rats but a small number of osteosarcomas occurred in higher-dose male rats. Thus, there was equivocal evidence for carcinogenicity of sodium fluoride in male rats.

An epidemiological study in New York State compared the incidence of primary bone cancers, including osteosarcomas, in residents of areas with and without water fluoridation (*354*). Osteosarcoma incidence rates among both younger and older males and females have been essentially unchanged since 1970. Data from the period 1976–1987 indicated no difference in average annual age-adjusted incidence of osteosarcomas in fluoridated as compared to non-fluoridated areas.

Between 1960 and 1973, residents of the Ikeno district in Japan were accidentally exposed to drinking water containing 7.8 ppm fluoride. When changes in the appearance of teeth, suggestive of fluorosis, occurred in children in the area, the problem was recognized and an alternative water supply (<0.2 ppm fluoride) was provided. Data on age-specific incidence of fluorosis among children exposed at different ages and for different lengths of time revealed two "at risk" periods for development of moderate or severe fluorosis (*355*). One period started at birth and ended early in tooth development while the other period started later and ended at tooth eruption. Continuous exposure throughout tooth development caused severe changes in all tooth types.

Examinations of the teeth of 338 12-year-old children in an Australian city with fluoridated water (0.8 mg F/L) and 321 children from another area in Australia without fluoridated water demonstrated prevalences of fluorosis of 0.4 and 0.33, respec-

tively (*356*). Odds of fluorosis were greatest for those living longest in the fluoridated area and for those using fluoride supplements.

Since some populations living at high altitudes in Kenya have more severe dental fluorosis problems than lowland populations, a similar study was conducted in 3 communities in Tanzania, one at sea level and 2 others at 1500 m (*357*). All had drinking water sources with 0.1–1.0 ppm fluoride. Although residents in the village at sea level consumed more fish and tea, they had the lowest incidence of fluorosis. Surprisingly, one of the high-altitude villages had a much higher incidence of fluorosis than the other. Mothers in the affected village reported the frequent use of a salt deposit (for cooking) called "magadi" which had an average fluoride concentration of 2638 ppm. Magadi samples from the other high-altitude village contained 111 ppm fluoride.

A series of 10 patients with osteofluorosis, 10 with otosclerosis on sodium fluoride therapy (30 mg daily), 20 patients with non-ulcer dyspepsia, and 10 controls with non-gastrointestinal problems, were evaluated clinically for dyspeptic symptoms and history of fluoride exposure (*358*). All patients with osteofluorosis and 11 with non-ulcer dyspepsia lived in areas with high fluoride levels (maximum of 11.36 ppm) in drinking water while none of the controls lived in such areas. Histological evaluation and scanning EM studies of gastric and duodenal mucosa revealed gastritis and significant cytomorphologic abnormalities in all the otosclerosis and osteofluorosis patients, in over half of the dyspepsia patients and in none of the controls. Ingested fluoride appeared to damage gastrointestinal mucosa leading to dyspeptic symptoms.

Red blood cells from 10 Indian patients with severe skeletal fluorosis were examined and compared with red blood cells from healthy controls of similar age and socioeconomic status (*359,360*). The patients had been drinking water containing 7.2–10.7 ppm fluoride while fluoride levels in drinking water of controls ranged from 0.5 to 1.0 ppm. In these cells, chronic high fluoride exposure appeared to inhibit glycolysis by nearly 70%, decreased total ATPase activity by about 24%, and nearly doubled lipid peroxidation levels.

Several different microdiffusion procedures for the determination of free and ionizable fluoride in milk were evaluated (*361*). A modified version of the hexamethyldisiloxane–acid diffusion technique, utilizing increased amounts of perchloric acid and sodium hydroxide and changes in the configuration of the fluoride-sensitive electrode, was found to have improved accuracy and precision. This method was free of interferences and capable of measuring fluoride concentrations from 0.02 to 10.0 mg dm^{-3}.

LEAD

Reports given at a Society of Toxicology symposium entitled "An Update on the Exposure and Effects of Lead" in 1991 have been summarized and published (*362*). An overview was presented on critical issues associated with lead toxicity ranging from fundamental mechanisms of toxicity to assessments of the effectiveness of lead abatement measures.

Exposure to lead can occur through a variety of media and this fact complicates hazard evaluation of this toxicant. An integrated exposure/pharmacokinetic-based approach to risk assessment for lead has been developed by the EPA (*363*). This analysis evaluates the relative contributions of various media to elevated blood lead levels in children and identifies site- and situation-specific strategies for lead abatement.

Sources of lead in the human diet

As overall levels of dietary lead decrease, the relative importance of the lead present in chemicals added to foods increases. The role of the Committee on Food Chemicals Codex in lowering dietary lead consumption has been reviewed (*364*). The Committee plans to lower recommended lead limits for food chemicals based on their level of consumption or reported use. For example, because of the high level of consumption of sweeteners, salt, and edible oils, reducing lead levels in these chemicals could significantly decrease dietary intake of lead.

Lead concentrations were measured in consumable tissues of cattle from an industrial and a rural area of northern Greece (*365*). Mean lead levels in muscle, liver, and kidney of 97 animals from the industrial area were 0.64, 0.81, and 1.22 mg/kg wet weight, respectively, while corresponding values from 62 animals from the rural area were 0.51, 0.64, and 0.65 mg/kg. Except for the kidney, lead levels in the tissues did not increase with age. Although these lead concentrations did not exceed regulatory limits, continued monitoring is recommended.

Transfer of ingested lead to milk was studied in dairy cattle who were accidentally, acutely exposed to lead by licking burnt storage batteries left in their pasture (*366*). Nine cows died of lead poisoning within 3 days of exposure, and another 8 without evident symptoms were monitored for 18 weeks. Lead concentrations in kidney, liver, and muscle of the cows who died were 70–330 mg/kg, 10–55 mg/kg, and 0.23–0.5 mg/kg, respectively. (Normal tissue levels of lead in Sweden were reported to be 0.1, 0.05, and <0.005 mg/kg, respectively.) Mean lead levels in the milk and blood of surviving cows, two weeks after exposure, were 0.08 and 0.36 mg/kg, respectively. An exponential relationship was found between blood lead and milk lead concentrations, with lead levels in milk increasing sharply at higher blood concentrations (>0.25 mg/kg). The apparent half-life of lead in blood was about 9 weeks.

Blood lead levels were measured in a total of 222 Montana cattle representing 8 herds grazing within 10.5 km of a 103-year-old primary lead smelter and one control herd living 43 km from the smelter in another valley (*367*). All 45 animals in the control herd and 141 animals from the herds near the smelter had blood lead levels <22 µg/dL. Twenty-one cattle had elevated lead levels (22–34 µg/dL) and 15 animals (all immature) had toxic levels (>35 µg/dL). Higher blood lead levels were found in herds closer to the smelter, as expected.

Organic lead compounds, originating from mining, combustion of coal, and gasoline additives, are 10–100 times more toxic than inorganic lead. Ionic alkyl lead, tetraalkyl lead, and total lead were determined in fresh, frozen, and canned shellfish, fresh lobster, canned crab meat, and canned cod liver obtained in Canada (*368*). Total lead levels were generally low (<5.4–626 ng/g) except for one sample of cockles in a soldered can (2850 ng/g) and one sample of mussels in a welded can (1070 ng/g). Ionic alkyl leads were found in 60% of the samples, with trimethyl- and dimethyl-lead accounting for 89% of the alkyl lead residues. No tetraalkyl leads were detected in any samples. Alkyl leads accounted for >5% of the total lead in lobster hepatopancreas and cod liver but for only 0.02–1.1% of the total lead in the other samples.

Of two wet digestion procedures evaluated for the determination of lead in plant materials by electrothermal atomic absorption spectrometry (ETA–AAS), the combination of HNO_3, H_2O_2, and HF gave results which corresponded best with reference values (*369*). A mixture of sulfuric, nitric, and perchloric acids gave results that were too low in some cases because of the formation of a mixed precipitate $(Pb,Ba)SO_4$. Determination of lead in cola drinks by ETA–AAS did not require destruction of organic matter if samples were first reacted with lanthanum and nitric acid to reduce interferences (*370*). Using this direct method, lead concentrations as low as 9.77 ng/mL could be detected.

Ethanol, tartaric acid, and other compounds interfere with the detection of lead in wine by hydride generation atomic absorption spectrometry (371). Experiments designed to overcome these problems indicated that optimal values for pH, peroxide, and $NaBH_4$ were 0.86, 7.5% H_2O_2, and 21% $NaBH_4$. Reaction time between peroxide and lead in wine should be 3 min. Under these conditions, detection limit for lead was 24 ppb and analyses of 14 wines by this method and the standard AOAC method gave similar results.

A method for the determination of lead in frying oils by direct current plasma–atomic emission spectrometry has been developed and applied to analyses of used frying oil samples collected from different locations in Cairo, Egypt (*372*). Lead levels in frying oil (cottonseed oil) collected during frying in quiet areas and heavy traffic areas did not differ significantly, averaging 0.42 µg/g. However, oil samples obtained from pans cooled in open air for several hours in the heavy traffic area had about twice as much lead as those from quiet areas (averages of 1.57 compared to 0.71 µg/g). Apparently the oil is recontaminated from dust fall during cooling.

A local cooking salt used by some villagers in Nigeria has been found to contain high levels of lead (433 µg/L) and manganese (2340 µg/L) as compared to common salt containing 1 µg Pb/L and 8.7 µg Mn/L (373). The origin of this lead is unknown. However, the village is near old mines where lead, silver, and iron ores were mined in the 1940s. This cooking salt is recovered from a local hot spring which may have naturally high mineral levels leached from surrounding rocks and ores.

Of 50 infants (<12 months of age) with mean blood lead levels of 39 µg/dL seen at a lead referral program in Massachusetts during a 4-year period, the apparent source of lead for 9 infants was formula prepared with lead-contaminated water (*374*). Three hazardous aspects of formula reconstitution were identified: (a) Use of contaminated tap water which had been boiled for 10–20 minutes. Three such samples of boiled water contained 1000, 117 and 142 ppb lead. (b) Use of contaminated first-draw water (150 ppb lead) to make the day's supply of formula. (c) Use of a leaded vessel for boiling water (1,700–3,500 ppb lead). These vessels included an antique copper-covered lead vessel, a cooking vessel brought from the Middle East, and a pot manufactured in the USA. Another case of lead poisoning in an infant in Canada was traced to an electric urn of Iranian origin with visible areas of spot solder on the inside of the pot (*375*). Tap water, boiled in this urn and used for reconstituting infant formula, contained 89.9 µmol Pb/L.

Use of automobile radiators containing lead-soldered parts for the distillation of alcohol (moonshine) is an important source of lead poisoning in some rural areas of the USA. During 1990–1991, nine persons in Alabama were diagnosed with elevated blood lead levels (16-259 µg/dL; average, 67 µg/dL) associated with consumption of 0.2-1.5 L moonshine/day (*376*). All patients had been evaluated at a hospital for alcohol-related symptoms. No specimens of the implicated moonshine were available for analysis but samples of moonshine from 2 radiator stills confiscated in the same county in 1991 contained 7400 and 9700 µg Pb/L compared with undetectable levels (<1.0 µg Pb/L) from municipal water from the area. These 9 cases are believed to underrepresent the number of lead toxicity cases in this area.

Investigation of blood lead levels and lifestyle habits of 99 women in Mexico City revealed that the use of lead-glazed ceramics was a major determinant of blood lead levels (377). Mean blood lead level was 10.6 µg/dL, with a range of 1–52 µg/dL. Age, time spent outdoors, and consumption of tap water and/or canned foods were not important correlates of blood lead. However, there was a significant increasing trend in blood lead concentrations with increasing frequency of consumption of food prepared in lead-glazed ceramic ware.

Plastic wrappers from 14 national brands of bread purchased in 1990 were analyzed for lead content in the print on the bags (378). Lead was detected in 17 of 18 bread bags analyzed, with an average of 26 mg lead/bag (range 0.9–84 mg/bag). Of 106 families surveyed 41% reported reusing the bags and 16% said they turned the bags inside out before reuse. A weak acid, such as vinegar, could readily leach 100 µg lead from one of these bags in 10 minutes. In addition paint sometimes flaked off the bag and onto stored food. In October 1991, industry representatives assured the FDA that lead inks had been off the market in the USA and Canada for a year, so lead on bread bags should no longer be a concern (379).

Indices of human exposure to lead

Surveillance reports of elevated blood lead levels in adults from 14 states from 1989, 1990, and 1991 were published (380). States differ in their reporting requirements, some requiring that results of all blood lead tests be reported and others mandating the reporting only of test results exceeding 10, 15, 25, or 40 µg/dL. Although the data indicate a slight decrease in the number of reports of >25 µg Pb/dL during these 3 years, the data for some years are incomplete, so that there is no reliable indication of a trend.

A total of 940 households in three selected high-risk areas in California were surveyed to determine lead levels in blood of resident children, in household paint, and in soil near the house (381). The most contaminated area was in Oakland: lead in interior paint, exterior paint, and soil samples averaged (geometric mean) 2540 ppm, 13,545 ppm, and 897 ppm, respectively. Blood lead levels in 67% of the children in these houses were ≥10 µg/dL and in 5% were ≥20 µg/dL.

In 1990–1991 a total of 1408 people, aged 6 months to 50 years, in Singapore were surveyed to determine blood lead levels and important environmental or lifestyle factors affecting these levels (382). Mean blood level for the whole group was 7.66 µg/dL, while for children under 5 the level was <6 µg/dL. Factors correlated with higher blood lead concentrations were older age, active smoking, exposure to passive smoke, exposure to road traffic, living in an apartment below the 10th story, and exposure to recent paint work.

Lead accumulates in teeth and bones and these tissues may be analyzed to assess lead exposure. Recent analyses of teeth from 143 individuals (aged 14–60 years) in Israel (383), 1466 people (about 5–80 years of age) in Germany (384), and 6 people (aged 67–96 years) in California (385) demonstrated that lead concentrations increase with age but, within the same population, do not differ between the sexes. Incisors generally have higher concentrations of lead than molars and premolars. Analyses of teeth and bones from the California subjects using stable Pb isotopic tracers indicated that the residence time of Pb is longer in teeth than in bones.

Comparison of lead levels in 753 shed teeth from primary school children in Taiwan with 2331 shed teeth from children in Boston revealed overlapping lead concentrations (386). Incisors had the highest lead levels (4.5 µg/g in Taiwan; 3.4 µg/g in Boston). Pb concentrations in canines and molars from Taiwan were 3.8 and 2.9 µg/g, respectively, and corresponding values from Boston were 2.3 and 3.3 µg/g. Examination of the surface enamel of incisor teeth from 318 Belgian children, mostly from urban areas, and 60 rural Kenyan children of about the same age revealed that the Belgian children had about an 8.5-fold higher lead concentration in their teeth (1236 ppm vs. 145 ppm) (387).

Teeth and bones from 23 persons living 700 to 1000 years ago in the American Southwest were analyzed for Ca, Pb, and Ba (*388*). Data indicated that mean natural body burden of Pb among these prehistoric people was about 40 µg Pb for a 70-kg human. This is approximately one-thousandth of the mean body burden of an adult American today and may indicate that even exposure to general background levels of lead may have caused some dysfunctions in most Americans.

Biological effects and toxicity of lead

A number of reports have documented an association between low levels of lead in blood of children and various adverse neurophysiological effects. Effects of an array of socio-demographic, behavioral, caregiving, and environmental risk factors were investigated in a cohort of 270 socio-economically disadvantaged mother–child pairs in Cleveland (*389*). Strong persistent pairwise relationships were observed between lead levels in blood and teeth of children and maternal IQ, parental education, examination ratings of the condition and cleanliness of the environment, and the HOME scale, which assesses the quality of the caregiving environment. These results emphasized the importance of adjusting for these factors when interpreting correlational data on lead levels and cognitive function in children.

Problems in evaluating the effects of confounding factors were also addressed in a Danish study involving 1291 first-grade children (*390*). Elevated dentin lead levels in shed teeth were inversely related to performance on the Bender gestalt test scored by the Göttingen system. Within this cohort, a group of 200 children were examined in detail. Twenty-nine of these children, primarily from the low-lead group, had encountered obstetrical complications or other medical risks for neurobehavioral dysfunction. Because lead-related neurobehavioral problems are non-specific, inclusion of these children in the data analysis would distort the results toward the null hypothesis. Such non-specific effects, in addition to problems of irregular exposure, existence of a threshold, and compensation and repair mechanisms, were discussed with suggestions for possible epidemiological strategies for minimizing these effects.

Another complicating factor in interpreting data on the effects of lead is the apparent existence of genetic factors which may predispose some individuals to lead toxicity. Two populations, 202 lead factory workers in Germany and 1278 children environmentally exposed to lead in New York, were examined to determine erythrocyte δ-aminolevulinate dehydratase (ALAD) phenotype (*391*). In both groups, people with the ALAD 1–2 or 2–2 isozyme phenotype (11% of the children and 21% of the workers) had significantly higher blood lead levels than individuals with the ALAD 1–1 phenotype. In fact, 53% of the children with the 1–2 and 2–2 phenotypes had blood lead levels ≥25 µg/dL while only 29% of the children with the 1–1 phenotype had such elevated lead levels. These results support the hypothesis that ALAD 2 polypeptide has a stronger affinity for lead than ALAD 1 and, therefore, that persons with the ALAD 2 allele may be more susceptible to lead poisoning.

Even well-designed studies of the risks of lead exposure may be jeopardized by missing data for some subjects. It is likely that non-response on some occasions or to some tests is related to the variables of interest. In an analysis of categorical variables subject to non-response in studies of prenatal lead levels and learning difficulties in children, statistical methods for incorporating incomplete data into analyses were discussed and evaluated (*392*). Different conclusions as to the effects of lead will be reached when the incomplete data is included compared to analyses when the incomplete data is discarded.

When 9 volunteers ingested a high level of lead in beer (350–490 µg/L) during a 28-day period, increase in blood lead varied by a factor of 2 (*393*). Each individual consumed 0.5 L/day of the "leaded" beer, and blood lead levels were observed to rise during the first 21 days and then to gradually decrease. A similar two-fold variation was observed in the whole-body uptake (average 14%) of a single oral dose of ^{203}Pb.

Data on blood lead levels and height of 1454 Mexican–American children, aged 5–12 years, living in southwestern USA indicated that moderately elevated lead levels (0.14–1.92 µmol/L) were directly correlated with reduced stature (*394*). After the effects of other variables were statistically controlled for, children whose blood lead concentrations were above the median for their age and sex were about 1.2 cm shorter than those whose blood lead concentrations were below the median. Another study of the relationship between prenatal and early childhood exposure to lead in Cincinnati (235 subjects) also reported an inverse relationship between mean blood lead level and height at 33 months (*395*). This relationship was only evident in children whose mean blood lead concentration between 3 and 15 months was above the median (10.77 µg/dL). Results also suggested that the effects of prenatal or early childhood exposure to lead on growth were transient, provided that subsequent exposure to lead was not excessive.

However, a study of 185 children in Cleveland found no significant relationship between growth in early childhood (up to 58 months) and maternal blood lead levels during pregnancy or preschool blood lead levels in children (*396*). The children's blood lead levels averaged 15.92 µg/dL. The authors noted that reported number of cigarettes smoked by the mother during pregnancy was quite strongly correlated to weight and length of their infants.

Examination of data on 3545 subjects, aged 6–19 years, who participated in the Hispanic Health and Nutrition Survey revealed that elevated blood lead levels were associated with minor hearing impairment (*397*). An increase in blood lead from 6 to 18 µg/dL was associated with a 2-dB loss in hearing at all frequencies. Although effects were small, after controlling for a number of covariates, higher prenatal, neonatal, and postnatal blood lead levels in the Cincinnati cohort (n=259) were significantly related to poorer central auditory processing abilities on the Filtered Word Subtest of the SCAN (a screening test for auditory processing abilities) (*398*). These children were about 5 years old when tested.

Psychomotor development of a group of 81 6-year-old children from a rural area in France was compared with lead exposure in utero as estimated by maternal hair lead levels (*399*). Scores on the general cognitive, verbal, quantitative, and memory subscales of the McCarthy psychometric scale were significantly and negatively related to maternal hair lead concentrations. Lead levels in shed teeth of 764 children in Taiwan in grades 1–3 were found to be negatively correlated with scores of children on Raven's Colored Progressive Matrices Test (*400*). Adjustment of the data to account for other risk factors decreased, but did not eliminate, the importance of the role of lead on performance on this intelligence test.

Investigation of the influence of lead on classroom behavior of these Taiwanese children, as determined by teachers' responses to a modified version of the Rutter's Child Behavior Check List, revealed only 2 measures which appeared to be related to lead exposure (*401*). Among boys, those in the highest quartile of lead exposure as compared to those in the lowest quartile were 4.2 times more likely to be hyperactive and 8.4 times more likely to have difficulty with tasks.

Lead exposure (1.0 mg lead acetate/kg/day from birth to one year of age) appeared to affect the behavior of young rhesus monkeys (*402*). Play behavior, observed at 3–10 months and again at 16–19 months was particularly susceptible to lead. Total play, both social and nonsocial, was significantly suppressed, and fearful behaviors increased in lead-treated monkeys.

Two recent articles reviewed the reproductive toxicology of lead in humans. Information regarding lead levels during gestation in humans and evidence relating lead exposure to various health and developmental parameters of the fetus and newborn were summarized and evaluated (*403*). Available data on possible effects of in utero exposure to lead on all delayed outcomes in the human child, including effects on health, growth, and functional and behavioral outcomes were also summarized and discussed (*404*). Both reviews emphasize that more carefully designed and controlled research needs to be done before unequivocal conclusions can be drawn about the effects of low-level lead exposure.

Thirty-five survivors of childhood lead poisoning in the period 1930–1944 were surveyed in 1990 to determine effects of childhood plumbism on reproductive history (*405*). Compared to 22 matched controls, female plumbism subjects reported a higher proportion of spontaneous abortions and stillbirths among pregnancies and a higher proportion of children with learning disabilities among school-age children. There was no evidence of confounding by parents' educational level. Although the results were of borderline significance, the 35 participants had a history of less severe plumbism than 37 other cases of childhood plumbism in the Boston area who did not participate in the study.

Female cynomolgus monkeys orally dosed with 1500 µg lead acetate/kg body weight/day from birth to 10 years (lifetime), from birth to 400 days (childhood), or from 300 days to 10 years (adolescent) were assessed for reproductive function between 9–10 years (*406*). No overt toxic effects of lead were observed on general health or menstrual function, although blood lead levels of the adolescent- and lifetime-exposed monkeys were approximately 35 µg/dL at ages 9–10 years. However, lead did decrease circulating levels of estradiol, follicle-stimulating hormone, and luteinizing hormone, but not of progesterone, during the menstrual cycle without producing overt signs of menstrual irregularity.

Epidemiological studies in a population of 2150 men, aged 49–65 years, demonstrated an inverse correlation between blood lead levels and ADP-induced platelet aggregation measured by optical density in platelet-rich plasma (*407*). Blood lead levels in this group, the Caerphilly Collaborative Heart Disease Study, averaged 15.38 µg/dL, with a range of 4–56 µg/dL. Blood lead levels were not related to thrombin-induced aggregation.

MERCURY

Sources of dietary exposure to mercury

The most famous outbreak of mercury intoxication occurred at Minamata Bay, Japan, where industrial wastes severely contaminated fish. Recent reviews have discussed the importance of non-point sources of pollution in contaminating fish (*408,409*). Large quantities of mercury are released from fossil fuel combustion, smelters and incinerators and are transported by air to aquatic ecosystems. For example, many lakes in northern Wisconsin, remote from obvious sources of Hg contamination, contain fish exceeding state health guidelines for Hg contamination (0.5 µg/g). Total atmospheric Hg deposition readily accounts for the Hg in the fish and lake water. Therefore, contamination of fish may occur in unexpected places.

Recent analyses of different types of fish have demonstrated Hg levels: (a) averaging 0.15–1.8 µg Hg/g dry weight in 8 species of fish (160 specimens) from Kuwait (*410*); (b) averaging 0.4–2.38 mg/kg wet weight in lesser spotted dogfish from 11 sampling sites in the northeast Irish Sea (*411*); (c) averaging 0.035–0.476 mg/kg wet weight in flounder from 18 sampling sites in the northeast Irish Sea (*412*); (d) averaging 3.41 µg/g dry weight in 14 specimens of bluefin tuna from the northwest Atlantic (*413*); and (e) averaging 0.3–13.7 nmol/g fresh weight in 5 species of fish from several lakes in northern Manitoba which were enlarged to form hydroelectric reservoirs. The same species of fish from lakes in the same area which were not affected by the Churchill River diversion had mercury levels averaging 0.1–1.9 nmol/g fresh weight (*414*). Mercury levels were found to vary with size (age) of fish, their eating habits, and proximity to some source of pollution.

Seven freshwater and eight saltwater species of fish and several species of marine invertebrates comprising a total of 229 samples were analyzed to determine levels of total mercury, monomethyl mercury, and dimethyl mercury in edible muscle tissue (*415*). No sample contained detectable dimethyl mercury while total mercury and monomethyl mercury levels varied between 0.011 and 2.78 µg/g wet weight. Methyl mercury constituted 69–132% of total mercury, with a relative standard deviation for quintuplicate analyses of about 10%. Greater variability in results was obtained with poorly homogenized samples. These results indicate that, for the species studied, nearly all the mercury present is methyl mercury.

Several gas chromatographic columns were evaluated for their sensitivity in determining methyl mercury in aqueous solution (*416*). Of the packed columns, AT-1000, which was used previously in headspace GC with microwave-induced plasma detection, yielded the best results. However, better results were obtained in preliminary tests with two wide-bore thick-film fused-silica open tubular columns (FSOT). With the FSOT columns methyl mercury could be detected at sub-picogram levels. However, in assays with real tissue samples, the FSOT column was only slightly more sensitive than the AT-1000 column. Furthermore, reconditioning of the FSOT column was a disadvantage for routine measurements.

A procedure utilizing microwave dissolution in a closed Teflon bomb followed by cold vapor atomic absorption spectrometry was developed for the routine analysis of mercury in samples of sugar cane, sweet corn, potato, green bean, banana, lettuce, and tomato (*417*). Detection limit was 0.195 ng/mL, with recoveries of 99.8–101.7% in spiked samples. Of 51 crop samples surveyed, residues ranged from 0.005 µg/g (lettuce and tomato) to 0.215 µg/g (sweet corn). Factors affecting the determination of total mercury in biological samples by acidic reduction of Hg using continuous-flow cold vapor atomic absorption spectrometry were investigated (*418*). Results indicated that acidic reduction of mercury by Sn in this system required prior breakdown of organomercurials. This breakdown could be achieved by tissue digestion using $HNO_3/H_2SO_4/HCl$ followed by the addition of $K_2Cr_2O_7$ to stabilize Hg^{2+}. Using this method good analytical sensitivity and convenience of operation were achieved.

Occurrence and effects of mercury in humans

Over 20,000 people are thought to have been poisoned by methyl mercury contaminating fish in Minamata Bay, Japan, since the outbreak was first recognized in 1956. A recent review describes the situation immediately after its initial discovery and updates it with current information (*419*). In 1969, fish in Minamata Bay contained up to 50 mg Hg/kg compared to the WHO recommended maximum level of 0.5 mg/kg. Although these concentrations have decreased and the government is considering reopening the bay for fishing, it is likely that some species and sizes of fish still contain excessive levels of mercury. Approximately 95% of ingested compounds are absorbed from the gastrointestinal tract, and mercury tends to accumulate in the brain, liver and kidneys. Three major symptoms of intoxication are sensory disturbances, constriction of visual fields, and ataxia. Nearly 30% of infants born in the Minamata area during 1955–1958 were mentally retarded and many had poor motor coordination. During 15 years of followup, motor function has improved in the milder cases but intelligence was unimproved in all cases. In 1987, a retrospective study revealed that only 12% of 1084 people from the general population in the Minamata Bay area had none of the 3 classical symptoms of this disease.

Red blood cells from 1178 residents of a coastal town near Minamata Bay were determined to have mean geometric levels of 27.8 ng Hg/g (males) and 20.4 ng/g (females) in 1988 (*420*). These concentrations are similar to those observed in other areas of Japan and are considerably less than the minimum clinical effective mercury level of 200 ng/g in whole blood (about 400 ng/g in red blood cells), reported by the WHO.

Comparison of pathological features of arteries and arterioles in specific areas of the bodies of 22 victims of Minamata disease and 36 controls with no residential or occupational history indicative of methyl mercury (Me-Hg) poisoning revealed that arteriosclerotic changes in both groups were similar (*421*). This indicates that Me-Hg does not induce or exacerbate arteriosclerosis in humans.

Another mercury poisoning disaster is apparently just beginning to become evident in Brazil (*422*). During the past 30 years goldminers have dumped 2000 tons of mercury into opencast or riverbed mines (as part of the gold-separating process) throughout Amazonia. This mercury has drained into the river or has been burnt off into the atmosphere. Hair samples with mercury levels 15-fold higher than the recommended maximum limit have been obtained from gold miners and gold buyers and also from residents of riverside communities far removed from gold mines.

Hair samples obtained from 77 women in Seville, Spain, near the end of their pregnancy demonstrated an average concentration of 1.18 µg Hg/g (range 0.3-2.16 µg/g) (*423*). Maternal and umbilical venous blood samples contained averages of 6.23 and 6.43 µg Hg/g, respectively. A great deal of interindividual variability was noted in the group but despite relatively high Hg levels in some mothers, no toxic effects or fetal abnormalities were observed in newborns.

Use of hair analyses to detect mercury intoxication has been reviewed (*424*). Concentrations of >5 ppm Hg in scalp hair indicate mercury intoxication. Consumption of fish represents the main non-occupational exposure to mercury and, in fact, a positive linear correlation has been established between fish consumption and hair Hg levels. During chronic ingestion, the hair/blood ratio for mercury is in the range of 200:1 to 300:1.

Exposure of human spermatozoa to 20 µM Me-Hg for 30 min inhibited motility of 95% of the sperm (*425*). The Me-Hg was apparently not taken up by the cells but did induce coiled tails and kinks in the mid-piece region. These deleterious effects were not attenuated by the addition of 5 µM sodium selenite.

Effects of mercury in experimental animals and cell cultures

Interactions between mercury and selenium were recently reviewed with particular emphasis given to the "protective action" of selenium against mercury toxicity at the subcellular, organ/tissue, and organism level (*426*). Selenium neither inhibits uptake of Hg nor enhances its elimination but is believed to rechannel Hg from one organ to another and from one subcellular fraction to another. Selenium may also act by preventing oxidative damage, converting toxic forms of Hg to nontoxic or less toxic forms, combining with Hg to form a complex, and by competing with Hg for binding sites. In a few instances Se and Hg (as mercuric chloride) act synergistically in exerting toxic effects.

In rats exposed to 5 or 10 ppm methyl mercury hydroxide in drinking water a unique urinary porphyrin profile was observed after only 1 or 2 weeks' exposure (*427*). Highly elevated levels of 4- and 5-carboxyl porphyrins and another atypical porphyrin (with an undetermined structure) were characteristic of this profile. Levels of these porphyrins increased progressively during 30 weeks of mercury treatment and were highly correlated with renal Hg levels. If a similar unique urinary porphyrin profile is present in humans, it may serve as a useful biomarker for mercury exposure.

In an investigation of the mechanism of neurotoxicity of Hg, rat cerebellar granule cells were incubated with 20 µM methyl mercury (Me-Hg) (*428*). After 3 h exposure, >85% of the cells were dead and Me-Hg was observed to cause a concentration-dependent increase in membrane lipoperoxidation. Hydrogen peroxide (5 mM) closely mimicked the cytotoxic effects of Me-Hg, suggesting that oxidizing conditions produced by Me-Hg caused cell death.

Rats were exposed to low doses of Me-Hg during gestation and lactation (3.9 mg Hg/kg diet fed to their dams) and then in their own diet up to 50 days of age to study possible detrimental effects of Me-Hg on development of the central nervous system (*429*). At this level of exposure no general toxic effects were observed and no discernable general morphological alterations were seen in the brain or in maturation of the neurons and astrocytes. However, some differences from controls were observed in specific neurotransmitter-identified systems, such as noradrenaline input to the cerebellum.

In similarly exposed rats who were examined at 15 days post-partum, white blood cell counts were increased and natural killer cell activity was reduced by 42% (*430*). The lymphoproliferative response to T-cell mitogen was increased in thymocytes (by 30–48%) and decreased in splenocytes (by 30–32%). Thus, exposure to Me-Hg during gestation and lactation adversely affected the developing immune system of rats.

Me-Hg is known to be predominantly excreted from the body via the bile. The role of the gall bladder in this process was investigated in guinea pigs, hamsters, and macaque monkeys using radiolabelled Me-Hg (*431*). When labelled Me-Hg was instilled into the gall bladders of hamsters and guinea pigs, only 42.5% and 27.6%, respectively, remained in the gall bladder after 2 h. However, in similar experiments, 90–95% of inorganic mercury was retained in the gall bladder. Gall bladder bile from monkeys who had been chronically dosed with Me-Hg for 2 years always contained a lower concentration of Me-Hg than hepatic bile. Results of these experiments demonstrated that Me-Hg is extensively absorbed by the gall bladder. This suggests a biliary–hepatic cycling of Me-Hg which probably contributes to the long biological half-life and toxicity of Me-Hg.

SELENIUM

A relatively narrow range in dietary selenium concentrations is essential for health, with both selenium excess and selenium deficiency known to have toxic effects. In an area in central Africa where myxedematous cretinism is endemic, diets are deficient in iodine and selenium. It was hypothesized that Se deficiency, resulting in decreased levels of glutathione peroxidase (GPX, a Se-containing enzyme), enhanced peroxidative damage by H_2O_2 to the thyroid gland. Therefore, a selenium supplementation trial was conducted in northern Zaire in which 9 cretins were given a tablet containing 50 μg Se daily for 2 months (432). These supplements increased serum Se and GPX to normal levels but also significantly decreased the already subnormal levels of thyroxine (T4) and thyroid-stimulating hormone. Thus, it appears that Se deficiency protects against some consequences of iodine deficiency, and programs that aim to correct Se deficiency before improving iodine status may actually be dangerous.

Recently it has been shown that type I iodothyronine 5'-deiodinase, the enzyme which converts T4 to its active form T3, contains Se (433). Therefore, the fall in T4 levels observed in the dietary supplementation trial with the cretins can be explained by increased levels of this enzyme. Se deficiency has at least two major effects on thyroid metabolism.

In some Se-deficient areas in China, a disease called Kashin–Beck syndrome is endemic. Average dietary Se levels in two such areas in China, as determined by analyses of duplicate diets, were 0.009 and 0.006 μg/g (434). For comparison, dietary Se levels in areas in the same provinces where Kashin–Beck is not endemic were 0.021 and 0.027 μg/g. Following application of a Se-supplemented fertilizer, dietary Se levels rose from 0.009 to 0.0336 μg/g in one area. This corresponds to an increase in daily dietary intake from 4.6 to 16.8 μg.

A Se supplementation trial in another Se-deficient area in China which had a high incidence of Keshan disease demonstrated that selenomethionine caused more rapid increases in plasma and erythrocyte Se concentrations than did selenate (435). GPX levels in plasma and erythrocytes increased similarly in response to both supplements but with selenate a higher percentage of total plasma and erythrocyte Se was associated with GPX.

Experiments with 18 healthy Norwegian women fed 100, 200, or 300 μg Se daily in wheat containing relatively high levels of selenomethionine demonstrated that serum Se levels increased in a dose-dependent manner (436). This is in contrast to marginal effects, observed in previous studies, when diets were supplemented with selenite or pea Se. Previous studies had also shown that GPX levels did not change when a Se-replete population is given additional Se. The blood response and renal clearance results from this experiment indicate that selenomethionine from the diet is incorporated into a non-specific amino acid pool.

A kinetic model for human selenium metabolism has been proposed. Appearance and disappearance of labelled selenium in plasma, urine, and feces of 6 adults given a single oral dose of ^{74}Se as L-selenomethionine were measured for several weeks following dosing and used to construct a model (437). Selenomethionine was completely and rapidly absorbed from the gastrointestinal tract, and turnover time in peripheral tissues ranged from 61–86 days. This slow turnover appears to result from efficient recycling and reutilization of selenomethionine. This could be advantageous in cases of low Se intake but could result in excessive tissue accumulation and toxicity if intakes were high.

Cattle fed Se supplements (0.25 µg/kg dry matter), as plant selenium, in feed were found to experience a 7–8-fold increase in muscle levels of Se compared to those on a basal diet (*438*). However, supplementation at the same level with selenite resulted in only a 3–4-fold increase in muscle Se levels. Since meat and meat products are an important dietary source of Se, feed supplements should be formulated with care.

Three methods have been described for the determination of Se in human diets. A method using radiochemical neutron activation analysis selectively separated Se from other radioactive dietary constituents by volatilization as selenium tetrabromide and then precipitation in elemental form using sulfur dioxide prior to analytical determination (*439*). In a second method concentrated nitric acid and hydrogen peroxide were used to oxidize food samples prior to Se determination by Zeeman effect graphite furnace atomic absorption spectrometry (*440*). Finally, an inductively coupled plasma mass spectrometer with a newly designed continuous flow hydride generator was also used to successfully determine Se in biological samples (*441*).

TIN

Tributyl tin compounds (TBT) have been used as antifouling paints for hulls and fishing nets and have been detected in fish and shellfish from various areas. Of 25 samples of commercial fish (eel, rainbow trout, sweetfish) cultured in fresh water in Japan, TBT was detected in 21 fish at concentrations of 0.03–0.20 µg/g (*442*). Further investigations at 5 rainbow trout fisheries revealed no detectable TBT in water but TBT was present in 13 of 15 fish (0.01–0.05 µg/g) and in all samples of trout feed (0.06–0.15 µg/g). Fish meal, constituting 54–63% of the feed, was believed to be the source of TBT.

A flame photometric detector optimized for the generation of a quartz surface-induced tin luminescence was constructed and found to be significantly more sensitive than the commonly used SnH gas-phase luminescence for the detection of butyl tins in mussel tissue (*443*.) TBT was first extracted with toluene, pentylated, preseparated from lipids, and then separated by GC. Minimum detectable amount of TBT in mussel tissue was about 150 pg/g tissue.

An analytical method based on hexane extraction and methylation followed by cleanup by column chromatography and detection by GC with flame photometric detection was developed to determine residues of triphenyltin (TPT) in fish (*444*). Limit of detection was 0.8 ng/g for 0.1 g fish samples, and recoveries from spiked fish averaged 77%.

Serum levels of several elements and fatty acid composition of red blood cell membranes were determined in 36 subjects with Alzheimer's disease (AD), in 6 subjects with multi-infarct dementia (MID), and in 49 controls of similar age (*445*). Serum aluminum, tin, and vanadium levels were higher in the AD patients than in the MID patients. In addition, there was a significant negative correlation between tin and 6 of the 20- and 22-carbon essential fatty acids of the *n*-6 and *n*-3 series. Since organotin compounds produce neurotoxic symptoms in laboratory animals and some other metals are known to alter essential fatty acid metabolism, it may be that tin is involved in peroxidation of membrane lipids in AD patients.

Subchronic toxicity studies of TBT acetate and TPT acetate demonstrated that these compounds caused histopathologic lesions in lungs, liver, intestine, and kidney of rats even at the lowest doses used: 4 mg TBTA/kg and 5 mg TPTA/kg (*446*). Rats were dosed orally three times a week for 5 weeks. High doses of TPTA reduced mean counts of lymphocytes and monocytes but other hematologic parameters were unchanged.

Teratogenic effects of di-*n*-butyltin chloride (DBT) were investigated in a series of experiments in rats (*447,448*). Pregnant rats gavaged on days 7–15 of pregnancy with 5–10 mg DBT/kg produced fetuses with a variety of malformations, including cleft jaw, ankyloglossia, club foot, and anal atresia. Maternal toxicity was also evident at the two highest doses (7.5 and 10 mg/kg). Further experiments with rats dosed on different days during days 6–15 of pregnancy revealed that the fetuses were only susceptible to the teratogenic effects of DBT on days 7 and 8 of gestation.

In one-month feeding trials with 5 and 25 ppm TBT oxide (TBTO) and TBT chloride (TBTC), TBTO accumulated to a greater extent in the rats and caused greater immunotoxic effects than TBTC (*449*). Seven days after starting treatment with TBTO, marked atrophic changes were seen in the thymus and alterations occurred in the spleen but only minor changes were evident in the peripheral lymph nodes. By 28 days, the thymus, although smaller, was histologically normal and the spleen looked completely normal but there were marked changes in the lymph nodes. Other experiments in which rats were exposed to 150 ppm TBTO in the diet for 6 weeks demonstrated that these apparent immunotoxic effects of TBTO did not increase the susceptibility of rats to experimental infections with pneumonia virus of mice or *Mycoplasma pulmonis* (*450*).

VANADIUM

Vanadium is released to the environment in relatively large quantities by the burning of fossil fuels and may be locally abundant in some areas due to industrial processes. One such case occurred in Czechoslovakia where sludge containing about 1% soluble vanadium and wastewaters containing 0.5–1.0 g V/L contaminated a brook and local water supplies. Although people were forbidden to drink water from local wells, it was suspected that children accidentally consumed some contaminated water. Vanadium levels in hair and blood samples from 23 potentially exposed children and from 17 non-exposed children from another, non-polluted area were analyzed for vanadium by instrumental neutron activation analysis and neutron activation analysis with radiochemical separation (*451*). No differences were detected in V levels in hair: medians of 98 and 88 µg/kg for normal and exposed groups, respectively. However, significantly increased V concentrations were found in blood of exposed children (0.078 µg/L) com-

pared to control children (0.042 µg/L) and unexposed adults (0.056 µg/L). Significantly higher V concentrations were detected in the blood of 9 industrially exposed workers, ranging from 3.1 to 217.0 µg/L.

Distribution and half-life of retention of vanadium was determined in the organs of rats (*452*). Rats provided with drinking water containing 0.6–0.8 mg vanadate/mL for 6 weeks or 1 mg vanadyl/mL for 10 weeks were found to accumulate vanadium primarily in the kidney, with average levels of 185 nmol/g wet weight. Liver and spleen had about 3 times less vanadium, and lowest levels were detected in lung, blood plasma, and blood cells. A time course study with rats fed vanadyl sulfate trihydrate (0.75 mg/mL) for 3 weeks and normal drinking water thereafter indicated that the half-life for elimination of V from the body was about 12 days.

Rats gavaged with radioactive [^{48}V] as vanadate (1.8 mg/kg) were found to have absorbed only 4.2% of the dose after 24 h (*453*). Approximately 66% of the absorbed dose was excreted in the urine during the 2 weeks after dosing. Only slightly more than 1% of the absorbed dose was present in the kidneys and in the liver at 2 weeks, and 31% remained in the carcass.

After 4 weeks' exposure to drinking water containing 0.15 mg ammonium metavanadate/mL, erythrocyte and hemoglobin levels in rat blood were significantly decreased (*454*). Neutrophilic granulocyte and lymphocyte counts were significantly elevated and vanadium appeared to inhibit the phagocytic activity of granulocytes.

Teratogenic effects of vanadium were investigated in fetuses of mice gavaged with sodium orthovanadate (7.5, 15, 30, and 60 mg/kg) on gestational days 6–15 (*455*). Mice were sacrificed and fetuses examined on day 18 of gestation. Maternal toxicity was caused by the highest doses—increased maternal deaths at 30 and 60 mg/kg/day and reduced weight gain and food consumption at 15 and 30 mg/kg/day. Significant delays in the ossification process were observed in some areas of the fetuses in the group dosed with 30 mg/kg/day. The no-observed-adverse-effect levels for maternal toxicity and developmental toxicity were 7.5 mg/kg and 15 mg/kg, respectively, under the conditions of this experiment.

OTHER INORGANIC RESIDUES AND CONTAMINANTS

Copper

Since mutton constitutes an important part of the diet in Saudi Arabia, muscle, liver, kidney, heart, and intestine samples of Australian, Syrian, and Najdi lambs were analyzed to determine concentrations of 23 metals (*456*). Cadmium was detected at very low levels in some liver and kidney samples and lead was not detectable in any sample. Copper, present in Australian lamb liver at a mean concentration of 79.1 mg/kg (range, 21.8–160.6 mg/kg), was the only metal of toxicological concern. Copper supplements in feeds may have caused these high levels as Najdi lambs, which graze on desert pastures, had a mean of only 6.2 mg Cu/kg in liver. Frequent consumption of the Australian lamb liver might induce symptoms of copper toxicity.

Germanium compounds

Since 1982, 18 cases of acute renal dysfunction, including 2 deaths, linked to oral intake of germanium elixirs have been reported. Nephrotoxicity and neurotoxicity to humans of organogermanium compounds and germanium oxide were recently reviewed (*457*). Germanium is widely distributed in edible foods usually at very low levels, with levels in tomato juice and baked beans (nearly 5 ppm) and in canned seafood (2.28–3 ppm) being about the highest. No living organism has a known physiological requirement for germanium. Nevertheless, in recent years some germanium compounds have been sold as "nutritional supplements." Reported intakes of germanium by the cases with renal dysfunction were between 100 and 2000 times the average intake of 1.5 mg/day. Because germanium-containing preparations are widely available over-the-counter, it is likely that there are additional cases of germanium poisoning.

Iodine

Premilking teat preparations may leave iodine residues which then contaminate milk. Contrary to expectations, teat dipping with a 0.25% iodophor teat dip resulted in higher iodine residues in milk than treatment with a 0.5% iodophor dip (*458*). Wiping of teats with cotton towels for 20 seconds after dipping removed most of the iodine from the teat surface and resulted in milk with insignificant iodine residues (9 µg/L) as compared to wiping with cotton for 6 seconds (62 µg/L).

Three sensitive procedures for the determination of iodine in foods have been recently described. A spectrophotometric kinetic assay based on measurement of the iodide-catalyzed reduction of Ce(IV) to Ce(III) by As(III) was monitored at 370 nm and the initial velocity was used to quantitate iodine levels (*459*). This method had a detection limit of 0.4 ng, and recoveries of iodine added to foods ranged from 94% to 102%. Of several ashing methods used to prepare the food samples, successive treatments with KOH and then with zinc sulfate gave the best results.

Another kinetic assay, based on the inhibitory effect of iodide on the Pd(II)-catalyzed reaction between EDTA-Co(III) and the hypophosphite ion, achieved a limit of detection of 1.2 ng/mL (*460*). Recoveries of iodide added to milk samples were in the range 97.1%–101.1%. Trace levels of iodine in table salt, edible seaweed, and eggs have also been determined by cathodic stripping voltammetry using the quaternary ammonium salt Zephiramine as the ionic associating agent (*461*). Samples were pretreated by combustion in an oxygen flask prior to iodine determination. Limit of determination was 0.1 ng/mL.

Iron

In contrast to hemochromatosis in European populations which is believed to be hereditary, iron overload in sub-Saharan Africa was believed to be a result of consumption of a traditional home-brewed beer fermented in steel drums. Average iron content of this beer is 80 mg/L, and some people may consume several liters/day on weekends. A total of

236 members of 36 African families, each of which contained a member with iron overload, were tested to determine serum iron levels and total iron-binding capacity (*462*). Among family members reporting high levels of consumption of traditional beer, mean serum ferritin concentrations and transferrin saturation in serum were distributed bimodally. This indicates that iron overload in Africa probably results from an interaction between a genetic factor and high dietary levels of iron.

To assess whether dietary iron supplementation is a precipitating factor for hemochromatosis in the USA, trends in hematologic screening parameters during the past 20 years were examined (*463*). Data from several sources, including NHANES I and II, Medicaid data, and the National Hospital Discharge Survey, provided no strong evidence of an increase in hemochromatosis since dietary iron supplementation began in 1940.

Chronic iron overload in humans results in hepatocellular damage and fibrosis. Experiments with rats fed a chow containing 3% by weight of carbonyl iron for 1, 4, or 8 weeks revealed that moderate and high degrees of iron loading significantly reduced hepatic mitochondrial oxidative metabolism and calcium sequestration (*464*). At all 3 levels of iron loading (1360, 2060, and 3170 μg/g) there were significant decreases in microsomal cytochrome P450 levels and calcium sequestration. These alterations may impair intracellular calcium homeostasis leading to cellular injury.

Nickel

To determine whether foods can leach nickel from stainless steel pots during cooking, three acidic foods, rhubarb, spinach, and sauerkraut, were cooked in several types of stainless steel pots manufactured by 4 different companies (*465*). Analyses of nickel levels in the foods before and after cooking revealed no significant changes, indicating that nickel was not released from the pots.

Within 12–16 h after swallowing a 1967 Canadian nickel, a 6-year-old boy was brought to an emergency room with generalized erythema (*466*). His white blood cell count was elevated with 85% neutrophils, and serum nickel level, about 24 h after

ingestion, was measured at 20.2 μg/L (normal: 0.2–3.0 μg/L). The coin was removed and 1 month later his serum nickel level had returned to normal. The boy had a previous history of local contact metal allergy and this coin, made of 100% nickel, triggered a systemic allergic reaction.

Effects of dietary nickel (2.7 g nickel sulfate/kg diet) on humoral and cellular immunity were investigated in female SJL mice (*467*). Mice were fed the supplemented diets from 4 to 8 weeks of age and then injected with keyhole limpet hemocyanin (KLH) at 8 weeks. Eight days later IgG and IgM responses to KLH were significantly depressed in Ni-fed mice as compared to controls. Response of splenocytes from Ni-fed mice to KLH in vitro was also depressed compared to those from control animals. Proliferative responses of B cells in response to the mitogen lipopolysaccharide were also significantly depressed in Ni-fed mice.

Platinum

Although metallic platinum is non-toxic and non-allergenic, some of its soluble compounds are known to be toxic and others are suspected carcinogens. Platinum concentrations in a variety of Australian foods were found to range from 0.13 μg/kg in whole milk to 8.11 μg/kg in liver (*468*). Using these data the typical diet of an Australian adult was estimated to contain 1.44 μg Pt/day. Absorption of dietary platinum was estimated to be at least 42% and, therefore, diet apparently makes a substantial contribution to total Pt intake. Median Pt concentrations in Australian adults were whole blood, 0.56 μg/L; hair, 3.84 μg/kg; and urine 0.23 μg Pt/g creatinine.

Zinc

Amyotrophic lateral sclerosis, endemic in Guam and some areas of the western Pacific, is associated with some environmental factors but the exact causative agent remains elusive. Consumption of the cycad is one implicated factor but the toxic amino acid in cycad appears to be present in levels too low to be neurotoxic. Tests with 17 samples of cycad flour prepared the traditional Guamian way revealed that four demonstrated dose-dependent neurotoxic effects on mesencephalic and cerebellar granule cell cultures (*469*). Toxic amino acid levels in the flours were low, but one flour analyzed for metals contained very high levels of zinc: 360 µg Zn/100 g flour compared to concentrations of 0.55–0.99 µg/100 g in unprocessed cycad flour, nontoxic processed cycad flour, and household wheat flour. Toxicity to the cell cultures was related to zinc concentrations in the flours, and EDTA, a chelating agent, protected against neurotoxic effects. During processing of cycad tissue in a galvanized pail in the laboratory there was a time-dependent increase in zinc content, with a concentration of 1.2 mg Zn/g tissue achieved after 7 days of soaking. These results suggest that traditional methods of cycad flour preparation may introduce high levels of zinc.

Concentrations of zinc were measured in hair samples from 57 mothers who delivered infants with neural tube defects (NTD), from 30 healthy mothers with normal offspring, and from 37 nonpregnant women from middle-income background (*470*). Mean hair zinc level in the NTD mothers was 128.2 µg/g compared to levels of 180 and 192 µg/g in the two control groups. However, mean hair zinc level in infants with NTD was elevated (250.4 µg/g) compared to that in normal infants (193.4 µg/g). It may be that maternal zinc deficiency is one of the factors responsible for NTD in Turkey.

During the period of 1875–1913 there was a significant decline in fertility in western Europe. A recent article discussed various explanations for this phenomenon, including availability of contraceptives, a decline in infant mortality motivating parents to have fewer children, and increasing industrialization and urbanization motivating people to change their spending habits and have fewer children (*471*). However, none of these explanations appears to be adequate since, among other things the available data do not support them and the incidence of illegitimate births decreased at the same rate as legitimate births. An alternative hypothesis, that zinc deficiency was the cause of decline in fertility, was proposed and relevant data were discussed. Around 1875, wheat became more available and it was being processed to remove the germ which contained most of the minerals and vitamins natural to wheat. Zinc is known to be essential for reproduction and thus the decline in dietary zinc may have reduced fertility.

RADIONUCLIDES

Levels in humans and toxicological effects

Distribution of uranium, a naturally occurring radioactive heavy metal, varies in different areas of the earth's crust, depending on rock types. In a recent review, the nephrotoxicity and radiotoxicity of uranium were discussed (*472*). Toxicological data from studies with dogs indicated that the no-observed-effect level of uranium was approximately 1 mg U/kg body weight/day. As for radiotoxicity, the maximum estimated dietary intake in Switzerland (40 µg or 1 Bq/person/day) was estimated to result in a fatal cancer lifetime risk of about 10^{-4}. Criteria for the determination of cancer risks and their applicability to regulatory controls were discussed and compared with criteria used in estimating risks from chemical carcinogens in foods.

A total of 413 hypertensive subjects from Scotland and the Western Isles were studied to determine their whole body levels of ^{137}Cs and their intake of foods which might contain radioactivity (*473*). Patients from the Western Isles had a median body concentration of 2.54 Bq/gK of ^{137}Cs as compared to concentrations of 0.42–0.47 Bq/gK from those on the Scottish mainland. Dietary sources of this radioactivity in the islanders were mainly mutton (16 Bq/kg) and milk (1.6 Bq/L). Higher levels of radioactivity were also detected in fish, seaweed, and grasses from the islands as compared to the mainland. ^{134}Cs, which is produced by reprocessing nuclear fuels, was also detected in most of the samples, indicating that a nuclear reprocessing plant located in northern England was the probable source of the excess radioactivity in the Western Isles. (All these measurements were done prior to the Chernobyl accident.)

Total body burdens of ^{137}Cs in 14 adults in Athens ranged from 593 to 2801 Bq in 1989 and from 205 to 659 Bq one year later (*474*). These results, as compared to the known half-life of this isotope, indicated that these individuals were consuming 0–3.7 Bq/day of this isotope in their food. The Chernobyl reactor accident deposited comparatively high levels of radionuclides in Greece and was the likely source of this contaminated food.

Radionuclides in foods and transfer in the food chain

Results of radioactivity measurements made in 1990 on foods collected in regions of Russia, Byelorussia, and the Ukraine, heavily contaminated by the Chernobyl accident, were reported and used to estimate safety of the foods (*475*). Total radiocesium contamination ranged from 1–170 Bq/kg in samples of milk, cheese, buttermilk, kasja, potatoes, calabash, carrots, and beets. ^{90}Sr levels in milk, kasja, and cheese were 1.8–30 Bq/kg. Mushrooms and reindeer moss were very highly contaminated, with radiocesium levels of 103,000 to 284,000 Bq/kg and ^{90}Sr levels of 7.8 to 1,550 Bq/kg in the fresh product. Except for mushrooms, all the food products investigated can be regarded as safe with respect to radioactive contamination. The radioactive burden associated with consumption of these foods was estimated to be 0.2 mSv/year.

Mushrooms collected in woods in central Italy from August 1986 to November 1989 were found to contain increasing amounts of radiocesium, up to a plateau averaging about 70 Bq/kg fresh weight (*476*). Different species of mushrooms varied considerably in the amount of radiocesium accumulated, with average concentrations ranging from 6 to 540 Bq/kg. Concentrations of ^{137}Cs in 60 samples of dried Japanese mushrooms collected in the autumn of 1989 ranged from <3 to 1,520 Bq/kg (*477*). In edible mushrooms, concentrations were normally <50 Bq/kg and therefore the effective dose equivalent due to the dietary intake of mushrooms was estimated to be 1.6×10^{-7} Sv.

Following the Chernobyl accident in April 1986, radiocesium levels were monitored in brown trout in a Norwegian subalpine lake situated in an area of high fallout (*478*). Average total cesium levels after icebreak in 1986 rose rapidly from 300 to 7000 Bq/kg by the end of August. Mean values fell to 4700 Bq/kg during the summer of 1987 and to 3000 Bq/kg in June 1989. Considerable variation in radioactivity levels was observed between individual fish. Based on the changes observed during this period, half-lives for ^{137}Cs and ^{134}Cs in trout were estimated to be 3.0 and 1.3 years, respectively.

Prior to Chernobyl, reindeer and pike in Sweden had ^{137}Cs levels of 57–180 and 14–24 Bq/kg, fresh weight, as a result of earlier nuclear bomb tests (*479*). After Chernobyl, animals in the northernmost region had similar amounts of radioactivity while those in the southernmost locality contained up to 80-times higher levels. The highest value recorded was 18,425 Bq/kg in reindeer muscle, while the highest value in pike was 567 Bq/kg.

Samples of food imported into Iraq early in 1986 prior to the Chernobyl accident did not contain detectable radiocesium levels, but of foods imported after the accident, all lamb meat, 81% of lentils, 44% of powdered milk and chick peas, and 17% of the roast beef samples tested were contaminated with ^{134}Cs and/or ^{137}Cs (*480*). Highest levels of ^{137}Cs in these foods were 82, 147, 420, 6, and 4 Bq/kg, respectively. Only one sample (powdered milk) contained a concentration higher than the Iraqi intervention level of 370 Bq/kg.

Various foods typical of a Southeast Asian community were collected from markets in Hong Kong in 1992 and analyzed for ^{137}Cs (*481*). Mean concentrations were low, ranging from 0.1 Bq/kg in freshwater fish and fruit to 0.6 Bq/kg in rice. Annual intake of this radionuclide was estimated, from a simple food model, to be 160 Bq/person.

Uptake of radionuclides from contaminated soil (*482*) and contaminated irrigation water (*483*) into crop plants has been studied in greenhouse and small plot experiments. Transfer factors (activity in plant dry weight/activity in soil dry weight) for cucumber, tomato, parsley, radish, and lettuce growing on ^{137}Cs-contaminated peat varied from 0.66 to 1.8. Transfer factors for wheat, alfalfa, and beets irrigated with water containing ^{238}U, ^{232}Th, ^{226}Ra, ^{210}Pb, and ^{210}Po varied with the species of plant and the type of irrigation. Sprinkling irrigation apparently deposited more radioactivity on plants than that absorbed from flooding type of irrigation.

An area in Brazil with elevated levels of naturally occurring uranium, thorium, and radon was investigated to determine comparative bioavailability of these isotopes to adult steers, pigs and chickens (*484*). Muscle-to-soil concentration ratios for U and Th ranged from 0.4×10^{-4} (pigs) to 1×10^{-4} (chickens). Mean values for Ra were about 3–5 times higher. Bone-to-soil concentration ratios were higher than those for muscle, especially those for radon, which were about 10^{-1} for chickens and steers.

Some transfer parameters used in models for predicting the migration of radionuclides in the environment were evaluated using data collected at various Italian sites following the Chernobyl accident (*485*). Data reported here and that in previous literature indicate that the variability of some parameters is very wide. This variability is due, at least in part, to uncertainties in sampling and measurement techniques. Therefore, the uncertainty of generic model predictions appears to be at least an order of magnitude.

Decontamination of radioactive foods

Although it appears from recent data that radiation contamination of humans from radioactive foods is actually less than predicted, decontamination of some foods, such as milk intended for infants, may be necessary. In a recent review different methods for decontamination of food were summarized and evaluated (*486*). For fruits and vegetables surface-contaminated by radioactive fallout, washing and peeling removes a high percentage of the radioactivity. Foods that are totally contaminated, e.g. plants which have absorbed radionuclides from the soil and milk from cows which have consumed contaminated feed, are much more difficult to clean up, and the methods used may remove valuable constituents from the foods as well as the radioactivity. Thus, the most important strategy is to prevent the radionuclides from entering the food chain by protecting or treating the soil and by removing surface contamination carefully and as quickly as possible.

Efficiency of measures aimed at decreasing contamination of agricultural products in areas con-taminated by the Chernobyl accident was described and discussed (*487*). The types of measures taken included: (a) prohibitions—preventing the use of heavily contaminated fields for crops or pasture; (b) survey of contaminated areas to determine degree of contamination and types of radionuclides present; (c) determination of soil parameters governing transfer of radionuclides to plants and of ways to treat soils and pastures to reduce this transfer. Concentration of ^{137}Cs in crop plants has been shown to vary 10–100-fold depending the plant species and the soil type. Liming and fertilizing of meadows was shown to increase the yield of grass and reduce the transfer of radionuclides to cow's milk by up to 3.5-fold.

Soaking of meat and fish (*488*) and cheese (*489*) in water or brine solutions for varying lengths of time was tested as a method for removing radionuclides. After 2 days of soaking in water, 5% brine, or 10% brine, the radioactive cesium remaining in meat samples was 42.2%, 38.7%, and 35.9%, respectively. Successive treatments with water or brine or increasing the brining temperature improved the removal of radioactive cesium. Soaking fish in 5% brine or water for 4 h removed >50% of its radioactivity. An 18% NaCl solution effectively removed $\geq$45% of ^{131}I and ^{137}Cs from feta cheese after 24 h.

Consumption of winkles (shellfish) is a major contributor to the radiation dose (plutonium, americium, and cesium) received by local consumers in West Cumbria, near a nuclear fuels reprocessing plant. Solubilization of these radionuclides in cooked winkles by in vitro digestion was investigated to determine their potential bioavailability (*490*). For winkles containing different levels of inorganic particulate matter (presumably ingested sediment), 1–7% of the plutonium was solubilized with no direct relationship between particulate matter and solubilization. In contrast, there was a strong inverse relationship between the particulate content and the amount of radiocesium solubilized. Between 13 and 63% of the cesium was solubilized. It appears that only about 50% of the cesium in winkles is available for absorption, and thus the radiation dose received by seafood consumers in this area may be overestimated by a factor of 2.

LITERATURE CITED

1. International Dairy Federation. *Monograph on Residues and Contaminants in Milk and Milk Products.* Brussels, International Dairy Federation (1991).

2. Pearson, A.M., and T.R. Dutson (eds.). *Meat and Health. Adv. Meat Res.* 6 (1990).

3. Comerford, J.W. Heavy metal and hydrocarbon residues in tissue and blood of beef steers bedded on waste newspapers. *Bull. Environ. Contam. Toxicol.* 49:18–22 (1992).

4. Price, R.J. Residue concerns in seafoods. *Dairy Food Environ. Sanit.* 12:139–143 (1992).

5. Hollstein, A. Rückstände von organochlorpestiziden, PCB's und chlorphenolen in fischen aus teichwirtschaften und fischwirtschaftlich genutzten gewässern im gebiet um Frankfurt (Oder). *Nahrung* 35:1029–1040 (1991).

6. Galal-Gorchev, H. Dietary intake of pesticide residues: cadmium, mercury, and lead. *Food Addit. Contam.* 8:793–806 (1991).

7. Kannan, K., S. Tanabe, A. Ramesh, et al. Persistent organochlorine residues in foodstuffs from India and their implications on human dietary exposure. *J. Agric. Food Chem.* 40:518–524 (1992).

8. Tanabe, S., K. Kannan, M.S. Tabucanon, et al. Organochlorine pesticide and polychlorinated biphenyl residues in foodstuffs from Bangkok, Thailand. *Environ. Pollut.* 72:191–203 (1991).

9. Cairns, T., and E.G. Siegmund. Confirmation of trace level residues in the food supply. *Crit. Rev. Food Sci. Nutr.* 30:397–402 (1991).

10. O'Daly, J.P., J. Zhao, P.A. Brown, and R.W. Henkens. Electrochemical enzyme immunoassay for detection of toxic substances. *Enzyme Microb. Technol.* 14:299–302 (1992).

11. Rodriguez, O.M., P.G. Desideri, L. Lepri, and L. Checchini. Simultaneous separation and determination of hydrocarbons and organochlorine compounds by using a two-step microcolumn. *J. Chromatogr.* 555:221–228 (1991).

12. World Health Organization. Evaluation of certain veterinary drug residues in food. Thirty-eighth report of the joint FAO/WHO expert committee on food additives. *Weekly Epidemiol. Rec.* 67:134 (1992).

13. Anonymous. Toxicological evaluation of certain veterinary drug residues in food. *Vet. Hum. Toxicol.* 34:92 (1992).

14. Multiple authors. *Symposium on Biological Models to Determine the Safety of Bound Residues in the Tissues of Food-producing Animals. Drug Metab. Rev.* 22(6–8):585–906 (1990).

15. Suhren, G., A. Hoffmeister, J. Reichmuth, and W. Heeschen. Incidence of inhibitory substances in milk for consumption from various European countries. *Milchwissenschaft* 45:485–490 (1990).

16. Wilson, D.J., B.B. Norman, and C.E. Franti. Detection of antibiotic and sulfonamide residues in bob veal calf tissues: 967 cases (1987–1988). *J. Am. Vet. Med. Assoc.* 199:759–766 (1991).

17. Nagata, T., and M. Saeki. Simultaneous determination of five antibacterials in swine muscle by high performance liquid chromatography. *J. Liq. Chromatogr.* 14:2551–2561 (1991).

18. Teh, W.L., and A.S. Rigg. Possible penicillin allergy after eating chicken. *Lancet* 339:620 (1992).

19. Dewdney, J.M., L. Maes, J.P. Raynaud, et al. Risk assessment of antibiotic residues of β-lactams and macrolides in food products with regard to their immuno-allergic potential. *Food Chem. Toxicol.* 29:477–483 (1991).

20. Plakas, S.M., A. DePaola, and M.B. Moxey. *Bacillus stearothermophilus* disk assay for determining ampicillin residues in fish muscle. *J. Assoc. Off. Anal. Chem.* 74:910–912 (1991).

21. Meetschen, U., and M. Petz. Gaschromatographische analysenmethode für rückstände von sieben penicillinen in lebensmitteln tierischen ursprungs. *Z. Lebensm. Unters. Forsch.* 193:337–343 (1991).

22. Moats, W.A. High-performance liquid chromatographic determination of penicillin G, penicillin V and cloxacillin in beef and pork tissues. *J. Chromatogr.* 593:15–20 (1992).

23. Moats, W.A., and R. Malisch. Determination of cloxacillin and penicillin V in milk using an automated liquid chromatography cleanup. *J. AOAC Int.* 75:257–260 (1992).

24. Fletouris, D.J., J.E. Psomas, and A.J. Mantis. Determination of some monobasic penicillins in milk by ion-pair liquid chromatography. *J. Agric. Food Chem.* 40:617–621 (1992).

25. Voyksner, R.D., K.L. Tyczkowska, and A.L. Aronson. Development of analytical methods for some penicillins in bovine milk by ion-paired chromatography and confirmation by thermospray mass spectrometry. *J. Chromatogr.* 567:389–404 (1991).

26. Takahashi, Y., A.A. Said, M. Hashizume, and Y. Kido. Sulfadimethoxine residue in broiler-chicken skin. *J. Vet. Med. Sci.* 53:33–36 (1991).

27. Ellerbroek, L.I., and G. Steffen. Effect of pasteurization and fermentation on residues of sulphonamides in sausages. *Int. J. Food Sci. Technol.* 26:479–483 (1991).

28. Medina, M.B., R.A. Barford, M.S. Palumbo, and L.D. Rowe. Evaluation of commercial immunochemical assays for detection of sulfamethazine in milk. *J. Food Protect.* 55:284–290 (1992).

29. Hoffmeister, A., G. Suhren, and W. Heeschen. Enzyme immunoassays for screening sulfadimidine and sulfanilamide residues in milk. *Milchwissenschaft* 46:712–717 (1991).

30. Sheth, H.B., and P. Sporns. Development of a single ELISA for detection of sulfonamides. *J. Agric. Food Chem.* 39:1696–1700 (1991).

31. Agarwal, V.K. Detection of sulfamethazine residues in milk by high performance liquid chromatography. *J. Liq. Chromatogr.* 13:3531–3539 (1990).

32. Hoffmeister, A., G. Suhren, and W. Heeschen. High-pressure liquid chromatographic determination of sulfadimidine residues in milk—Incidence in consumer milk from various European countries. *Milchwissenschaft* 46:770–774 (1991).

33. Diserens, J.-M., C. Renaud-Bezot, and M.-C. Savoy-Perroud. Simplified determination of sulfonamides residues in milk, meat and eggs. *Dtsch. Lebensm.-Rundsch.* 87:205–211 (1991).

34. Van Poucke, L.S.G., G.C.I. Depourcq, and C.H. Van Peteghem. A quantitative method for the detection of sulfonamide residues in meat and milk samples with a high-performance thin-layer chromatographic method. *J. Chromatogr. Sci.* 29:423–427 (1991).

35. Takeda, N., and Y. Akiyama. Pre-column derivatization of sulfa drugs with fluorescamine and high-performance liquid chromatographic determination at their residual levels in meat and meat products. *J. Chromatogr.* 558:175–180 (1991).

36. Walker, L.V., J.R. Walsh, and J.J. Webber. High-performance liquid chromatography of sulphonamides extracted from bovine and porcine muscle by solid-phase disperson. *J. Chromatogr.* 595:179–184 (1992).

37. Pleasance, S., P. Blay, M.A. Quilliam, and G. O'Hara. Determination of sulfonamides by liquid chromatography, ultraviolet diode array detection and ionspray tandem mass spectrometry with application to cultured salmon flesh. *J. Chromatogr.* 558:155–173 (1991).

38. Ackermans, M.T., J.L. Beckers, F.M. Everaerts, et al. Determination of sulphonamides in pork meat extracts by capillary zone electrophoresis. *J. Chromatogr.* 596:101–109 (1992).

39. Anderson, K., and R.C. Bayer. A rapid method for determination of oxytetracycline levels in the American lobster. *Progressive Fish-Culturist* 53:26–28 (1991).

40. Walsh, J.R., L.V. Walker, and J.J. Webber. Determination of tetracyclines in bovine and porcine muscle by high-performance liquid chromatography using solid-phase extraction. *J. Chromatogr.* 596:211–216 (1992).

41. Aoyama, R.G., K.M. McErlane, H. Erber, et al. High-performance liquid chromatographic analysis of oxytetracycline in chinook salmon following administration of medicated feed. *J. Chromatogr.* 588:181–186 (1991).

42. Ueno, R., K. Uno, and T. Aoki. Determination of oxytetracycline in blood serum by high-performance liquid chromatography with direct injection. *J. Chromatogr.* 573:333–335 (1992).

43. Agasøster, T., and K.E. Rasmussen. Fully automated high-performance liquid chromatographic analysis of whole blood and plasma samples using on-line dialysis as sample preparation. Determination of oxytetracycline in bovine and salmon whole blood and plasma. *J. Chromatogr.* 570:99–107 (1991).

44. Kindack, D.G., A. Macintosh, M. Lebelle, et al. Separation, identification and determination of lumichrome in swine feed and kidney. *Food Addit. Contam.* 8:737–748 (1991).

45. Carlsson, A., and L. Björck. Liquid chromatography verification of tetracycline residues in milk and influence of milk fat lipolysis on the detection of antibiotic residues by microbial assays and the Charm II test. *J. Food Protect.* 55:374–378 (1992).

46. Kijak, P.J., M.G. Leadbetter, M.H. Thomas, and E.A. Thompson. Confirmation of oxytetracycline,

tetracycline and chlortetracycline residues in milk by particle beam liquid chromatography/mass spectrometry. *Biol. Mass Spectrom.* 20:789–795 (1991).

47. Matsuka, M., and J. Nakamura. Oxytetracycline residues in honey and royal jelly. *J. Apicultural Res.* 29:112–117 (1990).

48. Argauer, R.J., and E.W. Herbert, Jr. Stability of oxytetracycline residues in pollen pellets harvested from medicated research colonies of the honey bee. *Am. Bee J.* 132:332–334 (1992).

49. van der Heeft, E., A.P.J.M. de Jong, L.A. van Ginkel, et al. Conformation and quantification of chloramphenicol in cow's urine, muscle and eggs by electron capture negative ion chemical ionization gas chromatography/mass spectrometry. *Biol. Mass Spectrom.* 20:763–770 (1991).

50. Keukens, H.J., M.M.L. Aerts, W.A. Traag, et al. Analytical strategy for the regulatory control of residues of chloramphenicol in meat: preliminary studies in milk. *J. AOAC Int.* 75:245–256 (1992).

51. Samaha, I., L. Ellerbroek, A. Ebrecht, et al. Pharmacokinetics and tissue residues of flumequine in chickens. *Arch. Lebensmittelhyg.* 42:32–36 (1991).

52. Samaha, I., A. Ebrecht, L. Ellerbroek, et al. Flumequine residues in eggs. *Arch. Lebensmittelhyg.* 42:37–39 (1991).

53. Boon, J.H., J.M.F. Nouws, M.H.T. van der Heijden, et al. Disposition of flumequine in plasma of European eel (*Anguilla anguilla*) after a single intramuscular injection. *Aquaculture* 99:213–223 (1991).

54. Steffenak, I., V. Hormazabal, and M. Yndestad. Reservoir of quinolone residues in fish. *Food Addit. Contam.* 8:777–780 (1991).

55. Björklund, H.V., C.M.I. Råbergh, and G. Bylund. Residues of oxolinic acid and oxytetracycline in fish and sediments from fish farms. *Aquaculture* 97:85–96 (1991).

56. Larocque, L., M. Schnurr, S. Sved, and A. Weninger. Determination of oxolinic acid residues in salmon muscle tissue by liquid chromatography with fluorescence detection. *J. Assoc. Off. Anal. Chem.* 74:608–611 (1991).

57. Carignan, G., L. Larocque, and S. Sved. Assay of oxolinic acid residues in salmon muscle by liquid chromatography with fluorescence detection: interlaboratory study. *J. Assoc. Off. Anal. Chem.* 74:906–909 (1991).

58. Jarboe, H.H., and K.M. Kleinow. Matrix solid-phase dispersion isolation and liquid chromatographic determination of oxolinic acid in channel catfish (*Ictalurus punctatus*) muscle tissue. *J. AOAC Int.* 75:428–432 (1992).

59. Steffenak, I., V. Hormazabal, and M. Yndestad. Rapid assay for the simultaneous determination of residues of oxolinic acid and flumequine in fish tissues by high-performance liquid chromatography. *J. Liq. Chromatogr.* 14:61–70 (1991).

60. Hormazabal, V., A. Rogstad, I. Steffenak, and M. Yndestad. Rapid assay for monitoring residues of enrofloxacin and sarafloxacin in fish tissues by high performance liquid chromatography. *J. Liq. Chromatogr.* 14:1605–1614 (1991).

61. Lynch, M.J., F.R. Mosher, R.P. Schneider, et al. Determination of carbadox-related residues in swine liver by gas chromatography/mass spectrometry with ion trap detection. *J. Assoc. Off. Anal. Chem.* 74:611–618 (1991).

62. Nouws, J.F.M., and J. Laurensen. Postmortal degradation of furazolidone and furaltadone in edible tissues of calves. *Vet. Q.* 12:56–59 (1990).

63. Hoogenboom, L.A.P., M. van Kammen, M.C.J. Berghmans, et al. The use of pig hepatocytes to study the nature of protein-bound metabolites of furazolidone: a new analytical method for their detection. *Food Chem. Toxicol.* 29:321–328 (1991).

64. Soliman, M.M., A.R. Long, and S.A. Barker. Method for the isolation and liquid chromatographic determination of furazolidone in chicken muscle tissue. *J. Liq. Chromatogr.* 13:3327–3337 (1990).

65. Parks, O.W., and L.F. Kubena. Liquid chromatographic determination of incurred nitrofurazone residues in chicken tissues. *J. AOAC Int.* 75:261–262 (1992).

66. Matusik, J.E., M.G. Leadbetter, C.J. Barnes, and J.A. Sphon. Identification of dimetridazole, ipronidazole, and their alcohol metabolites in turkey tissues by thermospray tandem mass spectrometry. *J. Agric. Food Chem.* 40:439–443 (1992).

67. Carignan, G., K. Carrier, and S. Sved. The identification and assay of 2-methyl-5-nitroimidazole in pigs treated with dimetridazole. *Food Addit. Contam.* 8:467–475 (1991).

68. Assil, H.I., and P. Sporns. ELISA and HPLC methods for analysis of fumagillin and its decomposi-

tion products in honey. *J. Agric. Food Chem.* 39:2206–2213 (1991).

69. Moats, W.A. Determination of lincomycin in milk and tissues by reversed-phase liquid chromatography. *J. Agric. Food Chem.* 39:1812–1816 (1991).

70. Cravedi, J.P., M. Baradat, and G. Choubert. Digestibility, tissue distribution and depletion kinetics of [^{14}C]-virginiamycin and related factors fed to rainbow trout. *Aquaculture* 97:73–83 (1991).

71. Prabhu, S.V., T.A. Wehner, and P.C. Tway. Determination of ivermectin levels in swine tissues at the parts per billion level by liquid chromatography with fluorescence detection. *J. Agric. Food Chem.* 39:1468–1471 (1991).

72. Wyhowski de Bukanski, B., J.-M. Degroodt, and H. Beernaert. Determination of levamisole and thiabendazole in meat by HPLC and photodiode array detection. *Z. Lebensm. Unters. Forsch.* 193:545–547 (1991).

73. Facino, R.M., M. Carini, and P. Traldi. Application of collisionally activated decomposition mass-analysed ion kinetic energy spectrometry to a survey of sheep milk for benzimidazole residues in relation to withdrawal periods. *Biol. Mass Spectrom.* 21:195–201 (1992).

74. Schenck, F.J., S.A. Barker, and A.R. Long. Matrix solid phase dispersion (MSPD) isolation and liquid chromatographic determination of clorsulon in milk. *J. Liq. Chromatogr.* 14:2827–2834 (1991).

75. Multiple authors. *International Meeting on Anabolics. Ann. Rech. Vét.* 22(3):249–328 (1991).

76. Laganà, A., and A. Marino. General and selective isolation procedure for high-performance liquid chromatographic determination of anabolic steroids in tissues. *J. Chromatogr.* 588:89–98 (1991).

77. Bagnati, R., and R. Fanelli. Determination of 19-nortestosterone, testosterone and trenbolone by gas chromatography–negative-ion mass spectrometry after formation of the pentafluorobenzylcarboxymethoxime-trimethylsilyl derivatives. *J. Chromatogr.* 547:325–334 (1991).

78. Pulce, C., D. Lamaison, G. Keck, et al. Collective human food poisonings by clenbuterol residues in veal liver. *Vet. Hum. Toxicol.* 33:480–481 (1991).

79. World Health Organization. Foodborne clenbuterol poisoning. *Weekly Epidemiol. Rec.* 67:279–280 (1992).

80. Meyer, H.H.D., and L.M. Rinke. The pharmacokinetics and residues of clenbuterol in veal calves. *J. Anim. Sci.* 69:4538–4544 (1991).

81. Degand, G., A. Bernes-Duyckaerts, and G. Maghuin-Rogister. Determination of clenbuterol in bovine tissues and urine by enzyme immunoassay. *J. Agric. Food Chem.* 40:70–75 (1992).

82. Di Muccio, A., I. Camoni, L. Vergori, et al. Screening for coumatetralyl in soft drinks by solid-matrix extraction and high-performance liquid chromatography with diode-array detection. *J. Chromatogr.* 553:305–309 (1991).

83. Ferrer, A., and R. Cabral. Toxic epidemics caused by alimentary exposure to pesticides: a review. *Food Addit. Contam.* 8:755–776 (1991).

84. Lander, F., A. Brock, E. Pike, and K. Hinke. Chronic subclinical intake of dietary anticholinesterase agents during the spraying season. *Food Chem. Toxicol.* 30:37–40 (1992).

85. Garabrant, D.H., J. Held, B. Langholz, et al. DDT and related compounds and risk of pancreatic cancer. *J. Natl. Cancer Inst.* 84:764–771 (1992).

86. Rupa, D.S., P.P. Reddy, and O.S. Reddi. Clastogenic effect of pesticides in peripheral lymphocytes of cotton-field workers. *Mutat. Res.* 261:177–180 (1991).

87. Akhtar, M.H., S.U. Khan, and S. Kacew. Bioavailability of bound pesticide residues and potential toxicologic consequences. *Proc. Soc. Exp. Biol. Med.* 199:13–21 (1992).

88. Akay, M.T., G. Yilmazoglu, S. Yasacan, et al. Bioavailability and toxicological potential of wheat-bound pirimiphos-methyl residues in rats. *Xenobiotica* 22:293–302 (1992).

89. Food and Drug Administration Pesticide Residue Monitoring Program. Residues in foods. *J. Assoc. Off. Anal. Chem.* 74:121A–140A (1991).

90. Papadopoulou-Mourkidou, E. Postharvest-applied agrochemicals and their residues in fresh fruits and vegetables. *J. Assoc. Off. Anal. Chem.* 74:745–765 (1991).

91. Hotchkiss, J.H. Pesticide residue controls to ensure food safety. *Crit. Rev. Food Sci. Nutr.* 31:191–203 (1992).

92. Winter, C.K. Pesticide tolerances and their relevance as safety standards. *Reg. Toxicol. Pharmacol.* 15:137–150 (1992).

93. Hogendoorn, E.A., R. Hoogerbrugge, C.E. Goewie, et al. Development of a rational optimisation procedure for the automated sample clean-up with column switching in pesticide residue analysis. *J. Chromatogr.* 552:113–135 (1991).

94. Kadenczki, L., Z. Arpad, I. Gardi, et al. Column extraction of residues of several pesticides from fruits and vegetables: a simple multiresidue analysis method. *J. AOAC Int.* 75:53–61 (1992).

95. García, A.V., E.G. Pradas, J.M. Vidal, and A.A. López. Simple and efficient multiresidue screening method for analysis of nine halogen-containing pesticides on peppers and cucumbers by GLC-ECD. *J. Agric. Food Chem.* 39:2188–2191 (1991).

96. Hsu, R.C., I. Biggs, and N.K. Saini. Solid-phase extraction cleanup of halogenated organic pesticides. *J. Agric. Food Chem.* 39:1658–1666 (1991).

97. Long, A.R., M.D. Crouch, and S.A. Barker. Multiresidue matrix solid phase dispersion (MSPD) extraction and gas chromatographic screening of nine chlorinated pesticides in catfish (*Ictalurus punctatus*) muscle tissue. *J. Assoc. Off. Anal. Chem.* 74:667–670 (1991).

98. Hopper, M.L., and J.W. King. Enhanced supercritical fluid carbon dioxide extraction of pesticides from foods using pelletized diatomaceous earth. *J. Assoc. Off. Anal. Chem.* 74:661–666 (1991).

99. France, J.E., and J.W. King. Supercritical fluid extraction/enzyme assay: a novel technique to screen for pesticide residues in meat products. *J. Assoc. Off. Anal. Chem.* 74:1013–1016 (1991).

100. Mortimer, R.D., and B.A. Dawson. Using ^{19}F NMR for trace analysis of fluorinated pesticides in food products. *J. Agric. Food Chem.* 39:1781–1785 (1991).

101. Tuinstra, L.G.M.T., F.R. Povel, and A.H. Roos. Multi-matrix–multi-pesticide method for agricultural products. *J. Chromatogr.* 552:259–264 (1991).

102. Hsu, J.P., H.J. Schattenberg III, and M.M. Garza. Fast turnaround multiresidue screen for pesticides in produce. *J. Assoc. Off. Anal. Chem.* 74:886–892 (1991).

103. Leoni, V., A.M. Caricchia, and S. Chiavarini. Multiresidue method for quantitation of organophosphorus pesticides in vegetable and animal foods. *J. AOAC Int.* 75:511–518 (1992).

104. Hopper, M.L. Analysis of organochlorine pesticide residues using simultaneous injection of two capillary columns with electron capture and electrolytic conductivity detectors. *J. Assoc. Off. Anal. Chem.* 74:974–981 (1991).

105. Ting, K.-C., and P. Kho. GC/MIP/AED method for pesticide residue determination in fruits and vegetables. *J. Assoc. Off. Anal. Chem.* 74:991–998 (1991).

106. Lee, S.M., and P.L. Wylie. Comparison of the atomic emission detector to other element-selective detectors for the gas chromatographic analysis of pesticide residues. *J. Agric. Food Chem.* 39:2192–2199 (1991).

107. Gansewendt, B., U. Foest, D. Xu, et al. Formation of DNA adducts in F-344 rats after oral administration or inhalation of [^{14}C]methyl bromide. *Food Chem. Toxicol.* 29:557–563 (1991).

108. Fallico, R., and M. Ferrante. Exposure to inorganic bromides from greenhouse crops where methyl bromide was applied for soil fumigation. *Zbl. Hyg.* 191:555–562 (1991).

109. Scheffrahn, R.H., L. Bodalbhai, and N.-Y. Su. Residues of methyl bromide and sulfuryl fluoride in manufacturer-packaged household foods following fumigation. *Bull. Environ. Contam. Toxicol.* 48:821–827 (1992).

110. Ford, J.H., M.G. Legendre, D.L. Ladner, et al. Automated closed-system headspace determination of methyl bromide in a variety of raw and processed nuts. *J. AOAC Int.* 75:328–333 (1992).

111. Kulkarni, A.P., J. Edwards, and I.S. Richards. Metabolism of 1,2-dibromoethane in the human fetal liver. *Gen. Pharmacol.* 23:1–5 (1992).

112. Chhabra, R.S., S. Eustis, J.K. Haseman, et al. Comparitive carcinogenicity of ethylene thiourea with or without perinatal exposure in rats and mice. *Fund. Appl. Toxicol.* 18:405–417 (1992).

113. Kurttio, P., K. Savolainen, A. Naukkarinen, et al. Urinary excretion of ethylenethiourea and kidney morphology in rats after continuous oral exposure to nabam or ethylenethiourea. *Arch. Toxicol.* 65:381–385 (1991).

114. Gonzalez, A.R., A. Mauromoustakos, E.R. Elkins, and E.S. Kim. Removal of carbamate residues from leafy greens with water and detergent solutions. *J. Environ. Sci. Health* A25:1009–1017 (1990).

115. Lehotay, J., E. Brandsteterová, and D. Oktavec. High-performance liquid chromatographic determination of ethylenethiourea in food. *J. Liq. Chromatogr.* 15:525–534 (1992).

116.   Patsakos, P.G., K. Liapis, G.E. Miliadis, and K. Zafiriou. Mancozeb residues on field sprayed apricots. *Bull. Environ. Contam. Toxicol.* 48:756–761 (1992).

117.   Doerge, D.R., and C.J. Miles. Determination of ethylenethiourea in crops using particle beam liquid chromatography/mass spectrometry. *Anal. Chem.* 63:1999–2001 (1991).

118.   Friar, P.M.K., and S.L. Reynolds. The effects of microwave-baking and oven-baking on thiabendazole residues in potatoes. *Food Addit. Contam.* 8:617–626 (1991).

119.   Corti, P., E. Dreassi, N. Politi, and C. Aprea. Comparison of an HPTLC and an HPLC procedure for the determination of chlorpropham, propham and thiabendazole residues in potatoes. *Food Addit. Contam.* 8:607–616 (1991).

120.   Motohashi, N., H. Nagashima, and R. Meyer. High-performance liquid chromatography of fungicides in citrus fruits. *J. Liq. Chromatogr.* 14:3591–3602 (1991).

121.   Bushway, R.J., H.L. Hurst, J. Kugabalasooriar, and L.B. Perkins. Determination of carbendazim in blueberries by reversed-phase high-performance liquid chromatography. *J. Chromatogr.* 587:321–324 (1991).

122.   Bushway, R.J., J. Kugabalasooriar, L.B. Perkins, et al. Determination of methyl 2-benzimidazolecarbamate in blueberries by competitive inhibition enzyme immunoassay. *J. AOAC Int.* 75:323–327 (1992).

123.   Gilvydis, D.M., and S.M. Walters. Gas chromatographic determination of captan, folpet, and captafol residues in tomatoes, cucumbers, and apples using a wide-bore capillary column: interlaboratory study. *J. Assoc. Off. Anal. Chem.* 74:830–835 (1991).

124.   Quest, J.A., K.L. Hamernik, R. Engler, et al. Evaluation of the carcinogenic potential of pesticides. 3. Aliette. *Reg. Toxicol. Pharmacol.* 14:3–11 (1991).

125.   Chichila, T.M., and S.M. Walters. Liquid chromatographic determination of paraquat and diquat in crops using a silica column with aqueous ionic mobile phase. *J. Assoc. Off. Anal. Chem.* 74:961–967 (1991).

126.   Gaynor, J.D., D.C. MacTavish, and A.S. Hamill. GC/MSD detection of the metabolic residues of metolachlor in tomato fruit. *Chromatographia* 33:147–150 (1992).

127.   Wigfield, Y.Y., and M. Lanouette. Residue analysis of glyphosate and its principal metabolite in certain cereals, oilseeds, and pulses by liquid chromatography and postcolumn fluorescence detection. *J. Assoc. Off. Anal. Chem.* 74:842–847 (1991).

128.   Szeto, S.Y., and P.M. Price. High-performance liquid chromatography method for the determination of dinoseb: application to the analysis of residues in raspberries. *J. Agric. Food Chem.* 39:1614–1617 (1991).

129.   Drake, S.R., T.A. Eisele, and J.D. Baranowski. Daminozide residue present in apple fruit after long and short term exposure. *J. Food Safety* 11:247–253 (1991).

130.   Pylypiw, H.M., Jr., G.W. Harrington, R. Kozeniauskas, and D. Diaz. The formation of N-nitrosodimethylamine and N-nitrodimethylamine from the plant growth regulator daminozide (Alar). *J. Food Protect.* 55:218–219 (1992).

131.   Faughnan, K.T., and M.A. Woodruff. Modified gas chromatographic/mass spectrometric method for determination of daminozide in high protein food products. *J. Assoc. Off. Anal. Chem.* 74:682–692 (1991).

132.   Vadukul, N.K. Determination of maleic hydrazide in onions and potatoes using solid-phase extraction and anion-exchange high-performance liquid chromatography. *Analyst* 116:1369–1371 (1991).

133.   Galoux, M., M. De Proft, and A. Bernes. Aldicarb in edible potato crops: agronomic interest and residues in tubers during growth and after cooking. *J. Agric. Food Chem.* 40:139–141 (1992).

134.   Skerritt, J.H., A.S. Hill, H.L. Beasley, et al. Enzyme-linked immunosorbent assay for quantitation of organophosphate pesticides: fenitrothion, chlorpyrifos-methyl, and pirimiphos-methyl in wheat grain and flour-milling fractions. *J. AOAC Int.* 75:519–528 (1992).

135.   Ahmed, M.T., M. Morsy, and S. Awny. Residues of pirmiphos-methyl on lettuce and endive. *Dtsch. Lebensm.-Rundsch.* 88:150–151 (1992).

136.   Prabhu, S.V., R.J. Varsolona, T.A. Wehner, et al. Rapid and sensitive high-performance liquid chromatographic method for the quantitation of abamectin and its delta 8,9-isomer. *J. Agric. Food Chem.* 40:622–625 (1992).

137.   Bagheri, H., and C.S. Creaser. Determination of carbaryl and 1-naphthol in English apples and strawberries by combined gas chromatography–fluorescence spectrometry. *J. Chromatogr.* 547:345–353 (1991).

138.   Cabras, P., M. Melis, C. Tuberoso, et al. High-performance liquid chromatographic determination of

fenbutatin oxide and its persistence in peaches and nectarines. *J. Agric. Food Chem.* 40:901–903 (1992).

139.   Aly, M.A.S., and W.C. Dauterman. Bioavailability, biological activity and characterization of bound residues of fenvalerate in wheat. *J. Environ. Sci. Health* B27:223–233 (1992).

140.   Boyer, A.C., P.W. Lee, and J.C. Potter. Characterization of fenvalerate residues in dairy cattle and poultry. *J. Agric. Food Chem.* 40:914–918 (1992).

141.   Akhtar, M.H., C. Danis, H.L. Trenholm, and K.E. Hartin. Deltamethrin residues in milk and tissues of lactating dairy cows. *J. Environ. Sci. Health* B27:235–253 (1992).

142.   Di Muccio, A., A. Ausili, R. Dommarco, et al. Solid-matrix partition for separation of organochlorine pesticide residues from fatty materials. *J. Chromatogr.* 552:241–247 (1991).

143.   France, J.E., J.W. King, and J.M. Snyder. Supercritical fluid-based cleanup technique for the separation of organochlorine pesticides from fats. *J. Agric. Food Chem.* 39:1871–1874 (1991).

144.   Prapamontol, T., and D. Stevenson. Rapid method for the determination of organochlorine pesticides in milk. *J. Chromatogr.* 552:249–257 (1991).

145.   Kim-Kang, H. Volatiles in packaging materials. *Crit. Rev. Food Sci. Nutr.* 29:255–271 (1990).

146.   Ema, M., T. Itami, and H. Kawasaki. Effect of period of exposure on the developmental toxicity of butyl benzyl phthalate in rats. *J. Appl. Toxicol.* 12:57–61 (1992).

147.   Ema, M., T. Itami, and H. Kawasaki. Embryolethality and teratogenicity of butyl benzyl phthalate in rats. *J. Appl. Toxicol.* 12:179–183 (1992).

148.   Thomas, W.C., L.F. McGrath, K.A. Baarson, et al. Subchronic oral toxicity of cellulose acetate in rats. *Food Chem. Toxicol.* 29:453–458 (1991).

149.   Til, H.P., V.J. Feron, and H.R. Immel. Lifetime (149-week) oral carcinogenicity study of vinyl chloride in rats. *Food Chem. Toxicol.* 29:713–718 (1991).

150.   Sugita, T., H. Ishiwata, and A. Maekawa. Intestinal absorption and urinary excretion of melamine in male Wistar rats. *J. Food Hyg. Soc. Japan* 32:439–443 (1991).

151.   Ishiwata, H., T. Sugita, and M. Takeda. Effect of long-term use of melamine tableware on the release of monomers and some other changes. *J. Food Hyg. Soc. Japan* 33:52–57 (1992).

152.   Petersen, J.H. Survey of di-(2-ethylhexyl)-phthalate plasticizer contamination of retail Danish milks. *Food Addit. Contam.* 8:701–706 (1991).

153.   Castle, L., A.J. Mercer, and J. Gilbert. Migration from plasticized films into foods. 5. Identification of individual species in a polymeric plasticizer and their migration into foods. *Food Addit. Contam.* 8:565–576 (1991).

154.   Grob, K., A. Artho, M. Biedermann, et al. Batching oils on sisal bags used for packaging foods: analysis by coupled LC/GC. *J. AOAC Int.* 75:283–287 (1992).

155.   Grob, K., M. Biedermann, A. Artho, and J. Egli. Food contamination by hydrocarbons from packaging materials determined by coupled LC-GC. *Z. Lebensm. Unters. Forsch.* 193:213–219 (1991).

156.   Castle, L., M. Kelly, and J. Gilbert. Migration of mineral hydrocarbons into foods. 1. Polystyrene containers for hot and cold beverages. *Food Addit. Contam.* 8:693–700 (1991).

157.   Tan, S., T. Tatsuno, and T. Okada. Gas chromatographic/mass spectrometric determination of α-methylstyrene in styrene-based polymers and food simulants. *J. Assoc. Off. Anal. Chem.* 74:815–818 (1991).

158.   Jickells, S.M., J.W. Gramshaw, L. Castle, and J. Gilbert. The effect of microwave energy on specific migration from food contact plastics. *Food Addit. Contam.* 9:19–27 (1992).

159.   Begley, T.H., J.E. Biles, and H.C. Hollifield. Migration of an epoxy adhesive compound into a food-simulating liquid and food from microwave susceptor packaging. *J. Agric. Food Chem.* 39:1944–1945 (1991).

160.   Losada, P.P., P.L. Mahía, L.V. Odériz, et al. Sensitive and rapid reversed-phase liquid chromatography–fluorescence method for determining bisphenol A diglycidyl ether in aqueous-based food simulants. *J. Assoc. Off. Anal. Chem.* 74:925–928 (1991).

161.   Sivaswamy, S.N., B. Balachandran, and S. Balanehru. South Indian foods: contaminants and their effects. *Bull. Environ. Contam. Toxicol.* 47:251–260 (1991).

162.   Wild, S.R., and K.C. Jones. Polynuclear aromatic hydrocarbon uptake by carrots grown in sludge-amended soil. *J. Environ. Qual.* 21:217–225 (1992).

163.   Mothershead, R.F., II, R.C. Hale, and J. Greaves. Xenobiotic compounds in blue crabs from a highly

contaminated urban subestuary. *Environ. Toxicol. Chem.* 10:1341–1349 (1991).

164. Tanacredi, J.T., and R.R. Cardenas. Biodepuration of polynuclear aromatic hydrocarbons from a bivalve mollusc, *Mercenaria mercenaria* L. *Environ. Sci. Technol.* 25:1453–1461 (1991).

165. Dennis, M.J., R.C. Massey, G. Cripps, et al. Factors affecting the polycyclic aromatic hydrocarbon content of creals, fats and other food products. *Food Addit. Contam.* 8:517–530 (1991).

166. Hattemer-Frey, H.A., and C. C. Travis. Benzo-a-pyrene: environmental partitioning and human exposure. *Toxicol. Indust. Health* 7:141–157 (1991).

167. Buckley, T.J., and P.J. Lioy. An examination of the time course from human dietary exposure to polycyclic aromatic hydrocarbons to urinary elimination of 1-hydroxypyrene. *Br. J. Indust. Med.* 49:113–124 (1992).

168. Barnea, E.R., and R. Shurtz-Swirski. Modification of pulsatile human chorionic gonadotrophin secretion in first trimester placental explants induced by polycyclic aromatic hydrocarbons. *Hum. Reprod.* 7:305–310 (1992).

169. Holz, O., T. Krause, and H.W. Rüdiger. Differences in DNA adduct formation between monocytes and lymphocytes after in vivo incubation with benzo[a]pyrene. *Carcinogenesis* 12:2181–2183 (1991).

170. Safe, S. Polychlorinated dibenzo-*p*-dioxins and related compounds: sources, environmental distribution and risk assessment. *Environ. Carcinogen. Ecotoxicol. Rev.* C9:261–302 (1991).

171. Ahlborg, U., R.E. Clement, J. Duinker, et al. (eds.). Chlorinated dioxins and related compounds 1990–Part 1. *Chemosphere* 23(8–10):957–1550 (1991).

172. Ahlborg, U., R.E. Clement, J. Duinker, et al. (eds.). Chlorinated dioxins and related compounds 1990–Part 2. *Chemosphere* 23(11–12):1551–1966 (1991).

173. Phillips, L.J., and G.F. Birchard. Regional variations in human toxics exposure in the USA: an analysis based on the National Human Adipose Tissue Survey. *Arch. Environ. Contam. Toxicol.* 21:159–168 (1991).

174. Wagner, S.L., L.R. Durand, R.D. Inman, et al. Residues of pentachlorophenol and other chlorinated contaminants in human tissues: analysis by electron capture gas chromatography and electron capture negative ion mass spectrometry. *Arch. Environ. Contam. Toxicol.* 21:596–606 (1991).

175. Ferrer, A., M.A. Bona, M. Castellano, et al. Organochlorine residues in human adipose tissue of the population of Zaragoza (Spain). *Bull. Environ. Contam. Toxicol.* 48:561–566 (1992).

176. Hovinga, M.E., M.F. Sowers, and H.E.B. Humphrey. Historical changes in serum PCB and DDT levels in an environmentally-exposed cohort. *Arch. Environ. Contam. Toxicol.* 22:362–366 (1992).

177. Mussalo-Rauhamaa, H. Partitioning and levels of neutral organochlorine compounds in human serum, blood cells, and adipose and liver tissue. *Sci. Total Environ.* 103:159–175 (1991).

178. Mes, J. Organochlorine residues in human blood and biopsy fat and their relationship. *Bull. Environ. Contam. Toxicol.* 48:815–820 (1992).

179. Sasaki, K., T. Ishizaka, T. Suzuki, et al. Organochlorine chemicals in skin lipids as an index of their accumulation in the human body. *Arch. Environ. Contam. Toxicol.* 21:190–194 (1991).

180. Sasaki, K., Y. Kawasaki, K. Sekita, et al. Disposition of β-hexachlorocyclohexane, *p,p′*-DDT, and *trans*-chlordane administered subcutaneously to monkeys (*Macaca fascicularis*). *Arch. Environ. Contam. Toxicol.* 22:25–29 (1992).

181. Kannan, K., S. Tanabe, H.T. Quynh, et al. Residue pattern and dietary intake of persistent organochlorine compounds in foodstuffs from Vietnam. *Arch. Environ. Contam. Toxicol.* 22:367–374 (1992).

182. Fricker, C., and J.K. Hardy. Characterization of commercially available coffee filter papers. *J. Environ. Sci. Health* A25:927–936 (1990).

183. Borlakoglu, J.T., and K.D. Haegele. Comparative aspects on the bioaccumulation, metabolism and toxicity with PCBs. *Comp. Biochem. Physiol.* 100C:327–338 (1991).

184. Lang, V. Polychlorinated biphenyls in the environment. *J. Chromatogr.* 595:1–43 (1992).

185. Swain, W.R. Effects of organochlorine chemicals on the reproductive outcome of humans who consumed contaminated Great Lakes fish: an epidemiological consideration. *J. Toxicol. Environ. Health* 33:587–639 (1991).

186. Gladen, B.C., and W.J. Rogan. Effects of perinatal polychlorinated biphenyls and dichlorodiphenyl dichloroethene on later development. *J. Pediatr.* 119:58–63 (1991).

187. Falck, F., Jr., A. Ricci, Jr., M.S. Wolff, et al. Pesticides and polychlorinated biphenyl residues in human breast lipids and their relation to breast cancer. *Arch. Environ. Health* 47:143–146 (1992).

188. Kalina, I., R.J. Srám, H. Konecná, and A. Ondrusseková. Cytogenetic analysis of peripheral blood lymphocytes in workers occupationally exposed to polychlorinated biphenyls. *Teratogen. Carcinogen. Mutagen.* 11:77–82 (1991).

189. Brown, J.F., Jr., R.W. Lawton, M.R. Ross, and J. Feingold. Assessing the human health effects of PCBs. *Chemosphere* 23:1811–1815 (1991).

190. Williams, D.T., and G.L. LeBel. Coplanar polychlorinated biphenyl residues in human adipose tissue samples from Ontario municipalities. *Chemosphere* 22:1019–1028 (1991).

191. Dewailly, E., J.P. Weber, S. Gingras, and C. Laliberté. Coplanar PCBs in human milk in the province of Québec, Canada: are they more toxic than dioxin for breast fed infants? *Bull. Environ. Contam. Toxicol.* 47:491–498 (1991).

192. Bachour, G., S. Georgii, I. Elmadfa, and H. Brunn. "Dioxin-analoge" PCB-kongenere in frauenmilch. *Dtsch. Lebensm.-Rundsch.* 88:18–19 (1992).

193. Hong, C.-S., B. Bush, J. Xiao, and E.F. Fitzgerald. Isolation and determination of mono-ortho and non-ortho substituted PCBs (coplanar PCBs) in human milk by HPLC porous graphitic carbon and GC/ECD. *Chemosphere* 24:465–473 (1992).

194. Golub, M.S., J.M. Donald, and J.A. Reyes. Reproductive toxicity of commercial PCB mixtures: LOAELs and NOAELs from animal studies. *Environ. Health Perspect.* 94:245–253 (1991).

195. Poul, J.-M. Time course reversibility of liver and blood changes induced in weanling rats after polychlorinated biphenyl exposure during lactation. *Arch. Environ. Contam. Toxicol.* 21:528–535 (1991).

196. Poul, J.M. Long term effects of PCBs (phenoclor DP5) on rat microsomal enzymes, liver, and blood lipids after peri- and postnatal exposure. *Bull. Environ. Contam. Toxicol.* 48:313–320 (1992).

197. Lilienthal, H., and G. Winneke. Sensitive periods for behavioral toxicity of polychlorinated biphenyls: determination by cross-fostering in rats. *Fund. Appl. Toxicol.* 17:368–375 (1991).

198. Eriksson, P., U. Lundkvist, and A. Fredriksson. Neonatal exposure to 3,3',4,4'-tetrachlorobiphenyl: changes in spontaneous behaviour and cholinergic muscarinic receptors in the adult mouse. *Toxicology* 69:27–34 (1991).

199. Shain, W., B. Bush, and R. Seegal. Neurotoxicity of polychlorinated biphenyls: structure–activity relationship of individual congeners. *Toxicol. Appl. Pharmacol.* 111:33–42 (1991).

200. Seegal, R.F., B. Bush, and W. Shain. Neurotoxicology of ortho-substituted polychlorinated biphenyls. *Chemosphere* 23:1941–1949 (1991).

201. Buchmann, A., S. Ziegler, A. Wolf, et al. Effects of polychlorinated biphenyls in rat liver: correlation between primary subcellular effects and promoting activity. *Toxicol. Appl. Pharmacol.* 111:454–468 (1991).

202. Hemming, H., L. Wärngård, and U.G. Ahlborg. Inhibition of dye transfer in rat liver WB cell culture by polychlorinated biphenyls. *Pharmacol. Toxicol.* 69:416–420 (1991).

203. Jenke, H.-S., G. Michel, S. Hornhardt, and J. Berndt. Protooncogene expression in rat liver by polychlorinated biphenyls (PCB). *Xenobiotica* 21:945–960 (1991).

204. Tryphonas, H., M.I. Luster, K.L. White, Jr., et al. Effects of PCB (Aroclor® 1254) on non-specific immune parameters in rhesus (*Macaca mulatta*) monkeys. *Int. J. Immunopharmacol.* 13:639–648 (1991).

205. Meserve, L.A., B.A. Murray, and J.A. Landis. Influence of maternal ingestion of Aroclor 1254® (PCB) or FireMaster BP-6® on unstimulated and stimulated corticosterone levels in young rats. *Bull. Environ. Contam. Toxicol.* 48:715–720 (1992).

206. Brouwer, A. Role of biotransformation in PCB-induced alterations in vitamin A and thyroid hormone metabolism in laboratory and wildlife species. *Biochem. Soc. Trans.* 19:731–737 (1991).

207. Jan, J., and M. Adamic. Polychlorinated biphenyl residues in foods from a contaminated region of Yugoslavia. *Food Addit. Contam.* 8:505–512 (1991).

208. Kipcic, D., and J. Vukusic. Polychlorinated biphenyls in fresh and canned fish from the Central Adriatic. *Food Addit. Contam.* 8:501–504 (1991).

209. Falandysz, J., N. Yamashita, S. Tanabe, and R. Tatsukawa. Isomer-specific analysis of PCBs including toxic coplanar isomers in canned cod livers commercially processed in Poland. *Z. Lebensm. Unters. Forsch.* 194:120–123 (1992).

210. Hong, C.-S., B. Bush, and J. Xiao. Coplanar PCBs in fish and mussels from marine and estuarine waters of New York State. *Ecotoxicol. Environ. Safety* 23:118–131 (1992).

211. Grove, H.-H., H. Schmidt, and H.-O. Knöppler. Zum gehalt an polychlorierten biphenylen (PCB) bei in-vivo-proben und im fleisch von rindern. *Arch. Lebensmittelhyg.* 43:38–41 (1992).

212. Ye, Q., R.K. Puri, S. Kapila, et al. Studies on uptake of PCBs by *Hordeum vulgare* (barley) and *Lycopersicon esculentum* (tomato). *Chemosphere* 23:1397–1406 (1991).

213. Johnson, E.S. Human exposure to 2,3,7,8-TCDD and risk of cancer. *Crit. Rev. Toxicol.* 21:451–463 (1992).

214. Manz, A., J. Berger, J.H. Dwyer, et al. Cancer mortality among workers in chemical plant contaminated with dioxin. *Lancet* 338:959–964 (1991).

215. Tarone, R.E., H.M. Hayes, R.N. Hoover, et al. Service in Vietnam and risk of testicular cancer. *J. Natl. Cancer Inst.* 83:1497–1499 (1991).

216. Saracci, R., M. Kogevinas, P.-A. Bertazzi, et al. Cancer mortality in workers exposed to chlorophenoxy herbicides and chlorophenols. *Lancet* 338:1027–1032 (1991).

217. Calvert, G.M., R.W. Hornung, M.H. Sweeney, et al. Hepatic and gastrointestinal effects in an occupational cohort exposed to 2,3,7,8-tetrachlorodibenzo-para-dioxin. *JAMA* 267:2209–2214 (1992).

218. Bertazzi, P.A., C. Zocchetti, A.C. Pesatori, et al. Mortality of a young population after accidental exposure to 2,3,7,8-tetrachlorodibenzodioxin. *Int. J. Epidemiol.* 21:118–123 (1992).

219. Hoffman, R.E. Recent studies of the human immunotoxic effects of 2,3,7,8-tetrachlorodibenzo-*p*-dioxin. In *Clinical Immunotoxicology.* D.S. Newcombe, N.R. Rose, and J.C. Bloom, eds. New York, Raven Press, Ltd. Pp. 339–347 (1992).

220. Koppe, J.G., H.J. Pluim, K. Olie, and J. van Wijnen. Breast milk, dioxins and the possible effects on the health of newborn infants. *Sci. Total Environ.* 106:33–41 (1991).

221. Pluim, H.J., J.G. Koppe, K. Olie, et al. Effects of dioxins on thyroid function in newborn babies. *Lancet* 339:1303 (1992).

222. Lipp, H.-P., D. Schrenk, T. Wiesmüller, et al. Assessment of biological activities of mixtures of polychlorinated dibenzo-p-dioxins (PCDDs) and their con-stituents in human HepG2 cells. *Arch. Toxicol.* 66:220–223 (1992).

223. Harper, P.A., R.D. Prokipcak, L.E. Bush, et al. Detection and characterization of the Ah receptor for 2,3,7,8-tetrachlorodibenzo-*p*-dioxin in the human colon adenocarcinoma cell line LS180. *Arch. Biochem. Biophys.* 290:27–36 (1991).

224. Keenan, R.E., D.J. Paustenbach, R.J. Wenning, and A.H. Parsons. Pathology reevaluation of the Kociba et al. (1978) bioassay of 2,3,7,8-TCDD: implications for risk assessment. *J. Toxicol. Environ. Health* 34:279–296 (1991).

225. Landers, J.P., and N.J. Bunce. The *Ah* receptor and the mechanism of dioxin toxicity. *Biochem. J.* 276:273–287 (1991).

226. Sutter, T.R., K. Guzman, K.M. Dold, and W.F. Greenlee. Targets for dioxin: genes for plasminogen activator inhibitor–2 and interleukin-1β. *Science* 254:415–418 (1991).

227. Wu, L., and J.P. Whitlock, Jr. Mechanism of dioxin action: Ah receptor-mediated increase in promoter accessibility *in vivo*. *Proc. Natl. Acad. Sci. USA* 89:4811–4815 (1992).

228. Holsapple, M.P., D.L. Morris, S.C. Wood, and N.K. Snyder. 2,3,7,8-Tetrachlorodibenzo-*p*-dioxin-induced changes in immunocompetence: possible mechanisms. *Annu. Rev. Pharmacol. Toxicol.* 31:73–100 (1991).

229. Holsapple, M.P., N.K. Snyder, S.C. Wood, and D.L. Morris. A review of 2,3,7,8-tetrachlorodibenzo-*p*-dioxin-induced changes in immunocompetence: 1991 update. *Toxicology* 69:219–255 (1991).

230. Lundberg, K., L. Dencker, and K.-O. Grönvik. 2,3,7,8-Tetrachlorodibenzo-*p*-dioxin (TCDD) inhibits the activation of antigen-specific T-cells in mice. *Int. J. Immunopharmacol.* 14:699–705 (1992).

231. Tomar, R.S., and N.I. Kerkvliet. Reduced T-helper cell function in mice exposed to 2,3,7,8-tetrachlorodibenzo-*p*-dioxin (TCDD). *Toxicol. Lett.* 57:55–64 (1991).

232. Funseth, E., and N.-G. Ilbäck. Effects of 2,3,7,8-tetrachlorodibenzo-*p*-dioxin on blood and spleen natural killer (NK) cell activity in the mouse. *Toxicol. Lett.* 60:247–256 (1992).

233. Morris, D.L., N.K. Snyder, V. Gokani, et al. Enhanced suppression of humoral immunity in DBA/2 mice following subchronic exposure to 2,3,7,8-

tetrachlorodibenzo-*p*-dioxin (TCDD). *Toxicol. Appl. Pharmacol.* 112:128–132 (1992).

234. Safe, S., B. Astroff, M. Harris, et al. 2,3,7,8-Tetrachlorodibenzo-*p*-dioxin (TCDD) and related compounds as antioestrogens: characterization and mechanism of action. *Pharmacol. Toxicol.* 69:400–409 (1991).

235. DeVito, M.J., T. Thomas, E. Martin, et al. Antiestrogenic action of 2,3,7,8-tetrachlorodibenzo-*p*-dioxin: tissue specific regulation of estrogen receptor in CD1 mice. *Toxicol. Appl. Pharmacol.* 113:284–292 (1992).

236. Moore, R.W., C.W. Jefcoate, and R.E. Peterson. 2,3,7,8-Tetrachlorodibenzo-*p*-dioxin inhibits steroidogenesis in the rat testis by inhibiting the mobilization of cholesterol to cytochrome $P450_{scc}$. *Toxicol. Appl. Pharmacol.* 109:85–97 (1991).

237. Mably, T.A., R.W. Moore, and R.E. Peterson. *In utero* and lactational exposure of male rats to 2,3,7,8-tetrachlorodibenzo-*p*-dioxin. 1. Effects on androgenic status. *Toxicol. Appl. Pharmacol.* 114:97–107 (1992).

238. Mably, T.A., R.W. Moore, R.W. Goy, and R.E. Peterson. *In utero* and lactational exposure of male rats to 2,3,7,8-tetrachlorodibenzo-*p*-dioxin. 2. Effects on sexual behavior and the regulation of luteinizing hormone secretion in adulthood. *Toxicol. Appl. Pharmacol.* 114:108–117 (1992).

239. Mably, T.A., D.L. Bjerke, R.W. Moore, et al. *In utero* and lactational exposure of male rats to 2,3,7,8-tetrachlorodibenzo-*p*-dioxin. 3. Effects on spermatogenesis and reproductive capability. *Toxicol. Appl. Pharmacol.* 114:118–126 (1992).

240. Frommberger, R. Polychlorinated dibenzo-p-dioxins and polychlorinated dibenzofurans in fish from south-west Germany: River Rhine and Neckar. *Chemosphere* 22:29–38 (1991).

241. Hanberg, A., M. Ståhlberg, A. Georgellis, et al. Swedish dioxin survey: evaluation of the H-4-II E bioassay for screening environmental samples for dioxinlike enzyme induction. *Pharmacol. Toxicol.* 69:442–449 (1991).

242. Huestis, S.Y., and D.B. Sergeant. Removal of chlorinated diphenyl ether interferences for analyses of PCDDs and PCDFs in fish. *Chemosphere* 24:537–545 (1992).

243. Glidden, R.M., P.J. Brown, R.A. Sittig, et al. Determination of 2,3,7,8-tetrachlorodibenzo-p-dioxin and 2,3,7,8-tetrachlorodibenzofuran in cow's milk. *Chemosphere* 20:1619–1624 (1990).

244. Ryan, J.J., C. Shewchuk, B.P.-Y. Lau, and W.F. Sun. Polychlorinated dibenzo-*p*-dioxins and polychlorinated dibenzofurans in Canadian bleached paperboard milk containers (1988–1989) and their transfer to fluid milk. *J. Agric. Food Chem.* 40:919–923 (1992).

245. Rappe, C., G. Lindström, B. Glas, et al. Levels of PCDDs and PCDFs in milk cartons and in commercial milk. *Chemosphere* 20:1649–1656 (1990).

246. van Rhijn, J.A., W.A. Traag, W. Kulik, and L.G.M.Th. Tuinstra. Automated clean-up procedure for the gas chromatographic–high-resolution mass spectrometric determination of polychlorinated dibenzo-*p*-dioxins and dibenzofurans in milk. *J. Chromatogr.* 595:289–299 (1992).

247. Rappe, C., P.-A. Bergqvist, L.-O. Kjeller, et al. Levels and patterns of PCDD and PCDF contamination in fish, crabs, and lobsters from Newark Bay and the New York Bight. *Chemosphere* 22:239–266 (1991).

248. Lambert, G.H., D.A. Schoeller, H.E.B. Humphrey, et al. The caffeine breath test and caffeine urinary metabolite ratios in the Michigan cohort exposure to polybrominated biphenyls: a preliminary study. *Environ. Health Perspect.* 89:175–181 (1990).

249. Becker, M., T. Phillips, and S. Safe. Polychlorinated diphenyl ethers—a review. *Toxicol. Environ. Chem.* 33:189–200 (1991).

250. Murk, A.J., J.H.J. van den Berg, J.H. Koeman, and A. Brouwer. The toxicity of tetrachlorobenzyltoluenes (Ugilec 141) and polychlorobiphenyls (Aroclor 1254 and PCB-77) compared in Ah-responsive and Ah-nonresponsive mice. *Environ. Pollut.* 72:57–67 (1991).

251. Babineau, K.A., A. Singh, J.F. Jarrell, and D.C. Villeneuve. Surface epithelium of the ovary following oral administration of hexachlorobenzene to the monkey. *J. Submicrosc. Cytol. Pathol.* 23:457–464 (1991).

252. Goldey, E.S., and D.H. Taylor. Developmental neurotoxicity following premating maternal exposure to hexachlorobenzene in rats. *Neurotoxicol. Teratol.* 14:15–21 (1992).

253. Krishnan, K., J. Broudeur, and M. Charbonneau. Development of an experimental model for the study of hexachlorobenzene-induced hepatic porphyria in the rat. *Fund. Appl. Toxicol.* 17:433–441 (1991).

254. Bouthillier, L., E. Greselin, J. Brodeur, et al. Male rat specific nephrotoxicity resulting from subchronic administration of hexachlorobenzene. *Toxicol. Appl. Pharmacol.* 110:315–326 (1991).

255. Escribano, P.M., M.J. Díaz de Atauri, and M.A. Gómez Sánchez. Persistence of respiratory abnormalities four years after the onset of toxic oil syndrome. *Chest* 100:336–339 (1991).

256. Kilbourne, E.M., M. Posada de la Paz, I.A. Borda, et al. Toxic oil syndrome: a current clinical and epidemiologic summary, including comparisons with the eosinophilia-myalgia syndrome. *J. Am. Coll. Cardiol.* 18:711–717 (1991).

257. James, T.N., M.A. Gomez-Sanchez, F.J. Martinez-Tello, et al. Cardiac abnormalities in the toxic oil syndrome, with comparative observations on the eosinophilia-myalgia syndrome. *J. Am. Coll. Cardiol.* 18:1367–1379 (1991).

258. Silver, R.M., S.E. Sutherland, P. Carreira, and M.P. Heyes. Alterations in tryptophan metabolism in the toxic oil syndrome and in the eosinophilia-myalgia syndrome. *J. Rheumatol.* 19:69–73 (1992).

259. Khan, M.F., B.S. Kaphalia, A. Palafox, et al. Toxicity of oleic acid anilide in rats. *Arch. Environ. Contam. Toxicol.* 21:571–577 (1991).

260. Khan, M.F., B.S. Kaphalia, A. Palafox, et al. Heated linoleic acid anilide: toxicity and relevance to toxic oil syndrome. *Toxicology* 68:143–155 (1991).

261. Posada de la Paz, M., R.M. Philen, I.A. Borda, et al. Manufacturing processes at two French rapeseed oil companies: possible relationships to toxic oil syndrome in Spain. *Food Chem. Toxicol.* 29:797–803 (1991).

262. Hidaka, T., T. Kirigaya, M. Kamijo, et al. Simultaneous determination of residual chlorine and volatile chlorinated organic compounds in vegetables by the head space method. *Shokuhim Eiseigaku Zasshi* 32:308–314 (1991).

263. Norman, K.N.T. Determination of tetrachloroethylene in olive oil by automated headspace gas chromatography. *Food Addit. Contam.* 8:513–516 (1991).

264. Hahn, H., E. Eder, and C. Deininger. Genotoxicity of 1,3-dichloro-2-propanol in the SOS Chromotest and in the Ames test. Elucidation of the genotoxic mechanism. *Chem.-Biol. Interact.* 80:73–88 (1991).

265. Bache, C.A., D.J. Lisk, and G.S. Stoewsand. Cyclohexylamine residue in vegetables blanched with primary steam. *J. Food Safety* 12:161–166 (1992).

266. Chadha, K., and F. Lawrence. Ion chromatographic determination of cyanide contamination in fruit and evaluation of a colorimetric test kit. *Int. J. Environ. Anal. Chem.* 44:197–202 (1991).

267. Chadha, R.K., F. Bryce, J.F. Lawrence, et al. Toxicity of potassium cyanide added to fresh fruit and juice. *Food Chem. Toxicol.* 29:681–684 (1991).

268. Restani, P., and C.L. Galli. Oral toxicity of formaldehyde and its derivatives. *Crit. Rev. Toxicol.* 21:315–328 (1991).

269. Barry, J.L., and D. Tomé. Formaldehye content of milk in goats fed formaldehyde-treated soybean oilmeal. *Food Addit. Contam.* 8:633–640 (1991).

270. Newton, J.M., B.S. Rothman, and F.A. Walker. Separation and determination of diesel contaminants in various fish products by capillary gas chromatography. *J. Assoc. Off. Anal. Chem.* 74:986–990 (1991).

271. Krone, C.A., J.E. Stein, and U. Varanasi. Estimation of levels of metabolites of aromatic hydrocarbons in fish tissues by HPLC/fluorescence analysis. *Chemosphere* 24:497–510 (1992).

272. Grob, K., A. Artho, M. Biedermann, and J. Egli. Food contamination by hydrocarbons from lubricating oils and release agents: determination by coupled LC–GC. *Food Addit. Contam.* 8:437–446 (1991).

273. Momcilovic, B., ed. *Trace Elements in Man and Animals. 7.* Monography, proceedings, round tables and discussions of the Seventh International Symposium on Trace Elements in Man and Animals (TEMA-7). May 20–25, 1990. Zagreb, Croatia, Yugoslavia, Institute for Medical Research and Occupational Health, University of Zagreb (1991).

274. Dabeka, R.W., and A.D. McKenzie. Total diet study of lead and cadmium in food composites: preliminary investigations. *J. AOAC Int.* 75:386–394 (1992).

275. Becker, W., and J. Kumpulainen. Contents of essential and toxic mineral elements in Swedish market-basket diets in 1987. *Br. J. Nutr.* 66:151–160 (1991).

276. Meah, M.N., G.A. Smart, A.J. Harrison, and J.C. Sherlock. Lead and tin in canned foods: results of the UK survey 1983–1987. *Food Addit. Contam.* 8:485–496 (1991).

277. Zurera-Cosano, G., R. Moreno-Rojas, F. Rincon-Leon, and M. Amaro-Lopez. Cadmium and lead content in fresh and canned peas. *J. Sci. Food Agric.* 57:565–572 (1991).

278. Bache, C.A., M. Rutzke, and D.J. Lisk. Absorption of vanadium, nickel, aluminum and molybdenum by swiss chard grown on soil amended with oil fly ash or bottom ash. *J. Food Safety* 12:79–84 (1991).

279. Taylor, R.W., I.O. Ibeabuchi, K.R. Sistani, and J.W. Shuford. Accumulation of some metals by legumes and their extractability from acid mine spoils. *J. Environ. Qual.* 21:176–180 (1992).

280. Boon, D.Y., and P.N. Soltanpour. Lead, cadmium, and zinc contamination of Aspen garden soils and vegetation. *J. Environ. Qual.* 21:82–86 (1992).

281. Madden, J.D., R.M. Grodner, S.E. Feagley, et al. Minerals and xenobiotic residues in the edible tissues of wild and pond-raised Louisiana crayfish. *J. Food Safety* 12:1–15 (1991).

282. Schwarz, Th., A. Busch, and R. Lenk. First studies on lead, cadmium and arsenic contents of feed, cattle and food of animal origin coming from different farms in Saxonia. (Summary in English.) *Dtsch. Tierärztl. Wochenschr.* 98:369–372 (1991).

283. Schulz-Schroeder, G. Lead and cadmium contents in meat, liver, and kidney samples from lambs and sheep. (Summary in English.) *Fleischwirtschaft* 71:1435–1438 (1991).

284. Salisbury, C.D.C., W. Chan, and P.W. Saschenbrecker. Multielement concentrations in liver and kidney tissues from five species of Canadian slaughter animals. *J. Assoc. Off. Anal. Chem.* 74:587–591 (1991).

285. Cibulka, J., T. Turecki, D. Miholová, et al. Cadmium, lead and mercury levels in feeding yeast produced in Czechoslovakia. *Sci. Total Environ.* 114:73–86 (1992).

286. De Gregori, I., D. Delgado, H. Pinochet, et al. Toxic trace elements in Chilean seafoods: development of analytical quality control procedures. *Sci. Total Environ.* 111:201–218 (1992).

287. Alvarez, G.H., and S.G. Capar. Continuous hydride generation–atomic absorption method for the determination of selenium and arsenic in foods. *Anal. Lett.* 24:1695–1710 (1991).

288. Vahter, M., M. Berglund, S. Slorach, et al. Methods for integrated exposure monitoring of lead and cadmium. *Environ. Res.* 56:78–89 (1991).

289. Krishnan, U., and S.S. Que Hee. Ear wax: a new biological monitoring medium for metals? *Bull. Environ. Contam. Toxicol.* 48:481–486 (1992).

290. Ericson, J.E., D.R. Smith, and A.R. Flegal. Skeletal concentrations of lead, cadmium, zinc, and silver in ancient North American Pecos Indians. *Environ. Health Perspect.* 93:217–223 (1991).

291. Magos, L. Epidemiological and experimental aspects of metal carcinogenesis: physicochemical properties, kinetics, and the active species. *Environ. Health Perspect.* 95:157–189 (1991).

292. Riordan, J.F., and B.L. Vallee, eds. *Metallobiochemistry. Part B. Metallothionein and Related Molecules. Methods in Enzymology, Vol. 205.* New York, Academic Press, Inc. (1991).

293. Lote, C.J., and H. Saunders. Aluminium: gastrointestinal absorption and renal excretion. *Clin. Sci.* 81:289–295 (1991).

294. Ecelbarger, C.A., and J.L. Greger. Dietary citrate and kidney function affect aluminum, zinc and iron utilization in rats. *J. Nutr.* 121:1755–1762 (1991).

295. Domingo, J.L., M. Gomez, J.M. Llobet, and C. Richart. Effect of ascorbic acid on gastrointestinal aluminium absorption. *Lancet* 338:1467 (1991).

296. Anonymous. Water pollution at Lowermoor, North Cornwall. Second report of the Lowermoor Incident Health Advisory Group. *Commun. Dis. Environ. Health Scotland Weekly Rep.* 26(1):3 (1992).

297. Garruto, R.M., M.J. Strong, and R. Yanagihara. Experimental models of aluminum-induced motor neuron degeneration. In *Amyotrophic Lateral Sclerosis and Other Motor Neuron Diseases.* L.P. Rowland, ed. *Adv. Neurol.* 56:327–340 (1991).

298. Yasui, M., Y. Yase, K. Ota, and R.M. Garruto. Evaluation of magnesium, calcium and aluminum metabolism in rats and monkeys maintained on calcium-deficient diets. *Neurotoxicology* 12:603–614 (1991).

299. Yasui, M., Y. Yase, K. Ota, and R.M. Garruto. Aluminum deposition in the central nervous system of patients with amyotrophic lateral sclerosis from the Kii Peninsula of Japan. *Neurotoxicology* 12:615–620 (1991).

300. Crapper McLachlan, D.R., T.P. Kruck, W.J. Lukiw, and S.S. Krishnan. Would decreased aluminum ingestion reduce the incidence of Alzheimer's disease? *Can. Med. Assoc. J.* 145:793–804 (1991).

301. Neri, L.C., and D. Hewitt. Aluminium, Alzheimer's disease, and drinking water. *Lancet* 338:390 (1991).

302. Forbes, W.F., L.M. Hayward, and M. Agwani. Dementia, aluminium, and fluoride. *Lancet* 338:1592–1593 (1991).

303. Wettstein, A., J. Aeppli, K. Gautschi, and M. Peters. Failure to find a relationship between mnestic skills of octogenarians and aluminum in drinking water. *Int. Arch. Occup. Environ. Health* 63:97–103 (1991).

304. Quarles, L.D. Paradoxical toxic and trophic osseous actions of aluminum: potential explanations. *Miner Electrolyte Metab.* 17:233–239 (1991).

305. Goodman, W.G., and M.E.L. Duarte. Aluminum: effects on bone and role in the pathogenesis of renal osteodystrophy. *Miner Electrolyte Metab.* 17:221–232 (1991).

306. Zaman, K., M. Mukhtar, H. Siddique, and H. Miszta. The effect of aluminum on the stomal cells (*in vitro*) on bone marrow in rats. *Toxicol. Indust. Health* 8:103–109 (1992).

307. Jorhem, L., and G. Haegglund. Aluminium in foodstuffs and diets in Sweden. *Z. Lebensm. Unters. Forsch.* 194:38–42 (1992).

308. Baxter, M.J., J.A. Burrell, H. Crews, and R.C. Massey. Aluminium levels in milk and infant formulae. *Food Addit. Contam.* 8:653–660 (1991).

309. Bloodworth, B.C., C.T. Hock, and T.O. Boon. Aluminium content in milk powders by inductively-coupled argon plasma–optical emission spectrometry. *Food Addit. Contam.* 8:749–754 (1991).

310. Davenport, A., and R. Goodall. Aluminium and dementia. *Lancet* 339:1236 (1992).

311. Duggan, J.M., J.E. Dickeson, P.F. Tynan, et al. Aluminium beverage cans as a dietary source of aluminium. *Med. J. Aust.* 156:604–605 (1992).

312. Tennakone, K., W.A.C. Perera, and A.C. Jayasuriya. Aluminium contamination via assisted leaching from metallic aluminium utensils at neutral pH. *Environ. Monitor. Assess.* 21:79–81 (1992).

313. Vaessen, H.A.M.G., C.G. van de Kamp, and B. Szteke. Aluminium determination in food matrices. IUPAC check sample survey of analytical performance. *Z. Lebensm. Unters. Forsch.* 194:456–460 (1992).

314. Roses, O.E., J.C. García Fernández, E.C. Villaamil, et al. Mass poisoning by sodium arsenite. *Clin. Toxicol.* 29:209–213 (1991).

315. Bates, M.N., A.H. Smith, and C. Hopenhayn-Rich. Arsenic ingestion and internal cancers: a review. *Am. J. Epidemiol.* 135:462–476 (1992).

316. Stöhrer, G. Arsenic: opportunity for risk assessment. *Arch. Toxicol.* 65:525–531 (1991).

317. Börzsönyi, M., A. Bereczky, P. Rudnai, et al. Epidemiological studies on human subjects exposed to arsenic in drinking water in Southeast Hungary. *Arch. Toxicol.* 66:77–78 (1992).

318. García-Vargas, G.G., A. García-Rangel, M. Aguilar-Romo, et al. A pilot study on the urinary excretion of porphyrins in human populations chronically exposed to arsenic in Mexico. *Hum. Exp. Toxicol.* 10:189–193 (1991).

319. Ostrosky-Wegman, P., M.E. Gonsebatt, R. Montero, et al. Lymphocyte proliferation kinetics and genotoxic findings in a pilot study on individuals chronically exposed to arsenic in Mexico. *Mutat. Res.* 250:477–482 (1991).

320. Stijve, T., and B. Bourqui. Arsenic in edible mushrooms. *Dtsch. Lebensm.-Rundsch.* 87:307–310 (1991).

321. Sabbioni, E., M. Fischbach, G. Pozzi, et al. Cellular retention, toxicity and carcinogenic potential of seafood arsenic. I. Lack of cytotoxicity and transforming activity of arsenobetaine in the BALB/3T3 cell line. *Carcinogenesis* 12:1287–1291 (1991).

322. Navarro, M., H. López, M.C. López, and M. Sánchez. Determination of arsenic in fish by hydride generation atomic absorption spectrometry. *J. Anal. Toxicol.* 16:169–171 (1992).

323. Momplaisir, G.M., J.-S. Blais, M. Quinteiro, and W.D. Marshall. Determination of arsenobetaine, arsenocholine, and tetramethylarsonium cations in seafoods and human urine by high-performance liquid chromatography–thermochemical hydride generation–atomic absorption spectrometry. *J. Agric. Food Chem.* 39:1448–1451 (1991).

324. Robards, K., and P. Worsfold. Cadmium: toxicity and analysis. A review. *Analyst* 116:549–568 (1991).

325. Moreiras, O., and C. Cuadrado. Theoretical study of the intake of trace elements (nutrients and contaminants) via total diet in some geographical areas of Spain. *Biol. Trace Elem. Res.* 32:93–103 (1992).

326. Jackson, A.P., and B.J. Alloway. The bioavailability of cadmium to lettuce and cabbage in soils previously treated with sewage sludges. *Plant Soil* 132:179–186 (1991).

327. Thomas, G.M., and H.C. Harrison. Genetic line effects on parameters influencing cadmium concentrations in lettuce (*Lactuca sativa* L.). *J. Plant Nutr.* 14:953–962 (1991).

328. Florijn, P.J., J.A. Nelemans, and M.L. van Beusichem. Cadmium uptake by lettuce varieties. *Neth. J. Agric. Sci.* 39:103–114 (1991).

329. Muramoto, S., and I. Aoyama. Effects of fertilizers on the vicissitude of cadmium in rice plant. *J. Environ. Sci. Health* A25:629–635 (1990).

330. Strmisková, G., F. Strmiska, and J. Dubravicky. Mineral composition of oyster mushroom. *Nahrung* 36:210–212 (1992).

331. Antoniou, V., and N. Zantopoulos. Cadmium concentrations in plants and goats tissues from various areas of Chalkidiki, Greece. *Bull. Environ. Contam. Toxicol.* 48:515–519 (1992).

332. Smith, R.M., R.M. Leach, L.D. Muller, et al. Effects of long-term dietary cadmium chloride on tissue, milk, and urine mineral concentrations of lactating dairy cows. *J. Anim. Sci.* 69:4088–4096 (1991).

333. Morcombe, P.W., P. Ross, H.G. Masters, et al. Cadmium concentrations in the kidneys of Western Australian pigs. *Aust. Vet. J.* 69:113–114 (1992).

334. King, R.H., W.G. Brown, V.C.M. Amenta, et al. The effect of dietary cadmium intake on the growth performance and retention of cadmium in growing pigs. *Anim. Feed Sci. Technol.* 37:1–7 (1992).

335. Iwata, K., H. Saito, M. Moriyama, and A. Nakano. Association between renal tubular dysfunction and mortality among residents in a cadmium-polluted area, Nagasaki, Japan. *Tohoku J. Exp. Med.* 164:93–102 (1991).

336. Iwata, K., H. Saito, and A. Nakano. Association between cadmium-induced renal dysfunction and mortality: further evidence. *Tohoku J. Exp. Med.* 164:319–330 (1991).

337. Nishino, H., T. Tanaka, K. Shiroishi, et al. Increase of urinary and serum hydroxyproline in subjects exposed to cadmium. *Bull. Environ. Contam. Toxicol.* 47:609–616 (1991).

338. Aoshima, K., and M. Kasuya. Preliminary study on serum levels of 1,25-dihydroxyvitamin D and 25-hydroxyvitamin D in cadmium-induced renal tubular dysfunction. *Toxicol. Lett.* 57:91–99 (1991).

339. Staessen, J., A. Amery, A. Bernard, et al. Blood pressure, the prevalence of cardiovascular diseases, and exposure to cadmium: a population study. *Am. J. Epidemiol.* 134:257–267 (1991).

340. Staessen, J., A. Amery, A. Bernard, et al. Effects of exposure to cadmium on calcium metabolism: a population study. *Br. J. Indust. Med.* 48:710–714 (1991).

341. Staessen, J.A., G. Vyncke, R.R. Lauwerys, et al. Transfer of cadmium from a sandy acidic soil to man: a population study. *Environ. Res.* 58:25–34 (1992).

342. Hajem, S., P. Hannaert, T. Moreau, et al. Cadmium and membrane ion transport in a French urban male population. *Bull. Environ. Contam. Toxicol.* 47:850–857 (1991).

343. Näyä, S., H. Korpela, L. Pyy, and J. Hassi. Effect of Soviet industry on blood cadmium in Finns. *Lancet* 338:1593 (1991).

344. Morselt, A.F.W. Environmental pollutants and diseases. A cell biological approach using chronic cadmium exposure in the animal model as a paradigm case. *Toxicology* 70:1–132 (1991).

345. Cosma, G.N., D. Currie, K.S. Squibb, et al. Detection of cadmium exposure in rats by induction of lymphocyte metallothionein gene expression. *J. Toxicol. Environ. Health* 34:39–49 (1991).

346. Groten, J.P., E.J. Sinkeldam, J.B. Luten, and P.J. van Bladeren. Cadmium accumulation and metallothionein concentrations after 4-week dietary exposure to cadmium chloride or cadmium–metallothionein in rats. *Toxicol. Appl. Pharmacol.* 111:504–513 (1991).

347. Min, K.-S., Y. Fujita, S. Onosaka, and K. Tanaka. Role of intestinal metallothionein in absorption and distribution of orally administered cadmium. *Toxicol. Appl. Pharmacol.* 109:7–16 (1991).

348. Felley-Bosco, E., and J. Diezi. Dietary calcium restriction enhances cadmium-induced metallothionein synthesis in rats. *Toxicol. Lett.* 60:139–144 (1992).

349. Murphy, V.A., E.C. Embrey, J.M. Rosenberg, et al. Calcium deficiency enhances cadmium accumulation in the central nervous system. *Brain Res.* 557:280–284 (1991).

350. Groten, J.P., E.J. Sinkeldam, T. Muys, et al. Interaction of dietary Ca, P, Mg, Mn, Cu, Fe, Zn and Se with the accumulation and oral toxicity of cadmium in rats. *Food Chem. Toxicol.* 29:249–258 (1991).

351. Saygi, S., G. Deniz, O. Kutsal, and N. Vural. Chronic effects of cadmium on kidney, liver, testis, and

fertility of male rats. *Biol. Trace Elem. Res.* 31:209–214 (1991).

352. Hamilton, M. Water fluoridation: A risk assessment perspective. *J. Environ. Health* 54(6):27–32 (1992).

353. Bucher, J.R., M.R. Hejtmancik, J.D. Toft II, et al. Results and conclusions of the National Toxicology Program's rodent carcinogenicity studies with sodium fluoride. *Int. J. Cancer* 48:733–737 (1991).

354. Mahoney, M.C., P.C. Nasca, W.S. Burnett, and J.M. Melius. Bone cancer incidence rates in New York State: time trends and fluoridated drinking water. *Am. J. Public Health* 81:475–479 (1991).

355. Ishii, T., and G. Suckling. The severity of dental fluorosis in children exposed to water with a high fluoride content for various periods of time. *J. Dent. Res.* 70:952–956 (1991).

356. Riordan, P.J., and J.A. Banks. Dental fluorosis and fluoride exposure in Western Australia. *J. Dent. Res.* 70:1022–1028 (1991).

357. Mabelya, L., K.G. König, and W.H. van Palenstein Helderman. Dental fluorosis, altitude, and associated dietary factors. *Caries Res.* 26:65–67 (1992).

358. Susheela, A.K., T.K. Das, I.P. Gupta, et al. Fluoride ingestion and its correlation with gastrointestinal discomfort. *Fluoride* 25:5–22 (1992).

359. Kumari, D.S., and P.R. Rao. Red cell membrane alterations in human chronic fluoride toxicity. *Biochem. Int.* 23:639–648 (1991).

360. Saralakumari, D., and P.R. Rao. Red blood cell glucose metabolism in human chronic fluoride toxicity. *Bull. Environ. Contam. Toxicol.* 47:834–839 (1991).

361. van Staden, J.F., and S.D. Janse van Rensburg. Improvement on the microdiffusion technique for the determination of ionic and ionizable fluoride in cows' milk. *Analyst* 116:807–810 (1991).

362. Beck, B.D. An update on exposure and effects of lead. *Fund. Appl. Toxicol.* 18:1–16 (1992).

363. DeRosa, C.T., H. Choudhury, and W.B. Peirano. An integrated exposure/pharmacokinetic based approach to the assessment of complex exposures. Lead: a case study. *Toxicol. Indust. Health* 7:231–248 (1991).

364. Bigelow, S.W. Role of the *Food Chemicals Codex* in lowering dietary lead consumption: a review. *J. Food Protect.* 55:455–458 (1992).

365. Zantopoulos, N., H. Tsoukali-Papadopoulou, P. Epivatianos, et al. Lead concentrations in consumable beef tissues. *J. Environ. Sci. Health* A25:487–494 (1990).

366. Oskarsson, A., L. Jorhem, J. Sundberg, et al. Lead poisoning in cattle—transfer of lead to milk. *Sci. Total Environ.* 111:83–94 (1992).

367. Neuman, D.R., and D.J. Dollhopf. Lead levels in blood from cattle residing near a lead smelter. *J. Environ. Qual.* 21:181–184 (1992).

368. Forsyth, D.S., R.W. Dabeka, and C. Cléroux. Organic and total lead in selected fresh and canned seafood products. *Food Addit. Contam.* 8:477–484 (1991).

369. Temminghoff, E.J.M., and I. Novozamsky. Determination of lead in plant tissues: a pitfall due to wet digestion procedures in the presence of sulfuric acid. *Analyst* 117:23–26 (1992).

370. Barbera, R., R. Farré, and P. Garcia Andión. Direct determination of lead in cola beverages by electrothermal atomic absorption spectrophotometry. *Nahrung* 36:202–204 (1992).

371. Cacho, J., V. Ferreira, and C. Nerín. Determination of lead in wines by hydride generation atomic absorption spectrometry. *Analyst* 117:31–33 (1992).

372. Ibrahim, H. Determination of lead in frying oils by direct current plasma atomic emission spectrometry. *J. Am. Oil Chem. Soc.* 68:678–679 (1991).

373. Dim, L.A., A.M. Kinyua, J.M. Munyithya, and J. Adetunji. Lead and other metals distribution in local cooking salt from the Fofi salt-spring in Akwana, Middle Benue Trough, Nigeria. *J. Environ. Sci. Health* B26:357–365 (1991).

374. Shannon, M.W., and J.W. Graef. Lead intoxication in infancy. *Pediatrics* 89:87–90 (1992).

375. Lockitch, G., B. Berry, E. Roland, et al. Seizures in a 10-week-old infant: lead poisoning from an unexpected source. *Can. Med. Assoc. J.* 145:1465–1468 (1991).

376. Centers for Disease Control. Elevated blood lead levels associated with illicitly distilled alcohol—Alabama, 1990–1991. *Morbid. Mortal. Weekly Rep.* 41:294–295 (1992).

377. Hernandez Avila, M., I. Romieu, C. Rios, et al. Lead-glazed ceramics as major determinants of blood lead levels in Mexican women. *Environ. Health Perspect.* 94:117–120 (1991).

378. Weisel, C., M. Demak, S. Marcus, and B.D. Goldstein. Soft plastic bread packaging: lead content

and reuse by families. *Am. J. Public Health* 81:756–758 (1991).

379. Anonymous. Bread bags are lead free, industry tells FDA. *Food Protect. Rep.* 7(12):8 (1991).

380. Centers for Disease Control. Surveillance of elevated blood lead levels among adults—United States, 1992. *Morbid. Mortal. Weekly Rep.* 41:285–288 (1992).

381. Centers for Disease Control. Blood lead levels among children in high-risk areas—California, 1987–1990. *Morbid. Mortal. Weekly Rep.* 41:291–294 (1992).

382. World Health Organization. Environmental pollution. Biological monitoring of human exposure to environmental lead. *Weekly Epidemiol. Rec.* 67:265–272 (1992).

383. Bercovitz, K., and D. Laufer. Age and gender influence on lead accumulation in root dentine of human permanent teeth. *Arch. Oral Biol.* 36:671–673 (1991).

384. Manuwald, O., W. Mey, V. Herzog, et al. Levels of lead in permanent teeth of the population of Erfurt and surroundings. *Zbl. Hyg.* 192:76–93 (1991).

385. Maena-Krichten, M., C. Patterson, G. Miller, et al. Comparative increases of lead and barium with age in human tooth enamel, rib and ulna. *Sci. Total Environ.* 107:179–203 (1991).

386. Rabinowitz, M.B., D. Bellinger, A. Leviton, and J.D. Wang. Lead levels among various deciduous tooth types. *Bull. Environ. Contam. Toxicol.* 47:602–608 (1991).

387. Cleymaet, R., D.H. Retief, E. Quartier, et al. A comparative study of the lead and cadmium content of surface enamel of Belgian and Kenyan children. *Sci. Total Environ.* 104:175–189 (1991).

388. Patterson, C., J. Ericson, M. Manea-Krichten, and H. Shirahata. Natural skeletal levels of lead in *Homo sapiens sapiens* uncontaminated by technological lead. *Sci. Total Environ.* 107:205–236 (1991).

389. Greene, T., C.B. Ernhart, and T.A. Boyd. Contributions of risk factors to elevated blood and dentine lead levels in preschool children. *Sci. Total Environ.* 115:239–260 (1992).

390. Grandjean, P., T. Lyngbye, and O.N. Hansen. Lessons from a Danish study on neuropsychological impairment related to lead exposure. *Environ. Health Perspect.* 94:111–115 (1991).

391. Wetmur, J.G., G. Lehnert, and R.J. Desnick. The δ-aminolevulinate dehydratase polymorphism: higher blood lead levels in lead workers and environ-mentally exposed children with the 1–2 and 2–2 isozymes. *Environ. Res.* 56:109–119 (1991).

392. Conaway, M.R., D. Waternaux, E. Allred, et al. Pre-natal blood lead levels and learning difficulties in children: an analysis of non-randomly missing categorical data. *Statistics Med.* 11:799–811 (1992).

393. Newton, D., C.J. Pickford, A.C. Chamberlain, et al. Elevation of lead in human blood from its controlled ingestion in beer. *Hum. Exp. Toxicol.* 11:3–9 (1992).

394. Frisancho, A.R., and A.S. Ryan. Decreased stature associated with moderate blood lead concentrations in Mexican–American children. *Am. J. Clin. Nutr.* 54:516–519 (1991).

395. Shukla, R., K.N. Dietrich, R.L. Bornschein, et al. Lead exposure and growth in the early preschool child: a follow-up report from the Cincinnati Lead Study. *Pediatrics* 88:886–892 (1991).

396. Greene, T., and C.B. Ernhart. Prenatal and preschool age lead exposure: relationship with size. *Neurotoxicol. Teratol.* 13:417–427 (1991).

397. Schwartz, J., and D. Otto. Lead and minor hearing impairment. *Arch. Environ. Health* 46:300–305 (1991).

398. Dietrich, K.N., P.A. Succop, O.G. Berger, and R.W. Keith. Lead exposure and the central auditory processing abilities and cognitive development of urban children: The Cincinnati Lead Study cohort at age 5 years. *Neurotoxicol. Teratol.* 14:51–56 (1992).

399. Huel, G., P. Tubert, N. Frery, et al. Joint effect of gestational age and maternal lead exposure on psychomotor development of the child at six years. *Neurotoxicology* 13:249–254 (1992).

400. Rabinowitz, M.B., J.-D. Wang, and W.T. Soong. Dentine lead and child intelligence in Taiwan. *Arch. Environ. Health* 46:351–360 (1991).

401. Rabinowitz, M.B., J.-D. Wang, and W. T. Soong. Children's classroom behavior and lead in Taiwan. *Bull. Environ. Contam. Toxicol.* 48:282–288 (1992).

402. Laughlin, N.K., P.J. Bushnell, and R.E. Bowman. Lead exposure and diet: differential effects on social development in the rhesus monkey. *Neurotoxicol. Teratol.* 13:429–440 (1991).

403. Ernhart, C.B. A critical review of low-level prenatal lead exposure in the human: 1. Effects on the fetus and newborn. *Reproduct. Toxicol.* 6:9–19 (1992).

404. Ernhart, C.B. A critical review of low-level prenatal lead exposure in the human: 2. Effects on the developing child. *Reproduct. Toxicol.* 6:21–40 (1992).

405. Hu, H. Knowledge of diagnosis and reproductive history among survivors of childhood plumbism. *Am. J. Public Health* 81:1070–1072 (1991).

406. Foster, W.G. Reproductive toxicity of chronic lead exposure in the female cynomolgus monkey. *Reproduct. Toxicol.* 6:123–131 (1992).

407. Sharp, D.S., A. Beswick, S. Renaud, et al. Blood lead and platelet aggregation—evidence for a causal association. *Thromb. Haemostasis* 66:604–608 (1991).

408. D'Itri, F.M. Mercury contamination—What we have learned since Minamata. *Environ. Monitor. Assess.* 19:165–182 (1991).

409. Fitzgerald, W.F., and T.W. Clarkson. Mercury and monomethylmercury: present and future concerns. *Environ. Health Perspect.* 96:159–166 (1991).

410. Al-Hashimi, A.H., and M.A. Al-Zorba. Mercury in some commercial fish from Kuwait: a pilot study. *Sci. Total Environ.* 106:71–82 (1991).

411. Leah, R., S. Evans, and M. Johnson. Mercury in muscle tissue of lesser-spotted dogfish (*Scyliorhinus caniculus* L.) from the north-east Irish Sea. *Sci. Total Environ.* 108:215–224 (1991).

412. Leah, R.T., S.J. Evans, and M.S. Johnson. Mercury in flounder (*Platichthys flesus* L.) from estuaries and coastal waters of the north-east Irish Sea. *Environ. Pollut.* 75:317–322 (1992).

413. Hellou, J., L.L. Fancey, and J.F. Payne. Concentrations of twenty-four elements in bluefin tuna, *Thunnus thynnus* from the Northwest Atlantic. *Chemosphere* 24:211–218 (1992).

414. Jackson, T.A. Biological and environmental control of mercury accumulation by fish in lakes and reservoirs of northern Manitoba, Canada. *Can. J. Fish. Aquat. Sci.* 48:2449–2470 (1991).

415. Bloom, N.S. On the chemical form of mercury in edible fish and marine invertebrate tissue. *Can. J. Fish. Aquat. Sci.* 49:1010–1017 (1992).

416. Lansens, P., C.C. Laiño, C. Meuleman, and W. Baeyens. Evaluation of gas chromatographic columns for the determination of methylmercury in aqueous head space extracts from biological samples. *J. Chromatogr.* 586:329–340 (1991).

417. Navarro-Alarcón, M., M.C. López-Martinez, M. Sánchez-Viñas, and H. López-García de la Serrana.

Determination of mercury in crops by cold vapor atomic absorption spectrometry after microwave dissolution. *J. Agric. Food Chem.* 39:2223–2225 (1991).

418. Scheuhammer, A.M., and D. Bond. Factors affecting the determination of total mercury in biological samples by continuous-flow cold vapor atomic absorption spectrophotometry. *Biol. Trace Elem. Res.* 31:119–129 (1991).

419. Davies, F.C.W. Minamata disease: a 1989 update on the mercury poisoning epidemic in Japan. *Environ. Geochem. Health* 13:35–38 (1991).

420. Sakamoto, M., A. Nakano, Y. Kinjo, et al. Present mercury levels in red blood cells of nearby inhabitants about 30 years after the outbreak of Minamata disease. *Ecotoxicol. Environ. Safety* 22:58–66 (1991).

421. Oyanagi, K., A. Furuta, E. Ohama, and F. Ikuta. Does methylmercury intoxication induce arteriosclerosis in humans? A pathological investigation of 22 autopsy cases in Niigata, Japan. *Acta Neuropathol.* 83:217–227 (1992).

422. Byrne, L. Brazil's mercury poisoning disaster. *Br. Med. J.* 304:1397 (1992).

423. Soria, M.L., P. Sanz, D. Martínez, et al. Total mercury and methylmercury in hair, maternal and umbilical blood, and placenta from women in the Seville area. *Bull. Environ. Contam. Toxicol.* 48:494–501 (1992).

424. Katz, S.A., and R.B. Katz. Use of hair analysis for evaluating mercury intoxication of the human body: a review. *J. Appl. Toxicol.* 12:79–84 (1992).

425. Ernst, E., and J.G. Lauritsen. Effect of organic and inorganic mercury on human sperm motility. *Pharmacol. Toxicol.* 68:440–444 (1991).

426. Cuvin-Aralar, M.L.A., and R.W. Furness. Mercury and selenium interaction: a review. *Ecotoxicol. Environ. Safety* 21:348–364 (1991).

427. Woods, J.S., M.A. Bowers, and H.A. Davis. Urinary porphyrin profiles as biomarkers of trace metal exposure and toxicity: studies on urinary porphyrin excretion patterns in rats during prolonged exposure to methyl mercury. *Toxicol. Appl. Pharmacol.* 110:464–476 (1991).

428. Sarafian, T., and M.A. Verity. Oxidative mechanisms underlying methyl mercury neurotoxicity. *Int. J. Dev. Neurosci.* 9:147–153 (1991).

429. Lindström, H., J. Luthman, A. Oskarsson, et al. Effects of long-term treatment with methyl mercury on

the developing rat brain. *Environ. Res.* 56:158–169 (1991).

430. Ilbäck, N.-G., J. Sundberg, and A. Oskarsson. Methyl mercury exposure via placenta and milk impairs natural killer (NK) cell function in newborn rats. *Toxicol. Lett.* 58:149–158 (1991).

431. Dutczak, W.J., T.W. Clarkson, and N. Ballatori. Biliary-hepatic recycling of a xenobiotic: gallbladder absorption of methyl mercury. *Am. J. Physiol.* 260:G873–G880 (1991).

432. Contempre, B., D. Je, N. Bebe, et al. Effect of selenium supplementation in hypothyroid subjects of an iodine and selenium deficient area: the possible danger of indiscriminate supplementation of iodine-deficient subjects with selenium. *J. Clin. Endocrinol. Metab.* 73:213–215 (1991).

433. Arthur, J.R. The role of selenium in thyroid hormone metabolism. *Can. J. Physiol. Pharmacol.* 69:1648–1652 (1991).

434. Liquiang, X., S. Wangxing, X. Qinhua, et al. Selenium in Kashin-Beck disease areas. *Biol. Trace Elem. Res.* 31:1–9 (1991).

435. Xia, Y., X. Zhao, L. Zhu, and P.D. Whanger. Metabolism of selenate and selenomethionine by a selenium-deficient population of men in China. *J. Nutr. Biochem.* 3:202–210 (1992).

436. Meltzer, H.M., G. Norheim, E.B. Løken, and H. Holm. Supplementation with wheat selenium induces a dose-dependent response in serum and urine of a Se-replete population. *Br. J. Nutr.* 67:287–294 (1992).

437. Swanson, C.A., B.H. Patterson, O.A. Levander, et al. Human [^{74}Se]selenomethionine metabolism: a kinetic model. *Am. J. Clin. Nutr.* 54:917–926 (1991).

438. Ekholm, P., P. Varo, P. Aspila, et al. Transport of feed selenium to different tissues of bulls. *Br. J. Nutr.* 66:49–55 (1991).

439. El-Hallaq, Y.H., I.G. Gökmen, N.K. Aras, and A. Gökmen. Determination of selenium in human diets by radiochemical neutron activation analysis. *Analyst* 117:447–451 (1992).

440. Ari, U., M. Volkan, and N.K. Aras. Determination of selenium in diet by Zeeman effect graphite furnace atomic absorption spectrometry for calculation of daily dietary intakes. *J. Agric. Food Chem.* 39:2180–2183 (1991).

441. Buckley, W.T., J.J. Budac, D.V. Godfrey, and K.M. Koenig. Determination of selenium by inductively coupled plasma mass spectrometry utilizing a new hydride generation sample introduction system. *Anal. Chem.* 64:724–729 (1992).

442. Iijima, M., Y. Hoshino, and N. Nose. Studies on tributyl tin contamination in fish cultured in fresh water. *Eisei Kagaku* 37:296–299 (1991).

443. Jiang, G.B., P.S. Maxwell, K.W.M. Siu, et al. Determination of butyltins in mussel by gas chromatography with flame photometric detection using quartz surface-induced luminescence. *Anal. Chem.* 63:1506–1509 (1991).

444. Tas, J.W., and A. Opperhuizen. Analysis of triphenyltin in fish. *Marine Environ. Res.* 32:271–278 (1991).

445. Corrigan, F.M., A.G. Van Rhijn, G. Ijomah, et al. Tin and fatty acids in dementia. *Prostaglandins Leukotrienes Essential Fatty Acids* 43:229–238 (1991).

446. Attahiru, U.S., T.T. Iyaniwura, A.O. Adaudi, and J.J. Bonire. Subchronic toxicity studies of tri-N-butyltin and triphenyltin acetates in rats. *Vet. Hum. Toxicol.* 33:499–502 (1991).

447. Ema, M., T. Itami, and H. Kawasaki. Teratogenicity of di-*n*-butyltin dichloride in rats. *Toxicol. Lett.* 58:347–356 (1991).

448. Ema, M., T. Itami, and H. Kawasaki. Susceptible period for the teratogenicity of di-*n*-butyltin dichloride in rats. *Toxicology* 73:81–92 (1992).

449. Bressa, G., R.H. Hinton, S.C. Price, et al. Immunotoxicity of tri-*n*-butyltin oxide (TBTO) and tri-*n*-butyltin chloride (TBTC) in the rat. *J. Appl. Toxicol.* 11:397–402 (1991).

450. Carthew, P., R.E. Edwards, and B.M. Dorman. The immunotoxicity of tributyltin oxide (TBTO) does not increase the susceptibility of rats to experimental respiratory infection. *Hum. Exp. Toxicol.* 11:71–75 (1992).

451. Kucera, J., A.R. Byrne, A. Mravcová, and J. Lener. Vanadium levels in hair and blood of normal and exposed persons. *Sci. Total Environ.* 115:191–205 (1992).

452. Ramanadham, S., C. Heyliger, M.J. Gresser, et al. The distribution and half-life for retention of vanadium in the organs of normal and diabetic rats orally fed vanadium(IV) and vanadium(V). *Biol. Trace Elem. Res.* 30:119–124 (1991).

453. Al-Bayati, M.A., O.G. Raabe, S.N. Giri, and J.B. Knaak. Distribution of vanadate in the rat following

subcutaneous and oral routes of administration. *J. Am. Coll. Toxicol.* 10:233–241 (1991).

454. Zaporowska, H., and W. Wasilewski. Haematological results of vanadium intoxication in Wistar rats. *Comp. Biochem. Physiol.* 101C:57–61 (1992).

455. Sanchez, D., A. Ortega, J.L. Domingo, and J. Corbella. Developmental toxicity evaluation of orthovanadate in the mouse. *Biol. Trace Elem. Res.* 30:219–226 (1991).

456. Sadiq, M., and I. Alam. Metal concentrations in different body parts of Saudi lambs. *J. Environ. Sci. Health* A26:607–619 (1991).

457. Schauss, A.G. Nephrotoxicity and neurotoxicity in humans from organogermanium compounds and germanium dioxide. *Biol. Trace Elem. Res.* 29:267–280 (1991).

458. Rasmussen, M.D., D.M. Galton, and L.G. Petersson. Effects of premilking teat preparation on spores of anaerobes, bacteria, and iodine residues in milk. *J. Dairy Sci.* 74:2472–2478 (1991).

459. Mahesh, D.L., Y.G. Deosthale, and B.S. Narasinga Rao. A sensitive kinetic assay for the determination of iodine in foodstuffs. *Food Chem.* 43:51–56 (1992).

460. Soledad Garcia, M., C. Sanchez-Pedreño, M.I. Albero, and C. Sanchez. Kinetic determination of iodide in pharmaceutical and food samples. *Analyst* 116:653–656 (1991).

461. Yang, S., S. Fu, and M. Wang. Determination of trace iodine in food and biological samples by cathodic stripping voltammetry. *Anal. Chem.* 63:2970–2973 (1991).

462. Gordeuk, V., J. Mukiibi, S.J. Hasstedt, et al. Iron overload in Africa. Interaction between a gene and dietary iron content. *New Engl. J. Med.* 326:95–100 (1992).

463. Gable, C.B. Hemochromatosis and dietary iron supplementation: implications from US mortality, morbidity, and health survey data. *J. Am. Diet. Assoc.* 92:208–212 (1992).

464. Britton, R.S., R. O'Neill, and B.R. Bacon. Chronic dietary iron overload in rats results in impaired calcium sequestration by hepatic mitochondria and microsomes 1, 2, and 3. *Gastroenterology* 101:806–811 (1991).

465. Vrochte, H., M. Schätzke, E. Dringeberg, et al. Untersuchungen zur frage der nickelfreisetzung aus edelstahlkochtöpfen. *Z. Ernährungswiss.* 30:181–191 (1991).

466. Ewing, S., and R. Miller. Generalized nickel dermatitis in a 6-year-old boy as a result of swallowing a Canadian nickel. *J. Am. Acad. Dermatol.* 25:855–856 (1991).

467. Schiffer, R.B., F.W. Sunderman, Jr., R.B. Baggs, and J.A. Moynihan. The effects of exposure to dietary nickel and zinc upon humoral and cellular immunity in SJL mice. *J. Neuroimmunol.* 34:229–239 (1991).

468. Vaughan, G.T., and T.M. Florence. Platinum in the human diet, blood, hair and excreta. *Sci. Total Environ.* 111:47–58 (1992).

469. Duncan, M.W., A.M. Marini, R. Watters, et al. Zinc, a neurotoxin to cultured neurons, contaminates cycad flour prepared by traditional Guamanian methods. *J. Neurosci.* 12:1523–1537 (1992).

470. Çavdar, A.O., M. Bahçeci, N. Akar, et al. Maternal hair zinc concentration in neural tube defects in Turkey. *Biol. Trace Elem. Res.* 30:81–85 (1991).

471. Matossian, M.K. Fertility decline in Europe, 1875–1913. Was zinc deficiency the cause? *Perspect. Biol. Med.* 34:604–616 (1991).

472. Bosshard, E., B. Zimmerli, and Ch. Schlatter. Uranium in the diet: risk assessment of its nephro- and radiotoxicity. *Chemosphere* 24:309–321 (1992).

473. Isles, C.G., I. Robertson, J.A.J. Macleod, et al. Body concentration of caesium-137 in patients from Western Isles of Scotland. *Br. Med. J.* 302:1568–1571 (1991).

474. Louizi, A., C. Proukakis, S.E. Simopoulos, and M.G. Angelopoulos. Effect of dietary intake on the ^{137}Cs retention model. *Health Physics* 61:885–888 (1991).

475. de Ruig, W.G., and T.D.B. van der Struijs. Radioactive contamination of food samples in the areas of the USSR affected by the Chernobyl disaster. *Analyst* 117:545–548 (1992).

476. Borio, R., S. Chiocchini, R. Cicioni, et al. Uptake of radiocesium by mushrooms. *Sci. Total Environ.* 106:183–190 (1991).

477. Muramatsu, Y., S. Yoshida, and M. Sumiya. Concentrations of radiocesium and potassium in basidiomycetes collected in Japan. *Sci. Total Environ.* 105:29–39 (1991).

478. Brittain, J.E., A. Storruste, and E. Larsen. Radiocesium in brown trout (*Salmo trutta*) from a subalpine lake ecosystem after the Chernobyl reactor accident. *J. Environ. Radioactivity* 14:181–191 (1991).

479. Forberg, S., T. Odsjö, and M. Olsson. Radiocesium in muscle tissue of reindeer and pike from northern Sweden before and after the Chernobyl accident. A retrospective study on tissue samples from the Swedish Environmental Specimen Bank. *Sci. Total Environ.* 115:179–189 (1992).

480. Marouf, B.A., A.K. Al-Hadad, N.A. Toma, et al. Radionuclide contamination of foods imported into Iraq following the Chernobyl nuclear reactor accident. *Sci. Total Environ.* 106:191–194 (1991).

481. Man, C.-K., S.-Y. Lau, P. Chan, and M.K. Tsang. Cesium-137 intake from food in Hong Kong. *J. Environ. Radioactivity* 16:255–260 (1992).

482. Malm, J., A. Rantavaara, A. Uusi-Rauva, and O. Paakkola. Uptake of caesium-137 from peat and compost mould by vegetables in a greenhouse experiment. *J. Environ. Radioactivity* 14:123–133 (1991).

483. Fevraleva, L.T., T.A. Fedorova, and Y.T. Bobrikova. Uptake of natural radionuclides from irrigation water by crops. [Translated from *Agrokhimiya* 2:87-91 (1991)]. *Soviet Soil Sci.* 23:26–30 (1991).

484. Linsalata, P., R. Morse, H. Ford, and M. Eisenbud. Th, U, Ra and rare earth element distributions in farm animal tissues from an elevated natural radiation background environment. *J. Environ. Radioactivity* 14:233–257 (1991).

485. Monte, L. Analysis of radiocontamination data, collected in Italy following the Chernobyl accident, for the evaluation of transfer parameters of radionuclides in the deposition–vegetation–cow–milk pathway. *J. Environ. Radioactivity* 14:317–329 (1991).

486. Hecht, H. Decontamination of radio-active foods. Meat, meat products and milk. *Fleischwirtschaft* 72:751–755 (1992).

487. Prister, B., N. Loshchilov, L. Perepelyatnikova, et al. Efficiency of measures aimed at decreasing the contamination of agricultural products in areas contaminated by the Chernobyl NPP accident. *Sci. Total Environ.* 112:79–87 (1992).

488. Petäjä, E., A. Rantavaara, O. Paakkola, and E. Puolanne. Reduction of radioactive caesium in meat and fish by soaking. *J. Environ. Radioactivity* 16:273–285 (1992).

489. Vosniakos, F., A. Kesidou, A. Moumtzis, and P. Karakoltsidis. ^{131}I and ^{137}Cs removal from cheese, upon immersion in a sodium chloride solution. *Toxicol. Environ. Chem.* 31–32:241–246 (1991).

490. McKay, W.A., and S.D. Memmott. An investigation of the availability of ^{137}Cs and $^{239+240}$Pu for gut absorption in winkles following cooking and *in vitro* simulated gastro-intestinal digestion. *Food Addit. Contam.* 8:781–786 (1991).

9

Naturally Occurring Toxicants and Food Constituents of Toxicological Interest

Seafood toxins
Biogenic amines
Mutagens and carcinogens in heated foods
Coffee and methylxanthines
Alkaloids
Glucosinolates
Cyanogenic compounds
Urethane
Protease inhibitors
Phytate
Toxic amino acids
Other antinutritional compounds in legumes
Phenolic compounds
Toxicity and carcinogenicity of mushrooms
Food allergy and food intolerance
Other food-related toxins

Toxic substances in crop plants are comprehensively reviewed in a recent book (*1*). Topics covered include toxic amino acids, lectins, protease inhibitors, antigenic proteins, glucosinolates, alkaloids, tannins, cyanogens, mycotoxins, fibrous polysaccharides, and saponins. The antinutritional effects of these compounds in animals and humans and the potential for detoxification were discussed, and information was provided on their distribution and ecological significance.

SEAFOOD TOXINS

Naturally occurring seafood poisonings, including ciguatera, scombroid fish poisoning, paralytic shellfish poisoning (PSP), neurotoxic shellfish poisoning (NSP), diarrhetic shellfish poisoning (DSP), amnesic shellfish poisoning (ASP), and puffer fish poisoning were recently reviewed (*2*). For each illness, the symptoms, geographical distribution, incidence in the USA, toxins and toxic organisms were described. All of these toxins are heat resistant and their presence is not detectable by organoleptic means. Except for scombroid, which results from temperature abuse of fish after capture, fish and shellfish containing the other toxins acquire them through the food chain. During 1978–1987, 791 cases of ciguatera, 757 of scombroid, and 137 of PSP were reported to the Centers for Disease Control (CDC). Only two deaths, due to PSP, were recorded during this period.

Recent LC analyses of extracts of Gulf Coast oysters demonstrated the presence of the DSP toxin, okadaic acid (OA), at a concentration of 0.162 µg/g shellfish (*3*). *Dinophysis caudata*, a possible source of OA, was present in nearby seawater samples. Phytoplankton samples also contained the diatom *Nitzschia pungens* f. *multiseries*, which has been associated with ASP. Domoic acid concentrations in these diatoms averaged 2.1 pg/cell. Although these toxin concentrations do not constitute a public health hazard, they should be monitored regularly to prevent outbreaks of shellfish poisoning.

Ciguatoxin and OA are structurally related polyether toxins. Experiments with monoclonal antibodies prepared against ciguatoxin and against OA show that the toxins are also immunologically related (*4*). Use of the ciguatoxin antibody in a stick enzyme immunoassay procedure gave peak titers of 1.5 ng/mL and 50 ng/mL for ciguatoxin and OA, respectively. With the OA antibody, peak responses were 50 ng/mL for OA and 10 ng/mL for fragment B-C of ciguatoxin.

Tetrodotoxin (TTX, from puffer fish) and saxitoxin (STX, the PSP toxin) are also immunologically related. Antiserum prepared from rabbits injected with TTX–formaldehyde–keyhole limpet hemocyanin conjugate reacted with both toxins and was able to inhibit toxin-induced death of Neuro-2A cells in culture (*5*). Injections of 350 ng TTX or of 400 ng STX were lethal to all mice tested. But prior incubation of the toxins with the antiserum resulted in survival of 9 of 15 TTX-treated mice and 7 of 10 STX-treated mice. Preincubation of TTX with a monoclonal antibody against TTX prepared in mice immunized with the same conjugate completely prevented lethality.

It has been suggested that low concentrations of PSP toxins may be extracted and concentrated by the organic solvent extraction method used to prepare DSP toxins. Of 247 Norwegian mussel samples found positive for PSP toxins during 1986–1989, 15 were also extracted for assay of DSP toxins (*6*). These extracts did not cause symptoms of PSP poisoning, indicating that PSP toxins were not present in the DSP extracts.

Ciguatera

Two patients with biopsy-proven polymyositis were found to have suffered severe episodes of ciguatera poisoning 6 and 11 years previously (*7*). Since polymyositis is quite rare (0.8/100,000 per year), it may be that ciguatoxin is causally related to the disease in these people. Studies of large populations of persons exposed to ciguatoxin would provide more data to evaluate this hypothesis.

A severe intoxication with ciguatera occurring in a woman at 16 weeks of pregnancy had no apparent ill effects on her child delivered at term (*8*). After consuming a large portion of barracuda contaminated with ciguatoxin (CTX) the woman experienced a great increase in fetal movements which lasted for a few hours. She herself suffered multisystemic symptoms typical of ciguatera for 8 weeks. The newborn had normal neurological and respiratory reflexes at birth and developed normally in his first 10 months.

A case of suspected ciguatera poisoning following consumption of saupe (*Sarpa salpa*) on the Mediterranean coast of Israel may instead have been due to a saupe which had consumed the green alga *Caulerpa* sp. (*9*). These algae produce a sesquiterpenoid which has strong toxic properties producing some of the same symptoms as ciguatoxin. Since other more commonly ciguatoxic fish did not carry ciguatera at that time and saupe is known to eat *Caulerpa* sp., this is more probably a case of *Caulerpa* poisoning.

Since ciguatera occurs sporadically and may affect a variety of fish, much research is devoted to investigating factors responsible for its appearance. Examination of 14 strains of the dinoflagellate *Gambierdiscus toxicus* from Australia, Hawaii, Polynesia, the Virgin Islands, and Kiribati showed that only 3 of them produced putative ciguatoxin precursors named gambiertoxins (*10*). Changes in nutrient media did not induce the other strains to produce gambiertoxins, thereby suggesting that only certain strains are genetically capable of producing these toxins.

Environmental factors (temperature, salinity, and light intensity) were found to significantly affect toxin synthesis by 8 dinoflagellate species associated with ciguatera (*11*). Temperature optima varied from 25 to 29°C while salinity optima were <35% for all species except one. A light intensity of <10% full sunlight was optimal for most species. Thus, both genetic and environmental factors affect toxin production.

Some ciguatera-associated dinoflagellates are highly toxic to brine shrimp while others may be consumed by these crustaceans without severe effects (*12*). Cichlid fish fed brine shrimp which had eaten toxic dinoflagellates developed symptoms typical of ciguatera poisoning. Therefore, studies of the ciguatera food chain should be expanded to include crustaceans.

Paralytic shellfish poisoning

Although PSP toxins are not destroyed by ordinary, short cooking methods, thermal degradation of gonyautoxins (GTX) 1-4 was investigated to determine whether these toxins could be denatured by longer periods of heating (*13*). A mixture of GTX 2 and GTX 3 dissolved in water and heated for 180 min at 100, 110, and 120°C retained 39, 17, and <3%, respectively, of its initial toxicity. A mixture of GTX 1 and GTX 4 was more heat sensitive, retaining little toxicity when heated at 120°C for 60 min. However, oysters containing PSP toxins became twice as toxic when heated at these temperatures for 30 or 60 min. Further heating of the oysters resulted in toxin degradation. Several unknown compounds, presumably degradation products, were detected by TLC and HPLC in heated toxin samples.

Analyses of 64 rock scallop samples collected along the coasts of British Columbia, California, and Washington during 1980–1990 for PSP toxins indicated that this species is a potential health hazard and should be monitored regularly (*14*). Of the viscera, adductor muscles, and whole body samples tested, 87%, 24%, and 38%, respectively, were unsafe (>80 µg STX equivalents/100 g tissue). Maximum concentrations detected in these three types of samples were 26,000, 2,000, and 13,593 µg STX equivalents/100 g tissue, respectively.

Shore crabs (*Hemigrapsus oregonesis*) resistant to PSP toxins synthesize a unique, high-molecular-weight protein called saxitoxin-induced protein (SIP). Butter clams, collected along the northern British Columbia coast, were examined for the presence of PSP toxins and for proteins similar to SIP (*15*). Clams with a wide range of toxicities (<80–2000 µg STX equivalents/100 g tissue) were studied. STX was the principal toxin in most samples although some samples also had high levels of neosaxitoxin. Several soluble proteins that cross-reacted with crab anti-SIP serum were detected in toxic but not in non-toxic clams. Soluble proteins with distinctly different molecular weights were found in the siphon and in the foot. These toxin-induced proteins may be useful as a screen to identify toxic shellfish.

Lest it be thought that butter clams accumulate PSP toxins simply to annoy humans, the evidence indicates that they make themselves toxic as a defense against natural predators. Both sea otters (*16*) and staghorn sculpins (marine fish; *17*) are apparently able to distinguish non-toxic from toxic butter clams and avoid the latter while feasting on the former. The mechanism by which they detect toxicity is unknown.

The northern quahog (*Mercenaria mercenaria*) can also detect PSP toxicity in its food—dinoflagellates of the genus *Alexandrium* (*18*). The clams readily ingest a monospecific diet of strains with low toxicity while ingesting toxic species at a low rate and only when non-toxic dinoflagellates are also present. Natural populations of quahogs rarely accumulate substantial levels of PSP toxins, but as these experiments demonstrate they can become very toxic (up to 10,543 µg STX equivalents/100 g tissue) after feeding for two weeks on toxic species of *Alexandrium*.

Polyclonal antibodies against neosaxitoxin (neo-STX) were isolated from rabbits following injections with neo-STX conjugated to either keyhole limpet hemocyanin (KLH) or to bovine serum albumin (*19*). Competitive indirect ELISA using the neo-STX–KLH antiserum revealed that although the antibodies were specific for neo-STX, they also reacted well with STX. As little as 0.5 ng/mL of either toxin (in buffer solution) could be measured with this indirect ELISA. A radioimmunoassay developed during this study proved to be less sensitive than the ELISA. This assay could be an effective means of monitoring shellfish for PSP toxins.

A direct immunoassay using polyclonal antibodies against STX has also been developed for the detection of saxitoxin in shellfish (*20*). Two assay formats were devised: a microtitration plate ELISA and a test strip enzyme immunoassay (EIA). Detection limits for saxitoxin (in buffer solution) were 7 pg/mL for the ELISA and 200 pg/mL for the test strip EIA using visual evaluation. Detection limits of these methods for STX in extracts of shellfish tissue were 3 and 4 ng/g, respectively. Recovery of STX from spiked (10–1000 ng/g) mussel and clam tissue was 75–88%.

An improved LC method for determination of PSP toxins was described in which the toxins were converted to fluorescent purines by prechromatographic oxidation with periodate (*21*). Addition of ammonium formate to the periodate oxidation reaction greatly improved the yield of fluorescent derivatives. As little as 3–6 ng of the nonhydroxylated toxins and 7–12 ng of the hydroxylated compounds per gram of shellfish could be detected. Because the oxidation products of neosaxitoxin and B-2 could not be separated, the parent toxins were separated before oxidation using an SPE–COOH ion exchange cartridge. The repeatability coefficient of variation varied from 3 to 11% depending on the toxin and its concentration in the extract. Analytical results from this assay were comparable to results obtained with the mouse bioassay.

Of 17 oyster extract tablets (a so-called health food) tested, 11 apparently contained PSP toxins in the range of 3.9–12.5 mouse units/g (*22*). However, further analysis of these samples by TLC and HPLC did not confirm the presence of the toxins. Instead, mouse toxicity was correlated with calcium content of the tablets. It appears that the calcium carbonate in the tablets was converted to calcium chloride during the acid extraction step and that this compound was toxic to the mice.

Domoic acid intoxication (amnesic shellfish poisoning, ASP)

An extensive investigation into the cause of an unusually large number of sick and dying pelicans and cormorants along the California coast in September, 1991, identified the neurotoxin domoic acid (DA) in anchovies and shellfish (*23*). Levels of DA in razor clams were as high as 154 ppm, with the highest concentrations in the foot of the clam. At least 25 cases of human DA intoxication occurred in November following consumption of razor clams. Contrary to some earlier outbreaks of ASP, all of these cases exhibited only mild, transitory symptoms.

Mussels normally contain relatively large amounts of the more common excitatory amino acids, aspartic and glutamic acids (5.15 µmol/g wet weight) (*24*). Toxic mussels contain similar concentrations of these amino acids and, in addition, 0.64 µmol/g of DA, a rare excitatory amino acid. Toxic effects of mussel extracts containing DA on primary cultures of rat cerebellar neurons were significantly greater than similar concentrations of purified DA. This increased toxicity is apparently the result of synergism between DA and the other excitatory amino acids. Even subtoxic concentrations of DA could potentiate aspartic and glutamic acid neurotoxicity.

Experiments with nonaxenic (*25*) and axenic (*26*) cultures of *Nitzschia pungens* f. *multiseries* revealed that this diatom synthesizes maximal levels of DA during stationary phase of growth. Highest cellular concentrations of DA were 2 and 7 pg/cell in axenic and nonaxenic cultures, respectively. Three conditions were required for DA production in the nonaxenic cultures: cessation of cell division, availability of nitrogen, and the presence of light.

A one-compartment computer model has been developed to study the flux of DA through a mussel population near the Canadian coast (*27*). Comparison of the simulation results with data from field studies on toxic diatom populations and DA levels in the diatoms and in mussel tissues indicated that some unexpected physiological feedback processes were occurring. When mussel DA levels were very high (close to 300 ppm), the time for depuration of DA from the mussels was considerably longer than the usual 2–3 days observed in laboratory studies at lower DA concentrations. This suppression of depuration may explain the abnormal buildup of DA in mussels during some toxic blooms of *N. pungens*.

Neither salinity (18 or 28%) nor starved vs. fed condition of mussels affected depuration rate in mussels containing up to 50 ppm DA (*28*). Depuration was faster at 11 than at 6°C and in small (45–55 mm) than in large (60–70 mm) mussels. Generally, 50% of the toxin was eliminated within 24 h and after 72 h mussels were either clean or contained <5 ppm DA.

A greatly improved procedure has been devised for the extraction of DA from mussel tissues and from phytoplankton (*29*). More than 90% of DA was recovered from two extractions with a mixture of chloroform:methanol (1:2). DA and other water-soluble compounds were present in the aqueous methanol layer while lipids were dissolved in chloroform and denatured proteins remained at the interface. Since the extracted DA was relatively pure, elaborate cleanup was not necessary to obtain a product suitable for preparative HPLC. In fact, when analyzed by HPLC, UV–VIS absorption detection and amino acid analyses, the DA prepared by this procedure was as pure as and as toxic as DA obtained from commercial sources.

Following a collaborative study by 10 laboratories, an LC method using the AOAC PSP extraction procedure for determination of DA in mussels has been adopted official first action by AOAC (*30*). DA was extracted with 0.1 N HCl and then aliquots of the supernatant were diluted, filtered and analyzed by reverse-phase LC with a mobile phase of acetonitrile:water adjusted to about pH 2.5. Mean recovery of DA from spiked extracts (14.1 and 18.9 µg DA/g) was 75%. Relative standard deviations between laboratories ranged from 7.5 to 19.4%. Detection limit was about 1 µg DA/g.

A simple chemical confirmatory technique using butyl isothiocyanate has been developed (*31*). Following extraction of DA from mussel tissue with water and methanol, analysis was carried out by reverse-phase LC with UV absorption. For confirmation, aliquots of the extract were evaporated to dryness and reacted with butyl isothiocyanate to form a thiourea derivative which elutes later than underivatized DA. In mussel extracts, this derivative was obtained with a yield of 86–91% compared to a pure solution of DA. Detection limit for the derivative was about 5–10 µg/g of equivalent DA in extracts of mussels, clams, or oysters.

Diarrhetic shellfish poisoning

Plankton tows from a commercial mussel cultivation site on the Atlantic coast of Canada yielded numerous species of algae including a relatively small number of *Prorocentrum lima* (*32*). This species was identified by morphological characteristics and brought into unialgal culture. Analysis of culture extracts using HPLC with fluoresence detection revealed the presence of the diarrhetic shellfish poisoning (DSP) toxins okadaic acid (OA) and dinophysistoxin-1 (DTX-1) in about equal proportions (both at 25 ng/mL culture). *P. lima* is the first North American dinoflagellate species obtained from an area where DSP had occurred which has been shown to produce DSP toxins in culture.

Comparison of mussels from two different shellfish farms in the northern Adriatic Sea demonstrated a lower level of DSP toxicity in the area which was deeper and had abundant freshwater inflow (*33*). Phytoplankton samples revealed the presence of 8 species of *Dinophysis* in the area of both farms. A high positive correlation existed between the onset of mussel toxicity during a DSP outbreak in Slovenia in 1989 and the appearance of *Dinophysis* spp.

Okadaic acid (OA), one of the DSP toxins, was found to exert potent neurotoxic effects on rat cerebellar neurons in culture (*34*). At a concentration of 0.5 nM, OA did not affect non-neuronal cells but was toxic to neurons causing disintegration of neurites and swelling of cell bodies followed by cellular death. Endogenous excitatory amino acids do not appear to be involved in the mechanism of toxicity.

A higher toxicity was detected in mussel samples by the standard mouse bioassay than could be explained by their content of OA and DTX-1 as determined by HPLC (*35*). Since different extraction solvents (acetone vs. aqueous methanol) were used to prepare samples for HPLC and for the mouse assay, there may have been a difference in extraction efficiency, thereby explaining the difference in toxicity. However, extraction experiments using both solvents indicated that this was not the case. Therefore, it appears that some other toxin is present in these Norwegian mussels.

Several aspects of the mouse bioassay, as applied to mussel extracts for the detection of DSP toxins, have been evaluated (*36*). Mice of different sizes injected with the same amount of mussel extract were found to vary in their response. Even mice of the same size show some individual variation in response to the toxic extracts. The authors suggest that two mice be given size-adjusted doses of extracts followed by a 4-h surveillance period and a limit of one hour for acceptable time variation between parallel samples. An HPLC method was developed for the determination of OA and free fatty

acids in mussels (*37*). OA and the fatty acids were extracted from mussels and derivatized with 9-chloromethylanthracene prior to HPLC. This compound enhances the fluorescent detection sensitivity of very small amounts of OA. Analyses of mussels from the Gulf of Trieste revealed the presence of toxic fatty acids (e.g. linolenic acid) which may interfere with the mouse bioassay of DSP toxins, but OA was not detected in these samples.

Tetrodotoxin

Tetrodotoxin (TTX) is a potent neurotoxin most commonly associated with puffer fish (*Fugu* spp.) consumed in Japan. It has been generally accepted that artificially hatched and cultured puffer are nontoxic. But recently low levels of TTX (about 0.2 MU/g of tissue as TTX) were discovered in the intestines of 60-day- and one-year-old cultured puffer fish (*F. rubripes*) (*38*). Neither mouse bioassay nor HPLC detected TTX in the liver of these fish.

Freshwater puffer fish (*Tetraodon fangi* and *T. palembangensis*) from a region in Thailand where an outbreak of *T. fangi* poisoning had occurred were found to be toxic throughout most of the year (*39*). Mouse bioassay revealed a marked variation in toxicity among individuals, with the highest levels found in the skin (907 MU/g), eggs (336 MU/g), muscle (331 MU/g), liver (225 MU/g), and intestine (159 MU/g).

Six puffer-related fish species consumed in Japan were examined for toxicity and for tetrodotoxin and its derivatives (*40,41*). Of 31 specimens of the pufferfish *Arothron firmamentum*, toxicity was detected in the skin of 6 and in the ovaries of 11 but not in the muscle, liver, or digestive tract of any fish. Maximum lethal potency was 30.6 MU/g in males (skin) and 888 MU/g in females (ovaries). No toxicity in the mouse bioassay was exhibited by liver extracts of spiny puffer (*Diodon holacanthus*), sunfish (*Mola mola*), puffer (*Triodon bursarius*), or the filefish (*Stephanolepis cirrhifer* and *Navodon modestus*). HPLC and GC–MS analyses detected TTX and anhydroTTX in small amounts in the liver of the spiny puffer but not in any other fish.

Only one of 6 species of marine gastropods collected from fish markets in Taiwan tested negative for TTX (*42,43*). Of 112 specimens of calf moon shell (*Natica vitellus*), 56 of bladder moon shell (*Polinices didyma*), 20 of pear-shaped moon shell (*P. tumidus*), 17 of *Rapana rapiformis*, and 28 of *R. venosa venosa,* 34%, 71%, 5%, 24%, and 21%, respectively, were toxic and contained TTX. Maximum toxicities of whole specimens of each species were 711, 1563, 6, 400, and 477 MU/specimen, respectively.

Various strains of marine bacteria are known to produce TTX, and previous reports indicated that TTX accumulates in marine sediments off the coast of Japan. Of 10 actinomycetes isolated from various marine sediments (inshore as well as 3569 and 5974 m offshore), pure cultures of 9 produced TTX (*44*). Tissue culture assay, HPLC, and GC–MS confirmed the identity of the toxins.

A monoclonal antibody reacting with TTX has been prepared and used in a direct competitive ELISA to detect TTX in biological samples (*45*). Sensitivity of the assay as determined by concentrations required for 50% and 20% inhibition were 6–7 ng/mL and 2–3 ng/mL, respectively. Results obtained with this assay were comparable to those obtained with HPLC, and the immunoassay was more sensitive and required less sample preparation, less time, and a reduced investment in equipment.

Neurotoxic shellfish poisoning

Neurotoxic shellfish poisoning (NSP), characterized by paresthesia, reversal of hot and cold temperature sensation, myalgia, and vertigo, results from eating shellfish containing brevetoxins produced by marine dinoflagellates during red tide blooms. In 1987, 48 persons in North Carolina who had consumed oysters reported symptoms of NSP (*46*). The illnesses were generally mild and there were no deaths. Median incubation period was 3 h and median duration of illness was 17 h. Only 4 persons had bought oysters at fish markets; the remainder reported eating oysters harvested by themselves or friends. In all but one instance, the oysters had been cooked prior to eating. Although the dinoflagellates were detected in the water for several months after the first NSP case was reported, the number of cases dropped sharply on November 2 when the first closure of affected shellfish waters occurred.

Polyclonal antibodies were prepared from rabbits immunized with a brevetoxin B immunogen (*47*). In a competitive binding assay using these antibodies, brevetoxin B alcohol was six times more effective as an inhibitor than brevetoxin B while brevetoxin B was 500 times more effective than brevetoxin A.

Palytoxin

Thirteen people on Guam who consumed a seaweed, *Polycavernosa tsudai*, reported a range of gastrointestinal and neurological symptoms (*48*). Persons who only tasted the seaweed or ate a few spoonfuls were mildly affected while 3 others who ate about half a cereal bowl of the seaweed died about 31–120 h after ingestion. The implicated seaweed was purchased from a single vendor who had collected it during high tide (contrary to the usual practice of collecting at low tide). Preliminary toxicological analysis detected a compound similar to palytoxin in seaweed obtained from one affected household. Further studies are underway to determine how this toxin came to contaminate normally edible seaweed. Two methods for determination of palytoxin by high-performance-capillary electrophoresis (HPCE) and by HPLC were devised (*49*). Detection limits for these two techniques were 0.5 pg/injection and 125 ng/injection, respectively. Detection sensitivity at 230 nm was twofold higher than at 263 nm. Sample analysis time for both methods was about 10 min. The HPCE method allows detection of low concentrations of palytoxin in small sample volumes which is not possible by HPLC.

Blue-green algal toxins in mussels

A seasonal blue-green algal bloom (*Nodularia*) in a brackish/marine water estuary in western Australia raised the question of toxicity in edible mussels growing there (*50*). Extracts of a series of mussels collected during a bloom period were toxic in a mouse bioassay. Toxicity was associated only with the gastrointestinal tract and associated organs from the mussels. Autopsy of the tested mice revealed hepatocyte necrosis and degeneration characteristic of poisoning by *Nodularia*. Approximately 1 g of the gastrointestinal tract of the most toxic mussel sample was a lethal dose for 1 kg live weight of mice.

BIOGENIC AMINES

Biogenic amines, such as histamine, tyramine, and β-phenylethylamine, have been implicated as etiological agents in several outbreaks of food poisoning, in dietary-induced migraine headaches, and in cases of hypertensive crisis in some patients. In a recent review, the importance of biogenic amines in cheese (particularly histamine) and other fermented foods was discussed (51). Clinical aspects and epidemiology of histamine poisoning, methods of analysis, and the regulatory situation relative to histamine in the U.S. were also briefly covered.

Tyramine content of a variety of preserved and fermented foods and condiments of Far Eastern cuisine was determined by HPLC with fluorescence detection (52). Nearly all items tested contained some tyramine, with the highest levels found in a soybean condiment from Taiwan, soy sauce from Taiwan, fermented soybeans from Singapore, Swiss soy sauce, and a fermented soybean paste from Korea (939, 878, 713, 293, and 206 mg/kg or mg/L, respectively). Total tyramine content of 7 complete meals offered at typical restaurants in Zurich varied from 1.61 mg at a large Chinese restaurant to 20.94 mg at a large Korean restaurant.

Seafood

Ingestion of marlin fillets was responsible for the largest Canadian outbreak of scombroid poisoning affecting 12 persons (53). The fish, which was imported from Ecuador, was purchased at two grocery stores in Ontario and consumed 1–6 days later after cooking. Four pieces of leftover cooked marlin were found to contain an average of 360 mg histamine/100 g while raw marlin from the store contained an average of 331 mg histamine/100 g. Since

this is 3–4 times the amount of histamine known to cause illness, the onset of symptoms (flushing, rash, headache, diarrhea, and weakness) was rapid—within a few minutes in some cases. Duration of illness was 4–96 h.

Controversy continues concerning the importance of histamine in the etiology of scombrotoxicosis. A total of 86 mackerel fillets associated with an outbreak of toxicosis were analyzed for their contents of histamine, cadaverine, putrescine, spermine, spermidine, and tyramine and were then fed to informed healthy volunteers under medical supervision. Only 30 of the fillets rapidly induced symptoms. No statistically significant differences could be found between the amine contents of the fillets causing scombrotoxicosis and those which did not. Nor was there a significant relationship between the amine doses and volunteer reactions (54). Volunteers appeared to fall into susceptible and non-susceptible groups. Further experiments with susceptible volunteers predosed with either a placebo or an antihistamine (chlorpheniramine, 4 mg) demonstrated that the antihistamine could abolish the vomiting and diarrhea associated with the ingestion of scombrotoxic fish (55). Therefore, it appears that endogenous histamine released by mast cell degranulation may be a primary factor in scombrotoxicosis while the role of dietary histamine is minor. The substance responsible for mast cell degranulation is now being investigated.

After 24 h at ambient temperature (24–28°C) or 8 days on ice, the surface bacteria on freshly caught sardines grew rapidly and invaded the muscle tissue (56). Histamine and cadaverine accumulated to levels of 2350 and 1050 ppm, respectively. Fresh fish had a high histidine content and this decreased during storage. Salting of fish at 8% delayed bacterial and chemical changes in iced, but not in ambient temperature, fish.

The Greenland shark (*Somniosus microcephalus*) has long been known to be toxic to dogs and humans. Recent analyses of the toxic fractions of shark flesh revealed the presence of large amounts of trimethylamine oxide (TMAO): 1.05–1.3 g TMAO/100 g frozen shark flesh (57). Symptoms of shark poisoning appear to be due to acute trimethylamine poisoning resulting from intestinal reduction of

TMAO to trimethylamine. High concentrations of trimethylamine block contractions of the rat phrenic nerve–diaphragm preparation.

Dairy products

Histamine production by *Lactobacillus buchneri* strain St2A, isolated from Swiss cheese implicated in an outbreak of histamine poisoning, occurs readily in Swiss cheese in which NaCl levels never exceed 3%. However, higher salt concentrations partially inhibit (3.5%) or greatly inhibit (5.5%) histamine production by this strain. Cheddar cheese, with 5% salt in the moisture phase, usually contains very little or no histamine. To assess the potential for histamine production in low-salt cheddar cheese, pasteurized milk was inoculated with 10^2–10^4 cells of *L. buchneri*/mL and then manufactured into low-salt cheddar cheese (*58*). After 180 days of aging at 7°C, these bacteria had increased 100-fold and proteolysis increased about 4-fold but histamine levels remained low, <6 mg/100 g. It appears that relatively low levels of proteolysis and low temperature of storage inhibit histamine production in this type of cheese.

A survey of 17 low-salt cheeses and of 50 Swiss cheeses revealed that 2 of the former (both low-salt Swiss varieties) and 9 of the latter contained >45 mg histamine/100 g cheese (*59*). Over 800 randomly chosen bacterial colonies isolated from these cheeses were screened for histamine production. None of the isolates from the low-salt cheeses and only 5 from Swiss cheese (identified as species of *Lactobacillus, Lactococcus,* and *Entero-coccus*) produced histamine in MRS broth supplemented with L-histidine. Therefore, it appears that histamine-producing bacteria are not widespread.

An improved procedure for extraction of 8 biogenic amines in cheese and their determination by HPLC has been developed (*60*). The procedure involved two extractions with 0.1 M HCl, addition of solid sodium carbonate to raise the pH above 12, and finally an extraction with *n*-butanol–chloroform. The extract was reacted with dansyl chloride, and the dansyl derivatives of the amines were separated by reversed-phase LC followed by UV detection at 254 nm. Recoveries were good (70–100%)

for all the amines except putrescine, spermine, and spermidine. Detection limits varied from 0.02 to 0.08 for the different compounds.

Alcoholic beverages

Samples corresponding to various stages of beer brewing were obtained from a Spanish brewery and assayed for histamine and tyramine (*61*). Increases in histamine during brewing were negligible but tyramine levels increased from 2.5 mg/L in the wort to 40 mg/L in the final product. Most of this increase occurred during the first 5 days of manufacture, coinciding with the most rapid increase in alcohol content. Analyses of 64 samples of 4 types of beer from the Spanish market revealed averages of 0.38–1.49 mg histamine/L (maximum of 4.9 mg/L) and 3.48–7.68 mg tyramine/L (maximum of 30.6 mg/L).

An LC method for the determination of 16 biogenic amines in wine was developed (*62*). Wine samples were first cleaned up on an Amberlite CG-50 column and then the amines were derivatized with dansyl chloride. LC analyses were performed on Finepak SIL C18S and LiChrosorb RP-8 columns with an acetonitrile–water elution gradient. Recoveries of the amines from spiked samples averaged 91–105% except for tryptamine, which was only 59%. A survey of 75 commercial red and white wines using this method detected 12 amines in most samples, with total concentrations ranging from undetectable to 31.5 µg/mL. The amines present in highest concentrations in red and white wines, respectively, were putrescine (4.84 µg/mL) and isoamylamine (5.11 µg/mL).

An HPLC method for the determination of the 6 most important wine amines (histamine, tyramine, putrescine, cadaverine, isoamylamine, and β-phenethylamine) has been automated with pre-column derivatization with *o*-phthalaldehyde and fluorescence detection (*63*). Wine samples were derivatized directly without a cleanup step. Detection limits for the amines ranged from 0.006 to 0.05 mg/L but, due to background interference, the determination limits for the amines in wine ranged from 0.5 to 1.0 mg/L. Analyses of 16 red and 5 white wines by this method demonstrated that putrescine was the most abundant amine (2–72 mg/L) in all samples except for 1 white wine with 3.7 mg isoamylamine and 2 mg putrescine/L.

Other foods

A series of experiments was carried out to assess the importance of certain factors on histamine levels in eggs (64). Egg yolks of good layers (egg production rate >75%) had a much higher histamine content (778 ng/g) than those with an egg production rate <60% (589 ng/g). Stress caused by crowding hens in cages did not significantly affect histamine levels in eggs. Significant decreases, of 100–141 ng/g, in histamine concentrations were observed in eggs stored for 3–5 days at 10–13°C or incubated at 41°C for 30 or 60 min. Even greater decreases of 381–416 ng/g occurred when the yolks were boiled for 5–10 min.

Effects of heat treatment and storage temperature on the concentrations of 6 biogenic amines in straw mushrooms (*Volvariella volvacea*) were studied (65). The total amine content in fresh straw mushrooms was reduced by about 80% from 147.7 mg/kg to 28.1 mg/kg after boiling for 5 min. Commercial canned mushrooms contained very low levels (7.1 mg/kg) of only 3 amines (putrescine, tyramine, and 2-phenylethylamine). Levels of all 6 amines increased with storage time (up to 5 days) at both 4 and 25°C, with a more rapid increase at 25°C.

MUTAGENS AND CARCINOGENS IN HEATED FOODS

Heterocyclic amines

During the last decade a series of mutagenic and carcinogenic heterocyclic amines has been isolated from cooked foods. In a recent review, data on the tryptophan pyrolysis products was summarized (66). These compounds can be detected in cooked meat and fish as well as in cigarette smoke, diesel exhaust, and rainwater. They are strongly mutagenic in the Ames test, induce chromosomal aberrations, chromatid exchanges, and cell transformation in cultured cells and induce hepatocellular carcinoma and adenomas in rodents. Their presence in human plasma, urine, and bile indicates that they may also pose a health risk to humans.

A series of three papers in *Cancer Research* reviewed some recent research on heterocyclic amines produced under ordinary cooking conditions. The chemistry of these compounds, their relative abundance in different cooked foods, and their carcinogenic potential in rodents was summarized (67). Since a linear relationship exists between a wide range of heterocyclic amine doses and DNA adduct levels in animals, even low doses in humans may form DNA adducts and be implicated in carcinogenicity. Another report highlighted results from studies in nonhuman primates, primarily cynomolgus monkeys, and from in vitro experiments examining the metabolism and genotoxicity of heterocyclic amines (68). Both 2-amino-3-methyl-imidazo[4,5-*f*]quinoline (IQ) and 2-amino-1-methyl-6-phenylimidazo[4,5-*b*]pyridine (PhIP) form high levels of DNA adducts in a number of organs, particularly the liver, kidney, and heart. In the case of IQ this correlates well with long-term carcinogenicity studies in monkeys, in which 50% of those orally dosed with 20 mg IQ/kg, 5 days/week, developed hepatocellular carcinomas. Similar long-term studies with PhIP and 2-amino-3,8-dimethyl-imidazo[4,5-*f*]quinoxaline (MeIQx) are in progress. Formation of MeIQx and 2-amino-3,4,8-trimethyl-imidazo[4,5-*f*]quinoxaline (4,8-DiMeIQx) in commercial fried-beef patties can be substantially reduced by prior microwave treatment of the meat and pouring off the resulting liquid before frying (69). This procedure reduced mutagenic activity in *Salmonella* assays and MeIQx and 4,8-DiMeIQx levels to 5–10%, 12%, and 50% of that found in unmicrowaved meat. In rodents orally dosed with MeIQx (5 mg/kg to 500 ng/kg), a linear relationship was observed between dose and DNA adduct formation. Extrapolation from rodent carinogenicity data to humans gives a maximum credible risk from consumption of heterocyclic amines of approximately 1/1000 exposed individuals.

OCCURRENCE AND DETECTION IN FOODS. In a survey of basic extracts of 7 types of canned meat and fish in Taiwan, the highest mutagenicity, as determined by the Ames test, was associated with canned roasted eel (*70*). Further analysis of the mutagenic fractions from canned eel revealed the presence of approximately 1.1 ng MeIQx and 5.3 ng of 7,8-DiMeIQx. Frying of raw eel was found to increase its mutagenicity with a linear relationship observed between mutagenicity and cooking temperature and an exponential relationship between mutagenicity and frying time.

A sensitive method was devised for the determination of 2-amino-3,8-dimethylimidazo[4,5-*f*]-quinoline (MeIQ) in instant coffee and lyophilized home-brewed coffee (*71*). Samples were dissolved in water and treated with Amberlite XAD-2, Extrelut/copper phthalocyanine–Sephasorb, Sephasorb HP, and propanesulfonic acid/octadecyl silica to remove impurities. The purified extracts were then analyzed by HPLC. The estimated detection limit was 5-10 pg/g of coffee beans, and recoveries of 49-61% were achieved in samples spiked at picogram levels. Using this method, MeIQ was not detected in samples of instant or roasted coffee.

Determination of heterocyclic amines in cooked salmon was also achieved by HPLC following sample purification on Extrelut and propylsulfonic acid gel (*72*). Detection limits were in the low ng/g range, and recoveries from spiked samples varied from 45% to 90% for the different compounds. In salmon oven-cooked at 200°C for up to 40 min or pan-broiled (200°C) or barbecued (270°C) for less than 6 min, little or no production of MeIQx or PhIP was observed. However, pan-broiling or barbecuing for longer than 6 min resulted in up to a 10-fold increase in PhIP (but not in MeIQx) levels.

Since anticarcinogenic effects have been imputed to yogurt and lactic acid bacteria, some recent studies have investigated the ability of bovine milk caseins (*73*), α-lactalbumin and β-lactoglobulin (*74*), and lactic acid bacteria (*Streptococcus cremoris*, *Lactobacillus acidophilus*, and *Bifidobacterium bifidum*) (*75*) to bind to heterocyclic amines. Experiments with the milk proteins involved exposure of 2 mg protein to 20 μg of heterocyclic amine in 0.4 mL of phosphate buffer, pH 7.4 in a shaker for 10 min at 37°C. Whole casein and κ-casein bound >82% of the 3-amino-1,4-dimethyl-5*H*-

pyrido[4,3-*b*]indole (Trp-P-1), 3-amino-1-methyl-5*H*-pyrido[4,3-*b*]indole (Trp-P-2), and 2-amino-6-methyldipyrido[1,2-*a*:3',2'-*d*]imidazole (Glu-P-1) in the test solutions. The lactalbumins and lactoglobulins were more efficient at binding Trp-P-1 (78.7–90.4%) than Trp-P-2 (23.9–43.9%) and Glu-P-1 (40.8–57.4%). In both cases maximum binding was at pH 7.4. Cytoplasm of the lactic acid bacteria did not bind the heterocyclic amines but whole cells bound 85–87% and cell wall skeletons bound 69–71% of these amines. Trp-P-1 was bound more efficiently. In similar experiments, cells of 50 yeast isolates from a traditional alcoholic beverage brewed in Ghana were found to bind 78–99% of Trp-P-1 in test solutions (*76*). Binding to cell walls and the glucan fraction was better than to the mannan fraction. This binding was also pH dependent and was inhibited by metal salts. Binding of heterocyclic amines by these proteins and cells may reduce their bioavailability and therefore their toxicity.

Several experiments with model systems have demonstrated the importance of glucose or other sugars in the production of heterocyclic amines. When a mixture of creatine (0.9 mmol), phenylalanine (0.9 mmol), and glucose (0.45 mmol) was heated for 10 min at 180 or 225°C, at least three mutagens were produced: PhIP, MeIQx, and 3,4,8-TriMeIQx (*77*). Heating the system without glucose resulted in the formation of only PhIP, but in much smaller amounts. If glucose was present in greater than or equimolar amounts of the other two reactants, mutagen production was also greatly reduced.

In a system containing 100 mM creatinine and 100 mM phenylalanine and heated for 2 weeks at 60°C, PhIP was produced only if a sugar (glyceraldehyde, erythrose, arabinose, ribose, glucose, or galactose) or an aldehyde (acetaldehyde or formaldehyde) was present (*78*). Erythrose and glyceraldehyde were the most productive sugars. Incubation of this mixture with ribose or glucose at 37°C for 6 weeks also resulted in PhIP formation.

A new heterocyclic amine was isolated from a mixture of 1 g glutamic acid, 0.89 g creatine, and 0.61 g glucose heated dry for 2 h at 200°C (*79*). This compound was purified by HPLC and its structure was determined to be 2,6-diamino-3,4-dimethyl-7-oxo-pyrano[4,3-*g*]benzimidazole by NMR and IR spectral data. This new compound was mutagenic in the Ames test.

BIOLOGICAL EFFECTS. In order to estimate normal human exposure to carcinogenic heterocyclic amines, the concentrations of Trp-P-1, Trp-P-2, PhIP, and MeIQx were measured in 24-h urine samples from 10 healthy volunteers eating a normal diet (80). All 4 amines were detected in the urine of all subjects at levels of 0.04–1.43 ng Trp-P-1, 0.03–0.68 ng Trp-P-2, 0.12–1.97 ng PhIP, and 11–47 ng MeIQx. Since 1.8–4.9% of an oral dose of MeIQx has been reported to be excreted unchanged, the daily exposure of humans was estimated to be 0.2–2.6 µg/person. None of these amines were detected in the urine of 3 inpatients receiving parenteral alimentation.

HPLC analyses of plasma and red blood cell samples of 8 healthy subjects and of 8 patients with uremia (being treated with hemodialysis) revealed the presence of Trp-P-1 and Trp-P-2 in all of them (81). Both amines were present in greater concentrations in the plasma and red blood cells of uremic patients. In plasma, healthy subjects had 2.4 pg Trp-P-1/mL and 2.7 pg Trp-P-2/mL, respectively, while uremic patients had 12.6 and 7.8 pg/mL, respectively. In red blood cells, healthy subjects had 18.8 and 55.8 pg/g hemoglobin and uremic patients had 43 and 131 pg/g hemoglobin.

Metabolic activation of the heterocyclic amines IQ, MeIQx, PhIP, and Glu-P-1 by human liver microsomes and human liver and colon cytosols was investigated (82). All of these amines were readily activated by N-hydroxylation by the liver microsomes, with PhIP exhibiting the highest rate of oxidation. These N-OH amines bound covalently to calf thymus DNA in vitro. Further activation of the N-OH derivatives by O-acetylation occurred in liver and colon cytosol preparations. Some of the 8 cytosolic samples from different individuals were more rapid acetylators than others. Acetylation activity in colonic cytosols was generally less than in the liver cytosols, and the acetylation rate varied for the different N-OH heterocyclic amines. These data on metabolic activation of the heterocyclic amines are significant in light of recent epidemiological studies demonstrating an excess of rapid acetylator

individuals among colon cancer patients and of slow acetylator individuals among bladder cancer patients.

DNA adducts were formed with IQ and MeIQ in human mammary epithelial cell aggregates in vitro (83). Analysis by ^{32}P-postlabelling assays revealed that the adduct patterns obtained resemble those previously demonstrated in DNA of tissues of mice fed IQ or MeIQ. Mice and rats fed a single oral dose of 5–50 mg IQ/kg body weight were found to form 4 or 5 DNA adducts in various tissues, with the highest adduct levels in the liver and lower levels detected in the small intestine, large intestine, forestomach, and lungs (84,85). In all cases, adduct formation was related to dose and the major adduct, comprising 68–79% of the total, was N-(deoxyguanosin-8-yl)-IQ. An N^2-(2'-deoxyguanosin-8-yl)–PhIP adduct has been detected in the liver of a rat dosed orally with labelled PhIP (1 mg/kg) following induction with an injection of 200 mg PCB/kg (86).

DNA adducts have also been detected in the hearts of rats fed for 4 weeks with diets containing carcinogenic dose levels of IQ (0.03%), MeIQx (0.04%), Trp-P-1 (0.015%), or Glu-P-1 (0.05%) (87). All of these compounds formed adducts at 10–20% of the respective liver adduct levels. Heart DNA adducts with MeIQx increased linearly during 40 weeks of feeding and were not eliminated when the rats were fed MeIQx for 20 weeks and then the basal diet alone for another 20 weeks.

Rats gavaged with single doses of ^{14}C-PhIP (0.3–30 mg/kg) excreted most of the dose in feces within 48 h (88,89). Unchanged PhIP in the feces accounted for 51% of a 0.6 mg/kg dose at 24 h and 42% of a 3.0 mg/kg dose at 48 h. Blood contained a small fraction of the dose, some of which persisted in a form bound to hemoglobin. Pretreatment of rats with PCB or 3-methylcholanthrene resulted in a increase in 4'-hydroxylation of PhIP and increased binding of PhIP to the liver and kidney, while pretreatment with phenobarbital increased the amount of N-hydroxylation and generally reduced the binding of PhIP to body tissues.

Effects of a range of doses (0.01–20 mg/kg) on the metabolism of MeIQx in rats were investigated (90). Sulfamate and glucuronide conjugates of MeIQx were the predominant urinary metabolites detected in high-dose rats while at low doses, glucuronide formation was the most important metabolic pathway. Pretreatment with PCB enhanced *N*-hydroxylase activity about 20-fold in hepatic microsomes, thereby increasing excretion of the *N*-glucuronide conjugate in urine.

Many heterocyclic amines are known carcinogens in laboratory animals. Recently, PhIP, the most abundant heterocyclic amine in broiled meat and fish, was tested for carcinogenicity in rats (*91*). After 52 weeks of consuming a diet containing 400 ppm PhIP (equivalent to a daily intake of 400–500 kg of broiled beef), 16% of male rats developed colon adenocarcinomas and 14% of female rats developed mammary adenocarcinomas. No hepatic tumors were observed.

Hepatic tumors were observed in mice which had been given 3 injections of Glu-P-1, IQ, MeIQx, or PhIP during the first 15 days of life (*92*). At autopsy at 12 months, 11% of control mice had liver tumors, and 75%, 37%, 33%, and 50% of those receiving injections of the respective heterocyclic amines had liver tumors.

Since several heterocyclic amines may be present in cooked foods, experiments were conducted to determine the possibility of synergistic effects (*93*). Rats were fed diets containing possible carcinogenic doses of Trp-P-2 (500 ppm), Glu-P-1 (500 ppm), 2-amino-3-methyl-9*H*-pyrido[2,3-*b*]indole (MeAαC) (800 ppm), 2-amino-9*H*-pyrido[2,3-*b*]indole (AαC) (800 ppm), or PhIP (400 ppm), or at 1/5 or 1/25 of those doses, or all 5 compounds together, each at 1/5 or 1/25 of those doses for 8 weeks. As expected, all the amines except PhIP significantly increased the number of hepatic GST-P positive foci at the highest doses. With the combined treatment at the 1/5 dose level, a significant synergistic enhancement of the number and size of these foci occurred. This was not true for the combined 1/25 dose group.

Genotoxic effects of IQ and MeIQx were evaluated in an extensive series of assays, including mutagenicity tests in *Salmonella typhimurium* and Chinese hamster V79 cells, chromosome aberration assays in Chinese hamster ovary cells and cultured human lymphocytes, and toxicokinetic, tissue distribution, and micronuclei induction studies in mice

(*94*). Overall results indicate that these compounds are weakly genotoxic and carcinogenic. Both compounds are mutagenic to *S. typhimurium*, bind to mouse liver DNA and induce mutagenicity in urine of mice fed these compounds. Neither amine was mutagenic to V79 cells nor did they induce micronuclei in mice. IQ, but not MeIQx, was able to induce chromosomal aberrations in vitro.

Cholesterol oxides

Cholesterol oxidation products (COPS) have been implicated in the etiology of atherosclerosis and coronary heart disease. Recent literature on the chemistry of COPS, factors affecting their occurrence in foods, and in vitro and in vivo studies on their cytotoxic and atherogenic effects have been reviewed (*95*). Various animal food products, such as meat, egg and dairy products, have been reported to contain several COPS developed during certain processing treatments involving heat.

COPS present in fast-food French fried potatoes fried in animal–vegetable shortening varied from 11 to 50 ppm, in daily samples from two restaurants during a 30-day period (*96*). Six different COPS were identified by capillary GC and MS: 5α-cholestane-3β,5,6β-triol(triol); 7α-hydroxycholesterol; 7β-hydroxycholesterol; α-epoxide; β-epoxide; and 7-ketocholesterol. In restaurant A, the major COPS were the α- and β-epoxides (average of 11 ppm) with only traces of triol while in restaurant B, triol levels were high (average of 9 ppm) and epoxide levels were low. Triol is one of the most potent of the angiotoxic COPS.

Conditions favoring formation of COPS during spray-drying of egg yolk using a direct-heated spray dryer with an evaporative capacity of up to 7 kg water/h were investigated (*97*). The only two parameters with significant effects on COPS levels were the outlet air temperature and nitrogen oxides (NO_x) in the combustion gases. At 5 ppm NO_x, the total COPS concentrations formed at 75, 100, and 150°C were 21, 32, and 75 ppm, respectively. At 300 ppm NO_x, total COPS levels at these temperatures were 58, 72, and 213 ppm, respectively. Much of the increase in COPS detected at the higher NO_x concentrations is due to the 3.5- to 4.5-fold increase in β-epoxide. Generally, levels of all of the 5 individual COPS monitored were increased by higher temperatures and higher NO_x concentrations.

COPS formed during the production of ghee (clarified butter fat) and in ghee used for frying were investigated (98). No COPS were detected in fresh cream and only traces were observed in butter. Production of ghee at a temperature of 120°C induced the formation of 4 or 5 COPS with total levels of 15–21 mg/kg. After 3 one-hour cycles of frying wheat dough at 185–200°C, levels of all 7 individual COPS monitored increased dramatically, with a total COPS concentration of 332.5 mg/kg in the final sample.

Although COPS are present in higher levels in cooked foods, they have been detected at low concentrations in raw veal (340 ppb), beef (1330 ppb), pork (126 ppb), and chicken (253 ppb) (99). Meat samples were extracted by a modified dry column procedure using silicic acid in the trap of the column. Then sterols were isolated by preparative TLC and quantified by HPLC. All the meats contained 7-ketocholesterol (63–829 ppb), cholesterol 5α,6α-epoxide (33–134 ppb), and cholesterol 5β,6β-epoxide (41–367 ppb). During storage in a refrigerator (0–4°C), total COPS in beef increased with time, reaching a level of 3670 ppb after 3 weeks.

A rapid, single-run HPLC method has been devised to separate and quantify benzoate esters of 5 cholesterol oxides (100). A Novapak C_{18} column with a mobile phase of 85% isopropanol–water was used to separate 7-ketocholesterol, cholestane-triol, epoxy-cholesterol, 7-hydroxycholesterol, and 25-hydroxycholesterol. These compounds were detected by UV at 230 nm. Linearity was excellent, and as little as 500 ng cholesterol benzoate/20 μL of solution could be detected.

Because cholesterol can oxidize under relatively mild conditions to form a variety of oxidation products, the problem of producing COPS artifacts during procedures for COPS analysis in foods is serious. Deuterium-labelled cholesterol added to samples immediately upon isolation can be used to monitor artifactually produced COPS (101). Liver samples, thus labelled, were extracted and subjected to silica gel LC and reversed-phase HPLC to separate the COPS fraction. Then the ratios of labelled to unlabelled oxides and of labelled to unlabelled cholesterol were determined by capillary GC and MS. This method has been used successfully to accurately detect COPS at the ppm level and to correct for COPS produced under "harsh" analysis conditions.

Other lipid oxidation products

Some of the major mechanisms by which lipid oxidation products are generated during the processing of foods and the potential toxicological relevance of these oxidation products were recently reviewed (102). Lipid oxidation is initiated by free radical and/or singlet oxygen mechanisms and, depending on the nature of the food and environmental factors, results in the formation of a wide variety of oxidation products. The toxicity of these products depends on their own structure and on their interactions with other food components which may enhance their toxicity or limit their bioavailability.

Biological effects of coconut oil and of a vegetable oil which had been used for deep frying (180°C for 10 h/day for 3 consecutive days) were tested in *Salmonella typhimurium* and in rats (103). Polar fractions of both oils were mutagenic to *S. typhimurium* strain TA97, and the polar fraction of the vegetable oil was also mutagenic to strain TA100. Rats fed the heated oils as 10% of their diet for 4 weeks showed no increased mutagenicity in urine or feces to strain TA97 or increased fecal mutagenicity to strain TA100 compared to rats fed unheated oils. However, consumption of heated vegetable oil did significantly increase urinary excretion of TA100 mutagens relative to controls. Enhanced cell proliferation in the esophagus and alterations in some serum biochemical markers, indicating cellular damage to liver and kidneys, were also observed in rats fed the heated vegetable oil.

Consumption of fresh and thermally oxidized (heated for 100 h at 200°C, without food) olive and sunflower oils as 12% of the diet for 10 months altered desaturase activities and lipid composition of liver microsomes in rats (104). Although membrane composition and fluidity were affected by the heated oils, no signs of acute toxicity were observed.

Fourteen days following a single oral dose of 1000, 300, 100, 30, 10, or 0 mg *trans*-4-hydroxy-2-nonenal (HNE)/kg body weight, a dose-dependent increase in diffuse liver cell necrosis occurred (*105*). Two rats died within 8 h of receiving the highest dose of HNE, and autopsy revealed extensive necrosis of the kidney but little liver damage. Renal effects were mild in the other rats which survived to the end of the experiment (14 days). Small amounts of HNE have been detected in various foods and oils.

Heating of linoleic acid for 7 days at 37°C resulted in the formation of hydroperoxides (18%) and of secondary oxidation products (35%) (*106,107*). When these oxidation products were fed to rats, only the aldehyde fraction of the secondary oxidation products was incorporated into the liver. Although several hepatic enzymes are inhibited in vitro by dietary products of lipid oxidation, only mitochondrial NAD-dependent aldehyde dehydrogenase and glucose-6-phosphate dehydrogenase were inactivated in vivo in rats. It appears that, in vivo, the aldehydic fraction incorporated into the liver inhibits these enzymes as well as destroying coenzyme A and disturbing the synthetic system of glucokinase. Reversed-phase liquid chromatography was used to monitor formation of acrolein and other low-molecular-weight aldehydes (LMWA) from vegetable oil used for frying fish and doughnuts (*108*). Analyses for LMWA in the doughnuts, the coating of the fried fish, and the volatiles emitted during frying revealed that most of the LMWAs formed codistilled with steam during frying. Different frying temperatures (182 or 204°C) did not affect LMWA content in coatings from fried fish nor did freshness of the frying medium, frying time, or batch size affect LMWA content in doughnuts. Highest mean acrolein levels detected in fish coatings, yeast doughnuts, and cake doughnuts were, respectively, 0.1, 0.3, and 0.9 ppm.

Frying oil stability was found to be enhanced when the coating of batter-breaded beef nuggets contained defatted glandless cottonseed flour (GCF) (*109*). Cottonseed oil was used for continuous (2-day) frying of beef nuggets at 177°C. Oil used to fry nuggets with the GCF coating had lower free fatty acid levels, lower levels of TBA-reactive substances, and a lighter color compared to the control oil not exposed to GCF. The coating and the meat portion of the experimental nuggets also tended to have lower TBA levels.

Effects of microwave and thermal heating on the production of lipid oxidation products in fatty acid ester model systems were compared (*110*). Aqueous fresh and frozen solutions of ethyl arachidonate, ethyl linolenate, and ethyl linoleate were heated to boiling by both methods. Malonaldehyde and formaldehyde formed in the heated samples were derivatized and quantitated by capillary GC with a nitrogen–phosphorus detector. No significant differences were observed in malonaldehyde and formaldehyde concentrations in the solutions heated by the two methods. Malonaldehyde concentrations were related to the degree of unsaturation in the fatty acid.

Sun-drying and broiling of fish was found to promote lipid peroxidation and mutagenicity to *S. typhimurium* TA100 (*111*). Ether extracts of raw fish were not mutagenic but those from broiled and sun-dried fish were. HPLC analysis of the ether extract revealed the presence of methylglyoxal and other carbonyl compounds. Methylglyoxal appears to form from peroxidation of fish lipids.

A fluorometric method using diphenyl-1-pyrenylphosphine was developed for the determination of hydroperoxides in oil and food samples (*112*). This method is simple, requires only a small sample, and was highly sensitive. Recoveries of hydroperoxides from food samples averaged 93.8%–103.4%, and as little as 1–5 nano equivalents/tube could be detected. Peroxide levels determined by this method and by conventional iodometry were in good agreement.

Other compounds in heated foods

Production of a high-protein meal by extraction of canola seed with a mixture of methanol, hexane, and ammonia at elevated temperatures may form lysinoalanine (LAL), a potentially toxic cross-linked amino acid. Preparation of protein isolates under mildly alkaline conditions (without prolonged heating, pH 9–12) produced LAL concentrations of <500 μg/g (*113*). These concentrations were similar to those detected in commercially produced casein and soybean isolates. However, increased exposure to a strong alkali (0.1 N NaOH) at 75°C greatly increased LAL levels in canola, soybean, and casein meals: 14,400 μg/g, 13,500 μg/g, and >19,500 μg/g, respectively.

Heat-processing of milk-based infant formulas also produces LAL. In a pilot study, 12 healthy preterm babies were first fed for 10 days with human milk and then for 5 days each with preterm infant formulas sterilized by either ultra high temperature (UHT) or by a conventional retort process (*114*). The UHT formula contained <0.1 g LAL/kg while the in-can sterilized formula contained 0.53 g LAL/kg. Urinary excretion of LAL ranged from 6.2 to 9.3% of the ingested amount. The higher levels of LAL in the in-can sterilized formula had no apparent detrimental effects on glomerular function (as measured by creatinine clearance and electrolyte excretion) or on the proximal tubules in the kidney (as determined by urinary excretion of 4 kidney-derived enzymes).

Eight pyrolysates of carbohydrates were tested for initiating activity in the two-stage mouse skin tumorigenesis assay using 12-*O*-tetradecanoyl-phorbol-13-acetate (TPA) as the promoter (*115*). The 8 pyrolysates were topically applied to the dorsal skin twice weekly for 5 weeks with or without TPA for the following 47 weeks. No tumors appeared in any mice without TPA or in mice treated with methylglyoxal and TPA. The other 7 pyrolysates induced tumors in 10–40% of mice but statistical analysis indicated that only 4 (thiazolidine, furfural, levoglucosan, and levoglucosenone) possessed tumor-initiating ability.

COFFEE AND METHYLXANTHINES

Acute effects

Acute episodes of urticaria following ingestion of coffee, tea, and cola drinks were reported by a 53-year-old man (*116*). Itching, erythema, and wheals developed on his face, neck and upper trunk about 20 min after drinking one of these beverages and usually resolved without treatment 1 to 2 h later. Skin prick and intradermal tests with pure caffeine were negative but on two separate occasions, double-blind, placebo-controlled oral challenge with 25 mg pure caffeine produced itching and urticaria on face, neck, and trunk in 20 min. Such allergic-like reactions caused by caffeine are extremely rare.

A healthy 5-year-old boy became ill an hour after drinking part of a bottle of chocolate milk which had been standing open outdoors for three days (*117*). On admission to the hospital, he was subcomatose, with generalized muscular hypotonia and an increased heart rate. Serum caffeine and theobromine levels were very high, 15.6 and 3.5 μg/mL, respectively. Although chocolate drinks contain small amounts of these compounds, spoilage of the drink would not increase its alkaloid content. It may be that an error occurred during manufacture of this drink or that the child had consumed other foods or drinks containing caffeine. Only a few cases of acute caffeine poisoning have been reported in the literature.

In doses above 1 gram (equivalent to 5 or 6 cups of strong coffee), caffeine is anxiogenic, inducing restlessness, trembling, anxiety, and fear. To study the mechanism of this reaction, 15 healthy volunteers who were not abusers of coffee or caffeine-containing beverages were challenged with a 2-g dose of caffeine (*118*). Symptoms of anxiety occurred 30 to 60 min after caffeine ingestion. Plasma kyneurine levels were highest during peak anxiety and about 4.5–5 h later returned to normal levels. Kyneurine, a metabolite of tryptophan, is known to have anxiogenic effects in animals. Caffeine may act by stimulating synthesis of kyneurine or by inhibiting its breakdown.

Metabolism of caffeine

Caffeine biotransformation and 4 monooxygenase activities were studied in microsomes from 25 human liver samples obtained from organ donors immediately after death (*119*). There was a wide range in ability to oxidize caffeine in the liver samples from different individuals. Rate of formation of two caffeine metabolites, paraxanthine and theobromine, was correlated with the 4 monooxygenase activities and P-450IA2 levels. Inhibition of caffeine metabolism by phenacetin indicated that only the *N*-3 demethylation of caffeine was catalyzed by P450IA2. Thus, other P-450 enzymes must be involved in caffeine metabolism.

Effects on the digestive system

Lower esophageal sphincter pressure, gastric acid secretion and blood gastrin levels were measured in 8 healthy volunteers following consumption of 8 varieties of coffee (*120*). The 4 ground coffees included two types of decaffeinated coffee (extracted with ethyl acetate or methylene chloride), a coffee made from steam-treated beans (to remove cuticle wax), and an ordinary roasted, ground coffee. Instant coffees included two decaffeinated varieties treated with ethyl acetate (one of which was then extracted with 112°C water and freeze-dried) and two instant coffees made by extracting coffee solids with 300°C water (one of which was contacted with ethyl acetate). A sustained decrease in lower esophageal sphincter pressure was observed following consumption of all coffees except for 3 of those extracted with ethyl acetate. Caffeinated ground coffee stimulated more acid secretion than the decaffeinated ground coffees but not more than the steam-treated coffee. Consumption of the ground caffeinated coffee resulted in significantly higher blood gastrin levels than the other ground coffees. Caffeine itself did not seem to be responsible for any specific effects on the gastrointestinal system.

Carcinogenic effects

Following a critical assessment of numerous epidemiological and experimental studies, an International Agency for Research on Cancer (IARC) working group concluded that there was some evidence that coffee was a human bladder carcinogen (*121*). However, breast cancer risk was unrelated to coffee drinking and there was some evidence that coffee exerts a protective effect against colon and rectal cancer.

Cardiovascular effects

In a prospective epidemiological study in Sweden, 6765 men, aged 51–59 years at baseline and free of myocardial infarction, were questioned about family history of heart disease, smoking habits, psychological stress, physical activity and coffee consumption (*122*). During a 7.1-year followup, there were 230 non-fatal myocardial infarctions, 169 coronary deaths, and 478 deaths from all causes. Among smokers, there was no association between coronary disease and death and coffee consumption. Among non-smokers, a weak but insignificant trend was noted for an increasing incidence of coronary heart disease among heavy consumers of coffee. Coffee consumed in this population was predominantly of the filtered type.

PLASMA LIPID LEVELS. Two trials with healthy male volunteers in the USA focused on the effects of caffeinated and decaffeinated coffee on plasma lipid levels. In one study, 100 men (aged 20–59) went for 8 weeks with no caffeine-containing beverages (washout period) and then were randomly assigned to consume 720 mL/day of caffeinated coffee, 720 mL/day of decaffeinated coffee, 360 mL/day of caffeinated coffee, or no coffee for another 8 weeks (*123*). No other sources of caffeine were allowed during the experiment. Men who consumed 720 mL caffeinated coffee/ day experienced small but significant increases in mean plasma levels of total cholesterol (0.24 mmol/ L), low-density lipoprotein (LDL) cholesterol (0.17 mmol/L), and high-density lipoprotein (HDL) cholesterol (0.08 mmol/L) as compared to the men in the other 3 groups. In the other study, 181 middle-aged, non-smoking men consumed 3–6 cups of a standard caffeinated coffee/day for 8 weeks and then were randomized to drink the same amount of caffeinated coffee, the same amount of decaffeinated coffee, or no coffee for an additional 8 weeks (*124*). Subjects who changed to decaffeinated coffee experienced small but significant increases in LDL cholesterol (0.12 mmol/L) and in apolipoprotein B levels (0.06 g/L). However, plasma lipid levels were not changed significantly in the group which changed to no coffee. There may be some factor in decaffeinated coffee which affects plasma lipid levels.

Since brewing method has been suggested as a determining factor in the cardiovascular effects of coffee, some European studies have investigated the effects of boiled versus boiled-and-filtered coffee and the Italian brewing method (espresso) on serum lipid levels. Of 1625 middle-aged Swedish subjects (51% male), consumers of boiled coffee (about 50% of the study population) had significantly higher serum levels of total cholesterol than consumers of filtered coffee (125). Those who drank boiled coffee also reported a higher intake of fat but statistical analyses correcting for this indicated that boiled coffee was still significantly related to elevated serum cholesterol levels.

Twenty healthy middle-aged Finnish subjects consumed, in random order, 6–10 dL/day of strong boiled coffee and similarly boiled coffee which had been passed through a conventional paper filter, for periods of 4 weeks in a crossover design (126). Serum total cholesterol, LDL-cholesterol, triglyceride, and apoprotein B levels were all significantly higher during consumption of the boiled, unfiltered coffee. Filtering removed >80% of the lipid soluble substances present in boiled coffee; it may be that one or more of these substances has a hypercholesterolemic effect.

An epidemiological study in Italy involving 8983 subjects (aged 18–65 years, 83% male) found significantly higher serum cholesterol levels in coffee drinkers compared to non-drinkers (127). After the data were adjusted for age, body mass index, alcohol and cigarette consumption, increases in total cholesterol of 3.4, 5.8, and 9.6 mg/dL were observed in groups consuming 1–3, 4–5, and >5 cups of coffee per day. These values were essentially unchanged when smokers and non-smokers were analyzed separately. Although Italian coffee is not boiled as Scandinavian coffee often is, ground coffee is preheated by steam and the water which passes through the coffee is at a higher temperature than with other brewing methods. Thus, this method

of preparation may also extract some hypercholesterolemic agent from ground coffee.

BLOOD PRESSURE. In the same Italian study group, chronic coffee consumption was inversely associated with blood pressure, particularly in male subjects (128). Analysis of the data, correcting for age, body mass index, cigarette and alcohol consumption, and physical activity, revealed that male and female non-coffee drinkers had mean blood pressure levels of 130.8/83.1 and 121.7/78.0 mm Hg, respectively. Subjects consuming >5 cups of coffee/day had blood pressures of 127.5/81.9 and 119.6/77.3 mm Hg, respectively.

Acute hemodynamic effects of Italian coffee (40 mL dose, mean caffeine content 2.6 mg/mL) and a 200-mg dose of purified caffeine were measured in 15 healthy non-coffee-drinkers (129). Each volunteer consumed these liquids and two "control" beverages, a highly decaffeinated drink and caffeine-free china extract with the same bitter taste as the caffeine solution, at 10-day intervals. Blood pressure, rest flow, and peripheral resistance in the arm were measured during 2 h after consumption of these drinks. Both coffee and caffeine significantly decreased rest flow and increased peripheral resistance. Systolic blood pressure increased by 10% in the test groups. No significant effects were observed after placebo treatment.

To test the effects of boiled coffee, 64 Dutch volunteers first consumed 6 cups/day of boiled and filtered coffee (887 mg caffeine/L) for 17 days and then were randomly assigned to a group continuing consumption of the same coffee, consuming 6 cups/day of boiled, unfiltered coffee (860 mg caffeine/L), or consuming no coffee or tea for the next 79 days (130). Elimination of coffee and tea did not significantly affect heart rate or blood pressure compared to the run-in period on boiled, filtered coffee. However, consumption of the unfiltered coffee as compared to continued consumption of the filtered coffee significantly increased mean systolic blood pressure. Filtration may remove some hypertensive substance in the boiled coffee.

Effects of caffeine on blood pressure in persons at risk for hypertension were investigated in two studies. A total of 52 persons with untreated borderline or mild hypertension completed a randomized, crossover trial of 4 two-week dietary regimes: normal diet, caffeine-free diet, caffeine-free diet plus decaffeinated instant coffee, and caffeine-free plus caffeinated instant coffee (*131*). Mean 24-h ambulatory blood pressure did not differ during the different dietary periods, and no significant correlation was observed between plasma caffeine concentrations and blood pressure. Effects of caffeine on pressor regulation during rest and exercise were assessed in 20 men considered at high risk for hypertension (blood pressure of 135 to 154/85 to 94 mm Hg and parental hypertension) and in 14 men at low risk for hypertension (*132*). Subjects were dosed orally with placebo (unsweetened grapefruit juice) or caffeine (3.3 mg/kg in the same juice), and their blood pressure, vascular resistance, and cardiac index were measured at rest and during supine bicycle exercise. Compared with placebo, caffeine increased the number of low-risk men (0-36%) and high-risk men (35-50%) who attained abnormal exercise blood pressures and also blunted the normal increments in cardiac index at higher work loads among high-risk men.

Some studies have demonstrated an association between coffee consumption and various forms of arrhythmias. A cholinomimetic compound has been isolated from instant regular and decaffeinated coffees and purified 90-fold. Its probable structure is that of a charged pyridinium compound with a polyhydride aliphatic chain. Injection of this extract into rats produced an abrupt depression in blood pressure and heart rate (*133*). Pretreatment of the animals with atropine completely abolished this effect. The extract also caused relaxation of isolated rat and rabbit aortic ring preparations that were contracted under norepinephrine but did not inhibit acetylcholinesterase.

Reproductive and developmental effects

Results from several epidemiological studies indicate that heavy caffeine intake by a mother may have some effect on growth and development of her fetus but the effect is not very strong. Data from birth certificates and interviews with 1230 mothers in the USA revealed a positive association between heavy caffeine consumption (>300 mg/day) and intrauterine growth retardation and low birthweight (*134*). When the data were adjusted for cigarette and alcohol consumption and hypertension during pregnancy, odds ratios for the two conditions were 2.90 and 2.05, respectively. No association was observed between caffeine consumption and preterm delivery.

Information on the coffee-drinking habits of 40,445 Canadian women and outcome of their pregnancies demonstrated a slight increase in the risk for preterm delivery in women who drank more than 10 cups of coffee/day (odds ratio of 1.24) and in the risk for low birthweight for gestational age for women who drank 5–9 cups of coffee/day (odds ratio of 1.34) (*135*). These data were corrected for cigarette and alcohol consumption and maternal age, education, and employment. Analysis of 35,848 previous pregnancies in these Canadian women (*136*) indicated a weak association between coffee consumption and spontaneous abortion (odds ratio of 1.17 for women consuming 5–9 cups of coffee/day).

Followup studies of 500 children in the Seattle area during their first 7 years detected no relationship between prenatal caffeine exposure and height, weight, head circumference, or IQ and attention tests at 7 years (*137*). In this study, a total of 1529 women had been interviewed during pregnancy about their intakes of coffee, tea, soft drinks, and chocolate milk and candy, and their total caffeine intake from all these sources was calculated. Chocolate candy was the most frequently reported source of caffeine, and average daily caffeine intake from all sources was 193 mg/day (range of 0–2506 mg/day) during early pregnancy.

Previous studies with a group of 40 monkeys (*Macaca fascicularis*) revealed an increase in stillbirths and miscarriages among those receiving 0.15 or 0.35 mg caffeine/mL in their drinking water before and during pregnancy. Among the liveborn infants from these studies, body weights and somatic measurements of males were significantly reduced during the first 30 days, as were a number of initial somatic measurements in both male and female infants (*138*). However, these effects were not evident after one year of age, and no treatment-related effects on infant tooth eruption or milk consumption were observed.

Effects on mineral metabolism

As part of the Nurse's Health Study, 84,484 U.S. women aged 34–59 years completed a dietary questionnaire in 1980, with followup questionnaires sent out every two years thereafter. During the 6 years after the original questionnaire, 593 forearm and 65 hip fractures occurred in association with mild to moderate trauma. Analysis of dietary data while controlling for potentially confounding variables revealed that the relative risk of hip fracture for women in the highest quintile of caffeine consumption (>817 mg caffeine/day) was 2.95. Caffeine intake was not associated with incidence of forearm fractures. Increasing alcohol intake was independently associated with both hip and forearm fractures (139).

Data obtained from an age-stratified random sample of 290 women in Rochester, MN, indicated that there was no relationship between caffeine consumption and bone mineral levels at 5 skeletal sites (140). However, at one site, the femoral shaft, there was a statistically significant interaction between age and caffeine consumption so that high intakes of caffeine were associated with slight reductions in bone mineral among elderly subjects but with modestly increased bone mineral in younger women. These results suggest that caffeine is not an important risk factor for osteoporosis in most women, with the possible exception of elderly women in whom calcium balance performance is impaired.

In fact, in a group of 85 patients (aged 48-77 years) with postmenopausal crush fracture osteoporosis, coffee intake was found to significantly affect calcium metabolism (141). Individual records of the usual home diet were used to construct similar hospital diets served during the experimental period to assess 7-day combined calcium balance and ^{47}Ca tracer-kinetic turnover. Dietary calcium was measured in all meals and all urine and feces were collected for calcium analysis. Multiple backward linear regression analysis indicated that only calcium and coffee intakes, of the ten dietary constituents tested, significantly influenced calcium balance. A coffee intake of >1000 mL/day could induce an extra calcium loss of 1.6 mmol Ca/day.

Effects of caffeine on bone formation were investigated using a chick osteoblast culture system (142). Chronic doses of 0.1, 0.2, and 0.4 mM caffeine did not affect cell proliferation or cell numbers in secondary cultures of osteoblasts. However, osteocalcin levels, alkaline phosphatase activity and total calcium levels decreased in a dose-dependent manner in caffeine-treated cultures. The highest dose of caffeine also significantly depressed collagen levels. Caffeine appears to inhibit the formation of a competent extracellular matrix during osteoblast differentiation.

Determination of caffeine

Simple background correction methods were developed to enable determination of caffeine in coffee, tea, and other beverages by second-derivative ultraviolet spectrophotometry (143). Interfering compounds in coffee and soft drinks were minimized by treatment with NaOH, while tannins in tea were precipitated with cupric acetate. Second derivatives of caffeine were measured at 298.6 nm. Calibration graphs for the three types of beverages had slightly different slopes and linear ranges. Analysis of a number of soft drinks, coffees, and teas by this method yielded results similar to those obtained with HPLC.

Two accurate, precise and sensitive methods were described for the determination of caffeine, theobromine, and theophylline in chocolate, coffee, tea, and other beverages (144). One method utilized a reverse-phase HPLC column with a mobile phase of 0.01 M sodium acetate solution:acetonitrile (85:15%) at pH 4 with detection at 272 nm. The other method was based on derivative UV-spectrophotometry. A first derivative procedure was used for the determination of theobromine in the presence of theophylline and caffeine while a second derivative procedure was adopted for the determination of theophylline in the presence of caffeine and theobromine. Caffeine was determined by compensation method using zero-order spectrophotometry.

Simultaneous determination of caffeine and chlorogenic acid in coffee samples was achieved by high performance gel filtration chromatography using a TSK 3000-SW column (*145*). Samples were extracted with hot distilled water and then applied to the column. Mobile phase was bidistilled water containing 0.05% sodium azide. Results obtained using this method correlated well with those obtained by separate reversed-phase chromatography procedures for the two compounds. Average recoveries for caffeine and chlorogenic acid were 105% and 95%, respectively.

ALKALOIDS

Pyrrolizidine alkaloids

Results from several studies on the mutagenicity of pyrrolizidine alkaloids (PA) in the *Salmonella typhimurium*/mammalian microsome assay have been contradictory. A recent reassessment of mutagenicity with 5 different *S. typhimurium* strains, with and without preincubation of the alkaloids with rat liver S9, demonstrated that retrorsine was weakly mutagenic only to strain TA100 and only after a 20-min preincubation at 37°C (*146*). Senecivernine, seneciphylline, and extracts of 3 *Senecio* spp. were also weakly mutagenic to TA100 following preincubation.

Eight PA with differing stereochemistry and functional groups were tested for their ability to cross-link cellular DNA in cultured bovine kidney epithelial cells (*147*). Following a 2-h exposure to the alkaloids and an external metabolizing system (S9), all the alkaloids induced DNA cross-links but none induced detectable DNA single-strand breaks. PA containing a macrocyclic necic acid ester and an α,β-unsaturated ester function, such as seneciphylline, riddelline, retrorsine, and senecionine, were much more effective in inducing DNA cross-links than PA without these structures (heliosupine, monocrotaline, latifoline, and retronecine).

In spite of its known toxic effects, extracts of *Heliotropium curassavicum* var. *argentinum* are a commonly used medicinal herb in South America and in Africa where it is consumed during pregnancy and lactation. An aqueous extract (prepared according to the Argentine pharmacopeia) of this plant caused significant increases in the percentage of abnormal metaphases and in total chromosomal aberrations in Chinese hamster ovary (CHO) cells in culture (*148*). These effects were enhanced by addition of a rat liver S9 fraction. Three PA (heliovicine, curassavine, and coromandeline) were detected in the aqueous extract.

In experiments with C57BL/6 mice, monocrotaline (MCT) was found to alter the functional integrity of various immune effector responses in a dose-dependent manner (*149*). Mice were dosed orally with 0–100 mg MCT/kg/day for 14 days. Immunosuppressive effects included: a decrease in the percentage of activated macrophages following injection of sheep red blood cells; a decrease in antibody responses to two T-cell-independent antigens; a significant suppression of the blastogenic response to the T cell mitogen concanavalin A and to the B cell mitogen lipopolysaccharide.

An off-line supercritical fluid extraction (sfe) method was found to be superior to the classical MeOH Soxhlet extraction for the isolation of PA from *Senecio* spp. (*150*). This new method used MeOH/CO_2 as extraction medium at 55°C and 15 MPa. Sfe required a smaller amount of sample and provided a quicker extraction, a cleaner extract, and a higher recovery than the Soxhlet method. Following extraction, samples were analyzed by capillary GC.

Glycoalkaloids from Solanum *spp.*

Several potato glycoalkaloids and aglycones were evaluated in the frog embryo teratogenesis assay-*Xenopus* (FETAX) with and without metabolic activation by rat liver microsomes (*151*). Data indicated that α-chaconine was teratogenic and about 3-fold more toxic than α-solanine. The liver microsomes appeared to partially detoxify both compounds since the concentration–response curves for mortality, malformation and growth were shifted significantly to the left. The alkaloids caused a number of head and facial malformations in the *Xenopus* embryos. The aglycone derivatives demissidine, solanidine, and solasodine were less toxic.

An improved assay was developed to measure α-chaconine and α-solanine content of different potato varieties, different parts of potato plants, and commercial potato products (*152*). Samples were extracted with tetrahydrofuran–water–acetonitrile, then treated with 0.2 N HCl and centrifuged. The supernatant was neutralized with ammonium hydroxide and the resulting precipitate was dissolved in hot methanol and then filtered through a 0.45 μm filter membrane before HPLC analysis. Recoveries from spiked samples ranged from 89–95%. Total α-solanine and α-chaconine contents in different parts of a high glycoalkaloid strain (NDA 1725), in mg/100 g fresh weight, were tubers, 14.7; leaves, 145; and sprouts, 997. Total glycoalkaloid content determined by titration with bromophenol blue was 12–30% greater than the glycoalkaloid content determined by HPLC. Both glycoalkaloids were also detected in commercial potato products with totals (mg/100 g) in French fries of 0.08–0.84; in skins, 3.1–20.3; in potato chips, 2.4–10.9; and in potato pancake powders, 4.5-6.5. Whether the variation in alkaloid content of the potato products is due to the different potato cultivars used or to differences in processing conditions is unknown.

In an epidemiological study of esophageal cancer in Transkei, southern Africa, 100 cancer patients and 100 controls were interviewed to determine usual diet and social habits during the previous 10 years (*153*). Statistical analyses of the data demonstrated that smoking, use of traditional medicines, and consumption of *Solanum nigrum* as a food were significant risk factors, with relative risks of 2.6, 2.1, and 3.6, respectively. *S. nigrum*, garden or black nightshade, contains the alkaloid solanine in amounts which vary with climate, soil, and season. In season the leaves of this plant may be ingested daily, in large amounts, either fresh or made into a relish. Further investigations should be conducted to elucidate possible relationships between *Solanum* glycoalkaloids and esophageal cancer.

Atropine and scopolamine

Five incidents of poisoning with tropine alkaloids from *Datura* spp. were reported. An 82-year-old American male, who grew angel's trumpet (*D. innoxia*) near his herb garden, erroneously dug up a root of this plant from his horseradish bed. Thinking it was horseradish, he ate a nickel-sized bite. About 45 min later he experienced a dry mouth and during the next few hours he became progressively confused and disoriented, with a temperature of 38°C. With treatment he recovered in 1.5 days but remained amnestic for a period beginning shortly after the root ingestion and ending about 1 day later. Analysis of the rest of the root by TLC and GC/MS demonstrated the presence of both atropine and scopolamine (*154*).

Following ingestion of 3 teaspoons of a home-made wine, a 76-year-old American male experienced symptoms of respiratory distress and weakness (*155*). The wine had been made with 115 blossoms of "moon flower" (*D. suaveolens*), sugar, yeast, and water, and was fermented for about 3 months. Analysis of a sample of the wine by reversed-phase HPLC revealed the presence of scopolamine (29 mg/mL) but not of atropine. The scopolamine content was higher than expected and the authors suggest that the fermentation process may have concentrated the original extract.

A 17-year-old man in Guadeloupe was found unconscious, with a dry mouth, rash on the neck, and a temperature of 39°C (*156*). His white blood cell count was elevated (23,000 polynuclear neutrophils/cc) but no sign of infection was detected. The patient recovered after 3 days in the hospital and reported having drunk a tea made with 2 fresh flowers of *D. stramonium*. Symptoms appeared within 30 min. Although this is a common ornamental plant on Guadeloupe, there are few serious cases of poisoning because most people recognize it as toxic.

Ten agitated and psychotic patients were admitted to a hospital in Tanzania following ingestion of stiff porridge made from millet (*157*). Symptoms of dry mouth, tachycardia, fixed, dilated pupils, and hallucinations developed about an hour after a meal of porridge, fish, and spinach. Examination of the millet grain used to make the porridge revealed the presence of small, bean-shaped black seeds in a proportion of 5–20% in the grain. These were identified as seeds of *D. stramonium* and contained an atropine-like alkaloid. In another area of Tanzania, 7 patients with similar symptoms were treated at a local hospital (*158*). All these patients reported that they had recently eaten chapattis or bread made from locally grown wheat. Small black particles were observed in a sample of the flour used for baking. GC analysis revealed the presence of both atropine and scopolamine. Again, contamination with seeds of *D. stramonium*, a common weed in grain fields, was the cause of these cases of food poisoning. Fortunately, all patients recovered after a few days of supportive therapy.

A monoclonal antibody against scopolamine has been produced and characterized and used in a specific, sensitive ELISA for quantitation of this alkaloid (*159*). Detection limit was 0.1 ng scopolamine/mL of plant extract. Results obtained with this assay and with an HPLC assay of leaves from 18 individual *Duboisia* hybrid plants grown in a greenhouse were very similar. Scopolamine levels ranged from 0.55% to 5% in dry matter.

Lupin alkaloids

Although lupin seed has mainly been used for animal feeds, it is increasingly being used as a source of vegetable protein for people in Asia. Antinutritional factors are in lower concentration in lupin as compared to other legumes but the presence of several alkaloids limits the usefulness of some varieties of *Lupinus angustifolius*. An ELISA, utilizing polyclonal, anti-alkaloid antibodies has been developed for the determination of total alkaloids in lupin (*160*). The antisera were highly specific for (+)-lupanine and (+)-13-hydroxylupanine, the most important alkaloids. Results of analyses of the same samples by ELISA and by capillary GC were very similar (correlation coefficient of 0.94) over the range of 10–900 µg alkaloid/g seed.

Toxicology of argemone oil

Argemone mexicana grows wild in mustard fields and its seeds may be inadvertently mixed with mustard seeds and processed into oil. Consumption of such contaminated oil causes symptoms such as erythema, edema, breathlessness, tachycardia and hepatotoxicity. To determine the mechanism of hepatotoxicity, rats were given single or multiple intraparenteral injections of argemone oil (10 mL/kg body weight) and sacrificed 1–3 days later for examination of liver enzymes (*161*). Various effects were observed, including an inhibition of cytochrome P-450 and its dependent mixed-function oxidases and a depletion of endogenous glutathione with an increase in lipid peroxidation. The argemone alkaloids, sanguinarine and dihydrosanguinarine, apparently affect both membrane-bound and cytosolic enzymes.

GLUCOSINOLATES

Biological effects

Glucosinolates, which occur in cruciferous plants such as cabbage, broccoli, and rapeseed, exert goitrogenic effects in some animals and may be involved in the promotion or prevention of cancer. To determine possible harmful effects of brussels sprouts, rats were fed for 4 weeks with diets containing 0–30% of dry matter as cooked brussels sprouts (*162*). Total glucosinolate contents of the 2.5% and 20% diets were 147 and 1120 µmol/kg wet weight. An increase in prothrombin times was noted in rats fed the 2.5% diet while growth depression, impaired kidney function, and morphological activation of the thyroid gland were observed in rats fed the 10% diet. Decreased levels of blood hemoglobin and plasma thyroxin were found at the 15% dietary level.

Subacute oral toxicity of benzyl isothiocyanate, a hydrolysis product of benzyl glucosinolate (BITC) which naturally occurs in garden cress (*Lepidium sativum*), Indian cress (*Tropaeolum majus*), and melon tree (*Carica papaya*), was evaluated in rats (*163*). Animals were gavaged with daily doses of 0, 50, 100, or 200 mg BITC/kg body weight/day for 4 weeks. No mortality was caused by BITC but body weight gain was significantly decreased in all treatment groups. Other adverse effects noted were an increase in serum cholesterol and renal dysfunction as indicated by reduced urine volume, proteinuria, and enhanced urinary lactate dehydrogenase activity.

Occurrence in foods

Using HPLC, glucosinolate levels in 6 lines of green-curded cauliflowers, 6 lines of green-curded cauliflowers with pyramidal curds, and 9 lines of purple-headed broccoli were determined to be 18.4–42.8 mg/100 g, 27.0–41.6 mg/100 g, and 72.0–212.2 mg/100 g, respectively (164). The glucosinolate levels in green-curded varieties were lower than those previously determined in ordinary white-curded varieties. 3-Methylsulfinylpropyl and indolyl-3-methyl glucosinolates were the major glucosinolates in all three varieties of vegetables tested here.

Mechanical wounding of petioles of rapeseed plants was found to increase their content of indole glucosinolates and decrease levels of aliphatic glucosinolates (165). Infestation of rapeseed with cabbage stem flea beetles produced similar effects. Damaged kale and mustard plants also had elevated levels of total glucosinolates compared to undamaged plants.

Myrosinase, an endogenous enzyme in crucifers, hydrolyzes glucosinolates to yield products with potent goitrogenicity. Therefore, a wet heat treatment is used by processors to inactivate this enzyme. Optimum conditions for inactivation of this enzyme by microwave inactivation were recently investigated (166). A moisture content of 10–16% and medium to high microwave power appeared to give the best results. A regression equation was generated which could predict the extent of enzyme inactivation at practical levels of moisture and microwave power. Microwave treatment did cause significant increases in the yellow color and sulfur content of the seed oils.

Determination of glucosinolates

A rapid, simple method for the determination of total glucosinolates in rapeseed which did not require the use of expensive equipment was developed for use by plant breeders and for determination of glucosinolates in commercial rapeseed loads (167). First, glucosinolates were hydrolyzed by endogenous myrosinase at pH 9, and then the glucose produced was detected with commercially available glucose test strips. The intensity of color on the strip was measured with a portable reflectometer and was directly related to glucose levels.

Myrosinase immobilized on a nylon 6.6 membrane was used as a novel detector for glucosinolates in crude aqueous extracts of cruciferous materials (168). Since the hydrolysis of glucosinolates produces H^+ ions, a pH-stat technique was used to measure the reaction rate. Trials using sinigrin, progoitrin, and increasing amounts of crude extracts showed a linear correlation up to 3.5 μmol of glucosinolate. Recovery of sinigrin from a crude rapeseed extract ranged from 99 to 103%. The immobilized myrosinase was very stable if stored wet at 4°C and could be used for 1000 assays. This method is also applicable to rapid field and laboratory analyses.

Rapid determination of desulfated derivatives of rapeseed glucosinolates was achieved by isocratic liquid chromatography (169). Effects of different stationary phases, eluent compositions, and temperatures were evaluated. Using a Lichrospher CN column and water as the mobile phase, the chromatographic analysis could be completed in <12 min. Relative standard deviations for repeatability of this method ranged from 0.4 to 1.7%.

The X-ray fluorescence method for glucosinolate determination in rapeseed assumes a 21% protein content in the seeds and is based on the good correlation between total sulfur and total glucosinolate content in the seeds. However, protein content of the seeds was found to range from 16 to 22.6%, depending on the amount of nitrogen and sulfur fertilizer added to the fields (170). Therefore, a correction for seed protein content was found to significantly improve the quantitation of glucosinolates by X-ray fluorescence.

A liquid chromatographic method has been devised for the determination of 5-vinyl-1,3-oxazolidine-2-thione (5-VOT), a goitrogenic compound produced from progoitrin, the major rapeseed glucosinolate (171). This compound was extracted by complexation with phenyl mercury acetate under cyclohexanic conditions and then decomplexed by using aqueous sodium thiosulfate. Reversed-phase LC using an isocratic elution with UV detection detected 5-VOT in concentrations as low as 0.5 ppb.

CYANOGENIC COMPOUNDS

Cassava

Cassava, the most important staple food crop for millions of people in the tropics is, unfortunately, toxic unless correctly prepared, due to its content of cyanogenic glycosides, linamarin and methyl-linamarin. Three cases of acute cyanide poisoning were admitted to the University Teaching Hospital in Lagos, Nigeria (*172*). The patients had shared a meal based on "gari" (a cassava-based meal) and experienced abdominal pain and vomiting shortly after eating. Upon admission, all were experiencing renal failure and all died within 24 h following cardiopulmonary arrest. Cyanide levels in blood and urine samples of the patients averaged 1.12 and 0.54 mg/L, respectively. Although such severe poisoning cases are not very common, over 150 deaths from cyanide poisoning were reported in Nigeria in 1989.

Konzo, a tropical myelopathy characterized by abrupt onset of spastic paraparesis, occurs in epidemic form in some rural areas of Africa experiencing declining agricultural yields (as in drought periods). The rapidly growing populations in these areas can only survive by cultivating high-yielding, bitter cassava with high cyanogen levels. Epidemiological studies in Zaire (*173,174*) compared cassava consumption patterns in two villages affected by konzo with that in 4 villages without konzo cases. The affected populations consumed cassava porridge made of flour from roots soaked for only one day while the unaffected villagers consumed only a steam-boiled cassava paste made from roots soaked for at least 4 days. Cyanohydrin levels were much higher in the short-soaked cassava and this was reflected in much higher mean urinary thiocyanate levels in affected (757 µmol/L) than

unaffected (50 µmol/L) villagers. Relatively low levels of urinary inorganic sulfate (indicating a protein deficient diet) were observed in both areas. This protein deficiency most likely contributes to the toxicity of cassava since it limits endogenous detoxification reactions.

Seven cases of konzo in rural Mozambique were examined following an abrupt onset of symptoms during a period of food shortage (drought) (*175*). High urinary and serum levels of thiocyanate were measured in these patients. All patients reported that prior to disease onset, they had been eating a high-yielding, bitter variety of cassava which was sometimes processed for a short time or by non-traditional methods. Low urinary sulfate levels also indicated protein deficiency in this population.

The fermentation of peeled, chopped cassava roots in water as is done in Cameroon was found to effectively remove cyanogenic compounds from cassava (*176*). Fresh roots contained 91–1515 mg total cyanogens/kg. Traditional water fermentation followed by pressing and sun-drying or boiling reduced cyanogen levels to 0–11.3 mg/kg, even in bitter cassava varieties. Higher temperature during fermentation and greater comminution of cassava enhanced the rate of glycoside hydrolysis. Storage of the prepared cassava products for several months at ambient temperatures further reduced cyanogen levels.

Modifications to the enzymic assay for cyanogens in fresh and processed cassava were found to improve extraction efficiency and recoveries (*177*). Inclusion of 25% ethanol in the extraction solvent increased the volume of recovered extract and the extraction of cyanohydrin and eliminated the need for centrifugation. By buffering aliquots of the extraction mixture to pH 4, accurate determinations of free cyanide, formed by linamarase, could be achieved. Above pH 4, cyanohydrin degradation also occurs, producing more free cyanide and giving rise to misleading values. During a 2-month storage period at refrigeration temperatures, cyanogens in the ethanol/acid extraction medium were stable but free cyanide was not.

A rapid, inexpensive screening assay was developed to measure the cyanide content of cassava tubers (*178*). A small sample of a tuber was placed in a stoppered glass tube with a piece of filter paper spotted with tetra-base [4,4'-methylenebis-(*N,N*-dimethylaniline)] and cupric acetate. Depending on the amount of HCN liberated from the cassava, a blue color developed and intensified during a period of 5–60 min. The intensity of the color was rated on a visual scale of 0–5 after 1 h. A reasonably good correlation (0.77) was obtained between results from this rapid assay and those determined by acid hydrolysis.

Other foods and beverages

Raw bamboo shoots (*Dendrocalamus giganteus*) contain high levels of HCN (about 750 mg/kg) primarily in the form of taxiphyllin, a thermolabile cyanogenic compound. Four processing techniques have been compared for their efficiency in reducing HCN levels: still water maceration; batch cooking at room pressure; intermittent cooking at room pressure; and batch cooking at 0.5 atm (*179*). The maceration process was the least efficient, with only about 0.3% of the HCN eliminated after 12 h and 86% after 72 h. All the cooking processes reduced HCN levels to around 100 mg/kg after 40 min. Cooking under 0.5 atm decreased HCN levels more rapidly than the other cooking processes during the early stages.

In 14 stone fruit (cherries, peaches, plums, and apricots) varieties tested, a cyanogenic compound, amygdalin, was detected at levels of 0.003–6.5% by weight in seeds (*180*). Prunasin, a probable precursor of amygdalin, occurred in concentrations of 0.12–29.51 mg/kg in the pulp. Highest cyanogen levels were found in morello cherries and lowest levels were in some apricot cultivars. Since these cyanogenic compounds can be hydrolyzed to release HCN, factors affecting HCN content in unstoned, heat-processed fruits packed in 30% sucrose were investigated. The most important factors affecting HCN content in canned fruit were the glycoside content of the raw fruit and the conditions of heat processing. Long heating at low temperatures apparently activates glucosidase activity, increasing HCN levels. Therefore, HTST processing is recommended. The highest levels of HCN found in the edible portion of canned unstoned fruits were 3–4 mg CN⁻/kg. Although these levels are not acutely toxic, they are very close to the acceptable daily intake for 1 kg of fruit by an adult.

Sorghum, an important staple food in some parts of Africa, contains tannins and small amounts of cyanide. The fates of these antinutritional factors during various steps in preparation of sorghum-derived foods and beverages were monitored (*181*). Samples of brown sorghum seeds were soaked, sprouted for 24–96 h, fermented and boiled. Compared to unsoaked seeds, soaking reduced cyanide concentrations by about 75% (from 12.0 to 3.1 ppm). However, sprouting increased cyanide levels to a maximum of 156.1 ppm after 72 h. Fermentation of unsoaked, unsprouted seeds and of soaked, sprouted seeds reduced cyanide content by about 50%. Boiling of all fermented sorghum decreased cyanide concentrations to <6 ppm. This combination of cooking and fermentation also significantly reduced tannin levels.

Jojoba seeds yield a valuable oil but the hexane-extracted meal contains cyanogenic compounds (simmondsin and 3 of its derivatives) which limit its usefulness as an animal feed or protein isolate. Three methods for the detoxification of the seed meal were developed, first as laboratory-scale projects and then scaled up to produce enough meal for 8-week mouse feeding studies (*182*). All the processes tested, water extraction, enzymatic degradation utilizing endogenous enzymes, and fermentation by *Fusarium moniliforme*, produced jojoba meal which was apparently non-toxic and did not adversely affect growth in mice. Under current industrial processing conditions, fermentation appears to be the best choice for detoxification. However, since some strains of *F. moniliforme* produce mycotoxins, this process must be carefully monitored.

An ion chromatographic method with electrochemical detection has been developed for the detection of ferrocyanide in wine (*183*). Determination limit was 1 ng sodium ferrocyanide/mL of wine, with recoveries averaging 88–130% in spiked samples. Low levels of cyanide (trace to 4.7 ng/mL) were detected in 22 samples of Japanese red and white wines. The presence of low cyanide concentrations in musts for wines indicates that cyanide in wine is naturally occurring.

URETHANE

Ethyl carbamate (urethane), which occurs naturally in numerous fermented foods and beverages, is known to have genotoxic and carcinogenic effects. Recent experiments with mice confirmed the in vivo clastogenic effects of urethane (*184*) and of vinyl carbamate (*185*), a hypothetical metabolite of urethane. Oral and i.p. doses of both compounds induced significant levels of micronuclei in normochromatic erythrocytes in peripheral blood and in polychromatic erythrocytes in bone marrow, respectively. Fetal liver tissue from pregnant mice injected with urethane had very high levels of micronucleated polychromatic erythrocytes. Vinyl carbamate was about 40 times as potent as ethyl carbamate.

Since urea is one of the major precursors of urethane in wine, fermentation conditions were varied to assess their contribution to urea formation in fermenting grape juice (*186*). As noted in previous studies, high levels of amino acids, especially arginine, and the use of certain yeast strains resulted in relatively high urea concentrations. At first continuous aeration caused rapid production of urea but this was followed by a period of rapid utilization so that final urea concentrations were very low. However, if fermentation became anaerobic during the later stages, the urea was only partially utilized and a high urea concentration was found in the final wine. Fermentations which were anaerobic at the start and aerobic later also accumulated low levels of urea.

A series of 4 articles (*187–190*) detailed studies on ethyl carbamate formation in grain-based spirits. Freshly distilled grain whiskey normally contains <20 ppb urethane which forms, during fermentation, from a naturally occurring cyanogenic glycoside, epiheterodendrin. Depending on the presence of trace anionic precursors such as cyanate, cyanide, and copper cyanide complexes,

more urethane may form during normal maturation in oak casks.

A new procedure for determination of urethane in Italian grape distillate, aqua vitae (grappa), was based on the selective reaction of urethane and an internal standard (methyl urethane) with xanthydrol (*191*). The xanthylamides thus formed were quantified by GC–MS in the selected ion monitoring mode on an apolar DB 5 silica column. The calibration curve was linear from 10 to 1000 µg/mL and the minimum detection level was 1 µg urethane/mL. Analysis of 20 grappa samples revealed urethane levels ranging from 70 to 400 µg/mL, with an average of 87 µg/mL.

PROTEASE INHIBITORS

Physiological effects of Bowman-Birk (BBI) and Kunitz (KTI) protease inhibitors found in legumes and in other plants have been investigated to determine possible carcinogenic, anticarcinogenic, and nutritional activities. In addition to trypsin (inhibited by KTI and BBI) and chymotrypsin (inhibited by BBI), several other proteolytic enzymes are active in the human small intestine. In spite of the high concentrations of KTI present in duodenal juices during raw soybean instillation, extensive soybean degradation occurred immediately (*192*). Four different forms of trypsin were isolated from human duodenal juices and partially characterized by electrophoresis, isoelectric focusing, and Western immunoblotting. The relative proportion of the trypsin variant with the lowest molecular weight increased during raw soybean extract instillation and this variant was relatively insensitive to KTI.

Incubation of normal rat intestinal epithelial cells in vitro with BBI (1–25 µg/mL) demonstrated that BBI was nontoxic and had no effect on doubling time (*193*). BBI was taken up by the epithelial cells, and cell fractionation experiments revealed that most of the inhibitor was present in the cytosol. BBI from the treated cells was still active against chymotrypsin and would therefore be able to inhibit intracellular proteases and possibly suppress malignant transformations.

Three hours following an oral dose of [^{125}I]BBI, labelled BBI was widely distributed in various organs of the mouse (*194*). Approximately 55% of the recovered label was in the luminal contents, feces, bladder and urine. Labelled BBI isolated from tissue homogenates behaved chromatographically like BBI standard and was able to inhibit chymotrypsin, indicating that it was still intact.

Soya bean trypsin inhibitor concentrate (STIC) was fed to rats for periods of 4 weeks to 3 months to assess its ability to initiate or promote formation of putative preneoplastic lesions in the pancreas (*195*). In the first experiment where rats were initiated with a single azaserine injection, three months of 3.7% STIC in the diet was found to significantly increase the percentage volume of the pancreas occupied by atypical acinar cell foci. In the second experiment, STIC at a level of 3.7% in the diet was not sufficient to initiate the putative preneoplastic lesions.

Two types of acinar pancreatic lesions can be experimentally induced by 4-hydroxyaminoquinoline 1-oxide (HAQO) in rats: eosinophilic nodules, which are believed to be precursors of malignant tumors and basophilic foci, which mimic age-associated degenerative changes. Effects of dietary soybean trypsin inhibitor (SBTI) on development of these lesions were investigated in long-term experiments (*196*). Rats were given a single injection of HAQO (7 mg/kg) and then fed for 57 weeks with a control diet or diets containing 5 or 10% SBTI. At the end of the experiment, the incidence of eosinophilic nodules was significantly higher and that of the basophilic foci was less in the HAQO/SBTI-treated rats than in rats treated with HAQO alone. This is further evidence that SBTI is a promotor of neoplastic changes.

Effects of various domestic processing methods on trypsin inhibitor activity and tannin content of faba beans were investigated (*197*). Soaking and dehulling resulted in slight (4–10%), nonsignificant decreases in trypsin inhibitor activity while germination of seeds for 48 h, ordinary cooking, and autoclaving for 25 min reduced inhibitor activity by 64–65%, 75–76%, and 95–98%, respectively. Tannin levels were significantly reduced by soaking and dehulling (75–76%), cooking (76–81%),

sprouting for 48 h (90–91%), and autoclaving for 25 min (93–95%). It appears that ordinary preparation and cooking methods destroy a high percentage of these antinutritional factors.

Whole beans, bean flours, and bean albumin extracts from nine dry bean varieties commonly used in the USA were screened for heat-stable trypsin inhibitor activity (*198*). Boiling for 30 min inactivated 95–97.5%, 37–70%, and 0–3% of trypsin inhibitor activity in soaked whole beans, bean flour, and bean albumin extracts, respectively. Eleven isolated trypsin isoinhibitors were detected by isoelectric focusing of extracts from Great Northern beans. Some of these isoinhibitors also inhibited chymotrypsin. Amounts of the individual trypsin inhibitors varied in the 9 different strains tested.

A new serine protease inhibitor (MTI-2) was purified from seeds of white mustard (*Sinapis alba* L.) by affinity chromatography and reverse-phase HPLC (*199*). Amino acid analysis of this inhibitor showed that it consisted of 63 amino acids and had very little homology to other known serine protease inhibitors. MTI-1 inhibited the catalytic activity of bovine β-trypsin and bovine α-chymotrypsin, with dissociation constants of 1.6×10^{-10} M and 5.0×10^{-7} M, respectively, at pH 8.0 and 21°C.

Heat stability of trypsin inhibitors from rice, sweet potato, taro (*Colocasia esculenta* var. *esculenta*), giant taro (*Alocasia macrorrhiza*), and giant swamp taro (*Cyrtosperma chamissonis*) was investigated (*200*). Heating of the 3 varieties of taro to 80°C resulted in a large increase in trypsin inhibitor activity, probably caused by the breakdown of cellular structure making the inhibitor available for extraction. At this point the taro had a rubbery texture but was not fully cooked. Baking or boiling of brown rice, sweet potato, taro, and giant swamp taro until they were soft enough to eat fully inactivated their moderate levels of trypsin inhibitor activity. Giant taro, however, contained 10 to 100 times as much inhibitor as the other foods and required >30 min of boiling to inactivate it.

Five varieties of bananas grown in India were found to have more protease inhibitor activity when ripe than when unripe (*201*). Trypsin, chymotrypsin, and papain activities were all inhibited by crude extracts of these bananas. An alkaline pH destroyed the inhibitory activity towards papain but not that towards trypsin and chymotrypsin, indicating that there may be two distinct inhibitors. The nutritional effects of these protease inhibitors is unknown but should be studied because ripened bananas are not usually cooked before eating.

The structures (*202*) and inhibitory activities (*203*) of 3 trypsin/chymotrypsin inhibitors from fenugreek (*Trigonella foenum-graecum*) seeds have been elucidated. C-terminal residue analysis indicated that these inhibitors belong to the Bowman-Birk protease inhibitor family. The 3 inhibitors had different amino acids at their reactive sites, and these were related to differences in the binding of human and bovine trypsin and chymotrypsin. The inhibitor with arginine and leucine at its active site bound the greatest amount of the chymotrypsins while the inhibitor with two arginines at its active site bound the greatest amount of the trypsins.

PHYTATE

Phytic acid 'Daiichi' (PA), a natural food additive produced from rice bran and containing about 49% phytic acid, was fed to Fischer rats for 100–108 weeks to evaluate its carcinogenic potential (*204*). PA was added to drinking water at levels of 1.25 and 2.5%. A dose-dependent reduction in mean final body weights was observed for the treated rats but there were no treatment-related effects on measures of clinical chemistry or hematology. Necrosis and/ or calcification of renal papillae were observed in 27 females and 4 male rats at the high dose and in 12 females and 1 male at the low dose. Renal papillomas developed in 4 females and 3 males at the high dose and in 3 females at the low dose. Other tumors also developed in these rats but their incidence did not differ significantly from those previously reported for this strain of rats.

To test the effect of phytate on absorption of iron, human volunteers consumed rolls made from various types of whole grain flours and fermented in different ways and labelled with ^{55}Fe or ^{59}Fe (*205*).

Each volunteer also consumed labelled rolls made of white wheat flour (55% extraction) and served as his or her own control. With the exception of rolls made from whole rye flour and white wheat flour and fermented for 2 days + 1 h + 20 min (sour dough type), all the other experimental rolls decreased iron absorption significantly but to different extents. Different ingredients and fermentation times decreased phytate levels in flour by 40 to 94% with lowest levels in rolls made with whole rye + white wheat (5.7 mg P/roll) and highest levels in rolls made with wheat bran + white wheat (227 mg P/ roll). Not only phytate but also its inositol phosphate–degradation products inhibited iron absorption while fiber appeared to have no effect on iron absorption.

Distribution of phytic acid in milled fractions of Scout 66 hard red winter wheat was determined by HPLC (*206*). Samples of the different fractions were sonicated to extract phytic acid, then cleaned up and concentrated on silica-based anion-exchange columns, and analyzed by reversed-phase HPLC. Ground whole grain contained 1.03% phytate; among the milled fractions, reduction and break flours, shorts, and bran contained <0.08%, 1.05%, and 4.06% phytate, respectively. Screening of shorts and bran fractions to separate 5 size classes of particles revealed that the largest sized particles had the highest phytate levels.

Various methods to decrease phytate levels during breadmaking have been investigated. Increasing fermentation periods were found to increase phytate losses while increasing calcium levels (from dairy products) and the addition of sprouted wheat decreased phytate losses during the making of whole wheat bread (*207*). Phytate reduction in breads made from whole wheat and rye flours (*208*) and oat flour, oat bran and rye bran (*209*) was found to be optimal when the pH was between 4.4 and 5.1, as in the making of sourdough bread or in breads in which the bran or flour was scalded (55°C for 4 h) and then adjusted to the appropriate pH with lactic acid. In doughs at the optimal pH, an increase in temperature to about 55°C further enhanced phytate hydrolysis. Phytate levels were reduced from initial contents in flour by as much as 96% in soured breads.

Fermentation of wheat flour with buttermilk to produce a traditional northern Indian food, rabadi, also significantly reduces phytate levels (*210*). When carried out at 40°C for 48 h, such fermentations reduced phytate levels as much as 74% from initial levels. Starch and protein digestibility were also improved by this process.

Formation of soybean protein–phytate complexes during processing has been associated with a reduction in protein digestibility and in the bioavailability of minerals such as Ca, Zn, Fe, and Mg. To investigate associations between phytate and proteins and essential minerals, defatted soybean flakes were extracted, dialyzed and chromatographed on Sepharose 6B (*211*). Analysis of 8 fractions for their contents of protein, minerals, and phytate revealed that phytate was involved in some protein–mineral associations but not in others.

Treatment of acidic food extracts with EDTA (4 g/L) resulted in an improved determination of phytate by ion exchange chromatography (*212*). This concentration of EDTA eliminated the interference of metal ions in the extract and allowed separation and quantitation of phytic acid on an anion exchange column (Dionex AS-3). Following an in-line post-column derivatization with a ferric salt, phytic acid was detected at 300 nm. The use of a heated reaction coil (50°C) resulted in higher peaks in the chromatogram.

TOXIC AMINO ACIDS

Tryptophan and its derivatives

An outbreak of eosinophilia–myalgia syndrome (EMS) associated with the ingestion of L-tryptophan occurred in 1989 in the USA. Two elderly patients in the U.K. presenting with symptoms of eosinophilia but not myalgia were recently described (*213*). Symptoms could not be attributed to allergy, infection, or malignant disease. Both patients had been consuming 1.5–3.0 g of the same brand of L-tryptophan daily.

A contaminant ("peak E"), identified as 1,1'-ethylidenebis(tryptophan), was detected in lots of L-tryptophan associated with cases of EMS. Splenic T cells from a healthy donor incubated with peak E or some of the implicated tryptophan produced significantly greater levels of interleukin-5 than T cells incubated with pure tryptophan (*214*). These results indicate that peak E may induce eosinophilia by an interleukin-5-mediated mechanism.

Peak E was purified by HPLC and its behavior in an acid environment (simulated gastric juice) was investigated (*215*). Peak E was unstable in this environment and decomposed to form tryptophan and compounds called peak X/X'. Intermediate decomposition products, peak Y/Y', were also detected. The chemical structures of these compounds were determined by NMR and fast atom bombardment mass spectrometry. Use of these compounds may help elucidate the relationship between peak E and onset of EMS.

An infant with eosinophilia at birth which persisted for several months was born to a mother who had ingested 1 g L-tryptophan daily during the fourth through the ninth months of pregnancy (*216*). The infant's eosinophil count peaked at 4 weeks and then decreased rapidly at first and then more gradually to finally reach normal levels at about 40 weeks. Although it is impossible to prove that the infant's symptoms were caused by the mother's consumption of L-tryptophan, evidence from the recent EMS epidemic strongly suggests that the symptoms may have been caused by transplacental transfer of a contaminant or of elevated levels of a tryptophan metabolite.

Experiments in which pregnant rats were orally dosed with L-tryptophan (50–1000 mg/kg mother's body weight) demonstrated that tryptophan readily crosses the placental barrier (*217*). A dose-dependent increase in fetal brain tryptophan and serotonin levels was observed in treated rats.

Dietary tryptophan supplementation (0.4% of diet) was found to increase plasma lipid peroxidation in normal and hypercholesterolemic rats (*218*). Macrophage cholesterol uptake and esterification were also increased significantly by tryptophan supplementation. Thus excessive dietary tryptophan exerts atherogenic effects.

An assay system in which tryptophan was mixed with rat fecal suspensions revealed that the bacteria in the gastrointestinal tract were capable of metabolizing tryptophan to compounds that could bind to the aryl hydrocarbon (Ah) receptor (*219*). The suspensions were incubated at 37°C overnight and then analyzed for the presence of Ah receptor ligands. Oxygen was required for the production of such ligands from tryptophan but was not required for activation of indole-3-carbinol (a compound found in cruciferous vegetables). These ligands have the potential to significantly alter the metabolism of carcinogens in the intestine.

Lathyrism and Pacific amyotrophic lateral sclerosis

In a recent review, the etiology of long- and short-latency motor system disorders was discussed (*220*). Lathyrism, caused by excessive ingestion of seeds of *Lathyrus sativus*, usually during times of food shortage, is a form of spastic paraparesis particularly affecting the legs. The seeds contain about 1% of the free, toxic amino acid β-*N*-oxalylamino-L-alanine, which causes neurotoxic effects in laboratory animals. Consumption of 200–400 g of seeds daily for 1–3 months elicits symptoms in some persons while others appear to be less susceptible. Western Pacific amyotrophic lateral sclerosis (ALS) develops a longer time after exposure to cycad toxins either in food or from topical medicines applied to open sores. At least two toxins are present in cycad seeds: cycasin, a glucoside of methylazoxymethanol, and β-*N*-methyl-amino-L-alanine (BMAA). Both compounds cause neurotoxic effects in laboratory animals but controversy still continues as to whether either, both, or some other toxin is responsible for symptoms of ALS.

A recent review of the role of BMAA in the etiology of amyotrophic lateral sclerosis–Parkinsonism dementia complex in the western Pacific concluded that BMAA could not be the principal neurotoxin responsible for this disease (*221*). BMAA is apparently only found in cycads and in relatively low levels (0.29-1.56 mg/g in female gametophyte tissue). Significantly lower levels are present in cycad flour made from the

seeds. Animal studies indicate that BMAA is not very toxic, does not readily cross the blood–brain barrier, and is not stored in the body. It is difficult to explain how this toxin could cause a disease with a slow onset, culminating in a rapidly progressive illness.

The toxic amino acid associated with lathyrism, also called β-*N*-oxalyl-L-α,β-diaminopropionic acid (β-L-ODAP), has also been shown to have gliotoxic effects on cultures of neonatal rat astrocytes (*222*). β-L-ODAP induced a series of morphological changes in the cells including extensive vacuole formation, pale and swollen nuclei, and cellular swelling. About 50% of astrocytes were lysed after 48 h exposure to 2.1 mM β-L-ODAP.

Toxic hypoglycemic syndrome

Following reports in January and February, 1991, in Jamaica, of 8 cases (2 fatal) of toxic hypoglycemic syndrome (THS) associated with consumption of unripe ackee fruit, an epidemiologic investigation of all cases of THS seen in Jamaican hospitals in 1989–1991 was conducted (*223*). A total of 38 patients (of whom 8 died) met the case definition. Reported symptoms included vomiting (77%), coma (26%), and seizures (24%). Twenty-eight of the cases were attributed to ackee poisonimg, 1 to renta yam poisoning, and the others to idiopathic toxic hypoglycemia. THS is endemic in Jamaica, where ackee is the national fruit, because the unripe fruit contains a potent hepatotoxic amino acid, hypoglycin A (hyp A).

Using a reversed-phase HPLC system, ackee fruits representing a range of maturities were analyzed for hyp A content (*224*). At all stages of maturity the seeds contained appreciable hyp A, about 1000 ppm. Hyp A levels in large full-sized fruit only slightly yellow in color averaged just under 1500 ppm. As the fruits turned red or yellow and then split open to about 15 mm separation between the lobes, hyp A levels declined to an average of 21 ppm, with a range of 0–90 ppm. These fruits were still considered unripe. When the pods split further so that the seeds were visible, then hyp A levels were almost undetectable. These data indicate that unopened or partially opened ackee, even though bright red and full sized, should not be consumed.

OTHER ANTINUTRITIONAL COMPOUNDS IN LEGUMES

Factors affecting mineral bioavailability

In studies with neonatal pigs, the bioavailability of zinc from soy flour was found to be much less than that from nonfat dry milk or low-fat yogurt (*225*). Pigs were fed for 4 weeks with diets containing 4–16 µg Zn/g diet provided by zinc carbonate, dry milk, yogurt, or soy flour (food grade textured vegetable protein). When results from several measures of zinc bioavailability (femur Zn concentrations, plasma Zn levels, Zn balance studies) were pooled the bioavailabilities of Zn from milk, yogurt, and soy flour were 97%, 95%, and 7%, respectively, relative to zinc carbonate. This reduced availability of Zn in soy flour may be due to its phytate content.

Excretion of several minerals was monitored in rats fed for 10 days with diets containing raw faba bean meal (474–500 g/kg diet), hulls from dark or light varieties of faba beans (65 g/kg), or insoluble cotyledon residue (237 g/kg) from the same beans (*226*). Compared to control rats pair-fed with similar diets which did not contain faba beans, those rats fed the bean meal exhibited a reduced absorption of Zn and Mn and those fed the hulls absorbed less Fe from their diets. The cotyledon residue had no significant effect on mineral content of feces. Since phytate levels in these beans are low (6.7–7.8 g/kg), the elevated loss of Zn and Mn is probably due to other seed constituents, such as the soluble non-starch polysaccharides, while some insoluble structural hull components may reduce Fe absorption.

Occurrence and determination of antinutritional factors

Legume seeds contain a number of antinutritional factors (ANF), apparently to protect themselves against predators. Changes in levels of these ANF during germination have been reviewed (*227*). Proteinaceous factors, such as lectins, amylase- and protease-inhibitors, are partly degraded during germination but the extent of this degradation depends on the variety of legume, the kind of ANF, and the catabolic enzymes in the seed. Significant degradation of tannins has not been observed during germination.

Five high-yielding varieties of rice bean (*Vigna umbellata*) and one variety each of green gram and black gram were analyzed to determine their content of ANF (*228*). Trypsin inhibitor activity was similar in all 7 varieties, ranging from 35 to 49 units/g. There was some variation in tannin, phytate, and saponin levels among the rice bean varieties, with average concentrations of 1394, 2033, and 2285 mg/100 g, respectively. Lower levels of these ANF were present in the gram varieties: 1069–1073, 937–1321, and 1542–1683 mg/100 g, respectively. Hemagglutinating activity due to lectins was detected in all strains but was not quantified.

Seeds from three leguminous trees (*Acacia catechu, Parkinsonia aculeata,* and *Prosopsis chilensis*), which are consumed only by some tribal people in India, were investigated to determine their chemical composition and content of ANF (*229*). Trypsin inhibitor activity and tannin levels did not exceed those found in other edible legumes. Hemagglutinating activity was weak in *P. aculeata* and very strong in *A. catechu*. These underexploited tree pulses also contained high levels of protein and were rich sources of K, Mg, Ca, and Fe.

A combined method for analysis of trypsin inhibitors and lectins in white kidney beans has been developed (*230*). Both ANF were extracted with buffered saline and were then purified by affinity chromatography with trypsin–Sepharose 4B (for trypsin inhibitors) and with porcine thyroglobulin–agarose (for lectins). Protein content of the purified extracts was determined by standard methods. This procedure was used to monitor the decrease of both ANF during germination of seeds at 20°C for 7 days. Repeatability coefficients of variation were 2–10%. After 7 days' germination, trypsin inhibitors and lectins were reduced by 72% and 92%, respectively.

Effects of cooking and processing on antinutritional factors

Fate of some antinutritional factors during different cooking methods (100–125°C for 1–12 h) was monitored in faba beans (*231*). Optimal heat treatments for easy-to-cook and hard-to-cook beans were, respectively, 125°C for 1 h and 120°C for 2 h. Less than 10% of tannins were degraded but up to 48% were leached into the cooking water. About 31% of the original trypsin inhibitor activity remained in the beans while another 18% was retained in the cooking water. Less than 15% of phytate was destroyed, with 66–72% remaining in the cooked beans.

Another study with faba beans demonstrated that soaking and dehulling could reduce phytate by 4% and saponins by 26–29% (*232*). Cooking further reduced phytate by 28–31% and saponins by 8–10%, while autoclaving of soaked, dehulled seeds removed a further 21–24% of phytate and 31–37% of saponins. Cooking and autoclaving of seeds completely removed hemagglutinating activity.

The raffinose family of sugars occurs widely in legume seeds and reduces their acceptability by promoting flatulence. Effects of processing temperature and moisture content in the barrel during high-temperature extrusion of pinto bean starch on the levels of these sugars were investigated (*233*). The extrusion process at 163°C reduced raffinose and stachyose levels to 33–37% of those found in the bean starch. Higher temperatures removed more sugars but moisture content in the extruder barrel did not significantly affect sugars in the samples.

Lectins

Effects of purified native and heated lectins from navy and red kidney beans on pancreatic α-amylase activities were investigated (*234*). Since legume starches are digested at a lower rate than cereals, it has been hypothesized that lectins or some other ANF inhibit α-amylase. However, in these experiments, all purified lectins, whether native or heated, significantly increased α-amylase activity in vitro. One semi-purified lectin preparation inhibited α-amylase activity. But this was probably due to some

contaminant, since further purification of this lectin eliminated the inhibitory activity.

Hemagglutinating activity of 10 varieties of dry beans (*Phaseolus vulgaris*) was found to range from 128 to 512×10^4 units/g of whole, raw bean flour (*235*). Small red beans and red kidney beans had the highest levels. Germination reduced hemagglutinating activity, while cooking for 30 min completely destroyed it in all beans tested. For most bean varieties, even cooking for 15 min was sufficient to eliminate this activity.

Lectin from a northern Mexican bean variety, Ojo de Cabra, was partially purified and characterized (*236*). Following purification by affinity chromatography on immobilized fetuin, two lectin subunits were detected and found to be immunologically related to red kidney bean lectin. The lectin had a very high hemagglutinating ability but this was decreased by 84% by dry heating and by 99.8% by cooking. Raw, but not cooked, beans were toxic to rats.

PHENOLIC COMPOUNDS

Coumarins and furocoumarins

Scopoletin (6-methoxy-7-hydroxy coumarin) was determined in gari (a traditional cassava food) and in cassava flour purchased at markets in Nigeria (*237*). Cassava flour had higher levels of this coumarin (76.8 mg/100 g dry sample) than gari (57.6 mg/100 g), which probably reflects the different processing methods for these foods. Scopoletin levels were not significantly affected by post-processing treatments such as refrigeration and storage for 4 weeks. Cassava has been implicated as an etiological agent in a slowly developing tropical neuropathy endemic in populations subsisting on cassava diets. The authors suggest that scopoletin, rather than or in addition to cyanogenic glycosides, may be responsible for this syndrome.

Two comparative studies on the metabolism of coumarin by rat, gerbil, and human liver microsomes concluded that the gerbil is a better model for human liver coumarin metabolism than the rat (*238,239*). Several pathways for coumarin metabolism were found in all species. *o*-Hydroxyphenylacetaldehyde 7-hydroxycoumarin was a major metabolite in all 3 species, but only gerbil and human liver microsomes produced 7-hydroxycoumarin as a major metabolite.

Natural furocoumarins are widespread, frequently consumed dietary components, some of which may exert toxic effects. A recent analysis of data on dietary intake of different foods in the USA and furocoumarin levels in these foods indicated that per capita exposure is about 1.3 mg furocoumarin/day (*240*). Most of the exposure is from limes, with smaller amounts from other citrus and umbelliferous food plants. At this time it is impossible to assess the health risk from this level of intake but exposure can be reduced by controlling stress in growing plants and stored food products.

The risk of phototoxic skin reactions in response to UV irradiation caused by consumption of vegetables containing furocoumarins was assessed in human volunteers (*241*). Following ingestion of 300 g of celery roots (total phototoxic furocoumarin content, 28.2 µg/g), blood levels of the furocoumarins were below the analytical detection limit of 2 ng/mL and no skin reactions were observed after UVA exposure ($1.5–9$ J/cm^2). Ingestion of 15 mg each of 8-methoxypsoralen (8-MOP) and 5-methoxysporalen (5-MOP), the two most important furocoumarins in vegetables, induced a strong and persistent erythema in 3 of 4 subjects exposed to $3–25$ J/cm^2 UVA. At a lower dose (10 mg of each compound) only mild to moderate erythema was induced in one subject. This appears to be the phototoxic threshold dose and resulted in blood levels of $12–15$ ng/mL for 8-MOP and 5-MOP. Although normal levels of consumption of celery and other vegetables would not contain this high a dose of furocoumarins, the safety factor between possible actual intake of furocoumarins and the phototoxic threshold dose is only about 2–10.

Flavonoids

In experiments with human and rabbit gastrointestinal tract microsomes, α-naphthoflavone was found to greatly enhance (by 7- to 45-fold) the metabolism of the heterocyclic amine MeIQ to a mutagen as determined by the Ames test (*242*). This effect was observed in human jejunal and ileal microsomes but in only one of four colonic microsome preparations tested. P4503A proteins were detected by Western blots of microsomes prepared from both human and rabbit small intestine. These data demonstrate that flavonoids can markedly increase the activation of heterocyclic amines but the significance of this interaction in the etiology of human cancer is unclear.

Mutagenicity of 13 bioflavonoids was examined using the L-arabinose forward mutation assay of *Salmonella typhimurium* (*243*). All flavonoids induced statistically significant numbers of mutants, in some cases with metabolic activation by an S9 mixture and in other cases without activation. Minimum mutagenic doses varied from 4 nmol for quercetin to 1626 nmol for taxifolin. Flavonols were the strongest mutagens.

A total of 16 flavonoids were identified from 10 samples of Spanish honey (*244*). Filtration through Amberlite XAD-2 eliminated sugars and polar compounds from the honey and then the flavonoid fraction was purified with Sephadex LH-20 and analyzed by HPLC. Sunflower honey from France was found to contain 5 major and 2 minor flavonoids (*245*). This honey was first treated with petroleum ether and then the phenolic compounds were extracted with ethyl acetate and analyzed by reverse-phase TLC, reverse-phase HPLC using post-column derivatization, and GC/MS.

Reversed-phase HPLC methods were developed for the preparative isolation and analytical separation of quercetin and kaempferol rhamnodiglucosides, two characteristic phenolic compounds in tea (*246*). The structures of these compounds were determined by NMR spectroscopy, fast atom bombardment MS, and GC/MS. Analysis of 7 varieties of black tea revealed quercetin and kaempferol rhamnodiglucoside levels of $0–0.95$ g/kg and $0.05–1.25$ g/kg, respectively.

Effects of quercetin on lipid peroxidation and DNA damage were studied in isolated rat liver nuclei under aerobic conditions (*247,248*). Quercetin, at levels of 20 to 100 µM, induced significant, concentration-dependent nuclear lipid peroxidation and DNA degradation. These effects were enhanced by iron and copper ions and inhibited by mannitol. Results of experiments testing the effects of catalase, superoxide dismutase, glutathione, and diallyl sulfide suggested that reactive oxygen species, especially hydroxyl radicals, were responsible for the damage caused by quercetin.

Gossypol

Outbreaks of unexplained infertility in some areas of China during the 1930s and 1940s were traced to gossypol, a component of cottonseed oil used as a cooking oil by these people. Since then gossypol levels in foods derived from cottonseed and in food animals fed cottonseed meal have been of concern. In experiments using membranes and dispersed cells from rat and human adrenal glands, gossypol was found to increase microviscosity of the membranes as measured by an increase in fluorescence polarization (*249*). Along with this change in the membranes, gossypol inhibited the activities of two adrenal enzymes and the ACTH-stimulated cAMP and cortisol levels. The corticosterone response to ACTH in rats was also inhibited in rats gavaged with 25 mg gossypol/kg/day for 7 weeks. It appears that gossypol has multiple effects on adrenal function.

Gossypol also exerts genotoxic effects in mammalian cell cultures and has been shown to bind to calf thymus DNA, which may lead to strand breaks (*250*). Superoxide anions and singlet oxygen, detectable in aqueous solutions of gossypol, may cause the strand breakage in DNA.

Liquid chromatographic methods for the determination of gossypol in chicken liver have been developed (*251,252*). In the first paper, an HPLC method with a detection limit of 0.5 ppm determined free gossypol levels in homogenized, deproteinized chicken liver. The pure gossypol was partitioned into chloroform and analyzed by gradient elution (methanol:water) on a Spherisorb ODS 2, 10 µm column. Overall recovery of gossypol from spiked samples was 81.1%. This method was modified to enable determination of bound as well as free gossypol by hydrolysis of bound gossypol in the presence of ascorbic acid. Addition of octane-1-sulfonate to the methanol–water mobile phase improved separation and determination of gossypol.

Chickens fed a normal balanced ration mixed with unground cottonseed for 1 and 2 weeks were found to have 4.6–7.0 ppm and 17.7–26 ppm gossypol, respectively, in their liver tissues.

Tannins

TEA. Tannin levels in over-the-counter Indian tea, in green coffee beans, and in roasted coffee beans were determined with a radial diffusion–protein precipitation technique and with a spectrophotometric method (*253*). Both methods provided an easy analysis and gave good results. Tannin concentrations in green and roasted coffee were, respectively, 6.6–6.8 and 17–18 mg/g. Tea contained 37 mg/g and 24 mg/g as determined by spectrophotometry and by the protein precipitation method, respectively.

Effects of tea on apparent utilization of niacin, thiamin, and protein were measured in 10 adult volunteers (*254*). The subjects were fed the same diet during two 14-day experimental periods except that during one period they also consumed instant tea (8 g/day on a dry weight basis). During the tea period, urinary thiamin losses were depressed but niacin losses were increased. Serum concentrations of thiamin were also decreased but niacin levels remained about the same. These results suggest that tea consumption inhibits the utilization of thiamin. Tea apparently had no effect on protein status.

Effects of tea on iron and aluminum metabolism in rats were monitored during a 28-day feeding study (*255*). Rats were maintained on a semi-synthetic diet containing normal (38 µg/g) or low (9 µg/g) levels of iron with or without tea infusion (20 g leaves/L water) to drink. At the end of the experiment all rats on the low-iron diet were severely anemic but those in the tea group showed even greater iron depletion. Blood and liver aluminum levels were not increased by tea even though aluminum intake was increased.

LEGUMES. Soaked beans of ten varieties were cooked for 60, 90, and 120 min and the cooking broth was analyzed for tannins (*256*). Tannin levels in broth increased with cooking time and were higher in broth from beans with red seed coats as compared to those with white or yellow seed coats. However, none of these differences were significant. Tannin levels in broth after 60 min of cooking varied from 1.994 to 8.739 g catechin equivalents/ kg dry matter.

Freezing of alfalfa leaf juice produces a curd, called freezing curd, which contains 60% of the protein and 50% of the dry matter in the original juice. Since this curd has been proposed as a high-protein supplement in human diets, the types and amounts of polyphenols in the curd have been determined (257). Total polyphenols constituted 1.034% of the dry matter in the curd. Extraction of the curd with 2-propanol reduced polyphenol content by 65% while washing the curd prior to 2-propanol extraction completely eliminated polyphenols.

Several assay procedures for the determination of polyphenols in black beans were compared and validated (258). Polyphenols were fractionated by adsorption chromatography into tannins and non-tannins and then were assayed with Prussian blue, Folin-Denis, and corrected and uncorrected vanillin tests. In spite of its low specificity, the Prussian blue assay was the most convenient and its results correlated well with other procedures. Neither vanillin test performed well because of interference by non-tannin compounds present in raw bean extracts.

Although acorns are not widely used today, they have been a staple food in many areas of the northern hemisphere in the past. A traditional method for reducing the activity of tannic acid, the primary astringent and toxic constituent of these nuts, in both California and Sardinia (Italy) involves mixing acorn meal with a locally obtained red clay. In recent experiments (259), acorn bread was prepared according to these methods using clay from these areas and then the tannic acid available after acidic digestion was measured. Cooking by itself reduced tannic acid release from digestion by up to 66% while addition of clay before cooking resulted in a reduction of available tannic acid to about 10–16% of that in raw acorn meal. Tannic acid adsorbs to clay particles, and this apparently accounts for at least part of the detoxification caused by clay.

Wide variations in levels of phenolic compounds in whole seeds, hulls, and cotyledons of 4 tropical varieties of rapeseed were determined (260).

Hulls of all cultivars contained higher levels of catechin, procyanidine, proanthocyanidine, and flavan-4-ols and, generally, lower amounts of sinapine, tannic acid, and total phenols than cotyledons. Therefore, simple dehulling does not remove all polyphenols from rapeseed, but a combination of dehulling and solvent extraction removes most of the polyphenols.

Relatively high levels of phytate and polyphenols in pearl millet significantly reduce the digestibility of its proteins and carbohydrates. Sequential fermentation of millet by yeast and then by lactobacilli for 72 h each at 30°C significantly reduced levels of both of these antinutrients (261). The best combinations were *Saccharomyces cerevisiae* and *Lactobacillus brevis* for polyphenol reduction of 22% and *S. diastaticus* and *L. brevis* for phytate reduction of 78%.

The Prussian blue method for determination of polyphenols has two main drawbacks: formation of a precipitate after short incubation periods and an increase in color density with time. In experiments testing 3 chelating agents and 6 protective colloids, a combination of gum acacia (or Reten, an anionic polyacrylamide) and phosphoric acid was found to be most effective in preventing color change and precipitation for up to 60 h (262).

OTHER PHENOLIC COMPOUNDS. Both F344 rats and C57BL/6N × C3H/HeN F_1 mice were used to test the long-term carcinogenic effects of 2% caffeic acid in the diet (263). After 96 (mice) or 104 (rats) weeks of exposure, detailed histopathological examination revealed the presence of forestomach squamous cell papillomas or carcinomas at high incidence in rats (77–80%) and at low incidence in mice (3–13%). Statistically significant incidences of renal tubular cell hyperplasias were observed in male rats (73%) and in female mice (97%) and of alveolar type II cell tumors in male mice (27%). Although caffeic acid is widely distributed in vegetables, fruits, and beverages, it is usually ingested at very low levels so that the carcinogenic risk to humans may be negligible.

Using a simple spectrophotometric method, levels of sinapic acid, the predominant phenolic acid in rapeseed, were determined in 3 varieties of rapeseed and 1 variety of mustard seed meals (*264*). In hexane-extracted meals sinapic acid constituted 65–85%, 71–97%, and 7–32% of free, esterified, and insoluble bound phenolic compounds, respectively. Treatment of defatted meals with 10% ammonia in 95% methanol removed 41–75% of total free phenolics and 82–93% of esterified phenolics and enhanced the flavor and nutritional value of the meals.

Both wine (white, red, and rosé) and brandy tested positive in the Ara forward mutagenicity assay with *Salmonella typhimurium* in the absence of mammalian microsomal activation (*265–267*). Preincubation with an S9 mix abolished most of the mutagenic activity, and catalase was identified as the component of the S9 mix most likely responsible for destroying mutagenicity. Phenolic compounds naturally present in the wine and extracted from the wood during maturation of brandy in barrels may be responsible for the mutagenicity through an autoxidative process leading to production of hydrogen peroxide.

Since hydrogen peroxide is present in coffee infusions but is not detectable in green coffee beans, an investigation was conducted to determine the factors affecting hydrogen peroxide formation (*268*). Greater concentrations of hydrogen peroxide were found in coffee prepared using a filter rather than a coffee maker and in coffee at higher temperatures in the light. Several components of coffee were found to contain very low levels of hydrogen peroxide before heating but higher levels after roasting. Formation of hydrogen peroxide from caffeic acid was particularly marked.

TOXICITY AND CARCINOGENICITY OF MUSHROOMS

During 1989, 9208 cases of mushroom exposure were reported to the American Association of Poison Control Centers "National Data Collection System" in the USA (*269*). It is estimated that this is approximately 73% of all cases which actually occurred during that year. In only 313 cases was the mushroom identified, with 48 different species reported. Three fatalities occurred, all associated with *Amanita* spp. For 78.4% of cases only a minimal effect or no effect was reported, while in 2.6% of cases a moderate or major effect occurred. Besides *Amanita* spp., mushrooms associated with moderate effects were *Chlorophyllum molybdites* (14 cases), *Lycoperdon candidum* (1 case), *Gyromitra esculenta* (1 case), *Morchella augusticeps* (1 case), *Pleurotus ostreatus* (1 case), and *Scleroderma citrinum* (1 case). In 81% of cases the patient was <6 years old, and 95% of cases were accidental.

Effects of *Amanita pantherina/muscaria* poisoning in children (age 1–6 years) were reported for a series of 9 cases occurring in Washington State during 1979–1989 (*270*). Symptoms occurred 30–180 min after ingestion, with the onset of central nervous system depression, ataxia, waxing and waning obtundation, hallucinations, intermittent hysteria or hyperkinetic behavior. Vomiting was rare. Seizures or twitching occurred in 4 patients. Following treatment with ipecac (6 cases), charcoal and gastric lavage (6 cases), diazepam (4 cases), phenobarbital (2 cases), and/or atropine (2 cases), all patients recovered uneventfully within 14 h.

Toxicity of phalloidin and α-amanitin (*Amanita* spp. toxins) and of DL-propargylglycine (identified from *A. abrupta*) was compared in isolated rat hepatocytes (*271*). Phalloidin was the most potent compound in significantly increasing cytosolic Ca^{2+} and altering phosphoinositide turnover. This resulted in activation of phosphorylase *a* and glycogenolysis. α-Amanitin had similar but weaker effects while DL-propargylglycine had no significant effect on these parameters.

A reversed-phase HPLC method allowing the simultaneous determination of up to 8 amatoxins and phallotoxins was devised (*272*). Toxins extracted from fruiting bodies of *A. phalloides* were separated, identified, and determined by gradient elution with 0.02 M aqueous ammonium acetate–acetonitrile and simultaneous monitoring of absorbances at 214 and 295 nm. Limit of detection for each toxin was 10 ng/mL extraction medium. This assay also correctly identified toxins in *Galerina marginata*, a species containing only amatoxins. The method is relatively simple and should be suitable for detection of these toxins in other mushroom species and may be scaled up to a preparative level.

Another mushroom which has caused severe poisonings and even death in humans is *Gyromitra esculenta*, the false morel. A recent review described characteristics of poisoning by this mushroom, the toxins involved, and in vivo and in vitro toxicity tests (*273*). Intoxications occur within 48 h after consumption of raw or poorly cooked mushrooms and are manifested primarily by vomiting and diarrhea, followed by jaundice, convulsions, and coma in severe cases. Frequent consumption has caused hepatitis and neurological diseases. The toxins, gyromitrin and its homologues, are water soluble and heat sensitive. In vivo they are converted into *N*-methyl-*N*-formylhydrazine (MFH) and then into *N*-methylhydrazine (MH). Experiments with laboratory animals and cell cultures indicate that these compounds are hepatotoxic and carcinogenic. Possible mechanisms of toxicity were discussed.

A variety of tumors were induced in mice fed raw (previously frozen) false morels ad libitum for 3 days/week and a semisynthetic diet for 4 days/week for up to 130 weeks (*274*). Tumors in the lungs (70-80%) and blood vessels (32-50%) were most common, followed by those in the cecum, stomach, nasal cavity and liver. Tumor types included adenomas, adenocarcinomas, hemangiosarcomas, hemangiomas, hepatomas, and squamous cell papillomas. The concentrations of gyromitrin and MFH in these mushrooms were 44 and 4 mg/kg, respectively.

Swiss mice gavaged once a week for 52 weeks with 50 or 100 μg hexanal methylformylhydrazone (HMFH)/g body weight developed tumors primarily in the lungs but also in the liver and preputial glands (*275*). In the high-dose group, 90% of females and 70% of males had adenomas or adenocarcinomas of the lungs at autopsy while 86% of males had adenomas, carcinomas or squamous cell papillomas of the preputial gland. This compound is the sixth carcinogenic constituent found in *Gyromitra esculenta*.

It has been suggested that the carcinogenicity of gyromitrin and related toxins is due to methylation of guanine residues in DNA of target tissues.

To investigate this reaction, rats and mice were injected i.p. with gyromitrin (12.6 mg/kg, rats; 2.6 mg/kg, mice) or with *N*-methylhydrazine (MMH) (6.4-7.5 mg/kg) and then liver, kidney, and lung tissues were analyzed (*276*). No O^6MeGu was detected in any tissues using an HPLC method with fluorimetric detection, which allowed detection of pmol quantities of O^6MeGu in the presence of 1000-fold larger amounts of guanine. Mice consuming drinking water containing 0.01% MMH for two weeks had 66 μmol O^6MeGu in liver cells and 37 μmol in kidney cells. No O^6MeGu was detected in lung samples. It appears that these mushroom toxins present a relatively low carcinogenic risk except to individuals with a decreased detoxification rate (acetylation) of MMH.

Long-term feeding experiments with rats failed to demonstrate any carcinogenic effects of *Agaricus bisporus*, the most frequently commercially cultivated mushroom in the West (*277*). The rats were fed for 500 days with a basal diet with or without 30% dry powder of *A. bisporus*. At autopsy, mammary tumors, thymomas, adrenal adenomas, and pituitary adenomas were observed in both experimental and control groups with no significant differences between the two groups. The body weights of the treated animals were substantially lower than those of controls throughout the experiment but all animals survived until the end of the experiment.

Acromelic acid (ACRO), recently isolated from the poisonous mushroom *Clitocybe acromelalga*, has been found to induce selective neuron damage in the rat spinal cord (*278*). Injection of 5 mg ACRO/kg caused frequent cramps and generalized convulsions. Two rats which survived this dose developed long lasting spastic paraparesis and degenerative changes in small interneurons in the lumbosacral cord.

Toxicity of the deadly mushroom *Cortinarius speciosissimus* has been reported to be due to fluorescent cyclic decapeptides called cortinarins. However, recent analyses (using TLC, GC-MS, and NMR) of *C. speciosissimus* collected in different places over a period of 9 years failed to detect any cortinarins (*279*). Instead, the results indicated that the fluorescent compounds were primarily steroids along with some decomposition products of orellanine, a nephrotoxin previously isolated from some species of *Cortinarius*.

Three new triterpene glycosides, hebevinosides XII, XIII, and XIV, were recently isolated from the poisonous mushroom *Hebeloma vinosophyllum* (*280*). The toxins were isolated by HPLC and characterized by NMR. Related toxins present in these mushrooms have neurotoxic effects.

FOOD ALLERGY AND FOOD INTOLERANCE

Case reports

Three incidents of severe reactions to sesame seeds or sesame oil occurred recently. A 23-year-old woman arrived at a casualty unit in Switzerland with anaphylactic symptoms after eating a falafel-burger, consisting of a wheat-flour bun filled with chickpea balls and served with a red and white sauce (*281*). Following treatment with intravenous corticosteroids and antihistamines, she recovered and was discharged. Skin tests were negative for common inhalant and food allergens but were strongly positive for the white sauce containing sesame seed paste and for sesame seeds alone. Her sensitivity was probably due to use of a commercial spice mixture containing sesame seeds because she reported rhinitis, itching eyes, and burning skin every time she added the spice during cooking. The allergens in the spice mixture were apparently destroyed during cooking because she had no reaction to the cooked, spiced food.

A 46-year-old businessman reported a series of severe food reactions during the past 18 years, many of which were attributed to the ingestion of sesame products, particularly sesame oil (*282*). Symptoms included pin-and-needle sensation on his face, chills, abdominal cramps, and occasionally facial and lip swelling. Skin testing revealed a 4+ Multitest response to whole commercial sesame seed oil and only a 2+ response to commercial sesame seed antigen at 1:1000 concentration. RAST was only marginally positive to sesame seeds, oil, and commercial antigens. However, BHR (basophil histamine release) tests demonstrated significant histamine release with sesame antigen (90%) prepared by the authors, cooked sesame seed extract (80%), commercial sesame seed oil (40%), and whole sesame seeds (70%) but only a small reaction (6.3%) to commercial sesame seed antigen.

A 26-year-old man occupationally exposed to sesame seed dust reported symptoms of rhinitis, urticaria, and IgE-mediated asthma (*283*). The patient was in charge of a mill in which waste bread was ground for animal feed. Dust levels in the area were as high as 22 mg/m^3. Skin tests and Phadezym RAST were negative for flours and storage mites but positive for crushed sesame seeds. After the patient handled crushed sesame seeds for 30 min, he had an immediate asthmatic attack with wheezing, a marked nasal reaction, and urticaria on the face, breast and hands.

Two infants developed atopic dermatitis after consuming the same milk formula (*284*). Prick tests were strongly positive to peanut allergens, and oral challenges of 1 g of peanut oil brought on generalized rashes within 15 min in both infants. The vegetable lipid content of the milk formula was found to be 10%, 80% of which was peanut oil. Although previous research has indicated that peanut oil is non-allergenic even to peanut-allergic patients, these results demonstrate that allergenic proteins are present in peanut oil and that this oil should not be used in milk formulae.

Immunological reactions and history of exposure were evaluated in 20 females, aged 27–73 years, who reported anaphylactic reactions to a psyllium-containing cereal, Heartwise (*285*). Symptoms developed within 2–30 min after ingestion of <1 cup of cereal and included moderate to severe wheezing, throat and chest tightness, and urticaria. All the women required medical treatment. All but 3 of the women had prior exposure to psyllium, either by ingestion or dispensing of psyllium-containing products, such as the laxative Metamucil. Specific IgE and IgG antibodies to psyllium protein fractions were present in all 20 subjects.

Although chicken soup has been considered a panacea for all kinds of illnesses, a case of anaphylaxis following ingestion of chicken soup recently occurred in an 18-year-old man (*286*). Following consumption of a bowl of packaged chicken soup reconstituted with water, he suffered symptoms of chest pain, dyspnea, and facial edema. Treatment at an emergency room relieved symptoms and the patient recovered. Later, skin tests revealed a marked response to the packaged chicken soup and moderate responses to peanut, parsley, carrot, celery, cucumber, and grapefruit but not to chicken. A brief and amusing history of the chicken in medicine was included in this report.

A case report of allergic contact dermatitis caused by exposure to several species of the mushroom genus *Suillus* was described (*287*). Symptoms of reddening, swelling and itching appeared after contact with the pileus cuticle mucilage and the pore layer tissues but not with spores. Similar cases of contact allergy associated with the mushroom genera *Agaricus, Boletus, Lactarius, Paxillus, Ramaria,* and *Suillus* were summarized from literature reports.

An adverse reaction to pomegranate ingestion occurred in an 85-year-old woman (*288*). A few hours after eating this fruit her tongue became swollen and she sought medical care. The swelling responded to methylprednisolone. Tests to demonstrate an IgE-mediated mechanism (prick test, histamine release test, and RAST with pomegranate) were all negative. However, her sensitivity to pomegranate was proven in a double-blind challenge test in which fresh pomegranate seeds were mixed with strawberry yogurt. The patient did not react to the yogurt alone but did experience tongue angioedema after ingesting 40 g pomegranate seeds in yogurt.

An unusual association of two rare allergies to latex and to certain fruits (banana, avocado, and chestnuts) was reported in 5 patients (*289,290*). Following surgery for bladder cancer, a 67-year-old man started having recurrent anaphylactic reactions after ingestion of banana and avocado. Skin prick and RAST tests with these fruits were positive. Later medical examinations where latex gloves were used also provoked anaphylaxis, and skin prick and RAST tests with latex were also positive. Two nurses with histories of contact urticaria to rubber gloves at work suffered symptoms of anaphylaxis after eating banana, avocado, and chestnut. A fourth patient

had a severe reaction with urticaria and loss of consciousness after eating a fresh chestnut. This man had also experienced conjunctivitis and itching of the lips after inflating a rubber balloon. The fifth patient, a 12-year-old boy, suffered severe symptoms after ingesting bananas, chestnuts, figs, passion fruit, or celery and also after inflating rubber balloons. RAST tests with latex were positive in these patients and all three patients tested by skin prick with banana had positive reactions as did the two patients tested by skin prick with chestnuts.

Reviews

A recent issue of *Immunology and Allergy Clinics of North America* was devoted to food allergy (*291*). Topics reviewed included immunologic reactions, including IgE-mediated reactions, anaphylaxis, and oropharyngeal and gastrointestinal symptoms, to a variety of foods; non-immunologic food reactions which may be confused with food allergy; food and migraine headache; developmental aspects of food allergy through infancy and childhood; food challenge testing; and in vitro assays for the evaluation of immunologic reactions to foods.

A special clinical section in *Nutrition Research* (*292*) reviewed a number of topics related to food allergy in childhood: strategies for prevention of atopic disease; hypoallergenic formulas; cow's milk allergy; gastrointestinal and extraintestinal manifestations of food allergy in infants and children; food allergy diagnosis; and management of atopic dermatitis. Although it is not possible to prevent all food allergies, preventative strategies such as breast feeding and delayed introduction of solid foods, particularly egg, peanut, and fish, are extremely cost-effective.

An overview in *Food Technology* (*293*) discussed the nature and mechanisms of food allergies; manifestations and diagnosis of food hypersensitivity; chemistry and detection of food allergens; and occupational reactions in the food industry.

Allergies to specific foods

In order to identify the allergic components of honey, 22 subjects with a history of systemic allergic symptoms following honey ingestion were given skin tests and RAST with 3 varieties of Swiss honey (dandelion, forest, and rape), pollen of Compositae species, celery tuber, extract of bee pharyngeal glands, honey bee venom, and bee whole body extract (*294*). Of the honey-allergic subjects, 17 were sensitive to dandelion honey and in some cases to one or both of the other honeys also. Allergy to Compositae pollen, honey bee venom, bee pharyngeal glands, and bee body extract was observed in 13, 9, 3, and 3 persons, respectively. These results suggest that honey-allergic patients are most frequently sensitized to either pollen- or bee-related antigens. Some other allergens, such as mold spores, yeast, or algae may be responsible for sensitization in some people but this did not appear to be the case with these subjects because none of them reacted only to the forest honey (the only one containing algae and mold spores).

To aid in diagnosis of milk-protein allergies, 13 children with strongly suspected milk-protein allergy and some adults were given skin prick tests with purified samples of the main cow's milk proteins: α-lactalbumin, β-lactoglobulin A+B, α_s-casein, β-casein, and κ-casein (*295*). Positive skin reactions occurred rarely in adults while 11 children had distinct skin reactions to one or more of the proteins. The highest prevalence and intensity of skin reactions was observed with α-lactalbumin and β-lactoglobulin B, with a significantly lower incidence and intensity of reactions to casein.

Recently, hydrolyzed cow's milk proteins have been used to produce hypoallergenic infant formulas. In tests with 36 atopic children and 20 children with cow's milk protein allergy, the hydrolyzed cow's milk demonstrated a decreased but partially conserved allergenic potency compared to unhydrolyzed milk (*296*). Histamine release from basophil leukocytes after incubation with the hydrolysate was observed in 5 atopic and 2 cow milk–allergic children. IgE binding to the hydrolysate was detectable in 5 of 10 allergic children tested.

Seventy patients with positive skin tests to birch and/or mugwort pollens and celery were given scratch tests to determine their sensitivity to a series of powdered commercial spices (*297*). Spices from the same botanical family as celery (Apiaceae), viz. cumin, coriander, fennel and anise, induced positive responses in more than 24 subjects, with anise being the most allergenic (46 positive responses). Spices from different families (cinnamon, nutmeg, ginger, red pepper, and white pepper) rarely provoked skin reactions; the most common was red pepper with 11 reactions. Positive RAST results occurred mainly in those patients with allergies to both celery and mugwort.

Eleven children and young adults with histories consistent with IgE-mediated fish hypersensitivity were skin-prick tested with extracts of 10 fish species to determine whether they could safely eat any fish (*298*). Positive results were obtained with all fish extracts in 8 subjects. However, positive oral challenges occurred to only one fish species in 7 subjects, to two fish species in 1 subject, and to three fish species in 2 subjects. Immunoblot analyses with sera from fish-allergic patients demonstrated specific IgE binding to proteins from fish which did not induce a positive response on oral challenge. Thus, skin prick test and IgE binding did not correlate well with symptomatic fish allergy. All of these fish-hypersensitive patients could consume one or more other fish species without adverse reactions.

Isolation and characterization of allergens

A major peanut allergen, Ara h I, has been identified and partially purified by the use of serum from peanut-allergic patients who responded positively to a double-blind, placebo-controlled food challenge with peanuts (*299*). Anion exchange chromatography yielded several fractions which bound IgE from the serum of allergic patients. By measuring anti-peanut-specific IgE in an ELISA and IgE-specific immunoblotting, an allergenic protein was identified by electrophoresis. This allergen is a glycoprotein with a molecular weight of 63.5 kD and a mean pI of 4.55.

A major allergen from Oriental mustard seeds, Bra j I, has been isolated and characterized (*300*). Two different ELISAs demonstrated that this allergen reacts with IgE from mustard-sensitive individuals. Amino acid analysis and immunodiffusion assays indicated that this allergen is a 2S albumin protein very similar to the allergen Sin a I, previously isolated and purified from yellow mustard.

Using sera from soybean-sensitive patients with atopic dermatitis, at least 16 soybean proteins were identified as potential allergens (*301*). IgE antibodies from the allergic individuals bound most strongly to a protein of molecular weight 30,000 in the 7S-globulin fraction. This appeared to be the major allergen in soybeans and was named Gly m Bd 30K.

Immunoblotting analysis, histamine release from human leukocytes, and RAST inhibition assays have identified a 16-kD protein from rice as a major allergen (*302*). In RAST inhibition assays using sera with positive RAST for 5 cereal grains (rice, wheat, corn, Japanese millet, and Italian millet), this rice allergen inhibited IgE binding to all cereal disks in a dose-dependent manner. Similarly, extracts of all 5 cereals inhibited IgE binding to rice allergen disks. These results demonstrate cross-allergenicity between these cereal grain extracts.

OTHER FOOD-RELATED TOXINS

Toxicity of licorice

Fifty-nine cases of glycyrrhizin (licorice)-induced hypokalemic myopathy were reviewed with respect to conditions leading to the onset, clinical manifestations, muscle biopsy findings, and treatment (*303*). Average age of cases was 55.2 years (range of 15–86) and many patients reported habitual licorice ingestion or long-term use of anti-tuberculosis agents or other medicines containing licorice. Factors which aggravate hypokalemia, such as diuretics, alcoholism, and diarrhea, increase the risk of developing this disease. Symptoms included muscular weakness and pain with numbness in the extremities. Myopathic changes, including phagocytosis, necrotic changes, and sporadic neurogenic changes, were observed in muscle biopsies. In 57 cases a complete cure was attained after discontinuation of licorice use.

Two cases of licorice-induced arrhythmia were reported from Germany in patients who consumed 300–400 g licorice/day (*304*). Both patients had underlying heart problems and licorice caused a marked hypokalemia followed by arrhythmia. Following treatment, both were discharged without symptoms.

Licorice, as a component of an herbal medicine, was the suspected cause of a sudden increase in high blood pressure in a 43-year-old nurse (*305*). The nurse had essential hypertension which was controlled by drugs, but suffered headaches, dizziness, and increased blood pressure following use of an herbal remedy for allergic rhinitis. Another component of the herbal medicine, ephedrine, may also have affected her blood pressure.

Effects of licorice on 11β-hydroxysteroid dehydrogenase activity and the renin-aldosterone system were studied in a 70-year-old patient with chronic licorice intoxication (*306*). The patient was admitted with hypertension and hypokalemia and gave a history of eating 60–100 g licorice candy, containing approximately 0.3% glycyrrhizic acid, daily for the past 4–5 years. Urine from this patient contained elevated levels of cortisol and a decreased ratio of cortisone to cortisol metabolites, thus confirming that licorice impaired normal cortisol metabolism. Suppression of 11β-hydroxysteroid dehydrogenase persisted for two weeks after licorice withdrawal while the basal activity of the renin–aldosterone system remained low for several months after licorice withdrawal.

In experiments with 6 healthy male volunteers, a daily dose of 7.5 g of a pure derivate of licorice appeared to cause transient effects on cortisone metabolism in some subjects and a decrease in serum potassium, an increase in body weight and a suppression of the renin–angiotensin–aldosterone axis in all subjects (*307*). Blood pressure was not affected during the 7 days of treatment.

Two new phenolic compounds, glicoricone and licofuranone, were isolated from a species of licorice from northwestern China (*308*). These compounds, along with 4 other licorice constituents, were found to inhibit monoamine oxidase.

Grayanotoxins

Grayanotoxins occur in various parts of certain plants, notably rhododendrons, and may also be present in pollen and honey made from nectar of these plants. In humans the most common symptoms of grayanotoxin poisoning are severe bradycardia, other cardiac arrhythmias, and hypotension. To elucidate the mechanism of toxicity, anesthetized rats were injected intracerebroventricularly or intraperitoneally with extracts of a Turkish honey involved in a case of grayanotoxin poisoning (*309*). Marked bradycardia was observed in these animals but not in similarly injected rats which had been bilaterally vagotomized. These results indicate that grayanotoxins act at a site within the central nervous system and that the bradycardic effect of grayanotoxin is mediated by vagal stimulation at the periphery.

Amaranth

Seeds and leaves of *Amaranthus* spp. have high levels of protein and carotene, respectively, and are an important food source in some areas with low rainfall and poor soil. The foliage of 61 varieties of *Amaranthus,* including 10 species, was analyzed to determine their content of some antinutritional factors such as nitrate and oxalate (*310*). Nitrate levels varied from 1.8 to 9.2 mg/kg fresh weight and oxalate levels varied from 3 to 19.2 mg/kg. Nitrate levels were fairly constant in all leaves of a single variety but oxalate levels tended to increase as the leaves aged.

Some wild-growing species of *Amaranthus* spp. in Brazil were reported to be toxic to young pigs (*311*). Within 48 h of consuming leaves of these plants the pigs became acutely ill, with weakness and muscle tremors and finally death. Symptoms were caused by acute renal tubular injury but the toxin involved was not identified.

Oxalic acid in tea

Oxalate and calcium concentrations were determined in teas made from black tea leaves and from 4 varieties of Japanese green tea (*312*). Oxalate and calcium levels in 3 of the green teas and the black tea ranged from 3.06 to 11.02 g/100 mL and from 0.29 to 0.67 mg/100 mL, respectively. Higher levels were found in the other green tea. Since oxalate complexes with calcium, a calcium deficit may occur in those drinking a lot of tea unless milk is also consumed to counterbalance the effects of tea drinking.

Cashew nut shell oil

Oil derived from the shell of cashew nuts contains compounds which can cause allergic dermatitis following contact or accidental consumption. Using the murine 2-stage skin tumorigenesis model, this oil was found to have a weak tumor-promoting effect (*313*). Mice were initiated with DMBA and the cashew nut oil was applied 3 times a week for 20 weeks. Croton oil (1% in acetone), the positive control, induced about 2.5 times as many tumors as 2% cashew nut oil in acetone.

Flour infested with beetles

Flour in which beetles (*Tribolium castaneum*) have built up a large population becomes pink in color but may still be consumed during times of food shortage. Carcinogenic effects of this flour, of biscuits made from this flour, and of 1,4-benzoquinone (a quinoid secretion of this beetle) were investigated in mice fed these substances 2 or 3 times a week for 13 months (*314*). Animals fed infested flour developed tumors in the liver and spleen (lympholeukemia) and those fed the biscuits developed liver and breast (adenocarcinoma) tumors. The purified quinoid produced effects similar to the infested flour. Tumor incidences varied from 29% to 35.2% in the different groups.

Literature Cited

1. D'Mello, J.P.F., C.M. Duffus, and J.H. Duffus (eds.). *Toxic Substances in Crop Plants*. Cambridge, Royal Society of Chemistry. (1991).

2. Ahmed, F.E. Naturally occurring seafood toxins. *J. Toxicol.—Toxin Rev.* 10:263–287 (1991).

3. Dickey, R.W., G.A. Fryxell, H.R. Granade, and D. Roelke. Detection of the marine toxins okadaic acid and domoic acid in shellfish and phytoplankton in the Gulf of Mexico. *Toxicon* 30:355–359 (1992).

4. Hokama, Y., T.W.P. Hong, M. Isobe, et al. Cross-reactivity of highly purified okadaic acid (OA), synthetic, spiroketal East sphere of OA and ciguatoxin. *J. Clin. Lab. Anal.* 6:54–58 (1992).

5. Kaufman, B., D.C. Wright, W.R. Ballou, and D. Monheit. Protection against tetrodotoxin and saxitoxin intoxication by a cross-protective rabbit anti-tetrodotoxin antiserum. *Toxicon* 29:581–587 (1991).

6. Stabell, O.B., M. Yndestad, and B. Heidenreich. Paralytic shellfish toxins seem absent in extracts of diarrhetic shellfish toxins. *Environ. Toxicol. Chem.* 10:331–334 (1991).

7. Stommel, E.W., J. Parsonnet, and L.R. Jenkyn. Polymyositis after ciguatera toxin exposure. *Arch. Neurol.* 48:874–877 (1991).

8. Senecal, P.-E., and J.D. Osterloh. Normal fetal outcome after maternal ciguateric toxin exposure in the second trimester. *Clin. Toxicol.* 29:473–478 (1991).

9. Chevaldonné, P. Ciguatera and the saupe, *Sarpa salpa* (L.), in the Mediterranean: a possible misinterpretation. *J. Fish Biol.* 37:503–504 (1990).

10. Holmes, M.J., R.J. Lewis, M.A. Poli, and N.C. Gillespie. Strain dependent production of ciguatoxin precursors (gambiertoxins) by *Gambierdiscus toxicus* (Dinophyceae) in culture. *Toxicon* 29:761–775 (1991).

11. Morton, S.L., D.R. Norris, and J.W. Bomber. Effect of temperature, salinity and light intensity on the growth and seasonality of toxic dinoflagellates associated with ciguatera. *J. Exp. Mar. Biol. Ecol.* 157:79–90 (1992).

12. Kelly, A.M., C.C. Kohler, and D.R. Tindall. Are crustaceans linked to the ciguatera food chain? *Environ. Biol. Fishes* 33:275–286 (1992).

13. Nagashima, Y., T. Noguchi, M. Tanaka, and K. Hashimoto. Thermal degradation of paralytic shellfish poison. *J. Food Sci.* 56:1572–1575 (1991).

14. Beitler, M.K. Toxicity of adductor muscles from the purple hinge rock scallop (*Crassadoma gigantea*) along the Pacific coast of North America. *Toxicon* 29:889–894 (1991).

15. Kitts, D.D., D.S. Smith, M.K. Beitler, and J. Liston. Presence of paralytic shellfish poisoning toxins and soluble proteins in toxic butter clams (*Saxidomus giganteus*). *Biochem. Biophys. Res. Commun.* 184:511–517 (1992).

16. Kvitek, R.G., A.R. DeGange, and M.K. Beitler. Paralytic shellfish poisoning toxins mediate feeding behavior of sea otters. *Limnol. Oceanogr.* 36:393–404 (1991).

17. Kvitek, R.G. Paralytic shellfish toxins sequestered by bivalves as a defense against siphon-nipping fish. *Marine Biol.* 111:369–374 (1991).

18. Bricelj, V.M., J.H. Lee, and A.D. Cembella. Influence of dinoflagellate cell toxicity on uptake and loss of paralytic shellfish toxins in the northern quahog *Mercenaria mercenaria. Marine Ecol. Progr. Ser.* 74:33–46 (1991).

19. Chu, F.S., X. Huang, and S. Hall. Production and characterization of antibodies against neosaxitoxin. *J. AOAC Int.* 75:341–345 (1992).

20. Usleber, E., E. Schneider, and G. Terplan. Direct enzyme immunoassay in microtitration plate and test strip format for the detection of saxitoxin in shellfish. *Lett. Appl. Microbiol.* 13:275–277 (1991).

21. Lawrence, J.F., and C. Ménard. Liquid chromatographic determination of paralytic shellfish poisons in shellfish after prechromatographic oxidation. *J. Assoc. Off. Anal. Chem.* 74:1006–1012 (1991).

22. Tadano, K., K. Yasuda, H. Ushiyama, and T. Nishima. Effect of calcium on the mouse bioassay method for paralytic shellfish poison (hygienic studies on health food (III)). *Shokuhim Eiseigaku Zasshi* 32:402–407 (1991).

23. Health and Welfare Canada. Domoic acid intoxication. *Can. Commun. Dis. Rep.* 18:118–120 (1992).

24. Novelli, A., J. Kispert, M.T. Fernández-Sánchez, et al. Domoic acid-containing toxic mussels produce neurotoxicity in neuronal cultures through a synergism between excitatory amino acids. *Brain Res.* 577:41–48 (1992).

25. Bates, S.S., A.S.W. de Freitas, J.E. Milley, et al. Controls on domoic acid production by the diatom *Nitzschia pungens* f. *multiseries* in culture: nutrients and irradiance. *Can. J. Fish. Aquat. Sci.* 48:1136–1144 (1991).

26. Douglas, D.J., and S.S. Bates. Production of domoic acid, a neurotoxic amino acid, by an axenic culture of the marine diatom *Nitszchia pungens* f. *multiseries* Hasle. *Can. J. Fish. Aquat. Sci.* 49:85–90 (1992).

27. Silvert, W., and D.V. Subba Rao. Dynamic model of the flux of domoic acid, a neurotoxin, through a *Mytilus edulis* population. *Can. J. Fish. Aquat. Sci.* 49:400–405 (1992).

28. Novaczek, I., M.S. Madhyastha, R.F. Ablett, et al. Depuration of domoic acid from live blue mussels (*Mytilus edulis*). *Can. J. Fish. Aquat. Sci.* 49:312–318 (1992).

29. Nijjar, M.S., B. Grimmelt, and J. Brown. Purification of domoic acid from toxic blue mussels (*Mytilus edulis*) and phytoplankton. *J. Chromatogr.* 568:393–406 (1991).

30. Lawrence, J.F., C.F. Charbonneau, and C. Ménard. Liquid chromatographic determination of domoic acid in mussels, using AOAC paralytic shellfish poison extraction procedure: collaborative study. *J. Assoc. Off. Anal. Chem.* 74:68–72 (1991).

31. Lawrence, J.F., and C. Ménard. Confirmation of domoic acid in shellfish using butyl isothiocyanate and reversed-phase liquid chromatography. *J. Chromatogr.* 550:595–601 (1991).

32. Marr, J.C., A.E. Jackson, and J.L. McLachlan. Occurrence of *Prorocentrum lima*, a DSP toxin-producing species from the Atlantic coast of Canada. *J. Appl. Phycol.* 4:17–24 (1992).

33. Sedmak, B., and N. Fanuko. Occurrence of *Dinophysis* spp. and toxic shellfish in the Northern Adriatic. *J. Appl. Phycol.* 3:289–294 (1991).

34. Fernández, M.T., V. Zitko, S. Gascón, and A. Novelli. The marine toxin okadaic acid is a potent neurotoxin for cultured cerebellar neurons. *Life Sci.* 49:PL-157–PL-162 (1991).

35. Stabell, O.B., I. Steffenak, K. Pedersen, and B. Underdal. Diversity of shellfish toxins of "diarrhetic" type revealed by biological and chemical assays. *J. Toxicol. Environ. Health* 33:273–282 (1991).

36. Stabell, O. B., I. Steffenak, and T. Aune. An evaluation of the mouse bioassay applied to extracts of 'diarrhoetic' shellfish toxins. *Food Chem. Toxicol.* 30:139–144 (1992).

37. Zonta, F., B. Stancher, P. Bogoni, and P. Masotti. High-performance liquid chromatography of okadaic acid and free fatty acids in mussels. *J. Chromatogr.* 594:137–144 (1992).

38. Sato, S., K. Komaru, T. Ogata, and M. Kodama. Occurrence of tetrodotoxin in cultured puffer. *Nippon Suisan Gakkaishi* 56:1129–1131 (1990).

39. Saitanu, K., S. Laobhripatr, K. Limpakarnjan-arat, et al. Toxicity of the freshwater puffer fish *Tetraodon fangi* and *T. palembangensis* from Thailand. *Toxicon* 29:895–897 (1991).

40. Fuchi, Y., H. Narimatsu, S. Nakama, et al. Tissue distribution of toxicity in a pufferfish, *Arothron firmamentum* ("Hoshifugu"). *Shokuhim Eiseigaku Zasshi* 32:520–525 (1991).

41. Saito, T., T. Noguchi, Y. Shida, et al. Screening of tetrodotoxin and its derivatives in puffer-related species. *Nippon Suisan Gakkaishi* 57:1573–1577 (1991).

42. Hwang, D.F., K.P. Tai, C.H. Chueh, et al. Tetrodotoxin and derivatives in several species of the gastropod Naticidae. *Toxicon* 29:1019–1024 (1991).

43. Hwang, D.F., S.C. Lu, and S.S. Jeng. Occurrence of tetrodotoxin in the gastropods *Rapana rapiformis* and *R. venosa venosa*. *Marine Biol.* 111:65–69 (1991).

44. Do, H.K., K. Kogure, C. Imada, et al. Tetrodotoxin production of actinomycetes isolated from marine sediment. *J. Appl. Bacteriol.* 70:464–468 (1991).

45. Raybould, T.J.G., G.S. Bignami, L.K. Inouye, et al. A monoclonal antibody-based immunoassay for detecting tetrodotoxin in biological samples. *J. Clin. Lab. Anal.* 6:65–72 (1992).

46. Morris, P.D., D.S. Campbell, T.J. Taylor, and J.I. Freeman. Clinical and epidemiological features of neurotoxic shellfish poisoning in North Carolina. *Am. J. Public Health* 81:471–474 (1991).

47. Levine, L., and Y. Shimizu. Antibodies to brevetoxin B: serologic differentiation of brevetoxin B and brevetoxin A. *Toxicon* 30:411–418 (1992).

48. Haddock, R.L., and O.L.T. Cruz. Foodborne intoxication associated with seaweed. *Lancet* 338:195–196 (1991).

49. Mereish, K.A., S. Morris, G. McCullers, et al. Analysis of palytoxin by liquid chromatography and capillary electrophoresis. *J. Liq. Chromatogr.* 14:1025–1031 (1991).

50. Falconer, I.R., A. Choice, and W. Hosja. Toxicity of edible mussels (*Mytilus edulis*) growing naturally in an estuary during a water bloom of the blue-green alga *Nodularia spumigena*. *Environ. Toxicol. Water Qual.* 7:119–123 (1992).

51. Stratton, J.E., R.W. Hutkins, and S.L. Taylor. Biogenic amines in cheese and other fermented foods: a review. *J. Food Protect.* 54:460–470 (1991).

52. Da Prada, M., and G. Zürcher. Tyramine content of preserved and fermented foods or condiments of Far Eastern cuisine. *Psychopharmacology* 106:S32–S34 (1992).

53. Health and Welfare Canada. Scombroid poisoning - an outbreak in two Ontario communities. *Can. Commun. Dis. Rep.* 18:17–18 (1992).

54. Clifford, M.N., R. Walker, P. Ijomah, et al. Is there a role for amines other than histamines in the aetiology of scombrotoxicosis? *Food Addit. Contam.* 8:641–652 (1991).

55. Ijomah, P., M.N. Clifford, R. Walker, et al. The importance of endogenous histamine relative to dietary histamine in the aetiology of scombrotoxicosis. *Food Addit. Contam.* 8:531–542 (1991).

56. Ababouch, L., M.E. Afilal, H. Benabdeljelil, and F.F. Busta. Quantitative changes in bacteria, amino acids and biogenic amines in sardine (*Sardina pilchardus*) stored at ambient temperature (25–28°C) and in ice. *Int. J. Food Sci. Technol.* 26:297–306 (1991).

57. Anthoni, U., C. Christophersen, L. Gram, et al. Poisonings from flesh of the Greenland shark *Somniosus microcephalus* may be due to trimethylamine. *Toxicon* 29:1205–1212 (1991).

58. Stratton, J.E., R.W. Hutkins, and S.L. Taylor. Histamine production in low-salt Cheddar cheese. *J. Food Protect.* 54:852–855,867 (1991).

59. Stratton, J.E., R.W. Hutkins, S.S. Sumner, and S.L. Taylor. Histamine and histamine-producing bacteria in retail Swiss and low-salt cheeses. *J. Food Protect.* 55:435–439 (1992).

60. Moret, S., and R. Bortolomeazzi. Improvement of extraction procedure for biogenic amines in foods and their high-performance liquid chromatographic determination. *J. Chromatogr.* 591:175–180 (1992).

61. Izquierdo-Pulido, M.L., M.C. Vidal-Carou, and A. Mariné-Font. Histamine and tyramine in beers. Changes during brewing of a Spanish beer. *Food Chem.* 42:231–237 (1991).

62. Ibe, A., K. Saito, M. Nakazato, et al. Quantitative determination of amines in wine by liquid chromatography. *J. Assoc. Off. Anal. Chem.* 74:695–698 (1991).

63. Lehtonen, P., M. Saarinen, M. Vesanto, and M.-L. Riekkola. Determination of wine amines by HPLC using automated precolumn derivatisation with *o*-phthalaldehyde and fluorescence detection. *Z. Lebensm. Unters. Forsch.* 194:434–437 (1992).

64. Moudgal, R.P., J.N. Panda, and J. Mohan. Histamine in egg yolk: heat resistance and relation to production status. *Br. Poult. Sci.* 32:865–869 (1991).

65. Yen, G.C. Effects of heat treatment and storage temperature on the biogenic amine contents of straw mushroom (*Volvariella volvacea*). *J. Sci. Food Agric.* 58:59–61 (1992).

66. Manabe, S., O. Wada, and Y. Kanai. Pharmacotoxicological aspects of carcinogenic tryptophan pyrolysis products in the environment. *J. Environ. Sci. Health* A26:1449–1469 (1991).

67. Wakabayashi, K., M. Nagao, H. Esumi, and T. Sugimura. Food-derived mutagens and carcinogens. *Cancer Res.* 52(Suppl.):2092S–2098S (1992).

68. Snyderwine, E.G., H.A.J. Schut, R.H. Adamson, et al. Metabolic activation and genotoxicity of heterocyclic arylamines. *Cancer Res.* 52(Suppl.):2099S–2102S (1992).

69. Felton, J.S., M.G. Knize, M. Roper, et al. Chemical analysis, prevention, and low-level dosimetry of heterocyclic amines from cooked food. *Cancer Res.* 52(Suppl.):2103S–2107S (1992).

70. Lee, H., and S.-J. Tsai. Detection of IQ-type mutagens in canned roasted eel. *Food Chem. Toxicol.* 29:517–522 (1991).

71. Gross, G.A., and U. Wolleb. 2-Amino-3,4-dimethylimidazo[4,5-*f*]quinoline is not detectable in commercial instant and roasted coffees. *J. Agric. Food Chem.* 39:2231–2236 (1991).

72. Gross, G.A., and A. Grüter. Quantitation of mutagenic/carcinogenic heterocyclic aromatic amines in food products. *J. Chromatogr.* 592:271–278 (1992).

73. Yoshida, S., and Ye-Xiuyun. The binding ability of bovine milk caseins to mutagenic heterocyclic amines. *J. Dairy Sci.* 75:958–961 (1992).

74. Yoshida, S., Ye-Xiuyun, and T. Nishiumi. The binding ability of α-lactalbumin and β-lactoglobulin to mutagenic heterocyclic amines. *J. Dairy Sci.* 74:3741–3745 (1991).

75. Zhang, X.B., and Y. Ohta. Binding of mutagens by fractions of the cell wall skeleton of lactic acid bacteria on mutagens. *J. Dairy Sci.* 74:1477–1481 (1991).

76. Zhang, X.B., B. Demuyakor, N. Asahara, and Y. Ohta. Binding of heterocyclic amines by yeast cells and their fractions. *J. Sci. Food Agric.* 57:253–262 (1991).

77. Skog, K., and M. Jägerstad. Effects of glucose on the formation of PhIP in a model system. *Carcinogenesis* 12:2297–2300 (1991).

78. Manabe, S., N. Kurihara, O. Wada, et al. Formation of PhIP in a mixture of creatinine, phenylalanine and sugar or aldehyde by aqueous heating. *Carcinogenesis* 13:827–830 (1992).

79. Knize, M.G., E. Hopmans, and J.A. Happe. The identification of a new heterocyclic amine mutagen from a heated mixture of creatine, glutamic acid and glucose. *Mutat. Res.* 260:313–319 (1991).

80. Ushiyama, H., K. Wakabayashi, M. Hirose, et al. Presence of carcinogenic heterocyclic amines in urine of healthy volunteers eating normal diet, but not of inpatients receiving parenteral alimentation. *Carcinogenesis* 12:1417–1422 (1991).

81. Manabe, S., M. Suzuki, E. Kusano, et al. Elevation of levels of carcinogenic tryptophan pyrolysis products in plasma and red blood cells of patients with uremia. *Clin. Nephrol.* 37:28–33 (1992).

82. Turesky, R.J., N.P. Lang, M.A. Butler, et al. Metabolic activation of carcinogenic heterocyclic aromatic amines by human liver and colon. *Carcinogenesis* 12:1839–1845 (1991).

83. Pfau, W., M.J. O'Hare, P.L. Grover, and D.H. Phillips. Metabolic activation of the food mutagens 2-amino-3-methylimidazo[4,5-*f*]quinoline (IQ) and 2-amino-3,4-dimethylimidazo[4,5-*f*]quinoline (MeIQ) to DNA binding species in human mammary epithelial cells. *Carcinogenesis* 13:907–909 (1992).

84. Zu, H.-X., and H.A.J. Schut. Formation and persistence of DNA adducts of 2-amino-3-methylimidazo[4,5-*f*]quinoline in male Fischer-344 rats. *Cancer Res.* 51:5636–5641 (1991).

85. Zu, H.-X., and H.A.J. Schut. Sex differences in the formation and persistence of DNA adducts of 2-amino-3-methylimidazo[4,5-*f*]quinoline (IQ) in CDF1 mice. *Carcinogenesis* 12:2163–2168 (1991).

86. Frandsen, H., S. Grivas, R. Andersson, L. Dragsted, and J.C. Larsen. Reaction of the N^2-acetoxy derivative of 2-amino-1-methyl-6-phenylimidazo[4,5-*b*]pyridine (PhIP) with 2'-deoxyguanosine and DNA. Synthesis and identification of N^2-(2'-deoxyguanosin-8-yl)–PhIP. *Carcinogenesis* 13:629–635 (1992).

87. Övervik, E., M. Ochiai, M. Hirose, et al. The formation of heart DNA adducts in F344 rats following dietary administration of heterocyclic amines. *Mutat. Res.* 256:37–43 (1991).

88. Watkins, B.E., H. Esumi, K. Wakabayashi, et al. Fate and distribution of 2-amino-1-methyl-6-phenylimidazo[4,5-*b*]pyridine (PhIP) in rats. *Carcinogenesis* 12:1073–1078 (1991).

89. Watkins, B.E., M. Suzuki, H. Wallin, et al. The effect of dose and enzyme inducers on the metabolism of 2-amino-1-methyl-6-phenylimidazo[4,5-*b*]pyridine (PhIP) in rats. *Carcinogenesis* 12:2291–2295 (1991).

90. Turesky, R.J., J. Markovic, I. Bracco-Hammer, and L.B. Fay. The effect of dose and cytochrome P450 induction on the metabolism and disposition of the foodborne carcinogen 2-amino-3,8-dimethylimidazo[4,5-*f*]quinoxaline (MeIQx) in the rat. *Carcinogenesis* 12:1847–1855 (1991).

91. Ito, N., R. Hasegawa, M. Sano, et al. A new colon and mammary carcinogen in cooked food, 2-amino-1-methyl-6-phenylimidazo[4,5-*b*]pyridine (PhIP). *Carcinogenesis* 12:1503–1506 (1991).

92. Dooley, K.L., L.S. Von Tungeln, T. Bucci, et al. Comparative carcinogenicity of 4-aminobiphenyl and the food pyrolysates, Glu-P-1, IQ, PhIP, and MeIQx in the neonatal B6C3F$_1$ male mouse. *Cancer Lett.* 62:205–209 (1992).

93. Hasegawa, R., T. Shirai, K. Hakoi, et al. Synergistic enhancement of glutathione *S*-transferase placental form-positive hepatic foci development in diethylnitrosamine-treated rats by combined administration of five heterocyclic amines at low doses. *Jpn. J. Cancer Res.* 82:1378–1384 (1991).

94. Loprieno, N., G. Boncristiani, and G. Loprieno. An experimental approach to identifying the genotoxic risk from cooked meat mutagens. *Food Chem. Toxicol.* 29:377–386 (1991).

95. Kumar, N., and O.P. Singhal. Cholesterol oxides and atherosclerosis: a review. *J. Sci. Food Agric.* 55:497–510 (1991).

96. Zhang, W.B., P.B. Addis, and T.P. Krick. Quantification of 5α-cholestane-3β,5,6β-triol and other cholesterol oxidation products in fast food French fried potatoes. *J. Food Sci.* 56:716–718 (1991).

97. Morgan, J.N., and D.J. Armstrong. Quantification of cholesterol oxidation products in egg yolk powder spray-dried with direct heating. *J. Food Sci.* 57:43–45,107 (1992).

98. Kumar, N., and O.P. Singhal. Effect of processing conditions on the oxidation of cholesterol in ghee. *J. Sci. Food Agric.* 58:267–273 (1992).

99. Zubillaga, M.P., and G. Maerker. Quantification of three cholesterol oxidation products in raw meat and chicken. *J. Food Sci.* 56:1194–1196,1202 (1991).

100. Fillion, L., J.A. Zee, and C. Gosselin. Determination of a cholesterol oxide mixture by a single-run high-performance liquid chromatographic analysis using benzoylation. *J. Chromatogr.* 547:105–112 (1991).

101. Wasilchuk, B.A., P.W. LeQuesne, and P. Vouros. Monitoring cholesterol autoxidation processes using multideuteriated cholesterol. *Anal. Chem.* 64:1077–1087 (1992).

102. Kubow, S. Routes of formation and toxic consequences of lipid oxidation products in foods. *Free Rad. Biol. Med.* 12:63–81 (1992).

103. Hageman, G., H. Verhagen, B. Schutte, and J. Kleinjans. Biological effects of short-term feeding to rats of repeatedly used deep-frying fats in relation to fat mutagen content. *Food Chem. Toxicol.* 29:689–698 (1991).

104. Ruiz-Gutierrez, V., and F.J.G. Muriana. Effect of ingestion of thermally oxidized frying oil on desaturase activities and fluidity in rat-liver microsomes. *J. Nutr. Biochem.* 3:75–79 (1992).

105. Nishikawa, A., R. Sodum, and F.-L. Chung. Acute toxicity of *trans*-5-hydroxy-2-nonenal in Fischer 344 rats. *Lipids* 27:54–58 (1992).

106. Kanazawa, K. Hepatic dysfunction caused by dietary products of lipid peroxidation. *Int. J. Tissue Reactions* 13(2):67–78 (1991).

107. Kanazawa, K., and H. Ashida. Target enzymes on hepatic dysfunction caused by dietary products of lipid peroxidation. *Arch. Biochem. Biophys.* 288:71–78 (1991).

108. Lane, R.H., and J.L. Smathers. Monitoring aldehyde production during frying by reversed-phase liquid chromatography. *J. Assoc. Off. Anal. Chem.* 74:957–960 (1991).

109. Rhee, K.S., S.E. Housson, and Y.A. Ziprin. Enhancement of frying oil stability by a natural antioxidative ingredient in the coating system of fried meat nuggets. *J. Food Sci.* 57:789–791 (1992).

110. Wong, J.W., H.C.H. Yeo, and T. Shibamoto. Determination of malonaldehyde and formaldehyde formed from fatty acid ethyl esters upon microwave and thermal heating. *J. Agric. Food Chem.* 39:2260–2262 (1991).

111. Tomita, I., K. Shimoi, M. Suzuki, et al. Changes in the levels of lipid peroxidation and mutagenicity of fish after sun-drying and broiling. *Shokuhim Eiseigaku Zasshi* 32:543–547 (1991).

112. Akasaka, K., I. Sasaki, H. Ohrui, and H. Meguro. A simple fluorometry of hydroperoxides in oils and foods. *Biosci. Biotech. Biochem.* 56:605–607 (1992).

113. Deng, Q.Y., R.R. Barefoot, L.L. Diosady, et al. Lysinoalanine concentrations in rapeseed protein meals and isolates. *Can. Inst. Food Sci. Technol. J.* 25:140–142 (1990).

114. Langhendries, J.P., R.F. Hurrell, D.E. Furniss, et al. Maillard reaction products and lysinoalanine: urinary excretion and the effects on kidney function of preterm infants fed heat-processed milk formula. *J. Pediatr. Gastroenterol. Nutr.* 14:62–70 (1992).

115. Miyakawa, Y., Y. Nishi, K. Kato, et al. Initiating activity of eight pyrolysates of carbohydrates in a two-stage mouse skin tumorigenesis model. *Carcinogenesis* 12:1169–1173 (1991).

116. Gancedo, S.Q., P. Freire, M.F. Rivas, et al. Urticaria from caffeine. *J. Allergy Clin. Immunol.* 88:680–681 (1991).

117. Jorens, P.G., J.M. Van Hauwaert, M.I. Selala, and P.J.C. Schepens. Acute caffeine poisoning in a child. *Eur. J. Ped.* 150:860 (1991).

118. Orlikov, A., and I. Ryzov. Caffeine-induced anxiety and increase of kynurenine concentration in plasma of healthy subjects: a pilot study. *Biol. Psychiatry* 29:391–396 (1991).

119. Berthou, F., J.-P. Flinois, D. Ratanasavanh, et al. Evidence for the involvement of several cytochromes P-450 in the first steps of caffeine metabolism by human liver microsomes. *Drug Metab. Dispos.* 19:561–567 (1991).

120. Van Deventer, G., E. Kamemoto, J.T. Kuznicki, et al. Lower esophageal sphincter pressure, acid secretion, and blood gastrin after coffee consumption. *Digest. Dis. Sci.* 37:558–569 (1992).

121. International Agency for Research on Cancer. IARC monographs on the evaluation of carcinogenic risks to humans. Vol. 51. Coffee, tea, maté, and methylxanthines and methylglyoxal. Lyon, IARC (1991).

122. Rosengren, A., and L. Wilhelmsen. Coffee, coronary heart disease and mortality in middle-aged

Swedish men: findings from the Primary Prevention Study. *J. Intern. Med.* 230:67–71 (1991).

123. Fried, R.E., D.M. Levine, P.O. Kwiterovich, et al. The effect of filtered-coffee consumption on plasma lipid levels. *JAMA* 267:811–815 (1992).

124. Superko, H.R., W. Bortz, P.T. Williams, et al. Caffeinated and decaffeinated coffee effects on plasma lipoprotein cholesterol, apolipoproteins, and lipase activity: a controlled, randomized trial. *Am. J. Clin. Nutr.* 54:599–605 (1991).

125. Lindahl, B., I. Johansson, F. Huhtasaari, et al. Coffee drinking and blood cholesterol—effects of brewing method, food intake and life style. *J. Intern. Med.* 230:299–305 (1991).

126. Ahola, I., M. Jauhiainen, and A. Aro. The hypercholesterolaemic factor in boiled coffee is retained by a paper filter. *J. Intern. Med.* 230:293–297 (1991).

127. Salvaggio, A., M. Periti, L. Miano, et al. Coffee and cholesterol, an Italian study. *Am. J. Epidemiol.* 134:149–156 (1991).

128. Salvaggio, A., M. Periti, L. Miano, and C. Zambelli. Association between habitual coffee consumption and blood pressure levels. *J. Hypertens.* 8:585–590 (1990).

129. Casiglia, E., S. Bongiovì, C.D. Paleari, et al. Haemodynamic effects of coffee and caffeine in normal volunteers: a placebo-controlled clinical study. *J. Intern. Med.* 229:501–504 (1991).

130. van Dusseldorp, M., P. Smits, J.W.M. Lenders, et al. Boiled coffee and blood pressure. A 14-week controlled trial. *Hypertension* 18:607–613 (1991).

131. MacDonald, T.M., K. Sharpe, G. Fowler, et al. Caffeine restriction: effect on mild hypertension. *Br. Med. J.* 303:1235–1238 (1991).

132. Pincomb, G.A., M.F. Wilson, B.H. Sung, et al. Effects of caffeine on pressor regulation during rest and exercise in men at risk for hypertension. *Am. Heart J.* 122:1107–1115 (1991).

133. Tse, S.Y.H. Cholinomimetic compound distinct from caffeine contained in coffee. II. Muscarinic actions. *J. Pharm. Sci.* 81:449–452 (1992).

134. Fenster, L., B. Eskenazi, G.C. Windham, and S.H. Swan. Caffeine consumption during pregnancy and fetal growth. *Am. J. Public Health* 81:458–461 (1991).

135. McDonald, A.D., B.G. Armstrong, and M. Sloan. Cigarette, alcohol, and coffee consumption and prematurity. *Am. J. Public Health* 82:87–90 (1992).

136. Armstrong, B.G., A.D. McDonald, and M. Sloan. Cigarette, alcohol, and coffee consumption and spontaneous abortion. *Am. J. Public Health* 82:85–87 (1992).

137. Barr, H.M., and A.P. Streissguth. Caffeine use during pregnancy and child outcome: a 7-year prospective study. *Neurotoxicol. Teratol.* 13:441–448 (1991).

138. Gilbert, S.G., and D.C. Rice. Somatic development of the infant monkey following *in utero* exposure to caffeine. *Fund. Appl. Toxicol.* 17:454–465 (1991).

139. Hernandez-Avila, M., G.A. Colditz, M.J. Stampfer, et al. Caffeine, moderate alcohol intake, and risk of fractures of the hip and forearm in middle-aged women. *Am. J. Clin. Nutr.* 54:157–163 (1991).

140. Cooper, C., E.J. Atkinson, H.W. Wahner, et al. Is caffeine consumption a risk factor for osteoporosis? *J. Bone Min. Res.* 7:465–471 (1992).

141. Hasling, C., K. Sóndergaard, P. Charles, and L. Mosekilde. Calcium metabolism in postmenopausal osteoporotic women is determined by dietary calcium and coffee intake. *J. Nutr.* 122:1119–1126 (1992).

142. Tassinari, M.S., L.C. Gerstenfeld, G.S. Stein, and J.B. Lian. Effect of caffeine on parameters of osteoblast growth and differentiation of a mineralized extracellular matrix in vitro. *J. Bone Min. Res.* 6:1029–1036 (1991).

143. Lau, O.-W., S.-F. Luk, O.-M. Cheng, and T.P.Y. Chiu. Background-correction methods for the determination of caffeine in beverages, coffee and tea by using second-derivative ultraviolet spectrophotometry. *Analyst* 117:777–783 (1992).

144. Abuirjeie, M.A., M.S. El-Din, and I.I. Mahmoud. Determination of theobromine, theophylline, and caffeine in various food products using derivative UV-spectrophotometric techniques and high-performance liquid chromatography. *J. Liq. Chromatogr.* 15:101–125 (1992).

145. Trugo, L.C., C.A.B. De Maria, and C.C. Werneck. Simultaneous determination of total chlorogenic acid and caffeine in coffee by high performance gel filtration chromatography. *Food Chem.* 42:81–87 (1991).

146. Rubiolo, P., L. Pieters, M. Calomme, et al. Mutagenicity of pyrrolizidine alkaloids in the *Salmonella typhimurium*/mammalian microsome system. *Mutat. Res.* 281:143–147 (1992).

147. Hincks, J.R., H.-Y. Kim, H.J. Segall, et al. DNA cross-linking in mammalian cells by pyrrolizidine alkaloids: structure–activity relationships. *Toxicol. Appl. Pharmacol.* 111:90–98 (1991).

148. Carballo, M., M.D. Mudry, I.B. Larripa, et al. Genotoxic action of an aqueous extract of *Heliotropium curassavicum var. argentinum. Mutat. Res.* 279:245–253 (1992).

149. Deyo, J.A., and N.I. Kerkvliet. Tier-2 studies on monocrotaline immunotoxicity in C57BL/6 mice. *Toxicology* 70:313–325 (1991).

150. Bicchi, C., P. Rubiolo, C. Frattini, et al. Off-line supercritical fluid extraction and capillary gas chromatography of pyrrolizidine alkaloids in *Senecio* species. *J. Nat. Prod.* 54:941–945 (1991).

151. Friedman, M., J.R. Rayburn, and J.A. Bantle. Developmental toxicology of potato alkaloids in the frog embryo teratogenesis assay—Xenopus (FETAX). *Food Chem. Toxicol.* 29:537–547 (1991).

152. Friedman, M., and L. Dao. Distribution of glycoalkaloids in potato plants and commercial potato products. *J. Agric. Food Chem.* 40:419–423 (1992).

153. Sammon, A.M. A case–control study of diet and social factors in cancer of the esophagus in Transkei. *Cancer* 69:860–865 (1992).

154. Hanna, J.P., J.W. Schmidley, and W.E. Braselton, Jr. *Datura* delirium. *Clin. Neuropharmacol.* 15:109–113 (1992).

155. Smith, E.A., C.E. Meloan, J.A. Pickell, and F.W. Oehme. Scopolamine poisoning from homemade 'moon flower' wine. *J. Anal. Toxicol.* 15:216–219 (1991).

156. Strobel, M., J. Chevalier, and B. de Lavarelle. Coma fébrile avec polynucléose dû à une intoxication par *Datura Stramonium.* (Letter.) *Presse Médicale* 20:2214 (1991).

157. Rwiza, H.T. Jimson weed food poisoning. An epidemic at Usangi rural government hospital. *Trop. Geog. Med.* 43:85–90 (1991).

158. van Meurs, A., A. Cohen, and P. Edelbroek. Atropine poisoning after eating chapattis contaminated with *Datura stramonium* (thorn apple). *Trans. Roy. Soc. Trop. Med. Hyg.* 86:221 (1992).

159. Hagemann, K., K. Piek, J. Stöckigt, and E.W. Weiler. Monoclonal antibody-based enzyme immunoassay for the quantitative determination of the tropane alkaloid, scopolamine. *Planta Med.* 58:68–72 (1992).

160. Greirson, B.N., D.G. Allen, N.F. Gare, and I.M. Watson. Development and application of an enzyme-linked immunosorbent assay for lupin alkaloids. *J. Agric. Food Chem.* 39:2327–2331 (1991).

161. Upreti, K.K., M. Das, and S.K. Khanna. Biochemical toxicology of argemone oil. I. Effect on hepatic cytochrome P-450 and xenobiotic metabolizing enzymes. *J. Appl. Toxicol.* 11:203–209 (1991).

162. de Groot, A.P., M.I. Willems, and R.H. de Vos. Effects of high levels of Brussels sprouts in the diet of rats. *Food Chem. Toxicol.* 29:829–837 (1991).

163. Lewerenz, H.-J., D.W.R. Bleyl, and R. Plass. Subacute oral toxicity study of benzyl isothiocyanate in rats. *Nahrung* 36:190–198 (1992).

164. Lewis, J.A., G.R. Fenwick, and A.R. Gray. Glucosinolates in brassica vegetables: green-curded cauliflowers (*Brassica oleracea* L. Botrytis group) and purple-headed broccoli (*B. oleracea* L. Italica group). *Lebensm. Wiss. Technol.* 24:361–363 (1991).

165. Koritsas, V.M., J.A. Lewis, and G.R. Fenwick. Glucosinolate responses of oilseed rape, mustard and kale to mechanical wounding and infestation by cabbage stem flea beetle (*Psylliodes chrysocephala*). *Ann. Appl. Biol.* 118:209–221 (1991).

166. Owusu-Ansah, Y.J., and M. Marianchuk. Microwave inactivation of myrosinase in canola seeds: a pilot plant study. *J. Food Sci.* 56:1372–1374,1406 (1991).

167. Truscott, R.J.W., and J.T. Tholen. Total glucosinolate content in rapeseed using reflectance. *Fat Sci. Technol.* 92:272–274 (1990).

168. Leoni, O., R. Iori, and S. Palmieri. Immobilization of myrosinase on membrane for determining the glucosinolate content of cruciferous material. *J. Agric. Food Chem.* 39:2322–2326 (1991).

169. Quinsac, A., D. Ribaillier, C. Elfakir, et al. A new approach to the study of glucosinolates by isocratic liquid chromatography. Part I. Rapid determination of desulfated derivatives of rapeseed glucosinolates. *J. Assoc. Off. Anal. Chem.* 74:932–939 (1991).

170. Zhao, F., E.J. Evans, P.E. Bilsborrow, et al. Correction for protein content in the determination of the glucosinolate content of rapeseed by the X-RF method. *J. Sci. Food Agric.* 58:431–433 (1992).

171. Quinsac, A., and D. Ribaillier. Analysis of 5-vinyl-1,3-oxazolidine-2-thione by liquid chromatography. *J. AOAC Int.* 75:529–536 (1992).

172. Akintonwa, A., and O.L. Tunwashe. Fatal cyanide poisoning from cassava-based meal. *Hum. Exp. Toxicol.* 11:47–49 (1992).

173. Tylleskär, T., M. Banea, N. Bikangi, et al. Epidemiological evidence from Zaire for a dietary etiology of knozo, an upper motor neuron disease. *Bull. WHO* 69:581–589 (1991).

174. Tylleskär, T., M. Banea, N. Bikangi, et al. Cassava cyanogens and konzo, an upper motoneuron disease found in Africa. *Lancet* 339:208–211 (1992).

175. Essers, A.J.A., P. Alsen, and H. Rosling. Insufficient processing of cassava induced acute intoxications and the paralytic disease konzo in a rural area of Mozambique. *Ecol. Food Nutr.* 27:17–27 (1992).

176. O'Brien, G.M., L. Mbome, A.J. Taylor, and N.H. Poulter. Variations in cyanogen content of cassava during village processing in Cameroon. *Food Chem.* 44:131–136 (1992).

177. O'Brien, G.M., A.J. Taylor, and N.H. Poulter. Improved enzymic assay for cyanogens in fresh and processed cassava. *J. Sci. Food Agric.* 56:277–289 (1991).

178. Bradbury, J.H., and S. V. Egan. Rapid screening assay of cyanide content of cassava. *Phytochem. Anal.* 3:91–94 (1992).

179. Ferreira, V.L.P., K. Yotsuyanagi, R.O.T. Neto, et al. Elimination of cyanogenic compounds of bamboo-shoots (*Dendrocalamus giganteus* Munro) by different processes. *Rev. Esp. Cienc. Tecnol. Aliment.* 32:175–184 (1992).

180. Voldrich, M., and V. Kyzlink. Cyanogenesis in canned stone fruits. *J. Food Sci.* 57:161–162,189 (1992).

181. Obizoba, I.C., and J.V. Atii. Effect of soaking, sprouting, fermentation and cooking on nutrient composition and some anti-nutritional factors of sorghum (Guinesia) seeds. *Plant Foods Hum. Nutr.* 41:203–212 (1991).

182. Abbott, T.P., L.K. Nakamura, G. Buchholz, et al. Processes for making animal feed and protein isolates from jojoba meal. *J. Agric. Food Chem.* 39:1488–1493 (1991).

183. Yoshihira, K., Y. Goda, K. Hashimoto, et al. Analysis of ferrocyanide in wine by ion chromatography. (Abstract in English.) *Shokuhim Eiseigaku Zasshi* 32:559–563 (1991).

184. Balansky, R., P. Blagoeva, and Z. Mircheva. Clastogenic activity of urethane in mice. *Mutat. Res.* 281:99–103 (1992).

185. Wild, D. Micronucleus induction in bone marrow by vinyl carbamate, a hypothetical metabolite of the carcinogen urethane (ethyl carbamate). *Mutat. Res.* 260:309–310 (1991).

186. Henschke, P.A., and C.S. Ough. Urea accumulation in fermenting grape juice. *Am. J. Enol. Vitic.* 42:317–321 (1991).

187. Aylott, R.I., G.C. Cochrane, M.J. Leonard, et al. Ethyl carbamate formation in grain based spirits. Part I: Post-distillation ethyl carbamate formation in maturing grain whisky. *J. Inst. Brew.* 96:213–221 (1990).

188. MacKenzie, W.M., A.H. Clyne, and L.S. MacDonald. Ethyl carbamate formation in grain based spirits. Part II. The identification and determination of cyanide related species involved in ethyl carbamate formation in Scotch grain whisky. *J. Inst. Brew.* 96:223–232 (1990).

189. Cook, R., N. McCaig, J.M.B. McMillan, and W.B. Lumsden. Ethyl carbamate formation in grain-based spirits. Part III. The primary source. *J. Inst. Brew.* 96:233–244 (1990).

190. McGill, D.J., and A.S. Morley. Ethyl carbamate formation in grain spirits. Part IV—Radiochemical studies. *J. Inst. Brew.* 96:245–246 (1990).

191. Giachetti, C., A. Assandri, and G. Zanolo. Gas chromatographic–mass spectrometric determination of ethyl carbamate as the xanthylamide derivative in Italian aqua vitae (grappa) samples. *J. Chromatogr.* 585:111–115 (1991).

192. Thorsen, L.I., H. Holm, J.E. Reseland, et al. Characterization of a human trypsin resistant to Kunitz soybean trypsin inhibitor. Studies of duodenal juices after tube instillation of raw soybean extract. *Scand. J. Gastroenterol.* 26:589–598 (1991).

193. Billings, P.C., D.L. Brandon, and J.M. Habres. Internalisation of the Bowman–Birk protease inhibitor by intestinal epithelial cells. *Eur. J. Cancer* 27:903–908 (1991).

194. Billings, P.C., W.H. St. Clair, P.A. Maki, and A.R. Kennedy. Distribution of the Bowman Birk protease inhibitor in mice following oral administration. *Cancer Lett.* 62:191–197 (1992).

195. Myers, B.A., J. Hathcock, N. Shiekh, and B.D. Roebuck. Effects of dietary soya bean trypsin inhibitor

concentrate on initiation and growth of putative preneoplastic lesions in the pancreas of the rat. *Food Chem. Toxicol.* 29:437–443 (1991).

196. Furukawa, F., K. Imaida, T. Imazawa, et al. Modifying effects of soybean trypsin inhibitor on development of eosinophilic nodules and basophilic foci in the exocrine pancreas of male Sprague-Dawley rats treated with 4-hydroxyaminoquinoline 1-oxide. *Jpn. J. Cancer Res.* 83:40–44 (1992).

197. Sharma, A., and S. Sehgal. Effect of domestic processing, cooking and germination on the trypsin inhibitor activity and tannin content of faba bean (*Vicia faba*). *Plant Foods Hum. Nutr.* 42:127–133 (1992).

198. Rayas-Duarte, P., D. Bergeron, and S.S. Nielsen. Screening of heat-stable trypsin inhibitors in dry beans and their partial purification from Great Northern beans (*Phaseolus vulgaris*) using anhydrotrypsin–Sepharose affinity chromatography. *J. Agric. Food Chem.* 40:32–42 (1992).

199. Menegatti, E., G. Tedeschi, S. Ronchi, et al. Purification, inhibitory properties and amino acid sequence of a new serine proteinase inhibitor from white mustard (*Sinapis alba* L.) seed. *FEBS Lett.* 301:10–14 (1992).

200. Bradbury, J.H., B.C. Hammer, and I. Sugani. Heat stability of trypsin inhibitors in tropical root crops and rice and its significance for nutrition. *J. Sci. Food Agric.* 58:95–100 (1992).

201. Rao, N.M. Protease inhibitors from ripened and unripened bananas. *Biochem. Int.* 24:13–22 (1991).

202. Weder, J.K.P., and K. Haußner. Inhibitors of human and bovine trypsin and chymotrypsin in fenugreek (*Trigonella foenum-graecum* L.) seeds. Reactive sites and C-terminal sequences. *Z. Lebensm. Unters. Forsch.* 193:242–246 (1991).

203. Weder, J.K.P., and K. Haußner. Inhibitors of human and bovine trypsin and chymotrypsin in fenugreek (*Trigonella foenum-graecum* L.) seeds. Reaction with the human and bovine proteinases. *Z. Lebensm. Unters. Forsch.* 193:321–325 (1991).

204. Hiasa, Y., Y. Kitahori, J. Morimoto, et al. Carcinogenicity study in rats of phytic acid 'Daiichi', a natural food additive. *Food Chem. Toxicol.* 30:117–125 (1992).

205. Brune, M., L. Rossander-Hultén, L. Hallberg, et al. Iron absorption from bread in humans: inhibiting effects of cereal fiber, phytate and inositol phosphates with different numbers of phosphate groups. *J. Nutr.* 122:442–449 (1992).

206. Lehrfeld, J., and Y.V. Wu. Distribution of phytic acid in milled fractions of Scout 66 hard red winter wheat. *J. Agric. Food Chem.* 39:1820–1824 (1991).

207. Snider, M., and M. Liebman. Calcium additives and sprouted wheat effects on phytate hydrolysis in whole wheat bread. *J. Food Sci.* 57:118–120 (1992).

208. Fretzdorff, B., and J.-M. Brümmer. Reduction of phytic acid during breadmaking of whole-meal breads. *Cereal Chem.* 69:266–270 (1992).

209. Larsson, M., and A.-S. Sandberg. Phytate reduction in bread containing oat flour, oat bran or rye bran. *J. Cereal Sci.* 14:141–149 (1991).

210. Gupta, M., N. Khetarpaul, and B.M. Chauhan. Rabadi fermentation of wheat: changes in phytic acid content and *in vitro* digestibility. *Plant Foods Hum. Nutr.* 42:109–116 (1992).

211. Honig, D.H., and W.J. Wolf. Phytate–mineral-protein composition of soybeans: gel filtration studies of soybean meal extracts. *J. Agric. Food Chem.* 39:1037–1042 (1991).

212. Bos, K.D., C. Verbeek, C.H.P. van Eeden, et al. Improved determination of phytate by ion-exchange chromatography. *J. Agric. Food Chem.* 39:1770–1772 (1991).

213. Adamson, D.J.A., and J.S. Legge. L-tryptophan-induced eosinophilia without myalgia. *Lancet* 337:1474–1475 (1991).

214. Yamaoka, K.A., N. Miyasaka, and S. Kashiwazaki. L-tryptophan contaminant "peak E" and interleukin-5 production from T cells. *Lancet* 338:1468 (1991).

215. Ito, J., Y. Hosaki, Y. Torigoe, and K. Sakimoto. Identification of substances formed by decomposition of peak E substance in tryptophan. *Food Chem. Toxicol.* 30:71–81 (1992).

216. Hatch, D.L., J.E. Garona, L.R. Goldman, and K.O. Waller. Persistent eosinophilia in an infant with probable intrauterine exposure to L-tryptophan-containing supplements. *Pediatrics* 88:810–813 (1991).

217. Arevalo, R., D. Afonso, R. Castro, and M. Rodriguez. Fetal brain serotonin synthesis and catabolism is under control by mother intake of tryptophan. *Life Sci.* 49:53–66 (1991).

218. Aviram, M., U. Cogan, and S. Mokady. Excessive dietary tryptophan enhances plasma lipid peroxidation in rats. *Atherosclerosis* 88:29–34 (1991).

219. Perdew, G.H., and C.F. Babbs. Production of *Ah* receptor ligands in rat fecal suspensions containing tryptophan or indole-3-carbinol. *Nutr. Cancer* 16:209–218 (1991).

220. Spencer, P.S., C.N. Allen, G.E. Kisby, et al. Lathyrism and western Pacific amyotrophic lateral sclerosis: etiology of short and long latency motor system disorders. *Adv. Neurol.* 56:287–299 (1991).

221. Duncan, M.W. Role of the cycad neurotoxin BMAA in the amyotrophic lateral sclerosis–parkinsonism dementia complex of the western Pacific. *Adv. Neurol.* 56:301–310 (1991).

222. Bridges, R.J., C. Hatalski, S.N. Shim, and P.B. Nunn. Gliotoxic properties of the *Lathyrus* excitotoxin β-*N*-oxalyl-L-α,β-diaminopropionic acid (β-L-ODAP). *Brain Res.* 561:262–268 (1991).

223. Centers for Disease Control. Toxic hypoglycemic syndrome—Jamaica, 1989–1991. *Morbid. Mortal. Weekly Rep.* 41:53–54 (1992).

224. Brown, M., R.P. Bates, C. McGowan, and J.A. Cornell. Influence of fruit maturity on the hypoglycin A level in ackee (*Blighia sapida*). *J. Food Safety* 12:167–177 (1992).

225. Bobilya, D.J., M.R. Ellersieck, D.T. Gordon, and T.L. Veum. Bioavailabilities of zinc from nonfat dry milk, lowfat plain yogurt, and soy flour in diets fed to neonatal pigs. *J. Agric. Food Chem.* 39:1246–1251 (1991).

226. Rubio, L.A., G. Grant, S. Bardocz, et al. Mineral excretion of rats fed on diets containing faba beans (*Vicia faba* L.) or faba bean fractions. *Br. J. Nutr.* 67:295–302 (1992).

227. Savelkoul, F.H.M.G., A.F.B. Van der Poel, and S. Tamminga. The presence and inactivation of trypsin inhibitors, tannins, lectins and amylase inhibitors in legume seeds during germination. A review. *Plant Foods Hum. Nutr.* 42:71–85 (1992).

228. Kaur, D., and A.C. Kapoor. Nutrient composition and antinutritional factors of rice bean (*Vigna umbellata*). *Food Chem.* 43:119–124 (1992).

229. Rajaram, N., and K. Janardhanan. Studies on the underexploited tree pulses, *Acacia catechu* Willd., *Parkinsonia aculeata* L. and *Prosopis chilensis* (Molina) Stunz: chemical composition and antinutritional factors. *Food Chem.* 42:265–273 (1991).

230. Roozen, J.P., and J. de Groot. Analysis of trypsin inhibitors and lectins in white kidney beans (*Phaseolus vulgaris*, var. Processor) in a combined method. *J. Assoc. Off. Anal. Chem.* 74:940–943 (1991).

231. Ziena, H.M., M.M. Youssef, and A.R. El-Mahdy. Amino acid composition and some antinutritional factors of cooked faba beans (*Medammis*): effects of cooking temperature and time. *J. Food Sci.* 56:1347–1349,1352 (1991).

232. Sharma, A., and S. Sehgal. Effect of processing and cooking on the antinutritional factors of faba bean (*Vicia faba*). *Food Chem.* 43:383–385 (1992).

233. Borejszo, Z., and K. Khan. Reduction of flatulence-causing sugars by high temperature extrusion of pinto bean high starch fractions. *J. Food Sci.* 57:771–772,777 (1992).

234. You, X.-M., and S.K.C. Chang. Effect of purified lectins on pancreatic α-amylase activities. *J. Agric. Food Chem.* 40:638–641 (1992).

235. Deshpande, S.S., and R.K. Singh. Hemagglutinating activity of lectins in selected varieties of raw and processed dry beans. *J. Food Process. Preserv.* 15:81–87 (1991).

236. Almeida, N.G., A.M. Calderón de la Barca, and M.E. Valencia. Effect of different heat treatments on the antinutritional activity of *Phaseolus vulgaris* (variety Ojo de Cabra) lectin. *J. Agric. Food Chem.* 39:1627–1630 (1991).

237. Obidoa, O., and S.C. Obasi. Coumarin compounds in cassava diets: 2 health implications of scopoletin in gari. *Plant Foods Hum. Nutr.* 41:283–289 (1991).

238. Lake, B.G., H. Gaudin, R.J. Price, and D.G. Walters. Metabolism of [3-^{14}C]coumarin to polar and covalently bound products by hepatic microsomes from the rat, Syrian hamster, gerbil and humans. *Food Chem. Toxicol.* 30:105–115 (1992).

239. Fentem, J.H., and J.R. Fry. Metabolism of coumarin by rat, gerbil and human liver microsomes. *Xenobiotica* 22:357–367 (1992).

240. Wagstaff, D.J. Dietary exposure to furocoumarins. *Reg. Toxicol. Pharmacol.* 14:261–272 (1991).

241. Schlatter, J., B. Zimmerli, R. Dick, et al. Dietary intake and risk assessment of phototoxic furocoumarins in humans. *Food Chem. Toxicol.* 29:523–530 (1991).

242. McKinnon, R.A., W.M. Burgess, P. de la M. Hall, et al. Metabolism of food-derived heterocyclic amines in human and rabbit tissues by P4503A proteins in the presence of flavonoids. *Cancer Res.* 52(Suppl.):2108S–2113S (1992).

243. Jurado, J., E. Alejandre-Durán, A. Alonso-Moraga, and C. Pueyo. Study on the mutagenic activity of 13 bioflavonoids with the Salmonella Ara test. *Mutagenesis* 6:289–295 (1991).

244. Ferreres, F., F. A. Tomás-Barberán, M.I. Gil, and F. Tomás-Lorente. An HPLC technique for flavonoid analysis in honey. *J. Sci. Food Agric.* 56:49–56 (1991).

245. Sabatier, S., M.J. Amiot, M. Tacchini, and S. Aubert. Identification of flavonoids in sunflower honey. *J. Food Sci.* 57:773–774,777 (1992).

246. Finger, A., U.H. Engelhardt and V. Wray. Flavonol glycosides in tea—kaempferol and quercetin rhamnodiglucosides. *J. Sci. Food Agric.* 55:313–321 (1991).

247. Sahu, S.C., and M.C. Washington. Quercetin-induced lipid peroxidation and DNA damage in isolated rat-liver nuclei. *Cancer Lett.* 58:75–79 (1991).

248. Sahu, S.C., and M.C. Washington. Effects of antioxidants on quercetin-induced nuclear DNA damage and lipid peroxidation. *Cancer Lett.* 60:259–264 (1991).

249. Wu, Y.-W., C.L. Chik, B.D. Albertson, et al. Inhibitory effects of gossypol on adrenal function. *Acta Endocrinol. (Copenh.)* 124:672–678 (1991).

250. Zaidi, R., and S.M. Hadi. Interaction of gossypol with DNA. *Toxicol. in vitro* 6:71–76 (1992).

251. Botsoglou, N.A. High-performance liquid chromatographic method for the determination of free gossypol in chicken liver. *J. Chromatogr.* 587:333–337 (1991).

252. Botsoglou, N.A., and A.B. Spais. Ion-pair, liquid chromatographic analysis of total gossypol in chicken liver. *Chromatographia* 33:174–176 (1992).

253. Savolainen, H. Tannin content of tea and coffee. *J. Appl. Toxicol.* 12:191–192 (1992).

254. Wang, R.S.(A.), and C. Kies. Niacin, thiamin, iron and protein status of humans as affected by the consumption of tea (*Camellia sinensis*) infusions. *Plant Foods Hum. Nutr.* 41:337–353 (1991).

255. Fairweather-Tait, S.J., Z. Piper, S.J.A. Fatemi, and G.R. Moore. The effect of tea on iron and aluminium metabolism in the rat. *Br. J. Nutr.* 65:61–68 (1991).

256. Lyimo, M., J. Mugula, and T. Elias. Nutritive composition of broth from selected bean varieties cooked for various periods. *J. Sci. Food Agric.* 58:535–539 (1992).

257. Hernández, T., A. Hernández, and C. Martinez. Polyphenols in alfalfa leaf concentrates. *J. Agric. Food Chem.* 39:1120–1122 (1991).

258. Carmona, A., D.S. Seidl, and W.G. Jaffé. Comparison of extraction methods and assay procedures for the determination of the apparent tannin content of common beans. *J. Sci. Food Agric.* 56:291–301 (1991).

259. Johns, T., and M. Duquette. Traditional detoxification of acorn bread with clay. *Ecol. Food Nutr.* 25:221–228 (1991).

260. Bibi, N., A. Sattar, and M.A. Chaudry. Phenolic constituents in major fractions of tropical rapeseed. *Nahrung* 35:1053–1059 (1991).

261. Khetarpaul, N., and B.M. Chauhan. Sequential fermentation of pearl millet by yeasts and lactobacilli—effect on the antinutrients and *in vitro* digestibility. *Plant Foods Hum. Nutr.* 41:321–327 (1991).

262. Graham, H.D. Stabilization of the Prussian blue color in the determination of polyphenols. *J. Agric. Food Chem.* 40:801–805 (1992).

263. Hagiwara, A., M. Hirose, S. Takahashi, et al. Forestomach and kidney carcinogenicity of caffeic acid in F344 rats and C57BL/6N × C3H/HeN F_1 mice. *Cancer Res.* 51:5655–5660 (1991).

264. Naczk, M., P.K.J.P.D. Wanasundara, and F. Shahidi. Facile spectrophotometric quantification method of sinapic acid in hexane-extracted and methanol–ammonia–water-treated mustard and rapeseed meals. *J. Agric. Food Chem.* 40:444–448 (1992).

265. Ariza, R.R., and C. Pueyo. The involvement of reactive oxygen species in the direct-acting mutagenicity of wine. *Mutat. Res.* 251:115–121 (1991).

266. Ariza, R.R., A. Serrano, and C. Pueyo. Direct-acting mutagenic activity in white, rosé, and red wines with the Ara test of *Salmonella typhimurium. Environ. Molec. Mutagen.* 19:14–20 (1992).

267. Ariza, R.R., A. Serrano, and C. Pueyo. Study on the mutagenicity of brandy with the Ara test. *Mutagenesis* 7:77–81 (1992).

268. Tsuji, S., T. Shibata, K. Ohara, et al. Studies on the factors affecting the formation of hydrogen peroxide in coffee. (Abstract in English.) *Shokuhim Eiseigaku Zasshi* 32:504–512 (1991).

269. Trestrail, J.H., III. Mushroom poisoning in the United States—An analysis of 1989 United States Poison Center data. *Clin. Toxicol.* 29:459–465 (1991).

270. Benjamin, D.R. Mushroom poisoning in infants and children: the *Amanita pantherina/muscaria* group. *Clin. Toxicol.* 30:13–22 (1992).

271. Kawaji, A., K. Yamauchi, S. Fujii, et al. Effects of mushroom toxins on glycogenolysis; comparison of toxicity of phalloidin, α-amanitin and DL-propargylglycine in isolated rat hepatocytes. *J. Pharmacobio-Dyn.* 15:107–112 (1992).

272. Enjalbert, F., C. Gallion, F. Jehl, et al. Simultaneous assay for amatoxins and phallotoxins in *Amanita phalloides* Fr. by high-performance liquid chromatography. *J. Chromatogr.* 598:227–236 (1992).

273. Michelot, D., and B. Toth. Poisoning by *Gyromitra esculenta*—a review. *J. Appl. Toxicol.* 11:235–243 (1991).

274. Toth, B., K. Patil, H. Pyysalo, et al. Cancer induction in mice by feeding the raw false morel mushroom *Gyromitra esculenta. Cancer Res.* 52:2279–2284 (1992).

275. Toth, B., J. Taylor, and P. Gannett. Tumor induction with hexanal methylformylhydrazone of *Gyromitra esculenta. Mycopathologia* 115:65–71 (1991).

276. Bergman, K., and K.-E. Hellenäs. Methylation of rat and mouse DNA by the mushroom poison gyromitrin and its metabolite monomethylhydrazine. *Cancer Lett.* 61:165–170 (1992).

277. Matsumoto, K., M. Ito, S. Yagyu, et al. Carcinogenicity examination of *Agaricus bisporus*, edible mushroom, in rats. *Cancer Lett.* 58:87–90 (1991).

278. Kwak, S., H. Aizawa, M. Ishida, and H. Shinozaki. Systemic administration of acromelic acid induces selective neuron damage in the rat spinal cord. *Life Sci.* 49:PL-91–PL-96 (1991).

279. Matthies, L., and H. Laatsch. Cortinarins in *Cortinarius speciosissimus*? A critical revision. *Experientia* 47:634–640 (1991).

280. Fujimoto, H., K. Maeda, and M. Yamazaki. New toxic metabolites from a mushroom, *Hebeloma vinosophyllum*. III. Isolation and structures of three new glycosides, hebevinosides XII, XIII and XIV, and productivity of the hebevinosides at three growth stages of the mushroom. *Chem. Pharm. Bull.* 39:1958–1961 (1991).

281. Kägi, M.K., and B. Wüthrich. Falafel-burger anaphylaxis due to sesame seed allergy. *Lancet* 338:582 (1991).

282. Chiu, J.T., and I.B. Haydik. Sesame seed oil anaphylaxis. *J. Allergy Clin. Immunol.* 88:414–415 (1991).

283. Keskinen, H., P. Ostman, E. Vaheri, et al. A case of occupational asthma, rhinitis and urticaria due to sesame seed. *Clin. Exp. Allergy* 21:623–624 (1991).

284. Moneret-Vautrin, D.A., R. Hatahet, G. Kanny, and Z. Ait-Djafer. Allergic peanut oil in milk formulas. *Lancet* 338:1149 (1991).

285. James, J.M., S.K. Cooke, A. Barnett, and H.A. Sampson. Anaphylactic reactions to a psyllium-containing cereal. *J. Allergy Clin. Immunol.* 88:402–408 (1991).

286. Saff, R.H., and J.N. Fink. Anaphylaxis to chicken soup: A case report and a brief history of the chicken in medicine. *J. Allergy Clin. Immunol.* 89:1061–1062 (1992).

287. Bruhn, J.N., and M.D. Soderberg. Allergic contact dermatitis caused by mushrooms. A case report and literature review. *Mycopathologia* 115:191–195 (1991).

288. Igea, J.M., J. Cuesta, M. Cuevas, et al. Adverse reaction to pomegranate ingestion. *Allergy* 46:472–474 (1991).

289. Lavaud, F., C. Cossart, V. Reiter, et al. Latex allergy in patient with allergy to fruit. *Lancet* 339:492–493 (1992).

290. Ceuppens, J.L., P. van Durme, and A. Dooms-Goossens. Latex allergy in patient with allergy to fruit. *Lancet* 339:493 (1992).

291. Anderson, J.A., ed. *Food Allergy. Immunol. Allergy Clin. North Am.* 11(4) (1991).

292. Chandra, R.K. Food allergy: 1992 and beyond. *Nutr. Res.* 12:93–99 (1992).

293. Metcalfe, D.D. The nature and mechanisms of food allergies and related diseases. *Food Technol.* 46(5):136–156 (1992).

294. Helbling, A., Ch. Peter, E. Berchtold, et al. Allergy to honey: relation to pollen and honey bee allergy. *Allergy* 47:41–49 (1992).

295. Kaiser, C., H. Reibisch, R. Fölster-Holst, and H. Sick. Cow's milk protein allergy—Results of skin-prick test with purified milk proteins. *Z. Ernährungswiss.* 29:123–128 (1990).

296. Stephan, V., J. Kühr, G. Sawatzki, and R. Urbanek. Untersuchung zur Immunogenität und

Allergenität eines experimentellen Kuhmilchprotein-Hydrolysates. *Z. Ernährungswiss.* 29:112–121 (1990).

297. Stäger, J., B. Wüthrich, and S.G.O. Johansson. Spice allergy in celery-sensitive patients. *Allergy* 46:475–478 (1991).

298. Bernhisel-Broadbent, J., S. M. Scanlon, and H.A. Sampson. Fish hypersensitivity. I. In vitro and oral challenge results in fish-allergic patients. *J. Allergy Clin. Immunol.* 89:730–737 (1992).

299. Burks, A.W., L.W. Williams, R.M. Helm, et al. Identification of a major peanut allergen, *Ara h* I, in patients with atopic dermatitis and positive peanut challenges. *J. Allergy Clin. Immunol.* 88:172–179 (1991).

300. González de la Peña, M.A., L. Menéndez-Arias, R.I. Monsalve, and R. Rodríguez. Isolation and characterization of a major allergen from oriental mustard seeds, *Bra j* I. *Int. Arch. Allergy Appl. Immunol.* 96:263–270 (1991).

301. Ogawa, T., N. Bando, H. Tsuji, et al. Investigation of the IgE-binding proteins in soybeans by immunoblotting with the sera of the soybean-sensitive patients with atopic dermatitis. *J. Nutr. Sci. Vitaminol.* 37:555–565 (1991).

302. Urisu, A., K. Yamada, S. Masuda, et al. 16-Kilodalton rice protein is one of the major allergens in rice grain extract and responsible for cross-allergenicity between cereal grains in the Poaceae family. *Int. Arch. Allergy Appl. Immunol.* 96:244–252 (1991).

303. Shintani, S., H. Murase, H. Tsukagoshi, and T. Shiigai. Glycyrrhizin (licorice)-induced hypokalemic myopathy. Report of 2 cases and review of the literature. *Eur. Neurol.* 32:44–51 (1992).

304. Böcker, D. and G. Breithardt. Arrhythmia aggravation due to licorice ingestion. (Abstract in English.) *Z. Kardiol.* 80:389–391 (1991).

305. Itami, N., K. Yamamoto, T. Andoh, and Y. Akutsu. Herbal medicine can induce hypertension. *Nephron* 59:339–340 (1991).

306. Farese, R.V., Jr., E.G. Biglieri, C.H.L. Shackleton, et al. Licorice-induced hypermineralo-corticoidism. *New Engl. J. Med.* 325:1223–1227 (1991).

307. Pratesi, C., M. Scali, V. Zampollo, et al. Effects of licorice on urinary metabolites of cortisol and cortisone. *J. Hypertens.* 9(Suppl. 6):S274–S275 (1991).

308. Hatano, T., T. Fukuda, T. Miyase, et al. Phenolic constituents of licorice. III. Structures of glicoricone and licofuranone, and inhibitory effects of licorice constituents on monoamine oxidase. *Chem. Pharm. Bull.* 39:1238–1243 (1991).

309. Onat, F., B.C. Yegen, R. Lawrence, et al. Site of action of grayanotoxins in mad honey in rats. *J. Appl. Toxicol.* 11:199–201 (1991).

310. Prakash, D., and M. Pal. Nutritional and antinutritional composition of vegetable and grain amaranth leaves. *J. Sci. Food Agric.* 57:573–583 (1991).

311. Salles, M.S., C.S. Lombardo de Barros, R.A. Lemos, and C. Pilati. Perirenal edema associated with *Amaranthus* spp. poisoning in Brazilian swine. *Vet. Hum. Toxicol.* 33:616–617 (1991).

312. Kamiya, C., M. Ogawa, and H. Ohkawa. Oxalic acid and calcium contents in tea. *Shokuhin Eiseigaku Zasshi* 32:291–300 (1991).

313. Banerjee, S., and A.R. Rao. Promoting action of cashew nut shell oil in DMBA-initiated mouse skin tumour model system. *Cancer Lett.* 62:149–152 (1992).

314. El-Mofty, M.M., V.V. Khudoley, S.A. Sakr, and N.G. Fathala. Flour infested with *Tribolium castaneum*, biscuits made of this flour, and 1,4-benzoaquinone induce neoplastic lesions in Swiss albino mice. *Nutr. Cancer* 17:97–104 (1992).

Part III: Foodborne Microbial Illness

10

Mycotoxins

In a recent review, Kuiper-Goodman discussed approaches to assess the potential hazard to human health from the consumption of mycotoxins (aflatoxins, ochratoxin A, and zearalenone) in animal-derived foods (*1*). When animals consume mycotoxin-contaminated feeds, some carryover of the toxins into animal tissues and products (eggs and milk, for example) occurs. Wide variations in carryover ratios (sometimes as much as two orders of magnitude) have been reported in the literature. In addition to clarifying the extent of carryover, more research is required to determine the concentrations, bioavailability, and toxicity of mycotoxin metabolites in animal-derived foods. Finally, in risk assessment, there is always the problem of inter-species extrapolation and of extrapolation to low doses.

An overview of the major mycotoxins responsible for illnesses following ingestion of contaminated food was recently published (*2*). The compounds included were aflatoxins, cyclopiazonic acid, diplodiatoxin, diplosporin, fumonisins, ochratoxin A, patulin, tenuazonic acid, trichothecenes, wortmannin, and zearalenone. Toxin structures and the foods in which they commonly occur were described along with toxic effects, particularly in humans.

A total of 14 species of *Penicillium* were identified from 33 isolates from dairy products and a dairy environment in India (*3*). Six mycotoxins were produced by these isolates: citrinin, ochratoxins, patulin, penicillic acid, cyclopiazonic acid, and PR-toxin. Citrinin was the most commonly detected toxin.

A survey of 168 retail samples of nuts in Spain (including almonds, peanuts, hazelnuts, pistachio nuts, and sunflower seeds) revealed that all were contaminated to some extent by molds (*4*). *Penicillium* spp. and *Aspergillus* spp. were the most frequent isolates. Aflatoxins (AFB_1 and AFB_2) were detected in one sample of almonds (95 ppb AFB_1, 15 ppb AFB_2) and in one sample of peanuts (<10 ppb AFB_1). However, isolates of the different mold species were able to produce aflatoxins B_1, B_2, G_1, and G_2, sterigmatocystin, ochratoxin A, patulin, citrinin, griseofulvin, penicillic acid, and zearalenone in vitro. Although the incidence of mycotoxin contamination was low, in all samples there was a mycoflora present which was capable of producing mycotoxins under appropriate conditions.

A survey of 36 retail samples of Brazilian cheeses (hard Parmesan, grated Parmesan, Prato, and processed cheeses) revealed the presence of molds in all types of cheese except the processed cheese (*5*). *Aspergillus* spp. were detected only in grated Parmesan cheese while *Penicillium* spp. and other mold genera were found in all 3 unprocessed cheeses. However, no mycotoxins were detected in any of the cheeses. Only 3 of 21 *Penicillium* isolates and neither of the two *Aspergillus* isolates produced mycotoxins in vitro. Experiments with different types of cheese indicated that citrinin could be produced in cheese with high water activity but patulin appears to be unstable in cheese even with high water activity.

The antimycotic agent imazalil, when added to low density polyethylene film (LDPE), was found to markedly inhibit the growth of *Penicillium* sp. and *Aspergillus toxacarius* inoculated on potato dextrose agar and cheddar cheese (*6*). A concentration of 1 g imazalil/kg LDPE completely inhibited detectable mold growth on cheese for at least 10 days while cheese wrapped in LDPE alone exhibited mold growth after 3–4 days. Higher concentrations of imazalil were required to inhibit growth of *A. toxacarius* on potato dextrose agar.

In mutagenicity tests using the newer tester strain, TA102, of *Salmonella typhimurium*, neither ochratoxins A and B, citrinin, patulin nor combinations of citrinin and ochratoxin A induced reverse mutations with or without metabolic activation (*7*). Therefore, these mycotoxins apparently do not cause oxidative damage or crosslinks in DNA of this tester strain.

In renal cortical explants from male minipigs, ochratoxin A was a more potent inhibitor of macromolecular biosynthesis (at 0.001 mM) than citrinin while citrinin was a more potent inhibitor of respiration and organic ion transport (at 1.0 and 0.01 mM, respectively) (*8*). The mycotoxins were tested at concentrations of 0.001 to 1.0 mM. Increased protein leakage from cells was not caused by either toxin, indicating the absence of serious membrane damage.

To test subacute toxicity in vivo, citrinin and ochratoxin A were administered by gavage to 14 pigs during a 57-day period (*9*). Daily doses of 0.02 mg/kg body mass of one toxin or 0.01 mg/kg of both toxins were given. The concentrations used correspond to levels of contamination detected in Central Europe. No significant clinical or pathomorphological changes occurred in the pigs. However, significant mycotoxin levels were detected in plasma samples: averages of 302 ng/mL and 91 ng/mL in pigs given 0.02 mg ochratoxin A/kg and 0.02 mg citrinin/kg, respectively. These mycotoxin levels may have toxic effects on humans if swine blood is processed for food.

MYCOTOXINS PRODUCED BY *ASPERGILLUS* SPP.

Aflatoxins

AFLATOXINS IN HUMANS AND THEIR ASSOCIATION WITH ILLNESS. A severe outbreak of food poisoning affecting 62 ethnic Chinese (primarily children) and resulting in 13 deaths occurred in Malaysia during a Chinese festival late in 1988 (*10*). All cases had consumed a rice- and corn-flour based noodle from a common source. Autopsy results from 11 victims revealed high levels of aflatoxins B_1, B_2, G_1, M_1, and M_2 and aflatoxicol in various organs. These levels were at least 10-fold higher than those detected previously in healthy persons. Boric acid, which was added to the noodles to improve their color, flavor, and texture, was detected in all urine samples, with 16 samples containing >20 mg boric acid/dL. Pathological observations of toxic liver injury resulting in fulminant liver failure were attributable to aflatoxicosis, while metabolic acidosis and acute renal failure were most likely a result of boric acid poisoning.

While most research on the biological effects of aflatoxins is concerned with their carcinogenic potential, some evidence points to a role for aflatoxins in the disease kwashiorkor. This disease occurs seasonally in restricted geographical areas and has been associated with protein-deficient diets. But kwashiorkor is not simply a deficiency disease, as a variety of unique endocrinological, biochemical, and immunological changes occur in affected children. A recent review (*11*) summarized evidence correlating aflatoxin exposure with development of this disease and discussed future research needs.

Since aflatoxin exposure early in life may result in disease later on, it is important to assess such exposures. Of 30 new mothers tested in Gambia aflatoxin–albumin adducts were detected in maternal venous blood of 29 and in umbilical cord blood of 21 of their infants (*12*). Cord adduct levels were up to 10-fold less than maternal adduct levels, indicating that the albumin adduct does not easily cross the placenta. These aflatoxin–albumin adducts predominantly reflect dietary exposure during the previous 2–3 months. Dietary intake of aflatoxins by 5 lactating Gambian women was correlated with aflatoxin M_1 levels in breast milk (*13*). This toxin was detected in milk from all subjects (highest concentration, 1.4 ppt), and aflatoxin G_1 was also present in milk from 3 subjects. Estimates of dietary aflatoxin excreted as aflatoxin M_1 in milk ranged from 0.09 to 0.43%. Thus, infants whose mothers consume aflatoxin-tainted foods may themselves be exposed both prenatally as well as postnatally through their mothers' milk.

Controversy continues over the role, if any, of aflatoxins in the development of hepatocellular carcinoma (HCC). While many epidemiological studies have suggested that aflatoxin ingestion is a factor in carcinogenesis, one recent study in Thailand reported no apparent increase in liver cancer associated with higher dietary levels of aflatoxins (*14*). Sixty-five case–control pairs were interviewed to estimate aflatoxin exposure from possibly contaminated food. Aflatoxin–albumin adduct levels in blood samples were also determined for a majority of subjects. Although recent aflatoxin exposure did not appear to increase cancer risk, the authors caution that the patients' diets may have changed since the beginning of their illness.

Analysis of 27 pairs of tumor and adjacent non-tumor liver tissues from HCC patients in Taiwan revealed that 30% and 26%, respectively, were positive for AFB_1–DNA adducts (*15*). Hepatitis B surface antigen (HBsAg) was present in 37% of the tumor samples and in 81% of the adjacent non-tumorous tissues. These results implicate both afla-toxin exposure and carrier status of HBsAg in the induction of HCC in Taiwan.

In an effort to correlate dietary intake of afla-toxins with the amounts of the major aflatoxin–DNA adduct and other aflatoxin metabolites excreted in urine, the diets of 42 adults in Guangxi Autono-mous Region were monitored for 1 week and indi-vidual daily intakes of aflatoxins were calculated (16). Starting on the fourth day, consecutive 12-hour urine volumes were obtained and analyzed by HPLC and competitive radioimmunoassay. Average daily intakes of AFB_1 for men and women were 48.4 µg and 77.4 µg, respectively. Initial analyses using data from the radioimmunoassay yielded a correla-tion coefficient of only 0.26 for the association between the daily intake of AFB_1 and daily excre-tion of total aflatoxin metabolites. Further analyses using immunoaffinity/analytical HPLC for individual metabolites revealed correlation coefficients of 0.65 and 0.80 when AFB_1 intake was plotted against aflatoxin $N7$-guanine on a daily basis and for the total period, respectively.

Results from an ongoing prospective study of 18,244 middle-aged men in Shanghai provide fur-ther support for a link between aflatoxin exposure and HCC (17). Initially each subject completed a detailed food frequency questionnaire and provided blood and urine samples. After about 2 years' follow up, 22 cases of HCC were identified and each was matched with 5–10 controls from the cohort (total of 140 controls). Cases were more likely than con-trols to have detectable levels of urinary aflatoxin metabolites. When the data were adjusted for effects of HBsAg seropositivity, level of education, ciga-rette smoking, and alcohol consumption, relative risk of HCC associated with urinary aflatoxin me-tabolites was 3.8.

It has been suggested that aflatoxins may induce HCC by causing a mutation in codon 249 of the tumor suppressor gene *p53*. In one study of 167 HCC specimens from 14 countries, 17% of tumors (12/72) from countries in southern Africa and South-east Asia (regions with a high risk of exposure to aflatoxins) contained such mutations (18). None of the specimens from Europe, North America and the

Middle East contained mutations in the *p53* gene. Another study (19) found 2 of 47 HCC tumor speci-mens from countries with low aflatoxin exposure (U.K. and Egypt) and 2 of 8 HCC tumors from countries with high risk of aflatoxin exposure with codon 249 mutations. Neither study measured afla-toxin or aflatoxin metabolites in the tumor tissue samples.

Analysis of 9 tumors (4 HCC, 1 other liver tumor, 3 bile duct tumors and 1 tibial tumor) induced by AFB_1 in rhesus and cynomolgus mon-keys revealed no changes in codon 249 of gene *p53* (20). These data indicate that a mutation in gene *p53* may not be necessary for aflatoxin-induced carcinogenesis.

METABOLISM AND BIOLOGICAL EFFECTS OF AFLATOXINS. In vitro experiments with human liver microsomes demonstrated that both aflatoxin Q_1 (AFQ_1) and AFB_1 8,9-epoxide (measured as the glutathione conjugate) were major products of the oxidation of AFB_1 (21). Two lines of evidence indi-cate that cytochrome P-450 3A4 is the primary enzyme involved in both oxidations: (1) Rates of formation of both AFQ_1 and AFB_1 8,9-epoxide were highly correlated with rates of nifedipine oxidation, a marker for P-450 3A4. (2) Antibodies to P-450 3A4 effectively inhibited the formation of both AFQ_1 and AFB_1 8,9-epoxide by human liver micro-somes. Since AFQ_1 8,9-epoxide was 10-fold less effective than AFB_1 8,9-epoxide both in forming DNA adducts and in causing revertants in *S. typhimurium*, it appears that P-450 3A4 is involved in both the activation and detoxication of AFB_1. Further research is necessary to determine the role of this enzyme in vivo with chronic low dose expo-sure to aflatoxins.

Chemical synthesis of AFB_1 8,9-epoxide has been found to yield a 10:1 mixture of AFB_1 exo-8,9-epoxide:AFB_1-endo-8,9-epoxide (22). The endo-epoxide was also formed (as a minor product) by human and rat microsomes in vitro. Although the endo-epoxide is present in much smaller amounts, its genotoxicity and biological activity may be greater than that of the exo-epoxide.

Experiments using AFB_1–dichloride (AFB_1–Cl_2) as a more stable model for AFB_1 8,9-epoxide have shown that it has mutagenic, carcinogenic, and DNA-binding properties similar to those of the epoxide. Recent experiments with AFB_1–Cl_2 have provided strong evidence that this compound can covalently bind to cytosine as well as to guanine in DNA (*23*). Following incubation of DNA with AFB–Cl_2, cytosine–AFB_1 adducts were detected by HPLC.

A combined multiple monoclonal antibody immunoaffinity chromatography/HPLC method has been developed to isolate and quantify aflatoxin–DNA adducts and other metabolites in urine samples (*24*). Eleven different monoclonal antibodies recognizing AFB_1, AFQ_1, AFG_1, AFM_1, and aflatoxicol were produced, and three of these were selected for use in the immunoaffinity column. Using this column, 90–95% of total aflatoxin metabolites could be isolated from urine of rats orally dosed with 0.03–1.0 mg AFB_1/kg body weight. The following metabolites and their percentage composition of total aflatoxins were detected: AFM_1 (34.5%), AF-$N7$-guanine (9.6%), AFP_1 (8%), AFQ_1 (1.8%), AF-dihydrodiol (1.5%), and AFB_1 (1%). AFM_1 and AF-$N7$-guanine concentrations in urine were found to be closely correlated with AFB_1 dose ingested (correlation coefficients of 0.99 and 0.93, respectively). Furthermore, there was an excellent correlation between AF-$N7$-guanine excreted in urine and residual levels of aflatoxin binding to DNA.

AFB_1 is known to induce hepatocellular carcinoma in parenchymal but not in other liver cells in laboratory animals. Recent in vitro experiments showed that a 10-fold higher concentration of AFB_1 was required for non-parenchymal liver cells to produce a level of mutagenic metabolites similar to that of parenchymal cells (*25*). The level of AFB_1–DNA adducts formed in vivo in rat parenchymal cells was 3–5 times that observed in non-parenchymal cells following a single i.p. dose of labelled AFB_1 (*26*). These results may explain why non-parenchymal cells are less susceptible to the carcinogenic effects of AFB_1.

In a study to analyze AFB_1-induced hepatic changes in progeny of treated pregnant and lactating rats, extensive cystic lesions of the biliary and hepatic type were observed in the young (*27*). Six doses of 100 µg AFB_1 were administered to pregnant and to lactating rats. Some progeny of normal

and treated dams were cross-fostered while others remained with their own mothers. Hepatic lesions were more frequent and appeared earlier in progeny of treated dams fed by their own mothers. Lesions were much less frequent in progeny of normal dams fed by treated dams. Progeny of treated dams fostered by normal dams exhibited an intermediate effect of AFB_1.

Since protein kinase C can serve as a receptor for tumor promoters, some recent studies have investigated protein kinase activity in AFB_1-treated cells. A greater total amount of protein kinase C_α was detected in an AFB_1-transformed cell line than in the parent cell line and this was correlated with an altered response to phorbol ester treatments (*28*). Incubation of human platelet suspensions with AFB_1 resulted in increased protein kinase activity (*29*). Following activation, the enzyme is translocated from the cytosol to the particulate fraction. These results indicate that protein kinase activation may be related to the carcinogenic effects of aflatoxins.

Since aflatoxins have been reported to be immunotoxic, short-term cultures of mouse myeloid progenitor cells and mouse long-term bone marrow cultures were used to investigate the effects of AFB_1 on granulopoiesis and myelopoiesis (*30*). The short-term cultures were highly suppressed by 5 µg AFB_1/mL and slightly suppressed by 0.5 µg/mL. However, both of these concentrations exerted a strong suppression of myelopoiesis in the long-term bone marrow cultures. Thus, the long term culture appeared to be more sensitive and discriminatory in evaluating the toxic effects of AFB_1 on hemopoiesis.

Rabbit red blood cells incubated at 37°C for 16 hours with several concentrations of AFB_1 showed a concentration-dependent hemolysis between 1.4 and 3.1 µg/mL (*31*). Treated cells appeared swollen and spherical with the degree of swelling also related to AFB_1 concentration.

BIOSYNTHESIS OF AFLATOXINS. Molecular cloning of genes associated with aflatoxin biosynthesis is being pursued to study the mechanisms of gene expression in *Aspergillus parasiticus* and to further elucidate the biosynthetic pathway. Nineteen clones, which were positively correlated with and presumably enriched with genes associated with aflatoxin production, were isolated by a differential hybridization technique (*32*). A genomic library, formed between nuclear DNA and the pUC19 plasmid, was screened with 3 different cDNA probes transcribed from poly(A)+RNA isolated from: (a) mycelia grown in non-permissive media; (b) mycelia grown in permissive media but harvested well before significant aflatoxin production; and (c) mycelia grown in permissive medium and harvested just as aflatoxin production started to increase sharply. Of 20,000 colonies screened, 19 which hybridized strongly with cDNA from (c), weakly with cDNA from (b), and very weakly with cDNA from (a) were selected. Two of the clones when used as probes were found to hybridize only with poly(A)+RNA from mycelia grown at permissive temperatures. In another experiment, genomic DNA from *A. parasiticus* was inserted into a cosmid vector containing a nitrate reductase gene as a selectable marker (*33*). One cosmid was selected which caused an aflatoxin-negative, nitrate-nonutilizing mutant to produce aflatoxin. A 1.7-kb restriction fragment from this cosmid was found to be responsible for renewed aflatoxin production.

Two new mutants of *A. flavus* with altered patterns of aflatoxin production were recently isolated and characterized (*34*). One mutant was able to synthesize aflatoxin in the absence of carbohydrate (normally a non-permissive condition) during growth without a lag period. Another mutant produced no aflatoxin either in the presence or absence of carbohydrate. Chemical mutagenesis of this latter strain produced mutants which could synthesize aflatoxin in carbohydrate-containing media after a lag period during log phase growth. These mutants may be useful in studying the regulation of aflatoxin synthesis.

Two aflatoxin-negative *A. parasiticus* strains (SRRC 163 and SRRC 2043), when grown together in synthetic liquid media or on seeds were found to complement each other (*35*). SRRC 2043 was found to accumulate O-methylsterigmatocystin, a late precursor in AFB_1 synthesis, whereas SRRC 163 accumulated averantin, an early precursor. No mycelial contact was required between these two mutants for

aflatoxin synthesis to occur, indicating that a chemical rather than a genetic mechanism of complementation was involved

An aflatoxin-negative mutant of *A. parasiticus* (NIAH-26) was found to contain desaturase activity which converts versicolorin B (VB) to versicolorin A (VA) (*36*). When the mold was fed VA, it was capable of synthesizing AFB_1 and AFG_1; when fed VB or VC, the mold produced AFB_2 and AFG_2 as well as AFB_1 and AFG_1. These results indicate that the branching step between AFB_1 and AFB_2 corresponds to the desaturation reaction from VB to VA.

NIAH-26 can also produce aflatoxins when fed versiconal hemiacetal acetate (VHA), versiconol acetate (VOAc), and versiconol (VOH) (*37*). The insecticide dichlorvos was able to inhibit aflatoxin production from VHA and VOAc but not that from VOH or VB. From these and other metabolic studies, it appears that VHA and versiconal (VHOH) are reversibly converted to VOAc and VOH, respectively, by dehydrogenase enzymes which are insensitive to dichlorvos. VHA and VOAc are converted to VHOH and VOH, respectively, by esterase enzymes which are sensitive to dichlorvos.

OCCURRENCE AND CONTROL OF AFLATOXINS IN FOODS AND FOOD COMPONENTS. In a recent article, the occurrence of aflatoxins in foods and their biosynthesis and toxic effects on living organisms were comprehensively reviewed (*38*). Methods for detection and for control of these toxins were described and discussed along with future research needs, including alternative methods of control and mathematical modeling of factors influencing aflatoxin production.

Another review focused on food safety issues related to bound residues of aflatoxins in feeds and tissues of food-producing animals (*39*). Ammoniation appears to be a safe and effective method for decontamination of feeds containing aflatoxin residues but there is still some concern about the toxicity and potential carcinogenicity of aflatoxin/ammonia reaction products in human foods derived from animals fed ammoniated aflatoxin-contaminated feed. Evaluation of the safety of these reaction products and of other bound residues of aflatoxins in animal tissues was discussed.

High incidences and levels of aflatoxin contamination (up to 400 ppb) occurred in corn grown in some regions of midwestern and southern USA in 1988. To assess the potential for contamination in edible tissues of food-producing animals, samples of liver and muscle tissue were analyzed in January 1989 (from hogs fed corn soon after harvest) and in April 1989 (from hogs fed corn which was stored and then fed in the spring (*40,41*). Three of 60 liver samples from January and 9 of 100 taken in April were found to contain AFB$_1$ at levels of 0.01–0.24 ppb. Four of these samples also had detectable levels of AFM$_1$ (0.03–0.44 ppb). No aflatoxins were detected in any muscle tissue. These results demonstrate that aflatoxin levels in meat were low and unlikely to pose a health hazard even in this year when high aflatoxin levels would be expected in feed.

The most interesting and aromatic varieties of Spanish ham are cured for some time during which a superficial mold growth develops. *Aspergillus* and *Penicillium* were the most common genera isolated from 65 such dry-salted hams (*42*). Of 16 strains of *A. flavus* tested, only 9 produced aflatoxins in vitro. To examine whether aflatoxins can be produced in ham, samples of ham were inoculated with *A. parasiticus* NRRL-2999 and incubated at 5, 15, 25, and 30°C for 20 days. No growth occurred at 5°C and growth but no aflatoxins were seen at 15°C. Low levels of AFB$_1$ and AFG$_1$ were detected at the higher temperatures: 0.72 and 1.73 µg/kg at 25 and 30°C, respectively.

A survey of 168 rabbits, 94 pheasants and 56 deer living in the wild in Czechoslovakia revealed the presence of aflatoxins in their livers and kidneys (*43*). Average concentrations of 0.407, 0.329, and 0.696 µg/kg were found in liver and of 0.658, 0.679, and 0.794 µg/kg were found in the kidneys of these animals, respectively. Higher values were generally found in those animals living near silage trenches, haybarns, and slurry pits.

The pharmacokinetics and tissue distribution of ^{14}C-labelled AFB$_1$ were investigated after an oral dose (250 µg/kg body weight) in farm-raised channel catfish (*44*). Peak plasma and tissue concentrations (596 ppb and 40 ppb, respectively) occurred about 4 hours after dosing and then rapidly declined

to 32 and <5 ppb, respectively, after 24 hours. AFB$_1$ and its metabolites were detected at low levels in urine and bile (<5% of the administered dose), indicating incomplete absorption. These data demonstrate a very low potential for the accumulation of AFB$_1$ and its metabolites in channel catfish following consumption of contaminated feed.

In a survey of 376 samples of raw milk from farms in Czechoslovakia, 87.8% of the samples contained no AFM$_1$ and only 2 samples had concentrations >0.1 µg/mL (*45*). Commercial immunokits with a detection limit of 0.025 µg/mL were used to analyze the milk samples.

Hydrated sodium calcium aluminosilicate (HSCAS), used as an anticaking agent in agricultural feeds, was evaluated for its potential to reduce AFM$_1$ residues in milk of cows fed aflatoxin-contaminated feed (*46*). Inclusion of 0.5% HSCAS in feed containing 200 µg aflatoxin/kg reduced average AFM$_1$ secretion into milk by about 24% (from pretreatment of 1.85 µg/L to 1.41 µg/L). Addition of 1% HSCAS to feed containing 100 µg aflatoxin/kg reduced AFM$_1$ secretion by 44% (from 0.91 µg/L to 0.51 µg/L). These results indicate that HSCAS may be useful in preventing high levels of secretion of AFM$_1$ into milk.

Climatic conditions in the tropics along with late harvesting of crops and inadequate storage facilities are conducive to mycotoxin contamination of foodstuffs. During a 3-year survey in Bihar state (India), 162 of 416 samples of wheat, gram, and maize flours tested positive for aflatoxins (*47*). In all, 58% of maize, 33% of wheat, and 28% of gram flour samples were contaminated, with maximum concentrations of 2048, 1056, and 682 µg/kg, respectively, of AFB$_1$ detected. Some samples also contained AFB$_2$ and AFG$_1$. The high incidence of contamination may be related to high moisture levels (14%) in the flour. Of 100 samples of a variety of foods tested in Nigeria, 18 contained detectable levels of aflatoxins (*48*). The highest incidences were found in yam flour and in cassava flour with 7.6 and 5.4 µg/g, respectively, as the greatest concentrations.

AFB$_1$ was detected by enzyme-linked immunosorbent assay (ELISA) in 11 of 14 samples of maize imported into Japan (*49*). Highest levels were found in 2 lots from Thailand (23.3 and 31.2 ng/g); 4.3 and 7.3 ng/g were the highest concentrations determined in samples from the USA and the People's Republic of China, respectively.

In a recent review, various aspects of aflatoxin contamination of preharvest corn were discussed: the infection process, direct infection of corn, involvement of insects in infection, sources of inoculum, and factors affecting aflatoxin production (50). Management practices to reduce aflatoxin contamination, breeding for resistant varieties, and other control strategies were also discussed.

Another review focused on the role of insects in preharvest aflatoxin contamination of corn and genetic aspects of resistance to aflatoxin production in corn (51). High aflatoxin levels in corn have been associated with infestations of the corn earworm, fall armyworm, and the European corn borer. Numerous attempts to produce resistant corn varieties were described, but to date no known genotypes of corn are resistant to aflatoxin production. One proposed control strategy involves the prior inoculation of corn kernels with atoxigenic strains of *A. flavus*. In a field plot experiment in Louisiana, coinoculation of atoxigenic with toxigenic strains decreased aflatoxin production to 21–24% of the control levels (toxigenic strain only) (52). Inoculation with the atoxigenic strain 24 hours prior to inoculation with the toxigenic strain reduced aflatoxin levels to about 5% of control in preharvest corn.

Several fungal species which coexist with *A. flavus* in nature were evaluated for their influence on aflatoxin synthesis by *A. flavus* on corn seeds incubated at 28°C for 10 days (53). All 13 fungal associations inhibited AFB_1 and AFG_1 synthesis by 34.3 to 100%. Associations of *A. flavus* with *A. niger*, with *A. candidus* and *Fusarium oxysporum*, with *F. oxysporum* and *Rhizopus nigricans*, and with *A. niger* and *Penicillium chrysogenum* resulted in >88% inhibition of aflatoxin synthesis.

Aflatoxin synthesis by *A. flavus* was also markedly inhibited in vitro by culture media on which *A. niger* had grown (54). Use of pH-adjusted controls indicated that this was not simply a pH effect but was probably due to some metabolites produced by *A. niger*.

Both water activity (a_w) and temperature are known to influence aflatoxin synthesis. In a series of experiments to examine these parameters, *A. flavus* and *A. parasiticus* were grown on batches of irradiated maize kernels maintained at 25, 30, and 35°C and at 0.90, 0.95, and 0.98 a_w (55). Maximum aflatoxin production for *A. parasiticus* was at 25°C and 0.98 a_w and for *A. flavus* was at 30°C and 0.98 or 0.95 a_w. At 0.90 a_w, both species produced low levels of aflatoxins at all temperatures.

During an 8-year period (1982–1989), a total of 2510 randomly chosen, commercially available samples of peanut butter in Virginia were tested for aflatoxin contamination (56). Although 74% of the samples tested had detectable levels of aflatoxins, only 9.8% had levels exceeding the USDA action level for total aflatoxin (20 ppb). Of the samples testing positive, 8.6% contained 20–50 ppb, 3.7% contained 50–100 ppb, and 2.2% contained >100 ppb total aflatoxins. Highest levels of aflatoxin were detected in 1987 with 90% of the samples testing positive, nearly 30% having concentrations >20 ppb, and one sample with 215 ppb total aflatoxins. In some other years (1982 and 1989), there was a low incidence of positive samples (28% and 44%) and none of the samples had >20 ppb aflatoxins.

As with other foods, tropical climatic conditions present a challenge to the safe storage of groundnuts. In a 3-year study in Côte d'Ivoire, nearly all locally stored groundnuts were contaminated with aflatoxins (57). Nearly 8% of the stocks exceeded the toxicity level threshold of 250 ppb and 4.4% exceeded 1000 ppb. Significant correlations were found between aflatoxin contamination and several damage and rainfall parameters.

From a pool of 1107 groundnut genotypes screened for natural seed infection by *A. flavus* in India, genotypes with a seed infection rate of <2% were evaluated for resistance to field infection of seed by *A. flavus* in India and in Senegal (58). Twenty strains were resistant to field infection and some of these also had acceptable pod yields and commercial quality.

Aflatoxins were detected in 5.8% of 34 soybean samples harvested in 1986 and in 11.6% of 60 samples harvested in 1987 in Argentina (59).

Contamination levels were low, ranging from traces to 36 µg/kg. To examine the potential for aflatoxin production, 13 varieties of soybeans were inoculated with 1 strain of *A. parasiticus* and 2 strains of *A. flavus* and incubated at 25°C for 7 days. More AFB_1 was produced by *A. parasiticus* (7,500–20,800 µg/kg) than by *A. flavus* (25–7,000 µg/kg), with considerable differences for different varieties of soybeans. These results indicate that significant levels of aflatoxins can be produced on soybeans under optimal conditions.

AFB_1 was also detected in chickpeas stored in jute bags (up to 205 µg/kg) and in metal bins (up to 130 µg/kg) in Bihar, India (60). Chickpeas entering storage had a moisture content of 13% and a variety of "field" fungi were detected. During storage, moisture levels rose to 15.2% (jute bags) and 14% (metal bins). "Field" fungi gradually died off and "storage" fungi, including *Aspergillus* spp. and *Penicillium* spp., appeared. AFB_1 was detected after 3 months' storage in jute bags and after 6 months in metal bins. Of 61 isolates of *A. parasiticus*, 84% were toxigenic while only 64% of 569 isolates of *A. flavus* were toxigenic in culture.

Raw and parboiled rice from major rice producing/milling areas in Sri Lanka were surveyed for aflatoxin contamination (61). In general, the 329 parboiled rice samples had a greater incidence of contamination and higher levels of aflatoxins than the raw rice (156 samples). Some moldy parboiled rice samples with a fermented odor contained >1000 µg AFB_1/kg. Inoculation of commercially parboiled rice with a toxigenic strain of *A. flavus* resulted in 60–92 µg AFB_1/kg while much lower levels (12–29 µg/kg) were found in traditional "cottage" processed rice (62). AFB_1 content increased in proportion to the duration of soaking (24–144 hours).

Aflatoxins were detected in 13 of 24 lots of sunflower seeds in Pakistan (63). Highest concentrations of AFB_1 and AFB_2 were 437 and 14 µg/kg, respectively. Of 41 isolates of *A. flavus*, 29 produced aflatoxins in culture—up to 467 µg/L of AFB_1 and 234 µg/L of AFB_2.

Examination of 20 samples each of cocoa, roasted coffee, and tea powders collected from markets in Egypt revealed that nearly all of them were contaminated with *Aspergillus* spp. and many also contained *Penicillium* spp. (64). Many other genera of fungi were also identified. Six samples (2 of cocoa and 4 of tea) were toxic to brine shrimp and proved to be contaminated with aflatoxins (2.8–21.7 µg/kg). To test the potential for each of these powders to serve as substrates for aflatoxin production, samples of each were inoculated with *A. flavus* and incubated at 28°C for 2 weeks and then at 10°C for a further 2 weeks. Aflatoxin production was 1.4, 30, and 72 µg/kg dry substrate for coffee, cocoa, and tea, respectively.

Research since 1986 on mycotoxin contamination of herbs and spices and methods for reducing fungal and toxin levels was recently reviewed (65). Of 21 varieties of spices examined, those most commonly contaminated were "chillie" (capsicum) and nutmeg, with mean aflatoxin levels of 10 and 13 µg/kg, respectively. Caraway, clove, cumin, and thyme oil inhibited growth of *A. parasiticus* and aflatoxin production. Other studies indicated that irradiation can substantially reduce fungal counts and decompose AFB_1.

Mold contamination was observed in all 31 kinds of spices and herbs collected from markets in Spain (66). Some, such as whole nutmeg and ground cloves, cumin, and tarragon, were only slightly contaminated while others were very highly contaminated with $>10^5$ spores/gram. AFB_1 and AFB_2 were detected in only 4 cultures (two of mint, 1 of ground mustard, 1 of artemisia) at concentrations up to 0.55 and 0.27 µg/g.

AFB_1 was detected in 12 of 32 samples of betel nut collected in markets in several northern Indian cities (67). The range of aflatoxin concentrations in positive samples was 18–208 µg/kg. Incubation of betel nuts with propionic acid (0.5%), boric acid (0.5%), or potassium metabisulfite (1%) resulted in an inhibition of aflatoxin production during 4 weeks at 27°C. Propionic acid was the most effective preservative by causing an 85% inhibition of AFB_1 production at 4 weeks as compared to the control.

Treatment of poultry diet with 6 kGy of gamma irradiation completely inhibited growth and aflatoxin production by *A. flavus* for 10 days at 27°C (68). Growth and toxin production were also completely inhibited by 0.64% sodium propionate, 0.134% potassium sorbate, and 0.1% sodium bisulfite. Equally effective combination treatments were 0.48% sodium propionate, 0.022% potassium sorbate, or 0.0334% sodium bisulfite with 3 kGy of gamma-irradiation.

Experiments with two cassava products, gari and lafun, indicated that both hydrogen peroxide and sodium metabisulfite could partially degrade AFB_1 present in them (69). Sodium metabisulfite (1%) reduced AFB_1 levels in bitter cassava from 348 to 131 µg/kg during gari production and hydrogen peroxide (9%) reduced AFB_1 levels in sweet cassava from 150 to 75 µg/kg during lafun production.

Three natural coumarins, xanthotoxin, bergapten, and psoralene, and two natural chromones, khellin and visnagin, were evaluated for their ability to inhibit mycelial growth and aflatoxin production by *A. flavus* in rice/corn steep liquor medium after 6 days at 25°C (70). Mold growth was only slightly inhibited by all of these compounds but xanthotoxin and khellin at 5 mM completely inhibited aflatoxin production. At this concentration, the other 3 compounds reduced aflatoxin production to only 12 to 16% of the control level.

Growth and toxin production by *A. flavus* was also inhibited by eucalyptus oil (0.05, 0.1, and 0.2 mL/50 mL medium) during 6 days at 28°C in sucrose growth medium (71). However, after 12 days' incubation, AFB_1 concentrations were higher in media with eucalyptus oil than in the control. The medium with the highest concentration of eucalyptus oil contained 0.12 µg AFB_1/mg dry weight compared to the control, with 0.046 µg/mg.

AFB_1 production in corn and cottonseed by *A. flavus* was completely inhibited by 20 µL of the C_6 to C_9 alkenals in the atmosphere of the culture flasks (72). At the same levels, these alkenals caused only about a 30% inhibition of aflatoxin production on peanuts. These alkenals are decay products of poly-unsaturated fatty acids in plants and are produced when leaves are injured.

DETECTION AND DETERMINATION OF AFLA-TOXINS. A quality assurance program for non-governmental laboratories involved in the determination of aflatoxins in agricultural products intended for export was recently instituted in India (73). Twelve such laboratories were provided with check samples of naturally contaminated groundnut meal and of aflatoxin-free maize meal along with authentic reference standards of AFB_1 and AFB_2. Any standard international method routinely used in these laboratories could be used for the analyses. Eight laboratories returned analytical results to the coordinating laboratory. Seven reported no aflatoxin in the maize. Coefficients of variation for analyses of AFB_1 and AFB_2 in groundnut meal ranged from 11 to 29% and from 5 to 42%, respectively.

Several commercially available analytical systems for aflatoxin determination were evaluated. Mycosep, a multifunctional cleanup column for one-step extract purification, was successfully used in the analysis of 10 different grain and nut products and for cottonseed, fig paste, and mixed feeds (74). Samples were extracted with acetonitrile–water (9+1) and then forced through the Mycosep column for cleanup. AFB_1 and AFG_1 were converted to their hemiacetals and analyzed by liquid chromatography (LC) with fluorescence detection. Average recoveries were >95% for aflatoxins B_1, B_2, G_1, and G_2, and coefficients of variation were <3%.

Analysis of a series of 8 contaminated maize samples (approximately 0.16–22.0 ppb total aflatoxins) using the Aflatest immunoaffinity method yielded results which were not significantly different from those achieved with a traditional chemical method for aflatoxin extraction (75). The traditional method was lengthy, requiring more than 1 day to complete, and consumed large quantities of organic solvents (methanol, chloroform, and hexane). In contrast, an Aflatest analysis can be completed in 30 minutes and only about 150 mL of methanol and 1 mL of Aflatest developer are used.

Of 51 samples of aflatoxin-contaminated corn analyzed by LC and by CITE PROBE (an ELISA screening test with a positive/negative cutoff of 5 ng AFB_1/g), CITE PROBE correctly identified 47 (76). Each test probe was read by two analysts to assess the ability of the human eye to properly discern color intensity. (This can be difficult with samples near the cutoff concentration.) Two tests incorrectly interpreted by both analysts contained

4.4 and 4.1 ng AFB_1/g. The other two incorrect responses were correctly interpreted by one of the two analysts. This ELISA method appears to be very reliable.

A solid phase extraction/HPLC method for the determination of aflatoxins in groundnut meal has been developed and validated (*77*). Samples were extracted with acetone:water (85:15) and then cleaned up on a phenyl-bonded column prior to HPLC quantitation. Higher recoveries (101.3%) of AFB_1 were achieved using this system as compared to the official AOAC method. Limits of detection for AFB_1 and AFB_2 were 7.4 and 2.62 µg/kg, respectively. This proposed procedure was also far less time consuming and more economical on solvents.

Although ELISA methods for detection of aflatoxins in agricultural products have proven useful in developed countries, their relatively high cost and requirement for refrigeration limits their use in developing countries. A less expensive alternative for field analyses is an aflatoxin detection kit containing activated pressure minicolumns, aflatoxin standard columns, a blank, and a UV viewing chamber in addition to a grinder, a balance, solvents and glassware. A field evaluation in India of 88 groundnut samples and 20 groundnut meal samples using this kit gave results comparable to those obtained in a laboratory by conventional thin-layer chromatography (TLC) for 89% of the groundnut and for 100% of the groundnut meal samples (*78*). Aflatoxins were overestimated in 5% and underestimated in 6% of the groundnut samples. Further field trials should be carried out in other developing countries.

Using a new procedure for determination of aflatoxins in palm kernel extracts by TLC, consistent recoveries of >90% were achieved for spiked samples (*79*). Detection limits were 3.7, 2.5, 3.0, and 1.3 µg/kg for AFB_1, AFB_2, AFG_1, and AFG_2, respectively. The proposed procedure was found to be more efficient and precise than the British standard method. Palm kernel samples were extracted with acetone–water (80+20) and then cleaned up by solid phase extraction using a phenyl-bonded phase cartridge. Aflatoxins were eluted with chloroform and then quantified using bidirectional high-performance TLC.

A one-step ELISA using a highly sensitive and specific antibody to AFB_1 was compared with other analytical methods (LC and TLC) for the detection of AFB_1 in naturally contaminated corn and mixed feeds (*80*). Detection limit of the ELISA was as low as 100 pg/assay. Analysis of 20 samples of corn by the three methods revealed correlation coefficients of 0.93 between ELISA and TLC and 0.96 between ELISA and LC. However, corresponding correlation coefficients for the mixed feed samples were only 0.57 and 0.46. Further purification of the feed samples by column chromatography prior to ELISA resulted in better correlation between results from the three methods of analysis (0.90).

Immuno precolumns, short columns packed with immobilized antibodies, can be very useful in pretreating samples prior to LC analysis. A column switching system using such a precolumn was developed to automate the determination of aflatoxins in biological samples (*81*). The system was comprised of 3 columns: (a) an anti-aflatoxin immuno precolumn which first adsorbed aflatoxins—aflatoxins were then desorbed with methanol:water (70:30); (b) a C-18 precolumn to reconcentrate the aflatoxins; (c) an LC separation column. Analysis time was about 45 minutes with a detection limit of 10 ng/L. Important steps in optimizing the procedure, regeneration and stability of the immuno precolumn and general applicability of the procedure were discussed. This system efficiently determined AFM_1 levels in milk but, unlike with aqueous samples, with milk a new immuno precolumn had to be used for each sample.

However, such immuno precolumns could be reused in milk analyses if a dialysis unit was incorporated into the system (*82*). A hollow-fibre dialysis unit working according to the stagnant donor-flowing acceptor principle gave better results than a flat membrane dialysis unit working according to the flowing donor-flowing acceptor principle. Interfering compounds were efficiently removed allowing detection of 10 ng AFM_1/L in milk and the use of a single immuno column for over 70 analyses. Recovery of AFM_1 from spiked milk samples was only 6% but this was not expected to be a problem in real samples because relatively large sample volumes could be processed.

An ELISA using antibody-coated polystyrene beads was compared with an HPLC method for the determination of AFM_1 in 46 samples of raw milk (*83*). AFM_1 concentrations measured by the two methods were not statistically significantly different. The upper value of the measuring range for the bead method was 30 pg AFM_1/mL and the lower detection limit was estimated to be 12 pg/mL. Repeatability of results was similar for both methods.

Recent experiments demonstrated that HPLC/Thermospray mass spectrometry can unequivocally identify the aflatoxins in peanuts (*84*). Artificially contaminated peanut samples were extracted using a methanol:water mixture and then cleaned up on series-connected SPE columns. Finally, the extracts were applied to a reversed-phase HPLC column with a thermospray mass detector. Distinct peaks were obtained for AFB_1, AFB_2, AFG_1, and AFG_2, demonstrating that this method may be used for confirmation of different aflatoxins.

Tremorgenic mycotoxins

Four fumitremorgins have previously been identified from rice and home-made miso infected with *Aspergillus fumigatus* and associated with neurotoxic symptoms in humans. A new fumitremorgin has been isolated from cultures of *A. fumigatus* and its structure characterized by mass spectroscopy and NMR (*85*). It was detected only in cells under resting conditions and was second in amount to verruculogen, a previously described fumitremorgin.

Territrems A, B, and C (TRA, TRB, and TRC), isolated from rice cultures of *A. terreus*, induce sustained whole body tremors when injected into rats and mice. In order to elucidate their metabolism in laboratory animals, the biotransformation of territrems by the hepatic S9 fraction of rats pretreated with phenobarbital, 3-methyl-cholanthrene, or polychlorinated biphenyl was investigated (*86*). In this system TRA yielded two metabolites (MA_1 and MA_2), TRB yielded 4 metabolites (MB_1–MB_4), and TRC yielded 1 metabolite, MC. MS and NMR analyses revealed that MB_4 = TRC and MC = MB_1. The various metabolites were identified as products of hydroxylation and *O*-demethylation reactions.

MYCOTOXINS PRODUCED BY *PENICILLIUM* SPP.

Ochratoxins

Ochratoxin A (OA), produced by several species of *Aspergillus* and *Penicillium*, induces nephropathy in some animal species and is suspected of being the main etiologic agent in Balkan endemic nephropathy and associated urinary tract tumors in humans. Since OA has also been reported to alter a variety of biochemical parameters in the blood of rats, experiments were carried out to test its effects on platelet aggregation (*87*). A dose-dependent, irreversible inhibition of agonist-induced platelet aggregation was observed in vitro. OA also inhibited serotonin secretion and arachidonic acid release and metabolism, suggesting that this toxin acts by disrupting the integrity of the plasma membrane.

Administration of high doses of OA to rats (6 mg/kg/day) by gavage for 8 weeks significantly reduced in vivo absorption of ^{14}C-glucose and ^{14}C-glycine (*88*). Activities of several membrane-bound enzymes were also reduced, providing further evidence that OA damages plasma membranes.

Methods for preparation of ^{14}C-labelled OA and ochratoxin B (OB) were developed, and the resulting labelled compounds were injected into rats to study their distribution patterns (*89*). Results were similar for OA and OB except that OA was retained longer in the blood and OB appeared to be metabolized in tissues while no metabolites of OA could be detected. It was expected that tissue distribution in rats would differ from that previously described in mice because rats are highly susceptible to OA-induced cancer while mice are not. But this was not so: distribution patterns for the two species were very similar.

Four Egyptian strains of *A. ochraceus* and one of *A. alliaceus* examined for OA production were found to produce greater amounts of ochratoxins when grown on a yeast extract–sucrose medium than on a wheat solid medium (*90*). One other strain of *A. ochraceus* was more productive on the wheat medium. Maximum yields of OA did not coincide with peak fungal growth and, in most cases, OA levels in culture filtrates exceeded those in the mycelia.

Irradiation (1 kGy) of *A. alutaceus* NRRL 3174 growing on barley produced several color mutants with altered levels of OA production (*91*). Greater levels of OA were detected in lighter colored mutants: white and yellow variants produced 9.3 and 4.6 times as much OA as the ochre parent while a red variant produced only 0.09 times as much OA as the parent strain. These mutants may be useful in elucidating the regulatory control of OA biosynthesis.

Samples of muscle tissue (63), serum (255), healthy kidneys (63), and kidneys with macroscopic lesions (96) from Czechoslovakian swine were collected at a slaughterhouse and analyzed for OA residues by use of a commercial immunoassay kit (*92*). Detection limits for this assay were 1 µg/kg for tissue and 0.1 µg/L for serum. None of the muscle tissues tested positive and only one healthy kidney sample contained >1 µg OA/kg. Twenty of the kidneys with lesions had detectable OA but only 2 of them were >5 µg OA/kg (the Czechoslovak tolerance level for OA in children's food). For the serum samples (all from healthy pigs), 57% had detectable OA with an average of 1.9 µg/L. Only 5 serum samples contained >5 µg/L.

Of 191 liver and kidney samples randomly selected from slaughter pigs in Germany, 2.6% of liver and 3.7% of kidney samples contained >25 ppb OA (*93*). Mean OA concentrations in liver and kidney were 2.01 and 2.45 ppb, respectively.

From October 1989 to September 1990, 706 serum samples from swine slaughtered at two locations in Sweden were monitored for OA residues (*94*). OA levels in the positive herds ranged from 2 to 45 ng/mL with a mean of 5.2 ng/mL. Samples of feed used for 22 contaminated and 21 non-contaminated herds were also examined. Although total mold content in all the feeds was similar, significantly higher levels of *Aspergillus* spp. and *Penicillium* spp., particularly *P. verrucosum*, were found in the feed of OA-contaminated herds.

Influence of moisture, acid, and alkali on heat-induced degradation and detoxification of OA was investigated in a series of experiments (*95*).

Decomposition was detected by thin-layer chromatography (TLC) and toxicity was assessed with HeLa cell cultures. Heating of OA to 200°C under dry conditions had little effect on OA. Heating of moist and watery samples under neutral and acidic conditions to 175°C appeared to cause some degradation of OA but did not reduce cytotoxicity. Heating to 175°C in 0.1 N NaOH, however, resulted in both decomposition and detoxification. Several decomposition products, including phenylalanine, were observed on TLC.

A rapid HPLC method for the determination of low concentrations of OA in serum has been developed (*96*). Samples of serum were extracted with chloroform, chromatographed isocratically on a C_{18} column with methanol:water:acetic acid (30:70:1) as the mobile phase, and then quantitated by fluorescence. Recovery of OA from spiked samples (5–50 ng/mL) was 87–94%. This procedure was faster and more sensitive than the enzymatic spectrofluorometric method.

A solid-phase extraction and cleanup procedure has also been used prior to liquid chromatography (LC) for the determination of OA (*97*). A SEP PAK C_{18} was used for swine serum and a SEP PAK silica cartridge for pig feed samples. Temperature controlled esterification of the toxin resulted in a mixture of free and methylated OA on the same chromatogram. The fluorescent peak height of OA was used for quantitation while the ratio of free to methylated forms was used for confirmation of OA.

Results from an interlaboratory study of a rapid, solvent-efficient LC method for determination of OA in barley, corn, and swine kidney tissue indicated that this method was suitable for barley and corn but not for kidney (*98*). Sixteen laboratories in Europe and North America analyzed identical sets of spiked barley and corn (10, 20, and 50 ng OA/g) and kidney (5, 10, and 20 ng/g) samples using a standard protocol. Mean recoveries were 72–74% for barley, 77–82% for corn, and 53–97% for kidney. Within-laboratory relative standard deviations were 7.9, 20.1, and 15.7% for barley, corn and kidney tissue, respectively. Interlaboratory relative standard deviations were 20–31.7% for all OA concentrations in barley and corn but

32.7–68% for kidney tissue. This method has been adopted official first action by AOAC as quantitative at the levels tested for OA determination in corn and barley.

A novel procedure to confirm OA-positive results from HPLC down to the HPLC detection limit of 0.1 ppb has been developed (*99*). OA in the sample extract was converted to its *O*-methylochratoxin A methyl ester derivative which was then identified by GC–MS negative ion chemical ionization and multiple ion detection modes using the hexadeuterated *O*-methyl-d$_3$ ester derivative as internal standard for quantitation. The procedure was found to be very accurate in analyses of more than 60 contaminated samples.

Cyclopiazonic acid

In a survey of maize to identify cultivars resistant to production of cyclopiazonic acid (CPA), surface-sterilized maize seeds of 15 cultivars were inoculated with *P. griseofulvum* and stored for 30 days at 27–29°C (*100*). After incubation, most of the strains contained 225–277 µg CPA/200 g seeds. The most resistant variety had 85 µg CPA/200 g.

A liquid chromatographic method with quantitation limits of 50 and 100 ng/g, respectively, for corn and peanuts has been developed for CPA determination (*101*). CPA was extracted with methanol–2% NaHCO$_3$ (7+3), then defatted with hexane, and cleaned up on a Sep-Pak silica cartridge. A reversed phase LC column with a linear gradient of 0–4 mM ZnSO$_4$ in methanol–water (85+15) and UV detection at 279 nm resolved and quantified CPA. The ZnSO$_4$ gradient separated CPA from an interfering substance which had a similar retention time on the LC column. Recoveries of CPA from samples spiked with 50–500 ng CPA/g were 72–84% for corn and 74–80% for peanuts.

A competitive ELISA using anti-CPA antisera from rabbits was capable of determining 30 pg to 2 ng CPA in samples and showed an interassay variability of 3.7% and a between-day variability of 14% (*102*). This method allowed detection of CPA even at low levels in agar surface cultures of *Penicillium* spp. and could be used for screening fungal isolates for CPA production.

Citrinin

Renal toxicity in pigs, poultry, and laboratory animals has been attributed to ingestion of citrinin-contaminated feed. Two recent investigations indicate that these toxic effects are mediated through disruption of mitochondrial respiration in renal cells. Exposure of rat renal proximal tubules and isolated renal cortical mitochondria to 63–500 µM citrinin for 1–4 hours caused multiple effects on mitochondrial function, including alterations in ATP content and oxygen consumption (103). Furthermore, citrinin (10–1000 µM) inhibited almost all of the enzymes linked to the respiratory chain and decreased the membrane potential of energized mitochondria in a concentration-dependent fashion (*104*).

Experiments to determine the thermal decomposition and detoxification of citrinin under various moisture conditions were described and discussed in two reports (*105,106*). Cytotoxicity was assessed using HeLa cells, and decomposition was monitored using TLC and UV and fluorescence spectrophotometry. Both decomposition and detoxification occurred when citrinin was heated to 175°C under dry conditions, to 160°C under wet conditions (200 µg citrinin + 150 µL water), or to 140°C under semi-moist conditions (200 µg citrinin + 8 µL water). Although citrinin in water was degraded at 140°C, its decomposition products were as toxic or more toxic than citrinin itself.

Patulin

In a survey of 64 wheat samples collected from flour factories in eastern Spain, no patulin was detected but a patulin-producing mold, *P. griseofulvum* was isolated from 19 samples (*107*). Samples were analyzed by TLC with fluorescence detection. When patulin was added to wheat it was very unstable, disappearing in just a few days. In culture media, however, as much as 11.9 mg patulin/100 mL broth could be produced by stationary cultures of a wheat isolate of *P. griseofulvum* at 28°C.

Cytotoxic effects of patulin were examined in an immortalized rat granulosa cell line (*108*). When cells were incubated with 0.1–1000 µM patulin, a dose- and time-dependent decrease in glutathione (GSH) was observed. Other effects included a dose-dependent influx of Ca^{2+}, a reduction in intercellular communication, and decrease in intracellular pH. Thus, patulin appears to affect plasma membranes as well as cellular GSH levels and mitochondrial function.

Luteoskyrin

Luteoskyrin (LS), a mycotoxin produced by *P. islandicum*, is known to be hepatocarcinogenic in rodents. The in vitro transforming activity of this mycotoxin was recently demonstrated using mouse embryonal Balb/3T3 A31-1-1 cells (*109*). LS (0.5 µg/mL) induced type III foci in the cell cultures, and transplantation of these transformants into nude mice confirmed their tumorigenicity. Examination of cloned transformants revealed transcriptional activation of *c-myc* and *c-HA-ras* oncogenes.

Because of the quinoid moiety in its structure, LS was expected to generate hydroxy radicals in vivo. Experiments with ddY mice gavaged with 100 mg LS/kg demonstrated some significant alterations in serum biochemistry indicative of hepatic and renal damage (*110*). Time- and dose-dependent increases in hepatic 8-OH-dG and hepatic lipid peroxides were also observed. Injections of α-tocopherol (100 mg/kg) given the same day as LS reduced the level of hepatic peroxides but not that of 8-OH-dG.

Secalonic acid D

To elucidate dose–response relationships between teratogenic, neurotoxic effects and secalonic acid D (SAD) exposure in infant mice, neonates were dosed orally with 0–5 mg SAD/kg/day from postnatal day 3 through 35 (*111*). Even doses as low as 0.625 mg/kg/day significantly delayed ontogeny of swimming and cliff avoidance while mice receiving higher doses (2.5 mg/kg/day) showed toxic signs such as body tremors, uncoordinated movements and terminal coma. Brain norepinephrine levels were unchanged by all doses of SAD but dopamine levels significantly increased on day 13 and decreased on day 20 in the olfactory lobe of mice dosed with 1.25 mg/kg/day.

Eremofortin C and PR toxin

Factors affecting production of eremofortin C (EC) and PR toxin by *P. roqueforti* were investigated (*112*). Of 17 ATCC strains screened, 13 produced both EC and PR toxin. Higher toxin levels were produced when fungi were grown on cereals rather than on legumes, and addition of aqueous corn extracts to culture media greatly stimulated toxin production. The most toxigenic strain (ATCC 48936) produced maximal toxin levels in stationary cultures at 24°C and pH 4.0 (2,100 µg EC/mL and 1,427 µg PR toxin/mL).

Pennigritrem

Penitrem tremorgenic mycotoxins, produced by *Penicillium* spp., usually occur as a complex mixture of penitrems A–F, with penitrem A as the principal component. A new and abundant analog of penitrem A, designated pennigritrem, has been isolated and characterized from culture filtrates of *P. nigricans* (*113*). Its structure, as determined by NMR, involves the terminal diterpenoid isoprene in a cyclization which is unique among fungal indolediterpenoid compounds. This new toxin was the principal mycotoxin formed in stationary cultures by *P. nigricans* but was not produced by *P. crustosum*. Pennigritrem is less tremorgenic than penitrem A, perhaps because the cyclization impairs its binding to functional sites of neurological disturbance.

MYCOTOXINS PRODUCED BY *FUSARIUM* SPP.

Trichothecenes

GENERAL

Biological effects. Different environmental conditions and different substrates potentiate the synthesis of various trichothecene mycotoxins, and often more than one trichothecene is found in a given food or feedstuff. To examine possible interactions among different trichothecenes, deoxynivalenol (DON), 15-acetyldeoxynivalenol (15-ADON), and HT-2 toxin were tested alone and in combination in the Chick Embryotoxicity Screening Test (*114*). Toxin concentrations tested were: HT-2, 0.074–0.48 µg/egg; 15-ADON, 3.3–7.2 µg/egg; DON, 2.9–5.3 µg/egg. The combined cytotoxic effects of any two toxins were generally additive but not synergistic.

Synergistic effects of some trichothecene combinations were observed on carbon dioxide production by yeast (*115*). Carbon dioxide release was inhibited by 50% in <65 minutes by 0.0625, 0.125, 1.25, and 12.5 µg/mL of verrucarin A, roridin A, T-2 toxin, and HT-2 toxin, respectively. Neither 0.0625 µg T-2 toxin/mL nor 0.000125 µg roridin A/mL alone affected carbon dioxide production but together they inhibited its release by 50% within 60 minutes. This study indicates that when several mycotoxins are present in a food, the permissible levels for single toxins may be unacceptable because of mycotoxin interactions.

Biosynthesis. Treatment of *F. culmorum* cultures with xanthotoxin suppresses trichothecene synthesis and results in the accumulation of large amounts of trichodiene (TDN). Feeding of (^{14}C)TDN to *F. culmorum* cultures for 6 hours produced several major radiolabelled toxins (*116*). Feeding of labelled TDN for only 30 minutes resulted in detection of a new labelled precursor. This new metabolite was isolated and identified by a combination of ^{1}H and ^{13}C NMR and mass spectroscopy as isotrichodiol. This compound is the first demonstrated post-trichodiene intermediate in the biosynthesis of trichothecenes.

Toxicity of trichothecenes is related to the epoxide ring in their structures. Using a cell-free system from *F. culmorum*, epoxidation of a TDN derivative was demonstrated (*117*). The epoxidase required NADPH and molecular oxygen and was inhibited by CO. Thus, the enzyme appears to be a cytochrome P-450-dependent mono-oxygenase.

Occurrence and determination of trichothecenes. A survey of cereals (wheat, barley, oats, maize) grown in New Zealand during 1986–1989 showed a higher incidence and also higher levels of *Fusarium* mycotoxins, primarily trichothecenes, in samples from North Island (*118*). Nivalenol (NIV) and deoxynivalenol (DON), the most common contaminants, were found in 83% of North Island and in 20% of South Island samples. Although levels were generally low, concentrations as high as 11.95 mg DON/kg and 3.6 mg NIV/kg were recorded from North Island. NIV and DON contamination in South Island crops never exceeded 0.1 mg/kg. Maize was the most commonly affected crop. Mycotoxins derived from scirpentriol and T-2 tetraol were rarely detected, as was moniliformin. Zearalenone was detected at low levels in about 40% of the samples tested.

Of 28 samples of Korean rice, barley, millet, corn, and Indian millet from the 1989 harvest tested, only 6 were contaminated with NIV and/or DON (*119*). Rice and millet were clean while DON levels of 168–506 µg/kg were found in 5 samples and NIV levels of 189–624 µg/kg were present in 4 samples of the other crops. No T-2 toxin was detected in any cereal tested.

Determination of the trichothecene mycotoxins DON, NIV, 3-acetyldeoxynivalenol (3-ADON), T-2 toxin, HT-2 toxin, and diacetoxyscirpenol (DAS) in cereals by gas chromatography with ion trap detection has been described (*120*). Samples of wheat, barley, oats and corn were extracted by standard methods, and the toxins were derivatized by trifluoroacylation with trifluoroacetic acid anhydride. A capillary gas chromatograph combined with a selective mass detector (ion trap) working in the CI mode with methanol as reagent gas was used to quantify and confirm the identity of the toxins. The quantitation limit was 1–5 µg/kg and recoveries from cereals spiked with 200–500 ng of each toxin were 78–89%. This method would be applicable to routine monitoring of large numbers of samples.

Thermospray, plasmaspray, and dynamic fast-atom bombardment LC–MS methods were compared for the identification of 6 trichothecenes [DON, DAS, monoacetoxyscirpenol (MAS), triacetoxyscirpenol (TAS), T-2 toxin, and HT-2 toxin] (*121*). Thermospray produced only a very abundant ammonium adduct ion while plasmaspray produced some fragment ions in addition to the ammonium adduct ions. Dynamic fast-atom bombardment produced a protonated molecule, a glycerol adduct ion, and numerous fragment ions formed by the losses of functional groups as neutrals in various combinations. While all three methods can be used for monitoring of trichothecenes, only fast-atom bombardment is suitable for structure characterization.

DIPAIN [2-(diphenylacetyl)-1,3-indanedione-1-hydrazone] derivatives have proven useful in enhancing the fluorescence of trichothecene mycotoxins (*122*). Use of these compounds allows detection of as little as 50 ng T-2 toxin and of 0.1–4 μg of HT-2 toxin, DAS, neosolaniol, and fusarenon-X. This fluorescence enhancement does not occur in solution, and the effect is not apparent on a solid support until the spray solvent evaporates. It is suggested that these reagents may be useful as coatings in optical waveguide devices to detect trichothecenes in aerosols or in kits designed to detect surface contamination by trichothecenes.

T-2 TOXIN

Acute neurobehavioral effects of single oral doses of 0.4 and 2.0 mg T-2 toxin/kg body weight were assessed in male Wistar rats (*123*). Neither dose caused overt physical signs of intoxication although the higher dose retarded body weight gain. No effects on motor coordination or nociception were observed in tests 7.5–8 hours after dosing. Decreased motor activity on the open field and an impairment in the passive avoidance test were noted at 4 and 8 hours, respectively, for the high dose group.

Under natural conditions animals (or humans) may consume more than one type of toxin in contaminated foods. Since exposure to T-2 toxin causes many symptoms similar to those induced by endotoxin, experiments were conducted to determine the interaction of these two toxins (*124*). Male Swiss mice were dosed orally with 4 mg T-2 toxin/kg and/or injected with 3 μg endotoxin. Mortality, hypothermia, TNF-α production and thymic atrophy were all increased in mice receiving both toxins compared to those receiving either toxin alone. Further investigation revealed that T-2 toxin increased the absorption rate of endotoxin, thus enhancing its toxic effects.

Of 8 human cell lines tested for cytotoxic effects of T-2 toxin in vitro, a melanoma cell line (SK-Mel/27), a second passage keratinocyte line (NHEK), and a hepatoma cell line (HepG2) were the most sensitive (*125*). The neutral red cell viability test was used to quantitate the potency of T-2 and its metabolites. In the HepG2 cell line, T-2 was the most toxic, followed by HT-2, T-2 triol, and T-2 tetraol.

Fluorescence detection of T-2 and its metabolites as coumarin-3-carbonyl chloride derivatives by HPLC was described (*126*). The procedure involves first the synthesis of the derivatizing agent and then its use in the esterification of the mycotoxins. A silica gel cartridge was used to remove excess reagents and then the esterified toxins were separated on a reversed-phase column with acetonitrile:water (65:35) containing 0.75% acetic acid as the mobile phase and detected by fluorescence. The minimum detectable amounts of T-2 and its metabolites were 2.0 and 0.83 ng, respectively. Recoveries ranged from 80 to 100%.

NIVALENOL AND DEOXYNIVALENOL

Carcinogenic promoting activity of nivalenol (NIV) was assessed in F344 male rats initiated with injections with 200 mg diethylnitrosamine (DEN) with or without injections of aflatoxin B_1 (AFB$_1$, 0.5 mg/kg) (*127*). Following these injections the rats were fed a diet containing 6 ppm NIV for 6 weeks. GST-P-positive liver cell foci, as a measure of hepatocarcinogenicity, were observed in all DEN-treated rats, with significantly higher numbers seen in DEN + AFB$_1$ rats but not in the DEN + NIV rats. However, dietary NIV did significantly increase the numbers and areas of GST-P-positive foci in rats injected with both DEN and AFB$_1$ compared to those receiving the injections but no NIV. Therefore, it appears that NIV can enhance AFB$_1$-induced hepatocarcinogenesis.

In human IgA nephropathy, mesangial IgA deposition and hematuria occur almost always with the accumulation of complement component C3 and the deposition of IgG and/or IgM. Since dietary DON (vomitoxin) causes nephropathy with some of the same symptoms in animals, a 12-week feeding study with 25 ppm vomitoxin was conducted to determine further similarities and differences between the two diseases (*128*). Sera and urine were collected at 4, 8, and 12 weeks for analyses for hematuria and immunoglobulin complexes, and rats were also sacrificed at these intervals to quantitate mesangial (kidney) IgA, IgG, IgM, and C3. DON induced elevated levels of IgA-IC, mesangial IgA and hematuria (similar to human IgA nephropathy) but not of mesangial C3 deposition—a major difference from the human disease.

During a 6-week feeding trial with 0.1 to 10 ppm dietary DON an impairment in intestinal transfer and uptake of some nutrients was observed in male NMRI mice (*129*). At the end of the 6 weeks the animals were sacrificed and their intestines were isolated and used for in vitro experiments in nutrient uptake. The only significant effects noted were a decrease in glucose transfer and in the transfer and tissue accumulation of 5-methyltetrahydrofolic acid in the jejunum of high-dose rats. The absorption of leucine, tryptophan, water and iron were not altered.

Five tricyclic metabolites, identified as transient intermediates in trichothecene biosynthesis, were isolated from *F. culmorum* cultures fed an excess of isotrichodermin (*130*). The structures of these metabolites were characterized by spectroscopy, and four of them were unequivocally shown to be biosynthetic precursors of 3-acetyldeoxynivalenol (3-ADON). The data indicated that the first oxygenation step after isotrichodermin was at the C-15 position.

Results of a series of three preliminary intercomparisons of methods for the detection of DON carried out between 1985 and 1988 were reported (*131*). During the first trial, ten laboratories, using three different analytical methods (TLC, GC, and HPLC), achieved similar results in analyzing blanks and ethyl acetate solutions of DON (1.5 µg/mL) without any need for sample preparation. During the second trial, 13 participants were provided with naturally contaminated wheat (600 mg DON/kg) and maize (500 mg/kg). This trial was designed to establish recovery values for spiked samples, to test the effects of a prolonged extraction on recoveries, and to measure DON in naturally contaminated samples. Recoveries of ≥70% were achieved using both acetonitrile/water and methanol/water

extractions. A long (>6 hours) extraction period did not significantly improve recovery of DON from the contaminated samples. TLC proved to be a less reliable method of analysis since several participants had problems of interference with the maize extracts. Similar samples were provided to 15 laboratories for the third intercomparison, which aimed to improve on the results of the second trial based on the experience gained. Fewer participants used TLC and several used a charcoal column to aid in cleanup. Recoveries were generally acceptable. Extraction and cleanup were identified as critical steps in the methodology, and the need to demonstrate the absence of any matrix effects in calibration steps was seen as a requirement.

Three systemic fungicides, triadimefon, propiconazole, and thiabendazole, were field tested for their efficacy in suppressing growth of *F. graminearum* and DON production on wheat (*132*). Heads of wheat plants were inoculated with mold spores two days following anthesis. The fungicides were sprayed on the plots at the recommended dosages two days before, two days after, or both before and after inoculation. Triadimefon and propiconazole decreased *F. graminearum* infection and DON production by 39–61% and 34–79%, respectively. Thiabenzadole significantly decreased toxin production but not mold growth. Fungicide residue levels in the wheat kernels were found to be less than the maximum legal limits.

Removal of the most highly DON-contaminated wheat kernels by gravity table fractionation was described (*133*). Commercially grown wheat samples affected with *Fusarium* head blight were fractionated and the most severely infected kernels (tombstone kernels) were highly concentrated in the least dense fractions. DON levels were as high as 43.2 µg/g in the least dense fraction and always <1 µg/g in the most dense fraction. Further optimization of this procedure could lead to reliable recovery of wheat with DON values within food tolerance limits.

Polyclonal antisera against DON and 3-ADON were used in a direct ELISA to detect these mycotoxins in buffer solutions (*134*). The anti-DON antiserum had a stong cross-reactivity to 3-ADON and 15-ADON and minor cross-reactivity to NIV and fusarenon-X. The anti-3-ADON antisera was most specific for 3-ADON and had only minor cross-reactivities to acetyl T-2, 15-ADON, and T-2 tetrol tetraacetate. The detection limit for 3-ADON in the 3-ADON ELISA was 0.1 ng/mL while that for DON in the DON ELISA was 1 ng/mL.

DIACETOXYSCIRPENOL

A total of 53 strains of *F. sambucinum* were tested for their ability to synthesize trichothecenes and to form fertile crosses (*135*). Eight new fertile strains were identified and diacetoxyscirpenol (DAS) was detected in culture filtrates of these and in cultures of 40 non-fertile strains. Variations in the levels of DAS produced suggest that these strains may be useful in investigating the DAS biosynthetic pathway and its regulation. Trichothecene production was correlated with sexual fertility and original isolation from a diseased plant.

NEOSOLANIOL DERIVATIVES

A strain of *F. sporotrichioides*, which produces neosolaniol as its major mycotoxin, has been found to also produce two new trichothecenes, 8-*n*-pentanoylneosolaniol and 8-*n*-hexanoylneosolaniol, when grown on corn grits (136). These new compounds were characterized by GC–MS, NMR and X-ray crystallography. The cytotoxicity of the new toxins, as assessed with baby hamster kidney cells (BHK-21), was about 33% that of T-2 toxin and about twice that of neosolaniol.

Non-trichothecenes

GENERAL

Production of fusarin C and fumonisin B_1 by 10 strains of *F. moniliforme* cultured on corn was found to vary greatly: a range of 7 to 346 μg fusarin C/g and of 0 to 1090 μg fumonisin B_1/g (*137*). In most cases, fungi producing large amounts of one mycotoxin produced relatively small amounts of the other. Aqueous extracts of the fungi were not lethal to hepatocyte cultures and did not cause lactate dehydrogenase release from the cells but did inhibit or completely block the uptake of valine. Organic extracts killed more cells but had less effect on valine incorporation. Results from

hepatocyte cultures exposed to purified toxins showed that these toxic effects could not be completely accounted for by these known toxins and suggested that *F. moniliforme* produces other compounds toxic to liver cells.

Use of Czapek solution agar containing 20% saccharose was found to be a simple and accurate way to distinguish *F. moniliforme* from *F. proliferatum* and *F. subglutinans* (*138*). On this medium, *F. moniliforme* was noticeably coarser than the other two species and was light orange in color compared to pale yellowish-pink for the other species. Differences in microconidial chain length between *F. moniliforme* and *F. proliferatum* could also be observed.

FUMONISINS

Occurrence and control. A recent issue of *Mycopathologia* (*139*) presented 17 reports from a 1991 symposium on fumonisins. These mycotoxins, produced by *F. moniliforme*, have been associated with several animal and human diseases. The papers in this issue discuss isolation, characterization, biosynthesis, and toxicity of fumonisins. Animal toxicoses, including equine leukoencephalomalacia (ELEM) and pulmonary edema in swine, were reviewed and the implications for human health were discussed.

During a 1990–1991 survey, a total of 124 retail samples of corn-based human foods (primarily from the USA and South Africa) were analyzed for fumonisin B_1 (FB_1) and fumonisin B_2 (FB_2) (*140*). Sixteen cornmeal and 10 corn grits products from the USA contained mean concentrations of 1048 ng FB_1/g and 298 ng FB_2/g and 601 ng FB_1/g and 375 ng FB_2/g, respectively. Similar products from South Africa had only 13–28% as much mycotoxin contamination. Only 1 of 4 Peruvian cornmeal samples and 1 of 2 Canadian cornmeal samples tested had detectable levels of fumonisins. The two Egyptian cornmeal samples tested were highly contaminated, with means of 2380 ng FB_1/g and 595 ng FB_2/g. None of 5 cornflake samples and only 1 of 5 alkali-treated samples contained detectable fumonisins.

Homegrown corn samples from areas with high and low rates of human esophageal cancer in

Transkei, South Africa, were surveyed for the presence of fumonisins and *Fusarium moniliforme* during six seasons (*141*). *F. moniliforme* was present in 41.2% of good corn samples and in 61.7% of moldy corn from the high-risk area compared to incidences of 8.9% and 21.4% in the low-risk areas. Significantly higher levels of both FB_1 and FB_2 were also detected in corn from the high-risk areas. The highest levels of FB_1 and FB_2 measured were 117,520 ng/g and 22,960 ng/g, respectively. These are some of the highest concentrations measured in naturally infected corn.

Ethanolic fermentation of mycotoxin-contaminated grains usually results in toxin-free distilled alcohol with toxin accumulation in the spent grains. In tests using corn naturally contaminated with FB_1 (15 and 36 ppm) similar results were obtained (*142*). Little degradation of fumonisin occurred during fermentation and most was recovered in distillers' grain and stillage. The high-fumonisin corn contained less starch and yielded 7.2% ethanol while the low-fumonisin corn and fumonisin-free corn produced 8.8% ethanol. Such a fermentation coupled with an effective method for decontaminating the spent grain may be a practical means for salvaging contaminated corn.

Since ammonia treatment has been shown to effectively detoxify aflatoxins, the effects of ammoniation on fumonisin levels in corn either cultured or naturally contaminated with *F. moniliforme* were investigated (143). FB_1 levels were reduced in the culture material and in naturally contaminated corn by about 30% and 45%, respectively, following treatment with 1% ammonia for 1 day. Neither a higher ammonia concentration nor a longer incubation period significantly increased the degradation of FB_1. The reduction of fumonisin levels by ammoniation, however, was not accompanied by a reduction in toxicity of the treated corn. Similar elevations in serum enzyme levels occurred in rats fed the treated and the untreated corn.

Analyses of 98 feed samples associated with ELEM, 83 feed samples associated with porcine pulmonary edema syndrome (PPE), and 51 feed samples not associated with either disease revealed FB_1 levels of <1 to 126 µg/g, <1 to 330 µg/g, and <1 to 9 µg/g, respectively (*144*). FB_1 concentra-tions >10 µg/g were detected in 75% of the ELEM feeds and in 71% of the PPE feeds. FB_1 appears to be related to these diseases but due to problems of homogeneity and representativeness of the samples, it is not possible to calculate a dose-response relationship.

Ninety strains of *F. moniliforme* originally isolated in Canada, Africa, Australia, Nepal, and the USA from corn, other grains, and cases of mycotic keratitis or cancer were tested for their ability to produce fumonisins in culture (*145*). No FB_1 was detected in 3 cultures and only trace amounts appeared in 26 others (including all of the Australian strains). Highest levels were produced by isolates from corn in the USA (6421 ppm) and in Nepal (6397 ppm). In general, there was considerable variation in amounts of FB_1 produced by different strains.

A survey of 158 strains of *Fusarium* representing 9 species demonstrated that none of the cultures of *F. subglutinans* (23), *F. annulatum* (1), *F. succisae* (2), or *F. becomiforme* (15) produced FB_1 on cracked corn during 30 days' incubation at 25°C (*146*). Of the other species, 61% of *F. proliferatum*, 18% of *F. anthophilum*, 56% of *F. dlamini*, 15% of *F. napiforme*, and 37% of *F. nygamai* produced FB_1 in concentration ranges of 155–2936 ppm, 58–613 ppm, 42–82 ppm, 16–479 ppm and 17–7162 ppm, respectively. *F. proliferatum*, *F. napiforme*, and *F. nygamai* are of the greatest significance since they are associated with edible crops such as corn, peanuts, millet and sorghum.

Biological effects. To assess the toxicity and carcinogenicity of FB_1, rats were fed a semi-purified corn-based diet containing 50 mg FB_1/kg for 26 months (*147*). Autopsy results from rats sacrificed at intervals during and at the end of the experimental period revealed that the liver was the main organ affected by this toxin. Micro- and macronodular cirrhosis developed followed by primary hepatocellular carcinoma during the later stages. Chronic interstitial nephritis was also present in kidneys of treated rats at 26 months. No lesions were observed in the esophagus, heart, or forestomach.

Further studies investigated the carcinogenicity of FB_1 in rats exposed to dietary 0.1% FB_1 for 26 days or given 1 or 2 doses (by gavage) of FB_1 and FB_2 (*148*). Cancer initiation only occurred after the prolonged feeding, indicating that fumonisins are weak cancer initiators. The fumonisins also lacked genotoxic effects in in vivo and in vitro DNA repair assays in primary hepatocytes.

Studies with vervets (primates) provided with a fumonisin-contaminated diet for 1631 days indicated that these mycotoxins also have atherogenic effects (*149*). Culture material from *F. moniliforme* was mixed with a high-carbohydrate, low-fat diet at a level of 0.25–1.0% of the feed. Later analysis revealed fumonisin concentrations in the feed ranged from 2.5 to 21.1 mg/kg. Treatment resulted in elevations of LDL-C and apoprotein B (similar to those seen in vervets fed an atherogenic diet) and in increased plasma fibrinogen activity and of blood coagulation factor VII. As indicated by liver biopsies and serum enzyme levels, some liver damage (fibrosis but not cirrhosis) also occurred.

A series of 24 cultured mammalian cell lines was evaluated for sensitivity to FB_1 and FB_2 and the structurally related AAL toxin produced by *Alternaria alternata* (*150*). Of 9 rat hepatoma cell lines tested, 7 were sensitive, with a toxic response visible within 2 days. Approximate IC_{50} values for the most sensitive hepatoma cell line, H4TG, were 4, 2, and 10 µg/mL for FB_1, FB_2, and AAL toxin, respectively. Of the other 15 cell lines, which included human, monkey, pig, dog, mouse, hamster, and rat cells, only dog kidney cells, MDCK, were sensitive to these toxins, with IC_{50} values of 2.5, 2.0, and 5 µg/mL, respectively.

Since the fumonisins are structurally similar to the long-chain base backbones of sphingolipids, their potential for altering sphingolipid biosynthesis was investigated (*151,152*). Exposure of rat hepatocyte cultures and of $LLC-PK_1$ (a renal epithelial culture) to fumonisins resulted in the accumulation of the biosynthetic intermediate, sphinganine. FB_1 also inhibited the activity of sphingosine *N*-acyltransferase in rat liver microsomes. After a 24-hour lag period, fumonisins inhibited proliferation of and were cytotoxic to renal cells. This inhibition of sphingolipid biosynthesis was shown to be reversible in the kidney cells when the fumonisins were removed. This disruption of

sphingolipid biosynthesis may be an important aspect in the toxicity of fumonisins.

Methods for determination of fumonisins. A sensitive, reproducible, and accurate method for the HPLC determination of FB_1 in plasma and urine has been developed (*153*). Contaminated plasma and urine were collected from rats following i.p. injections with 7.5 mg FB_1/kg body weight. Samples were partially purified on Bond-Elut SAX solid-phase extraction cartridges, derivatized with *o*-phthaldialdehyde (OPA), and applied to a reversed-phase HPLC column. The toxin was detected and quantified by fluorimetry. Detection limit for this procedure was about 50 mg/mL and recoveries from spiked samples (1.4–6.2 µg/mL) were 86–87%.

Optimization of several steps in the LC method for co-determination of FB_1, FB_2, and FB_3 in foods and feeds was investigated (*154*). Results from tests with different reagents, apparatus, and times led to the following recommendations: (1) Initial extraction should be done with methanol–water (3+1) using a Polytron homogenizer. (2) For cleanup on SAX cartridges, pH of samples should be adjusted before cleanup, flow rate on the cartridge should be 0.8 mL/min and 1% acetic acid in methanol is the eluent of choice. (3) Because of the instability of fumonisin–OPA derivatives, they should be injected into the LC column within 4 minutes of the addition of the OPA reagent. This improved procedure was used to analyze 13 feed samples associated with ELEM. Twelve samples contained FB_3 (50–2650 ng/g). This is the first report of the natural occurrence of FB_3.

Polyclonal antibodies reactive to FB_1, FB_2, and FB_3 were generated in mice using a new immunization procedure with cholera toxin as both a hapten carrier and adjuvant (*155*). A competitive indirect ELISA with a detection limit of 100 ng/mL was developed. The antiserum reacted with all 3 fumonisins. Concentrations required for 50% binding were 260, 300, and 650 ng/mL, respectively, for FB_1, FB_2, and FB_3.

Monoclonal antibodies derived from mice treated with FB_1–cholera toxin have also been produced and used in a direct ELISA (*156*). All six subclone immunoglobulins tested reacted primarily with FB_1, with mean cross-reactivities for FB_2 and

FB$_3$ being 38 and 33%, respectively. In analyses with spiked (5–25 µg/g) feed samples, average recovery was 103%, with intra- and interassay coefficients of variation of 11% and 15%, respectively.

Methods for the preparative isolation of fumonisins from corn cultures of *F. moniliforme* have been devised (*157*). The toxins were extracted with methanol–water (3+1) and then purified on Amberlite XAD-2, silica gel and reverse-phase C$_{18}$ chromatography. The C$_{18}$ column effectively separated the individual fumonisins (FB$_1$, FB$_2$, FB$_3$, FB$_4$) to >90% purity. Although the method described is not optimal with respect to the quantities of toxins purified, it does yield ample amounts of these toxins for further experimentation.

FUSAROCHROMANONES

An analytical procedure combining an ELISA with thin-layer chromatography (TLC) or liquid chromatography (LC) has proven effective in detecting fusarochromanones at levels as low as 5 ppb in barley and wheat and in *F. equiseti* cultures grown in rice and corn (*158*). The mycotoxins were first extracted with 100% methanol and then subjected to LC or TLC without further cleanup. Individual fractions were then acetylated and analyzed by ELISA. Recovery of fusarochromanone from spiked (5–20 ppb) samples was 106.9–113.2%. Analysis of extracts of *F. equiseti* R6137 revealed that diacetyl-fusarochromanone was also produced by this fungus.

Electron impact ionization tandem mass spectrometry was used to elucidate the structures of some fragment ions which will be used as probes in biosynthetic and metabolic studies (*159*). In addition, a sensitive LC technique using direct injection continuous-flow fast atom bombardment for the detection of fusarochromanone in corn was developed. The lowest detectable amount in corn extracts was 50 ppb.

Six new fatty acid derivatives of fusarochromanone produced by *F. equiseti* growing on rice culture have been isolated and characterized (*160,161*). Five of the compounds had an acetyl group at the 3' position while the sixth compound had a formyl group at that position. Each compound had a different substitution at the 4' position. The

structures were elucidated by MS, NMR, and infrared spectral data.

ZEARALENONE

To test the effect of environmental estrogens on the developing brain, neonatal rats were given injections of 100 or 1000 µg zearalenone (ZEN) on post-natal days 1–10 (*162*). At 42 days, exposed females showed a significantly decreased pituitary response to GnRH. After sacrifice on day 49, females in the high-dose group had a significantly larger sexually dimorphic nucleus (SDN) area in the anterior hypothalamus area of the brain. (The SDN is normally 3–5 times larger in male than in female rats.) Although the male rats were castrated on day 21, no significant treatment effects were observed in them.

Optimum incubation temperature for ZEN production varies with the strain of *Fusarium* used. Experiments with *F. graminearum* and *F. oxysporum* demonstrated that both synthesized more ZEN (1095 and 7.0 mg/kg, respectively) when maintained at a constant 25°C for 6 weeks compared to incubation at 25°C for 3 weeks followed by 3 weeks at 12–14°C (*163*). One strain of *F. crookwellense* was found to produce maximal ZEN levels at 11°C (6540 mg/kg dry weight) while 4 other isolates of this species produced maximal levels at 20°C (2,460–10,150 mg/kg) (*164*). In another experiment, *F. crookwellense* strains maintained at ambient temperatures produced about three times as much ZEN when kept under the light rather than in the dark. As with other *Fusarium* species there was no advantage to decreasing incubation temperatures during the last 3 weeks.

Enhancement of the fluorescence response of ZEN and zearalenol by post-column derivatization with aluminum chloride was found to result in a significant improvement in limits of detection compared with most commonly used procedures (*165*). At a concentration of 0.25 M AlCl$_3$ and reaction coil temperatures of 50–60°C, the peak for ZEN increased about 5-fold while most interfering compounds were unaltered. One potential interference was noted in extracts of maize and mixed feed but not in wheat.

A method for the determination of α- and β-zearalenol and ZEN in cereals by gas chromatography combined with a selective mass detector (ion trap) working in the electron impact mode has been developed (*166*). Samples (wheat, barley, oats, corn) were extracted with ethyl acetate, cleaned up using a base treatment, and partitioned with water. Then the toxins were derivatized by trimethylsilylation and analyzed by gas chromatography. Detection limit for all three mycotoxins was 1 µg/kg. Recoveries from cereal samples spiked with 100–500 ng toxin were 82–86%.

FUSARINS

For the first time, the malignant transformation of rat esophageal epithelial cells was induced by fusarin C in culture (*167*). Preliminary experiments revealed that fusarin C was very toxic to this epithelial cell line (RE-525). Maximum transformation frequency occurred at 10 µg fusarin C/mL but only about 20% of the cells survived exposure to this concentration of fusarin C. These transformed cells grew rapidly, had an increased number of chromosomes, and an enhanced expression of the oncogenes *c-myc* and *v-erb-B*. Innoculation of the transformants into nude mice caused development of squamous cell carcinomas. These results are of particular interest since *F. moniliforme* frequently contaminates corn grown in an area of China with a high incidence of esophageal cancer.

Zinc-deficient culture media have been shown to enhance production of fusarin C by *F. moniliforme*. Further experiments to determine optimal culture conditions for fusarin C production indicated that urea and ammonium sulfate (0.3 g N/L) were the best nitrogen sources and fructose, sucrose, and glucose (30 g/L) were the best carbon sources (*168*).

Two new fusarins have recently been isolated from cultures of *F. moniliforme* and characterized by MS and NMR. (8Z)-Fusarin C was identified from culture extracts of strain ATCC 38932 (*169*). Production of this new toxin was found to vary according to temperature (30°C optimum), culture medium (YNB was optimal) and strain. A mutant strain, SG62, produced 8 mg (8Z)-fusarin C/g dry weight of mycelia after 6 days growth on YNB at 30°C.

The newly isolated fusarin F was rather unstable and was found to readily isomerize to fusarin C when separated on a reversed-phase column with a methanol–water solvent system (*170*). Use of 2.5% methanol in CH_2Cl_2 as eluent prevented the rearrangement of fusarin F to fusarin C and allowed preparation of pure fusarin F. The highest producer of fusarin F was strain DAOM 212260 from Canada which produced 120 mg fusarin F/L when grown at 28°C on a yeast–peptone–malt extract–glucose medium.

MONILIFORMIN

Moniliformin was reliably detected in cereal samples at levels as low as 0.05 mg/kg by a recently developed method involving extraction with acetonitrile–water, cleanup on reverse-phase and strong anion exchange disposable cartridge columns, and analysis by ion-pair HPLC with UV detection (*171*). Recoveries of 81–96% were obtained from samples spiked with 0.25 or 0.5 mg/ kg. Using this method, three maize-product samples from the U.K. had no detectable moniliformin while 33 others were contaminated with 0.05–0.25 mg/kg. Of 64 samples from 10 other countries, 37 were apparently moniliformin-free but some others had relatively high levels of this mycotoxin, including samples from Gambia (3.16 mg/kg) and South Africa (2.73 mg/kg). Visibly moldy field samples of maize, oats, wheat, rye, and triticale from Poland contained moniliformin concentrations of 0.5–38.3 mg/kg associated with *F. avenaceum* and of 4.2–399.3 mg/kg associated with *F. subglutinans*.

WORTMANNIN

Extraction and purification procedures for wortmannin, a hemorrhagic toxin produced by *F. oxysporum* N17B growing on rice were described and several bioassay systems were compared (*172*). Rats fed rice infected with this fungus along with rat chow in proportions of 1:3, 1:1, or 3:1, were severely affected, with the majority dying after 4–5 days of feeding. The most prominent toxic effect was hematuria with some hemorrhage occurring in the stomach and intestines of some rats. Ethyl acetate was chosen as the best solvent for extraction of this toxic factor from rice. The extracts were then defatted with petroleum ether, applied to a Florasil column, and then subjected to TLC. An oral dose of 4 mg purified wortmannin/kg was lethal to rats within 20 hours. LC_{50} value for wortmannin applied to 3T3 cells was 50 µg/mL and to cultures of GM498, HeLa cells, and neonatal rat beating heart cells was >50 µg/mL.

A potent inhibitor of smooth muscle myosin light chain kinase, isolated from cultures of *Talaromyces wortmannin* KY12420, was purified and identified as wortmannin (*173*). The inhibition was found to be irreversible and to be specific for this protein kinase, as wortmannin had little or no effect on 4 other protein kinases tested. Wortmannin also inhibited both the phosphorylation of myosin light chain and contraction in rat thoracic aorta preparations.

MYCOTOXINS PRODUCED BY *ALTERNARIA* SPP.

Of a total of 99 samples of grains (wheat, barley, rice, oats, rye and maize) from 7 Mediterranean countries, barley, wheat and oats were most frequently infected with *Alternaria* spp. (*174*). Two species, *A. alternata* and *A. triticina* predominated among the isolates. Only the *A. alternata* strains synthesized mycotoxins in rice culture, with all isolates producing tenuazonic acid (TZA) and most also producing alternariol (AOH), alternariol monomethylether (AME), altenuene (ALT), and the altertoxins I and II. Very high levels of TZA (2555–8750 mg/kg) were detected; much lower amounts of the other toxins were produced: 2–52 mg AME/kg, 6–118 mg AOH/kg, 1–37 mg ALT/kg and 1–9 mg altertoxins/kg.

A toxigenic strain of *A. alternata* isolated from beet leaves was found to produce abundant quantities of TZA, about 150 mg/L in broth culture (*175*). TZA was extracted from the fungus as a Na-complex and was identified and quantified by TLC and spectroscopy.

Eighty-seven *Alternaria* strains, isolated from maize and stored hay were examined for myco-

toxin production (*176*). All these strains produced AME and TZA, while AOH and ALT were produced by 77% and 18%, respectively. Concentration ranges determined in liquid media were: AME (0.08–482), AOH (0.05–1862), ALT (0.1–34), and TZA (0.02–42) mg/100 mL. Culture extracts were purified by column chromatography on silica gel, and toxins were identified and quantified by TLC and HPLC (*177*).

Effects of gamma-irradiation (1–4 kGy), water activity (a_w; 0.90–0.98), and incubation temperature (15 and 25°C) on the synthesis of TZA by *A. alternata* in tomato paste and juice were investigated (*178*). A radiation dose of 4 kGy completely inhibited mold growth and toxin production. Highest TZA levels were detected in paste (57.5 µg/g) and juice (26.3 µg/g) at 25°C and 0.98 a_w. Only traces of TZA were detected in paste and none in juice following 3 kGy irradiation and incubation at 25°C and 0.98 a_w. Decreasing water activity and temperature and increasing levels of irradiation all depressed toxin production.

The antibiotic cerulenin (50–100 µg/mL) was found to be an effective inhibitor of AOH and AME production by *A. alternata* in liquid culture (*179*). Cerulenin irreversibly inhibits lipid synthesis by inhibiting a condensing enzyme and may also inhibit the condensation step in the synthesis of polyketide mycotoxins (AOH and AME).

OTHER MYCOTOXINS

The lolitrems are tremorgenic mycotoxins found in perennial ryegrass and synthesized by the endophytic fungus, *Acremonium lolii*. They are thought to be the principal causative agents of ryegrass staggers in cattle. Recently, some biosynthetic precursors of lolitrem B, lolitriol, and α- and β-paxitriol were synthesized, characterized by NMR, and assayed for tremorgenic effects in mice (*180*). Neither lolitriol nor the paxitriols induced significant tremors in mice. Paxilline, a related tremorgenic mycotoxin produced by these fungi, was about 5 times less tremorgenic than lolitrem B.

LITERATURE CITED

1. Kuiper-Goodman, T. Risk assessment to humans of mycotoxins in animal-derived food products. *Vet. Hum. Toxicol.* 33:325–332 (1991).

2. Blunden, G., O.G. Roch, D.J. Rogers, et al. Mycotoxins in food. *Med. Lab. Sci.* 48:271–282 (1991).

3. Singh, R.S., M.K. Sharma, and H. Chander. Incidence of penicillium toxins in milk and milk products. *Indian J. Anim. Sci.* 63:285–286 (1992).

4. Jiménez, M., R. Mateo, A. Querol, et al. Mycotoxins and mycotoxigenic moulds in nuts and sunflower seeds for human consumption. *Mycopathologia* 115:121–127 (1991).

5. Taniwaki, M.H., and A.G.F. van Dender. Occurrence of toxigenic molds in Brazilian cheese. *J. Food Protect.* 55:187–191 (1992).

6. Weng, Y.-M., and J.H. Hotchkiss. Inhibition of surface molds on cheese by polyethylene film containing the antimycotic imazalil. *J. Food Protect.* 55:367–369 (1992).

7. Würgler, F.E., U. Friederich, and J. Schlatter. Lack of mutagenicity of ochratoxin A and B, citrinin, patulin and cnestine in *Salmonella typhimurium* TA102. *Mutat. Res.* 261:209–216 (1991).

8. Braunberg, R.C., O. Gantt, C. Barton, and L. Friedman. *In vitro* effects of the nephrotoxins ochratoxin A and citrinin upon biochemical function of porcine kidney. *Arch. Environ. Contam. Toxicol.* 22:464–470 (1992).

9. Sándor, G., A. Busch, H. Watzke, et al. Subacute toxicity testing of ochratoxin A and citrinin in swine. *Acta Vet. Hung.* 39:149–160 (1991).

10. Chao, T.-C., S.M. Maxwell, and S.-Y. Wong. An outbreak of aflatoxicosis and boric acid poisoning in Malaysia: a clinicopathological study. *J. Pathol.* 164:225–233 (1991).

11. Hendrickse, R.G. Kwashiorkor: the hypothesis that incriminates aflatoxins. *Pediatrics* 88:376–379 (1991).

12. Wild, C.P., F.N. Rasheed, M.F.B. Jawla, et al. In-utero exposure to aflatoxin in West Africa. *Lancet* 337:1602 (1991).

13. Zarba, A., C.P. Wild, A.J. Hall, et al. Aflatoxin M_1 in human breast milk from The Gambia, West Africa, quantified by combined monoclonal antibody immunoaffinity chromatography and HPLC. *Carcinogenesis* 13:891–894 (1992).

14. Srivatanakul, P., D.M. Parkin, M. Khlat, et al. Liver cancer in Thailand. II. A case-control study of hepatocellular carcinoma. *Int. J. Cancer* 48:329–332 (1991).

15. Zhang, Y.-J., C.-J. Chen, C.-S. Lee, et al. Aflatoxin B_1–DNA adducts and hepatitis B virus antigens in hepatocellular carcinoma and non-tumorous liver tissue. *Carcinogenesis* 12:2247–2252 (1991).

16. Groopman, J.D., Z. Jiaqi, P.R. Donahue, et al. Molecular dosimetry of urinary aflatoxin-DNA adducts in people living in Guangxi Autonomous Region, People's Republic of China. *Cancer Res.* 52:45–52 (1992).

17. Ross, R.K., J.-M. Yuan, M.C. Yu, et al. Urinary aflatoxin biomarkers and risk of hepatocellular carcinoma. *Lancet* 339:943–946 (1992).

18. Ozturk, M. and collaborators. p53 mutation in hepatocellular carcinoma after aflatoxin exposure. *Lancet* 338:1356–1359 (1991).

19. Patel, P., J. Stephenson, P.J. Scheuer, and G.E. Francis. p53 codon 249[ser] mutations in hepatocellular carcinoma patients with low aflatoxin exposure. *Lancet* 339:881 (1992).

20. Fujimoto, Y., L.L. Hampton, L.-d. Luo, et al. Low frequency of *p53* gene mutation in tumors induced by aflatoxin B_1 in nonhuman primates. *Cancer Res.* 52:1044–1046 (1992).

21. Raney, K.D., T. Shimada, D.-H. Kim, et al. Oxidation of aflatoxins and sterigmatocystin by human liver microsomes: significance of aflatoxin Q_1 as a detoxication product of aflatoxin B_1. *Chem. Res. Toxicol.* 5:202–210 (1992).

22. Raney, K.D., B. Coles, F.P. Guengerich, and T.M. Harris. The *endo*-8,9-epoxide of aflatoxin B_1: a new metabolite. *Chem. Res. Toxicol.* 5:333–335 (1992).

23. Yu, F.-L., J.-X. Huang, W. Bender, et al. Evidence for the covalent binding of aflatoxin B_1-dichloride to cytosine in DNA. *Carcinogenesis* 12:997–1002 (1991).

24. Groopman, J.D., J.A. Hasler, L.J. Trudel, et al. Molecular dosimetry in rat urine of aflatoxin-N^7-guanine and other aflatoxin metabolites by multiple monoclonal antibody affinity chromatography and immunoaffinity/high performance liquid chromatography. *Cancer Res.* 52:267–274 (1992).

25. Jennings, G.S., F. Oesch, and P. Steinberg. *In vivo* formation of aflatoxin B_1–DNA adducts in parenchymal and non-parenchymal cells of rat liver. *Carcinogenesis* 13:831–835 (1992).

26. Schlemper, B., J. Harrison, R.C. Garner, et al. DNA binding, adduct characterisation and metabolic activation of aflatoxin B_1 catalysed by isolated rat liver parenchymal, Kupffer and endothelial cells. *Arch. Toxicol.* 65:633–639 (1991).

27. Naidu, N.R.G., S. Sehgal, K.V.S. Bhaskar, and B.K. Aikat. Cystic disease of the liver following prenatal and perinatal exposure to aflatoxin B_1 in rats. *J. Gastroenterol. Hepatol.* 5:359–362 (1991).

28. Dunn, J.A., M.B. Faletto, S.J. Kasper, and H.L. Gurtoo. Aflatoxin-transformed C3H/10T½ cells overexpress protein kinase C and have an altered response to phorbol ester treatments. *Cancer Res.* 52:990–996 (1992).

29. Van den Heever, L.H., and H.W. Dirr. Effect of aflatoxin B_1 on human platelet protein kinase C. *Int. J. Biochem.* 23:839–843 (1991).

30. Cukrová, V., E. Langrová, and M. Akao. Effects of aflatoxin B_1 on myelopoiesis in vitro. *Toxicology* 70:203–211 (1991).

31. Verma, R.J., and P.J. Raval. Cytotoxicity of aflatoxin on red blood corpuscles. *Bull. Environ. Contam. Toxicol.* 47:428–432 (1991).

32. Feng, G.H., F.S. Chu, and T.J. Leonard. Molecular cloning of genes related to aflatoxin biosynthesis by differential screening. *Appl. Environ. Microbiol.* 58:455–460 (1992).

33. Chang, P.K., C.D. Skory, and J.E. Linz. Cloning of a gene associated with aflatoxin B1 biosynthesis in *Aspergillus parasiticus*. *Curr. Genet.* 21:231–233 (1992).

34. Gendloff, E.H., F.S. Chu, and T.J. Leonard. Variation in regulation of aflatoxin biosynthesis among isolates of *Aspergillus flavus*. *Experientia* 48:84–87 (1992).

35. Cleveland, T.E., D. Bhatnagar, and R.L. Brown. Aflatoxin production via cross-feeding of pathway intermediates during cofermentation of aflatoxin pathway-blocked *Aspergillus parasiticus* mutants. *Appl. Environ. Microbiol.* 57:2907–2911 (1991).

36. Yabe, K., Y. Ando, and T. Hamasaki. Desaturase activity in the branching step between aflatoxins B_1 and G_1 and aflatoxins B_2 and G_2. *Agric. Biol. Chem.* 55:1907–1911 (1991).

37. Yabe, K., Y. Ando, and T. Hamasaki. A metabolic grid among versiconal hemiacetal acetate, versiconol acetate, versiconol and versiconal during aflatoxin biosynthesis. *J. Gen. Microbiol.* 137:2469–2475 (1991).

38. Ellis, W.O., J.P. Smith, B.K. Simpson, and J.H. Oldham. Aflatoxins in food: occurrence, biosynthesis, effects on organisms, detection, and methods of control. *Crit. Rev. Food Sci. Nutr.* 30:403–439 (1991).

39. Park, D.L., and S.M. Rua, Jr. Biological evaluation of aflatoxins and metabolites in animal tissues. *Drug Metab. Rev.* 22:871–890 (1990).

40. Honstead, J.P., D.W. Dreesen, R.D. Stubblefield, and O.L. Shotwell. Aflatoxins in swine tissues during drought conditions: an epidemiologic study. *J. Food Protect.* 55:182–186 (1992).

41. Stubblefield, R.D., J.P. Honstead, and O.L. Shotwell. An analytical survey of aflatoxins in tissues from swine grown in regions reporting 1988 aflatoxin-contaminated corn. *J. Assoc. Off. Anal. Chem.* 74:897–899 (1991).

42. Rojas, F.J., M. Jodral, F. Gosalvez, and R. Pozo. Mycoflora and toxigenic *Aspergillus flavus* in Spanish dry-cured ham. *Int. J. Food Microbiol.* 13:249–256 (1991).

43. Bukovjan, K., A. Hallmannová, and A. Karpenko. Konzentration von aflatoxin B_1 in organen frei lebenden wildes. *Fleischwirtschaft* 72:794–796 (1992).

44. Plakas, S.M., P.M. Loveland, G.S. Bailey, et al. Tissue disposition and excretion of ^{14}C-labelled aflatoxin B_1 after oral administration in channel catfish. *Food Chem. Toxicol.* 29:805–808 (1991).

45. Fukal, L., and P. Brezina. Verfolgung des aflatoxin-M_1-gehaltes in milch für die produktion von säuglings- und kindernahrung mittels immunoassay. *Nahrung* 35:745–748 (1991).

46. Harvey, R.B., T.D. Phillips, J.A. Ellis, et al. Effects on aflatoxin M_1 residues in milk by addition of hydrated sodium calcium aluminosilicate to aflatoxin-contaminated diets of dairy cows. *Am. J. Vet. Res.* 52:1556–1559 (1991).

47. Sinha, K.K., and A.K. Sinha. Monitoring and identification of aflatoxins in wheat, gram and maize

flours in Bihar state (India). *Food Addit. Contam.* 8:453–457 (1991).

48. Ibeh, I.N., N. Uraih, and J.I. Ogonor. Dietary exposure to aflatoxin in Benin City, Nigeria: a possible public health concern. *Int. J. Food Microbiol.* 14:171–174 (1991).

49. Hirano, K., Y. Adachi, M. Hara, et al. Detection of aflatoxin B_1 in imported maize kernel used as feed by enzyme-linked immunosorbent assay. *J. Vet. Med. Sci.* 53:767–768 (1991).

50. Payne, G.A. Aflatoxin in maize. *Crit. Rev. Plant Sci.* 10:423–440 (1992).

51. Gorman, D.P., and M.S. Kang. Preharvest aflatoxin contamination in maize: resistance and genetics. *Plant Breeding* 107:1–10 (1991).

52. Brown, R.L., P.J. Cotty, and T.E. Cleveland. Reduction in aflatoxin content of maize by atoxigenic strains of *Aspergillus flavus. J. Food Protect.* 54:623–626 (1991).

53. Choudhary, A.K. Influence of microbial co-inhabitants on aflatoxin synthesis of *Aspergillus flavus* on maize kernels. *Lett. Appl. Microbiol.* 14:143–147 (1992).

54. Paster, N., A. Pushinsky, M. Menasherov, and I. Chet. Inhibitory effect of *Aspergillus niger* on the growth of *Aspergillus ochraceus* and *Aspergillus flavus*, and on aflatoxin formation. *J. Sci. Food Agric.* 58:589–591 (1992).

55. Faraj, M.K., J.E. Smith, and G. Harran. Interaction of water activity and temperature on aflatoxin production by *Aspergillus flavus* and *A. parasiticus* in irradiated maize seeds. *Food Addit. Contam.* 8:731–736 (1991).

56. Gagliardi, S.J., T.F. Cheatle, R.L. Mooney, et al. The occurrence of aflatoxin in peanut butter from 1982 to 1989. *J. Food Protect.* 54:627–631 (1991).

57. Pollet, A., C. Declert, W. Wiegandt, et al. Three years' studies on relationships between traditional groundnut storage and aflatoxin problems in Côte-d'Ivoire. Main results. *Oléagineux* 47:71–85 (1992).

58. Mehan, V.K., A. Ba, D. McDonald, et al. Field screening of groundnuts for resistance to seed infection by *Aspergillus flavus. Oléagineux* 46:109–115 (1991).

59. Fernández Pinto, V.E., G. Vaamonde, S.B. Brizzio, and N. Apro. Aflatoxin production in soybean varieties grown in Argentina. *J. Food Protect.* 54:542–545 (1991).

60. Ahmad, S.K., and P.L. Singh. Mycofloral changes and aflatoxin contamination in stored chickpea seeds. *Food Addit. Contam.* 8:723–730 (1991).

61. Bandara, J.M.R.S., A.K. Vithanege, and G.A. Bean. Occurrence of aflatoxins in parboiled rice in Sri Lanka. *Mycopathologia* 116:65–70 (1991).

62. Bandara, J.M.R.S., A.K. Vithanege, and G.A. Bean. Effect of parboiling and bran removal on aflatoxin levels in Sri Lankan rice. *Mycopathologia* 115:31–35 (1991).

63. Dawar, S., and A. Ghaffar. Detection of aflatoxin in sunflower seed. *Pak. J. Bot.* 23:123–126 (1991).

64. Abdel-Hafez, A.I.I., and O.M.O. El-Maghraby. Fungal flora and aflatoxin associated with cocoa, roasted coffee and tea powders in Egypt. *Cryptogamie Mycol.* 13:31–45 (1992).

65. Llewellyn, G.C., R.L. Mooney, T.F. Cheatle, and B. Flannigan. Mycotoxin contamination of spices—an update. *Int. Biodeteriorat. Biodegradat.* 29:111–121 (1992).

66. Garrido, D., M. Jodral, and R. Pozo. Mold flora and aflatoxin-producing strains of *Aspergillus flavus* in spices and herbs. *J. Food Protect.* 55:451–452 (1992).

67. Raisuddin, S., and J.K. Misra. Aflatoxin in betel nut and its control by use of food preservatives. *Food Addit. Contam.* 8:707–712 (1991).

68. El-Far, F., N.H. Aziz, and S. Hegazy. Inhibition by gamma-irradiation and antimicrobial food additives of aflatoxin B_1 production by Aspergillus flavus in poultry diet. *Nahrung* 36:143–149 (1992).

69. Adegoke, G.O., A.K. Babalola, and A.I. Akanni. Effects of sodium metabisulphite, hydrogen peroxide and heat on aflatoxin B1 in lafun and gar--two cassava products. *Nahrung* 35:1041–1045 (1991).

70. Mabrouk, S.S., and N.M.A. El-Shayeb. Inhibition of aflatoxin production in *Aspergillus flavus* by natural coumarins and chromones. *World J. Microbiol. Biotechnol.* 8:60–62 (1992).

71. Ansari, A.A., and A.K. Shrivastava. The effect of eucalyptus oil on growth and aflatoxin production by *Aspergillus flavus. Lett. Appl. Microbiol.* 13:75–77 (1991).

72. Zeringue, H.J., Jr. Effect of C_6 to C_9 alkenals on aflatoxin production in corn, cottonseed, and peanuts. *Appl. Environ. Microbiol.* 57:2433–2434 (1991).

73. Sashidhar, R.B., H.V.V. Murthy, and V.R. Bhat. Analytical quality assurance for analysis of aflatoxins in

agricultural export produce. *Food Chem.* 43:403–405 (1992).

74. Wilson, T.J., and T.R. Romer. Use of the mycosep multifunctional cleanup column for liquid chromatographic determination of aflatoxins in agricultural products. *J. Assoc. Off. Anal. Chem.* 74:951–956 (1991).

75. Candlish, A.A.G., M.K. Faraj, G. Harran, and J.E. Smith. Immunoaffinity column chromatography for detection of total aflatoxins in experimental situations. *Biotechnol. Tech.* 5:317–322 (1991).

76. Beaver, R.W., and M.A. James. Comparison of an ELISA-based screening test with liquid chromatography for the determination of aflatoxins in corn. *J. Assoc. Off. Anal. Chem.* 74:827–829 (1991).

77. Roch, O.G., G. Blunden, R.D. Coker, and S. Nawaz. The development and validation of a solid phase extraction/HPLC method for the determination of aflatoxins in groundnut meal. *Chromatographia* 33:208–212 (1992).

78. Sudershan, R.V., G.S. Prasad, T.P. Krishna, and R.V. Bhat. Field level evaluation of aflatoxin detection kit. *J. Food Protect.* 55:392–394 (1992).

79. Nawaz, S., R.D. Coker, and S.J. Haswell. Development and evaluation of analytical methodology for the determination of aflatoxins in palm kernels. *Analyst* 117:67–74 (1992).

80. Hongyo, K.-I., Y. Itoh, E. Hifumi, et al. Comparison of monoclonal antibody-based enzyme-linked immunosorbent assay with thin-layer chromatography and liquid chromatography for aflatoxin B$_1$ determination in naturally contaminated corn and mixed feed. *J. AOAC Int.* 75:307–312 (1992).

81. Farjam, A., N.C. van de Merbel, H. Lingeman, et al. Non-selective desorption of immuno precolumns coupled on-line with column liquid chromatography: determination of aflatoxins. *Int. J. Environ. Anal. Chem.* 45:73–87 (1991).

82. Farjam, A., N.C. van de Merbel, A.A. Nieman, et al. Determination of aflatoxin M1 using a dialysis-based immunoaffinity sample pretreatment system coupled on-line to liquid chromatography. *J. Chromatogr.* 589:141–149 (1992).

83. Nieuwenhof, F.F.J., J.D. Hoolwerf, and J.W. van den Bedem. Evaluation of an enzyme immunoassay for the determination of aflatoxin M$_1$ in milk using antibody-coated polystyrene beads. *Milchwissenschaft* 45:584–588 (1990).

84. Hurst, W.J., R.A. Martin, Jr., and C.H. Vestal. The use of HPLC/thermospray MS for the confirmation of aflatoxins in peanuts. *J. Liq. Chromatogr.* 14:2541–2550 (1991).

85. Abraham, W.-R., and H.-A. Arfmann. 12,13-Dihydroxy-fumitremorgin C from *Aspergillus fumigatus*. *Phytochemistry* 29:1025–1026 (1990).

86. Ling, K.H., C.M. Chiou, and Y.L. Tseng. Biotransformation of territrems by S$_9$ fraction from rat liver. *Drug Metab. Dispos.* 19:587–595 (1991).

87. Omar, R.F., E. Randell, and A.D. Rahimtula. In vitro inhibition of rat platelet aggregation by ochratoxin A. *J. Biochem. Toxicol.* 6:211–220 (1991).

88. Subramanian, S., N. Balasubramanian, S. William, and S. Govindasamy. *In vivo* absorption of ^{14}C-glucose and ^{14}C-glycine by the rat intestine during ochratoxin A toxicosis. *Biochem. Int.* 23:655–661 (1991).

89. Breitholtz-Emanuelsson, A., R. Fuchs, K. Hult, and L.-E. Appelgren. Syntheses of ^{14}C-ochratoxin A and ^{14}C-ochratoxin B and a comparative study of their distribution in rats using whole body autoradiography. *Pharmacol. Toxicol.* 70:255–261 (1992).

90. El-Shayeb, N.M.A., S.S. Mabrouk, and A.M.M. Abd-El-Fattah. Production of ochratoxins by some Egyptian *Aspergillus* strains. *Zbl. Mikrobiol.* 147:86–91 (1992).

91. Chelack, W.S., J. Borsa, J.G. Szekely, et al. Variants of *Aspergillus alutaceus* var. *alutaceus* (formerly *Aspergillus ochraceus*) with altered ochratoxin A production. *Appl. Environ. Microbiol.* 57:2487–2491 (1991).

92. Fukal, L. Spontaneous occurrence of ochratoxin A residues in Czechoslovak slaughter pigs determined by immunoassay. *Dtsch. Lebensm.-Rundsch.* 87:316–319 (1991).

93. Köfer, J., M. Schuh, and K. Fuchs. Ochratoxin A residues in Styrian slaughter pigs. (Summary in English.) *Tierärztl. Umschau* 46:657–660 (1991).

94. Holmberg, T., A. Breitholtz-Emanuelsson, P. Häggblom, et al. *Penicillium verrucosum* in feed of ochratoxin A positive swine herds. *Mycopathologia* 116:169–176 (1991).

95. Trivedi, A.B., E. Doi, and N. Kitabatake. Detoxification of ochratoxin A on heating under acidic and alkaline conditions. *Biosci. Biotech. Biochem.* 56:741–745 (1992).

96. Beker, D., and B. Radic. Fast determination of ochratoxin A in serum by liquid chromatography: comparison with enzymic spectrofluorimetric method. *J. Chromatogr.* 570:441–445 (1991).

97. Takeda, N., Y. Akiyama, and S. Shibasaki. Solid-phase extraction and cleanup for liquid chromatographic analysis of ochratoxin A in pig serum. *Bull. Environ. Contam. Toxicol.* 47:198–203 (1991).

98. Nesheim, S., M.E. Stack, M.W. Trucksess, and R.M. Eppley. Rapid solvent-efficient method for liquid chromatographic determination of ochratoxin A in corn, barley, and kidney: collaborative study. *J. AOAC Int.* 75:481–487 (1992).

99. Jiao, Y., W. Blaas, C. Rühl, and R. Weber. Identification of ochratoxin A in food samples by chemical derivatization and gas chromatography–mass spectrometry. *J. Chromatogr.* 595:364–367 (1992).

100. Reddy, V.K., and S.M. Reddy. Cyclopiazonic acid production by *Penicillium griseofulvum* in relation to different cultivars of maize. *World J. Microbiol. Biotechnol.* 8:208–209 (1992).

101. Urano, T., M.W. Trucksess, and J. Matusik. Liquid chromatographic determination of cyclopiazonic acid in corn and peanuts. *J. AOAC Int.* 75:319–322 (1992).

102. Hahnau, S., and E.W. Weiler. Determination of the mycotoxin cyclopiazonic acid by enzyme immunoassay. *J. Agric. Food Chem.* 39:1887–1891 (1991).

103. Aleo, M.D., R.D. Wyatt, and R.G. Schnellmann. The role of altered mitochondrial function in citrinin-induced toxicity to rat renal proximal tubule suspensions. *Toxicol. Appl. Pharmacol.* 109:455–463 (1991).

104. Chagas, G.M., A.P. Campello, and M.L.W. Klüppel. Mechanism of citrinin-induced dysfunction of mitochondria. I. Effects on respiration, enzyme activities and membrane potential of renal cortical mitochondria. *J. Appl. Toxicol.* 12:123–129 (1992).

105. Trivede, A.B., E. Doi, and N. Kitabatake. Cytotoxicity of citrinin heated at temperatures above 100°C. *Biosci. Biotech. Biochem.* 56:423–426 (1992).

106. Kitabatake, N., A.B. Trivedi, and E. Doi. Thermal decomposition and detoxification of citrinin under various moisture conditions. *J. Agric. Food Chem.* 39:2240–2244 (1991).

107. Jiménez, M., R. Mateo, J.J. Mateo, et al. Effect of the incubation conditions on the production of patulin by *Penicillium griseofulvum* isolated from wheat. *Mycopathologia* 115:163–168 (1991).

108. Burghardt, R.C., R. Barhoumi, E.H. Lewis, et al. Patulin-induced cellular toxicity: a vital fluorescence study. *Toxicol. Appl. Pharmacol.* 112:235–244 (1992).

109. Ueno, Y., W. Habano, H. Yamaguchi, et al. Transformation of mammalian cells by luteoskyrin. *Food Chem. Toxicol.* 29:607–613 (1991).

110. Masuda, T., N. Miyasaka, T. Kato, and Y. Ueno. Formation of the 8-hydroxydeoxyguanosine moiety in hepatic DNA of mice orally administered with luteoskyrin, a bis-anthraquinoid mycotoxin. *Toxicol. Lett.* 58:287–295 (1991).

111. Montella, P.G., and C.S. Reddy. Neurotoxic effects of secalonic acid D in mice during subchronic postnatal exposure. *Pharmacol. Biochem. Behav.* 40:241–247 (1991).

112. Chang, S.-C., Y.-H. Wei, D.L. Wei, et al. Factors affecting the production of eremofortin C and PR toxin in *Penicillium roqueforti*. *Appl. Environ. Microbiol.* 57:2581–2585 (1991).

113. Penn, J., J.R. Biddle, P.G. Mantle, et al. Pennigritrem, a naturally-occurring penitrem A analogue with novel cyclisation in the diterpenoid moiety. *J. Chem. Soc. Perkin Trans. 1*, pp. 23–26 (1992).

114. Rotter, B.A., B.K. Thompson, D.B. Prelusky, and H.L. Trenholm. Evaluation of potential interactions involving trichothecene mycotoxins using the chick embryotoxicity bioassay. *Arch. Environ. Contam. Toxicol.* 21:621–624 (1991).

115. Koshinsky, H.A., P.J. Hannan, and G.G. Khachatourians. HT-2 toxin, roridin A, T-2 toxin, and verrucarin A mycotoxins inhibit carbon dioxide production by *Kluyveromyces marxianus*. *Can. J. Microbiol.* 37:933–938 (1991).

116. Hesketh, A.R., L. Gledhill, D.C. Marsh, et al. Biosynthesis of trichothecene mycotoxins: identification of isotrichodiol as a post-trichodiene intermediate. *Phytochemistry* 30:2237–2243 (1991).

117. Gledhill, L., A.R. Hesketh, B.W. Bycroft, et al. Biosynthesis of trichothecene mycotoxins: cell-free epoxidation of a trichodiene derivative. *FEMS Microbiol. Lett.* 81:241–246 (1991).

118. Lauren, D.R., M.P. Agnew, W.A. Smith, and S.T. Sayer. A survey of the natural occurrence of *Fusarium* mycotoxins in cereals grown in New Zealand in 1986–1989. *Food Addit. Contam.* 8:599–605 (1991).

119. Park, J.C., M.S. Zong, and I.-M. Chang. Survey of the presence of the *Fusarium* mycotoxins nivalenol, deoxynivalenol and T-2 toxin in Korean cereals of the 1989 harvest. *Food Addit. Contam.* 8:447–451 (1991).

120. Schwadorf, K., and H.-M. Müller. Determination of trichothecenes in cereals by gas chromatography with ion trap detection. *Chromatographia* 32:137–142 (1991).

121. Kostiainen, R. Identification of trichothecenes by thermospray, plasmaspray and dynamic fast-atom bombardment liquid chromatography–mass spectrometry. *J. Chromatogr.* 562:555–562 (1991).

122. Novak, T.J., and K. Quinn-Doggett. 2-(Diphenylacetyl)-1,3-indanedione-1-hydrazone (DIPAIN) derivatives for detection of trichothecene mycotoxins. *Anal. Lett.* 24:913–924 (1991).

123. Sirkka, U., S.A. Nieminen, and P. Ylitalo. Acute neurobehavioural toxicity of trichothecene T-2 toxin in the rat. *Pharmacol. Toxicol.* 70:111–114 (1992).

124. Taylor, M.J., C. Lafarge-Frayssinet, M.I. Luster, and C. Frayssinet. Increased endotoxin sensitivity following T-2 toxin treatment is associated with increased absorption of endotoxin. *Toxicol. Appl. Pharmacol.* 109:51–59 (1991).

125. Babich, H., and E. Borenfreund. Cytotoxicity of T-2 toxin and its metabolites determined with the neutral red cell viability assay. *Appl. Environ. Microbiol.* 57:2101–2103 (1991).

126. Cohen, H., and B. Boutin-Muma. Fluorescence detection of trichothecene mycotoxins as coumarin-3-carbonyl chloride derivatives by high-performance liquid chromatography. *J. Chromatogr.* 595:143–148 (1992).

127. Ueno, Y., T. Yabe, H. Hashimoto, et al. Enhancement of GST-P-positive liver cell foci development by nivalenol, a trichothecene mycotoxin. *Carcinogenesis* 13:787–791 (1992).

128. Dong, W., J.E. Sell, and J.J. Pestka. Quantitative assessment of mesangial immunoglobulin A (IgA) accumulation, elevated circulating IgA immune complexes, and hematuria during vomitoxin-induced IgA nephropathy. *Fund. Appl. Toxicol.* 17:197–207 (1991).

129. Hunder, G., K. Schümann, G. Strugala, et al. Influence of subchronic exposure to low dietary deoxynivalenol, a trichothecene mycotoxin, on intestinal absorption of nutrients in mice. *Food Chem. Toxicol.* 29:809–814 (1991).

130. Zamir, L.O., K.A. Devor, and F. Sauriol. Biosynthesis of the trichothecene 3-acetyldeoxynivalenol. Identification of the oxygenation steps after isotrichodermin. *J. Biol. Chem.* 266:14992–15000 (1991).

131. Gilbert, J., A. Boenke, and P.J. Wagstaffe. Deoxynivalenol in wheat and maize flour reference materials. 1. An intercomparison of methods. *Food Addit. Contam.* 9:71–81 (1992).

132. Boyacioglu, D., N.S. Hettiarachchy, and R.W. Stack. Effect of three systemic fungicides on deoxynivalenol (vomitoxin) production by *Fusarium graminearum* in wheat. *Can. J. Plant Sci.* 72:93–101 (1992).

133. Tkachuk, R., J.E. Dexter, K.H. Tipples, and T.W. Nowicki. Removal by specific gravity table of tombstone kernels and associated trichothecenes from wheat infected with fusarium head blight. *Cereal Chem.* 68:428–431 (1991).

134. Usleber, E., E. Märtlbauer, R. Dietrich, and G. Terplan. Direct enzyme-linked immunosorbent assays for the detection of the 8-ketotrichothecene mycotoxins deoxynivalenol, 3-acetyldeoxynivalenol, and 15-acetyldeoxynivalenol in buffer solutions. *J. Agric. Food Chem.* 39:2091–2095 (1991).

135. Beremand, M.N., A.E. Desjardins, T.M. Hohn, and F.L. VanMiddlesworth. Survey of *Fusarium sambucinum* (*Gibberella pulicaris*) for mating type, trichothecene production, and other selected traits. *Phytopathology* 81:1452–1458 (1991).

136. Bekele, E., A.A. Rottinghaus, G.E. Rottinghaus, et al. Two new trichothecenes from *Fusarium sporotrichioides. J. Nat. Prod.* 54:1303–1308 (1991).

137. Norred, W.P., C.W. Bacon, R.D. Plattner, and R.F. Vesonder. Differential cytotoxicity and mycotoxin content among isolates of *Fusarium moniliforme. Mycopathologia* 115:37–43 (1991).

138. Clear, R.M., and S.K. Patrick. A simple medium to aid the identification of *Fusarium moniliforme, F. proliferatum,* and *F. subglutinans. J. Food Protect.* 55:120–122 (1992).

139. Riley, R.T., and J.L. Richard, eds. *Fumonisins: A current perspective and view to the future. Mycopathologia* 117:1–124 (1992).

140. Sydenham, E.W., G.S. Shephard, P.G. Thiel, et al. Fumonisin contamination of commercial corn-based human foodstuffs. *J. Agric. Food Chem.* 39:2014–2018 (1991).

141. Rheeder, J.P., W.F.O. Marasas, P.G. Thiel, et al. *Fusarium moniliforme* and fumonisins in corn in relation to human esophageal cancer in Transkei. *Phytopathology* 82:353–357 (1992).

142. Bothast, R.J., G.A. Bennett, J.E. Vancauwenberge, and J.L. Richard. Fate of fumonisin B$_1$ in naturally contaminated corn during ethanol fermentation. *Appl. Environ. Microbiol.* 58:233–236 (1992).

143. Norred, W.P., K.A. Voss, C.W. Bacon, and R.T. Riley. Effectiveness of ammonia treatment in detoxification of fumonisin-contaminated corn. *Food Chem. Toxicol.* 29:815–819 (1991).

144. Ross, P.F., L.G. Rice, R.D. Plattner, et al. Concentrations of fumonisin B$_1$ in feeds associated with animal health problems. *Mycopathologia* 114:129–135 (1991).

145. Nelson, P.E., R.D. Plattner, D.D. Shackelford, and A.E. Desjardins. Production of fumonisins by *Fusarium moniliforme* strains from various substrates and geographic areas. *Appl. Environ. Microbiol.* 57:2410–2412 (1991).

146. Nelson, P.E., R.D. Plattner, D.D. Shackelford, and A.E. Desjardins. Fumonisin B$_1$ production by *Fusarium* species other than *F. moniliforme* in section *Liseola* and by some related species. *Appl. Environ. Microbiol.* 58:984–989 (1992).

147. Gelderblom, W.C.A., N.P.J. Kriek, W.F.O. Marasas, and P.G. Thiel. Toxicity and carcinogenicity of the *Fusarium moniliforme* metabolite, fumonisin B$_1$, in rats. *Carcinogenesis* 12:1247–1251 (1991).

148. Gelderblom, W.C.A., E. Semple, W.F.O. Marasas, and E. Farber. The cancer-initiating potential of the fumonisin B mycotoxins. *Carcinogenesis* 13:433–437 (1992).

149. Fincham, J.E., W.F.O. Marasas, J.J.F. Taljaard, et al. Atherogenic effects in a non-human primate of *Fusarium moniliforme* cultures added to a carbohydrate diet. *Atherosclerosis* 94:13–25 (1992).

150. Shier, W.T., H.K. Abbas, and C.J. Mirocha. Toxicity of the mycotoxins fumonisins B$_1$ and B$_2$ and *Alternaria alternata* f. sp. *lycopersici* toxin (AAL) in cultured mammalian cells. *Mycopathologia* 116:97–104 (1991).

151. Wang, E., W.P. Norred, C.W. Bacon, et al. Inhibition of sphingolipid biosynthesis by fumonisins. *J. Biol. Chem.* 266:14486–14499 (1991).

152. Yoo, H.-W., W.P. Norred, E. Wang, et al. Fumonisin inhibition of *de novo* sphingolipid biosynthesis and cytotoxicity are correlated in LLC-PK$_1$ cells. *Toxicol. Appl. Pharmacol.* 114:9–15 (1992).

153. Shephard, G.S., P.G. Thiel, and E.W. Sydenham. Determination of fumonisin B$_1$ in plasma and urine by high-performance liquid chromatography. *J. Chromatogr.* 574:299–304 (1992).

154. Sydenham, E.W., G.S. Shephard, and P.G. Thiel. Liquid chromatographic determination of fumonisins B$_1$, B$_2$, and B$_3$ in foods and feeds. *J. AOAC Int.* 75:313–318 (1992).

155. Azcona-Olivera, J.I., M.M. Abouzied, R.D. Plattner, et al. Generation of antibodies reactive with fumonisins B$_1$, B$_2$, and B$_3$ by using cholera toxin as the carrier-adjuvant. *Appl. Environ. Microbiol.* 58:169–173 (1992).

156. Azcona-Olivera, J.I., M.M. Abouzied, R.D. Plattner, and J.J. Pestka. Production of monoclonal antibodies to the mycotoxins fumonisins B$_1$, B$_2$, and B$_3$. *J. Agric. Food Chem.* 40:531–534 (1992).

157. Cawood, M.E., W.C.A. Gelderblom, R. Vleggaar, et al. Isolation of the fumonisin mycotoxins: a quantitative approach. *J. Agric. Food Chem.* 39:1958–1962 (1991).

158. Yu, J., and F. S. Chu. Immunochromatography of fusarochromanone mycotoxins. *J. Assoc. Off. Anal. Chem.* 74:655–660 (1991).

159. Pawlosky, R.J., and C.J. Mirocha. Mass spectral analysis and fragment ion structure of fusarochromanone. *Biol. Mass Spectrom.* 20:743–749 (1991).

160. Xie, W., C.J. Mirocha, Y. Wen, et al. Isolation and structure elucidation of four fatty acid derivatives of the mycotoxin fusarochromanone produced by *Fusarium equiseti. J. Agric. Food Chem.* 39:1757–1761 (1991).

161. Xie, W., C.J. Mirocha, and Y. Wen. Formyl fusarochromanone and diacetyl fusarochromanone, two new metabolites of *Fusarium equiseti. J. Nat. Prod.* 54:1165–1167 (1991).

162. Faber, K.A., and C.L. Hughes, Jr. The effect of neonatal exposure to diethylstilbestrol, genistein, and zearalenone on pituitary responsiveness and sexually dimorphic nucleus volume in the castrated adult rat. *Biol. Reprod.* 45:649–653 (1991).

163. Milano, G.D., and T.A. Lopez. Influence of temperature on zearalenone production by regional strains

of *Fusarium graminearum* and *Fusarium oxysporum* in culture. *Int. J. Food Microbiol.* 13:329–334 (1991).

164. Di Menna, M.E., D.R. Lauren, and W.A. Smith. Effect of incubation temperature on zearalenone production by strains of *Fusarium crookwellense*. *Mycopathologia* 116:81–86 (1991).

165. Hetmanski, M.T., and K.A. Scudamore. Detection of zearalenone in cereal extracts using high-performance liquid chromatography with post-column derivatization. *J. Chromatogr.* 588:47–52 (1991).

166. Schwadorf, K., and H.-M. Müller. Determination of α- and β-zearalenol and zearalenone in cereals by gas chromatography with ion-trap detection. *J. Chromatogr.* 595:259–267 (1992).

167. Lu, F.-X., M.-X. Li, and S.-J. Cheng. *In vitro* transformation of rat esophageal epithelial cells by fusarin C. *Sci. China* 34:1469–1477 (1991).

168. Jackson, M.A., and S.N. Freer. The influence of carbon and nitrogen nutrition on fusarin C biosynthesis by *Fusarium moniliforme*. *FEMS Microbiol. Lett.* 82:323–328 (1991).

169. Barrero, A.F., J.F. Sánchez, J.E. Oltra, et al. Fusarin C and 8Z-fusarin C from *Gibberella fujikuroi*. *Phytochemistry* 30:2259–2263 (1991).

170. Savard, M.E., and J.D. Miller. Characterization of fusarin F, a new fusarin from *Fusarium moniliforme*. *J. Nat. Prod.* 55:64–70 (1992).

171. Sharman, M., J. Gilbert, and J. Chelkowski. A survey of the occurrence of the mycotoxin moniliformin in cereal samples from sources worldwide. *Food Addit. Contam.* 8:459–466 (1991).

172. Abbas, H.K., D.J. Mirocha, W.T. Shier, and R. Gunther. Bioassay, extraction, and purification procedures for wortmannin, the hemorrhagic factor produced by *Fusarium oxysporum* N17B grown on rice. *J. AOAC Int.* 75:474–480 (1992).

173. Nakanishi, S., S. Kakita, I. Takahashi, et al. Wortmannin, a microbial product inhibitor of myosin light chain kinase. *J. Biol. Chem.* 267:2157–2163 (1992).

174. Logrieco, A., A. Bottalico, M. Solfrizzo, and G. Mule. Incidence of *Alternaria* species in grains from Mediterranean countries and their ability to produce mycotoxins. *Mycologia* 82:501–505 (1990).

175. Robeson, D.J., and M.A.F. Jalal. Tenuazonic acid produced by an *Alternaria alternata* isolate from *Beta vulgaris*. *J. Inorg. Biochem.* 44:109–116 (1991).

176. Müller, M. Toxin production of moulds of the genus *Alternaria*. (Abstract in English.) *Zbl. Mikrobiol.* 147:207–213 (1992).

177. Müller, M., and P. Lepom. Analysis of *Alternaria* mycotoxins in laboratory cultures. (Abstract in English.) *Zbl. Mikrobiol.* 147:197–206 (1992).

178. Aziz, N.H., S. Farag, and M.A. Hassanin. Effect of gamma irradiation and water activity on mycotoxin production of Alternaria in tomato paste and juice. *Nahrung* 35:359–362 (1991).

179. Hiltunen, M., and K. Söderhäll. Inhibition of polyketide synthesis in *Alternaria alternata* by the fatty acid synthesis inhibitor cerulenin. *Appl. Environ. Microbiol.* 58:1043–1045 (1992).

180. Miles, C.O., A.L. Wilkins, R.T. Gallagher, et al. Synthesis and tremorgenicity of paxitriols and lolitriol: possible biosynthetic precursors of lolitrem B. *J. Agric. Food Chem.* 40:234–238 (1992).

11

Foodborne Bacterial Intoxications and Infections

Surveillance and epidemiology
Staphylococcus
Clostridium
Bacillus cereus
Salmonella
Shigella
Escherichia coli
Yersinia
Vibrio
Aeromonas
Campylobacter
Listeria
Other microbial pathogens
General (multiple pathogens)
Prevention and control

SURVEILLANCE AND EPIDEMIOLOGY

Whereas consumers are most concerned with food-safety issues related to food additives, preservatives, processing aids, and pesticide residues, food microbiologists and the U.S. FDA place top priority on microbiological hazards (*1*). An estimated 5–6 million cases of foodborne illness may cause >9000 deaths in the USA each year, at a cost of 10^1–10^6 million dollars. Seafood, red meat, and poultry were the implicated vehicles in nearly 60% of outbreaks reported in 1977–1984. *Salmonella* caused the greatest number of confirmed outbreaks in 1977–1982, followed by *Staphylococcus aureus, Clostridium perfringens,* and *Clostridium botulinum.* Organisms more recently recognized as serious threats because of either the high incidence of outbreaks or the severity of illness they cause include *Listeria monocytogenes, Campylobacter jejuni,* and *Yersinia enterocolitica.* Improper cooling was a major factor contributing to outbreaks; excessive time lapse between preparation and serving and contamination by infected persons were also frequently involved. The home kitchen was the most likely site of food abuse.

Roberts and Foegeding discussed the process of risk assessment for estimating the costs of foodborne microbial illness (*2*). They identified and evaluated sources of partial estimates, suggesting plausible ranges of estimates and a "best estimate" for the number of cases of acute illness caused by specific organisms. The probability of a foodborne disease being identified is influenced by the disease's severity, novelty, temporal relation to ingestion of the contaminated food, and name recognition; the availability of diagnostic tests; and the number of persons affected. The authors also discussed the fragmentary literature on costs of such illness, including the possibly large costs associated with chronic sequelae. Social costs incurred by individuals, government, or industry include medical, rehabilitation, legal, surveillance, investigative, and cleanup costs; and lost time, income, productivity, or sales. Some costs, such as suffering or nonmonetary costs to persons who are not wage earners, are not easily quantitated. Estimates for the cost per case of foodborne bacterial disease ranged from $200 for *Bacillus cereus* to $135,000 for *L. monocytogenes,* in cases requiring hospitalization.

Jay critically reviewed trends in the causative organisms and food vehicles in outbreaks of foodborne disease (*3*). He discussed new and historical methods for controlling foodborne pathogens, with special reference to innovations in packaging and minimal processing. Development and use of the Hazard Analysis Critical Control Point (HACCP) system was described. Another report compiled data on foodborne illness in West Germany and described the WHO program for European surveillance of foodborne illnesses (*4*). Meat, milk, and eggs were the major food vehicles of disease. The annual incidence of *Salmonella* infections and the meteoric rise of *Salmonella enteritidis* as a foodborne pathogen were traced.

Schofield discussed *L. monocytogenes, Y. enterocolitica, Plesiomonas shigelloides, C. botulinum, Aeromonas* spp., and *Bacillus* spp. as emerging foodborne pathogens of potential significance in chilled and extended-shelf-life foods (*5*). She argued that although it is possible for truly "new" pathogens to arise through acquisition of new virulence factors or antigenic profiles, what is more likely "emerging" is new hazards from changes in packaging and processing technology. Methods for monitoring, controlling, and identifying microbial contaminants were briefly mentioned.

Since the CDC published a "final" list of infectious and communicable diseases transmitted through handling the food supply (*Federal Register*, 16 August 1991), problems from *Taenia solium* have been recognized (*6*). The list and the methods of transmission have been up-dated. Most contamination occurs from infected food animals or during processing, but some pathogens are frequently transmitted to food by infected persons. These are hepatitis A virus, Norwalk and Norwalk-like viruses, *Salmonella typhi, Shigella* spp., *S. aureus,* and *Streptococcus pyogenes.* Species usually transmitted by source contamination or during processing but occasionally transmitted by infected food handlers are *C. jejuni,* enterohemorrhagic and enterotoxigenic *Escherichia coli, Y. enterocolitica, Vibrio cholerae*

O1, nontyphoidal *Salmonella*, rotavirus, *Entamoeba histolytica*, *Giardia lamblia*, and *T. solium*.

Guerrant and Bobak reviewed the epidemiology of bacterial and protozoal gastroenteritis, including traveler's diarrhea and foodborne and waterborne illness (*7*). They discussed food poisoning syndromes and the potential for widespread dissemination of foodborne pathogens. The pathophysiology, diagnosis, and therapy of these illnesses were summarized.

A review of reported outbreaks of foodborne disease in New York State found a 4-fold rise between 1980 and 1990, reflecting some actual increase but primarily an improvement in the state's reporting system (*8*). Data were presented in 10 figures and 5 tables; the text summarized specific findings, recommendations, and actions. Two appendixes presented guidelines for confirming a foodborne disease outbreak and a new classification for implicated foods. In 1990, 131 outbreaks involving 2425 cases and 3 deaths were reported. *Salmonella* was the agent most often implicated and shellfish was the most frequently reported vehicle. An innovation in the reporting classification was to utilize two categories in reporting the food vehicle: a "General Food Category" that includes methods of preparation (e.g., cook/serve foods, salads with raw ingredients, baked goods) and an "Ingredient Food Category" that specifies the source (e.g., raw egg added just before service). An additional "Contributing Factors Category" lists items such as improper hot-holding, toxic container, and cross-contamination.

Analysis of Canadian data on foodborne disease reported from 1975 to 1984 revealed a gradually increasing incidence (*9*). *Salmonella*, *S. aureus*, *C. perfringens*, and *B. cereus* were the commonest etiologic agents, although unspecified molds and yeasts were also regularly implicated; viral illness was reported only in 1983. *Salmonella*, *C. botulinum*, and *L. monocytogenes* were responsible for most of the 56 deaths during this period. Meat and poultry were the major food vehicles; the largest outbreak (>2700 cases) involved *Salmonella* contamination of cheese. The incidence of illnesses caused by *Salmonella*, *S. aureus*, *Campylobacter*, and *B. cereus* tended to peak during the summer

and, in some cases, in December. Most incidents of microbial illness were related to mishandling of food at foodservice establishments.

A surveillance summary from the CDC reviewed waterborne disease outbreaks reported in 1989–1990 (*10*). One outbreak in 1989 involved two persons in the same household in Idaho who drank bottled water exclusively. They stopped drinking the water after noting foreign objects in it and felt better within a few days. Samples from freshly opened bottles had high standard plate counts, and diatoms were present. The water came from a river in Washington, was chlorinated at a municipal plant, and passed through charcoal filters in the milk plant where it was bottled. On the day the implicated water was bottled the filters were bypassed because they were clogged with diatoms. The "waterborne" classification includes outbreaks of diarrheal illness on cruise ships. Two outbreaks on one ship were associated with exposures on land. An outbreak on another ship was associated with eating freshly cut fruit and stuffed eggs, and was probably viral. Two ships from the same cruise line experienced three outbreaks on three separate cruises during a 2-week period; cold seafood dishes containing scallops were the implicated vehicle and enterotoxigenic *E. coli* was the putative etiologic agent. Outbreaks occurred on four consecutive week-long cruises on another ship but the source of infection was not determined. In the first foodborne outbreak of shigellosis on a cruise ship investigated by CDC, German potato salad was the probable vehicle and multiresistant *Shigella flexneri* 4a was the etiologic agent. Consumption of water and ice was associated with illness in an unrelated outbreak but food histories were not available and the causative agent was not identified.

Outbreaks of foodborne disease in nursing homes are of growing concern because of the increase in institutionalized long-term care for the elderly and the great vulnerability of this population. Levine et al. described the epidemiology of outbreaks occurring in the USA from 1975 through 1987 and suggested where preventive action could be targeted (*11*). During the period studied, 26 states reported 115 outbreaks involving between 6 and 173 persons. Overall 4944 persons became ill,

213 were hospitalized, and 51 died. No trend was detected over time. Nursing home outbreaks accounted for 2% of the total illnesses and hospitalizations reported to CDC, but 19% of the deaths. Where the causative agent was established, *Salmonella* was involved in 52% of outbreaks and 44% of cases and *S. aureus* in ~23%; 6 outbreaks caused by *C. perfringens* accounted for another 22% of cases. High death rates (7–12%) were associated with outbreaks of *Salmonella montevideo, S. enteritidis,* and *E. coli* O157:H7. The most frequently implicated vehicles were foods containing poultry or eggs, and salads not containing beef, eggs, or poultry. Multiple vehicles were identified in 13 outbreaks. Improper storage or holding temperatures contributed to 37 of the 59 outbreaks in which one or more food-handling or preparation deficiencies were identified; poor personal hygiene of a food handler was involved in 21, contaminated equipment in 13, inadequate cooking in 12, and food from an unsafe source in 3. The authors believe that nursing home outbreaks, cases, and deaths are underreported because many of these institutions have very limited infection control programs, many of the frequent clusters of gastrointestinal illness are not identified as outbreaks, and epidemiologic investigations are seldom conducted. Enforcement by public health agencies of sanitation guidelines for institutional food services lags far behind that for commercial food services. The authors recommended steps that institutions could take to prevent outbreaks of foodborne illness and control them when they have occurred.

Zottola and Smith reviewed the sources, characteristics, and control of pathogenic bacteria associated with meat and meat products (*12*). *Salmonella, E. coli* O157:H7, *L. monocytogenes, Y. enterocolitica,* and *C. jejuni* were specifically discussed. Because these pathogens are widely distributed on and in meat animals and throughout the environment, the authors emphasized that education of consumers, food handlers, and food processors is a necessary adjunct to even the most stringent control measures. Mossel painted a gloomy picture of the incidence and impact of human illness transmitted by foods of animal origin (*13*). He argued that any attempt to manage foodborne diseases by current systems of inspecting end products is bound to fail miserably because the microbiological integrity of a food can only be assured by intervention. This philosophy became the basis of HACCP systems. However, such analysis and intervention must extend beyond the industrial processing of foods, to which it is most often applied, to the "longitudinal integration of safety assurance" (acronym LISA). This involves the HACCP approach at all stages from the farm to the table. As an example, Mossel described application of LISA to meat and poultry and discussed the interactive roles of science, industry, and government in consumer protection through LISA.

Seafood poses particular problems because of its potential for contamination by a broad range of microbial pathogens and its popularity when eaten raw or undercooked (*14–18*). Excerpts from a report by the Committee on Evaluation of the Safety of Fishery Products of the Food and Nutrition Board, Institute of Medicine, National Academy of Sciences, summarized the hazards of seafood consumption, deficiencies in their control, and proposed corrective measures (*14*). Because environmental contamination is global and most health risks associated with seafood originate in the environment, these risks are best dealt with by control of harvest or at the point of capture. Very few risks can be identified by organoleptic inspection. Although inspection is necessary at the processing level, it is unlikely that increasing it would significantly reduce the incidence of seafoodborne illness. There is need to improve protection for consumers of products derived from recreational and subsistence fishing, which are not subject to health-based control. Recommendations were made for improving public education and national surveillance systems. A volume on the microbiology of marine food products comprises sections on seafood quality, seafood safety, and special processing and packaging (*15*). The first section addressed problems related to the harvest and handling of finfish, bivalve molluscs, and crustaceans and discussed seafood inspection and HACCP. Papers in the second section reviewed water quality indicators, indigenous and nonindigenous bacterial pathogens, seafoodborne parasites and viruses, and toxins. The third covered pasteurization and minimally processed seafoods, modified atmosphere packaging, shellfish depuration, and irradiation. The chapter on nonindigenous bacterial pathogens focused on pathogens frequently found in seafoods but not common in the marine environment (*16*). Their presence in seafood is the result of fecal transmission from human or animal reservoirs or of poor sanitation and temperature abuse after harvest. They include *Salmonella, Campylobacter, Shigella, L. monocytogenes, Y. enterocolitica, S. aureus,* and pathogenic forms of *E. coli. Clostridium botulinum,* which may occur in the water column or sediments, was also discussed. Vibrios were discussed elsewhere in the book. A study was made of cockles (*Cardium edule*) and striped venus (*Chamelea gallina*) to establish relationships between classical indicator organisms and the main pathogens involved in shellfishborne illness (*17*). Animals were collected from five sampling stations in the estuary of the Guadalhorce River, Malaga, Spain, at different depths and seasons of the year. Factorial ANOVA showed a significant relationship only between season of the year and concentrations of total anaerobes, coliphage, and *Aeromonas hydrophila*. Classical indicators were not significantly correlated with pathogen levels in shellfish samples, casting doubt on the validity of any universal indicator of shellfish hygiene. However, linear correlations between detection percentages of pathogens and the medians of the lognormal distribution of the indicator organisms suggested that use of *E. coli,* fecal streptococci, and coliphages can estimate the hazard associated with *Salmonella, Vibrio parahaemolyticus,* and *S. aureus* in shellfish samples. In addition, the authors recommended direct determination of *Salmonella* in the samples. Pancorbo and Barnhart also warned of the need for better indicators of human fecal pollution in estuarine environments, particularly as markers of microbial pathogens in shellfish and shellfish beds (*18*). They reviewed the major shellfishborne microbial illnesses and the fate of bacteria and viruses in the estuarine environment. Further study of potential new indicators of human fecal pollution, such as *Bacteroides fragilis* bacteriophages and F+-specific coliphages belonging to serogroups II and III, was recommended.

STAPHYLOCOCCUS

A section in the proceedings of an international symposium on staphylococci was devoted to taxonomy and identification (*19*). Two papers discussed characteristics of *Staphylococcus aureus* associated with bovine mastitis and isolated from mastitic milk.

Outbreaks

Although a fatal outcome of staphylococcal food poisoning is rare, four elderly patients died during an outbreak in a Swedish hospital (*20*). Altogether about 50 patients became ill after eating spinach soup containing hard-boiled eggs. The eggs had been cooked and pealed two days earlier and refrigerated at a probable temperature of 10°C. Under experimental conditions at this temperature, small numbers of the implicated strain of *S. aureus* multiplied rapidly in cooked eggs, easily reaching populations of 10^6/g within 48 h. About 8×10^5 *S. aureus* organisms per gram were recovered from samples of left-over eggs. Enterotoxin A–producing *S. aureus* of the same phage type as that in the eggs was isolated from stools of 12 patients and from the hands and noses of two staff members who had handled the eggs. It was concluded that the eggs had become contaminated during peeling. Two patients died of generalized gastroenterocolitis within 12 h after the onset of symptoms; two patients died of other direct causes about 72 h after onset of symptoms, but intestinal infection was considered contributory. This indicates that consumption of food contaminated with *S. aureus* can rapidly lead to intestinal colonization and death in elderly persons.

On two consecutive days, a total of 12 persons became ill 2–4 h after the main meal on flights from Los Angeles to London (*21*). Similar illness had affected 14 persons flying from Los Angeles to Tokyo a day earlier. The three flights were serviced from the same catering establishment in the USA. An *S. aureus* strain that produced enterotoxins A and C was isolated from a dessert item served on the flights.

During the winter of 1988–1989, 155 persons suffered gastrointestinal symptoms associated with eating Stilton cheese (22). Thirty-six outbreaks were reported. The cheese was produced from unpasteurized cow's milk in the English midlands. Although the symptoms were suggestive of staphylococcal illness, extensive testing failed to detect any pathogen, toxin, or chemical in milk, cheese, or environmental samples from the suspect dairy. One sample of cheese associated with illness yielded a single strain of enterotoxin D–producing S. aureus, but only after enrichment. The implicated Stilton was withdrawn from the market and a decision was made to use pasteurized milk in subsequent cheese production.

Occurrence, growth, and toxin production in foods

It has been reported that ~40% of foodborne staphylococcal illnesses occur after consumption of meat and meat products and ~40% of these are associated with pork; in addition, S. aureus has frequently been isolated from equipment and the hands of staff in meat-processing plants. For these reasons, investigators in Switzerland determined the extent to which pig hindquarters used in producing cured raw ham were contaminated with S. aureus, thus contributing to dissemination of this pathogen in meat-processing plants (23). Of 4357 hindquarters tested, 22.7% were contaminated. Of these, 89% had counts of 10^1–10^3 cfu/cm^2 on the rind surface and 11% had counts of 10^3–10^6 cfu/cm^2. High levels of contamination were associated with particular abattoirs and were attributed to the technique and hygiene of slaughter and the subsequent refrigeration.

The enterotoxigenicity of 185 S. aureus isolates from meat products and various meat-industry sources in Belgium and Zaire was investigated (24). The isolates were biotyped, phage-typed, and tested for production of staphylococcal enterotoxin (SE). Of the 30 strains producing one or more enterotoxins, 23 belonged to the human biotype. Most SE-positive strains belonged to phage group III or mixed, or were not typable. No strains of poultry-like biotype (which were frequent in nasal carriers at meat plants and in minced meat) or avian biotype

produced SE. The authors concluded that their system for biotyping S. aureus would be useful in epidemiologic investigation, the human biotype is a high SEA and SEB producer and is thus of public health concern, and the avian and poultry-like biotypes are probably harmless. Other investigators evaluated the enterotoxigenicity of Staphylococcus strains isolated from Spanish dry-cured hams (25). Using the reversed passive latex agglutination method, they found that 86% of 135 strains produced SE and more than half of these produced SEA. One of two Staphylococcus epidermidis strains produced SEC. In the approximately one-third of enterotoxigenic strains that produced more than one SE, the most frequent combination was SEA and SEB. The different results found during fast and slow dry-curing were discussed.

A study of bacterial growth in Polish vacuum-packed, frozen cooked hams showed a decrease in numbers of aerobic, psychrophilic, and lipolytic bacteria after 2 months, followed by a continuous increase (26). However, no pathogenic staphylococci were found in these hams even after prolonged storage.

In his Wiley Award address, Bennett reviewed the mounting evidence that contrary to the older view, staphylococcal enterotoxins in thermally processed foods can be a health hazard (27). He discussed the lack of correlation between serological and biological activities of SE and the paradox that although ingestion of heated toxin causes a lower rate of illness than ingestion of unheated toxin, persons who do become ill may become *more* ill after ingesting heated toxin. Reevaluation of the thermal stability of staphylococcal enterotoxins revealed how the conformation of preformed SE can be altered in heat-treated foods so that the molecule no longer reacts with antibody but still retains biological activity; in some cases, renaturation of the toxin with urea restores its serological activity. From this, Bennett developed a concept of how thermal processing affects the serological and biological fate of SE, based on thermal denaturation and renaturation conditions and mechanisms underlying the toxin molecule's conformational changes. The illustrative case of food poisoning from Chinese canned mushrooms was presented.

Domenech et al. evaluated the ability of organic acids used by the food industry to prevent staphylococcal growth and enterotoxin production (*28*). The *S. aureus* test strains were FRI-100, S6, FRI-137, and FRI-472, which produced SEA, SEA plus SEB, SEC, and SED, respectively. They were grown in BHI broth to which lactic, citric, ascorbic, acetic, pyruvic, or propionic acid was added. The results varied with the strain and acid tested. Pyruvic acid was most inhibitory to growth of FRI-100 and FRI-472, whereas lactic acid was most inhibitory for FRI-137. Lactic acid was an effective inhibitor of SE synthesis, but acetic and citric acids had virtually no effect. SEB was most resistant to inactivation at low pH.

Tempeh is an Indonesian fermented product prepared by growing *Rhizopus oligosporus* on dehulled, cooked soybean cotyledons or various other legumes. Although pathogens in tempeh are generally killed during frying or boiling, there is risk of cross-contamination, undercooking, or persistence of heat-stable toxins. Therefore a study was made of the growth of *S. aureus* in fermenting tempeh and its inhibition by *Lactobacillus plantarum* (*29*). Samples of horsebeans, peas, chickpeas, and soybeans were soaked in tap water or tap water acidified with glacial acetic acid and cooked in the liquid used for soaking. After draining and cooling, they were inoculated with *R. oligosporus* spores, mixed with a suspension of *S. aureus*, and divided into two portions, one of which was further mixed with an *L. plantarum* suspension. *S. aureus* grew rapidly in all non-acid-soaked fermenting tempehs, reaching final counts of $\geq 10^8$ cfu/g. *Lactobacillus plantarum* sharply reduced growth of *S. aureus* in tempehs made from non-acid-soaked horsebean, pea, and chickpea and completely inhibited it in soybean tempeh. Acid-soaking reduced the initial growth rate in all tempehs, but after 18 h mycelial growth raised the pH and the growth rate recovered. Inoculation of acid-soaked samples with *L. plantarum* completely inhibited *S. aureus* growth in soybean tempeh and reduced final counts in the other products to $<10^4$ cfu/g. Inoculation of beans with *L. plantarum* may control *S. aureus* growth and enterotoxin production during commercial tempeh production.

In Morocco, the fermented product "Iben" is made from raw milk. Because Moroccan raw milk frequently has high bacterial counts, including *S. aureus*, the behavior of an SEC-producing strain during manufacture of Iben was assessed (*30*). With an inoculum of 10^3/mL, *S. aureus* reached a maximum of 7–8×10^4/mL within 24 h and there was no accumulation of thermonuclease. With a larger inoculum, 10^5/mL, *S. aureus* reached a maximum of ~3–4×10^7/mL; thermonuclease was detected after 8–12 h and enterotoxin was detected after 12–24 h. Although bacterial counts decreased between 24 and 72 h, thermonuclease and enterotoxin persisted. Control of initial *S. aureus* levels and screening for thermonuclease as an indicator of enterotoxin production were recommended to reduce the risk of staphylococcal food poisoning from Iben. Another product frequently made from raw milk is Manchego cheese, produced in Spain from ewe's milk (*31*). Batches of Manchego cheese were prepared with 0.1 and 1% lactic acid culture and inoculated with various strains of SE-producing *S. aureus*. Mean staphylococcal counts in cheeses from 0.1% cultures were generally >1 log higher than counts of the same strain in cheeses from 1% cultures. All counts declined sharply after 35–42 days; no organisms were detected in some cheeses after this time. Three cheeses prepared with 0.1% cultures and two prepared from 1% cultures contained detectable SEA or SED, at levels of 33–769 ng/100 g. Although results varied considerably from batch to batch, it was apparent that *S. aureus* can survive the ripening process of Manchego-type cheese and that enterotoxins may be present in the final product.

Because the human nares, skin, and hair are major reservoirs of *S. aureus* and large numbers of people have access to the foods on salad bars, the ability of two *S. aureus* strains to grow and produce enterotoxin on selected salad bar ingredients was evaluated (*32*). Clam chowder was also tested. The organism did not survive in salad dressing at pH 4.3 or in black olives. The SEA-producing strain did not survive in blue cheese crumbles. After 24 h, both strains declined in most ingredients. Active growth occurred for 24 h in green pepper and some growth occurred in moist and dry croutons, but no enterotoxin was detected. In clam chowder inoculated with 10^3 or 10^4 cfu/g, *S. aureus* counts exceeded 10^8 cfu/g after 12 h at 42°C; production of SE began shortly after 3 h, reaching maxima of 0.29 ng/g (SEA) and 1.6 ng/g (SED). The authors stressed that although many strains of *S. aureus* produce enterotoxins in culture media under all conditions that support growth, this is not necessarily true in foods. In this study, croutons and green pepper contained sufficient moisture and nutrients for growth but not for toxin production.

After at least four outbreaks of staphylococcal food poisoning were associated with eating canned mushrooms imported from the PRC, Brunner and Wong tested whether *S. aureus* could grow and produce SE under conditions simulating the storage, handling, and processing of mushrooms (*33*). An SEA-producing strain was inoculated onto mushrooms and incubated under simulated pre- and post-canning conditions. The organism grew and produced low levels of SEA in mushrooms incubated at 25°C in 10–20% NaCl. Growth and SEA production also occurred when mushrooms were stored in plastic bags at 37°C (but not at 25°C), or when they were heat-processed at 121.1°C and then inoculated. No SEA was recovered when mushrooms were inoculated with 1 or 10 ng/g of SEA and heated at 121.1°C for 4.5 min, but at inoculum levels of 100 and 1000 ng/g SEA was detectable after 10 min of heating. The authors concluded that SE could occur in canned mushrooms as a result of preprocessing contamination, but that postprocessing contamination is more likely.

The rate at which seafood is cooled after cooking is an important determinant of microbiological quality (*34*). In many processing plants, blue crabs (*Callinectes sapidus*) are debacked after cooking and refrigerated overnight. The microbiological quality of cooked blue crabs was evaluated under two cooling systems, forced air and static air. The rate of cooling was significantly faster in the forced-air system; psychrotrophic and aerobic plate counts were roughly 1 log lower and *S. aureus* counts were lower by a factor of 4.

Some staphylococcal strains produce very low levels of SE in laboratory media; their role as food pathogens has been unclear. To learn whether these organisms pose a health hazard, investigators inoculated sterile and nonsterile samples of cream pie and cooked ham with four low-SED-producing strains of *S. aureus* (*35*). A standard SED-producing strain was also tested. Enterotoxin was detected in all samples after 24 h at 37°C with an inoculum of 10^3/g. With an inoculum of 10^4/g, enterotoxin was detected in all sterilized and most unsterilized samples after 24 h at 30°C, and in most sterilized samples after incubation at 25°C. The authors concluded that strains producing SE in culture media at levels too low for detection by gel diffusion (ng/mL) can produce enough SE in foods (ng/g) to cause food poisoning.

Toxins and virulence factors

Staphylococcus aureus is thought to possess a variety of virulence factors—extracellular toxins and enzymes, and components of the capsular material and cell wall—whose expression is influenced by growth conditions (*36*). Clinical isolates and isolates grown under in vivo conditions may differ in antigenic composition from organisms propagated in laboratory media. The virulence properties of 6 bovine mastitis isolates of *S. aureus* were compared after growth in tryptic soy broth (TSB) and milk whey. In a mouse mastitis model, *S. aureus* grown in whey caused more severe lesions than homologous strains grown in TSB. With one strain, lethality in subcutaneously inoculated mice was 75% for whey cultures and 5% for TSB cultures. Mastitis strains lacked a true cellular capsule. Five of the 6 strains showed diffuse-type colony morphology, which changed to compact upon subculture on a variety of laboratory media but reverted to diffuse upon subsequent growth in whey. The authors suggested that diffuse growth is genetically regulated and associated with elevated release of one or more extracellular factors, which might be triggered by growth in whey. α-Toxin was shown not to be responsible for the enhanced virulence of organisms grown in whey.

It is difficult to obtain the relatively large amounts of SEs necessary for antibody production and other studies. The sac culture method was evaluated for enhanced production of SEA, SED, and SEE, which typically are formed at low levels (*37*). Optimum yields were obtained using 100 mL of medium per sac (Union Carbide sausage casing) at a shaking speed of 150 rpm. The media of choice were brain heart infusion (BHI) broth for SEA production by strain FRI-722 and SED production by strain 1151m, and Biosate plus yeast extract for SEE production by strain FRI-326.

To learn about the major type-specific and minor cross-reacting epitopes located on SEA and SEE, murine monoclonal antibodies (MAbs) against SEA and SEE were prepared and partially characterized (*38*). Of 5 MAbs to SEA, 2 reacted only with SEA and 3 reacted with both SEA and SEE. One MAb specific only for SEE was produced. Competitive binding assays with SEA or SEE and horse-radish peroxidase–conjugated MAbs using unconjugated MAbs as inhibitors suggested that multiple epitopes are located on SEA. Some of them may be associated with the minor cross-reacting epitopes between SEA and SEE. The availability of an MAb reacting with both SEA and SEE permitted this research group to purify these enterotoxins by immunosorbent chromatography (*39*). Conditions were described for obtaining yields of 76% for SEA and 70% for SEE. The purified SEs were immunologically and electrophoretically homogeneous. Similar studies of SED were conducted (*40*). MAbs were produced and used to purify SED by immunoaffinity chromatography. Again, the method easily provided a high yield of electrophoretically and antigenically pure enterotoxin.

Binek et al. reported localization of the mitogenic epitope of SEB (*41*). Limited tryptic digestion generated a 12-kDa N-terminal fragment and a 17-kDa C-terminal fragment, which were isolated by preparative isoelectric focusing. The C-terminal fragment showed significant mitogenic activity for murine splenocytes, whereas the N-terminal fragment was inactive. MAbs specific for the C-terminal fragment neutralized most of the mitogenic activity of the intact toxin and the active fragment. MAbs specific for the N-terminal fragment had no neutralizing activity. The authors concluded that the epitope or epitopes responsible for mitogenicity are located in the C-terminal region of SEB.

SEC produced by *S. aureus* FRI-909 was crystallized using a combination of ammonium sulfate and polyethylene glycol 400 with a small amount of detergent (*42*). Two crystal forms were obtained: one triclinic and one tetragonal. Both contained one toxin molecule per asymmetric unit. The results of X-ray diffraction analysis of these two crystal forms were presented.

Detection and identification

In *S. aureus*, membrane injury is generally expressed and studied as the loss of salt tolerance. The repair and enterotoxin production of heat-injured *S. aureus* FRI-472 was studied in three liquid media (*43*). Salt tolerance was repaired faster at 37 than at 22°C in all media. Powdered skim milk was the best medium for repair, followed by minimal medium and complex medium. However, no enterotoxin production was ever observed, no matter how rapidly and completely repair took place.

Bergdoll reviewed the analytical methods for detecting SEs (*44*). The methods fall into two categories: those for detecting SE-producing staphylococcal strains and those for detecting enterotoxins in foods. The most frequently used of the former are gel diffusion methods, in which the enterotoxin produced by a strain is compared with known enterotoxins. The sensitivity of gel diffusion techniques is not high, but is usually satisfactory for determining the enterotoxigenicity of staphylococcal strains. Methods applied to foods should be able to detect 1 ng of enterotoxin per gram of food without use of complicated extraction–concentration procedures. The radioimmunoassay (RIA), enzyme-linked immunosorbent assay (ELISA), and reversed passive latex agglutination (RPLA) method meet these criteria. Commercial ELISA and RPLA kits for detection of enterotoxins in foods are available. The development of an ELISA-based kit for detecting SE was described (*45*). Through use of polyclonal antibodies, it can identify and quantitate SEA, SEB, SEC_1, SED, and SEE in one test system within 50 min. The lower limit of detection is 0.5 ng/mL and the precision is 90%. Wieneke compared four commercial kits, three based on sandwich ELISA and one on RPLA, for detection of SE in foods from outbreaks of food poisoning (*46*). One ELISA kit detected enterotoxin in 14 of 18 foods. The other three kits detected enterotoxin in

9 of 10 foods. The advantages and disadvantages of each method were discussed.

It would be highly desirable to have standard reference materials for use in SE testing (47). Successful detection of SEs in foods hinges on many factors, and results have not always been reliable. Notermans et al. described the production of a reference material for SEA, potentially useful for testing laboratory performance, comparing various detection methods and results from different laboratories, and providing quantitative information on the recovery of SE from food. Preliminary evaluation of the reference material clearly indicated its suitability for practical application.

Brooks et al. reported increasing the sensitivity of an enzyme-amplified colorimetric immunoassay for protein A–bearing *S. aureus* in foods (48). The basis of amplification was the catalytic coupling of alkaline phosphatase to a substrate cycle involving $NAD^+/NADH$, using ethanol as the reductant. By adding semicarbazide hydrochloride to remove acetaldehyde, an end product of the reaction, the authors were able to increase the sensitivity of detection from $4–6 \times 10^3$ to 20 cfu/g (or cfu/mL). Although the new method is satisfactory for detecting *S. aureus* directly in foods, even greater sensitivity is necessary for detecting foodborne pathogens such as *Salmonella* and *Listeria monocytogenes*, which are of concern at levels of <1 per gram.

Detection of SEB by a sandwich ELISA was reported (49). The ELISA was insensitive to protein A, which is produced concurrently with enterotoxins by most *S. aureus* strains and frequently gives false-positive results with RIAs, ELISAs, and RPLA tests. The new test used rat MAbs of the IgG2a isotype, which showed no reactivity with protein A even at concentrations >1000 ng/mL. It detected SEB at levels <1 ng/mL.

MAbs capable of binding all SE serovars would be very useful for analysis of food samples because the individual enterotoxins would not have to be assayed separately. Therefore the homologous and heterologous reactivity of MAbs against SEA was studied using a standard indirect ELISA technique and a semiautomated electrophoresis system (50). Eight murine MAbs to SEA were prepared using standard hybridoma techniques. Their reactivities and cross-reactivities were studied by indirect ELISA and immunoblotting. Two of the MAbs reacted with all five SEs (A–E) in both systems and thus could be used to detect all five serovars in a single assay. One MAb reacted specifically only with SEA, and four reacted with SEA and SEE.

Shinagawa et al. described the detection of SEA by a double-antibody sandwich ELISA system, with at least one of the two MAbs reacting only with SEA (51). The method was specific for SEA and sensitive, detecting as little as 0.25 ng/mL of enterotoxin. Its adaptation for each individual SE and its use with clinical specimens as well as with foods incriminated in outbreaks of staphylococcal food poisoning appear feasible. However, it is necessary to remove protein A before the sandwich ELISA is used to detect SEs in culture supernatants.

The GENE-TRAK *S. aureus* kit was adapted for use in detecting *S. aureus* as an agent of bovine mastitis (52). By modifying the method of sample preparation, specific diagnosis of *S. aureus* in milk from udder quarters could be made within 6 h. The method was 100% specific and highly sensitive. The procedure was recommended for screening dairy products for staphylococcal contamination.

A dot blot hybridization technique with oligonucleotide probes was developed for specific detection of the TSST-1, SEA, SEB, SEC, SED, and SEE genes (53). A probe sequence was chosen from the previously determined sequence of each toxin gene. The genotypic method was compared with two phenotypic methods (gel immunodiffusion and ELISA) for 133 *S. aureus* strains and 12 coagulase-negative staphylococci. A correlation of 96% was observed between the genotypic and phenotypic assays. DNA from two coagulase-negative strains hybridized with a probe without detection of the corresponding toxin, and one SEC-producing *S. aureus* strain was not detected by the *entC* gene probe.

The polymerase chain reaction (PCR) was used to amplify the staphylococcal *entB, entC1,* and *nuc* genes (54). Nested primers were required to detect low copy numbers of purified DNA in diluent. With single primer pairs, 100 pg of target DNA was necessary for detection, whereas with nested primers as little as 1 fg could be detected. Enterotoxigenic *S. aureus* was detected in artificially contaminated dried skim milk samples at levels of ~10^5 cfu/mL within 8 h. No cross-reactivity between the highly homologous *entB* and *entC1* genes was observed; the method was 100% specific for *entC1* when tested against a wide variety of *S. aureus* and other *Staphylococcus* strains and *E. coli*. The authors recommend this as a rapid, sensitive, specific, and reliable method for detecting enterotoxigenic *S. aureus* in milk. Because it demonstrates the genetic potential for enterotoxin production it could serve as both a screening test and a confirmatory test for enterotoxins detected by RPLA or ELISA. It may prove useful in epidemiologic studies as well.

CLOSTRIDIUM

Schantz and Johnson reviewed the properties and medical use of botulinum toxin and other microbial neurotoxins (*55*). Their review provides information on mechanisms of action of botulinum toxin, preparation of botulinum toxin type A, botulism in humans, toxin production by various serotypes of *Clostridium botulinum*, and the structure and properties of toxic and nontoxic components of the toxin complex.

Clostridium botulinum

OUTBREAKS AND OCCURRENCE IN FOODS. An outbreak of type E botulism in New Jersey was linked to consumption of an ethnic uneviscerated, salt-cured fish product (*56*). Four members of a family of Egyptian descent were hospitalized 3 days after eating uncooked, unheated moloha allegedly purchased from a local retail market. Upon investigation, no moloha or similar fish product was found at the market and the owner denied selling that type of fish.

A case of unusual sensory symptoms associated with botulism was reported from Spain (*57*). A woman became ill 6 days after eating home-canned green beans. A serum specimen and sample of the beans were positive for type B botulinum toxin. Along with the typical evolution of botulism she developed a decreased pinprick sensation on the left half of her body and face, which disappeared with the resolution of her other symptoms.

To determine whether corn syrup and other syrups on the U.S. food market are sources of *C. botulinum* spores for infants, 738 bottles of various kinds of syrup were tested (*58*). Two were presumptively positive for *C. botulinum* type A spores, but on further testing proved negative. The authors concluded that corn syrup and other syrups are not food sources of *C. botulinum* spores for infants, and state further that suggestions of a statistical association between corn syrup consumption and infant botulism, perhaps because sticky corn syrup catches dust containing *C. botulinum* spores, remain unproven.

Because menhaden are often harvested in areas where *C. botulinum* may occur and menhaden surimi supports *C. botulinum*'s growth and toxin production, the incidence and heat resistance of *C. botulinum* type E spores in menhaden surimi was investigated (*59*). Seven of 565 raw surimi samples (1.2%) were positive for type E spores. Thermal death time studies of sterile surimi inoculated with type E spores indicated that although survival of spores at the higher temperatures was slightly greater than previously reported, the currently established time/temperature processing conditions provide an adequate margin of safety. Because *C. botulinum* type E spores do exist in raw menhaden surimi, manufacturers must ensure that processing conditions are sufficient to destroy them.

GROWTH AND TOXIN PRODUCTION. Lambert et al. studied toxin production by *C. botulinum* types A and B in modified-atmosphere-packaged (MAP), irradiated pork (*60,61*). Their work was motivated by questions concerning how O_2 and CO_2 influence toxin production in MAP foods. In one study, fresh pork was inoculated with *C. botulinum*, and five initial levels of CO_2 and three irradiation doses were tested using a factorial design (*60*). Headspace CO_2 levels increased in all samples during storage at 15°C. Under most conditions, spoilage preceded toxigenesis. Toxin production was more rapid in samples initially packaged with 15 or 30% CO_2 than with 45, 60, or 75%. Irradiation with 0.5 or 1.0 kGy delayed toxin production at all levels of CO_2. Including a CO_2 absorbent in the package enhanced toxin production, perhaps because the absorbent generated H_2 that could lower the oxidation–reduction potential of the meat. These findings demonstrated the complexity of *C. botulinum*'s requirements for germination, growth, and toxin production. The second study evaluated the effects of irradiation, initial O_2 and CO_2 concentration (0 or 20%, balance N_2), and O_2 and CO_2 absorbents on toxin production in inoculated pork stored at 15°C (*61*). All samples spoiled before they became toxic. Toxin production was faster in samples originally packaged with 20% O_2 than in samples packaged with 100% N_2. Headspace CO_2 was not an important factor in determining the time to toxin detection. Irradiation significantly delayed toxin production only in samples packaged with 20% O_2. This study confirmed that an initial level of 20% O_2 accelerates toxin production in this system, whereas packaging with CO_2 was not a significant factor. The effect of irradiation was not clarified.

The effect of headspace O_2 concentration on growth and toxin production by *C. botulinum* type B was also studied in broth media, at pH values of 5–7 and NaCl concentrations of 0–4% (*62*). Under these conditions, the critical (maximum) level of oxygen for germination and growth was ~1%. Growth and toxin production were favored by high pH and low salt levels and were related to inoculum size.

Clostridium botulinum type E occurs in seawater and sediments, and there is no assurance that pasteurized oysters are clostridia-free (*63*). Chai and Liang evaluated the thermal resistance of *C. botulinum* type E spores in homogenates of oysters from the Chesapeake Bay. Five isolates from Chesapeake Bay crabs and seafood botulism outbreaks in Alaska and Minnesota were tested. Although the organisms were less heat-resistant in oyster homogenate than in other seafood products, current oyster pasteurization procedures are not adequate to guarantee safety from type E *C. botulinum* spores.

The heat resistance of *Clostridium sporogenes* PA3679 and *C. botulinum* 213B spores was studied as a function of the pH of the heating medium and the NaCl concentration in the recovery medium (*64*). Heat resistance, expressed as $D_{112.8}$ or $D_{107.2}$ value, decreased as pH decreased from 7.0 to 5.0. For all levels of pH in the heating medium, addition of NaCl to the recovery medium at levels of 0.0, 0.5, 1.0, 1.5, and 2.0% progressively reduced the number of colony forming units in a population of heated spores. These results clearly demonstrated that reported D values are only apparent D values, which are influenced by both heating and recovery conditions.

Studies of the radiation resistance of *C. botulinum* and *Bacillus subtilis* spores in honey and sugar syrups found it to be a function of water content (*65*). Although D values for *C. botulinum* spores in honey were relatively high (8.1–12.8 kGy), the authors concluded that gamma irradiation could be used to reduce spore levels in honey and this might prevent up to ~14 cases of infant botulism per year.

Prompted by outbreaks of botulism caused by unacidified chopped garlic bottled in oil, Solomon et al. evaluated the ability of a wide range of unacidified products bottled in oil or water to support growth and toxin production by *C. botulinum* type A (*66*). Products were inoculated with about 50 spores per gram or milliliter of a mixture of five clostridial strains isolated from fresh garlic skins, onion skins, potato salad, green peppers in jars, and coleslaw. Samples were incubated at room temperature. Organoleptic acceptability was evaluated monthly for 4 months and portions were diluted and injected intraperitoneally into mice. None of the 120 samples exhibited toxicity at any time. The authors warned that although the products tested did not support outgrowth and toxin production by *C. botulinum* type A spores under the experimental conditions, other strains might grow or a combination of optimum conditions might induce growth in these products.

The relationship between the biotype of *C. botulinum* strains and their sensitivity to nisin and other bacteriocins was assessed (*67*). Although considerably different nisin sensitivities were found among the 18 strains tested, these differences were not associated with biotype. The extremes were spores from strain 56A, which required 2500 IU/mL of nisin to inhibit growth for 30 days and strain 169, which was inhibited for 30 days by only 10 IU/mL. Both strains were completely inhibited at the 10,000 IU/mL limit permitted in processed cheeses. When these strains and a strain with intermediate nisin sensitivity were tested for bacteriocin-mediated inhibition by *Lactococcus lactis*, *Pediococcus pentosaceus*, and *Lactobacillus plantarum*, no statistically significant differences in sensitivity were found.

The effectiveness of a combination of lactic acid starter culture and a sugar in preventing botulinum toxigenesis was first demonstrated in reduced-nitrite bacon, and this is the only application for which it is currently approved by the USDA (*68*). In theory, however, this "biocontrol preservation" technology should be applicable to many other low-acid refrigerated foods that receive less than a 12*D* thermal treatment. Hutton et al. tested it in chicken salad. They added a combination of *Pediococcus acidilactici* and dextrose to chicken salad inoculated with mixed spores of types A, B, and E and incubated the samples at 10–35°C. When the salad was temperature-abused, the lactic acid bacteria catabolized the dextrose to lactic acid at a rate sufficient to prevent botulinum toxigenesis. Another study evaluated the ability of *L. lactis*, *P. pentosaceus*, *L. plantarum*, and *Lactobacillus acidophilus* to inhibit *C. botulinum* spores at refrigeration and abuse temperatures (*69*). Modified deferred and simultaneous antagonism methods were used. All strains except *L. acidophilus* N2 produced inhibition zones on lawns of *C. botulinum* spores at 30°C. *Lactobacillus plantarum* BN, *L. lactis* ATCC 11454, and *P. pentosaceus* ATCC 43200 and 43201 were bacteriocinogenic at 4, 10, and 15°C as well. Supplementation of BHI agar with 0–5% NaCl increased the radii of the inhibition zones in a dose-related way in simultaneous antagonism assays. These results suggest that certain strains of lactic bacteria, in the presence of 3–4% NaCl, could be formulated into minimally processed refrigerated foods to protect against botulism.

Miller and Menichillo studied the antibotulinal efficacy of nitrite in several model beef sausage formulations (*70*). They demonstrated that use of blood fractions that increase iron levels in the sausage to >30 µg/g reduced the antibotulinal effect of sodium nitrite.

MOLECULAR STUDIES. Highly specific and sensitive sandwich ELISAs for detecting botulinum toxins A and B have been developed (*71*). As little as 0.5 ng/mL of either toxin can be detected. The ELISA for toxin A does not cross-react with toxin B, D, or E and the ELISA for toxin B does not cross-react with toxin A, D, or E at concentrations up to 1000 ng/mL. Use of this method might greatly reduce the need for mouse bioassays. Other investigators assessed the correlation between the mouse neurotoxin test and an ELISA for determining *C. botulinum* types A and B toxin (*72*). Although both tests detected toxin in a meat system inoculated with *C. botulinum* and various other aerobic and anaerobic bacteria, they gave quite different pictures of the relative toxigenicity of the samples. This suggested that some strains of *C. botulinum* produce antigens that react in the ELISA but have no neurotoxicity. Trypsin treatment tended to decrease the ELISA activity of most strains, whereas it increased activity in the mouse test. The authors recommended the ELISA for laboratory investigations utilizing known strains and large numbers of samples when fast results are desired; otherwise, ELISA results should be verified by the mouse test.

The PCR and a radiolabeled oligonucleotide probe were used to detect proteolytic and nonproteolytic *C. botulinum* type B (*73*). The test proved to be specific, sensitive, and rapid. Two synthetic primers deduced from the amino acid sequence of type B neurotoxin were used to amplify a 1500 base-pair fragment corresponding to the toxin's light chain. Although nonspecific priming occurred with other clostridia, only the PCR product from *C. botulinum* type B reacted with the radiolabeled internal probe. As little as 100 fg of DNA (representing ~35 cells) could be detected after 25 amplification cycles.

Genetic analysis of *C. botulinum* toxinogenesis has been hampered by lack of effective mutation and gene transfer systems and by restrictions on cloning of toxin gene fragments larger than 1000 bases and on certain other genetic manipulations (*74*). Lin and Johnson explored transposon mutagenesis as a way to obtain *C. botulinum* mutants with altered toxinogenetic or other important characteristics. The tetracycline-resistant transposon Tn*916* in *Enterococcus faecalis* was conjugatively transferred to *C. botulinum* strains Hall A and 113B. Southern blot analysis of *Eco*RI and *Hin*dIII chromosomal digests showed that the transposon inserted at different sites in the recipient chromosome, with a copy number of 1 to 3. Eleven auxotrophic mutants were studied for their specific amino acid requirements.

Botulinum neurotoxin A was isolated from liquid culture of *C. botulinum* and the purified toxin of M_r ~150,000 was crystallized in three crystal forms (*75*). Large enough crystals were obtained to permit preliminary X-ray analysis. The bipyramidal crystals demonstrated the trigonal space group $P3_121$ or $P3_221$ with one dimer per asymmetric unit. The unit cell dimensions were $a = b = 170.5$ Å, $c = 161.7$ A. The crystals diffract to 3 Å resolution.

Two λgt11 clones of *C. botulinum* type B toxin were identified by the monoclonal antibody specific to the heavy chain of the toxin (*76*). Restriction analysis and hybridization experiments revealed regions in the N-terminus of the heavy chain that were highly homologous with regions in type A botulinum neurotoxin and tetanus toxin.

There are many unanswered questions about the neurotoxigenicity of *Clostridium baratii* and *Clostridium butyricum*, which have been implicated in some cases of the toxicoinfectious form of botulism ("infant botulism") (*77*). Giménez et al. asked how the neurotoxin produced by a strain of *C. baratii* compares structurally with the neurotoxins of *C. botulinum*. They produced the toxin in dialysis bags, purified it, and analyzed it. The neurotoxin was a single-chain protein of ~140 kDa. Comparison of the sequence of the 19 N-terminal amino acids with the sequence of botulinum neurotoxins of serotypes A, B, and E showed 40–50% identical residues in comparable positions. Neurotoxicity of the *C. baratii* neurotoxin was not significantly enhanced by mild trypsinization, although the treatment did generate two primary fragments linked by an interchain disulfide bridge. These fragments resembled the well characterized light and heavy chains of *C. botulinum* neurotoxins A–F. It remains to be

learned whether or how non–*C. botulinum* species in the normal intestinal flora acquire and express the neurotoxin gene. Construction and use of DNA probes based on the reported sequence could help answer some of these questions.

The structural gene for the *C. botulinum* type E neurotoxin has been cloned and its sequence analyzed, and from this the complete amino acid sequence of the neurotoxin has been derived (*78*). With 1252 amino acids, it is the smallest of the botulinum neurotoxins characterized to date. The light chain has 40% sequence similarity to tetanus toxin and ~33% similarity to botulinum neurotoxins A, C, and D. Sequence similarity of the heavy E chain with heavy chains of the other toxins is 46% with type A, 36% with type C, 37% with type D, and 35% with tetanus. Alignment of the characterized sequences shows the toxins to be composed of highly conserved domains interspersed with sequences showing little overall similarity. For all the toxins, the most divergent region corresponds to the C-terminus. Other investigators determined the nucleotide sequences of the type E neurotoxin genes from two strains of *C. butyricum* isolated from cases of infant botulism (*79*). The two sequences were identical and differed at only 64 positions from the gene of *C. botulinum* E strain Beluga. This results in 97% identity at the amino acid level. The authors postulated transfer of the gene from *C. botulinum* to an initially nontoxigenic *C. butyricum*, followed by divergence through point mutations. If this process occurs readily, a neurotoxin-based classification of *C. botulinum* bears little relationship to the overall physiologic properties of the host strains. Similar studies determined similarities between the light chains of neurotoxins from *C. butyricum* strain BL6340 and *C. botulinum* type E strain Mashike (*80*). Of the 422 amino acids in the light chain, 17 differed between the strains; all of these were within 200 residues of the N-terminus. When compared with sequences of type A, C_1, and D toxins, five regions showed highly homologous sequences.

Besides the neurotoxin, *C. botulinum* strains also produce varying amounts of a thiol-activated hemolysin, "botulinolysin" (*81*). Botulinolysin was isolated from culture supernatants of *C. botulinum* strain C-203 Tox, purified to homogeneity, and characterized. The purified hemolysin gave a single protein band of M_r 58,000 with SDS–PAGE. In PAGE without SDS, hemolytic activity corresponded in position to the single protein band. The amino acid composition, hemolytic activity, cytotoxicity, and lethality for mice were evaluated. Two of three type D strains and one of five type E strains tested also produced relatively large amounts of botulinolysin. The methods developed in this study should be useful for further studies of the role of this hemolysin in botulinum infections and bacterial physiology and of relationships between structure and function of this and other thiol-activated cytolysins.

Clostridium perfringens

EPIDEMIOLOGY, OUTBREAKS, AND IDENTIFICATION. Labbé reviewed *Clostridium perfringens* as a foodborne pathogen (*82*). He considered the epidemiology and characteristics of foodborne infections, characteristics of the organism relevant to food poisoning, isolation and identification of the organism, and control measures. *Clostridium perfringens* food poisoning has most often been associated with meat and poultry products prepared in food-service establishments. Although fecal spore levels of $\geq 10^6$/g are considered indicative of food-poisoning, high spore levels are frequently found in healthy older persons. Fecal enterotoxin level may be more definitive, because it appears that not all strains of this organism can produce enterotoxin.

Multiple typing techniques were applied to a series of fecal specimens from persons involved in two *C. perfringens* food-poisoning outbreaks at the same institution, in an attempt to identify a common strain (*83*). Typing of 92 *C. perfringens* colonies was done with antisera and bacteriocins and by plasma analysis, and the colonies were tested for in vitro production of bacteriocin and enterotoxin. A strain of *C. perfringens* common to both outbreaks was found in the feces of affected persons. Enterotoxin was detected in 13 of 16 fecal specimens tested, of which 5 were from asymptomatic food handlers. A role of food handlers in these outbreaks was not proved, although five of them carried the

outbreak strain. Results of bacteriocin testing and serotyping correlated well, but plasma typing disrupted the relationship and was not helpful because the putative outbreak strain did not carry any detectable plasmids. The authors suggested that at least five colonies from each stool specimen be typed in investigations of this nature because more than one strain can be carried simultaneously in human feces.

Clostridium perfringens food poisoning is common wherever food is prepared in large quantities hours before serving. Large outbreaks occurred in two county jails in the state of Washington in autumn 1991 (*84*). In the first, 238 of 379 prisoners and staff became ill after eating a meal of "fiesta casserole," a dish containing ground meat. It had been prepared in large containers, cooled slowly, and reheated inadequately. Large numbers of spores were found in leftover food and fecal specimens. In the second, 320 of 400 inmates became ill after eating tacos with ground meat that had been improperly prepared.

A survey found *C. perfringens* in 64 of 118 ground beef samples (54%) and 40 of 55 ground turkey samples (73%) collected in northeast Kansas—a total of 104 positive samples (60%) (*85*). Three methods for detecting low numbers of the organisms were compared. Fung's double-tube procedure identified 94 positive samples, Oxyrase Enzyme identified 77, and Gas Pack Anaerobic System identified 73. After storage at 23°C for 6 days, the number of *C. perfringens* increased from 44/g to ~10^9/g; Fung's double-tube method gave the highest counts. The authors recommended Fung's double-tube procedure because it was simple, rapid, inexpensive, and gave the best results of the methods tested.

Clostridium perfringens food poisoning occurs when vegetative cells of an enterotoxin-producing strain are ingested and sporulate in the intestine. However, not all strains sporulate in the usual sporulation media, making identification of enterotoxin-producing strains by culture methods difficult (*86*). An alternative technique uses DNA probes to detect the enterotoxin gene. A survey in the Netherlands sampled intestinal contents of slaughter animals—50 cows, 50 pigs, and 59 broiler chickens—and fecal specimens of 50 horses.

Clostridium perfringens was detected in samples from 24% of horses, 36% of cattle, 80% of chickens, and 2% of pigs. The corresponding values for enterotoxigenic strains were 14, 22, 10, and 0%.

Clostridium perfringens is divided into five groups (A–E) based on the production of extracellular β, ε, and ι toxins; all groups produce α-toxin. Type A strains, which produce only α-toxin, are considered responsible for food poisoning in humans. An ELISA using antibodies specific to *C. perfringens* β, ε, and ι_b toxins was developed to type organisms in 192 isolates from food samples and 58 isolates from patients (*87*). Four food samples and 5 fecal specimens from patients with gastroenteritis proved to be *C. perfringens* type D; one type B and one type C were also detected in samples from patients with gastroenteritis. The sensitivity of the ELISA was 10–1000 times higher than that of the mouse lethality test and the guinea pig dermonecrosis test. Because of its greater sensitivity and speed, this ELISA could replace much animal testing.

GROWTH AND PATHOGENICITY. Methanol extracts of Japanese green tea (*Thea sinensis*) were fractionated and tested for growth-inhibitory activity against *Clostridium difficile* ATCC 9689 and *C. perfringens* ATCC 13124 (*88*). Several components of the polyphenol fraction were active at a level of 5 mg/disc. (+)-Catechin, (–)-epicatechin, (+)-gallocatechin, (–)-epicatechin gallate, and (–)-epigallocatechin gallate inhibited growth of *C. perfringens*, whereas only (–)-epicatechin gallate and (–)-epigallocatechin gallate were inhibitory for *C. difficile*.

The pathodynamics of lethal intoxication after i.v. administration of *C. perfringens* type A enterotoxin was studied in intact anesthetized rats and mice and in isolated organs (*89*). Death was apparently caused by hyperpotassemia elicited by the cytotoxic action of enterotoxin on hepatocytes, leading to cardiac failure.

The activity of enterotoxin from *C. perfringens* type A is enhanced about threefold by trypsinization, which cleaves the first 25 amino acids from the N-terminus. Because the small intestine in humans contains chymotrypsin as well as trypsin, Granum and Richardson tested whether chymotrypsin also

increases the activity of the enterotoxin (*90*). Treatment with chymotrypsin cleaved 36 amino acids from the N-terminus and 3 from the C-terminus, resulting in an increase of activity on Vero cells comparable to that found for trypsin treatment. The authors postulated that loss of 25–36 N-terminal amino acids facilitates structural changes necessary for membrane penetration. Shift from a β-sheet to an α-helix structure has also been suggested by others.

Platelet-activating factor is a potent inflammatory mediator that causes neutrophil adhesion and aggregation, chemotaxis, and increased vascular permeability. Investigators in Sweden demonstrated that phospholipase C from *C. perfringens* stimulates formation of platelet-activating factor in cultured intestinal epithelial cells (*91*). Exposure of INT cells to phospholipase C for up to 60 min caused a time-dependent formation and release of platelet-activating factor but did not affect cellular acetylhydrolase activity or the ability of the cells to metabolize exogenous ^{14}C-labeled platelet-activating factor. The authors postulated that when stimulated with an intestinal bacterial toxin in vivo, intestinal epithelial cells also generate and release platelet-activating factor and this may contribute to the pathophysiology of inflammatory bowel disease.

Investigators have studied the relationship between sporulation and enterotoxin production by *C. perfringens* type A under various conditions. When *C. perfringens* NCTC 8798 was grown in Duncan and Strong sporulation medium, spore formation was correlated with formation of both enterotoxin and the cytoplasmic inclusion body (*92*). The start of an exponential increase in enterotoxin production was associated with sporulation stage III, the time when forespore formation was first detected by electron microscopy. At stage IV, spore cortex became visible and the inclusion body appeared. Studies with mutants confirmed the tight coupling of sporulation and formation of enterotoxin and the cytoplasmic inclusion body. Nonsporulation mutants blocked at stage 0 or I produced neither enterotoxin nor inclusion bodies and had low protease activity. Mutants blocked at stage II or III produced enterotoxin but not the inclusion body, and had somewhat higher protease activity. Mutants blocked at stage IV or V produced both enterotoxin and inclusion bodies and their protease activity was near that of the wild-type strain. Other investigators reasoned that bile, which is continually secreted into the small intestine, might influence the growth, sporulation, and entertoxin production of *C. perfringens* (*93*). They studied the effect of human bile and bile salts on enterotoxin-positive and -negative strains of *C. perfringens* grown in liquid medium. Bile completely inhibited growth of all strains at a 1:320 dilution. A mixture of bile salts completely inhibited growth of the three enterotoxin-positive strains tested but not of the negative strain. However, bile salts stimulated sporulation of two of the positive strains and increased enterotoxin concentrations in the cell extracts. There was no effect on enterotoxin production in the enterotoxin-negative strain tested. Overall, bile and bile salts inhibited growth but stimulated sporulation and enterotoxin production of *C. perfringens*. The effects of individual bile acids varied. The effect of temperature on the growth, sporulation, enterotoxin production, and heat resistance of *C. perfringens* was evaluated in several enterotoxin-positive and -negative strains (*94*). The D_{85} or D_{95} of spores varied among strains but in all cases was directly related to sporulation temperature (32, 37, or 43°C). Enterotoxin and heat-resistant spores were produced in similar concentrations at 37 and 43°C, but production began and peaked sooner at 43°C. Similarly, growth was more rapid at 43°C than at 37 or 32°C.

MOLECULAR STUDIES. Rood and Cole reviewed the molecular genetics and pathogenesis of *C. perfringens* (*95*). They covered the bacteriophages, bacteriocins, and plasmids associated with the organism and determinants of antibiotic resistance. Genetic manipulation and chromosome mapping were reviewed. The α, β, ϵ, ι, θ, and μ toxins were discussed, as well as neuraminidase and several minor or questionable toxins and virulence factors. The production, biochemistry, and molecular genetics of enterotoxin were considered in some detail. The authors concluded that high levels of enterotoxin are produced in the cytoplasm after activation of the enterotoxin gene by transcriptional factors that also control sporulation genes. Accumulation of large amounts of enterotoxin then can result in aggregation, inclusion body formation, and trapping of small amounts of enterotoxin during spore biogenesis.

Hanna et al. located and analyzed the receptor-binding region of *C. perfringens* enterotoxin by cloning toxin fragments and creating synthetic peptides corresponding to specific nucleotide sequences (*96*). They found that a linear sequence of the C-terminal 30 residues was sufficient for recognizing and binding to the enterotoxin receptor in Vero cells. They then further mapped the functional regions of the *C. perfringens* type A enterotoxin (*97*). Removing the N-terminal 25 amino acids by trypsinization increased the enterotoxin's primary cytotoxic effect without affecting binding. Sequences required for four nonoverlapping epitopes recognized by MAbs were identified and mapped. Two epitopes were associated with the extreme C-terminal end of the enterotoxin.

BACILLUS CEREUS

Outbreaks, occurrence, and growth

Eight persons reported becoming ill after eating fried rice at a Chinese restaurant in Perth, Australia (*98*). High levels of *B. cereus* were found in a sample of vomit from one subject. A visit to the restaurant by two Environmental Health officers revealed four large bowls of boiled rice that had been cooked the day before and left overnight at ambient temperatures. This practice was routine. Instructions were given for safe storing of precooked rice at temperatures outside the danger zone of 5–63°C.

Meer et al. reviewed the psychrotrophic *Bacillus* species found in fluid milk products (*99*). They discussed the incidence of psychrotrophic spore-formers and the heat activation of *Bacillus* spores at pasteurization temperatures. Germination and growth of these organisms are strain- and source-dependent, and their heat resistance depends on characteristics of the strain and medium. The importance of *B. cereus* for public health was discussed in terms of the bacterial toxins and their detection and other aspects of pathogenesis. The authors stressed the dairy industry's need for an improved method for assessing either the heat-resistant psychrotroph population of raw milk and pasteurized products or their associated proteinases.

Bacillus cereus produces a variety of exo-products that contribute to its pathogenicity in varying degrees. Culture filtrates from 89 strains of *B. cereus* isolated from foods (chiefly dairy and bakery products) were tested to characterize the strains according to their production of enterotoxin, permeability and lethal factor, hemolysin, cytotoxin, and lecithinase (*100*). Three filtrates caused fluid accumulation in the ligated rabbit ileal loop; 71 caused an increase in vascular permeability in the rabbit skin test corresponding to moderate or strong toxin production; 59 were cytotoxic to Vero cells; 31 were lethal to mice; all 89 were hemolytic on agar plates containing 6% sheep blood and 81 hemolyzed 0.5% rabbit erythrocytes; 55 had lecithinase activity. The extent of the permeability reaction was correlated with cytotoxicity, lecithinase activity, and lethality, but not with hemolytic activity.

In Indonesian tapé fermentation, cooked rice is inoculated with traditional starter cultures and held at ambient temperatures for 1–3 days. The starter cultures may contain *B. cereus* that can grow during fermentation. The growth of *B. cereus* NCIB 8579 was studied in four varieties of rice with and without tapé fermentation (*101*). Both fermented and unfermented rice supported growth of the organism up to levels of 10^7–10^9 cfu/g. As fermentation progressed the pH fell, but populations remained at ~10^8 cfu/g except in the black glutinous rice, in which they dropped to ~10^6 cfu/g. Cells added at various times during fermentation fared less well. The authors postulated that after growth on rice is established, *B. cereus* survives fermentation as spores.

Investigators in Finland assessed the effects of drying, packaging, and storage conditions on the microbiological quality of herbs (*102*). Dill (*Anethum graveolens* L.), basil (*Ocimum basilicum* L.), marjoram (*Origanum majorana* L.), and wild marjoram (*Origanum vulgare* L.) were freeze- or air-dried and stored in glass jars under air at 23°C, or freeze-dried and stored in polyethylene–aluminum packs under vacuum or nitrogen at 23 or 35°C. After 1 and 2 years of storage samples were evaluated for aerobic plate count, yeast and mold counts, coliforms, aerobic and anaerobic spore-formers, and *B. cereus*. Although *B. cereus* was present in most herb samples, counts ranged from 50 to 3.9 × 10^3 per gram of dried herb, not high enough to cause food poisoning. Factors contributing significantly to the variance of *B. cereus* counts were herb, packaging, herb × packaging, herb × drying method, and storage temperature.

The effects of pressures up to 4000 bar on microorganisms in natural black pepper (*Piper nigrum* L.) and black pepper inoculated with *B. cereus* spores were tested (*103*). Treatment decreased the number of viable microorganisms by several orders of magnitude in liquid medium but was ineffective in dry pepper. There were minor changes in proportions of volatile oils and compounds responsible for the pungent taste of pepper.

Toxins

Shinagawa et al. have been studying the toxins of *B. cereus* by various methods (*104–106*). They purified a mouse lethal toxin, produced by a *B. cereus* strain isolated from a patient with vomiting-type food poisoning, by chromatography on DEAE–Sephadex A-25 and gel filtration on Sephadex G-75 (*104*). The purified toxin had an M_r of 33–34 × 10^3. It was lethal to mice and had hemolytic activity against sheep and rabbit erythrocytes but did not induce fluid accumulation in the mouse intestinal loop test. It was stable in the pH range of 6–9 and during storage at –20°C and was resistant to treatments with papain, cholesterol, lecithin, and dithiothreitol and to heating at 37°C for 5 min. Storage at 4 or 25°C for 2 weeks, treatment with trypsin, trypanblue, or ethanol, or heating at 60°C for 5 min destroyed most activity. The authors concluded that the mouse lethal toxin is similar to or identical with hemolysin II and different from the diarrheagenic toxin produced in diarrheal-type *B. cereus* food poisoning. They have also reported the development of three mouse MAbs against an enterotoxin involved in diarrheal-type food poisoning (*105*). These antibodies were evaluated for immunoaffinity-chromatographic purification of the enterotoxin, which had eluded attempts to purify it by conventional methods (*106*). Use of MAb B-10 gave a 25% yield of an electrophoretically and antigenically homogeneous enterotoxin that was active in the vascular permeability, mouse lethality, and mouse intestinal-loop fluid accumulation tests but did not possess hemolytic or lecithinase activity.

A nonhemolytic toxin from a strain of *B. cereus* isolated from radiation-pasteurized shrimps seemed to be associated with a 7.6-MDa plasmid (*107*). Cells grown in beef-infusion broth were examined for plasmids and the supernatant was tested for hemolytic and nonhemolytic toxins. Supernatants from plasmid-bearing cultures showed both toxin activities, but supernatants from plasmid-cured cultures had only hemolytic toxin activity. The authors concluded that the hemolytic toxin is regulated by DNA in the bacterial chromosome, whereas production of the nonhemolytic toxin depends on the presence of a plasmid.

Tomita et al. reviewed the sphingomyelinase of *B. cereus* (*108*). They discussed its physical, enzymatic, structural, and toxic properties, the sphingomyelinase gene, and the effects on sphingomyelinase–membrane interactions of altering critical amino acid residues in the enzyme or perturbing the membrane. The enzyme was compared with other bacterial sphingomyelinases such as the *S. aureus* β-toxin and other phospholipases C from *B. cereus* and *C. perfringens*.

Detection

Jackson discussed the criteria for diagnosing *B. cereus* food poisoning (*109*). She summarized properties and detection of the enterotoxin (diarrheal toxin) and the emetic toxin. Development of in vitro methods for enterotoxin detection has been hampered by difficulties in purifying the toxin. Jackson described a fluorescent immunodot assay that can detect as little as 50 ng of enterotoxin and is easy to use for large numbers of samples. She also

described a tissue-culture screening assay for the enterotoxin, which she is attempting to adapt for the emetic toxin.

The Oxoid BCET-RPLA kit was compared with the CHO and HEp-2 cell cytotonicity response for detection of the *B. cereus* diarrheal enterotoxin (*110*). Eleven strains of *B. cereus* and an enterotoxigenic strain of *Bacillus thuringiensis* were tested. CHO cells were consistently more sensitive than HEp-2 cells. Although there was general agreement between the cell culture method and the immunoassay method, results differed for certain strains. One strain was consistently negative with the immunoassay but was biologically active in both cell lines. Two other strains gave responses (one strong, one weak) with the kit but were negative in the cell tests. One strain was positive in CHO cells but negative in HEp-w cells and the immunoassay. In addition, activity in cell cultures was abolished by boiling the culture supernatants for 10 min, whereas the BCET-RPLA kit continued to detect significant levels of enterotoxin in boiled samples. The authors concluded that the specificity of the immunoassay needs further clarification and for the time being biological testing is still warranted.

SALMONELLA

Outbreaks and epidemiologic studies

Scope of the problem. Sockett reviewed the economic implications of salmonellosis in humans, with emphasis on industrialized countries (*111*). Costs are not only associated with investigating and treating illness but also affect the whole chain of food production. Sockett's review examined the rationale for economic evaluation of salmonellosis in terms of tangible and intangible costs to individuals and families, government, and industry. Economic analyses conducted in West Germany and Canada and a preliminary study in England and Wales were summarized. Details of the study in England and Wales were reported by Sockett and Roberts (*112*). Between August 1988 and March

1989, 1482 cases of salmonellosis were reported to environmental health departments in England and Wales. Ill persons and environmental health officers who investigated the cases were surveyed by questionnaire to obtain information on illness-associated costs to the public health sector, medical facilities, individuals and their families, and the wider economy. Costs of £996,339 were identified. Of this, £507,555 resulted from absence-related lost production and £392,822 represented costs of health care and investigation by local authorities. The remainder, £95,962, was the estimated impact on affected individuals and their families. These data do not include costs to businesses involved in the outbreak, such as those associated with withdrawal of products and closure of factories, or costs to the agricultural industry for treatment and containment. Tauxe reviewed *Salmonella* as a "postmodern" pathogen in the USA (*113*). The reported incidence of salmonellosis has risen inexorably since reporting began in 1943, and certain trends indicate that the increase will continue. First, a growing proportion of *Salmonella* isolates are resistant to multiple antimicrobial agents. Second, *Salmonella* bacteremia has become a serious complication in persons infected with the HIV virus. Third, infections caused by the egg-associated serotype of *Salmonella enteritidis* are increasing in number and geographic scope. Fourth, contamination of food produced in centralized facilities has caused extremely large and widespread outbreaks.

RISK FACTORS. Guam has a relatively high incidence of salmonellosis, and roughly half of the cases are in infants (3700 cases per 100,000 infants in 1984) (*114*). A case–control study was conducted to test the hypothesis that use of high-iron infant formulas is associated with this problem. Information on feeding practices and 16 physical, demographic, and socioeconomic variables was collected for 78 infants with laboratory-confirmed salmonellosis and 167 control infants. Case infants were less likely to have been breast-fed and more likely to have been fed infant formula containing ≥10 mg/L of iron. Although the route by which infants on Guam become infected is not known, consumption of high-iron infant formula was a significant risk factor.

The only other significant risk factor was complication of pregnancy or delivery.

Because of the increase in *S. enteritidis* infections in the northeastern USA and their potential severity, host risk factors were determined in a large nosocomial outbreak (*115*). The outbreak involved 274 of 965 patients in a New York hospital, 28 July–16 August 1987 (see *Food Safety 1991*, chapter 11, reference *157*). Patients who developed salmonellosis after eating the *S. enteritidis*–contaminated meal were more likely to be medication-dependent diabetics than those who did not develop the infection (17/75 vs. 7/80, Mantel-Haenszel adjusted odds ratio = 3.1, 95% confidence interval = 1.1, 8.6). Proposed mechanisms for diabetes as a risk factor for infection included decreased gastric acidity and an autonomic neuropathy of the small intestine that reduces intestinal motility, prolonging gastrointestinal transit time.

EPIDEMIOLOGIC STUDIES. Cloned DNA probes were used to analyze genomic relationships among 24 *S. enteritidis* isolates from the USA, Italy, Israel, and the U.K. (*116*). Seven subspecies of *Salmonella* were also examined to evaluate the discriminatory ability of the probes. Sequence divergence and rearrangements were determined in and around the *rfa, fim,* and *umuDC* loci and around insertion sites of the *Salmonella*-specific DNA insertion element IS*200*. Characteristic sequence divergence between subspecies was observed, but no intraserovar divergence was seen for *S. enteritidis*. The *umuDC* locus was not found in *S. enteritidis. Salmonella enteritidis* contained both a conserved and a variable insertion site of insertion sequence IS*200*. Analysis of the variable site revealed three evolutionary lines within isolates associated with human gastroenteritis. All U.K. isolates of epidemic phage type 4 belonged to a single clonal line. The authors concluded that the IS*200* profile is a well conserved molecular index of evolution, representing an interface of phylogenetics and epidemiology relevant to the medically important salmonellas. The same research group conducted similar studies of *S. enteritidis* strains isolated in Switzerland between 1965 and 1990 (*117*). Strains were selected to represent the preepidemic and current epidemic situation in Switzerland, with the dual objectives of establishing IS200 profiles as a method of typing a diverse group of *S. enteritidis* strains and of revealing the evolving epidemiology of this serovar. The phage type and plasmid profile of isolates were compared with the copy number and insertion loci of IS200. Three clonal lines of *S. enteritidis* were identified by IS200 profile, and each of these was specifically associated with particular phage types. All isolates from humans and poultry contained a 38-MDa plasmid that hybridized with a gene probe associated with mouse virulence. The authors concluded that for establishing very short-term evolutionary distance, phage typing is the most discriminatory method, whereas IS200 profiles provide a race-specific molecular marker of the chromosome and of vertical inheritance. IS200 profiles could complement plasmid profiling in epidemiologic applications, particularly when it is necessary to establish chromosomal genotypes.

Evaluation of *S. enteritidis* strains isolated from sporadic cases and outbreaks of salmonellosis in Maryland revealed changing clonal patterns from 1985 to 1990 (*118*). Ten plasmid profiles were identified. The predominant one, with a single plasmid of ~55 kilobases, was closely associated with phage type (PT) 8. It accounted for 42% of the 40 isolates from 1985 and 86% of 81 isolates from 1988–1989. Strains with this profile were identified in 4 of 9 outbreaks, including 1 of 3 in which eggs were implicated as a vehicle. Although plasmid profiles and phage typing provide complementary epidemiologic information, the apparent emergence of a predominant clone reduces the discriminatory ability of both typing systems. The shift in relative frequency of clones over time raises the possibility that certain strains of *S. enteritidis* have increased virulence or other characteristics that promote dissemination in human and chicken populations.

The phage typing scheme described by Ward et al. (*Epidemiol. Infect.* 99:291–294 [1987]) was used to type 573 strains of *S. enteritidis* isolated in the USA from humans, animals, food, and the environment (*119*). Most of the strains were collected from egg-related outbreaks in the Northeast in 1988 and 1989. Four of the 20 phage types identified accounted for 84% of the strains: PT8 (48.2%),

PT13a (20.1%) and PT13 and 14b (each 7.8%). Sixteen patterns were obtained for the 49 animal strains typed: 32% were PT8 (half of them from poultry), but no other type represented more than 8% of the animal strains. This system should be useful for studies of worldwide distribution of phage types and for monitoring the occurrence and spread of PT4.

The plasmid profiles, phage types, and antimicrobial resistance patterns were determined for *S. enteritidis* isolates in the USA (*120*). These represented sporadic isolates from national *Salmonella* surveillance studies conducted in 1979 (*n* = 28) and 1984 (*n* = 37), 43 isolates submitted to the CDC from outbreaks of salmonellosis between 1983 and 1987, and a random selection of 46 animal isolates submitted to the USDA Veterinary Services Laboratory in 1986 and 1987. Sporadic, outbreak, and animal isolates had similar rates of antimicrobial resistance (23, 14, and 24%, respectively); however, 11 of 12 resistant animal isolates were multiply resistant, whereas none of the human isolates were. Of the 16 plasmid profiles observed, two representing a single 36-MDa plasmid and a 36-MDa plus a 3.1-MDa plasmid accounted for the majority of isolates. Animal isolates had 14 phage types; human isolates had 5. PT13a and PT8 were the most common. A dominant plasmid profile was associated with each of the three most common phage types, although the most common plasmid profile could be subtyped into 7 phage types and PT8 could be subtyped into 5 plasmid profiles. The similar distribution of markers between sporadic and outbreak isolates suggested to the authors that they share a common reservoir.

Investigators in Sweden studied toxin production, hydrophobicity, and fibronectin-binding properties of 21 *Salmonella* strains isolated from Swedish travelers to different parts of the world (*121*). Five strains were *S. enteritidis*; the others were *S. newport, S. derby, S. braenderup, S. infantis, S. panama, S. bareilly, S. virchow, S. tees, S. typhimurium,* and *S. montevideo.* The noteworthy finding in this study was that *S. typhimurium* and *S. enteritidis* are not the only salmonellas that can produce enterotoxins and cytotoxins and interact with fibronectin. Strains of a wide variety of salmonellas worldwide possess these virulence properties. For example, cell sonicate supernatants from blood agar cultures of 80% of the strains induced induration and/or blueing in the rabbit skin permeability test and 19 were positive in the CHO cell test.

Salmon et al. discussed how analytical epidemiology can contribute to establishing the cause of food-poisoning outbreaks, stressing both strengths and limitations of this approach (*122*). As illustrative cases they examined three outbreaks of *S. enteritidis* PT4 food poisoning in Wales in 1989, in which epidemiological and microbiological investigation implicated eggs as the source but kitchen inspection and food preparation histories suggested other vehicles of infection. In only one of the three outbreaks was the organism actually isolated from a sample from the suspected meal. Nevertheless, the evidence implicating eggs in these outbreaks fulfilled 6 of 7 widely accepted criteria for establishing causation, and the authors conclude that if "proof" is possible at all, the cumulative evidence showed that eggs were a necessary, if not sufficient, cause.

A survey in a southwest coastal region of India found that cockroaches were reservoirs of antimicrobial-resistant salmonellas (*123*). Nine of 221 cockroaches collected in hospitals, houses, animal sheds, grocery stores, and restaurants yielded salmonellas belonging to *S. bovismorbificans, S. oslo, S. typhimurium, S. mbandaka*, and *S. braenderup*. All 9 strains were resistant to at least one antimicrobial agent tested and 7 showed multiple resistance. The authors concluded that by harboring potentially pathogenic drug-resistant salmonellas, these wandering arthropods pose an infective hazard to humans and animals.

Plasmid profile analysis of *S. berta* isolates from humans and food in England and Wales suggested that an increase in *S. berta* infections in humans is associated with imported poultry meat (*124*). From 1981 to 1985 only 3 isolates of *S. berta* from patients with food poisoning were identified, and 2 of these were from persons infected abroad. The picture then changed rapidly. From 1986 to 1990 only 20% of 279 isolates were from patients with a history of recent foreign travel. Moreover, until 1984 no isolates from human food had been received by the Central Public Health Laboratory,

whereas 40 food isolates have been identified since 1985: 35 of them from chicken carcasses, 28 of which were imported. Since 1988, 6 plasma profile types have caused infections in widely separated areas; 4 of these were identified in *S. berta* isolated from chicken carcasses imported from Denmark. Similar patterns of resistance to antimicrobial drugs have been observed in human and imported poultry isolates. These findings support the idea that from 1985 to 1990, contaminated Danish poultry has been a major source of *S. berta* strains that have caused an upsurge of salmonellosis in humans in England and Wales.

Salmonella arizonae is rarely isolated in the U.K. (*125*). From 1966 through 1990 there were 66 isolates from humans; 23 of these persons had recently traveled abroad and 32 were children ≤14 years old. Of animal isolates, 20 were from turkeys, 1 from a pig, 44 from sheep, 1 from a dog, 4 from tortoises, 25 from terrapins, and 2 from pet snakes. However, the turkey and sheep serotypes were rarely associated with human infection and in only one instance was the infection acquired in the U.K., whereas the reptilian serotypes were frequently encountered in human infections. The authors concluded that reptiles are potential sources of infection, particularly in children. Of 12 isolates from human foods, all were from imported foods and 7 were from Italian pasta.

OUTBREAKS. Fifteen persons who ate at a restaurant from October 17 to 25, 1991, developed gastroenteritis (*126*). Twenty-three of the restaurant's 78 employees also became ill. *Salmonella* group D was isolated from the feces of all 13 patrons who submitted stool specimens; the 8 isolates further typed were identified as *S. enteritidis*. *Salmonella enteritidis* was also isolated from stool samples of 15 of 22 ill employees and 6 of 44 asymptomatic employees. Fourteen of 15 ill patrons and none of 11 well patrons interviewed had eaten Caesar salad. Illness was not associated with eating any other uncooked egg dish. Only 3 culture-positive employees reported having eaten Caesar salad. However, confirmed *S. enteritidis* infection among employees was associated with exposure to raw eggs through consumption or handling at the restaurant. The Caesar salad dressing was prepared early in the morning   by combining yolks from hand-cracked eggs with olive oil, anchovies, garlic, and warm water. No lemon juice or vinegar was included. *Salmonella enteritidis* was isolated from one of 6 pools of eggs obtained from the supplier that provided the implicated shipment, and the source flock was identified. The restaurant had eliminated Caesar salad from the menu by the time the restaurant was inspected, and the implicated flock was destroyed before the outbreak was recognized. An unusual feature of this outbreak was that exposure to eggs was an occupational hazard for restaurant workers who did not eat the implicated food.

Of 114 residents of an old-people's home in Germany, 87 became ill after eating a lunch that included pudding with freshly prepared whipped egg white (*127*). Ten patients died. *Salmonella enteritidis* was isolated from the pudding at a level of 10^7/mL. Stool samples of residents and most personnel were negative, but 3 members of the kitchen staff excreted *S. enteritidis*. Samples from eggs, laying hens, feces, bedding, and feed from the incriminated farm were negative for salmonellas. Another outbreak of egg-associated *S. enteritidis* infection occurred in the U.K. in two adjoining nursing homes that shared kitchen facilities (*128*). Twenty-three residents and 6 staff members developed gastrointestinal symptoms during a 72-h period. *S. enteritidis* PT7a was isolated from stools of 15 of 16 case subjects who submitted specimens. There was a significant association between illness and consumption of a banana custard meringue. One young man on the staff ate three helpings of this food and became severely ill, suggesting a dose–response relationship. The banana custard meringue had been prepared the morning before it was served, using egg-free custard powder and the whites of 8 raw shell eggs. It was cooked for 10 min and then left to cool at room temperature. The kitchen was satisfactory and cross-contamination was considered unlikely.

In England, 36 people reported gastrointestinal illness after attending a Shabbaton held to teach children prayers, songs, and games organized around meals associated with the Jewish Sabbath (*129*). Most of the food for the weekend was prepared by a local kosher caterer. Of the 7 catering staff who completed questionnaires, none reported gastrointestinal symptoms. *Salmonella enteritidis* PT4 was isolated from 13 of 26 fecal specimens submitted by guests and 1 of 9 from the catering staff. Food was prepared on Friday morning and delivered that afternoon. Food for Friday's dinner was kept hot for several hours before serving; the rest was refrigerated. Illness was significantly associated with eating boiled gefilte fish, cake, mayonnaise, rice salad, and potato salad. After adjusting for the effect of other food items, only rice salad eaten at Saturday lunch remained independently significantly associated with illness. The salad contained rice, raisins, green peppers, mayonnaise, and seasoning. Two batches of mayonnaise had been prepared 4 or 5 days before it was served. The two batches, each using 30 shell eggs, were made in the same mixer. Two other outbreaks of *S. enteritidis* PT4 infection occurred during the same weekend and were associated with the same caterer: four people became ill after an engagement party and 5 became ill after a Jewish cultural event. The vehicle of infection could not be identified, but the caterer was advised to stop making mayonnaise from raw shell eggs.

The number of *S. enteritidis* PT4 infections is still increasing in the U.K., although the rate of increase has been reduced (*130*). Another egg-associated outbreak of *S. enteritidis* PT4 infection in England involved 7 of 9 people who ate a trifle topped with a mixture containing raw eggs. The organism was identified in feces of affected persons and in eggs from the same box as those used to prepare the topping. It was not possible to identify the flock or flocks that had produced the contaminated eggs.

In the USA, *S. enteritidis* infection is spreading beyond the Northeast, where the current pandemic has its geographic focus (*131*). A case–control study determined the source of a large outbreak of salmonellosis in Tennessee and traced the origin of the implicated eggs to a layer farm in Indiana. Eighty-one case patients were identified, 73 of whom had eaten egg-containing sauces at a local restaurant on the same evening. Eleven of 24 patients with culture-proved *S. enteritidis* infection were hospitalized. The 10 controls had eaten with the case patients but did not become ill. Hollandaise and bernaise sauces prepared with shell eggs were strongly associated with illness ($p < .001$). The sauces had been prepared at 5 o'clock and held at 38°C throughout the evening serving hours. Victims who required hospitalization ate their meals at a significantly later hour than those who were less severely ill. Testing of chickens and the environment at the farm in Indiana yielded *S. enteritidis* isolates with antimicrobial susceptibility patterns, phage type (PT8), and plasmid profiles indistinguishable from those of isolates from patients. Although infected hens seldom produce infected eggs, the Indiana flock was deprived of food and water shortly before the outbreak, which may have stressed the birds and increased excretion of the bacteria into the eggs.

In Scotland, consumption of duck eggs has been associated with *S. enteritidis* PT4 infection (*132*). Two infections occurred in members of the same family, one of whom was hospitalized while the other was symptom-free. A third case occurred in a different family two months later; this victim, too, had eaten duck eggs. Eggs implicated in these cases were purchased from different retail stores but had been supplied by the same farm. All egg samples from the farm were negative for *S. enteritidis*, but cloacal swabs yielded *S. enteritidis* PT4. Infection was widespread and the flock was destroyed.

Cross-contamination was involved in an extended hospital outbreak of *S. enteritidis* infection in Ontario (*133*). Between 18 September and 14 October 1991, 38 cases occurred. No food or food handler was associated with the outbreak, but health inspectors identified several poor food-handling practices in the kitchen. These were corrected. However, infection again broke out on 19 November, this time involving 57 cases. On 15 January 1992, *S. enteritidis* PT13 was identified in a sample of minced ham. The ham had been ground in a vertical food mixer also used to prepare other sandwich fillings and to blend raw shelled eggs for use in custard and French toast. *Salmonella enteritidis* PT13 was also found in samples of uncooked custard, minced beef, turkey, and tuna sandwiches that had been prepared in the mixer.

Seventy-eight of 123 people attending a wedding reception in southern England became ill with gastroenteritis, and two were hospitalized with salmonellosis (*134*). All guests were interviewed and 61 persons who became ill provided fecal specimens. Six secondary cases were subsequently identified. Gastrointestinal illness was significantly associated with eating turkey at the wedding: the attack rate for those who ate turkey was 84%, and turkey was the only risk factor independently associated with illness. The day before the wedding a nonprofessional caterer had prepared two large boned and rolled turkeys in her kitchen, cooking them until the juices ran clear. After cooling for an unknown length of time at room temperature, the turkeys were sliced and stored overnight in a cold room. Food was laid out the next morning and eaten during the afternoon and early evening. An experiment showed that when a 9-kg boned and rolled turkey was cooked until the "juices ran clear," the temperature at the center was only 55°C, insufficient to kill salmonellas.

Eighty-nine cases of confirmed or probable salmonellosis were identified among patrons who ate at a fast-food restaurant in Minnesota between 19 and 27 September 1989 (*135*). *Salmonella enteritidis* was isolated from fecal samples from 17 of 71 restaurant employees, and 7 employees reported gastrointestinal symptoms. By univariate analysis, quarter-pound beef patties, American cheese slices, curly-fried potatoes, and lettuce were associated with illness. Investigation indicated that the pathogen was being transmitted by one of the infected employees, who handled ice as well as curly-fried potatoes and sandwiches made from quarter-pound beef patties with his bare hands. Investigation of case-patrons and controls who ate at the restaurant during this employee's working hours showed that consumption of ice was also independently associated with illness and that the highest attack rates occurred during this employee's shifts. However, *every* shift during which case patients were exposed included at least one employee with confirmed or probable salmonellosis. No major deficiencies in the facility or cooking procedures were found. The authors concluded that one infected employee had transmitted his infection to other employees, who contaminated multiple food items causing further transmission of the infection to patrons.

During the years 1984–1988, *S. enteritidis* was repeatedly isolated from feces of ill persons who had consumed raw milk from the bulk tank at a dairy farm in southern Alberta (*136*). Investigation in 1988 identified *S. enteritidis* PT8 in samples from ill humans, milk-line filters, milk from the bulk tank, and milk from the right hindquarter of a 5-year-old cow on the farm. After the infected cow was removed from the herd she continued to shed *S. enteritidis* from this quarter during 7 months at an isolation facility. Such prolonged excretion of salmonella into milk is uncommon.

At a dairy farm in Scotland, *S. typhimurium* PT104 was isolated from 3 cows and a raw-milk filter sock, and from the dairy farmer, his wife, and a nearby housewife, all of whom had drunk raw milk from the farm (*137*). Besides drinking raw milk, the farmer had assisted his veterinarian with two ill cows, one of which died and one of which was slaughtered after confirmation of *S. typhimurium* PT104 infection. Unpasteurized milk from remaining symptomatic cows was also positive for salmonella.

Only 55 cases of infection with *S. mikawasima* were identified by the Laboratory of Enteric Pathogens between 1985 and 1991 in England and Wales, and 21 of these were associated with foreign travel (*138*). However, 21 cases were reported in different parts of England beginning in September 1992 (this account was dated 23 October). Eight people became ill after eating at the same fast-food restaurant in the South West Thames region; 6 cases were reported from Yorkshire and 1 from Oxford; 5 scattered cases were associated with travel to Spain.

Pets continue to be associated with salmonellosis in humans (*139–141*). Clusters of *S. hadar* infection in Connecticut, Maryland, and Pennsylvania in spring 1991 were linked with pet ducklings (*139*). The ducklings were traced to two hatcheries in Pennsylvania that distributed animals to retailers and by mail order. Although salmonellosis is generally a foodborne illness, most of these victims were children, who are less likely than adults to follow good hygienic practices. Children in two families in Scotland were infected with *S. java* (*140*). These infections were traced to tropical fish supplied by two pet shops in Lothian, although complete epidemiologic investigation was impossible in one case because the family dog ate the fish-food and its container. *S. java* is not considered a pathogen in tropical fish. It was thought likely that fish suppliers in Singapore were the source of infection, either the fish themselves or the transport water being the vector for transmission. In Utah in June 1992, a rare *S. poano* infection was diagnosed in an 8-week-old infant who was partially breast-fed and partially fed a high-iron infant formula (*141*) (see reference *114*). One month before the child became ill the family had exchanged their large pet lizard for a python. Specimens from the snake and its plastic cage were salmonella-free, but *S. poano* was recovered from feces left on the cage carpet and the water dish by the lizard nearly 3 months earlier. Only the father handled the lizard and the cage, but he walked around the cage in bare feet and washed heat rocks from the cage in the kitchen sink, practices which may have contributed to household contamination.

COMPLICATIONS AND UNUSUAL CLINICAL MANIFESTATIONS OF SALMONELLA ENTERITIS. Physicians in Austria reported a high frequency of pancreatitis in conjunction with salmonella enteritis (*142*). Within 18 months they treated 16 patients with *S. typhimurium* enteritis and 31 with *S. enteritidis* infection. Concomitant pancreatitis was found in 7 patients with *S. typhimurium* and 22 with *S. enteritidis* infections. The pathogenetic mechanisms involved in this are unknown but by analogy with other infections the authors suggested a hematogenous attack on parenchymal pancreatic cells. In sharp contrast, physicians in the U.K. reported no occurrences of pancreatitis associated with >500 cases of infective gastroenteritis, nearly all due to *S. typhimurium* or *S. enteritidis* (*143*). One man developed diarrhea during a holiday in a Majorcan resort and subsequently developed a pancreatic abscess (*144*). Only three previous cases of invasive salmonella infection of the pancreas had been reported. *S. bovismorbificans* was identified in surgical and vacuum-drain specimens; blood and stool cultures were negative for salmonellas.

Another salmonella serotype with an apparent propensity for abscess formation is *S. virchow* (*145*). Physicians in Scotland reported 5 cases of abscesses due to this organism within 5 years—a disproportionate number in relation to the number of *S. virchow* isolations. One patient reported fever, sweating, and vomiting but no diarrhea; no enteric pathogens were grown from the stool or urine, but blood cultures were positive for *S. virchow* after laparotomy. A bone scan showed features consistent with septic arthritis of the sacroiliac joint. A second patient reported a 3-day history of fever, abdominal pain and diarrhea. *S. virchow* was cultured from blood and stool samples, and ultrasound revealed an abscess in the right iliac fossa. Another woman had an abscess over the sternoclavicular joint, which yielded *S. virchow* upon culture; she had no gastrointestinal symptoms and stool samples were negative for the pathogen. A young man developed a testicular abscess 1 week after an episode of acute diarrhea and vomiting. *S. virchow* was isolated from pus and stool cultures. Another man had an *S. virchow*–positive abscess adjacent to his spleen, but stool and blood cultures were negative and he had no gastrointestinal symptoms. Although the source of these infections was not reported, the authors discussed the frequent association of salmonella abscesses with the gastrointestinal tract and the increase in *S. virchow* infections connected with poultry consumption. High incidences of bacteremia, septicemia, endovascular infection, and septic arthritis have also been associated with *S. virchow* infections.

Liver abscess is a rare complication of salmonella infection, but a case was reported from Spain (*146*). Nontyphoidal salmonella infections occasionally cause a chronic carrier state. This may have been the case in a 62-year-old man who had diarrhea and fever in 1988, when *S. enteritidis* was cultured from his stool. He did not receive antimicrobial therapy. Nearly 2 years later he developed a liver abscess from which *S. enteritidis* was cultured. Isolates from the initial gastroenteritis infection and the subsequent abscess had identical antimicrobial susceptibilities, phage types, and plasmid profiles.

Reactive arthritis is a fairly common complication of gastrointestinal salmonella infection. Mäki-Ikola and Granfors reviewed the etiology, diagnosis, and pathogenesis of this inflammation (*147*). They concluded that microorganisms that trigger reactive arthritis share three features: they cause infections on mucosal surfaces, they have lipopolysaccharide (LPS) on their outer membrane, and they are intracellular organisms. The interaction between host and microbe is thought to be abnormal in HLA-B27-positive subjects, who are prone to develop reactive arthritis. Microbial antigens are not efficiently eliminated after acute infections in these persons. Bacterial LPS enters joints and is important in the development of reactive arthritis. The authors' research group conducted a study of *Salmonella*-specific antibodies in 39 subjects who developed reactive arthritis after *Salmonella* infection and 58 who did not (*148*). Patients with reactive arthritis had higher levels of *Salmonella*-specific IgM, IgG, and IgA antibodies. IgA, IgA1, and IgG2 classes were especially well represented. Differences in antibody profiles between *Salmonella*- and *Yersinia*-triggered reactive arthritis suggest differences in the arthritogenic process induced by the two organisms.

Sun-dried rattlesnake meat in powder or capsule form is a popular folk remedy for many health problems—even AIDS—in Latin America and the southwestern USA (*149*). The customary method of preparation does not kill pathogenic organisms, of which *S. arizona* is especially worrisome because rattlesnakes are a principal reservoir of this organism. Kraus et al. described 6 patients with systemic lupus erythematosus (SLE) and one with dermatomyositis who developed severe *S. arizona* infections; all but one admitted consuming rattlesnake preparations. Four other immunosuppressed patients with nonrheumatic diseases also developed life-threatening *S. arizona* infections. One of these used rattlesnake preparations; the other three were unavailable for questioning (one died). What these 11 patients had in common was immunosuppressive drug therapy or a disease that could alter their immune response. A young man with a diagnosis of dermatomyositis developed sepsis at the site of a prosthetic hip joint. Two women with diagnoses of SLE developed sepsis of the knee. A 49-year-old woman with SLE underwent surgery for acute cholecystitis. *S. arizona* was isolated from bile and blood cultures. Another SLE patient developed painful knee and elbow effusions that yielded *S. arizona* on culture. A 29-year-old SLE patient with bilateral knee effusion and shoulder pain tested positive for *S. arizona* in blood, urine, and synovial fluid cultures. The only patient in this group who denied use of rattlesnake preparations was a 25-year-old SLE patient who complained of fever and urinary symptoms; a urine culture was positive for *S. arizona.* The organism was cultured from rattlesnake capsules provided by one of the patients.

Aphthous ulcers were reported in a young man with salmonella colitis (*150*). Cultures of feces and blood yielded *S. virchow* PTB. Although aphthous ulcers have been associated with other types of infective colitis, the authors believe theirs to be the first reported case associated with salmonella colitis.

Although most complications of pregnancy due to salmonella infection have involved typhoid, nontyphoid gastroenteritis can also cause sepsis and fetal loss (*151*). A 31-year-old woman in the 15th week of gestation became ill after eating a chicken and egg dish at a local delicatessen in the Washington, DC, area. Other members of her party also felt ill after this meal. The woman's gastrointestinal symptoms resolved after a week. However, they returned a few days later after she underwent amniocentesis for reasons unrelated to the illness. Blood samples and amniotic fluid contained group C1 *Salmonella*, and she delivered a stillborn fetus. The authors discussed *Salmonella*-induced abortion in animals and the implications of rising rates of foodborne salmonellosis for complication of pregnancy in humans.

Occurrence and control

OCCURRENCE. A comprehensive survey of *Salmonella* contamination in U.S. broiler chicken production and processing found little change since 1969 (*152*). *Salmonella* was found in 21% of samples from feed mills, 16% of samples from processing plants, 13% of samples from breeder/multiplier houses, 7% of samples from hatcheries, and 4% of samples from broiler houses. Sixty percent of meat and bone-meal samples from feed mills, 33% of samples collected from live-haul trucks, and 21% of whole processed broiler carcasses sampled at processing plants were contaminated. *S. typhimurium* was the most common serotype. Insects appeared to

be primarily mechanical carriers, but the gastrointestinal tract of 1 of 19 mice sampled was contaminated with *Salmonella*. *Salmonella* was most frequently isolated from feed and feed ingredients; pelleting reduced, but did not eliminate, this contamination. The ubiquity of *Salmonella* contamination in the broiler production system indicates that control efforts must be correspondingly comprehensive. In Canada, a nationwide survey of 294 commercial broiler flocks to estimate the prevalence of salmonellas identified 50 serovars in environmental (litter and water) samples (*153*). The most prevalent were *S. hadar*, isolated from 33.3% of flocks, *S. infantis*, isolated from 8.8%, and *S. schwarzengrund*, from 7.1%; *S. enteritidis* PT8 was isolated from 7 flocks and PT13a from 2 flocks. One or more litter samples from 75.9% of the flocks were positive; water samples were positive for 21.6% of the flocks; overall, one or more environmental samples from 76.9% of flocks were contaminated with *Salmonella*.

Salmonellas were isolated from 53% of 133 samples of frozen chicken giblets and offals in Berlin retail markets (*154*). The highest contamination rates were in hearts and giblets. High rates of contamination were also found in fresh chicken livers from a slaughterhouse: 93% of livers from one flock were positive, containing an average of 0.59 *Salmonella* organisms per gram. The serovars most frequently isolated were *S. virchow, S. typhimurium,* and *S. indiana.* Brilliant green–phenol red–lactose–saccharose agar was superior to mannitol–lysine–crystal violet–brilliant green agar as a selective plating medium.

The USDA Food Safety and Inspection Service monitored bacterial counts and prevalence of *Salmonella* on chicken throughout the slaughter, dressing, and chilling process in a modern plant (*155*). The procedures used significantly decreased bacterial contamination on the carcasses. *Salmonella* was determined as present or absent by culturing most of the rinse. Prevalence of salmonellas decreased from 58 to 48% during evisceration, then increased to ~75% during immersion chilling.

Salmonella enteritidis infection was diagnosed in a German laying flock that showed no decrease in egg production or other clinical evidence of infection (*156*). A study was then conducted of the primary and secondary transmission of the organism to eggs, in which the prevalence of infection was substantial. In one sample of 50 eggs, *S. enteritidis* was detected in the contents of 23 but not on any of the shells. In another sample of 640 fresh eggs, the organism was detected on the shell of 7, in the white of 3, in the yolk of 2, and in both white and yolk of 1. Based on these and other observations the authors proposed a model for transmission of *S. enteritidis* to eggs through penetration of the shell and by transovarian infection.

The prevalence of *S. enteritidis* and serovars not implicated in egg-associated outbreaks was determined in the ovaries of layer hens at the time of slaughter (*157*). Hens from 42 flocks from 7 southeastern states and Pennsylvania were sampled. Thirty-two flocks (76%) were positive at an infection rate >10% (mean percentage of infected samples = 27%). Fifteen serovars were identified, of which *S. heidelberg* was the most common (56% of isolates). *Salmonella agona, S. oranienburg, S. mbandaka, S. kentucky, S. montevideo, S. london, S. typhimurium, S. infantis, S. schwarzengrund, S. ohio, S. cerro, S. anatum,* and untypable serovars were also found. *Salmonella enteritidis* PT23 was recovered from one flock. The public health importance of systemic infections in layer flocks with these non–*S. enteritidis* serovars is not known.

A survey of 5700 eggs from 15 naturally infected flocks in England found *S. enteritidis* in the contents of 32 (0.6%) (*158*). The level of contamination of clean, intact shell eggs was <20 organisms per egg in most cases, even after >3 weeks of storage at room temperature. Two eggs, however, contained >10^4 *S. enteritidis* cells after prolonged storage. *Salmonella enteritidis, S. typhimurium,* and *S. hadar* were isolated from egg shells, whereas egg contents yielded only *S. enteritidis*. Contamination rates of shells and contents were similar, but albumen was contaminated more frequently than yolk.

In a 10-year study in Germany, >9000 eggs were examined for the presence of *S. enteritidis* (*159*). Most of the eggs were industrially produced and were sampled from retail markets; some were taken from producers or packers. The organism was found on the shells of 0.01–0.1% of eggs.

Thirty-seven of the contaminated eggs were obtained from private family flocks. Ten of these were contaminated on the shell only; 27 had *S. enteritidis* both on the shell and in the yolk. Another German study detected *S. enteritidis* on the shells of ~0.4% of grade A eggs randomly sampled, whereas 1.7% of shells and >3.0% of contents from eggs associated with outbreaks of salmonellosis were contaminated (*160*).

A survey was conducted of *Salmonella* contamination of 106 dozen eggs purchased from supermarkets in Oahu, Hawaii (*161*). Twelve brands were represented, 3 from U.S. producers on the mainland and 9 locally produced. Salmonellas were detected on egg shells from 10 of the 106 cartons sampled. No egg contents were positive. The serovars identified were *S. braenderup, S. oranienburg, S. cerro, S. ohio, S. mbandaka, S. havana, S. montevideo,* and *S. livingstone*. Positive eggs came from only 3 of the 12 brands; 7 of the 10 positive cartons were traced to a single processing plant, where malfunctioning egg-washing and sanitation equipment was found.

The first finding of *S. arizona* in an Austrian turkey flock was reported (*162*). An epidemic of acute illness in this flock was described.

In Sweden, a survey was conducted to determine the frequency of *Salmonella* outbreaks in wild and domestic animals and the occurrence of *Salmonella* in animal feed (*163*). Such reports have been published every five years since 1949. From 1983 through 1987, 760 animal outbreaks were reported, a substantial decrease from the 1266 reported in the previous period. Fifty-six serovars were identified; 17, of which 16 were isolated from reptiles, were new to Sweden. Twenty-eight outbreaks in swine and 86 in poultry were registered in 1983–1987, compared with 37 and 220, respectively, in 1978–1982. Testing of Swedish feed-producing plants yielded 236 isolates, the lowest number in 15 years.

The incidence of *Salmonella* in apparently healthy pigs slaughtered for human consumption was determined in a study in India (*164*). From 819 samples of liver, gall bladder, mesenteric lymph nodes, spleen, intestinal contents, and muscle collected from 149 pigs, 16 *Salmonella* isolates belonging to 3 serovars were obtained. Intestinal contents and lymph nodes were most frequently positive (5 isolates each). Most strains were relatively resistant to tetracycline but sensitive to the other antimicrobial agents tested. However, certain *S. typhimurium* strains showed multiple drug resistance, which was thought to be plasmid-mediated and potentially transferable to other enterobacteria in the gut when contaminated pork is eaten by humans.

The occurrence of fecal bacteria, salmonellas, and antigens associated with hepatitis A virus was investigated in shellfish taken from shellfish farming areas and natural beds along the French coast (*165*). Overall, salmonellas were detected in 5% of samples, but frequency of isolation was higher in areas heavily contaminated with fecal coliforms and fecal streptococci.

Field studies were conducted in a wastewater–aquaculture unit in Alabama to determine if silver carp (*Hypothalmichthys molitrix*) would become contaminated by *Salmonella* in the wastewater, if such contamination would lead to concentration of organisms or infection in the fish, if poor water quality affects the susceptibility of fish to salmonellosis, and if the fish could mount an immunologic response to *Salmonella* (*166*). *Salmonella* was isolated from 21 of 90 wastewater samples and 2 of 63 fish samples. The highest levels were 4.3 cells per 100 mL of wastewater and 5.5 cells per gram of fish intestine. All isolates tested with the Minitek *Enterobacteriaceae* II kit were confirmed as *S. enteritidis*. No agglutinating antibodies against *Salmonella* were detected in serum samples. Silver carp and channel catfish (*Ictalurus punctatus*) from a non-wastewater source were serologically negative 35 days after inoculation with *Salmonella* into the anterior intestine.

STUDIES IN POULTRY. A retrospective case–control study of risk factors for salmonellosis was conducted using data from 111 broiler breeder flocks (*167*). Multivariate models were developed based on results of univariate analyses. The final model indicated that flocks from farms having no disinfection tub and poor hygiene barriers and using feed from a small feed mill had a risk of being *Salmonella*-positive 46 times that of flocks from farms with a disinfection tub and good hygiene barriers and using feed from a large feed mill. This multivariate epidemiological approach may be applicable to integrated food-chain quality-control programs.

Feeding studies suggested that fructo-oligosaccharide causes a shift in gut microflora and in some situations reduces susceptibility to colonization by *Salmonella* (*168*). In vitro, none of 20 serotypes of *Salmonella* could grow when fructo-oligosaccharide was the only carbon source. For in vivo experiments, chicks were given feed containing 0, 0.375, or 0.75% fructooligosaccharide and then challenged with *S. typhimurium* after 7 days. At a level of 0.375%, fructooligosaccharide had little effect on colonization, but at 0.75% it enhanced the effectiveness of a competitive exclusion culture and reduced colonization in chicks stressed by deprivation of feed and water.

To determine the effects of formic and propionic acid on attachment of *S. typhimurium* in chick ceca, groups of chicks were fed broiler starter feed or this feed supplemented with 1% formic or propionic acid beginning on the day of hatch (*169*). On the second day they were inoculated orally with 10^6 cfu of *S. typhimurium*. Chicks from each group were killed for *Salmonella* recovery at the ages of 7, 14, and 21 days. The two fatty acids had comparable effects. At 7 days recovery of attached *Salmonella* was 1.4 log less in the fatty acid–fed groups than in controls and at 21 days it was 3.6 log less.

The effect of dietary lactose on incidence and levels of salmonellas on the carcasses of processed broiler chickens was determined by the most probable number (MPN) method (*170*). Most bacterial attachment mechanisms and receptor sites on animal tissues involve carbohydrates, and there is some evidence that lactose feeding decreases intestinal colonization by *Salmonella*. However, chickens are continually exposed to salmonellas from many sources and merely interfering with intestinal colonization may not reduce contamination of the processed carcass. Therefore, lactose was substituted for sand in the feed at levels of 0, 2.5, 5, and 7.5% beginning on day 1; birds were inoculated with *S. typhimurium* via their drinking water, and prechill carcasses were evaluated for incidence and levels of salmonellas in 24- and 50-day-old birds. There were no statistically significant differences in incidence of contamination, but the $\log_{10}$ MPN/mL of rinse fluid was significantly higher for chickens fed 7.5% lactose than for the other groups. Thus supplementing poultry diets with lactose is not an effective way to reduce the incidence or level of salmonella contamination on processed broiler carcasses. Another study by this research group evaluated the effects of bird density on salmonella contamination of prechill carcasses (171). Birds were reared in floor pens providing 557, 619, 697, 796, 929, or 1115 cm² per bird. Twenty percent of the chicks in each density group were inoculated with nalidixic acid–resistant *S. typhimurium* on day 2 and 20% of the uninoculated birds in each density group were processed at 42 days. Prechill carcasses were evaluated for nalidixic acid–resistant *Salmonella* by the whole-carcass rinse technique using a mechanical shaker. No consistent effect of bird density on contamination rate was seen at these densities.

Goodnough and Johnson investigated the control of *S. enteritidis* infections in poultry by antimicrobial agents (172). Of the compounds screened, polymyxin B showed the strongest antimicrobial activity in vitro, preventing growth of a virulent *S. enteritidis* strain at concentrations of ≤10 µg/mL. Administration of this substance in drinking water at a concentration of ≥50 µg/mL prevented infections in day-old chicks but did not eliminate established infections in 4-day-old chicks. Trimethoprim enhanced the in vivo activity of polymyxin: used together, the two agents effectively prevented colonization and eliminated existing *S. enteritidis* infections. However, when antimicrobial treatment was stopped, some chickens became reinfected, probably because the organism was present at infectious levels in the environment. This indicates the need for other exclusionary methods for control, such as good hygiene and nutrition and perhaps use of competitive exclusion cultures. Nevertheless, treatment with the polymyxin–trimethoprim system may by useful in preventing *S. enteritidis* colonization in poultry or eliminating the organism from infected flocks.

The influence of four antibiotics on the protective effects of an adult cecal flora against *Salmonella* contamination of chicks were evaluated (173). Avoparcin, bacitracin, flavomycin, and virginiamycin were individually incorporated into the basic feed at concentrations commonly used in the field. The competitive exclusion flora was administered by gavage to day-old chicks. Chicks were challenged orally with 10^4–10^5 rifampicin-resistant *S. typhimurium* cells when they were 2 days old. Ceca of chicks fed avoparcin had significantly more *Salmonella* than ceca of controls; chicks fed flavomycin had numbers similar to controls; and chicks fed bacitracin or virginiamycin had a significantly lower level of *Salmonella* carriage than controls. The authors concluded that further tests of the susceptibility of cecal anaerobic bacteria to commonly used antibiotics are needed.

Fowler and Mead discussed why some broiler breeder flocks protected by competitive exclusion from *S. enteritidis* PT4 infection early in life become positive when they are 30–40 weeks old and begin to lay (174). Mature hens may become particularly susceptible to infection under the stress of egg laying. An alternative explanation is a flare-up of a residual infection not eliminated by the early adult cecal flora treatment. Control of such infections was discussed.

A commercial product developed for competitive exclusion in chickens was compared with two similar preparations containing intestinal microorganisms from turkeys (175). All preparations were tested in both chicks and turkey poults. Birds were challenged with nalidixic acid–resistant *S. infantis* 24 h after treatment with the competitive exclusion flora and were killed 5 days later to assess cecal colonization by *S. infantis*. The commercial chicken preparation and the two turkey cecal cultures afforded similar, significant levels of protection against colonization in both species.

Suspensions or cultures of gut contents from adult birds can prevent or reduce colonization by salmonellas when given to day-old chicks (176). However, because these preparations have the disadvantage of being undefined and variable, a number of probiotic preparations have been used to control salmonella colonization. Hinton and Mead presented some illustrative results from their testing of *Bacillus, Lactobacillus,* and *Enterococcus* products, showing that probiotics as presently formulated confer little benefit in this application. They concluded that each product needs careful evaluation to determine its effectiveness for controlling salmonella infections in poultry. Only if it has a "protective factor" (calculated from the relative numbers of salmonellas in ceca of treated and untreated birds) >4 does it warrant testing on a commercial scale. Stavric et al. presented data from their testing of speciated and unspeciated *Lactobacillus* and *Bifidobacterium* probiotics, with and without supplemental fructooligosaccharides (*177*). Their findings affirmed the findings and conclusions of Hinton and Mead, and they too recommended that a probiotic have a protective factor value >4 to merit further investigation.

Some success has been reported with vaccines against *S. enteritidis*. Oral vaccination with live *S. enteritidis* PT4 *aroA* mutants reduced intestinal shedding and prevented seroconversion of chicks following challenge with a virulent strain (*178*). Vaccination of 24-week-old laying hens with a live attenuated strain of *S. gallinarum* 9R markedly reduced the number of isolates of the virulent *S. enteritidis* PT4 challenge strain from several organs, including ovaries, and from laid eggs (*179*). Vaccination with a rough *aroA* mutant of *S. enteritidis* PT4 reduced isolations from laid eggs but had little effect on isolations from the hen's organs. The vaccine strain itself was isolated from the ovaries in the case of the 9R strain, but not in the case of the *aroA* mutant. At a large German egg farm where *S. enteritidis* infections and contaminated eggs were a persistent problem, administration of an *S. typhimurium* vaccine approved for use in pigeons and waterfowl produced cross immunity against *S. enteritidis* (*180*). All chickens on the farm were then vaccinated at the age of 4, 6, and 7 weeks. Random samples tested until the end of the laying period demonstrated immunity against *S. typhimurium* in 98% of hens and against *S. enteritidis* in 95%. Other investigators showed that vaccination of chicks with an *S. typhimurium aroA* mutant produced the expected serum antibody response (*181*). Upon challenge with a lethal dose of virulent

S. typhimurium, all vaccinated chicks survived, whereas no unvaccinated chicks survived. When a nonlethal challenge of virulent *S. typhimurium* was given, vaccinated birds stopped excreting the challenge organism sooner than unvaccinated birds.

The phenotypic characteristics of *Salmonella* isolates from healthy and ill chickens were compared to determine whether isolates from clinically ill birds differed from isolates from their healthy counterparts (*182*). Paired isolates of *S. anatum, S. braenderup, S. enteritidis, S. hadar, S. heidelberg, S. infantis, S. litchfield, S. mbandaka, S. senftenberg, S. typhimurium,* and *S. kentucky* were compared for antibiotic resistance profile, production of colicins and siderophores, mannose-sensitive hemagglutination of erythrocytes, resistance to serum complement, utilization of carbon sources, presence and transmissibility of R plasmids, and invasiveness in primary chicken kidney cell cultures. Differences were found between pairs for utilization of carbon sources, mannose-sensitive hemagglutination, and invasiveness. These findings indicate that *Salmonella* possesses multiple virulence factors and that serotyping alone is insufficient for grouping salmonellas. The authors further suggested that because salmonellas from healthy birds seem to be relatively avirulent, the concern for salmonella contamination of poultry may be exaggerated; they did not, however, recommend that vigilance be relaxed.

Specific pathogen–free hens infected by inoculation of 10^3, 10^6, or 10^8 cells of *S. enteritidis* PT4 into the crop excreted the organism in feces for an average of 3.4, 16.4, and 36.8 days, respectively (*183*). The antibody response (IgG and IgM) was also dose-related. During the course of the experiment, 16 of the 20 birds laid 295 eggs. One bird laid two internally contaminated eggs; two birds laid shell-contaminated eggs. There was no relationship between egg contamination and antibody status, fecal excretion, or inoculum size. In experiments by Barrow and Lovell, most infected eggs laid by *S. enteritidis*–infected hens were surface-contaminated and did not result from infected ovaries (*184*). Intravenous inoculation of chickens with 10^5 or 10^6 organisms produced heavy infection of the ovaries, and some infection persisted for several weeks; however, none of the 810 eggs laid during this experiment contained *S. enteritidis*. Oral infection also caused ovarian infection, along with larger numbers of isolations from the cecum and cloaca. Two of 633 eggs from which only the contents were cultured and 36 of 614 eggs from which both shell and contents were cultured yielded *S. enteritidis*; most of the contaminated eggs were laid within 10 days after inoculation. However, high titers of IgG were still present after 27 weeks, when the experiment was terminated. Another study was conducted to determine the persistence and effect of the chicken's age on persistence of *S. enteritidis* PT13a in experimentally infected chickens (*185*). One-day-old and 7-day-old chicks were orally inoculated with 10^7 *S. enteritidis* cells. Groups of 4 infected birds and controls were killed at specified times and samples of liver, lung, spleen, testis or ovary, yolk sac, brain, duodenum, jejunum, ileum, cecum, and colon were collected for culture. Inoculation of day-old chicks caused high mortality, and all tissues of chicks that died were positive. In birds that survived, *S. enteritidis* was easily isolated from most organs until the end of the experiment (42 d, market age). In birds infected on day 7, the number of positive nonintestinal organs dropped sharply with time. Twenty-one days after infection, only liver, ileum, cecum, and colon were positive; at 42 d, *S. enteritidis* was isolated from 1 liver, 1 spleen, 2 ceca, 1 colon, and 1 yolk sac.

CONTROL OF *SALMONELLA* IN FOOD. Curtin and Krystynak summarized recent studies of the cost of foodborne diseases, proposed a unified framework for estimating such costs, and illustrated application of their proposed framework to the cost of salmonellosis in Canada (*186*). In addition to the costs of disease, a complete analysis includes a cost–benefit analysis of strategies for prevention and control. This was done at various levels for *Salmonella* control in the Canadian poultry industry. Results for each control measure were presented in terms of percent reduction of human salmonellosis, cost of the measure, and society-level benefits (avoided costs). According to these authors' reckoning, irradiation of poultry could reduce human salmonellosis by 90% at an annual cost of $18.5 million, avoiding a total societal cost of

$50.1 million; chlorination of chill water could cut salmonellosis in half at an annual cost of only $1.4 million, saving society $27.8 million; rigorous education of food service personnel could reduce salmonellosis by 52% at a cost of $1.9 million, saving $29 million. Other control measures proved less effective, more expensive, or both. The authors stressed that their analysis relied on previously published data and should be viewed as an illustration of a method rather than as a program evaluation and recommendations.

McCapes et al. used control of *Salmonella* in the U.S. turkey industry to illustrate the issues involved in the modern approach to controlling zoonotic disease agents for reasons related to public health, not animal health (*187*). They summarized *Salmonella* control in the turkey industry from its inception to the current control strategy. Sources and pathways of *Salmonella* infection and contamination were diagrammed and the hazard analysis critical control point (HACCP) system was discussed and illustrated.

Pilot tests and factory trials have confirmed the effectiveness of sodium diacetate treatment to control salmonellas and extend the shelf life of fresh poultry (*188*). When dry sodium diacetate is dusted onto the surface of poultry it dissolves in the surface moisture, dissociating into acetic acid and sodium acetate. This produces a high initial concentration of acid, a buffered pH of about 4.8 (appropriate for control of many bacterial species), and a relatively high osmotic pressure and correspondingly lower water activity. For whole chickens at an application rate of 1–3 mg/cm^2 (2–6 g per chicken), shelf life was extended by ~4 days at 2°C. For chicken pieces, shelf life was extended >10 days and *Salmonella* was significantly reduced. The process was also effective at higher storage temperatures. A feasible commercial technology based on electrostatics was demonstrated in factory trials at line speeds up to 140 carcasses per minute. Another promising new process for reducing *Salmonella* on poultry involves immersing or spraying whole birds with a solution of trisodium phosphate (*189*). The process is undergoing further testing and optimization, and after this has been completed final USDA approval will be sought.

The effects of γ-irradiation dose (0–1.8 kGy), irradiation temperature (–20 to +20°C), and preceding or subsequent heat treatment (0–3 min at 60°C) on survival of *S. typhimurium* in mechanically deboned chicken meat were evaluated (*190*). Heating the inoculated meat before irradiation did not sensitize the bacteria to subsequent irradiation, whereas irradiating inoculated meat made the *Salmonella* much more sensitive to subsequent heating. γ-Irradiation increased the heat sensitivity of *Salmonella* even when the irradiated meat was stored up to 6 weeks at 5°C before heating. When mechanically deboned chicken meat was irradiated at 0–2.50 kGy and then inoculated with *S. dublin, S. enteritidis,* or *S. typhimurium*, populations of inoculated organisms in some cases were larger in irradiated than in nonirradiated samples after storage at 10 or 20°C (*191*). The authors concluded that reduction of indigenous microflora by irradiation may create better conditions for growth of salmonellas when accidental contamination or temperature abuse occurs after radiation treatment. Therefore mechanically deboned chicken meat should be properly refrigerated and protected against contamination.

Electrical stimulation was evaluated as a method of reducing the number of *S. typhimurium* cells attached to chicken legs (*192*). The procedure utilized a square wave with an amplitude of 8.5–14.5 V, frequency of 9.33 Hz or 100 kHz, and duty cycle of 67%. Electrical stimulation killed bacteria in an electrolyte solution and reduced the number of salmonellas attached to chicken legs when the legs were connected to anodes. Some browning and increased firmness in meat in the immediate vicinity of the electrodes was noted. The killing of bacteria in solution suggests that this technique might be useful for killing bacteria in chill water. Although results were promising, numerous problems must be solved before the technique could become practical.

A study in Germany determined the incidence of *Salmonella* on frying chickens cooled by an air–water spray system (*193*). An overall contamination rate of 95% (107 of 113 birds) was found. The standard culture method detected 99 contaminated birds (88%) and a rapid-probe method detected 103

(91%). The authors concluded that the air–water spray system evaluated did not improve the hygienic status of the birds.

Investigators from the USDA evaluated the effects of chlorination of chill water on the bacteriologic profile of raw chicken carcasses and giblets (*194*). Placing the carcasses in chlorinated chill water reduced plate counts of aerobes, *Enterobacteriaceae*, and *Escherichia coli* by ~1 log, while the prevalence of carcasses with salmonellas remained about the same (~45%). Salmonellas were found on 12% of the giblets and necks sampled. The authors concluded that chlorination of chill water helps to control bacterial cross-contamination of carcasses, giblets, and necks.

D'Aoust reviewed disquieting reports on the survival and proliferation of *Salmonella* at refrigeration temperatures (*195*). Modified-atmosphere packaging extends the shelf life of chilled fresh meat. High levels of CO_2 inhibit growth of psychrotrophic spoilage bacteria and probably also of salmonellas, but have little effect on survival of salmonellas. The safety of chilled foods could be enhanced by exploiting the bacteriostatic potential of salt and low pH.

Using gradient gel plates, Thomas et al. studied the effects of multiple variables on the growth of various salmonellas (*196,197*). The first set of experiments evaluated the growth of *S. typhimurium* CRA663 (*196*). Under conditions of neutral pH and low salt, this organism grew well over the temperature range of 14–41°C; at acid pH or increased NaCl concentration, the optimum growth range was restricted to 21–29°C. Changes in growth rate occurred at specific points in the temperature–pH continuum. Increased salt concentration and acid pH enhanced the inhibitory effect of $NaNO_2$. The gradient gel plate appears to be a useful tool for rapidly screening the effect of multiple variables on the growth of microorganisms that may be found in food. The second set of experiments tested *S. panama, S. anatum, S. virchow,* and three strains of *S. typhimurium* (*197*). As in the first report, image analysis was used to present results as three-dimensional wire-frame graphs. On temperature–pH gradient plates the optimum growth range was 20–30°C and the minimum pH for visible growth was ~4 for all strains except *S. typhimurium* CRA63, which was more sensitive to temperature and pH conditions. On NaCl–pH gradient plates the maximum salt concentration at which growth was visible was 3.9–6.0%, and the minimum pH was 4.7–5.4, depending on strain. Addition of 0.02% $NaNO_2$ decreased the maximum salt concentration and increased the minimum pH at which growth occurred. The effects of nitrite under different conditions of salt concentration, pH, and temperature were more clearly shown by subtracting the data for plates containing nitrite from data for plates not containing nitrite.

Observations that *S. enteritidis* PT4 is isolated more frequently from egg albumen than from egg yolk and that the heat resistance of *S. enteritidis* may be enhanced by exposure to albumen (whose pH is ~9.2) led to tests of the hypothesis that habituation of *S. enteritidis* to alkaline conditions is accompanied by increased heat resistance (*198*). An egg isolate of *S. enteritidis* PT4 was tested. Incubation of the organism in broth at pH 9.2 ± 0.2 for ≥5 min significantly enhanced resistance to subsequent heating at 55°C at pH 7.0 but not to heating at pH 9.0. The enhanced heat resistance could not be explained by the appearance of a relatively heat-resistant subpopulation because little or no increase in cell number occurred during the incubation. Possible mechanisms associated with effects of alkali habituation on membrane properties and synthesis of heat-shock proteins were discussed.

The protective effect of common food constituents for a mixture of *Salmonella* species heated by microwave energy was evaluated (*199*). Combinations of sucrose, NaCl, caseinate, and corn oil, all at 1.0% (w/v) concentrations, were added to phosphate buffer producing a total volume of 100 mL, inoculated with *Salmonella*, and heated for 47 s in a 700-watt microwave oven. Mean final temperatures reached in the various mixtures did not vary by more than 4°C, but solutions containing NaCl gave up to 170 times the protection of the phosphate buffer control. Of the solutes studied, only NaCl afforded significant protection.

A model system simulating washing and sanitizing before and after evisceration, with and without spray-chilling, was evaluated for control of *Salmonella* on beef inoculated with a nalidixic acid–resistant strain of *S. california* (*200*). Inclusion of a 2% acetic acid sanitization step after washing with distilled water reduced surface populations of salmonellas by as much as 2 log. Increasing the acid temperature to 55°C reduced populations still further. Spray chilling, used in series with preevisceration and postevisceration treatments, appeared to permit recovery of some injured salmonellas.

A commercial buffered sodium hypochlorite solution, Bionox, was tested for efficacy in controlling *S. enteritidis* on cut poultry, fish fillets, fruits, and vegetables (*201*). Foods were immersed in a broth suspension of *S. enteritidis* and then air-dried for 10 s before exposure to the sanitizer. Count reductions of 2–4 log were achieved with all foods, although for fish fillets the sanitizer's performance was influenced by the background flora present before exposure to *Salmonella*. No adverse effects on proteins, lipids, or starches were detected by determinations of protein dispersibility and solubility, peroxide and iodine values, and changes in levels of reducing sugars.

Six new *N*-halamine compounds of potential value as disinfectants in the food-processing industry were tested against aqueous suspensions of *S. enteritidis, S. gallinarum, S. typhimurium,* and *Pseudomonas fluorescens* (*202*). Inactivation times for 10^6-fold reductions in bacterial counts were established at pH 6.5 and 25°C, and phenol coefficients for efficacy against *S. enteritidis* were determined. Considering stability, efficacy, and cost, two compounds—1,3-dichloro-2,2,5,5-tetramethyl-imidazolidin-4-one and 1-chloro-2,2,5,5-tetramethylimidazolidin-4-one—appeared promising as biocides for the food-processing industry.

Nisin, produced by *Lactococcus lactis lactis,* is used in some pasteurized cheese spreads to control growth and toxin production of *Clostridium botulinum.* It has a broad spectrum of activity against gram-positive bacteria, but its activity against gram-negative organisms is less well known. The inhibitory action of nisin in combination with Na_2EDTA against several *Salmonella* species and other gram-negative organisms was investigated (*203*). EDTA chelates magnesium ions in the outer membrane, increasing its permeability and rendering gram-negative organisms more sensitive to antibiotics and detergents. Neither nisin (50 µg/mL) nor Na_2EDTA (20 mM) alone significantly inhibited growth of any species tested. Together, however, they brought about a 2.5–4.7 log reduction in bacterial populations after a 30-min treatment and a 3.2–6.9 log reduction after 60 min. These results suggest possible applications of such combined treatments to control foodborne salmonellas and other gram-negative bacteria. Further studies by the same investigators indicated that the core oligosaccharide in lipopolysaccharide (LPS) is involved in nisin resistance (*204*). Tests of 8 outer-membrane LPS mutants and the parental strain of *S. typhimurium* LT2 showed that nisin sensitivity was associated with the extent of saccharide deletions from the core oligosaccharide. The results confirmed that the inhibitory activity of nisin can be extended to gram-negative bacteria if the outer cell membrane is altered so as to provide access to the cytoplasmic membrane, where nisin-mediated inactivation occurs.

Populations of *S. typhimurium* were monitored for 28 weeks in internal organs of experimentally infected swine (*205*). Mean populations in palatine tonsils, ileum, cecal wall and contents, ascending colon wall and contents, and mandibular and ileocolic lymph nodes were estimated using an MPN method. Fecal samples were 50–100% positive throughout the study. Mean populations fell sharply by as much as 6 log during the first 6–8 weeks after exposure, after which they maintained a fairly stable low level. These results confirm the possibility of a long-term carrier state in clinically normal pigs.

Detection and identification

The ability of Rambach agar to discriminate non-typhi *Salmonella* strains was tested on 190 *Salmonella* strains, 112 other strains of *Enterobacteriaceae*, 51 *Pseudomonas* strains, and 5 *Acinetobacter* strains (*206*). Of 170 non-typhi *Salmonella* strains, 82% gave bright red colonies after 24 h and 97% after 48 h. All other members of the family *Enterobacteriaceae* were of a different color. In addition to the salmonellas, red colonies were produced only by the acinetobacters and one *Pseudomonas* isolate produced red colonies. A C8 esterase test was conducted on 309 strains, including all the *Salmonella* isolates. All salmonellas were fluorescent under UV light, making this a useful test for the rare beige or colorless salmonellas. Another similar study using Rambach agar to identify *Salmonella* species yielded similar results (*207*). On this agar, 216 of 230 clinical isolates of *Salmonella* and 54 of 62 stock *Salmonella* cultures produced crimson-red colonies. Of the clinical isolates that displayed colors other than crimson, 8 were *S. typhi*, 2 were *S. paratyphi*, and 4 were other common serotypes. All 8 stock cultures that were not crimson belonged to rarely isolated serotypes. None of 83 non-*Salmonella* stock cultures representing 29 species produced crimson colonies. Five *Pseudomonas* and two *Acinetobacter* cultures produced scarlet-red growth but this color could be distinguished from the crimson of the salmonellas. Thus this medium can be used for presumptive identification and can assist in the definitive identification of the overwhelming majority of *Salmonella* isolates.

Semisolid Rappaport and modified semisolid Rappaport–Vassiliadis media were compared for the isolation of *Salmonella* from raw meat products, chicken feeds, and artificially contaminated low-moisture foods (chocolate, milk powder, grated coconut, and powdered cocoa) (*208*). The semisolid media were inoculated after a preenrichment step and also after enrichment. The enrichment broths were also streaked onto brilliant green and bismuth sulfite agars. Seven of 34 feed samples and 41 of 100 meat products were contaminated. The most frequently isolated of the 10 serotypes identified were *S. enteritidis*, *S. agona*, and *S. virchow*. Altogether, 62 of 154 samples were positive for *Salmonella* by one or more of the methods. Semisolid Rappaport medium detected all of them, but the productivity was greater (60 positive samples) when the medium was inoculated directly from the preenrichment broth. Modified semisolid Rappaport–Vassiliadis medium identified only 20 positive samples, but the recommended incubation temperature for this medium, 42°C, was found to be too high.

A new selective plating medium was evaluated for isolating *Salmonella* from samples containing large numbers of competing enteric bacteria (*209*). The medium incorporated a new inhibitor, 7-ethyl-2-methyl-4-undecanol-hydrogen sulfate, sodium salt (Tergitol 4), into the usual xylose–lysine agar base. This medium strongly inhibited *Proteus, Pseudomonas, Providencia*, and many other non-*Salmonella* species and provided good differentiation between *Salmonella* and *Citrobacter*. It was superior to the four other selective plating media tested (xylose–lysine–deoxycholate agar and brilliant green agar, with and without sodium novobiocin) for isolating *Salmonella* from chicken-farm environmental drag-swab samples. The authors recommended the new medium for clinical applications and for isolating non-typhi *Salmonella* from fecal-contaminated farm samples or other samples containing large numbers of competing bacteria. Another new medium for routine isolation of *Salmonella* from stool samples was also described (*210*). It incorporated novobiocin, brilliant green, glycerol, and lactose into an agar base. Brilliant green and novobiocin were added to inhibit saprophytes, and glycerol and lactose were used to discriminate between *Salmonella* and *Citrobacter*. This medium was used in parallel with *Salmonella–Shigella* agar and Hektoen agar to culture 2853 stool samples, 184 of which were confirmed to be *Salmonella*-positive. The new plating agar showed the highest sensitivity: 94% in direct plating, compared with 74% for *Salmonella–Shigella* and 65% for Hektoen, and 96% in enrichment broth plating, compared with 83 and 86%, respectively. The incidence of non-*Salmonella* black-centered colonies was very low.

The effect of a 48-h incubation on the productivity of various selective enrichment methods was compared with a standard 24-h incubation for detecting *Salmonella* in 797 high-moisture and 166 low-moisture naturally contaminated food samples (*211*). The enrichment broths used were tetrathionate brilliant green at 35 and 43°C, Muller–Kauffman tetrathionate brilliant green at 43°C, Rappaport–Vassiliadis at 43°C, and selenite cystine at 35°C. By one or more methods, 171 (21.5%) of the high-moisture and 80 (48.2%) of the

low-moisture food samples contained salmonellas. The 48-h incubation did not yield greater sensitivity than the 24-h incubation. Productivity after enrichment at 43°C exceeded productivity at 35°C, demonstrating the importance of an elevated temperature for enrichment. Other studies by the same research group found that 6-h selective enrichment in tetrathionate brilliant green (35 and 43°C), Rappaport–Vassiliadis (43°C), or selenite cystine (35°C) was consistently less productive than the standard 24-h enrichment (*212*). However, the difference was smaller for high-moisture foods (96 vs. 99% with a 1.0-mL transfer volume) than for low-moisture foods (92 vs. 100% with a 1.0-mL transfer volume). Again, the higher temperature was critical for repression of competitive microflora. The transfer volume (0.1 or 1.0 mL) had no important effect on sensitivity at either incubation time. Other authors also reported unsatisfactory results with a 6-h selective enrichment for samples of high-moisture foods (*213*). Significantly more positive samples were found after a 24-h enrichment in 2 of 8 experiments with artificially contaminated shredded cheese, 5 of 8 experiments with artificially contaminated lettuce, and tests of naturally contaminated chicken and pork sausage. From 200 samples of chicken, turkey, and pork sausage, 56 isolates representing 13 *Salmonella* serotypes were obtained. *S. derby* and *S. typhimurium* were most frequently isolated.

Distilled water and 0.85% NaCl were compared as rinse media for recovering total aerobic bacteria, total coliforms, *E. coli*, and salmonellas from broiler carcasses (*214*). Salmonellas were enumerated by an MPN procedure and by centrifugation and plating onto dulcitol novobiocin agar. Recovery of salmonellas was influenced by both rinse medium and enumeration technique. Using the MPN method, salmonellas were detected on 20% of carcasses rinsed with salt solution and 27% rinsed with distilled water. Centrifugation and culture on dulcitol novobiocin agar yielded salmonellas from 33% of salt-rinsed carcasses but none of the water-rinsed ones. With both enumeration methods the level of contamination was <1 cfu/mL of rinse medium. Rinse medium made no difference in the recovery of the other organisms of interest.

Investigators at the FDA compared the relative efficiency of preenrichment and direct selective enrichment procedures for recovery of *Salmonella* from liquid whole eggs, egg yolk, and egg albumen (*215*). They also determined the survival of *Salmonella* in refrigerated yolk and albumen and the efficiency of several preenrichment media for recovery of *Salmonella* from yolk. Preenrichment and direct selective enrichment performed similarly for liquid whole egg and yolk, but preenrichment in lactose broth gave significantly higher recoveries from albumen than did direct selective enrichment in selenite cystine or tetrathionate broth. Survival was determined over a 7-day period using the lactose preenrichment procedure. Counts of *S. enteritidis* inoculated into albumen decreased by 3 log, whereas counts in yolk did not change significantly. The authors therefore recommended that only egg yolks be examined for this pathogen. In a comparison of lactose broth, brain–heart infusion broth, trypticase soy broth, buffered peptone water, and nutrient broth as preenrichment media, trypticase soy broth gave the highest recovery of salmonellas and lactose broth the lowest. USDA scientists evaluated the incidence and numbers of *S. enteritidis* in fresh and stored eggs laid by experimentally infected hens between 4 and 14 days after inoculation (*216*). Determinations were made in homogenized whole eggs. The organism was found in the contents of only 3% of freshly laid eggs and 4% of eggs refrigerated for 7 days, whereas isolates were obtained from 16% of eggs held for 7 days at 25°C. The number of organisms in contaminated eggs was also highest in eggs stored at 25°C, although even in these, counts averaged only ~15/mL.

German law requires establishment of the interlaboratory precision of determining attributes of foods and other consumer goods (*217*). Two precision characteristics, repeatability (r) and reproducibility (R), of the *Limulus* microtiter test for detecting bacterial LPS in raw and heat-treated liquid eggs and their products were evaluated in an interlaboratory study. In analysis of liquid egg samples, r = .25 for LPS contents up to $10^{4.25}$ EU/g; R = .75 for LPS contents up to 10^3 EU/g and 1.00 for contents 10^3–$10^{4.25}$ EU/g.

An indirect ELISA was used to determine levels of LPS-specific IgG in yolks of eggs laid by hens from two flocks infected with *S. enteritidis* (*218*). Eggs from houses known to be free of *Salmonella* produced absorbance values <0.4 OD units, whereas 3–60% of values from infected houses were >0.4 OD units and some were >1.0 OD unit. This positive correlation between *Salmonella* infection and a high reading in the ELISA suggests that an ELISA using LPS as antigen could be useful in screening egg yolks for evidence of infection in chicken flocks.

An improved method for detecting and confirming salmonellas in high-fat, low-moisture food materials with low background flora, such as confectionery products, was described (*219*). A modified ornithine decarboxylase broth and a selenite–cystine–trimethylamine oxide–ribose medium improved selection and detection of salmonellas. Used with a lysine–iron–cystine–neutral red broth they were highly specific and sensitive in a screen of 80 *Salmonella* and 32 non-*Salmonella* strains. The new method gave confirmed negative and positive results within 48 h. Evaluation of 90 naturally and artificially contaminated product samples found complete agreement between the new method and the more time-consuming conventional method. A new 1-day procedure for enumerating salmonellas in milk powder was also described (*220*). A suspension of artificially contaminated milk powder was treated with trypsin and Tween 80 and centrifuged to sediment the bacterial cells. This sediment was plated onto xylose–lysine–deoxycholate agar for direct enumerating of *Salmonella*. Known populations of 1–200 cfu (representing 17 serotypes) per 25 g of milk-powder sample were recovered with an efficiency approaching 100% in 152 trials. This study confirms the authors' earlier report that centrifugation is an excellent method for concentration and physical enrichment of *Salmonella* cells in food suspensions.

A recently introduced commercial kit, the 1–2 Test®, was compared with a standard culture method for detecting *Salmonella* in 133 samples of chicken, turkey, pork, beef, ground meat, sausage, salads, and vegetables (*221*). Thirty-eight positive samples were identified by the culture method. The 1–2 Test had a sensitivity of 95% and a specificity of 98%: it gave a false-negative result for one chicken sample and a false-positive result for one turkey sample.

A rapid, sensitive method was developed for detecting salmonellas attached to chicken skin (*222*). Pieces of chicken skin were inoculated with *S. typhimurium*, incubated at room temperature for 30 min, washed, laid on a nitrocellulose membrane, and weighted to facilitate lifting of salmonellas from the skin. Pieces of control skin were treated identically except for the inoculation step. After 10 min at room temperature the membranes were removed and placed on xylose–lactose–deoxycholate agar, skin-contact side up, for 18 h at 37°C. Appearance of black colonies on the white membrane was considered a positive presumptive test for *Salmonella*. The presence of *Salmonella* was then confirmed by immunostaining of colonies on the membrane. This technique could detect *Salmonella* contamination of chicken skin within 24 h and was more sensitive than swabbing or washing techniques.

Although DNA hybridization techniques have been used to detect *Salmonella* in foods, they are not reliable in the presence of large populations of competing microorganisms (*223*). Culture conditions were tested for enrichment of salmonellas in foods with large populations of endogenous flora, in preparation for membrane hybridization with a nonradioactive DNA probe. Minced food samples were inoculated with $0–10^8$ cfu/g of various *Salmonella* serovars and non-*Salmonella* strains and preenriched in lactose–tetrathionate broth. The resulting cultures were streaked on *Salmonella–Shigella* agar and suspected colonies were spotted onto a nitrocellulose membrane for confirmation by colony hybridization. The biotin-labeled 1.8-kilobase DNA probe hybridized with all 324 *Salmonella* isolates, representing 26 serogroups and numerous serotypes, but with none of 51 non-*Salmonella* isolates tested. As few as 1.6 salmonellas per gram of food could be detected.

A new selective, differential culture medium for *Salmonella*, EF-18 agar, was evaluated for use in conjunction with the hydrophobic grid membrane filter (HGMF) (*224*). Thirty naturally contaminated samples and 880 inoculated samples from 25 food-product categories, and 2 uninoculated controls for

each inoculated sample, were tested. The conventional culture method (AOAC/BAM) was used as the standard for comparison. The HGMF/EF-18 method detected 653 *Salmonella*-positive samples, compared with 654 with AOAC/BAM. The presumptive false-positive rates were 0.3% for HGMF/EF-18 and 7.9% for AOAC/BAM. The new method was then tested in a multilaboratory collaborative study and has been accorded First Action status by AOAC.

A rapid procedure for detecting salmonellas by DNA hybridization and a fluorescent alkaline phosphatase substrate was evaluated (*225*). The probe was a biotinylated 600-base-pair fragment consisting of a tandem repeat of the insertion element IS*200*, common to most *Salmonella* species. Hybridization was carried out without prehybridization enrichment. Hybrids were detected by adding a streptavidin–alkaline phosphatase conjugate and an alkaline phosphatase substrate whose conversion to a fluorescent substance was evaluated in a fluorometer. Seventy-four strains of *Salmonella* representing 21 serovars and 98 strains of heterologous bacteria likely to occur in the *Salmonella* habitat were tested. All *Salmonella* strains but none of the heterologous strains gave positive results. The estimated sensitivity of the probe was 10^4 copies of target DNA, or 5×10^{-20} mol of DNA. Because each cell may have 10 or more copies of the IS*200* sequence, as few as 1000 cfu may be detected. In artificially contaminated chicken breast and hamburger, the method detected 5×10^3 cfu of *S. paratyphi* A.

Todd et al. reported a method for rapidly testing antibodies against numerous strains of *Salmonella* and other gram-negative organisms and reliably selecting the most specific ones (*226*). They replicated a library of *Salmonella* serovars and other strains arrayed on HGMFs, treated them with agents to expose their antigenic components, and reacted them with 46 monoclonal and polyclonal antibodies in an enzyme-linked antibody procedure. In this way they identified the antibodies giving the fewest false-positive and false-negative reactions. In the process they discovered that 5 of their MAbs were specific for group D *Salmonella*.

A rapid heat-stable caprylate esterase test for *Salmonella* was evaluated for screening stool samples cultured on deoxycholate–citrate agar (*227*). The reaction was considered positive if a bright color appeared on the filter paper inoculum site within 5 min. With 534 *Salmonella* strains and 535 other bacteria capable of growth on deoxycholate–citrate agar, the test was 100% sensitive for *Salmonella*, 99% specific, and more accurate than direct antiserum agglutination or a urease test (*228*).

The MUCAP test is a method for rapid identification of salmonellas, based on reaction of the 4-methylumbelliferyl caprylate reagent with the *Salmonella* C_8 esterase and release of fluorescent umbelliferone. Olsson et al. used the MUCAP test for 750 *Salmonella* strains and 130 strains of other *Enterobacteriaceae* species sent for identification as suspected *Salmonella* strains (*229*). They found MUCAP to be nearly 100% sensitive for *Salmonella*, the only false negative reaction coming from a single *Salmonella* subgroup V strain. One weakly positive *Hafnia alvei* strain was found. Thus MUCAP was a convenient complement to traditional biochemical identification methods, especially for atypical and unusual strains. In another study of 8634 H_2S-positive isolates from stool samples, all 794 colonies isolated on *Salmonella–Shigella* agar and all 752 colonies isolated on Hektoen agar and identified as *Salmonella* species by biochemical tests were positive in the MUCAP test (i.e., the sensitivity and negative predictive value were 100% for both media) (*230*). Six isolates identified as *Proteus vulgaris* by biochemical tests were positive by the MUCAP test, with a specificity of 99.8% and positive predictive value of 99.2% for both media. A comparison of the MUCAP, MicroScreen® latex slide agglutination, and Rambach agar rapid screening methods for *Salmonella* found sensitivities of 100, 96, and 91%, respectively, and specificities of 80, 96, and 100% (*231*). The 74 *Salmonella* strains were isolated from food, water, and clinical specimens and 101 non-*Salmonella* strains were food and water isolates. The relatively high number of false-positive reactions in the MUCAP test were given by strains of *Serratia, Aeromonas, Plesiomonas, Pseudomonas,* and *Chromobacter*, organisms that are easily distinguished from *Salmonella* by the cytochrome oxidase test or eliminated by use of selective media.

Development and testing of an ELISA for detecting antibodies against *S. enteritidis* in chickens was reported (*232*). Key to the performance of the assay was identification of outer-membrane protein antigens specific for this organism and highly sensitive to it. By protein immunoblotting, two *S. enteritidis* protein bands with M_r >40 kDa that did not react with antibodies to *S. pullorum* or *S. typhimurium* were selected. The assay was evaluated in experimentally infected chickens. It was more sensitive and specific than the conventional serum plate and microagglutination tests against which it was compared.

A sandwich capture ELISA based on an MAb against a genus-specific epitope in the outer core region of *Salmonella* LPS was used to detect common serotypes of *Salmonella* (*233*). Four-hour enrichment broth cultures of 31 *Salmonella* strains were positive by the method, whereas overnight broth cultures of 21 non-*Salmonella* strains were negative. As little as 1 ng/mL of Ra LPS or as few as 10^6 cells/mL of a smooth wild strain of *S. typhimurium* could be detected; 1120 cells of a smooth wild strain of *S. heidelberg* seeded into the enrichment broth were also detected after a 4-h incubation.

The ability of the Microscreen, Bactigen, and Spectate latex agglutination kits to detect *Salmonella* in pure cultures and naturally contaminated foods was examined (*234*). Tested against 190 salmonellas in pure culture, these systems correctly identified 90, 82, and 66%, respectively. However, the sensitivity of Spectate was 93% for somatic serogroups A–E plus G and strains harboring the Vi antigen. *Citrobacter fruendi* and *E. coli* produced numerous false-positive reactions, accounting for the kits' relatively poor specificity (3, 34, and 17% false-positive reactions, respectively). Tested against 24 naturally contaminated high- and low-moisture food samples, Microscreen detected 75% of culture-positive samples; Bactigen, 88%; and Spectate, 79%. Use of tetrathionate–brilliant green broth at 43°C in conjunction with the enrichment media recommended by the manufacturers enhanced the sensitivities of the kits to 83, 92, and 92%, respectively. Attempts to abbreviate the procedure failed.

The hybridization specificity of a 1.8-kilobase *Hind*III DNA fragment from *S. typhimurium* was confirmed by colony hybridization with 327 *Salmonella* strains and 56 closely related non-*Salmonella* strains (*235*). The fragment was highly specific for the *Salmonella* strains. Based on the nucleotide sequence of the fragment as determined by the dideoxynucleotide chain termination method, six oligonucleotide fragments were chemically synthesized and tested for hybridization specificity. Three of them were highly specific for the 327 *Salmonella* strains tested and could be used as probes for detecting salmonellas in foods or other types of samples.

MAbs to *S. enteritidis* outer-membrane proteins were screened against 57 *Salmonella* serovars and several related members of *Enterobacteriaceae* (*236*). MAbs with 100% specificity and sensitivity were used in a microtiter-plate antigen-capture ELISA to screen 2100 clinical samples. Of the 61 samples that yielded salmonellas by conventional culture after a 24-h incubation in selective media, 58 were detected by the ELISA. The ELISA also yielded 65 false positives, which were identified as *Enterobacter* spp. This ELISA could be used for presumptive salmonella-positive diagnosis after a 24-h selective enrichment incubation, but further refinement of the method is needed to reduce the number of false-positive results.

Two bioassays and three serological methods were compared for the detection of *Salmonella* enterotoxin (*237*). The serological tests were standardized with antiserum against the purified enterotoxin of *S. typhimurium* P/536. Thirty-seven strains of *Salmonella* belonging to 14 serotypes were tested. The most sensitive method was the CHO cell bioassay (86%) and the least sensitive was the rabbit ligated ileal loop bioassay (65%). The Biken test, an ELISA, and a staphylococcal coagglutination test showed 78–84% sensitivity. The same research group reported further on the coagglutination test (*238*). Using *Staphylococcus aureus* (Cowan type 1) cells coated with antiserum against purified *Salmonella* enterotoxin, they screened 101 cell-free culture supernatants from *Salmonella* strains of 15 serotypes. Of these, 76 were enterotoxigenic. The test could detect as little as 7.5 ng of toxin. The test was further adapted for detection of *Vibrio cholerae* and *E. coli* enterotoxins.

An efficient semiquantitative test for *Salmonella* in foods was developed (*239*). Homogenized samples of poultry, meat, milk, mayonnaise, flour, cheese, and chocolate were inoculated with *S. typhimurium* LT2 to give levels of 0, 1, 10, 100, and 1000 organisms per gram of food. The samples were then serially diluted in enrichment broth and incubated for ~20 h at 37°C. Deoxycholate-extracted *Salmonella* LPS was captured on polymyxin-coated polyester cloth and detected colorimetrically with an anti-*Salmonella* antibody–enzyme conjugate. The minimum dilution producing no detectable growth was correlated with the extent of contamination of the original food sample.

Two research groups described immunomagnetic separation of *Salmonella* from food samples (*240,241*). Skjerve and Olsvik coated immunomagnetic beads with affinity-purified antibodies against *Salmonella* common structural antigen-1 and added them to food samples artificially contaminated with *S. saint-paul* (*240*). The foods, bought from a local retail grocery, were soft cheese, pasteurized whole milk, whole milk powder, yogurt, chicken liver, vacuum-packed sliced ham, and a raw-vegetable blend. After immunomagnetic separation the beads were spread on brilliant green or MacConkey agar and incubated for 18 h at 37°C and colonies were counted. *S. saint-paul* was effectively isolated from pure cultures and mixed cultures with *E. coli*, even when *E. coli* cells outnumbered *Salmonella* by >1000:1. The success of the method with foods depended on the nature of the food matrix. Results were excellent for milk, milk powder, ham, and vegetable blend and good for cheese, but a substantial loss of beads occurred with yogurt and chicken liver. However, *Salmonella* was always detected when at least 2–10 cells/mL were present. Vermunt et al. used immunomagnetic methods to isolate *S. livingstone* from pure and mixed cultures (*241*). Nonspecific reactions with organisms such as *Aeromonas hydrophila* were reduced by substituting 4% skim milk for bovine serum albumin in the incubation medium. Loss of bacterial cells during washing, interference of other microorganisms with the separation, and optimum incubation conditions were determined. *Salmonella typhimurium* ORS and *S. stanleyville* were isolated from naturally contaminated samples of minced meat.

An automated conductance method for rapid detection of *Salmonella* in food was validated in a collaborative study involving 17 laboratories (*242*). Samples of coconut, fish meal, prawns, nonfat dried milk, liquid egg, and minced beef were artificially contaminated at two levels, 1–5 cells and 10–50 cells per 25 g. AOAC/BAM and conductance methods produced comparable results, and the conductance method was adopted by AOAC International as a first-action method.

ANTIBIOTIC RESISTANCE. Genes for antibiotic resistance in *Salmonella* are generally carried in plasmids. To establish a background profile of plasmid genes predating the widespread medical and agricultural use of antibiotics, Jones and Stanley analyzed 32 *Salmonella* strains from a collection of 279 isolated between 1917 and 1954 (*243*). They identified conjugative plasmids of the same incompatibility groups as contemporary enterobacterial plasmids. Forty-two plasmids of 23–72 MDa were found. Six groups were defined and tested by hybridization with probes from contemporary plasmids for genes involved in maintenance and incompatibility, DNA repair, and virulence. *Salmonella* virulence plasmids have not undergone detectable molecular evolution under the influence of antibiotic selection pressure. This finding was not unexpected because virulence plasmids are serotype-specific, poorly transferable, and not vectors of antibiotic resistance. In contrast, more readily transferable plasmids of the preantibiotic era were shown to have evolved into contemporary resistance plasmids by acquisition of new resistance genes, rather than by dissemination of resistance plasmids that existed before the introduction of antibiotics. Two plasmids failed to hybridize with any of the probes tested.

A study of the antibiotic resistance of agricultural and foodborne *Salmonella* isolates in Canada showed an overall increase in resistant strains from 29% in 1986 to 51% in 1989 (*244*). Strains representing 689 isolates from Canadian agricultural products and imported fish, shellfish, and reptiles

were tested for resistance to 11 antibiotics. Poultry was the major reservoir of resistant strains. Of 27 resistance patterns identified, all but 2 contained a resistance determinant for streptomycin, tetracycline, or both. Multiple resistance was highest in *Salmonella* strains belonging to somatic groups B and C. Five isolates exhibited resistance to 6 antibiotics: one was *S. indiana* from chicken gizzard, two were *S. typhimurium* from pork and one was *S. typhimurium* from beef, and one was *S. infantis* from pork. The authors concluded that this level of antibiotic-resistant *Salmonella* in the food chain demonstrates a need to reevaluate the use of subtherapeutically medicated feeds in animal agriculture. A survey of resistance to 14 antimicrobial agents in *Salmonella* isolates from cattle, poultry, sheep, and pigs in England and Wales, 1984–1987, produced different results (*245*). Little change has occurred during this time period or in comparison with earlier surveys. *Salmonella dublin* remained sensitive to most antimicrobial agents. In *S. typhimurium*, most resistance was associated with phage type DT204C; resistance to tetracycline and sulfonamides exceeded 60% in cattle, but *S. typhimurium* has grown more sensitive to neomycin and some other aminoglycosides. For other serotypes, resistance to sulfonamides and tetracycline has increased but resistance to other agents has remained low. In general, the level of resistance of isolates decreased in the order cattle > sheep > pigs > poultry.

Virulence and molecular studies

Selbitz presented an overview of the virulence factors of *Salmonella* (*246*). He discussed attachment of the organisms to target cells, invasion and intracellular parasitism, toxins, and virulence plasmids.

Chart et al. examined the expression of long-chain LPS by 44 type strains of *S. enteritidis* and 22 clinical and poultry-associated isolates of *S. enteritidis* PT23 and PT30 (*247*). Strains belonging to phage types 7, 23, and 30 were rough variants, a phenotype associated with avirulence for BALB/c mice; they did not produce LPS profiles with the "ladder" pattern typical of long-chain (smooth) LPS.

Salmonella bareilly has become the third most frequently isolated *Salmonella* in India (*248*).

Although it has been associated with cases of gastroenteritis in humans, its enterotoxigenicity and invasiveness have not been investigated in detail. Vashisht et al. evaluated the toxigenicity of 10 clinical isolates of *S. bareilly* in a variety of models. All whole-cell cultures, cell-free supernatants, and cell sonicates induced fluid accumulation in rat and rabbit ligated ileal loops. All strains also had an intracellular vascular permeability factor, and 5 strains were positive in the suckling mouse test, indicating the presence of a heat-stable type of toxin. The toxin or toxins were immunologically distinct from the *E. coli* heat-labile toxin and cholera toxin.

It is generally agreed that virulent salmonellas are invasive, but not all invasive strains of *S. typhimurium* are virulent. Douce et al. argued that the need to establish the role and mechanism of invasion of gut epithelium by salmonellas warrants efforts to establish in vitro methods that reflect the in vivo situation (*249*). To this end they explored conditions in an HEp-2 cell model that would distinguish virulent from avirulent strains of *S. typhimurium* by quantitative assessment of internalization. The effects of inoculum size, bacterium–cell interaction time, drop in pH of the medium, bacterial phenotype and growth phase, and treatments to increase the release and recovery of bacteria were investigated. Because invasiveness is measured by the number of bacteria recovered after treatment of cells with gentamicin and the number recovered increases with time, the authors stressed the importance of estimating how many bacteria actually invaded during the course of the experiment and how many resulted from intracellular multiplication after invasion.

The unidirectional fluxes of Na^+ and Cl^- were studied in rats treated with *S. typhimurium* enterotoxin to elucidate the mechanism of enterotoxin-induced diarrhea (*250*). In toxin-treated animals there was a net secretion of these ions, whereas there was a net absorption in controls. The Ca^{2+} ionophore A23187 induced secretion of Na^+ and Cl^- in controls and enhanced secretion in treated animals, whereas the calcium-channel blocker verapamil decreased toxin-induced secretion but could not change secretion to absorption.

Enterocytes from toxin-treated rats had significantly higher concentrations of intracellular free calcium than enterocytes from controls. Phorbol ester did not alter ion flux in treated rats but induced secretion in controls. Indomethacin and inhibitors of protein kinase C inhibited the effects of toxin. The authors postulated that *Salmonella* enterotoxin-mediated fluid secretion involves protein kinase C either directly or through stimulation of arachidonic acid metabolism, and may not involve extracellular calcium pools.

Liebold et al. reviewed the occurrence of cytotonic and cytotoxic enterotoxins in salmonellas and the methods by which toxicity was established (*251*). At present, cell culture assays are the method of choice for detecting these toxins, but the authors predicted that DNA hybridization will become important in the near future.

Fang et al. studied the regulation of a *Salmonella dublin* plasmid gene, *vsdC*, essential for virulence (*252*). They demonstrated that *vsdC* is selectively expressed during the stationary phase of bacterial growth. Carbon starvation induced *vsdC* expression by limiting bacterial growth. Expression depended on an upstream gene, *vsdA*, whose product has significant N-terminus homology with the LysR family of transcriptional activator proteins. The authors further showed that *vsdC* expression did not depend on the *Salmonella* chromosomal virulence regulatory loci *ompR, phoP,* and *cya-crp,* and that the gene could be expressed in a range of nontyphoid salmonellas including some in which introduction of the plasmid did not confer virulence in mice. This system is interesting as a model for studying transcriptional activation, for developing new expression vectors, and as a new mechanism of virulence gene regulation. The authors postulated that limitation of bacterial growth within phagosomes of host phagocytic cells is the environmental trigger that induces expression of plasmid-mediated virulence genes.

Valone and Chikami reported characterization of three proteins expressed from the virulence region of *S. dublin* plasmid pSDL2 (*253*). By sucrose-gradient cell fractionation, the 30-kDa protein was identified in the outer membrane fraction, the 76-kDa protein was in the cytosol, and the 27-kDa protein was found in both cytosolic and outer membrane fractions. Sequence data for the 4.1-kilobase *Eco*RI region showed that the two smaller proteins lack a typical sequence for export out of the cytoplasm. The authors suggested that the outer-membrane location of these proteins points to their export out of the cytoplasm by an unusual mechanism.

Studies of the plasmid-borne *mka* gene cluster, required for *S. typhimurium*'s virulence in mice, revealed the function of the MkaC protein (*254*). When the cloned genes *mkaA, mkaB, mkaC,* and *mkaD* were investigated, production of MkaC enhanced the expression of β-galactosidase from *mkaB-mkaA-lacZ, mkaB-lacZ,* and *mkaC-lacZ* gene fusions. Failure of MkaC to induce *mkaD-lacZ* and *mkaA-lacZ* fusions that did not contain the promoter-proximal region of *mkaB* indicated that *mkaB* and *mkaA* were induced together as an operon, and that the induction was transcriptional rather than translational. Although the Mka proteins are not expressed in detectable amounts in vitro, their production is thought to be enhanced during infection when their function is necessary. The authors suggested that because MkaC may promote its own production as well as production of the other *mka* genes, it is important in regulating the virulence genes and the environmental stimuli that lead to induction of *mkaC* are of special interest.

Studies of the 100-kilobase virulence plasmid of *S. typhimurium* by Tn*5* mutagenesis extended the previously defined virulence region (*255*). Eleven randomly selected *vir*::Tn*5* plasmids carried by a plasmid-free strain of *S. typhimurium* were mapped and tested in mice for LD$_{50}$ value and ability to induce splenomegaly and to achieve high populations in spleens of infected mice. Eight of 9 virulence-attenuated strains carried Tn*5* insertions that lay outside the known virulence region.

The *S. typhimurium* invasion locus was identified by transposon mutagenesis, by selection for hyperinvasive mutants that could enter HEp-2 cells even under repressing aerobic culture conditions (*256*). Three such classes of mutations were found. One of them was obtained only from mutagenesis with Tn*5*B50, suggesting that their increased invasiveness was due to constitutive expression of one or more genes from the exogenous *neo* promoter. Analysis of these mutants identified an *S. typhimurium* locus termed *hil*, which is essential for entry of bacteria into epithelial cells. The authors postulated that *hil* encodes an invasion factor or an activator of invasion-factor expression. The gene is in a region adjacent to other loci required for invasiveness and virulence.

Dewanti and Doyle investigated culture conditions for production of cytotoxic activity against Vero cells by *S. enteritidis* 11013 (*257*). The toxin could not be neutralized with antiserum to Shiga toxin or *E. coli* verotoxin-1 or -2; it was principally cell-associated and produced during the early stationary phase of growth. Toxin was produced in the pH range of 4.5 to 8.0, pH 7.0 being optimal, and in the temperature range of 12–42°C with the optimum at 37°C. Release of cytotoxin to the growth medium was induced by extremes of pH or a high incubation temperature. Although the importance of preformed *Salmonella* cytotoxin in human illness is not known, these results indicate that production of toxin could be prevented by refrigerating food at ≤7°C or acidifying it to a pH ≤4.0.

The role of type-1 and -3 fimbriae in adherence to epithelial cells was evaluated by using strains of *S. enteritidis* that possessed both types (strain A) or type 1 only (strain V) (*258*). Both strains, when grown in static broth, strongly agglutinated erythrocytes from horse, guinea pig, rat, and rabbit at room temperature and 4°C. Mouse, chicken, sheep, goat, and human erythrocytes were agglutinated moderately or weakly. Strain A attached to human buccal epithelial cells in numbers of ~160/cell, whereas only ~10 bacteria of strain V attached to each buccal cell. Strain A also bound more readily to epithelial cells of the mouse small intestine. Adherence of both strains was D-mannose-sensitive, and pretreating epithelial cells with tannic acid did not promote D-mannose-resistant binding of strain A bacteria. The highly fimbriated strain A was more virulent when mice were inoculated orally, whereas strain V was more virulent by intraperitoneal inoculation. The authors concluded that type 1 and type 3 fimbriae both contribute to adherence and to the virulence of *S. enteritidis*.

Nascimento et al. studied the relationship between egg-shell structure and the movement of *S. enteritidis* across the shell wall throughout the hen's laying cycle (*259*). They discussed the egg's defensive mechanisms to reduce invasion by microorganisms while maintaining other necessary functions. Ultrastructural examination of the cuticular layer, paired shell membranes, and mammillary layer revealed multiple ways in which the ability of a shell to block microbial penetration can be compromised; most of these were related to the hen's age. The authors developed a total structural score to index the shell's overall performance as a barrier to bacterial penetration. They concluded that the poultry industry's quality-control methods are largely subjective and assume a nonexistent uniformity of shell structure and function. The shell's defense can be breached at any point between the oviduct and the breakfast table. Other authors demonstrated airborne infection of laying hens with *S. enteritidis* PT4 (*260*). Exposure to contaminated aerosols produced systemic infections that in some birds persisted in a wide range of tissues, including ovaries and oviducts, throughout the 28-day experiment.

SHIGELLA

Epidemiology

A review of shigellosis surveillance data for the USA, 1967–1988, suggested that the infection has followed and will continue to follow a pattern of low-level transmission punctuated by periods of hyperendemic transmission (*261*). From 1986 to 1988, isolation rates of *Shigella sonnei* nearly doubled. The highest rates during 1987–1988 were reported from counties with large urban, ethnic minority, and poor populations; but the greatest *increases* in rates occurred in relatively wealthy, predominantly white counties. Between 1967 and 1988, the proportion of *Shigella* species isolated from persons ≥20 years old increased more than 7 times as fast as the proportion of this age group in the population. This indicates a shift toward infection at older ages, which may be due to changing levels of immunity to *S. sonnei*. In fact, cyclical changes in levels of immunity may explain the periodicity and transience of nationwide increases in shigellosis. Increasing use of day-care facilities might account for part of the nationwide increase in *Shigella* isolations but cannot explain the transient nature of nationwide increases in the early 1970s and late 1980s. Nor is there evidence for increased importation from abroad or the appearance of a new, widely disseminated vehicle. However, epidemiologic investigations have been limited by the paucity of methods for subtyping *S. sonnei*.

Multiple markers were used to investigate an epidemic of *S. sonnei* infections in Monroe County, New York, from July 1988 to July 1989 (*262*). During this time 304 cases were reported, more than 10 times the normal rate. Two foodborne outbreaks involved 10 women who acquired the infection at a music festival in Michigan and 43 Monroe County residents who attended a private funeral party. Potato salad prepared by a food handler who had diarrhea was implicated in the second outbreak. No common food or water source was identified for the remaining 251 cases. Resistance to ampicillin, tetracycline, or trimethoprim–sulfamethoxazole was encoded in a 70-MDa plasmid found in most isolates examined. Antibiotic resistance determinants apparently were deleted in some strains. Antibiograms clearly separated strains related to foodborne outbreaks from strains not related to foodborne outbreaks; they also distinguished more strains than plasmid profiles and were useful in tracing the dissemination of particular isolates in the community. Restriction analysis increased the discriminatory value of plasmid profiles and validated the antibiogram results. This study illustrated the potential complexity of shigellosis epidemics and the value of using several markers in the investigation.

Gastroenteritis was rampant in U.S. troops during the Persian Gulf war (*263*). After an average of 2 months in Saudi Arabia, 57% of the surveyed troops had had at least one episode of diarrhea. The pathogens most often identified were *E. coli* and *S. sonnei*, and the authors suggested that the prevalence of shigellosis was underestimated. Univariate analysis suggested an association between an episode of diarrhea and eating salad, dining in a mess hall, and drinking from a canteen. There was no association with obtaining food from local vendors, eating in a local restaurant, or drinking bottled water. Uncooked vegetables were suspected sources of enteric pathogens (*E. coli* was isolated from some lettuce samples).

Levine and Levine reviewed the evidence that houseflies (*Musca domestica*) are mechanical vectors of shigellosis (*264*). Some transmission of shigellosis is due to poor personal hygienic practices, even when environmental sanitation is good and water supplies safe; some occurs where sanitation is poor and no amount of hand-washing can make up for the sanitation deficit. The role of houseflies in transmitting shigellosis in developing areas needs to be evaluated. Houseflies can readily contaminate food and eating utensils, and fly-control programs in the USA have provided clear evidence for the role of houseflies in transmitting shigellas.

A study of 1211 shigellosis patients in India identified intestinal obstruction in 30 cases (2.5%) (*265*). The death rate in these patients was 4 times higher than in patients without obstruction. A case–control study found that patients with obstruction were less often breast-fed and had more often received antibiotics; they had a higher median blood leukocyte count, higher serum potassium and lower serum sodium and protein concentrations; and were more likely to have *Shigella dysenteriae* type 1 infection. The authors concluded that obstruction is an ominous complication of shigellosis and warrants therapy in addition to antimicrobial agents.

Antibiotic resistance is increasing in shigellas (*263,266–270*). In October 1989 an outbreak of gastroenteritis on a Caribbean cruise ship affected 14% of the 512 passengers and 3% of the 388 crew members who responded to a subsequent survey (*266*). Multiply antibiotic-resistant *Shigella flexneri* was isolated from 19 ill passengers and 2 ill crew members. Thirteen people were hospitalized, and therapy with an antibiotic to which the isolated strain was resistant was associated with a prolongation of their illness. German potato salad was implicated as the vehicle of transmission. It was prepared and probably infected by a food handler from a country where resistance of shigellas to multiple antibiotics is common, and limited toilet facilities

for the galley crew may have facilitated the organism's spread. This illustrates how antibiotic-resistant strains can be introduced into the USA, posing therapeutic problems, and highlights the continuing problem of foodborne gastrointestinal disease in settings such as cruise ships. As part of national epidemiologic surveillance in Canada, the antimicrobial susceptibility patterns of *Shigella* isolates at Ontario's Central Public Health Laboratory in 1990 was determined (*267*). Eighty percent of isolates were resistant to one or more antimicrobial agents, and 52% were resistant to 4 or more. Different prevalence and patterns of resistance were exhibited by *S. boydii*, *S. flexneri*, *S. dysenteriae*, and *S. sonnei*. *Shigella sonnei* is the most frequent cause of shigellosis in Canada. A study of antimicrobial susceptibilities of *S. sonnei* strains associated with outbreaks in Canada between 1988 and 1991 found that isolates from two outbreaks in Ontario were susceptible to all 18 antimicrobials tested, but isolates from the remaining six outbreaks were resistant to between 4 and 9 antibiotics (*268*). Each outbreak had a unique and consistent resistance pattern. The resistance patterns included resistance to one or more agents commonly used to treat shigellosis. *Shigella* isolates in the Netherlands have also been monitored for antibiotic resistance (*269*). About 10% of isolates from 1984 to 1989 were resistant to the combination of ampicillin, trimethoprim, and sulfamethoxazole. All strains were susceptible to the newer quinolones, but 5 nalidixic acid–resistant strains showed decreased susceptibility to norfloxacin. Because resistance to nalidixic acid appears not to be plasmid-mediated, the authors think it unlikely that plasmid-mediated resistance to nalidixic acid's quinolone analogues will occur. They do suggest monitoring selection of chromosomal mutants, which are likely to appear. In Bangladesh in 1983, 13% of *Shigella* isolates tested were resistant to ampicillin, 24% to trimethoprim-sulfamethoxazole, and 1% to both (*270*). By 1990, these values were 51, 48, and 40%, respectively. Resistance to nalidixic acid increased from 1% in 1986 to 20% in 1990. *Shigella dysenteriae* type 1 was particularly resistant to these drugs. Resistance patterns observed during community surveillance were similar to those of isolates at the Diarrhea

Treatment centre of Dhaka. In Bangladesh, ampicillin and trimethoprim–sulfamethoxazole are no longer considered useful for treating any *Shigella* infection, and nalidixic acid is no longer useful for treating infections due to *S. dysenteriae* type 1. Of 113 confirmed *Shigella* infections in U.S. troops during the Persian Gulf war, 85% were resistant to trimethoprim–sulfamethoxazole, 68% to tetracycline, and 21% to ampicillin (*263*). All isolates were sensitive to norfloxacin and ciprofloxacin.

Virulence and molecular studies

Yoshikawa and Sasakawa reviewed the molecular pathogenesis of shigellosis (*271*). They discussed virulence determinants on the large plasmid and on the chromosome, and the function, genetics, and regulation of virulence-associated loci. They concluded that the pathogenesis of shigellosis is complex, requiring numerous plasmid and chromosomal genes. These genes are under a complex regulatory network which itself involves genes on both the plasmid and the chromosome. Different virulence factors come into play during different stages of infection and are triggered by environmental stimuli such as temperature, oxygen pressure, osmolarity, and other biochemical and biophysical factors. Hale provided another review of the genetic basis of virulence in *Shigella* (*272*). He summarized the epidemiology, pathogenesis, and laboratory models of the infection before reviewing chromosomal and plasmid genes in more detail. The genetic and biochemical bases of virulence in enteroinvasive pathogens was discussed. The pathogenic mechanism of shigellosis has been characterized and the *Shigella* invasion plasmid identified; the next milestone may be biochemical characterization of the gene products to explain the cell biology of *Shigella* infection.

Louise and Obrig tested the hypothesis that Shiga toxin combines with endotoxin-elicited interleukin-1 or tumor necrosis factor alpha (TNFα) to facilitate the vascular damage characteristic of hemolytic uremic syndrome (HUS) (*273*). They found that both Shiga toxin and TNFα were cytotoxic to cultured human umbilical vein endothelial cells and that the two acted synergistically on cells sensitive to Shiga toxin. The effect was dose- and time-dependent for both agents and neutralized by MAbs against either agent. The synergistic response was maximal on the second day, and preincubating cells with TNFα sensitized them to Shiga toxin. The Shiga-toxin sensitivity of umbilical cell lines derived from different individuals varied, leading the authors to postulate the involvement of host genetic factors in development of HUS. Interleukin-1 was not cytotoxic, nor did it enhance the effect of Shiga toxin.

Sen et al. studied environmental signals that induce major changes in virulence of shigellas (*274*). Optimal expression of virulence required anaerobic growth to log phase. Brain–heart infusion broth and RPMI 1640 medium gave better results than yeast tryptone broth. As few as 2×10^5 cells of *S. dysenteriae* or *S. flexneri* grown under optimized conditions produced keratoconjunctivitis in guinea pigs in 15 h. Adherence to and invasion of Henle 407 cells at 37°C by these organisms were significantly greater than when organisms were grown aerobically. The authors concluded that expression of virulence in vivo and in vitro is a function of growth conditions. After anaerobic growth to log phase, infection proceeds efficiently under aerobic conditions. Thus growth conditions rather than proximity to host cells may serve as early signals for expression of at least some virulence gene products.

Twenty-three *Shigella* strains were analyzed by pulsed-field gel electrophoresis and their distribution of three insertion sequences (*275*). Nine *S. sonnei* isolates were closely related but distinguishable from each other and the four independent *S. flexneri* isolates showed clearly distinguishable DNA profiles. However, four epidemic *S. flexneri* isolates showed nearly total genetic identity by both methods. (The IS*911* probe proved too mobile in these epidemic strains to be of value in typing.) The five *S. dysenteriae* isolates comprised three completely different DNA profiles, demonstrating striking diversity within this species. These results demonstrated the potential usefulness of the methods employed for typing and molecular epidemiology studies of *Shigella*.

Restriction fragment length polymorphisms in highly conserved rRNA operons of chromosomal

DNA were used to subtype 100 strains of *S. sonnei* from 16 geographic locations and 4 outbreaks (*276*). The *Sal*I endonuclease differentiated six distinct rDNA patterns. All strains from the same outbreak had the same rDNA pattern. Strains from Minnesota and Michigan outbreaks, which gave the same pattern with *Sal*I, were differentiated by using the *Pvu*II enzyme. Strains from two outbreaks in Texas, which appeared identical with *Sal*I, were differentiated by *Sma*I. Use of the *Sst*I enzyme with strains from sporadic cases that appeared to have the same pattern divided these strains into two groups. From the patterns generated by the various endonucleases a dendrogram was constructed to show the approximate genetic relatedness of the strains. Ribotyping appears to be a useful tool for epidemiologic studies of *S. sonnei*, having the advantage of independence from plasmid-associated traits that are easily gained or lost.

ESCHERICHIA COLI

Epidemiology, outbreaks, and clinical features

Verotoxin-producing *E. coli* (VTEC) is receiving intense scrutiny as a new foodborne pathogen of major importance. The spectrum and epidemiology of disease caused by these organisms was briefly reviewed by Brook and Bannister (*277*). The first VTEC was identified in 1971 but its pathogenic significance was not appreciated until 11 years later, when verotoxin-producing *E. coli* serotype O157:H7 was linked to hemorrhagic colitis in an investigation of a gastroenteritis outbreak related to contaminated beef products. This and other verotoxin-producing serotypes have since been associated with hemolytic uremic syndrome (HUS). Griffin and Tauxe comprehensively reviewed the epidemiology of HUS and other infections caused by *E. coli* O157:H7 and similar enterohemorrhagic *E. coli* (EHEC) (*278*, with 221 references). They discussed the adherence and attachment of these organisms to the intestinal mucosal cell, their toxins, efforts to subtype *E. coli* O157:H7 strains, and serologic and

other methods of diagnosing infection. Risk factors and the many clinical manifestations of infection were considered in some detail. Epidemiologic investigations of outbreaks were summarized, including studies of the seasonal and geographic incidence of the various syndromes. A major section of the review was devoted to HUS. Other sections covered thrombotic thrombocytopenic purpura, animal reservoirs of the organisms, and food vehicles of infection. The authors concluded that *E. coli*, which in 1980 was a rapidly vanishing cause for concern in developed countries, has reappeared with the recognition of serotype O157:H7 as a problem of major proportions.

Fecal specimens are generally not cultured for VTEC unless there is clinical suspicion of this infection (*279*). Testing of feces from all patients hospitalized during a 6-month period at Seacroft Hospital, Leeds, with a diagnosis of gastroenteritis identified 9 of 161 bacterial strains isolated as VTEC; this was the same as the incidence of *Shigella*. Sorbitol-nonfermenting colonies were tested for agglutination with antiserum to *E. coli* O157:H7 and sorbitol-fermenting colonies were tested with antisera to type O26 and O111. Positive isolates of these serotypes were tested for toxicity to Vero cells. This procedure identified 7 strains as type O157 and 2 as type O26. Three of the patients developed HUS. The authors recommended that routine fecal microbiological testing include a search for VTEC in view of the incidence and wide clinical spectrum of this infection and the risk of HUS.

VTEC strains producing verotoxins designated VT1 and VT2 are generally pathogenic in humans, whereas strains producing VTe cause edema disease in piglets (*280*). Genes for the A subunits of VT2 and VTe are 94% homologous; the B-subunit genes are 78–80% homologous. While screening for VTEC in feces using a polymerase chain reaction (PCR) that amplified VT1, VT2, and VTe genes, investigators were surprised to find a VTe-producing strain of serotype O101:H9 in a diarrhetic man. This toxin has not been associated with symptoms in humans, nor is this serotype usually associated with porcine edema disease. Although VTe-producing strains could be present in pork and be transmitted to humans, this was the first report of a well documented isolation of such a strain from a person.

In Germany, from 1987 through 1990, 62 infections with VTEC other than serotype O157 were identified (*281*). The isolates belonged to 26 serotypes within 20 O groups; 10 were traditional enteropathogenic *E. coli* (EPEC) belonging to group O6. Serotypes O2:H5 and O91:H14 were exclusively associated with ulcerative colitis. VT1 was produced by 31 strains, VT2 by 26, and both by 5.

Rowe et al. conducted an epidemiologic study of childhood HUS in Canada to determine the risk factors for severe disease and the proportion of patients with stools positive for *E. coli* O157:H7 (*282*). The average annual incidence of HUS in children younger than 15 years was 1.44/100,000; in children younger than 5 years the incidence was 3.11/100,000. Risk in Alberta was nearly 3 times that in Ontario. *Escherichia coli* O157:H7 was isolated from 51% of 169 stool samples screened. Demographic variables, clinical presentation, and laboratory findings were discussed. The source of the infection was not considered. Other investigators have also tried to determine risk factors for severe HUS, because only a small proportion of infants and children with VTEC infections develop HUS and the disease varies in severity among those who do. Based on suggestions of an autosomally inherited susceptibility to HUS, Van de Kar et al. examined the HLA antigens of 31 Dutch and Flemish patients with chronic renal failure due to the epidemic form of HUS (*283*). They found an odds ratio of 2.5 (χ^2, $p = .04$) for patients having antigen type HLA-B40.

Of 22 children with acute HUS, 68% had evidence of VTEC infection by culture of the pathogen, detection of free verotoxin in the feces, or both (*284*). However, 91% of them had significantly elevated titers of serum antibodies to *E. coli* O157 LPS. Elevated titers were not found in healthy children or children with diarrhea caused by other enteric pathogens, or in 2 of 3 patients from whom non-O157 *E. coli* had been isolated. The high incidence of anti-O157 LPS antibodies in these patients indicates the predominance of this serogroup in HUS.

Apple cider is an unexpected vehicle of *E. coli* O157:H7 transmission (*285*). Although cider "ought

to be" too acid to support growth of pathogens, *E. coli* O157:H7 grows well in natural cider at refrigeration temperatures, which inhibit growth of competing molds and yeasts. This organism was implicated in an outbreak of HUS involving 6 children in Massachusetts in November 1991; altogether, 23 people with *E. coli*-related symptoms were identified during subsequent investigation. The small local mill that produced the cider was in violation of 10 production regulations, including failure to wash the apples. Like many producers, this one used apples that had fallen from the trees.

An outbreak of *E. coli* O157:H7 hemorrhagic colitis at a junior high school in Minnesota in October 1988 was associated with consumption of heat-processed meat patties in the school cafeteria (*286*). Thirty-two children became ill and 4 were hospitalized; none developed HUS. *Escherichia coli* was cultured from frozen patties manufactured at the same plant on the same dates as the implicated patties, but serotype O157:H7 was not isolated. In Scotland, outbreaks of hemorrhagic colitis due to *E. coli* O157 PT1 were reported in two nursing homes about 10 miles apart; an additional case occurred in the local community (*287*). No source of infection was confirmed despite intensive sampling of the food chain and environment. The two homes had a common meat supply source and both had served ground meat during the week preceding the outbreaks, but no food samples were available for testing. Intriguingly, the Scottish Agriculture College Veterinary Investigation Service was concurrently investigating a series of outbreaks of necrotic enteritis in suckling calves. The gross pathological findings resembled those in humans severely ill with *E. coli* O157 infections. At the time of the report, results of testing for this organism were not available. Surveillance of *E. coli* O157 infections in Scotland, which began in 1989, continues to show peaks during the summer; children and young adults are predominantly affected but incidence again rises in the elderly (*288*).

Investigators in Canada conducted a retrospective cohort study to identify risk factors for hemolytic anemia and HUS in children after sporadic *E. coli* O157:H7 gastrointestinal infection (*289*). Nine of 72 infected children developed hemolytic anemia and 6 of these had HUS. None of 72 age-matched controls with *Campylobacter jejuni* gastroenteritis developed hemolytic anemia. Female gender was the only statistically significant risk factor found: 8 of 29 girls developed hemolytic anemia, compared with 1 of 43 boys. Possible underlying genetic and immunoregulatory mechanisms for this finding, which is consistent with other reports, were discussed.

Seizures and abnormal EEG recordings are relatively common in HUS (*290*). The histories and EEG results of 11 children hospitalized at the University of Minnesota were discussed. Another neurologic lesion that can occur in HUS is pituitary hemorrhage (*291*). This complication was reported in a 5-year-old girl with HUS probably associated with *E. coli* O157:H7 infection. An 8-year-old boy with hemorrhagic colitis attributed to *E. coli* O157:H7 infection developed bacterial ileocecitis as a gastrointestinal manifestation of his infection (*292*). This case illustrates that O157:H7 infection that does not progress to HUS can produce prominent right-sided abdominal effects including involvement of the distal small bowel, with symptoms mimicking appendicitis.

Occurrence and growth in food

Sources of VTEC infection in Great Britain have been less well defined than in the USA, but meat and poultry are likely sources (*293*). Fresh and frozen whole chickens and fresh pork sausage from retail outlets in London were examined for VT1- and VT2-producing *E. coli* using DNA probes specific for these VT genes. Twenty-five percent of the 184 sausage samples hybridized with one or both probes, but none of 112 samples from 71 chickens hybridized with either probe. Because the samples were tested only after enrichment, these results demonstrate the presence but not the abundance of VTEC in the sausage. VTEC was isolated from 20 of the 46 probe-positive samples. The isolates represented eight O serogroups; six strains had an unidentifiable O antigen. Three of the serotypes (O91:H⁻, O115:H10, and O128ab:H2) have been isolated from cases of human infection; none of the isolates belonged to serotype O157.

Padhye and Doyle developed a rapid procedure for detecting *E. coli* O157:H7 in food and surveyed samples of raw milk and fresh ground beef for the organism (*294*). Food samples were enriched in a selective enrichment medium. The enrichment culture was applied to a sandwich ELISA that used a polyclonal antibody specific for *E. coli* O157 antigen as the capture antibody and an MAb specific for EHEC O157:H7 and O26:H11 as the detection antibody. The sensitivity for detecting *E. coli* O157:H7 in inoculated ground beef and dairy products was 0.2–0.9 cells per gram of food. A survey of 107 samples of fresh ground beef from retail stores in Madison, Wisconsin, detected the organism in 3 samples. Eleven of 115 raw milk samples from the bulk tanks of 69 farms were positive. By an MPN method, the estimated populations of *E. coli* O157:H7 in the contaminated ground beef were 0.4–1.5 cells per gram. Kim and Doyle reported modifying this procedure to give a sensitive and simple dipstick immunoassay for *E. coli* O157:H7 in ground beef (*295*). The organism could be detected in ground beef samples within 16 h, including the 12-h enrichment incubation. Faint but detectable reactions occurred with as few as 10^3 cfu/mL of pure cultures of the organism. The sensitivity of the method determined in artificially contaminated ground beef was 0.1–1.3 cells per gram, with a false-positive rate of 2.0%. A survey of retail ground beef using this method found 1 of 76 samples to be contaminated by *E. coli* O157:H7.

A survey for enteropathogenic *E. coli* (EPEC) was conducted in a food-serving establishment in Giza, Egypt (*296*). Ten samples were taken from each of the following sources: workers' hands, workers' clothing, tables, plates, towels, knives, raw meat, and cooked meat. Twenty-three serotypes were isolated; the EPEC serotype most frequently encountered was O26:K60 (B6). No serotype O157 was isolated.

The public health significance of preformed verotoxin in food is unknown, and factors governing its formation in foods are not well understood. Weeratna and Doyle developed a method for detecting VT1 in milk and ground beef and studied the conditions under which VT1 is formed in these foods (*297*). Their method was a sandwich ELISA that used a VT1-specific MAb as the capture antibody and a rabbit polyclonal antibody raised against VT2 as the detection antibody. This ELISA could detect as little as 0.5 ng/mL of VT1 in milk and 1.0 ng/g of VT1 in ground beef. In milk, maximum toxin production (306 ng/mL) occurred when samples were incubated at 37°C with agitation for 48 h. Very little production (1 ng/mL) occurred during 96 h of incubation at 25°C or 30°C. In beef, 452 ng/g of VT1 was produced at 37°C in 48 h; again, little toxin production occurred at the lower temperatures. The authors concluded that although milk and ground beef can support substantial VT1 synthesis, this is unlikely to occur under normal conditions of handling and storage.

Because *E. coli* O157:H7 is associated with raw milk, the fate of this organism was monitored during manufacture of cottage cheese from artificially contaminated pasteurized skim milk (*298*). The number of organisms increased 100-fold during the manufacturing process but all were killed during subsequent cooking of the curd. The same changes in pH and acidity occurred in contaminated and control samples, and the experiment clearly showed that *E. coli* O157:H7 can grow at the pH's generated by the lactic acid bacteria used in producing cottage cheese. Therefore if heat treatment of the curd were insufficient or contamination occurred after cooking the organism could survive in the subsequently refrigerated cottage cheese. This study involved artificial contamination with laboratory cultures of *E. coli* O157:H7; contamination of natural origin might give different results.

The lactoperoxidase system inhibits many bacterial species. Two of its three components, lactoperoxidase and thiocyanate, occur naturally in raw milk; and the complete system, which also includes H_2O_2, can temporarily preserve milk (*299*). El-Gazzar et al. studied the effect of the lactoperoxidase system on *E. coli* O157:H7 in artificially contaminated raw milk and semisynthetic medium. In both media, with inocula of 10^4 cfu/mL, a reduction in number of organisms was detected after as little as 20 h at 4°C, and complete inactivation occurred in 5 d. With inocula of 10^8 cfu/mL populations were reduced by 3.6–4.0 log after 5 d. The system was less effective at higher

temperatures; and after an initial inhibition, which was maximal at 6–12 h, growth resumed and populations reached control levels by 24 h. The authors concluded that control afforded by the lactoperoxidase system is influenced by level of contamination, exposure time, and temperature.

The effects of adult chickens' cecal microflora on in vitro growth of *E. coli* O157:H7 and *S. typhimurium* were examined (*300*). Two lactic acid–producing bacteria (*Enterococcus durans* and *Lactobacillus acidophilus*), one volatile fatty acid–producing bacterium (*Veillonella parvula*), and one starch-hydrolyzing bacterium (*Streptococcus morbillorum*) were isolated from cecal contents; their ability to inhibit growth of the pathogens on chicken-feed agar medium and to produce acetic, propionic, and lactic acid in chicken-feed broth medium was determined. *Streptococcus intermedius* was also tested. *Streptococcus morbillorum, S. intermedius, V. parvula*, and mixed inocula of the two did not inhibit growth of either pathogen. *Enterococcus durans* and a mixed culture containing *S. intermedius* and *V. parvula* produced very small zones of inhibition against both pathogens. Significantly larger inhibition zones were produced against both pathogens by pure and mixed cultures containing *L. acidophilus* and by a mixed culture containing *E. durans* and *V. parvula*. Growth inhibition was related to the production of acetic, propionic, and lactic acid in the culture medium. Production of these acids may partly explain how adult cecal microflora protects young chicks against colonization by enteropathogens. In in vitro experiments, treatment of chicks with adult fecal cultures on the day of hatching reduced intestinal colonization by *E. coli* O157:H7 upon subsequent challenge with the pathogen (*301*).

D- and *z*-values were determined for lean and fatty ground beef inoculated with ~10^7 cells/g of *E. coli* O157:H7 (*302*). As determined by enumeration on plate count agar plus pyruvate, *D*-values at 125°C were 78.2 and 115.5 min, respectively, for lean and fatty samples; corresponding values were 4.1 and 5.3 min at 135°F, and 0.3 and 0.5 min at 145°F. Results from the 2-h indole tests were similar. The *z*-values for lean and fatty beef using the plate count agar method were 8.3 and 8.4°F, respectively; the indole test gave a value of 7.8°F for lean beef but no value could be determined for fatty beef.

Murano and Pierson studied the effect of heat shock on the heat resistance of *E. coli* O157:H7 by growing cells to log phase at 30°C, heat-shocking them with various time–temperature combinations, subjecting them to heat treatment at 55°C, and determining the survivors (*303*). Heat-shocking at 42°C for 5 min caused the greatest increase in D_{55} value. Cells grown anaerobically, whether heat-shocked or not, had higher D_{55} values than aerobically grown cells. All anaerobically grown cells and aerobically grown heat-shocked cells contained a 71-kDa protein not found in non-heat-shocked aerobic controls. It was immunologically similar to a sigma^{32} subunit of RNA polymerase. The authors concluded that the stress of anaerobic growth can also cause synthesis of heat-shock proteins and increased survival of heat-treated cells.

Virulence and pathogenesis

When specific-pathogen-free mice were inoculated subcutaneously with 10^8 cfu of *E. coli* O157:H7 they displayed most of the symptoms and histological changes observed in human subjects (*304*). Histological changes in the intestine were mostly in the distal part of the small intestine and the cecum. Infected kidneys had swollen glomerular epithelial cells and thickened glomerular capillaries. Unexpectedly, sloughing of cells from bronchiolar walls partly or completely obstructed the lumens. Changes in the spleen, liver, and lymph nodes were also seen. Bacteria were recovered from a wide range of tissue samples and many tissues gave a positive immunoperoxidase reaction. These findings demonstrate the systemic nature of infection in this model.

Toxins. Pathogenic strains of *E. coli* produce four general types of toxins: verotoxins (also called Shiga-like toxins), hemolysins, cytotoxic necrotizing factors, and cytolethal distending toxin. De Rycke reviewed the biological and molecular properties of each of these, discussing their association with pathologic conditions in animals and the role of animals as reservoirs of strains pathogenic for people (*305*). Beutin reviewed the properties of the

hemolysins of *E. coli* and their role in pathogenicity (*306*). He discussed their synthesis, regulation, function, and activity, their genetics, their association with *E. coli* types and virulence markers, and their role in pathogenicity.

The culture conditions favoring maximum production of contact hemolysin by enteroinvasive *E. coli* (EIEC) and virulent and avirulent strains of four *Shigella* species were determined (*307*). The best medium for contact hemolysin activity of *Shigella* was tryptic soy broth, whereas for EIEC it was casamino acid–yeast extract broth with 1 mM $CaCl_2$. Both growth and hemolysin production were greatest at a slightly alkaline pH. Hemolysin production depended on the presence of a 140-MDa plasmid. Evidence suggested that the contact hemolysin was a protein and that a chitotriose-like moiety served as its receptor. It also appeared that metabolically active cells were required for contact hemolysin activity. The authors demonstrated the invasion of HeLa cells by EIEC and suggested that for these organisms, as for *S. flexneri*, contact hemolysin is essential for intracellular multiplication.

Tesh and O'Brien reviewed developments in research on the pathogenic mechanisms of Shiga toxin and Shiga-like toxins (verotoxins) (*308*). They presented evidence that these toxins damage vascular endothelial cells of target organs, disrupting their homeostatic capacity. Invasion of endothelial cells of the central nervous system produces neurologic complications; in the colon, the result is bacillary dysentery or hemorrhagic colitis; attack on the kidney can produce HUS. The authors outlined one mechanism by which Shiga toxin and the verotoxins could mediate the development of HUS: they participate in the initial insult, from which subsequent pathophysiologic alterations follow. However, there may be toxin-mediated damage to tubular epithelial cells as well as to glomerular endothelial cells, and the role of toxins in renal disease may be more complex than originally thought. Mainil reviewed the distribution of Shiga toxin and verotoxins in *Shigella* spp. and *E. coli*, discussing animal reservoirs of the organisms and biological activities of the toxins (*309*). Genetic aspects of the toxins and the use and specificity of genetic probes were discussed.

Shiga toxin, the verotoxins, and ricin are structurally similar in having an enzymatic A chain and a receptor-binding B chain. Comparison of the primary structures of the A subunits of VT1, VT2 and two of its variants, and ricin showed conserved regions at residues 51–55, 167–172, and 202–207 from the N-terminus of VT1 (*310*). All three regions corresponded to the active site of the ricin A chain deduced by X-ray crystal diffraction analysis. To determine the importance of these regions for VT1 activity, single amino-acid mutants were tested for Vero-cell cytotoxicity and inhibition of protein synthesis in a rabbit reticulocyte lysate. Substitutions in the 51–55 region had no important effect on toxicity. Both activities were drastically reduced by replacing glutamic acid–167 with glutamine or arginine-170 with leucine; fairly large reductions resulted from replacing arginine-170 with histidine or lysine or arginine-172 with leucine; and modest reductions occurred with substitutions at tryptophan-203. Glutamic acid–167 was known to be essential for activity; the authors concluded that arginine-170 is also important. They suggested a chemical mechanism for the *N*-glycosidase activity of VT1 based on the relative activities of the mutants tested. Other investigators used *Saccharomyces cerevisiae* to identify point mutations that abolished activity: induction of the wild-type cloned element in *S. cerevisiae* was lethal; mutations that permitted survival were likely to be at residues critical for catalytic activity (*311*). In this way the authors identified tyrosine-77 as critical for activity of VT1 and also tested other mutants. When active-site residues implicated in this and other studies were mapped to an energy-minimized computer model of the VT1 A-chain, a cleft was identified into which all of the implicated critical residues clustered, regardless of their distances from one another in the primary structure of the molecule. Many chemical features expected in the active site of an RNA *N*-glycosidase were present in the side chains of amino acids occupying the cleft.

Canadian researchers have crystallized the B-subunit of VT1 by vapor diffusion (*312*) and investigated its structure by X-ray crystallography (*312,313*). Surprisingly, the structure resembles that of the B oligomer of the cholera toxin–like heat-labile enterotoxin from *E. coli* even though the two proteins have no known sequence similarity. The authors postulated that the receptor-binding site lies in a cleft between adjacent subunits of the pentamer.

A third verotoxin, highly homologous to VT2 and several VT2 variants but immunologically distinct from VT1 and VT2, has been identified in a strain of *E. coli* O157:H7 (*314*). The genes for this toxin were cloned and sequenced. The predicted amino acid sequences of the A and B subunits and the toxin's activity against HeLa cells were compared with those of VT2 and several of its variants. Immunological differences and differences in toxicity were attributed to the small deviations identified within the primary structure of the B subunit.

Enterotoxigenic *E. coli* (ETEC) strains produce two kinds of heat-stable enterotoxin (STa and STb, also called STI and STII) that cause intestinal secretion and diarrhea. STa is methanol-soluble and active in the suckling mouse and porcine ligated ileum assays; STb is methanol-insoluble and reported to be active only in the porcine ligated ileum model. Fujii et al. purified STb to homogeneity (*315*). The purified toxin evoked a secretory response in the suckling mouse and ligated rat intestinal loop assays only in the presence of a protease inhibitor. The peptide contained 48 amino acid residues, in a sequence identical to that predicted from the nucleotide sequence of its gene. It contained 4 cysteine residues that formed intramolecular disulfide bonds at Cys-10–Cys-48 and Cys-21–Cys-36. When STb was applied to the serosa in isolated sections of mouse ileum, an acceleration of spontaneous motility and a weak contraction were observed after 2–3 min (*316*). This was not affected by atropine but was prevented by papaverine. Application of STb to the mucosa of the reversed ileum caused acceleration of spontaneous motility after 7–8 min but no contraction. The authors discussed these results in terms of the situation in an in vitro infection and suggested that STb acts directly on muscle cells of the ileum to enhance spontaneous intestinal motility.

de Sauvage et al. reported the cloning and expression of a gene encoding the human receptor for STa (*317*). The receptor contained an extracellular ligand-binding site and a cytoplasmic guanylyl cyclase catalytic domain, making it a member of the same family of receptors as the natriuretic peptide receptors. Stable mammalian cell lines over-expressing the STa receptor specifically bound ^{125}I-labeled STa and responded to STa by a ~50-fold increase in cellular cGMP. Sequence comparisons of rat and human STa receptors revealed less conservation in the extracellular domain than is shown by natriuretic peptide receptors of the two species. This may indicate species differences in ligand–receptor interaction. Comparisons of amino acid sequences of the STa and natriuretic peptide receptors showed the most conserved region to be the guanylyl cyclase domain; the low homology between extracellular domains suggests that natural ligands for the STa receptor would probably not belong to the natriuretic peptide hormone family. A second report by de Sauvage et al. described further characterization of a recombinant human STa receptor (*318*). They concluded that the STa receptor guanylyl cyclase identified by molecular cloning is the only receptor for STa present in the human T_{84} colonic cell line that endogenously expresses STa binding sites.

To determine the relative contribution of colon and ileum in STa-mediated diarrhea, toxin binding, guanylyl cyclase activation, and toxin-induced water flux were compared in rat colonocytes and ileocytes (*319*). The results suggested that STa-induced diarrhea results from increased fluid secretion in the small intestine accompanied by decreased absorptive capacity in the colon.

ETEC also produces a heat-labile enterotoxin (LT), which is similar to cholera toxin (CT). Both LT and CT are composed of an A subunit, where the biological activities reside, and a B subunit that binds to G_{M1} ganglioside receptors on target cells. A mutant strain of ETEC produced an abnormal LT whose A subunit had a single amino-acid substitution, glutamic acid–112 to lysine-112 (*320*). This mutant LT lacked ADP-ribosyltransferase activity. It had no ileal loop or vascular permeability activities, did not elongate CHO cells, and did not activate adenylate cyclase in target cells. The toxin's binding ability and the A chain's nicking site were unimpaired. The authors concluded that loss of ADP-ribosyltransferase activity was due to the substitution at position 112 and led to loss of the toxic activities. Although activation of adenylate cyclase may not be the mechanism for diarrhea, the authors determined that the sites for these effects are at least very close and glutamic acid–112 is involved in both of them.

X-ray studies of LT revealed two lanthanide (erbium and samarium) binding sites in the interface of the toxin's A subunit and the B pentamer and showed a conformational change induced by binding (*321*). The sequence of one site was very similar to that of CT. These findings were discussed in terms of the reported calcium ionophore activity of LT and CT and the effects of lanthanum ions on toxin activity.

By a checkerboard immunoblotting technique using polyclonal and monoclonal antibodies, investigators demonstrated immunologic heterogeneity in LTs from 133 ETEC strains of human origin (*322*). After defining optimum conditions for the procedure they identified 4 strains that produced an LT immunologically similar to LT1, 126 strains producing LT similar to LT2 or LT3, and 3 strains whose LT reacted like the LT produced by ETEC of porcine origin. They recommended their method for epidemiologic and serologic studies.

Murphy and Dallas analyzed two copies of the gene *elt* that encodes LT (*323*). The copies were located on the same 157-kilobase Ent plasmid; their physical arrangement was unlike that of the duplicated and amplified *ctx* genes of *V. cholerae*, which encode CT. The nucleotide sequences of the two *elt* alleles differed by 2 base-pairs. The DNA flanking *elt* appeared to be a hot-spot for insertion sequences.

ADHERENCE AND ATTACHMENT. A modified invasion assay was developed to take into account the variable ability of bacteria to adhere to cells, which is a prerequisite for invasion (*324*). The assay was used to study diarrheagenic strains of *E. coli* with differing ability to adhere to and invade HEp-2 cells. EIEC strains were the most invasive, followed by EPEC strains and then ETEC strains. These findings are consistent with what is known about the ability of *E. coli* to invade the intestinal tract in vivo. They indicate that the adhesins of diarrheagenic *E. coli* play no direct part in invasion, although they may facilitate the process by promoting the initial contact between bacteria and host cells.

The T_{84} human colonic epithelial cell line was shown to be a good model for studies of EHEC adherence (*325*). Twelve *E. coli* O157:H7 and other EHEC strains were incubated for 1–3 h with T_{84} cell monolayers grown on collagen-coated coverslips, unattached bacteria were removed, and attachment was quantitated microscopically. There were marked differences in adherence between strains—a range of 3–152 bacteria per oil-immersion field. Adherence of some strains was partially inhibited by mannose. One highly adherent strain formed microcolonies in the area of tight junctions. Attachment was correlated with the strain's ability to adhere to isolated rabbit colonocytes ($r = .91$, $p = .00004$, without mannose; $r = .60$, $p = .04$, with mannose). The advantages and possible applications of this model were discussed.

Barrett et al. pointed out that while cattle are a major reservoir of *E. coli* O157:H7, they also harbor non-O157 VTEC serotypes that are by far more common (*326*). People consuming beef and dairy products should also be exposed to non-O157 VTEC, yet the incidence of disease attributed to these organisms is low, suggesting that VT production alone is not sufficient for VTEC to cause disease in humans. Probes for VT1, VT2, and two factors that may affect virulence of VTEC (an EHEC plasmid and the *eae* gene necessary for production of attaching and effacing lesions) were used to screen isolates of *E. coli* O157:H7 from cattle and non-O157 isolates from cattle and humans. All 30 O157:H7 cattle isolates and 16 of 19 non-O157 human isolates reacted with both the *eae* and the plasmid probes; only 12 of 26 non-O157 cattle isolates reacted with both probes. The prevalence of toxin types did not differ between human and cattle non-O157 isolates. The authors suggested that because *eae* and plasmid sequences were present in all O157:H7 isolates and were more frequent in non-O157 isolates from humans than from cattle, they may represent virulence factors. However, large plasmids from VTEC exhibit considerable heterogeneity, so no single "EHEC plasmid" can be assumed. These data raise questions about what constitutes an EHEC and why non-O157 serotypes

with *eae* and plasmid sequences have not caused large outbreaks of illness. In the same area of inquiry, Pohl's review of studies of VTEC in cattle revealed an interesting distribution of serogroups (*327*). Among calves suffering from diarrhea or dysentery, VTEC of serogroups O5, O8, O20, O26, O111, and O118 were common. These organisms attach to the gut epithelium and efface the microvilli. Asymptomatic cattle most often carry VTEC of serogroups O22, O25, O116, O121, O157, and O171. Pohl postulated that these strains do not possess attaching–effacing properties. Of relevance to both of these papers is a report of the cloning and sequencing of a gene from *E. coli* O157:H7 that is highly homologous with the EPEC *eae* gene necessary for attaching–effacing activity (*328*). The EHEC sequence was 97% homologous to the EPEC *eae* gene over the first 2200 base-pairs and 59% homologous over the last 800 base-pairs. The receptor-binding domain of the *inv* gene product lies near the C-terminal, suggesting that the predicted sequence divergence at the C-terminal end of the *eae* gene products would produce different antigenic and receptor specificities.

ETEC isolated from diarrhetic patients in Burma, central Africa, and Peru were serotyped, checked for enterotoxin production, and screened by ELISA for colonization factor antigens (CFAs) and putative colonization factors (*329*). ETEC with identifiable colonization factors comprised 71% of Burmese strains, 69% of central African strains, and 52% of Peruvian strains. The proportions and types of colonization factors showed considerable geographic variation. The 29–48% of ETEC with no identifiable colonization factors were predominantly strains that produced only LT. This type of information is important for the formulation of vaccines.

The fimbrial morphology and location of the receptor-binding site of CFA/I, an adhesin of enterotoxigenic *E. coli* O78:H11, were analyzed (*330*). Stable fimbrial monomeric subunits were isolated. Antibodies obtained by immunization with purified subunits were more reactive with subunits than with fimbriae, predominantly labeling the fimbrial tips, whereas antibodies obtained by immunization with fimbriae reacted equally with fimbriae and subunits, densely labeling the fimbriae over their entire length. Antibodies to subunits strongly inhibited CFA/I-induced hemagglutination; antibodies to fimbriae inhibited agglutination only slightly. The authors concluded that CFA/I fimbriae consist of but one type of adhesive subunit, of which only the one at the tip is accessible to the receptor. Other investigators isolated and characterized CFA/I fimbriae from an ETEC strain, produced polyclonal antibodies against the fimbrial proteins, and developed an indirect ELISA for detection of CFA/I fimbriae (*331*). The ELISA was as sensitive as a DNA hybridization technique for detecting ETEC. A major subunit protein and one minor protein band were detected by SDS–PAGE.

Scanning electron microscopy showed that ETEC bearing CFA/I or CFA/II adhesive factors adhere to the brush border of cultured Caco-2 cells (*332*). Heat-killed *Lactobacillus acidophilus* strain LB, which also adhered to Caco-2 cells, inhibited adhesion of ETEC in a concentration-dependent manner. Because *L. acidophilus* does not express CFA adhesive factors, the authors postulated that the heat-killed cells inhibited ETEC attachment by steric hindrance of the Caco-2 cell's ETEC receptors.

Iron is one of the environmental factors that regulate production of virulence factors in some microorganisms. Karjalainen et al. found that the expression of CFA/I fimbriae by ETEC was responsive to fluctuations in iron concentration (*333*). Addition of 0.05 mM $FeSO_4$ to the growth medium decreased CFA/I antigen and fimbrial production by an ETEC strain as measured by quantitative ELISA and hemagglutination assay. The effect was prevented by addition of an iron chelator. In studies with ETEC strains containing wild-type and mutant genes for the metalloregulatory protein Fur, only the wild-type strain showed greater activity of the CFA/I subunit gene promoter in the presence of iron chelators. This suggested that Fur was involved in the iron-induced repression. Because several potential Fur-binding sites were identified in the promoter area, the authors postulated that Fur binds to the promoter of the CFA/I subunit gene.

Human ETEC isolates expressing CFA/IV produce plasmid-encoded CS5 fimbriae (*334*). Clark et al. determined the nucleotide sequence of the region that encodes the major CS5 fimbrial subunit. The only protein found in data-base searches to have statistically significant homology with the CS5 subunit was the major fimbrial subunit of the F41 porcine ETEC. The greatest homology was within the signal sequence and at the extreme ends of the mature protein. This suggests a common origin and highly conserved functional signal and C-terminal domains, but considerable evolutionary modification of antigenicity and adaptation to different host epithelial receptors.

An *E. coli* strain of serotype O127a:H2 was isolated from a diarrhetic child in Thailand (*335*). It was negative for virulence factors characteristic of ETEC, EPEC, EIEC, and EHEC and showed an aggregative pattern of adherence to HeLa cells. It was further investigated for adherence to a broad range of native and formalin-fixed human and animal mucosal cells. Adherence and hemagglutinating activity were resistant to D-mannose and were strictly regulated by environmental conditions. Adherence levels were compared with those of ETEC with CFA/I or CFA/II pili. The findings suggested unique adherence characteristics of the enteroaggregative strain and the possibility that adherence ability is a virulence factor.

Another recently described pattern of adherence is the diffuse type (DA). The adhesin mediating the DA phenotype of a diarrhea-associated *E. coli* O126:H27 strain has been isolated and characterized serologically (*336*). The DA phenotype is mediated by a 6-kilobase DNA fragment from a 100-kilobase plasmid. The fragment encodes a 100-kDa protein that was used to generate specific antisera in rabbits. Direct immunologic evidence was presented to show that this protein is the adhesin mediating the DA phenotype of this diarrhea-associated strain and represents a group of serologically related proteins in other DA strains.

Detection and identification

Conditions for optimal long-term preservation of LT-producing ETEC were investigated (*337*). Ten strains were preserved under 12 sets of conditions and examined for LT production after 1 month, 9 months, and 3 years. Seven media were tested at one or more temperatures. When kept on Dorset egg medium slants at 4°C or frozen in tryptic soy broth with 20% glycerol, all strains remained alive for 3 years with minimal loss of LT production.

Incorporation of rhamnose and cefixime into sorbitol–MacConkey agar improved its selectivity for verotoxigenic *E. coli* O157 (*338*). The standard sorbitol–MacConkey agar does not discriminate between *E. coli* O157 and other sorbitol-nonfermenting *E. coli* and *Proteus* strains, whereas most non-O157 *E. coli* do ferment rhamnose and the antibiotic cefixime is more active against *Proteus* than against *E. coli*.

A direct fecal VT assay was described for laboratory diagnosis of EHEC infection and used to screen stool samples submitted to health laboratories in British Columbia (*339*). Stool supernatants in 1:1 and 1:10 dilutions and supernatants treated with MAb mixtures to neutralize VT1 and VT2 were tested for cytotoxicity to Vero cells and the results compared with results from the standard cultural procedure using sorbitol-MacConkey agar. The direct method detected 10% more positive specimens than the culture method. Six of 80 positive specimens were positive only by the culture method: these were collected early in the illness, suggesting that free fecal toxin levels had not yet reached detectable levels. A notable finding was that VTEC of serotypes other than O157:H7 were causing disease in British Columbia.

Ability to ferment sorbitol, β-glucuronidase activity, and VT production were evaluated in 120 VT-producing strains of *E. coli* O157 (H type 7 or nonmotile) isolated from fecal specimens of patients in the U.K. and 169 other *E. coli* strains (*340*). The VT-producing O157 strains, which were diverse in their other properties, all failed to ferment sorbitol within 24 h and to hydrolyze 4-methylumbelliferyl-β-D-glucuronide (MUG). The two rare VT-negative strains of serotype O157:H7 also failed to ferment sorbitol and hydrolyze MUG, whereas no VT-negative strains of other serotypes were both sorbitol-nonfermenting and MUG-negative. The authors recommended that strains of *E. coli* O157:H7 identified by cultural methods or the MUG test be confirmed as VT-positive.

A large outbreak of illness due to enteroinvasive *E. coli* O143 provided opportunity for a molecular epidemiologic investigation of this organism (*341*). The outbreak affected 370 of 1350 persons who ate food catered by a restaurant in Houston, Texas, in September 1985. Plasmid patterns and chromosomal restriction endonuclease digestion patterns of EIEC from the outbreak, other *E. coli* of serogroup O143, and other EIEC isolated from patients with diarrhea were compared by pulsed-field gel electrophoresis. Striking restriction fragment length polymorphism was found. The restriction pattern of four outbreak isolates was identical to that of an O143 EIEC strain isolated 2 months earlier in Mexico and nearly identical to that of two other Mexican O143 EIEC isolates. These related strains also had the same plasmid pattern, although only a few plasmid bands were seen, in comparison with 21–30 chromosomal bands. The restriction patterns of all three non-O143 EIEC isolates, all five O143 non-EIEC isolates, and 6 of 15 O143 EIEC isolates were very different. The authors concluded that pulsed-field gel electrophoresis can distinguish among *E. coli* strains of the same serogroup and phenotype and can identify relatedness within the O143 serogroup. The data further suggested that the outbreak strain spread from Mexico to Houston.

Attempts to isolate *E. coli* O157:H7 sometimes fail because the target organism is lost through overgrowth of contaminants or serial dilution of the enrichment culture. A method was developed to capture and remove the target organisms from the mixed culture (*342*). Magnetic beads coated with *E. coli* O157 antibody were added to an enrichment culture of a meat product artificially contaminated with *E. coli* O157:H7, then removed from the culture with a magnetic concentrator, washed, and plated on sorbitol–MacConkey agar. Colonies were picked from these plates for biochemical and serological verification as *E. coli* O157:H7. The procedure permitted consistent recovery of the target organism from meat samples inoculated with 0.6–0.9 cfu/g. *Escherichia coli* O157 non-H7 and H7 competed with one another for sites on the beads, interfering to some extent with the isolation of O157:H7. Conditions for minimizing carryover of non-O157 cells were discussed.

An indirect immunodot assay employing anti-STb serum and a Western blotting chemiluminescence detection system was developed to detect STb in fecal specimens (*343*). Better than 90% correlation was observed between an intestinal ligated loop biological assay, a radioactive DNA probe, and the immunodot assay. The immunodot procedure could detect STb in the feces of a newborn pig inoculated with an STb-producing strain of *E. coli*.

SEROLOGICAL AND AGGLUTINATION TESTS. Investigators in Germany proposed a biotyping scheme for VT-producing *E. coli* O157 and listed serological cross-reactions between O157 and other gram-negative bacteria (*344*). The 41 strains investigated fell into 4 serovars—O157:H7, O157:H⁻, O157:H43, and O157:H45; but only O157:H7 and O157:H⁻ produced VT. These VTEC were biotyped based on their reactions with sorbitol, β-glucuronidase, dulcitol, rhamnose, raffinose, and sucrose. Antigenic relationships between the O157 antigen and the O antigens of other *E. coli* serogroups, and the antigens O:1B of *Yersinia pseudotuberculosis*, O:30 of *Salmonella*, and O:9 of *Yersinia enterocolitica* were demonstrated. The authors concluded that because of the phenotypic variability of VTEC, the diagnosis of O157 VTEC can be made only by ascertaining VT production. Complete determination of O and H antigens and biochemical testing may be necessary for confirmation. Other investigators investigated the antigenic relatedness of *E. coli* O157 and four sorbitol-negative species of *Escherichia*: *E. hermannii*, *E. fergusonii*, *E. vulneris*, and *E. blattae* (*345*). Their assays were a tube agglutination test using polyclonal antisera and a slide agglutination using latex reagents. Strains that cross-reacted with O157 in initial screening by the rapid slide procedure were tested by the tube method. Cultures positive for the O157 antigen were also tested for the H7 flagellar antigen. The only cross-reactivity detected by the tube method was with 4 of 24 *E. hermannii* isolates. The authors concluded that because of cross reactions, rapid serological tests cannot be relied on to identify *E. coli* O157:H7 without further biochemical and serological characterization.

Although VTEC of serotype O157:H7 are most frequently associated with HUS, VTEC belonging to other serotypes have also been isolated from patients with HUS (*346*). For this reason, attempts were made to purify LPS from VTEC isolated from cases of HUS and to develop a screening test for antibodies to LPS of VTEC other than *E. coli* O157:H7. The authors tested 64 HUS-patient sera that did not contain antibodies to LPS of *E. coli* O157:H7. Although they detected evidence of VTEC infection in only 12 sera, they were able to demonstrate antibodies to LPS of serogroups O5, O115, O145, O153, and O165, confirming that strains of non-O157 *E. coli* can cause HUS. Serology may be particularly valuable for detecting VTEC infection because the pathogen itself and its toxin are detectable in stool specimens only during a relatively short time soon after infection. The same authors reported improved detection of *E. coli* O157 infection in HUS patients in an assay using both IgA and IgM antibodies to LPS (*347*). They screened 125 serum samples for LPS antibodies by ELISA and immunoblotting. Forty-eight sera contained IgM antibodies and 42 contained IgA antibodies. Of these, 13 contained only IgM and 7 contained only IgA antibodies. Thus screening for both antibody classes increased the sensitivity of obtaining evidence of *E. coli* O157 infection. Other investigators reported high *E. coli* O157 LPS antibody titers by an indirect hemagglutination assay of sera from both culture-positive and culture-negative HUS patients (*348*). Titers ≥1:4096 were found in 22 of 27 HUS patients but in only 4 of 249 diarrhetic controls who did not develop HUS. The response was specific for LPS of *E. coli* O157.

Two commercial agglutination kits were compared with two cell-culture methods and a G_{M1} ganglioside ELISA for detecting *E. coli* LT (*349*). Twenty-three of 48 toxigenic strains were positive by all tests and 20 were negative by all tests. One was negative only by the staphylococcal coagglutination test. Four strains, all LT producers, were positive only by the Y-1 and Vero cell culture methods. The authors concluded that the coagglutination test was the least sensitive but simple and rapid; the reversed passive agglutination test was simple, sensitive, and a good substitute for cell culture or G_{M1}-ELISA.

ELISAs. By means of an ELISA, investigators in India demonstrated that 392 of 557 *E. coli* fecal isolates (70.4%) from patients with acute diarrhea produced ST (*350*). Serogroups O20, O78, and O128 each accounted for ≥21 isolates; serogroups O61, O149, O4, O55, O106, and O114 accounted for 8–19 isolates each. Characteristics of the ELISA were discussed. In assays of 100 strains, 88 were positive by ELISA whereas the suckling mouse assay identified only 80 positive strains. Thus the ELISA was more specific, rapid, and sensitive and did not require the use of animals.

French workers used the interaction between avidin and biotin to develop an ST–biotin ELISA in which the solid-phase ST was obtained by coupling the toxin to biotin and binding the resultant conjugate to avidin adsorbed to microtiter wells. Preparatory to adapting this ELISA for STa, they compared three toxin preparations at different stages of purification for their ability to measure anti-STa antibodies (*351*). They found that toxin obtained by gel filtration chromatography on Biogel P4 was sufficiently pure for use as an immunosorbent in this application.

Other French workers described two microtiter plate ELISAs for detecting free or extracted LT (*352*). One was a G_{M1}-ganglioside ELISA and the other was a sandwich ELISA using purified rabbit anti-LT immunoglobulins. Both used biotinylated anti-LT rabbit immunoglobulins with streptavidin-peroxidase and a commercial TMB substrate as the detection system. The detection limits for purified LT were 50 pg/mL for sandwich ELISA and 1.3 ng/mL for G_{M1} ELISA. Both methods could detect LT-positive strains using a single colony, but the sandwich ELISA gave the highest OD.

Law et al. developed an ELISA capable of recognizing low numbers of VTEC in mixed cultures (*353*). Their method detected both VT1 and VT2 after enhancement of toxin production by culture with mitomycin C. In tests with *E. coli* O157:H7 alone, in mixed culture with *E. coli* C600, and in mixed culture with *E. coli* C600, *Proteus mirabilis*, and *Enterococcus faecalis*, VT1 could be detected

when the proportion of toxigenic organisms represented 1% of the mixture; VT2 could be detected with a proportion as low as 0.025%. Examination of fecal samples with added *E. coli* O157:H7 detected VT2-producing strains when they comprised <0.1% of the coliform population.

To facilitate epidemiologic studies, Barrett et al. developed ELISAs for antibodies to VT1, VT2, and *E. coli* O157 LPS (*354*). ELISA results were compared with results of HeLa cell cytotoxicity neutralization assays. Serum samples from 83 patients in two outbreaks of *E. coli* O157:H7 diarrhea and 66 controls were tested. Forty-three patients (52%) had at least one serum sample positive for anti-O157 LPS antibodies, and 24 of 26 culture-confirmed patients had at least one positive sample. Two of 66 controls (3%) had positive anti-O157 LPS titers. Neutralization assays detected anti-VT1 antibodies in one or more serum samples from 20% of patients and 11% of controls; 19% of patients and 11% of controls had positive titers by anti-VT1 ELISA. All serum samples, including controls, showed nonspecific neutralization of VT2, but no positive antibody titers to VT2 were detected by either neutralization or ELISA. Thus both types of assay proved insensitive for detecting infected patients, although the ELISA for antibodies to *E. coli* O157 LPS was 92% sensitive and 97% specific, with a positive predictive value of 92%, for identifying culture-confirmed cases.

Speirs and Akhtar reported a sandwich ELISA for detecting VT (*355*). Sensitivities were roughly 100 cytotoxic doses for VT1 and 200 cytotoxic doses for VT2; ELISA results were in good agreement with Vero cell assays for the presence and type of toxin. In preliminary studies, the ELISA was moderately sensitive in detecting ground beef samples inoculated with VT2, but was unsatisfactory for stool specimens because inhibitory factors reduced the optical density readings.

DNA PROBES AND THE POLYMERASE CHAIN REACTION (PCR). Three types of adherence to tissue culture cells so far identified in *E. coli* are localized (LA), diffuse (DA), and aggregative (AggA). Organisms exhibiting LA are considered diarrheal pathogens, but the pathologic role of the other types is not clear (*356*). All three types are discernible in HEp-2 and HeLa cell assays used by the Center for Vaccine Development, Baltimore, but a method developed at the University of Texas Medical School recognizes only LA and DA types. Verifying their results by using LA, DA, and AggA strains identified by specific DNA probes, investigators in Bangladesh modified the University of Texas method so that it, too, identifies enteroaggregative *E. coli* (EAggEC). In London, investigators noted that 20% of 353 EPEC strains isolated from cases of diarrhea belonged to serotypes that did not hybridize with the EPEC adherence–factor (EAF) probe, considered diagnostic for EPEC (*357*). Further study of these EAF-nonreacting strains found that 7 of 13 O44:H18 isolates, all of 10 O111*ab*:H21 isolates, and 13 of 21 O126:H27 isolates were EAggEC that showed an aggregative pattern of attachment to HEp-2 cells and hybridized with the EAggEC probe. All of 15 O55:H7 strains and 7 of 8 O111*ab*:H25 strains showed the LA pattern of adherence to HEp-2 cells and gave the positive fluorescence actin-staining test that correlates with the attaching-and-effacing virulence mechanism of EPEC in vivo. Although all of these strains were isolated from patients with diarrhea, none would be identified in epidemiological surveys based solely on the EAF probe.

A method was described for detecting ETEC in fecal specimens using DNA probes labeled with acetylaminofluorene (AAF) to identify LT and ST (*358*). The preparation and use of the AAF probes were optimized to detect ETEC by colony hybridization or direct dot blot techniques, and results were compared with results from established biotinylated probes and bioassays. Although the AAF probes were less sensitive than radiolabeled or biotinylated probes, the authors considered their performance adequate and recommended them as a suitable alternative for clinical diagnosis of ETEC infections and for epidemiological studies in endemic areas. Investigators in Japan described detection of an LT gene in ETEC by densitometry, using highly specific alkaline phosphatase–conjugated oligonucleotide probes (*359*). The probes were antisense codon sequences, which are transcribed into mRNA, of the LT gene from a human isolate of ETEC. They were tested with 100 clinical isolates,

using a reflectance-type densitometer. Results agreed well with results from the Biken test and a ^{32}P-labeled DNA probe, and indicate a potential for densitometric evaluation of DNA hybridization.

DNA probes specific for ETEC LT and STaII, VTEC VT1 and VT2, and EPEC were labeled with digoxigenin and produced in large quantities by the PCR (*360*). Stool specimens were inoculated with control *E. coli* strains at a level of 10^5–10^6/g, plated onto MacConkey agar, and incubated overnight; they were then replica-plated and hybridized with the five probes. The number of positive colonies reflected the number of inoculated bacteria; uninoculated stool specimens showed no hybridization. The authors recommended this method for routine laboratory use. Jackson described another PCR, also utilizing a digoxigenin label, for detecting Shiga toxin–producing *Shigella dysenteriae* type 1 and VT1-producing *E. coli* (*361*). Target DNA liberated from whole cells was amplified using primer pairs homologous to the A-subunit genes of the toxins, incorporating the TTP analog digoxigenin-11-dUTP into the reaction mixture to nonradioactively label the amplified DNA. Labeled PCR reaction products were hybridized to specific gene sequences immobilized on a nitrocellulose membrane and detected with an alkaline phosphatase–conjugated antibody to digoxigenin. Toxin-producing strains of *E. coli* and *S. dysenteriae* type 1 appeared as colored spots on the membrane.

A PCR was developed for detecting a wide range of VTEC serotypes isolated from animal and food sources (*362*). A pair of oligonucleotide primers targeted conserved sequences common to VT1, VT2, and VTe genes. Supernatants of 223 VTEC isolates from meat, milk, and feces, 72 strains of non-VTEC *E. coli*, and 76 strains of other enteric and food bacteria were tested. All 223 VTEC isolates, comprising more than 50 serotypes, were detected by the PCR procedure and verified by Vero cell assay. *S. dysenteriae* type 1 was the only other organism yielding a positive test result. The assay could detect as little as 1 pg of VTEC DNA and as few as 17 cfu of VTEC.

A nested PCR followed by magnetic separation of amplified fragments was used to detect VT1 and VT2 genes in *E. coli* (*363*). The first PCR was carried out according to standard procedures and the double-stranded product was used as primer in the second PCR. In this procedure, one primer was biotin-labeled on one 5' end and the other was ^{32}P-labeled on the other 5' end. The test could differentiate between VT1 and VT2 in a positive/negative ratio of >20; it could detect 5 VT-positive *E. coli* organisms in the 5-μL test sample in the presence of 100-times larger populations of VT-negative strains. Another PCR protocol permitted the VTe-variant target sequence to be distinguished from closely related sequences in the same coding regions for VT1 and VT2 (*364*). This should be useful because the VTe variant has occasionally been associated with disease in humans.

Three new techniques for the detection of STb-positive *E. coli* were compared (*365*). Antiserum against purified STb was used to develop an ELISA, and STb-positive strains identified by ELISA were tested for bioactivity in rat jejunal loops. The new ELISA had the same sensitivity but less specificity than the bioassay. A digoxigenin-11-dUPT-labeled DNA probe for the STb gene was developed by the random primed labeling technique. It was more convenient to use than a radioactive probe, but it was less sensitive and specific than either the bioassay or the radioactive probe. The third new method was a PCR used to amplify a specific portion of the STb gene. This was an extremely specific and practical technique for identifying STb-positive strains. All *E. coli* strains tested that contained the STb gene also produced the STb toxin.

Meyer et al. reported a PCR protocol for detecting *E. coli* in surface water and soft cheese without preliminary cultivation of bacteria (*366*). The method was based on amplification of DNA sequences from the *E. coli* malB operon. Samples of surface water and soft cheese naturally contaminated with from 100 *E. coli* cells per gram to >10^5 cells per gram were analyzed by the PCR and standard culture techniques. The methods yielded comparable results. When artificially contaminated soft cheese samples were analyzed with a second PCR test specific for LT1, the detection limit was 1000 cfu/g. Two naturally contaminated soft cheeses having 2×10^5 and 6×10^5 cfu/g as determined by

culture were found by LT1-PCR to contain low levels of ETEC.

Another PCR approach was described for detecting low numbers of ETEC in minced meat (*367*). Two synthetic 29-mer oligonucleotides were used to specifically amplify a 195-base-pair fragment from the *E. coli* LT gene. When only 6 cfu were added to the reaction mixture as a template, the PCR yielded enough product for visualization on an agarose gel. Minced meat samples were subjected to enrichment culture for *E. coli* before PCR amplification. Three cfu of LT-producing *E. coli* added to 25-g samples before enrichment culturing gave positive results in the PCR assay. The authors concluded that this method meets the most important requirements for routine use: speed, simplicity, sensitivity, and specificity.

Keasler and Hill developed a PCR assay to identify EIEC seeded into raw milk (*368*). As few as 100 cells of EIEC per milliliter of milk were identified after amplification of a plasmid-borne gene required for invasion. Because only 10% of the final DNA preparation was used in the PCR, a sensitivity as low as 10 cells/mL may be possible.

ENZYME IMMUNOASSAY (EIA). A competitive EIA kit and the infant mouse assay were compared for detecting *E. coli* ST (*369*). Both assays detected STa in undiluted filtrates of 31 of 45 toxigenic strains tested; 14 strains were negative in both tests. A negative control was also negative in both assays. Nine of the negative strains were known to have produced STa before several years of storage, indicating possible loss of the plasmid encoding the toxin. The type of diluent influenced the performance of the EIA, but even under optimum circumstances the EIA remained less sensitive than the bioassay.

YERSINIA

El-Shenawy and Marth reviewed yersiniosis as a foodborne infection (*370*). They summarized the classification, distribution, and biological characteristics of yersinias. They described clinical manifestations of yersiniosis and methods for isolating the organism and discussed the occurrence, growth, and survival of the organism in foods. Papers presented at the 5th International Symposium on *Yersinia* were published as volume 12 of *Contributions to Microbiology and Immunology* (*371*). Major sections covered ecology and epidemiology, immunology, pathogenicity, bacteriology, and clinical aspects. Relevant individual papers are summarized in following sections of this chapter.

Epidemiological and clinical features

An incident of too hasty enthusiasm in attributing a case of yersiniosis to drinking raw goat's milk was described (*372*). *Yersinia enterocolitica* biotype 2, serotype O:9 was found in blood of a hospitalized patient and in raw goat's milk remaining in a bottle whose contents the patient and his wife had shared. The organism was not found in the wife's serum or in additional samples of goat's milk from the health-food store where the contaminated bottle was purchased. Questioning revealed that the milk had been purchased after the patient became ill and had probably been contaminated by him. The source of the infection was not established.

The finding that two serogroups of *Y. enterocolitica*, O:3 and O:6,30, were represented in a 1987–1988 Australian outbreak of enteritis prompted a search for environmental sources (*373*). Nine of 39 randomly chosen samples of pasteurized milk were positive for *Y. enterocolitica*, 1 yielded *Y. fredericksenii*, and 1 yielded *Y. intermedia*. All milk isolates belonged to biogroup 1; 6 were of serogroup O:6,30. In three tests for pathogenicity, autoagglutination, and serum resistance, human isolates were generally positive whereas no milk isolate was positive. However, SDS–PAGE outer membrane protein profiles of human and milk isolates were similar, suggesting an association. The environmental source of the O:3 isolates was not established.

Epidemiologic investigation of *Y. enterocolitica* O:3 has been difficult because the organism harbors few plasmids that are useful as strain markers and other methods, such as a phage-typing system, are not widely available (*374*). Blumberg et

al. adapted ribotyping to the study of 50 *Y. enterocolitica* isolates from humans and 11 from pork chitterlings. Altogether they distinguished 7 ribotypes; 4 were confined to the O:3 serogroup and clearly distinguished these strains from O:9, O:1,2,3, O:20, and O:5,27 strains. Ribotype patterns I and II corresponded to phage types 9b and 8, respectively. The finding of identical ribotype patterns in chitterling and human specimens from an Atlanta outbreak supported other evidence that pigs were the source of infection and are a major reservoir for *Y. enterocolitica* O:3. The results further suggested that a limited number of clones have become disseminated within the USA and globally.

Norwegian investigators used an ELISA to detect IgG antibodies against *Y. enterocolitica* O:3 in serum samples from 316 slaughterhouse employees, 171 veterinarians, and 813 military recruits, to learn whether exposure to pigs was associated with an increased prevalence of antibodies (*375*). The findings were suggestive but not conclusive. Within the pig-processing plants, the prevalence of antibodies was significantly greater in workers having direct contact with pigs (18%) than in office staff (2%). A similar tendency was seen among employees at poultry-processing plants, but no pathogenic yersinias were isolated from any poultry samples and the authors could only speculate on the reasons for these observations. Furthermore, there was a surprisingly high prevalence of antibodies in the military personnel (8%), particularly those from urban areas where contact with pigs would be very unusual. Antibodies were detected in 10% of veterinarians, but there was no difference between meat inspectors, general practitioners, and administrators. Thus the data from the pig-processing plants indicated an association between exposure to pigs and presence of IgG antibodies to *Y. enterocolitica*, but the overall study could not address the many confounding factors such as geographic distribution and food habits.

A cohort study of children in Santiago, Chile, found that asymptomatic infections with *Y. enterocolitica* were not uncommon (*376*). The organism was isolated from 6% of healthy children in the subgroup of children from whom weekly stool specimens were obtained. In addition, there was no correlation between illness and putative virulence factors: biogroup 1A strains, which lack traditional phenotypic and molecular markers for pathogenicity, were isolated from 7 children with diarrhea but from no healthy controls, whereas "pathogenic" strains in biogroup 4, serogroup O:3 were isolated from asymptomatic as well as symptomatic children.

Prentice et al. traced the epidemiology of *Y. enterocolitica* infection in the British Isles, 1983–1988 *(377)*. Sources of infection were not discussed, although pigs were mentioned as a reservoir. The number of pathogenic *Y. enterocolitica* isolates rose from 92 in 1983 to 158 in 1988. Serotype O:9 biotype 2 was first recorded in 1983, but by 1988 it represented 44% of all isolates typed; it was first recorded in pigs in the U.K. in 1990. The first Belgian isolate of *Y. enterocolitica* was documented in 1963 and a surveillance program was started in 1967 *(378)*. *Yersinia enterocolitica* surveillance in Belgium, 1979–1989, was summarized. The number of isolations peaked at 1469 in 1986 and fell to 1150 in 1989. Serotypes O:3 and O:9 have accounted for >90% of isolates since surveillance began. Again, sources of infection were not discussed.

Although the common features of acute *Y. enterocolitica* infection have been recognized for 20 years, reports of unusual acute and chronic manifestations of the infection keep appearing. In Norway, 458 patients hospitalized with a diagnosis of *Y. enterocolitica* infection were followed for 4–14 years *(379)*. Altogether, 64 patients suffered from chronic disease. Some developed rheumatic conditions; others developed chronic diseases of the liver, kidneys, heart, pancreas, thyroid, or nervous system. In 22 patients, chronic liver disease was associated with positive tests for antinuclear antibody and rheumatoid factor. Acute hepatic, renal, cardiac, pulmonary, pancreatic, or neurologic involvement was also frequently observed; several patients had multiple organs affected. Two patients had acute insulin-dependent diabetes, 2 had malignant mesothelioma, and 1 had specific lymph node inflammation. A second report by these authors provided more specific information on gastrointestinal manifestations of *Y. enterocolitica* infection in the same patient cohort *(380)*. Findings included

ulcerative colitis in 7 patients, Crohn's disease in 2, unspecific colitis in 11, and mesenteric lymphadenitis or ileitis in 43 (of 56, at laparotomy). Thirty-eight patients were readmitted with abdominal pain and 28 with diarrhea; these symptoms were correlated with the corresponding symptoms at first admission. Four patients had chronic colitis and 12 had chronic weight loss. Right iliac fossa pain during the acute infection was negatively associated with chronic abdominal problems. These two papers show that yersiniosis is a serious disease that frequently becomes chronic, affecting diverse organs.

Wenzel et al. presented a model for enteropathogenic *Y. enterocolitica* and organ-specific autoimmune diseases, specifically thyroid autoimmunity, in humans *(381)*. They proposed that a latent *Y. enterocolitica* infection triggers a macrophage response, which differs in autoimmune and normal persons. The bacterium responds by producing plasmid-coded release proteins, which have structural and functional similarities to heat-shock (stress) proteins. These release proteins also have epitope homologies with thyroid antigens, and an "altered self" immunoreaction results in both *Yersinia* release-protein antibodies and cross-reacting immunoresponses to thyroid antigenic epitopes.

In 1973, an epidemic of *Y. enterocolitica* infection affected 94 Finnish military personnel *(382)*. In a follow-up study in 1986, 37 of 75 men reported having a variety of problems: predominantly musculoskeletal disorders, but also symptoms involving the gastrointestinal tract, skin, eyes, and several other organs. The cause of the primary infection had been mainly *Y. enterocolitica* O:9, and patients with chronic, clinically evident disease had elevated antibody titers against this organism. There was also a close correlation between complications and the HLA-B27 antigen. Three cases of chronic connective tissue disorder and two cases of ankylosing spondylitis were diagnosed.

Although *Y. enterocolitica* generally causes self-limited gastroenteritis and mesenteric adenitis, persons with underlying conditions that cause iron overload are at increased risk for serious, even fatal, systemic infection. Complications associated with *Y. enterocolitica* infection were reported in two β-thalassemia patients who were treated with the iron chelator deferoxamine (*383,384*). This drug serves as an exogenous siderophore for the pathogen, which cannot produce its own siderophores to satisfy its iron requirement. One patient developed extensive abdominal disease and *Y. enterocolitica* was cultured from the peritoneal fluid (*383*); the other had an ileal perforation and required resection of the terminal ileum and right hemicolon (*384*).

Appendicitis-like syndromes are common in older children and young adults with *Y. enterocolitica* infections (*385*). A retrospective study of 2861 patients who underwent appendicectomy for clinically suspected appendicitis found that *Y. enterocolitica* type O:3 or O:9 had been isolated from 75; no pathogenic yersinias were isolated from appendixes of 326 gynecologic controls.

Mononuclear cells from synovial fluid of patients with reactive arthritis proliferate in vitro when challenged with bacteria associated with reactive arthritis; the maximum response occurs with the organism that caused the triggering infection. *Yersinia*-specific T cell clones were obtained from the synovial membrane and synovial fluid of an HLA-B27-positive man who worked as a butcher (*386*). This was the first report of isolating such T cell clones from the synovial membrane and characterizing them in detail. The clones could be useful for characterizing the *Y. enterocolitica* antigens that elicit T-cell immunity and for detecting antigen within the joints of patients with reactive arthritis.

Polyarteritis is another late manifestation of *Y. enterocolitica* O:3 infection (*387*). Two weeks after experiencing mild diarrhea, a 43-year-old man was hospitalized with severe generalized myalgia. Immunoperoxidase staining showed *Y. enterocolitica* O:3 antigen in the subendothelial layer of the blood vessels.

Occurrence and growth in foods and the environment

To estimate the prevalence of *Y. enterocolitica* O:3 in Danish pigs, tonsil swabs from 2218 freshly slaughtered pigs representing 99 herds were examined (*388*). The organism was found in 25% of pigs and 82% of herds; no herd-management factor could be associated with its presence. To determine the effect of slaughtering technique on surface contamination, 1256 pigs were eviscerated manually, by use of a mechanical bung cutter, or by enclosing the rectum and anus in a plastic bag and then using the bung cutter. With manual evisceration the rate of surface contamination was 26% on the medial hind limb and 13% in the area of the split sternum; mechanical cutting with the rectum closed off reduced these rates to ~2%. A survey of meat from retail butcher shops found *Y. enterocolitica* O:3 in 10 of 33 samples of minced pork, 3 of 24 samples of minced beef, and 0 of 32 low- to medium-salt vacuum-packaged meat products. Positive beef samples were collected at shops where minced pork samples were also positive, suggesting that *Y. enterocolitica* O:3 is common in pork and cross-contamination of other products is possible.

In Australia, a survey of meat and milk was made to determine the incidence of yersinias (*389*). Fifty samples each of beef, lamb, and pork from retail stores, 50 pasteurized cow's milk samples, and 150 raw bulk milk tank samples were examined. *Yersinia* was isolated from all types of samples except pasteurized milk, but none of the isolates harbored the virulence plasmid. Of 114 isolates, 90 were *Y. enterocolitica*, 9 were *Y. intermedia*, and 15 were *Y. frederiksenii*. During a 9-year period in the state of São Paulo, Brazil, and the city of Rio de Janeiro, 184 strains of *Yersinia* were obtained from raw and pasteurized milk, beef and pork, beef and chicken liver, chicken heart, gizzard, and lung sausage, hamburger, cheese, and lettuce (*390*). Of these, 46 were identified as *Y. enterocolitica*, 67 as *Y. intermedia*, 20 as *Y. frederiksenii*, and 8 as *Y. kristensenii*; 43 biochemically atypical strains could not be classified. No pathogenic types were detected. A survey of pork and related products in northern Taiwan found *Y. enterocolitica* in 29% of product samples (*391*). Contamination rates were especially high for pork ravioli (50%) and fresh pork (43%); <5% of pork sausage was contaminated, and the organism was not found in ham, canned paté, or bacon. The largest number of strains (10) belonged to serotype O:5. Detection rates were higher for refrigerated and frozen samples than for nonrefrigerated samples, suggesting that refrigeration favored growth of psychrotrophic *Y. enterocolitica* while suppressing other pathogenic bacteria. Seventeen of the 40 strains isolated were considered potentially pathogenic.

Japanese investigators studied colonization by *Y. enterocolitica* in the tonsils of 140 freshly slaughtered healthy pigs (*392*). *Yersinia enterocolitica* O:3 was isolated from 24% of 140 tonsils, 24% of 140 cecal content samples, 85% of 40 oral cavity swabs, and 36% of 25 masseter muscles. Bacterial counts were 10^2–10^3/g in masseter muscle, $<10^2$–10^5/g in cecal contents, and 10^5–10^6/g in tonsils. Although *Yersinia*-positive tonsils appeared grossly normal, histological examination revealed evidence of infection. The authors believe their results show that colonization of the tonsils by *Yersinia* is an important factor in contamination of the pig carcass and pork. Bülte et al. discussed the high prevalence of *Y. enterocolitica* in the mouth and head region of healthy pigs and the likelihood that this is frequently the source of contamination of the flesh (*393*). They suggested that alterations in slaughter technique could prevent much of the subsequent contamination of pork and pork products.

Eighty strains of *Yersinia* isolated from pigs and pork products in Saskatchewan were examined for virulence in 12 in vivo and in vitro assays (*394*). Some strains belonged to pathogenic bioserotypes of *Y. enterocolitica* and displayed virulence-associated characteristics in most or all tests. Others belonged to *Y. enterocolitica* biotype 1A and related species, which were avirulent in most of the assays. Salt aggregation and latex particle agglutination are both indexes of surface hydrophobicity, but salt aggregation proved the better indicator of virulence. Invasion of cells grown in culture was the best indicator of virulence. An isolate of *Y. kristensenii* from a pork product was lethal for 2 of 3 iron-overloaded mice, but the reference strain was not. The study confirmed that bioserotypes of *Y. enterocolitica* isolated from pigs and pork products in Saskatchewan include some that are pathogenic for humans and showed that testing for virulence phenotypes is a useful adjunct to speciation and bioserotyping.

Larkin et al. investigated the relationship between the incidence of *Y. enterocolitica* in raw milk and the bacteriological quality of the milk (*395*). Twenty-one high-quality samples (electronic somatic cell counts <200,000/mL) and 26 low-quality samples (counts >1,000,000/mL) were examined. *Y. enterocolitica* was detected in 24% of low-count samples and 11% of high-count samples. Samples of high-count milk were also inoculated with ~10^4 cells/mL of six strains of *Y. enterocolitica* and stored at 4°C; all strains survived 15 days of refrigerated storage. Thus *Y. enterocolitica* contaminated both high- and low-count milk and competed well with high populations of other microorganisms. Strains of serotype O:8 artificially inoculated into high-count milk maintained their virulence throughout the study, but no virulent strains were found in naturally contaminated samples. In other studies, Marth's research group found that the lactoperoxidase system reduced numbers of *Y. enterocolitica* strain 2635 NT in semisynthetic medium and raw milk after 2 h (*396*). In general, the degree of inactivation was inversely related to the initial inoculum size and directly related to temperature of exposure. At 30°C the initial decrease in cell numbers was followed by growth of surviving cells. The authors suggested use of the lactoperoxidase system for temporary control of *Y. enterocolitica* in raw milk as a public health measure.

Because *Listeria* and *Yersinia* are associated with raw milk and dairy products, a survey of Vermont's 34 dairy processing plants was conducted to identify environmental sources of these organisms (*397*). In 361 samples mainly from floors and other noncontact surfaces, the incidence of *Listeria monocytogenes* was low (1.4%) compared with the incidence of *Listeria innocua* (16.1%); 10.5% of samples were positive for *Y. enterocolitica*, whereas only 2.5% yielded other yersinias. Sites positive for either species were statistically more likely to be positive for the other as well. Fluid plants had a higher prevalence of *Listeria* and *Yersinia* than cheese or other types of dairy manufacturing plants. In the fluid plants, areas associated with case washers had the highest contamination rate. In all plants, contamination in wet areas was greater than in dry areas.

A mathematical model was developed to show the effect of pH, acidulant, and temperature on the growth rate of *Y. enterocolitica* (*398*). The growth inhibitory effects of acids tested were acetic > lactic > citric > sulfuric. The variation of growth rate with temperature could be represented by a square-root plot and the effect of pH could be incorporated by replacing the regression coefficient by its relationship with pH. The full model was represented by:

$$r^{1/2} = 0.0392(pH - pH_{MIN})^{1/2} (T - 269.0),$$

where r = growth rate, pH_{MIN} = pH at which no growth occurs, and T = temperature in °C. Values of maximum growth inhibitory pH derived from the model agreed well with experimental values for all acidulants when an acid-specific pH_{MIN} was used. The authors also studied the effects of these conditions on survival of *Y. enterocolitica* (*399*). Attempts to model the behavior of the organism found a negative square-root relationship between death rate and temperature at various combinations of pH and acidulant, but several other functions of death rate also described the data fairly well. The high coefficient of variation for T_0 precluded development of a combined temperature/pH model such as that described for growth.

During a survey of *Yersinia* in food in eastern France, 375 strains of *Y. enterocolitica* and related species were tested for antibiotic resistance (*400*). All carbenicillin-sensitive strains were either *Y. kristensenii* or biovar 3 of *Y. enterocolitica*. Isoelectric focusing studies of the β-lactamases of these and other *Yersinia* strains showed that lack of β-lactamase A explains the sensitivity to carbenicillin of susceptible strains of biovar 3 (serogroup 5,27) of *Y. enterocolitica*, of *Y. kristensenii*, and of most strains of *Yersinia* biovar 6, which are now included in two new species, *Y. mollaretii* and *Y. bercovieri*. The unique β-lactamase pattern of one of the food isolates, as well as its biochemical characteristics, supported its classification as *Y. bercovieri*.

On Honshu Island, Japan, *Yersinia* species were isolated from 65 of 223 free-living small mammals (*401*). One strain was *Y. enterocolitica* O:3; 8 were *Y. enterocolitica* O:5; 6 were *Y. enterocolitica* O:8; 3 were *Y. enterocolitica* O:9; and 1 was *Y. pseudotuberculosis* 4b. Five of the 6 O:8 strains were positive in virulence tests, contained the

45-MDa virulence plasmid, and showed high pathogenicity for mice. The authors postulated that these virulent O:8 strains originated in the USA because until recently they had not been found in Japan. In Shimane Prefecture, Japan, *Y. pseudotuberculosis* was isolated from 0.3% of patients with gastroenteritis; most of them lived in the mountains, where residents used well water or water from a mountain stream. Restriction endonuclease patterns of plasmid DNA from human isolates were compared with patterns of isolates from domestic and wild animals, food, soil, and water (*402*). The study confirmed that in mountainous areas, wild animals were a major reservoir of *Y. pseudotuberculosis* pathogenic for humans; pork and pet animals were common sources in all geographic regions. Restriction endonuclease analysis gave more definitive results than a serological approach.

Long-term survival of *Y. enterocolitica* in sterile spring water at 4°C was demonstrated (*403*). Water samples were inoculated with pure and mixed cultures of *Y. enterocolitica* and *E. coli*. During the first 3 weeks of storage at 4°C, populations of *Yersinia* increased by 2–3 log; even after 64 weeks, viable counts approximating initial numbers were obtained. *Escherichia coli* survived a maximum of 13 weeks in pure cultures; less, in mixed.

Isolation and identification

Because of disagreements over the usefulness of a cold-enrichment step in isolating pathogenic *Y. enterocolitica*, Bucci et al. compared the recovery of pathogenic and nonpathogenic strains from fecal specimens by direct plating on cefsulodin–irgasan–novobiocin (CIN) agar and by subculturing from cold enrichment onto CIN agar (*404*). *Yersinia* was isolated from stools of 3.2% of patients with intestinal disorders. Of the 163 *Yersinia* isolates, 27 belonged to serogroup O:3 and 2 to serogroup O:9. The O:3 isolates were biogroup 4 and phage type VIII; O:9 isolates were biogroup 2, phage type X_3. These are recognized human pathogens. Eighteen of the pathogenic strains were identified by both culture techniques, 6 were detected only by direct plating, and 5, only by cold enrichment followed by plating on CIN agar. In contrast, 126 of the 134 nonpathogenic strains were isolated only when the cold-enrichment step was employed; 3 were detected only by direct plating and 5 were detected by both methods. The authors concluded that the methods are equally sensitive for pathogenic strains (83% for direct plating, 79% for 3-week cold enrichment), and direct plating is more efficient and less expensive.

Zheng and Xie evaluated 10 media for studying differential colony morphology of virulent and avirulent clones of *Y. enterocolitica* (*405*). Among their observations was that emergence of small colonies of virulent strains was temperature-dependent but relatively independent of the richness of the medium. The role of absolute and relative Ca^{2+} and Mg^{2+} concentrations was not clearly defined. Other workers, however, reported a convenient agarose medium for simultaneous determination of the low-calcium response and Congo red binding by *Y. enterocolitica* clones bearing the virulence plasmid (*406*). At 37°C on the calcium-deficient agarose medium, the small, Congo red–binding colonies of plasmid-bearing clones were clearly distinguishable from the much larger, white colonies of plasmid-cured clones.

Ibrahim et al. developed a PCR-mediated digoxigenin-dUTP-labeled probe for the *Yersinia* heat-stable chromosomal enterotoxin gene (*407*). The probe was used in DNA–DNA colony hybridization to screen 113 strains of *Yersinia* isolated from red meat, milk, fish, humans, and animals. In *Y. enterocolitica*, even strains belonging to the same serotype were clearly identified as pathogenic or nonpathogenic. Of the other *Yersinia* species tested, only three strains of *Y. kristensenii* hybridized with the probe; these were readily distinguished from *Y. enterocolitica* by their pyrazinamidase activity. In artificially inoculated fecal specimens the probe easily detected the target gene sequence. Compared with probes that target a sequence in the *Yersinia* virulence plasmid, this probe had the advantages of specificity for *Y. enterocolitica* and closely related organisms and of not depending on the easily lost virulence plasmid.

Although pathogenic *Y. enterocolitica* is frequently isolated from the tonsils and mouths of pigs, and pork products are considered a major source of *Yersinia* infection in humans, Norwegian investigators were able to isolate *Y. enterocolitica* O:3 from only 1 of 127 raw pork products—a result that challenged the prevailing ideas. To resolve the issue, genotypic typing methods were used to compare human and porcine isolates, and retail pork products were again surveyed using a genetic probe for detecting the virulence plasmid of *Y. enterocolitica* (*408*). The same restriction endonuclease patterns of chromosomal and virulence-plasmid DNA were represented in isolates from human patients and pigs, regardless of serogroup, as were the same H antigens, biovars, phage types, and antibiograms. When 50 samples of raw pork products from 13 meat-processing plants were examined with the probe, pathogenic *Y. enterocolitica* was found in 30 (60%), whereas conventional isolation and enrichment procedures recovered the pathogen from only 9. The authors concluded that the prevalence of pathogenic *Y. enterocolitica* in Norwegian pork products is considerably higher than previously thought, and use of conventional isolation procedures may substantially underestimate it.

The biotype and antibiotic sensitivity of 100 clinical isolates of *Y. enterocolitica* were determined (*409*). All isolates were resistant to ampicillin but sensitive to ticarcillin–clavulanic acid and imipenem. Patterns of sensitivity to other β-lactam agents were biotype-specific (see also reference *400*).

Virulence and pathogenicity

In an interesting review, Brubaker discussed factors involved in the acute and chronic diseases caused by yersinias (*410*). He contrasted the metabolically restricted but strikingly lethal *Yersinia pestis* with enteropathogenic *Y. enterocolitica* and *Y. pseudotuberculosis* in terms of general properties, ecology, pathogenetic mechanisms, and virulence factors. The *Yersinia* Lcr virulence plasmid plays a basic role in all medically significant yersinias by promoting a form of immunosuppression that permits unrestrained growth accompanied by necrosis. Superimposed on this are effects mediated by plasmids unique to *Y. pestis* and the adhesive and invasive activities of the more robust enteropathogenic yersinias that favor chronic disease.

Brubaker concluded that just as it is "necessary" for *Y. pestis* to promote rapidly lethal disease, it is advantageous for *Y. enterocolitica* and *Y. pseudotuberculosis* not to kill their host—at least, not quickly.

Fifty *Yersinia* serogroup O:8 strains from human, animal, food, and environmental sources were characterized by species, biogroup, phage type, and potential virulence (*411*). A notable finding was that serogroup was not species-specific: factor O8 was found in both *Y. enterocolitica* and *Y. intermedia*. Nor could serogrouping reliably predict virulence. Biogrouping was useful for identifying pathogenic strains within *Y. enterocolitica* biogroup 1, but did not reveal a pattern for *Y. intermedia* O:8. Phage typing was of little epidemiologic value. All strains were negative for autoagglutination and calcium dependence and none were lethal for mice. None of the 8 "American" strains harbored the 42-MDa virulence plasmid; it may have been lost during laboratory cultivation. The authors emphasized that demonstration of plasmid DNA may not be a valid criterion on which to decide the public health significance of a bacterial strain.

The O side-chain of LPS proved to be essential for virulence of *Y. enterocolitica* O:3 in a mouse model of oral infection (*412*). The authors cloned the *rfb* gene cluster of *Y. enterocolitica* O:3 (which is responsible for biosynthesis of the O side-chain) and isolated an O side-chain-specific bacteriophage; they then isolated and characterized a *Y. enterocolitica* O:3 rough mutant that was resistant to the phage. As expected, LPS from the mutant lacked the O side-chain. Because both mutant and wild-type chromosomal DNA hybridized with an *rfb*-region probe, the authors concluded that a point mutation rather than a large deletion was involved. The mutant was ~50 times less virulent than the isogenic wild type. Transcomplementation experiments restored virulence and suggested that the *rfb* region is organized into at least two operons.

Using sera from patients with yersiniosis and hemolytic uremic syndrome (HUS), Chart et al. demonstrated one-way cross-reactivity with LPS of *Y. enterocolitica* O:9 and *E. coli* O157 (*413*). Sera from HUS patients reacted only with LPS of *E. coli* O157, whereas 80% of sera from yersiniosis patients contained antibodies to both *Y. enterocolitica* O:9 and *E. coli* O157 LPS. The authors postulated that the cross-reacting sera contained two groups of IgM antibodies that recognized distinct epitopes on the *Y. enterocolitica* LPS, one of which is also present on *E. coli* O157 LPS. Possible explanations for the differences in antibody response, such as differences in the physical structures of the two LPSs or aspects of pathogenesis, were discussed. Cross reactions such as this must be considered when serological testing provides the only evidence of infection.

To identify possible sources of *Y. pseudotuberculosis* infection in humans, restriction endonuclease patterns of virulence-associated plasmids from *Y. pseudotuberculosis* isolated from humans, pigs, pets, wild animals, soil, and water in Japan were examined (*414*). Nearly all of the 289 strains contained a single 40- to 50-MDa plasmid; a few also bore cryptic plasmids. Presence of the large plasmid was always associated with calcium dependence and autoagglutination. *Bam*HI digestion of plasmid DNA from serogroup 1b gave 5 types of patterns. Strains carrying the type-2 plasmid were isolated from humans, pigs, dogs, cats, rats, birds, raccoon dogs, and soil, indicating mutual transmission among these sources and the possibility of being infected through contaminated food or water. Strains carrying the type-3 plasmid were isolated only from humans, whereas types 1, 4, and 5 were never isolated from humans, although they had properties associated with virulence. Plasmids from other serogroups were similarly analyzed.

In his published thesis, Pærregaard discussed molecular components of *Y. enterocolitica* involved in adhesion (with special reference to plasmid-coded factors) and induction of the host's humoral immune response (*415*). Adhesion has been qualitatively studied in several ex vivo and in vitro models, to sort out the roles of chromosomal genes and the virulence plasmid. *Yersinia enterocolitica* antigens have been identified by crossed immunoelectrophoresis and serological cross-reactions between chromosome-coded *Y. enterocolitica* antigens and antigens from other bacteria quantitated. Antibodies against pYV-coded antigens were quantitated by ELISA.

Different sets of plasmid-mediated proteins are expressed in vivo and in vitro (*416*). Bacteria grown in the intestinal lumen produced all plasmid-coded proteins expressed in vitro except for the 26-kDa protein. They also synthesized an outer-membrane protein of 23 kDa that was not expressed in vitro, and synthesis of a 24-kDa protein, not a proteolytic product of the 26-kDa molecule, was enhanced. After penetration into the Peyer's patches two further proteins of 210 and 240 kDa were expressed, neither of which was detectable in the outer membrane of bacteria grown in vitro. Plasmid-coded proteins that are abundantly released in vitro in calcium-deficient media were not detected in the ileal lumen, suggesting that they are not important in pathogenesis. These results indicate that the intestinal milieu at least partly determines the composition of the outer membrane. The significance of the proteins produced in vivo but not in vitro is not known, but they may help plasmid-bearing bacteria to resist the host's immune response.

Video microscopy, immunofluorescence studies, and electron microscopy provided evidence that invasion of cultured eukaryotic cells by *Y. enterocolitica*, as mediated by the outer-membrane protein invasin, is associated with alterations in the cytoskeletal organization of the host cell (*417*). Polymerized actin and the actin-associated proteins filamin, talin, and the β_1 subunit of integrin accumulated around invading bacteria. Adherence and internalization were blocked by an antiserum directed against the β_1 chain of integrin cell-adherence molecule. Cytochalasin D also prevented bacterial entry, indicating that internalization involves actin microfilaments. No evidence was found for the involvement of tubulin.

The invasin protein of *Y. pseudotuberculosis* binds to β_1-subunit integrin receptors, promoting bacterial penetration into mammalian cells. The integrin-binding domain is coded by the C-terminal 192 amino acids. The structure of invasin was further characterized by studies with deletion derivatives and fusion proteins carrying different segments of invasin, using a set of 32 MAbs directed against invasin (*418*). Indirect immunofluorescence demonstrated two large regions of the protein containing epitopes exposed on the bacterial surface. All MAbs that recognized surface-exposed epitopes in the cell-binding domain inhibited both attachment to and penetration of cells; no other MAb inhibited either activity.

The outer-membrane protein YOP-1 of various serotypes of *Y. enterocolitica* and *Y. pseudotuberculosis* was studied by SDS–PAGE and peptide mapping (*419*). The apparent molecular weight of the protein ranged from 180,000 in O:8 to 206,000 in O:3. By peptide mapping the YOP-1 of "European" and "American" serotypes of *Y. enterocolitica* were assigned to three groups, which were conserved within a serotype. The similarity of peptide patterns in serotypes that predominate in certain regions suggests a common and independent evolution of YOP-1 in these serotypes and is evidence for the clonal nature of these pathogens.

Comprehensive in vitro studies were performed to delineate the role of temperature and the transcriptional activator VirF in the induction of pYV-coded virulence functions in *Y. enterocolitica* (*420*). The authors found that only some of the pYV genes involved in synthesis of Yops depend on VirF for their transcription. They found that temperature not only controls transcription of *virF* but also influences the interaction between VirF and the promoters of the target genes, presumably by modifying the DNA structure of the promoters. Specifically, the regulon controlled by *virF* includes at least the *yop* and *ysc* genes, *yadA,* and *ylpA* but appears not to include other genes involved in the production of Yops, such as *virA* and *virB*.

When highly pathogenic strains of yersinias are iron-starved, they synthesize two outer-membrane proteins of high molecular weight that are not synthesized by nonpathogenic or less pathogenic strains (*421*). Synthesis of these proteins depends on the *irp2* gene, which is located on a large unstable chromosomal fragment. The *irp2* gene was shown to be present only in highly pathogenic strains (*422*). Its promoter was iron-regulated in *E. coli*; specifically, the *irp2* promoter was controlled by the Fur repressor, so that repressibility of *irp2* by iron depended on a functional *fur* gene. Evidence was presented that the genes coding for these high-molecular-weight proteins constitute an operon where *irp2* is upstream of *irp1*, and that both proteins are required for expression of the high-pathogenicity phenotype.

VIBRIO

Rodrick reviewed the *Vibrionaceae* as indigenous pathogens in marine foods and the marine environment (*423*). Besides *Vibrio*, this family includes the genera *Aeromonas* and *Plesiomonas*. At least 11 species of *Vibrio* are pathogenic or considered potentially pathogenic to humans, causing wound infections, ear infections, gastroenteritis, and primary or secondary septicemia. The ecology of these species and the nature and epidemiology of the diseases associated with them were summarized. Kelly discussed surveys of pathogenic *Vibrionaceae* in infected patients and the environment, touching on the implications of the findings for divers (*424*).

Vibrio cholerae

EPIDEMIOLOGY AND OUTBREAKS. Two World Health Organization reports traced the spread of the pandemic of cholera El Tor from the time it reached Peru in late January 1991—the first cholera in the Western Hemisphere in the 20th Century (*425,426*). More than 80% of the 391,220 cases reported in South America during 1991 were in Peru; Ecuador reported ~46,000 cases and Colombia, ~12,000. In mid-June the epidemic reached Mexico, from where it spread to Guatemala, El Salvador, and Honduras; one case occurred in Nicaragua in November. In Africa, after remaining endemic since 1970 with seasonal increases during the rainy season, cholera affected greatly increased numbers of people in at least 21 African countries during 1991. The epidemic continued in Asia, and imported cases occurred in Canada, the USA, and western Europe. Contaminated food and water are considered the major sources of infection in this pandemic, rather than person-to-person spread. The same epidemic strain, *V. cholerae* O1 serotype Inaba biotype El Tor, has been confirmed at the Centers for Disease Control from 9 affected countries (*427*).

Microbiologic markers indicate a relationship of the Latin American epidemic strain with African and Asian strains—yet also differentiate the Latin American strain, suggesting its recent evolution. In Peru, documented sources of infection include foods and beverages purchased from street vendors and rice left at ambient temperatures for many hours before being eaten without reheating. Elsewhere, a broad variety of food and water vehicles have been implicated.

Officials of the Pan American Health Organization believe that the epidemic pathogen may have arrived in Peru on a foreign freighter that released contaminated bilge water into the harbor at Lima (*428*). The first people are thought to have been infected by eating contaminated ceviche, but the pathogen then quickly moved into the water supply. Ironically, its spread may have been facilitated by a decision not to chlorinate much of Peru's water supply because of reports that chlorination spawns carcinogens when chlorine reacts with byproducts of organic decay. This result demonstrates the importance of balanced risk assessment. Glass et al. summarized the origin and spread of the cholera epidemic in the Americas, citing major food vehicles of transmission in several countries (*429*). Contaminated public water supplies were a major problem in Peru. In Chile, consumption of uncooked vegetables irrigated with raw sewage was blamed for many cases. Contaminated shellfish were linked to spread of the disease in Ecuador. Cooked foods stored at ambient temperatures and eaten without reheating were also incriminated. In the USA, cases have occurred among travelers who were infected in epidemic areas, aboard an international flight, or by contaminated seafood brought back to the USA. The only Nicaraguan case reported through the end of 1991 was in a 2-month-old breast-fed baby (*430*).

Scientists from the CDC and WHO believe that lessons from the cholera epidemic in Africa are relevant to control of the disease in Latin America (*431*). Past public health practices such as quarantine, vaccination, and mass chemoprophylaxis are ineffective. The importance of food as a vehicle of transmission was emphasized and the role of such social phenomena as mass migration and burial practices must be better understood. Sanitary and behavioral interventions or improved vaccines might help to bring the current pandemic under control. In the same vein, Mossel et al. reviewed past patterns of cholera transmission and successful and unsuccessful strategies for its control (*432*). They then proposed a strategy for assessment and management of risks associated with foods from endemic areas in the current pandemic.

Conditions controlling the survival of *V. cholerae* in the environment have not been well defined (*433*). However, its ability to survive in both salt water and fresh water presents clear hazards. Frequent positive isolations of *V. cholerae* O1 from tropical and coastal regions of Peru have been made from the sea, rivers, and lakes, municipal and hospital sewage, irrigation water, plankton, skin and intestines of fish, and molluscs. Symptomless carriers may also spread the pathogen (*434*). *V. cholerae* O1 El Tor, Inaba, was isolated from 3% of rectal swabs taken from 5992 symptom-free persons living in the region of Piura, Peru. They had no recent history of cholera or diarrhea; many of them had had no contact with cholera patients. The Piura River, which runs through this area and provides water for domestic and agricultural uses, contained *V. cholerae* only after it reached Piura. This may explain why no symptomless carriers were identified upstream of the city, but carriers were found with similar frequency in Piura and downstream from it.

Genetic relationships between 23 toxigenic and 23 nontoxigenic human and environmental isolates of *V. cholerae* O1 from the U.S. Gulf Coast area were examined by multilocus enzyme electrophoresis (*435*). All toxigenic and 7 nontoxigenic strains had the same alleles at 16 enzyme loci; the remaining 16 nontoxigenic strains showed 9 distinct combinations of alleles. The authors postulated that the toxigenic strains belonged to a single clone to which some nontoxigenic strains were related, but most of the nontoxigenic strains were of diverse origin.

The current pandemic strain of *V. cholerae* O1 El Tor reached Bangladesh in 1973; El Tor and Ogawa serotypes both caused outbreaks of disease in 1991 (*436*). Analysis of Inaba isolates from Ecuador and Bangladesh by southern blots of *Hind*III

digests revealed the same cleavage patterns of their rRNA genes, suggesting genetic identity. This strengthens the contention that the South American cholera outbreak involves the *V. cholerae* strain that is causing the worldwide pandemic and is continuing to invade new territories.

Outbreaks of cholera have been associated with international air travel. On February 19, 1992, health agencies in California received the first reports of cholera in passengers on a flight from South America (*437*). The flight had left Buenos Aires, Argentina, on February 14, stopped in Lima, Peru, and then continued to Los Angeles. By 4 March, 76 cases had been associated with the outbreak: 51 from California, 14 from Nevada, 4 from Hawaii, 2 from Arizona, 4 from Japan, and 1 from Argentina (*438*). Three persons had eaten raw seafood within 3 days of the flight, 1 had bought food from a street vendor, and 2 had eaten in the Lima airport. At the time of reporting, the only menu item from the flight that was significantly associated with illness was a seafood salad supplied by a caterer in Lima (odds ratio, 6.18; 95% CI, 2.36–16.53).

The number of travel-associated cases of cholera in the USA is increasing (*439*). In 1991, 18 of the 26 cases reported were associated with travel to Latin America. Eleven of these were related to crabs brought back to the USA for consumption. By August 1992, 96 cases (with one death) had been reported, and all but one of them were associated with travel; 75 were in passengers on the Argentina–Los Angeles flight mentioned earlier (*437,438*). Fourteen cases were in other travelers to Latin America and 6 were related to travel to Asia. Seventeen cases occurred in persons who were visiting relatives and 2 were in Latin American residents visiting the USA.

Two cases of non-O1 *V. cholerae* enterocolitis were reported in residents of Quebec returning from the Dominican Republic (*440*). One man had been previously healthy; the other was immunocompromised. No source was implicated in either case, although the second patient reported eating cooked scampi that had an "unusual" taste.

The risk of *Vibrio* illness was estimated in adult residents of Florida who eat raw oysters (*441*). During 1981–1988, 333 cases of *Vibrio* illness were bacteriologically confirmed in this population; 197 patients (59%) had eaten raw oysters the week before they became ill. Of these 197, 38 had a liver disease, 13 had had gastric surgery, and 15 were diabetic. A population-based incidence rate was calculated for persons with these underlying conditions. The estimated age-standardized annual incidence of *Vibrio* illness per million was 95.4 for persons with liver disease who ate raw oysters, 9.2 for raw-oyster eaters without liver disease, and 2.2 for those who did not eat raw oysters. The incidence of *Vibrio* septicemia was 82.8 for persons with liver disease and 2.0 for persons without liver disease who ate raw oysters, compared with 0.4 for persons who did not eat raw oysters. Persons with previous gastric surgery had a moderately increased risk for *Vibrio* illness, but diabetes mellitus was not a significant risk factor. The greatest number of cases, 1981–1988, were caused by *V. cholerae* non-O1, *V. vulnificus*, and *V. parahaemolyticus*. *Vibrio hollisae* and *V. mimicus* each caused >15 cases of illness. Cases of gastroenteritis or septicemia were also attributed to *V. fluvialis, V. alginolyticus,* and *V. cholerae* O1.

An outbreak of cholera near Tokyo in 1991 was traced to a shipment of clams from Korea (*442*). About 20 cases were confirmed during the last week of August and the first week of September.

OCCURRENCE, GROWTH, AND IDENTIFICATION. The pandemic strain of *V. cholerae* serotype Inaba, biotype El Tor, was found in U.S. Gulf Coast samples for the first time in oysters and fish intestines collected on July 2, 1991 (*443*). An intensive sampling program was then undertaken. Three additional contaminated samples of oysters from Mobile Bay were found. All were toxigenic in DNA hybridization, ELISA, and CHO cell assays. They were indistinguishable from each other and different from the so-called Gulf Coast strain. They resembled Latin American epidemic strains by serotype, biotype, phage type, and multilocus enzyme electrophoresis type and in several genomic tests. This strain has not been implicated in cases of cholera associated with eating seafood from the U.S. Gulf Coast and whether it has established an ecological niche on the Gulf Coast has not been established, but its

appearance is of concern because of its demonstrated ability to cause widespread epidemic disease. Cargo ships are a likely source of the organism (*444*). Samples of ballast water, bilge water, and sewage from holding tanks were collected from 14 cargo ships docking at three ports in Alabama and Mississippi. Toxigenic *V. cholerae* O1 of the Latin American epidemic strain was recovered from samples from three ships whose last ports of call had been in Brazil, Colombia, and Chile. Routine discharge of ballast tanks or illegal discharge from holding tanks could thus contaminate the port. These findings illustrate the potential for global dissemination of pathogens by maritime activities.

The prevalence of the cholera toxin (CT) gene was determined in *V. cholerae* O1 isolates from food, humans, and the environment in Japan (*445*). All 225 isolates from natural waters were negative, but all 10 isolates from airplane toilets, septic tanks, rivers, and estuaries implicated in cholera cases were positive. Of 241 isolates from imported seafoods, 64 were positive for the CT gene, as were 43 of 45 strains from domestic cholera cases and 119 of 127 strains from imported cholera cases. The authors postulated that CT gene–positive strains were imported through seafoods and by travelers. Although sporadic cholera cases probably contaminated the surrounding environment, CT gene–positive strains may not have been able to persist in natural waters. Gene-positive strains were also positive for CT production, and the κ phage type was strongly correlated with the CT gene. The importance of CT gene–negative *V. cholerae* O1 in the environment is not known, but isolation of gene-negative strains from 5 travelers with mild diarrhea suggests the need to study the enterotoxigenicity of these organisms.

The first report was made of toxigenic *V. cholerae* non-O1 in farm animals in the Netherlands (*446*). Three goats from the same dairy herd died with no clinical signs of disease. Post-mortem examination of one of them yielded a diagnosis of enterotoxicosis, and a verotoxin-producing strain of *V. cholerae* non-O1 was isolated from the small intestine. Whether this organism was responsible for the pathologic findings could not be determined because *Clostridium perfringens* was also isolated.

No environmental source of infection was found. The authors posed questions regarding the prevalence and pathogenicity of *V. cholerae* non-O1 in farm animals, especially in areas with a rich waterfowl population.

In a survey of *V. cholerae* non-O1 in the aquatic environment of Hiroshima, 68% of 72 water samples and 36% of sediment samples were positive (*447*). The organism was most prevalent in summer, but its frequency of isolation was independent of salinity, pH, and other marine vibrios. All isolates were hemolytic on sheep blood agar and 60 of 102 were toxic to CHO cells. No isolate was capable of producing detectable cholera-like enterotoxin.

Because questions remain about the aquatic reservoir of *V. cholerae*, the potential for survival of the organism in association with amoebic trophozoites and within amoebic cysts was examined (*448*). Six clinical and environmental strains of *V. cholerae* were tested in laboratory microcosms preinoculated with trophozoites of *Naegleria gruberi* or *Acanthamoeba polyphaga*. All six strains survived with both species of amoeba; in most cocultures, the viable count of vibrios after 24 h was greater than in the original inoculum, whereas control *Vibrio* cultures showed a decrease in viable count. One of two strains tested for survival in cysts could be isolated from *N. gruberi* but not from *A. polyphaga* after encystment. The authors postulated that *V. cholerae* has an intracellular amoebal habitat. This would not require an invasive capacity because internalization would be effected by the amoebas.

Because the Peruvian Ministry of Health recommends that all drinking water be boiled as a cholera-control strategy, the minimum boiling time to ensure inactivation of *V. cholerae* was determined (*449*). Three strains of *V. cholerae* O1 Inaba, El Tor (a Peruvian epidemic strain, a nonhemolytic Gulf Coast strain, and an ATCC strain) were tested. Turbid suspensions of all three were totally inactivated by boiling for 30 s at 99.5°C. The thermal death points (minimum temperature to totally inactivate the organism in 10 min) were also measured in autoclaved dechlorinated tap water. These ranged between 60 and 62°C for the three strains. The authors conclude that even under turbid conditions

and at high altitudes where water boils at lower temperatures, holding at a rolling boil for 3 min would be more than adequate to ensure safety.

The sensitivity of two strains of *V. cholerae* O1 El Tor to disinfectants used in food processing, kitchens, and personal hygiene was compared with the sensitivity of a test strain of *E. coli* (*450*). In suspension, both *Vibrio* strains were slightly more sensitive than *E. coli*. Vibrios died rapidly during the initial drying phase in a hard-surface disinfectant test. The authors concluded that disinfectants that control the risks from pathogenic *Enterobacteriaceae* would also be effective for *V. cholerae*.

A selected antibody enzyme immunoassay for *Vibrio cholerae* O1 was developed and tested for sensitivity and specificity (*451*). It showed low cross-reactivity with other microorganisms, including *V. parahaemolyticus*. The detection limit was 4500 cells for all 13 strains examined. The method was used to measure growth of an El Tor strain in milk and solid foods cultured for 24 h. When mixed cultures of *E. coli* and *V. cholerae* were inoculated into food samples, growth of *E. coli* did not interfere with the assay.

Salles and Momen have defined a zymovar as strains or isolates possessing the same profile of enzyme variants and employed multilocus enzyme electrophoresis in the zymovar analysis of 260 *V. cholerae* strains (*452*). Using 13 structural loci, these strains and 3 *V. mimicus* reference strains were grouped into 73 zymovars. Fifty zymovars contained a single strain, and 12 contained 2; only 2 contained more than 4. Two findings illustrated the potential importance of this type of analysis: two strains from the USA, one CT$^+$ and the other CT$^-$, belonged to the same zymovar, and two strains were found in some supposedly pure collection cultures.

A dipstick ELISA was described for detecting *V. cholerae* O1 in oyster meat homogenate (*453*). Organisms were captured on antibody-coated membrane pads and detected using MAbs reactive with the O1 serovar–specific antigen A. Both Inaba and Ogawa O1 serovars were detected at concentrations of ~10^6 cfu per milliliter of enrichment broth. When alkaline peptone broth was seeded with 100 cells the organism was detected after a

6-h incubation, whereas other vibrios produced negative results after an 18-h incubation when seeded at levels as high as 10^8 cfu/mL. As few as 100 *V. cholerae* O1 cells per gram of oyster meat homogenate could be detected after a 30-min exposure in a 3-tube, 3-dilution MPN test.

Naka et al. reported a method for purifying the hemagglutinin/protease of *V. cholerae* non-O1 that is considerably simpler than their previously reported method (*454*). The new method employed immunoaffinity column chromatography using an MAb against the target protein. The major component of the hemagglutinin/protease purified by this method was a molecule of 34 kDa; there was a small amount of a 32-kDa component. Immunologically, the material was identical to the 32-kDa material isolated by the older method, suggesting that the larger molecule is an isoform or preform of the 32-kDa protein.

Canadian investigators reported that a bioassay for CT and heat-labile toxin from *E. coli* using human colonic adenocarcinoma HT29 cells could detect much lower concentrations of toxin than the CHO-cell assay (*455*). Both tests revealed the presence of toxin after 24–36 h of incubation; with HT29 cells the response became more obvious as incubation was continued, whereas the CHO-cell test became less distinctive after 4 days as cell monolayers became more confluent. The formation of large vacuoles in the HT29 cells appeared to depend on the ADP-ribosyltransferase subunit (B subunit) of the toxins.

A new bead ELISA consistently detected 40 pg/mL of CT under optimal buffer and pH conditions (*456*). No constituents of commonly used culture media interfered with the assay's performance. The bead ELISA was evaluated against the standard reversed passive latex agglutination test using 239 CT$^+$ and CT$^-$ strains of *V. cholerae* O1 of classical and El Tor biotypes. Both assays were highly specific, but the bead ELISA was more sensitive. The bead ELISA could be made quantitative by comparison with a standard curve.

Japanese investigators used a DNA probe for the CT A-chain gene to detect toxigenic *V. cholerae* in a rectal swab culture (*457*). The subject was a man who complained of diarrhea at the Osaka airport quarantine station upon his return from a 10-week visit to Indonesia. The authors believe this to be the first report of using such a probe in the clinical diagnostic laboratory.

A PCR for detecting the cholera enterotoxin (*ctx*) operon of *V. cholerae* was reported (*458*). Results for 47 *V. cholerae* O1 strains, 17 other *Vibrio* strains, and 5 *E. coli* LT$^+$ strains were identical with the PCR and a DNA colony hybridization test. The PCR could detect 1 pg of chromosomal DNA or three viable cells in a broth culture. It could also directly detect the *ctx* operon in stool samples from cholera patients with acute diarrhea.

Investigators in India reported finding widespread *V. cholerae* resistance to 2,4-diamino-6,7-diisopropylpteridine (*459*). This was always associated with resistance to multiple antimicrobial agents and nearly always linked to cotrimoxazole resistance. Furthermore, it occurred in Ogawa, Inaba, and non-O1 strains. The taxonomic implications of this were discussed.

Vibriophage VcA-3 was evaluated as an epidemic strain marker for the U.S. Gulf Coast *V. cholerae* O1 clone (*460*). Toxigenic and nontoxigenic U.S. and foreign strains were tested for phage production and the presence of phage and CT genes. Southern blot analysis of a *Hind*III chromosomal digest using the VcA-3 probe always separated toxigenic U.S. strains from foreign isolates and frequently separated them from nontoxigenic U.S. isolates. The phage production and colony hybridization assays had the same sensitivity as the Southern blot but were less specific.

VIRULENCE AND MOLECULAR STUDIES. The pathogenicity of wild-type and nonmotile mutant strains of *V. cholerae* El Tor, Inaba, and classical, Ogawa, was assessed in three animal models (*461*). Flagellate and aflagellate mutants were included. Classical wild-type and mutant strains did not differ in CT production either in vivo or in vitro; but in vivo, mutant El Tor strains produced less toxin than the wild type. In the animal models, however, motile strains were clearly more pathogenic than nonmotile, and nonmotile flagellate strains were more virulent than aflagellate, demonstrating a role for flagellar structures.

Several strains of *V. cholerae* El Tor isolated in India from patients with diarrhea showed atypical toxin production (*462*). In atypical strains, toxin production was enhanced only with anaerobic culture at 37°C, conditions simulating the intestinal environment. However, toxin did not remain membrane-bound under either aerobic or anaerobic conditions, indicating that toxin release is not the trigger for enhanced CT production as it is thought to be in anaerobically grown typical strains.

A brief news report in *Science* summarized recent progress and views on structure–function relationships in cholera toxin (*463*). Similarities and differences between CT and the *E. coli* LT toxin have also been established. These and other enterotoxins contain a B subunit that anchors itself to the target cell and effects entry of a second, enzymatic, A subunit into the cell. The A subunit turns on regulatory G proteins, initiating a series of events that poison the cell. Although CT and LT are very similar (80%), the 20% difference explains why CT can kill while LT merely makes the victim sick. The normal cell-surface receptor for the B subunit is ganglioside G_{M1} (*464*). When the oligosaccharide of ganglioside G_{M1} was attached to G_{M1}-deficient cells, the cells still bound large amounts of CT but did not accumulate cAMP. Treatment with chloroquine permitted the typical cAMP response. When the G_{M1} oligosaccharide was linked to human transferrin the molecule bound to the transferrin receptor on HeLa cells, again facilitating CT binding without cAMP accumulation—and again, chloroquine made these cells responsive to the toxin. These and other results led the authors to conclude that the pathway by which the A chain enters the cell and is processed differs according to whether the receptor is the oligosaccharide of G_{M1} in the presence of chloroquine or the natural G_{M1}.

The toxin-coregulated pilus (TCP) is positively regulated with CT and several outer membrane proteins by the transmembrane protein ToxR. TCP is important for intestinal colonization by *V. cholerae* O1 in humans. Immunoblotting and ELISA using MAbs and polyclonal antisera against TCP from classical vibrios revealed biotype-related epitope differences in TCP (*465*). TCP of classical strains has an epitope in the TcpA subunit that is

missing in El Tor, and a second epitope that is more strongly expressed. At the same time, there was evidence of major shared epitopes between classical and El Tor TcpA. These findings may provide clues to why El Tor vibrios express TCP poorly under most conditions.

Besides activating the promoter of the CT operon, ToxR also appears to control transcription of *toxT*, whose product activates several virulence genes under ToxR control (*466*). The *V. cholerae* *toxT* gene was cloned and its product, like ToxR, activated the *ctx* promoter in *E. coli*. It also activated *tcpA*, *tcpI*, *aldA*, and *tagA*, other members of the ToxR regulon, whereas ToxR did not. ToxT was able to partially suppress the ToxR⁻ phenotype. The level of toxT mRNA was greatly reduced in a *toxR* mutant of *V. cholerae*, and conditions reducing the expression of the ToxR regulon also reduced synthesis of toxT mRNA. For these reasons the authors concluded that ToxR controls transcription of *toxT*, which activates the genes listed above. In a short review, DiRita discussed this regulatory pathway further (*467*).

A new toxin produced by *V. cholerae* was discovered in non-CT-producing strains. It has been characterized (*468*) and its gene has been identified and cloned (*469*). The toxin increases the permeability of the small intestinal mucosa by affecting the structure of the intercellular tight junction and has been named ZOT, for zonula occludens toxin. Toxin activity is reversible, heat-labile, and sensitive to protease digestion. The toxin is found in culture supernatant fractions containing molecules 10–30 kDa in size. The *zot* gene consists of a 1.3-kilobase open reading frame with the potential to encode a 44.8-kDa polypeptide. It is located immediately upstream of the *ctx* operon that encodes CT. The authors postulated that this toxin accounts for the mild diarrhea caused by some CT-negative *V. cholerae* strains.

Moss and Vaughan reviewed CT- and LT-catalyzed ADP-ribosylation of G proteins, with emphasis on the role of a family of ADP-ribosylation factors (ARFs) (*470*). In vitro, in the presence of GTP, ARFs serve as allosteric activators of the toxin. Six mammalian ARF genes have been identified. They encode highly conserved proteins of 175–181 amino acids containing consensus domains responsible for guanine nucleotide binding. Sequence differences occur near the N-terminus and in the C-terminus half of the molecule. The ARFs have been immunologically localized to the Golgi apparatus, which is consistent with a postulated role in regulating the movement of newly synthesized proteins from the endoplasmic reticulum through the Golgi system to their destination. The reviewers speculated on other possible functions of the multiple yet very similar ARFs.

The *V. cholerae* neuraminidase gene (*nanH*) was cloned and sequenced and the role of neuraminidase in CT function was examined using culture filtrates from neuraminidase-positive and -negative strains of *V. cholerae* (*471*). Mouse fibroblasts exposed to positive filtrates bound 5–8 times as much CT as those exposed to negative filtrates. When enzyme-positive and -negative strains were inoculated into suckling mice, some difference in fluid accumulation was seen, but only at a high inoculum level (10^9 cfu) using nonfasted mice. The authors concluded that neuraminidase plays a subtle but significant role in the binding and uptake of CT under some conditions.

A further correlation of function with structure between the sequence-related cholera and pertussis toxin A subunits was demonstrated (*472*). In pertussis toxin, substitution of lysine for arginine at position 9 virtually abolishes ADP-ribosylation activity. Burnette et al. showed that a similar substitution of lysine for arginine at the equivalent 7-position of CT also eliminates catalytic activity of CT-A.

Site-directed mutagenesis was used to analyze the structure–function relationships of CT-B (*473*). Substitution of negatively charged or large hydrophobic residues for glycine-33 or charged residues for tryptophan-88 decreased binding of CT-B to its receptor and abolished toxicity. Substituting lysine or arginine for glycine-33 did not affect immunoreactivity or G_{M1}-binding activity, but lysine abolished and arginine reduced holotoxin activity. Substituting glutamate or aspartate for arginine-35 interfered with holotoxin formation, but no substitution at lysine-34 or arginine-35 affected binding to G_{M1}. The cysteine residues at positions 9 and 86

and tryptophan-88 were necessary to establish or maintain the native conformation of CT-B or to protect it from rapid degradation in vivo. The antigenicity of CT-B was further studied by mapping epitopic regions using polyclonal rabbit antisera and sera from convalescent cholera patients (*474*). Many epitopic regions were found, including a strongly reactive serine–glutamine–histidine–isoleucine sequence in the highly conserved region comprising residues 55–58. The nucleotide sequence of the CT operon, including promoter and terminating regions, was determined, verifying the previously published CT-B amino acid sequence (*475*). Differences at residues 18, 47, and 54 were found in three classical Ogawa and three El Tor strains.

Either the cholera holotoxin or its B chain induced formation of ionic channels in planar bilayer lipid membranes, but the A chain did not (*476*). The B subunit of the CT-B ionic channel measured 2.1 ± 0.2 nm and the channels exhibited voltage-dependent activity. The authors postulated that induction of ionic channels at low pH is essential for CT activity and that these channels facilitate entry of the A subunit into the cell.

The gene responsible for the Ogawa serotype of *V. cholerae* O1 has been identified and sequenced (*477*). It encodes a protein of 27 kDa. A plasmid carrying this gene converted serotype specificity from Inaba to Ogawa when introduced into *E. coli* cells harboring a *V. cholerae* genomic DNA fragment that expressed the O1 antigen of the Inaba serotype.

What determines the virulence of non-O1 *V. cholerae* is poorly understood, although colony morphology is frequently related to virulence. Phase variation between two colony morphologies may occur as virulence factors are turned on and off. Studies of one such virulence factor, a polysaccharide capsule, were reported (*478*). An encapsulated opaque form of strain NRT36S, a virulent clinical isolate, was protected from the bactericidal activity of serum, whereas a translucent variant was readily killed. The encapsulated variant also had increased virulence in mice. The authors thus showed that non-O1 *V. cholerae* can have a polysaccharide capsule, which may afford protection from host defenses and contribute to the ability of virulent strains to cause septicemia in susceptible hosts. Further studies with this strain using a modified removable intestinal tie adult rabbit diarrhea model provided clues to the pathophysiologic mechanisms underlying infection by non-O1 *V. cholerae* (*479*). Histologic examination showed dose-dependent necrosis of the colonic luminal epithelium and mild inflammatory cell infiltration in the adjacent lamina propria. High doses caused severe necrotizing colitis and enteritis followed by bacteremia and death. Invasion of the intestinal luminal epithelium was demonstrated by light and electron microscopy. Non-O1 strains that did not produce diarrhea in volunteers did not cause diarrhea or intestinal pathology in the rabbit model.

Another explanation has been proposed for the residual diarrhetic activity of some CT-negative strains of *V. cholerae* (*480*; see reference *468*). Classical isolates of *V. cholerae* have an 11-base-pair deletion in the structural gene for the El Tor hemolysin, leading to production of a truncated, nonhemolytic 27-kDa product. Studies with the truncated product suggested that the hemolytic domain of the El Tor hemolysin is at the C-terminus and that the N-terminus, which is conserved in classical strains, has enterotoxic activity. Investigation of transcription of the El Tor strain O17 *hlyA*, which encodes the hemolysin, showed that the transcript has a 430-nucleotide 5' untranslated region (UTR) preceding the coding sequence (*481*). This UTR may play a role in mRNA stability. After the 5' end of the transcript was located the authors searched for a promoter in that region. This led to identification of a previously undescribed regulatory locus, *hlyU*. How *hlyU* controls *hlyA* expression and perhaps affects expression of virulence factors is under investigation.

The structural gene *hap* for the extracellular hemagglutinin/protease of *V. cholerae* was cloned and sequenced (*482*). It contained a 1827-base-pair open reading frame potentially encoding a 609–amino acid polypeptide. The 46.7-kDa hemagglutinin/protease, which contains 414 amino acids, is processed to the 32-kDa form that is usually isolated. A hemagglutinin/protease-negative strain, HAP-1, was produced and the cloned fragment containing *hap* was shown to complement the

mutant strain. HAP-1 was then used to examine the role of hemagglutinin/protease in the virulence of *V. cholerae* (*483*). The mutants exhibited reversible variation in colony morphology similar to that of the parental strain; but unlike the parental strain, HAP-1 mutants were fully virulent in infant rabbits regardless of colony morphology. Thus the hemagglutinin/protease is not a major virulence factor for infant rabbits and is not responsible for the variation in colony morphology. From studies using cultured human intestinal cells the authors postulated, instead, that it is responsible for detachment of the vibrios from the cultured cells by digestion of several putative receptors for *V. cholerae* adhesins.

Vibrio parahaemolyticus

Vibrio parahaemolyticus can be divided into strains that hemolyze a high-salt blood agar medium (Kanagawa-positive strains) and strains that do not (Kanagawa-negative). The former are generally isolated from patients, whereas the latter are usually environmental. Investigators have found a difference in ability of Kanagawa-positive and -negative strains to adhere to rabbit intestinal cells in vitro (*484*). Ten positive clinical strains showed adherence ranging from 22 to 39%, whereas 10 negative environmental strains exhibited <1–10% adherence. All strains showed similar hydrophobicity, and neither hemolysin nor antihemolysin antiserum pretreatment influenced the adhesive capacity of any strain. The glycoprotein fetuin strongly inhibited adhesion; D-mannose and D-glucose were less effective; and *N*-acetyl glucosamine, *N*-acetyl galactosamine, and L-fucose had no effect. Thus, although Kanagawa-positive and -negative strains clearly differed in their adherence ability, the basis for this difference was not found.

Other investigators demonstrated a role for pili in colonization of the rabbit intestine by *V. parahaemolyticus* Na2, a Kanagawa-positive strain (*485*). Isolated pili adhered to the intestinal epithelium. The effect was blocked by treating the organisms with anti-pilus antibody.

Nearly half of Kanagawa-negative *V. parahaemolyticus* isolates from patients with diarrhea produce a hemolysin similar to but distinct from the thermostable direct hemolysin of Kanagawa-positive strains (*486*). To learn whether this hemolysin could be involved in seafoodborne diarrhea, four strains of *V. parahaemolyticus* isolated from frozen fish were tested for hemolysin production, using a clinical isolate as a positive control. All four environmental strains produced hemolysin identical to that of the clinical strain in hemolytic activity, antigenicity, reactivity in the rabbit ileal loop test, and N-terminal amino acid sequence. The authors concluded that this hemolysin is an important virulence factor.

The thermostable direct hemolysin is coded by two copies of the *tdh* gene, *tdh*1 and *tdh*2. By constructing a *tdh*2-deficient isogenic mutant of a Kanagawa-positive *V. parahaemolyticus* strain, Nishibuchi et al. showed that *tdh*1 contributes little to the Kanagawa phenomenon on blood agar (*487*). However, the mutant did synthesize hemolysin in broth medium, accounting for 0.5–9.4% of the total extracellular thermostable direct hemolysin produced by this strain. When four *tdh* genes (*tdh*1 and *tdh*2 from a hemolytic strain, *tdh*3 and *tdh*4 from a nonhemolytic strain) were cloned and analyzed, small differences in nucleotide sequences were found (*488*). The four gene products differed in electrophoretic mobilities under nondenaturing conditions, although all hemolyzed various animal erythrocytes, stimulated vascular permeability in the rabbit skin, and were lethal to mice. They were antigenically identical. The slight differences in potency were probably due to minor structural or charge differences, but overall the four genes have evolved to maintain a fundamental molecular structure and biological activity.

Japanese investigators isolated and characterized a new lecithin-dependent hemolysin produced by *V. parahaemolyticus* (*489*). On the basis of its catalytic activity the hemolysin should be classified as a phospholipase B. Phospholipase B, however, is usually not hemolytic because lysolecithin does not accumulate to damage erythrocyte membranes. The new hemolysin converted lysolecithin to glycerophosphocholine only slowly, permitting disruption of erythrocytes. The authors designated the new hemolysin as a phospholipase A_2/lysophospholipase.

Vibrio vulnificus

A serosurvey was conducted among 267 healthy volunteers living near the Chesapeake Bay to determine the prevalence of antibodies to *Vibrio* spp. (*490*). Groups with different levels of exposure to shellfish were compared: shellfish industry workers, people who attended a local seafood festival, and Seventh-Day Adventists (who traditionally do not eat shellfish). Although antibody response to *V. cholerae* was surprisingly high—up to 22% seropositive with a *V. cholerae* O1 Inaba vibriocidal assay and 14% with an ELISA for CT—there were no significant differences between groups. Shellfish industry workers did, however, have a significantly elevated antibody response to the unencapsulated phase variant of *V. vulnificus*, suggesting that *V. vulnificus* infection is relatively common among persons with high levels of exposure to shellfish.

To define the ecological relationship of *V. vulnificus* with the Gulf Coast oyster *Crassostrea virginica* and test the hypothesis that natural populations of the organism persist in the oyster's microbial flora, weathering traditional methods of purification, experiments were conducted in model depuration systems (*491*). Treatment consisted of UV light and filtration (0.2 μm pore size). *Vibrio vulnificus* was counted in the depuration water, oyster shell biofilms, oyster meat homogenates, and specific tissue homogenates (hemolymph, digestive region, gills, mantle, and adductor muscle). At 23°C, *V. vulnificus* counts increased—especially in the hemolymph, adductor muscle, and mantle. Counts in the depuration water remained high throughout the process, indicating that the organism was being released into the seawater faster than it was being killed. At 15°C the organism was not detected in the seawater and its multiplication in oyster tissues was inhibited. These results indicated that depuration and wet-storage operating conditions need reevaluation.

Persons with chronic iron overload are at increased risk of *V. vulnificus* infection. In in vitro tests, the organism was killed by normal human blood but grew rapidly in blood from patients with hemochromatosis (*492*). It also grew in normal blood if the saturation of the transferrin was increased or if hematin was added. These results are consistent with others suggesting that *V. vulnificus* requires a supply of readily available iron for growth in living tissue, and the increased availability of iron in persons with chronic iron overload enhances their susceptibility to *V. vulnificus* infection.

Oliver et al. studied 10 factors that might affect the nonculturable response of *V. vulnificus* (*493*). Cells taken from the stationary phase of growth required twice as long as log-phase cells to become nonculturable. The nonculturable response appeared related to the starvation response: 24 h of starvation at room temperature eliminated the nonculturable response upon subsequent incubation at 5°C. The authors postulated that synthesis of starvation proteins represses the viable-but-nonculturable program displayed during low-temperature incubation. Other manipulations of the medium, inoculum size, chill rate, and test strain had no significant effect on the nonculturable response. The ecological implications of these observations were discussed. The same research group also investigated resuscitation of *V. vulnificus* from the viable but nonculturable state (*494*). Total cell counts were monitored throughout the experiments. The authors were able to fully resuscitate nonculturable cells without adding nutrient, simply by manipulating the temperature. Nonculturable cells were cocci ~1.0 μm in diameter. Upon resuscitation they became large rods, with mid-log-phase cells 3.0 μm long. By four days after full resuscitation cells had decreased in size to 1.5 × 0.7 μm. Cells could undergo two cycles of nonculturability and subsequent resuscitation without change in total cell count; additional cycles were not investigated. By adding chloramphenicol and ampicillin to the medium, the authors showed that protein and peptidoglycan synthesis occurred at all stages of resuscitation.

Colistin–polymyxin B–cellobiose agar was evaluated for isolating *V. vulnificus* from naturally contaminated shellfish (*495*). It proved superior to SDS–polymyxin B–sucrose agar and thiosulfate–citrate–bile salts–sucrose agar in selecting for this species and differentiating it from other vibrios, as indicated by phenotypic examination and tests with

a gene probe and MAb specific for *V. vulnificus*. The former medium lacked selectivity for *V. vulnificus*, whereas the latter could not differentiate *V. vulnificus* from other sucrose-negative vibrios. Studies with artificially contaminated oysters also showed colistin–polymyxin B–cellobiose agar to be preferable to SDS–polymyxin B–sucrose agar as an isolation medium (*496*). Five enrichment broths recovered the organism in the order alkaline peptone water > marine broth > Horie's broth > Monsur's broth > glucose–salt–teepol. Based on these results, alkaline peptone water enrichment broth and colistin–polymyxin B–cellobiose isolation agar are the most efficient combination for recovery of *V. vulnificus* from oysters.

A PCR was developed to detect *V. vulnificus* DNA, eliminating the problem of nonculturability (*497*). The PCR primers flanked a 340-base-pair sequence within the hemolysin gene. As little as 72 pg of DNA from culturable cells and 31 ng from nonculturable cells could be detected. From the time of DNA extraction the procedure required <8 h. Possible reasons for the greater difficulty of amplifying DNA from nonculturable cells were discussed.

A serotyping scheme for *V. vulnificus* based on detection of LPS antigens was developed (*498*). MAbs identified 5 LPS serovars of *V. vulnificus* and one serovar each for *V. damsela* and *V. hollisae*. No cross-reactions were observed between *V. vulnificus* and *V. hollisae* or *V. damsela*.

Other vibrios

Strains of *V. mimicus*, *V. cholerae* O1, and *V. cholerae* non-O1 isolated from patients with diarrhea were evaluated for production of pili and cell-associated hemagglutinin and for adherence to formalin-fixed human and rabbit intestinal mucosa (*499*). Piliation and hemagglutinin production were comparable in the three organisms, but *V. mimicus* showed less ability to adhere to intestinal mucosa. This difference in adherence may help explain the lower pathogenicity of *V. mimicus*.

From a strain of *V. mimicus* isolated from a patient with traveller's diarrhea, investigators purified and characterized a hemolysin similar to the thermostable direct hemolysin of *V. parahaemo-*

lyticus (500). The M_r of the subunit was ~22,000, the isoelectric point was about pH 4.9, and hemolytic activity was stable upon heating at 100°C for 10 min. Hemolytic activity was similar to that of the *V. parahaemolyticus* hemolysin and immunological cross-reactivity was demonstrated between the two.

To learn whether environmental vibrios have the potential to cause diarrheal disease and serve as reservoirs of virulence factors, fresh-water *Vibrio* isolates were screened for production of hemolysin, cytotoxin, and enterotoxins *(501)*. Of 132 qualitatively hemolytic strains, 55% also showed hemolytic activity by a quantitative method. Seventeen strains of non-O1 *V. cholerae*, 2 strains of *V. fluvialis*, and 1 strain of *V. mimicus* produced >10² hemolytic units of hemolysin. About 70% of the hemolytic strains were either cytotoxic or cytotonic to RK-13 cells. Non-O1 *V. cholerae* and *V. mimicus* were predominantly cytotoxic, whereas *V. fluvialis* and other vibrios were cytotonic. The correlation between cytotoxin titers and hemolytic activity depended on the species of *Vibrio*. A new procedure for quantifying cytotoxic activity was described. The factor causing elongation in CHO cells did not correlate well with fluid accumulation in the conventional suckling mouse assay. The authors concluded that production of virulence factors by fresh-water environmental vibrios is of significance to mariculture in Japan.

Vibrio furnissii has been isolated from humans with diarrhea, and environmental isolates have caused accumulation of fluid in an animal model. With this in mind, a study was undertaken to determine the enterotoxicity of 14 strains isolated from ulcerated areas of eels *(502)*. All strains gave negative reactions in initial ileal loop tests but caused fluid accumulation after serial passage in ileal loops. Some strains caused fluid accumulation comparable to that with a toxigenic strain of *V. cholerae*. Most culture filtrates caused induration and increased vascular permeability in rabbit skin, but the activity was heat-labile. Some culture filtrates caused skin necrosis in addition to induration and increased vascular permeability; others caused only the necrotic reaction, suggesting that the necrotic factor is different from the enterotoxin. All culture filtrates

had high hemolytic indexes, indicating production of an extracellular hemolysin. The authors postulated that the ratio of toxigenic to nontoxigenic organisms is reduced under unfavorable conditions but enhanced by passage through a susceptible host. Since these toxigenic vibrios probably circulate through humans, animals, and the environment, they constitute a public health hazard.

Vibrio metschnikovii is another potentially pathogenic marine vibrio, but information on its occurrence in food and human disease is scanty. A survey of the prevalence of *V. metschnikovii* in a wide variety of finfish and shellfish purchased at retail markets found widespread contamination *(503)*. Overall, 26 of 59 fish samples, 18 of 121 shellfish samples, and 1 of 6 surimi samples contained the organism. Although at present there is no evidence that this organism is a serious health hazard related to seafood consumption, it is appropriate to document its occurrence in seafood and seafood products.

Another pathogenic vibrio, *V. alginolyticus*, was isolated from blood of a leukemic patient who had eaten oysters *(504)*. This infection was unusual in occurring during winter and in having a seafood-related digestive origin. (The organism is more commonly implicated in wound and ear infections after exposure to seawater.) This case illustrates the risk to immunocompromised patients of eating raw seafood even in winter.

The research group of Nishibuchi has analyzed a *V. hollisae* gene similar to the *tdh* genes of *V. parahaemolyticus (505)*. It contained a 567-base-pair open reading frame with 93.3–95.3% homology to the *tdh* genes of *V. parahaemolyticus, V. cholerae* non-O1, and *V. mimicus* that encode thermostable direct hemolysin or similar hemolysins. Nucleotide sequence analysis suggested that the *V. hollisae*-related *tdh* genes diverged from a common ancestral gene, that this was closely associated with the evolutionary divergence of *V. hollisae* from other vibrios, and that variation in the gene exists among strains of *V. hollisae*. Despite minor strain-to-strain variation, however, the *V. hollisae* gene is highly conserved, suggesting the importance of its product in this species. Another report from Nishibuchi's group provided evidence for insertion sequence–mediated spread of *tdh* among *Vibrio* spp. (*506*). All seven *tdh* genes cloned from *V. parahaemolyticus, V. mimicus*, and non-O1 *V. cholerae* were flanked by insertion sequence–like elements or related sequences derived from genetic rearrangements of insertion sequences. Several features of these regions, and similarities in their nucleotide sequences, suggest that they were derived from a common ancestral sequence. The authors discussed the possible mode of insertion sequence–mediated spread of the *tdh* gene from an evolutionary perspective.

AEROMONAS

Aeromonads remain puzzling "potential" food pathogens, widespread in food and water and capable of producing a variety of virulence factors yet difficult to incriminate in cases of foodborne illness. A multiauthor review discussed the taxonomy, isolation and identification, and virulence factors of aeromonads (*507*). Clinical aspects of *Aeromonas*-associated diarrhea, the enteropathogenicity of *Aeromonas caviae* in infants, *Aeromonas* and *Plesiomonas* infections in immunocompromised patients, and environmental studies of aeromonads were summarized. Janda also reviewed the taxonomy and pathogenicity of *Aeromonas* and infectious syndromes associated with this genus (*508*). Despite rapid advances in aeromonad research, no satisfactory animal model of *Aeromonas*-associated diarrhea exists and details of the polygenic virulence factors in these organisms and the complex interactions of bacterial and host factors are not understood. Until recently the motile aeromonads were considered food-spoilage organisms, but they are now respected as potential food-poisoning organisms (*509*). Bergann summarized the differential identification of motile aeromonads and the pathogenesis and clinical symptoms of *Aeromonas*-related enteritis. He documented the widespread occurrence of *Aeromonas* spp. in meat and poultry products and summarized conditions under which they grow, concluding that they should receive the same attention as other potential food pathogens.

A survey of 396 samples of ready-to-eat meat and poultry products, shellfish and finfish products, raw meat products, salads, and baked goods in New Zealand showed the highest incidence of motile aeromonads in shellfish (66%) (*510*). Vegetable products, luncheon meat, salami, paté, and poultry products had a very low incidence, and no motile aeromonads were found in 13 baked confectionery items, some of which contained whipped cream. More than 20% of red meat, sausage, and finfish products contained motile aeromonads. Most isolates were *A. hydrophila; A. caviae, A. sobria,* and atypical strains were also found. Similar results were obtained in a survey of foods in Uppsala, Sweden (*511*). Ten of 24 food samples contained *A. hydrophila* or *A. sobria. Aeromonas* was isolated from poultry, fish, beef, and pork but not from vegetables or raw milk. The majority of these isolates produced one or more virulence factors (hemolysin, cytotoxin, cytotonic toxin, enterotoxin, or protease), indicating that *Aeromonas* should be considered in cases of foodborne infection. Tested with a series of 8 antibiotics, *A. hydrophila* showed a high rate of multiple resistance; the five *A. sobria* strains tested were resistant to 7 of 8 antibiotics and only slightly sensitive to tetracycline. *Aeromonas hydrophila* isolates from a broiler processing operation in Georgia also showed multiple antibiotic resistance (46% of 119 isolates), although 76% of these were resistant only to ampicillin and cephalothin (*512*). Sixty-four percent of the isolates were cytotoxic to Y-1 mouse adrenal tumor cells. Cytotoxin-positive isolates were recovered from all stages of sampling—from chill water and from carcasses before and after evisceration, after immersion chilling, and after carcasses were boxed, iced, and refrigerated for 48 h. Highest cytotoxicity titers were in isolates from carcasses immediately after evisceration, suggesting bird feces as an important source of contamination in broilers and broiler processing plants. However, the percentage of cytotoxic isolates recovered did not show any striking relationship to the stage of sampling.

Twenty-five strains of *A. hydrophila* isolated from healthy and diseased fresh-water fish and fresh water were grouped by cluster analysis of plasmid profiles and other characteristics, to reveal possible relationships among these parameters (*513*). Ten strains contained no plasmids. The rest contained a 20-kilobase plasmid and 4 strains harbored one or two smaller plasmids as well. Differences in biochemical and physiological characteristics were small and were not related to the plasmid profile. However, some of the differences revealed by clustering could be associated with virulence.

A brief review of *Aeromonas* species emphasized their growth at refrigeration temperatures (*514*). The presence of *A. hydrophila* in water at 4°C suggests its ability to grow in aquatic organisms and organic debris at that temperature. Many isolates from water reservoirs, rivers, and chlorinated tap water grow well at 5 ± 2°C. Clinical isolates generally do not grow well at these temperatures, but in one study 13 of 25 that did were enterotoxigenic. Similarly, food isolates of *A. hydrophila* frequently grow and compete well with other psychrotrophic bacteria at 5°C. The effects of other variables on growth in foods at refrigeration temperatures were summarized. Palumbo et al. modeled the anaerobic growth of *A. hydrophila* K144 under various conditions of temperature, pH, and NaCl and $NaNO_2$ concentration (*515*). Logarithmic and square-root quadratic and cubic predictive models were developed for the Gompertz parameters B and M and tested against the derived kinetic parameters of lag time and generation time. The logarithmic quadratic polynomial response surface model gave the best fit. Results showed that pH, salt level, and nitrite level can be manipulated to decrease the growth of *A. hydrophila* when combined with low temperature incubation under anaerobic conditions. Palumbo and Williams reported the effect of several organic acids on growth of *A. hydrophila* K144 in brain–heart infusion broth, extending the work described in reference *515* (*516*). Again, type of acid, pH, NaCl level, and temperature interacted to influence lag time and generation time. Acetic acid inhibited growth most effectively, particularly at a relatively high pH, but both acetic and lactic acids effectively controlled growth at low temperatures. In general, organic acids were more effective than inorganic acids at higher pH values. Because of the inhibitory effect of lactic acid, the authors concluded that *A. hydrophila* should not be a problem in fermented foods.

The resistance of 106 strains of motile *Aeromonas* species to a panel of antibiotics was determined (*517*). Very little antibiotic resistance was noted, except for nearly total resistance to ampicillin. *Aeromonas sobria* strains showed less resistance than strains of *A. hydrophila* and *A. caviae*. The transfer of resistance by plasmids was demonstrated. One plasmid was transferable to *E. coli* and two were transferable only between strains of the same species or genus.

A dichotomous key was developed for identifying clinical aeromonads (*518*). Aerokey II is based on 7 highly discriminatory tests: esculin hydrolysis, production of gas from glucose, production of acid from arabinose, indole production, production of acid from sucrose, the Voges–Proskauer reaction, and resistance to 30 µg of cephalothin. In a blinded trial of 60 well characterized clinical strains of *A. hydrophila*, *A. caviae*, and *A. veronii* biovar sobria, 58 (97%) were correctly identified to the species level. Aerokey II also correctly identified 18 reference strains of the proposed taxa *A. schubertii*, *A. jandaei*, *A. trota*, and *A. veronii* biovar veronii.

Ribotyping was evaluated as a tool for epidemiological investigations of *Aeromonas* species (*519*). Purified chromosomal DNA was digested with restriction enzymes *Pst* I and *Sma* I and the fragments were separated, transferred to membranes, and probed with biotinylated plasmid pKK3535 DNA. Analysis of the rDNA patterns revealed heterogeneity among unrelated clinical and environmental strains, but homology among *A. caviae* isolates from three siblings with gastroenteritis and between *A. caviae* isolates from an infant and foster mother with acute gastroenteritis. Furthermore, multiple isolates of *A. caviae* from the same patient over >3 years produced homologous rDNA patterns that remained stable after 20 subcultures. When serotyping was possible, results were consistent with rDNA analysis.

During the course of molecular studies on the aerolysin gene of *Aeromonas* a species-specific gene probe for *A. trota* was discovered (*520*). Whereas the structural gene *aer*A contains sequences that were widespread among *Aeromonas* isolates, a probe from the regulatory region *aer*C was specific for a cluster of 14 presumed atypical *A. sobria* strains (identified by numerical taxonomy techniques) that were subsequently designated as the new species *A. trota*. The authors believe that these observations demonstrate selection pressure to maintain the clonality of the new species and have implications for the evolution of pathogenic profiles in *Aeromonas* species.

Studies of 54 clinical and 93 environmental isolates of *A. hydrophila, A. sobria,* and *A. caviae* revealed widespread enterotoxicity as evaluated by fluid accumulation in rabbit ileal loops (*521*). *Aeromonas hydrophila* and *A. sobria* produced significantly more fluid than *A. caviae*, although 55–65% of *A. caviae* strains provoked a positive response. Strains that were negative or weakly positive in initial experiments became increasingly active enterotoxin producers after 1–3 passages through rabbit ileal loops. The authors concluded that all strains of these species are potentially enterotoxigenic, whether from clinical or environmental sources.

Eighty-six clinical isolates of *A. hydrophila* were evaluated for their production of a hemolysin active against rabbit erythrocytes, cytotoxin and endotoxin active in Vero cell cultures, and the cholera toxin–like factor detected by ELISA (*522*). One or more of these exotoxins were produced by 80% of enteric and 96% of nonenteric isolates. Hemolysin and cytotoxin producers dominated the nonenteric isolates, whereas enterotoxin and cholera toxin-like factor were more common in enteric isolates. Enteric isolates displayed greater variety than nonenteric isolates in their exotoxin profiles. Another study found no correlation between exotoxin production and species (*A. hydrophila, A. sobria, A. caviae*) or source of isolation (clinical or environmental) (*523*). Hemagglutination of human O-group erythrocytes was not related to exotoxin production or the source of the isolate, but was associated with species. The commonest extracellular virulence phenotype was enterotoxin-, cytotoxin-, and hemolysin-positive. Hybridization experiments showed the *Aeromonas* cytotoxin and hemolysin to be distinct from verotoxin and the thermostable direct hemolysin of *Vibrio parahaemolyticus*. One clinical strain of *A. caviae* adhered diffusely to HeLa cells. The strains tested did not fall into any discernible pattern on the basis of enzyme profiles determined by

use of the API ZYM kit. The authors concluded that the mechanism of pathogenesis in *Aeromonas* is multifactorial and it is important to develop models for assessing the importance of putative *Aeromonas* virulence factors in causing diarrhea in humans.

Because for most enteric pathogens attachment to the intestinal epithelium is a prerequisite for infection, 273 isolates of *Aeromonas* from fecal, food, and environmental samples were assayed for mannose-resistant adhesion to INT407 cells (*524*). Seventeen of 102 fecal isolates adhered at a rate of >10 bacteria per cell, whereas only 2 of 118 isolates from foods and river water adhered to the INT407 cells. Eight highly adhesive strains (20 adhering organisms per cell) were further examined to determine their mechanism of adhesion. There was no apparent association between adhesion and hydrophobicity. Fucose inhibited both adhesion and hemagglutination in 4 strains. Flexible curvilinear fimbriae were seen by electron microscopy in 2 of the 8 strains. The authors suggested that adhesion to INT407 cells may help to discriminate between fecal and environmental strains of aeromonads.

Pili of *A. sobria* Ae1 were purified, characterized, and evaluated as a possible colonization factor (*525*). They were electrophoretically and immunologically distinct from the W pili of *A. hydrophila* Ae6, although morphologically indistinguishable from them. Strain Ae1 and its purified pili adhered to human and rabbit intestine and agglutinated human and rabbit erythrocytes. Hemagglutination was inhibited by D-galactose and D-mannose but not by L-fucose. Organisms pretreated with antipilus antibody failed to adhere, nor did they adhere to intestines pretreated with purified pili. The authors concluded that the pili are a colonization factor of *A. sobria* Ae1.

CAMPYLOBACTER

Epidemiology and clinical features

Since Scotland's surveillance of human campylobacter infection began, the number of isolates has increased steadily from 1170 (23 per 100,000) in 1978 to 3430 (67 per 100,000) in 1991 (*526*). *Campylobacter* isolates have exceeded *Salmonella* isolates each year since 1985. Most cases occurred as sporadic infections or within families and no source was identified. When available, epidemiologic evidence frequently implicated transmission by contaminated foods (cold meats, salads, raw milk), by handling raw meat or poultry, or by direct or indirect contact with pets, farm animals, or wild birds. Although uncommon, community outbreaks were reported in most years. The incidence of infection peaks sharply in spring and early summer, 6–8 weeks before the peak in *Salmonella* infections. The British saga of "birds, milk, and *Campylobacter*" continued (*527*). A case–control study in the Gateshead area found a very strong association between *Campylobacter* infection and consumption of milk from bottles whose caps had been pecked by jackdaws and magpies ($\chi^2 = 12.6, p < .0004$). Sixty-three isolates of campylobacters were made from the bill and cloaca of local jackdaws, magpies, and crows; and when target bottles were set out, campylobacters were isolated from 12 of 123 pecked bottles. Numerous serotypes were identified in isolates from birds, milk, and case-patients.

The epidemiology and pathogenesis of *Campylobacter fetus fetus* infection is poorly understood, but there is frequently evidence for gastrointestinal exposure. From April 1984 through May 1990, *C. fetus fetus* was isolated from five patients at the Mayo Clinic (*528*). Three of these had gastrointestinal symptoms, although the source of infection was not discovered. In two cases, the organism was identified using culture conditions geared to detect only *Campylobacter jejuni*.

In India, a study was conducted in animal handlers to determine the prevalence of *Campylobacter* spp. and to evaluate the enterotoxigenic potential of the isolates (*529*). *Campylobacter* was isolated from 19 of 90 stool samples from healthy handlers (21%) and 5 of 30 samples from handlers with diarrhea (17%). Ten strains of *C. jejuni*—5 from diarrhetic handlers and 5 from healthy handlers—were tested in the ligated ileal loop of rats. All strains from diarrhetic subjects and 2 from healthy subjects were enterotoxigenic in the first trial; the remaining 3 became positive after one or two passages through rat gut. Thus domestic animals are a reservoir for *Campylobacter* and contact with animals is a source of infection in humans. In addition, cycling of the organisms through the gut may enhance their enterotoxigenicity.

Two cases of septicemia caused by *Campylobacter laridis* and *Campylobacter mucosalis* were reported in Sweden (*530*). The *C. laridis* infection was in a man with a history of abdominal pain and diarrhea, who had eaten shellfish in Paris about 10 days before his symptoms began. The *C. mucosalis* infection was in an elderly, debilitated, immuno-compromised man. This organism causes chronic intestinal disease in pigs and lambs, but the authors believe theirs to be the first report of its involvement in human septicemia. Although no port of entry was evident and stool cultures were negative for *C. jejuni*, the authors considered the intestinal route most probable. Another study in Sweden reported acute rheumatic symptoms in 7 of 35 victims of an outbreak of *C. jejuni* food poisoning (*531*). The antibody response correlated well with the intensity of symptoms, and in the early phase of gastrointestinal disease patients with acute rheumatic symptoms had significantly higher serum IgM levels than other subjects. Thirty-one symptom-free subjects also had increased levels of antibodies to *C. jejuni*, and 4 of them suffered from chronic rheumatic disorders at follow-up 5.5 years later. An HLA-B27-positive woman developed reactive arthritis with a relapse 7 years later (see references *147,148,382* for other reports of the association of the HLA-B27 antigen and reactive arthritis). The authors concluded that *C. jejuni* enterocolitis is significantly associated with rheumatic symptoms in the early phase and may also cause chronic rheumatic disorders.

A case of bursitis associated with *C. jejuni* infection was reported in an 81-year-old man (*532*). The onset and cause of the bursitis were not determined, nor was the source of the *C. jejuni* infection discovered. However, the authors postulated the most likely sequence of events to be *C. jejuni* enteritis followed by bacteremia, with superinfection of an already damaged bursa. Upon presentation the man had reported chills, fever, nausea, and occasional vomiting but did not complain of diarrhea.

Various neuropathies are also sequelae of *Campylobacter* enteritis (*533–538*). A 12-year-old girl consulted a neurologist because of a horizontal diplopia (*533*). The previous week she had had an episode of diarrhea, anorexia, and abdominal cramps. Serological findings indicated *C. jejuni* infection, and a diagnosis of postinfectious bilateral abducens paresis following *C. jejuni* enteritis was made. A case of atypical acute axonal polyneuropathy followed *Campylobacter* enteritis in a 17-year-old man who had severe axonal loss restricted to the distal part of his limbs (*534*). Japanese workers investigated the HLA class I antigens in six patients with acute axonal polyneuropathy following *C. jejuni* infection (*535*). All six showed axonopathy causing pure motor dysfunction associated with IgG anti-G_{M1} antibodies, and all had the HLA-B35 antigen. There was no significant association of the disease with any other class I antigen. An acute neurologic disease in northern China known as "Chinese paralytic syndrome" resembles the Guillain-Barré syndrome (*536*). It most frequently occurs during the summer and predominantly involves rural children. These features are consistent with *C. jejuni* infection. A serologic study was conducted in 26 patients with Chinese paralytic syndrome, 10 U.S. soldiers with *C. jejuni* enteritis, and healthy controls. As expected, most of the soldiers showed evidence in their convalescent serum of recent *C. jejuni* infection, whereas most healthy controls did not. The Chinese cases had a significantly higher rate of seropositivity in all three Ig classes. IgG responses were more common within 2 weeks of onset of neurologic symptoms, whereas IgM responses were more common later. These data suggest but do not prove a role for *C. jejuni* infection in the Chinese paralytic syndrome. *Campylobacter jejuni* infection is also associated with Guillain-Barré syndrome. Japanese investigators reported a common serotype of *C. jejuni* in isolates from four patients with Guillain-Barré syndrome (*537*). All four belonged to serotype PEN 19:LIO 7. PEN 19 represents <2% of clinical isolates, suggesting that serotyping of *C. jejuni* strains may be important in determining the pathogenesis of this syndrome. Testing of 17 consecutive acute Guillain-Barré patients from the Boston area for antibodies to *C. jejuni*

identified 3 who were seropositive (*538*). All three had had severe enteritis before the onset of neurologic symptoms. The authors concluded that in this series of patients *Campylobacter* enteritis was an important antecedent illness for Guillain-Barré syndrome but *C. jejuni* did not precipitate the syndrome without enteritis.

Although *C. fetus* is a well known cause of septic abortion in animals, campylobacters have rarely been implicated as human placental pathogens. This may be partly because campylobacters have special culture requirements and are not routinely sought in cases of spontaneous abortion. Denton and Clarke reported a case of septic abortion due to *C. jejuni* in a previously healthy woman with diarrhea (*539*). On histologic examination the placenta showed focal infiltration of villi with acute and chronic inflammatory cells, with necrotic areas in the center of these lesions. There was also pronounced chorioamnionitis, but no evidence of infection of fetal organs. Feces, the retained products of conception, and a high vaginal swab were positive for *C. jejuni* biotype 1. No other bacterial pathogen was identified. Because unexplained villitis is not uncommon in spontaneous abortion, the authors warned that the incidence of campylobacters as human placental pathogens may be underestimated. Because the ability of organisms to grow or survive in amniotic fluid is important in the pathogenesis of abortion, premature labor, and neonatal infections, Gurgan and Diker evaluated the survival of campylobacters in human amniotic fluid (*540*). They found that amniotic fluids supported growth of *C. fetus fetus, C. jejuni*, and *C. coli* and cells remained viable for 11–12 weeks.

Occurrence and survival

Park and Sanders surveyed 1054 samples of fresh vegetables from supermarkets and outdoor farmers' markets in Canada for the occurrence of campylobacters (*541*). No campylobacters were found on supermarket samples, whether collected in summer or winter. However, 2 of 60 spinach samples, 2 of 67 lettuce samples, 2 of 74 radish samples, 1 of 40 green onion samples, 1 of 42 parsley samples, and 1 of 63 potato samples from outdoor summer markets were positive. Most of the isolates (88%) were *C. jejuni,* but *C. lari* and *C. coli* were also identified. Washing with chlorinated water destroyed the organisms. The authors recommended that vegetables from outdoor markets be either decontaminated or thoroughly cooked before being eaten.

The survival of *C. jejuni* and pathogenic *Escherichia coli* in artificially inoculated mahewu, a fermented cereal gruel in Zimbabwe, was evaluated (*542*). No strain of *C. jejuni* was detected 30 min after inoculation with 10^6–10^7 cfu. Some *E. coli* survived for 24 h but did not grow. The authors concluded that mahewu has antimicrobial properties and is unlikely to transmit these enteropathogens.

Fox reviewed campylobacteriosis and salmonellosis in wild, domestic, and laboratory animals and discussed the prevention and control of zoonotic infections (*543*). Chattopadhyay et al. discussed poultry as a reservoir of campylobacters and a source of human campylobacteriosis in India (*544*). Twenty-five of 80 fecal samples from fowls, 43 of 100 fecal samples from chicks, and 82 of 140 samples of intestinal contents from freshly slaughtered chickens were positive for *Campylobacter.* Most of the isolates were *C. jejuni* and slightly more than half were biotype 2. In a survey of refrigerated frying chicken conducted in Oregon, 42% of 288 raw birds were contaminated with cephalothin-resistant thermophilic campylobacters (*545*). There was no difference between birds sampled in summer and birds sampled in fall. The median cfu count was 200/g for tissue samples and 40/mL for rinse water. The authors concluded that *Campylobacter* continues to be a frequent contaminant of ready-to-cook poultry, representing a hazard if birds are undercooked or cross-contamination of ready-to-eat foods occurs.

Two selective enrichment broths (differing in their combination of antimicrobial agents) and two plating agars were compared for isolation of *C. jejuni* and *C. coli* from 92 fresh retail chicken samples in Mexico (*546*). Thirty-three samples (36%) were positive in one or both enrichment broths. Butzler agar gave comparable results for the two enrichment broths, but Skirrow agar was effective only when the inoculum was derived from broth containing the same antibiotics as the Butzler

agar. Although the antimicrobials proposed by Butzler (bacitracin, colistin, cephalothin, cycloheximide, and novobiocin) have not been commonly used to detect *Campylobacter* in foods, these results showed their superiority over those used in Skirrow agar (vancomycin, trimethoprim, polymyxin B).

A study of *Campylobacter* contamination of newly slaughtered broiler chickens and older hens from Swedish flocks known to harbor the organisms in their intestines found campylobacters in 89% of neck skin samples, 93% of peritoneal cavity swab samples, and 75% of subcutaneous samples (*547*). However, the numbers in subcutaneous samples were relatively low despite the high incidence, and the incidence of *Campylobacter* in muscles was only 3%. The authors suggested that the organisms are introduced into the subcutis layer through the feather follicles. When normal and abnormal livers from slaughtered broiler chickens were examined bacteriologically, 47 *Campylobacter* isolates were obtained from 223 livers with macroscopic lesions (21%) (*548*). Six *C. jejuni* isolates were obtained from 50 normal livers (12%). *Campylobacter jejuni* biotype 2 was the most frequent isolate from abnormal livers, whereas *C. jejuni* biotype 1 was isolated from 5 of the 6 normal livers. The authors concluded not only that campylobacters are part of the intestinal flora of chickens and thus are a potential source of contamination during slaughter, but also that they are involved in the pathogenesis of necrotic hepatitis lesions originating before slaughter.

Cudjoe and Kapperud investigated the effect of lactic acid sprays on *Campylobacter* populations of naturally and artificially contaminated broiler chicken carcasses (*549*). Lactic acid sprays had a significant bactericidal effect on *C. jejuni* that became evident several hours after treatment and depended on the concentration of the spray (1 or 2%) and the timing of spray treatment (10 min or 24 h after inoculation).

Cecum-colonizing bacteria were isolated from *C. jejuni*–free laying hens and screened for production of anti-*C. jejuni* metabolites (*550*). A mixture of 9 isolates possessing this characteristic was then administered to day-old chicks to see if it would protect them from colonization by campylobacters.

The treatment provided 41–85% protection. The mixture was then reduced to three strains based on the organism's ability to utilize mucin as a sole substrate for growth. Feeding trials with the combination of *Klebsiella pneumoniae*, *Citrobacter diversus*, and *Escherichia coli* O13:H⁻ afforded 43–100% protection. The dominant cecal bacterium from treated chicks was consistently *E. coli* O13:H⁻, and trials with this organism alone gave 49–72% protection from campylobacter colonization. In all trials, treatment reduced the numbers of *C. jejuni* present in chicks that were colonized.

ANTIBIOTIC RESISTANCE. The in vitro activities of 22 antimicrobial agents against 78 isolates of *Campylobacter cryaerophila* and *Campylobacter butzleri*, two aerotolerant species associated with diarrhea in human and nonhuman primates, were evaluated (*551*). Ten additional agents were tested at concentrations used in selective *Campylobacter* media. Differences in susceptibility between aerotolerant campylobacters and the more common *C. jejuni* suggest that different treatment strategies may be necessary depending on the organism involved. The results further suggested the desirability of modifying primary isolation methods for campylobacters to include the aerotolerant strains. Other investigators reported the emergence of fluoroquinolone resistance in *C. jejuni* and *C. coli* isolated from patients with campylobacteriosis in Finland, 1978–1990 (*552*). Susceptibility to erythromycin, gentamicin, and doxycycline did not change during that period. Fluoroquinolone resistance was also found in *C. jejuni* and *C. coli* isolated from human feces in Switzerland (*553*). One subject was thought to have acquired a resistant strain from another patient in the same household who had been treated with norfloxacin. In the U.K., a *C. jejuni* strain sensitive to both erythromycin and ciprofloxacin was isolated from a woman with severe enteritis, and she was treated with erythromycin (*554*). Four days later another fecal specimen yielded an isolate resistant to erythromycin but sensitive to ciprofloxacin, but the patient recovered temporarily with no change in therapy. Upon relapse a week later, however, a strain resistant to both erythromycin

and ciprofloxacin was recovered. As the patient had not received ciprofloxacin treatment, the development of ciprofloxacin resistance appeared to have been spontaneous.

Ansary and Radu studied the conjugal transfer of antibiotic resistance and plasmids in clinical isolates of *C. jejuni* (*555*). Multiple resistance to at least 3 of the 9 antibiotics tested was observed, tetracycline resistance being most common. En bloc transfer of donor resistances at frequencies of 10^{-8}–10^{-4} occurred in 5 of 6 isolates. Streptomycin resistance was lost in ~10% of transconjugants even though they carried the donor's complement of 3 plasmids. About 1% of transconjugants, which did not carry any plasmids, were resistant only to kanamycin.

Isolation and identification

Kist reviewed methods for studying organisms in the genera *Campylobacter* and *Helicobacter* (*556*). Topics covered were the pathologic importance of various campylobacters, techniques for obtaining and transporting specimens, media and procedures for isolating and identifying organisms, and biochemical and physiological properties of *Campylobacter* species. Helicobacters were discussed more briefly.

A comparative study was made of three selective media for isolating campylobacters from highly contaminated environmental samples (*557*). All media contained blood supplements. Twelve *C. coli* and 9 *C. jejuni* isolates from sewage and 15 sewage samples were used in the evaluation. Overall, all broth–agar combinations gave comparable median values for campylobacters. Variations between strains were thought to be caused by differences in sensitivity to the antibiotics incorporated into the media. Because of excessive bacterial overgrowth on CAR agar and problems in retrieving organisms from mCCD agar, combinations of Preston or CAR broth with Preston agar were considered most satisfactory.

A selective medium containing cefoperazone was formulated to detect *C. upsaliensis* in fecal samples from diarrheic dogs and cats (*558*). Strains were identified by DNA:DNA hybridization using digoxigenin-labeled total genomic DNA of 4 reference strains (*C. jejuni, C. coli, C. lari,* and *C. upsaliensis*) as probes. Sixty-six of 72 *Campylobacter* isolates could be identified to the species level in this way and the results agreed completely with results from conventional tests. Of the 72 strains isolated, 39 were thermophilic catalase-negative species. Thirty-three were *C. upsaliensis* and 6 catalase-negative strains phenotypically similar to *C. upsaliensis* did not hybridize with any of the probes. The authors concluded that if relative resistance to cefoperazone characterizes *C. upsaliensis* as a species, as appears possible from these results, this must be taken into account when isolating campylobacters on selective media.

Differences in performance of various broths and agars and in incubation times and temperatures can be critical for success in isolating campylobacters (*559,560*). Results with the semisolid selective motility medium of Goossens and Butzler depended both on major variables (e.g., incubation temperature) and on less obvious variables (e.g., brand of agar). These factors could explain some discrepant findings.

Thermophilic campylobacters grow best in an atmosphere containing 5–10% O_2 and 1–10% CO_2. For laboratories where more sophisticated procedures are not possible, incubation in a low-oxygen atmosphere produced by burning a measured amount of methylated spirit in a closed container is inexpensive and simple and produces excellent results (*561*). Other authors compared a modified internal gas generator system with the commercial Gaspak and mixtures from gas cylinders for isolating campylobacters (*562*). The internal gas generator system and Gaspak gave identical results, superior to those with the compressed-gas mixture. Because the chemicals required for the internal gas generator system are common and inexpensive, this method is more economical than the Gaspak method.

Twenty species or subspecies of *Campylobacter, Helicobacter,* and *Arcobacter* were used to assess the reproducibility of 25 phenotypic tests used to identify these organisms (*563*). Tests were performed three times on different batches of freshly prepared medium and the 22 tests that depended on growth inhibition were performed using three basal media. The best growth occurred on blood agar (100% recovery); 10 of the 20 strains grew reproducibly on nutrient agar; and only 1 strain grew reproducibly on brucella agar. The most reproducible results were obtained using blood agar (94%), followed by nutrient agar (92%) and brucella agar (89%). The discriminatory power of each test–medium combination was also evaluated. For example, no strain tolerated 1% bile with the nutrient agar base (no discrimination), but 55% were positive with the blood agar base (good discrimination). The authors concluded that the reproducibility of certain tests for certain taxa is questionable even when the inoculum and the test are carefully standardized. Although blood agar in general was the medium of choice, nutrient agar gave more reproducible results for the potassium permanganate, safranine O, and sodium arsenite tests. Similarly, the same authors evaluated the reproducibility of 9 enzyme detection tests used to identify campylobacters, helicobacters, and arcobacters (*564*). They found considerable variation in the ease of interpretation and reproducibility of the tests and slight procedural modifications affected test results. Nevertheless, they concluded that certain enzyme tests, performed according to their recommendations and used alone or in conjunction with a conventional identification protocol, rapidly provide data for presumptive identification.

Three commercial latex agglutination tests were compared for detection of campylobacters (*565*). All three showed clear agglutination with 5 test strains in both the spiral and coccoid forms. The number of cells needed for agglutination varied from 2×10^6 to 5×10^8, depending on the test and strain. Microscreen was roughly 10 times as sensitive as Campyslide and Meritec. When the tests were applied to enrichment broth cultures of chicken products, 69% of *Campylobacter*-positive cultures were positive with Microscreen and Meritec detected 63%. Campyslide detected only 15% and frequently showed nonspecific agglutination. There was only one false-positive reaction with minced meat but false-negative results occurred frequently in enrichment procedures when the cultures contained large numbers of competing microorganisms.

Twelve thermophilic *Campylobacter* isolates from human feces and seawater were biotyped and ribotyped (*566*). The strains were identified as *C. jejuni* and *C. coli*. All had distinctive ribotypes except for three identical fecal isolates of *C. jejuni* biotype 1. There was no correlation between Lior biotype and *Hae*III ribotype, but several bands within the ribopatterns were identified as possible species markers for use in diagnostic and epidemiologic work. A numerical analysis of the ribopatterns was carried out and a dendrogram was constructed.

Oligodeoxynucleotide probes were constructed for identification of *C. fetus* and *Campylobacter hyointestinalis* based on 16S rRNA sequences (*567*). The specificity of the probes was tested with type strains of 15 *Campylobacter* and *Arcobacter* species and field isolates of *C. fetus* and *C. hyointestinalis*. Two probes hybridized with 57 confirmed isolates of *C. fetus* but not with any other campylobacter. A *C. hyointestinalis* probe reacted with 47 of 48 confirmed isolates of this species but with no other campylobacter. Southern blot analysis of genomic DNA digests revealed multiple copies of genes encoding rRNA. Other analysis showed that a single base change differentiated *C. fetus fetus* from *C. fetus venerealis*, whereas 28 base mismatches distinguished *C. fetus* from *C. hyointestinalis*. The phylogenetic tree of these species was constructed based on 16S rRNA sequence data, showing their relationship to other campylobacters and to selected species of *Bacteroides, Wolinella, 'Flexispira', Helicobacter, Escherichia*, and *Proteus*.

Twenty-seven *C. coli* strains of serogroup 20, biotype 1 were studied by plasmid, protein, and restriction endonuclease analysis and multilocus enzyme electrophoresis (MEE) (*568*). Restriction endonuclease analysis using the HhaI (CfoI) enzyme permitted the best discrimination among these strains. Protein profiles were more similar than restriction endonuclease analysis patterns, but discriminated fairly well among strains. Three strains did not harbor plasmids; the remaining 24 fell into 11 groups according to their plasmid profile. On MEE, 10 enzymes showed easily distinguishable bands; only malate dehydrogenase migrated uniformly for all strains. Isocitrate

dehydrogenase was the most polymorphic, with 5 electromorphs. The 27 strains were assigned to 9 electrotypes.

Immunologic methods for identifying campylobacters have been investigated (*569–571*). Several protein antigens of *Campylobacter* spp. were identified by Western blot analysis (*569*). One, specific to *C. coli*, had an M_r of 38,000 and was recognized by sera and intestinal lavage fluids from parenterally immunized mice. Another, specific to *C. jejuni*, with an M_r of 27,000, was detected by sera from parenterally immunized mice. A third antigen of M_r 31,000 was common to *C. coli* and *C. jejuni*. Mills et al. reported a simplified procedure based on the O antigen for serotyping *C. jejuni* and *C. coli* (*570*). Erythrocytes were sensitized with an antigenic extract and used in a slide agglutination assay with specific antisera. The standard typing antisera were grouped into 9 pools for *C. jejuni* and 4 for *C. coli*, cross-reacting antisera being allocated to the same pool. Generally each reference strain reacted with only one pool; the specific serotype could be determined by further testing with the individual antisera in that pool. When 246 clinical isolates of *C. jejuni* and 57 of *C. coli* were typed by this technique and by the slower, more labor-intensive passive hemagglutination assay, the two gave very similar results although there were differences for a few isolates. Further investigation showed that variation of the O antigen can occur in vivo (*571*). O-serotyping of three *C. jejuni* isolates from the same patient showed marked differences between the first and third isolates in both passive hemagglutination assays and immunoblots of LPS from proteinase K–digested whole cells. The isolates were not distinguishable by restriction endonuclease analysis of genomic DNA, gel electrophoresis of whole-cell proteins, or silver-stained LPS gels, indicating that they belonged to the same strain.

The behavior of campylobacters in the environment is not well understood beyond the knowledge that the organisms survive and grow poorly outside the host's intestine. Environmental isolates rapidly develop a nonmotile "coccoid" form and become nonculturable, but under some circumstances these cells can recover and regain their infectivity (*572–574*). Suspensions of 4 *C. jejuni* strains that had become nonculturable after storage in pond water were fed to suckling mice (*572*). One strain colonized the intestine and yielded culturable isolates; a second strain regained its culturability and colonized the intestine after one mouse passage; two strains, which showed near-total degeneration upon electron microscopic study, failed to colonize. The authors pointed out that although the methods used in this study are not suitable for epidemiologic work (which is hampered by frequent inability to culture campylobacters from environmental and food samples), the existence of the viable but nonculturable state suggests the value of molecular detection techniques in epidemiology. Other investigators measured the ATP content of *Salmonella typhimurium* and *C. jejuni* cells held at 20°C in saline for 3 weeks (*573*). ATP levels remained fairly constant in both species, but *S. typhimurium* cells remained fully viable (culturable) while *C. jejuni* cells rapidly lost culturability. This suggested that energy remained available for initiating growth of *C. jejuni* if other conditions were favorable. Nevertheless, these authors could not demonstrate infectivity of the nonculturable cells in either animals or human volunteers. Fully virulent organisms were recovered, however, from 7 of 16 freeze-thaw-injured nonculturable stocks of *C. jejuni* after two or three passages through rat gut (*574*).

Virulence

A comparative study of two congenic strains of *C. jejuni*, one colonizing and one noncolonizing, was conducted to identify colonization mechanisms (*575*). The strains were indistinguishable by transmission electron microscopy, plasmid content, or DNA digestion patterns generated by 8 restriction enzymes. The strains showed the same chemotactic behavior to mucin and fucose and both caused necrosis of villus epithelial cells in chick cecal tissue cultures. However, only the colonizing strain was detected in crypt cells. These findings demonstrated the importance for colonization of infiltration into intestinal crypts.

Extracts from 75 *C. jejuni* and *C. coli* strains from poultry and other animal sources were examined for toxicity in in vitro cell assays (*576*). No source-related differences in toxigenicity were seen and no strain produced cytotonic enterotoxin. Extracts from most strains were toxic to CHO-KI and fetal calf lung cells; 69% of *C. jejuni* and 75% of *C. coli* strains were toxic to CEF cells; 51% of *C. jejuni* strains were toxic to Vero cells; and 46% of *C. jejuni* strains were toxic to HeLa cells. These results demonstrate the complexity of toxin production by thermophilic campylobacters and may explain some difficulties and inconsistencies of experimental studies of *Campylobacter* enteritis. A study of virulence markers in 49 clinical isolates of *C. jejuni* and *C. coli* in France and Tunisia identified 4 pathovars, based on association with HeLa cells and ability to elongate CHO cells (*577*). *Campylobacter jejuni* biotype 1 was more frequent among Tunisian strains, whereas biotype 2 predominated in French strains. Twenty-one strains elongated CHO cells and 24 associated with HeLa cells. These phenotypes were independently distributed and not related to biotype. The pathovar lacking both virulence markers was correlated with lack of clinical signs of diarrhea and fever ($p = .00004$).

Studies in rabbits demonstrated the importance of flagella in initiating colonization and eliciting protective immunity (*578*). Animals were immunized by gastric feeding with *Campylobacter* strains of various Lior and Penner serogroups. Immunization protected an animal against challenge with strains of a homologous Lior serotype, but not against a different serotype. Animals challenged with matched Penner but unmatched Lior strains showed marginal protection. Experiments with isogenic flagellated and nonflagellated strains of *C. coli* showed that multiple feedings of the mutant afforded complete protection against the isogenic flagellated strain but only weak protection against other strains of the same Lior serotype. The authors concluded that the flagellum is the cross-strain protective component of the Lior antigen complex. However, nonflagellar somatic antigens apparently elicited resistance to colonization by the same strain. The role of flagella in *C. jejuni*'s adhesion to and penetration of eukaryotic cells was studied by inactivation of the flagellin genes *flaA* and *flaB* (*579*). A defective *flaA* gene led to immotility, whereas *flaB* mutants remained motile. Nonmotile mutants lost their ability to adhere to and penetrate human intestinal cells in vitro. Invasive properties were partially restored by centrifuging the mutants onto the cultured cells, showing that motility is a major, but probably not the only, factor involved in invasion. Other investigators isolated a recombinant phage clone lambda gt11RK that expressed a 56-kDa *C. jejuni* flagellin protein that reacted specifically with antiflagellin antibody (*580*). The flagellin gene was sequenced. The parts of the flagellin antigen involved in motor and assembly functions are conserved, but nucleotide and amino acid sequence analysis identified a region showing hypervariability among species and strains of *Campylobacter*.

LISTERIA

Farber and Peterkin thoroughly reviewed the literature on *Listeria monocytogenes,* emphasizing its role as a foodborne pathogen (*581*, with 445 references). Farber also briefly reviewed the behavior of *L. monocytogenes* in foods, the organism's virulence factors and methods for its control, and human listeriosis (*582*). Another comprehensive review, written by the *L. monocytogenes* working group of the National Advisory Committee on Microbiological Criteria for Foods, was published as an issue of the *International Journal of Food Microbiology* (*583*). It includes an executive summary and recommendations for control strategies and future research. Doyle developed an argument for reconsidering the policy of zero tolerance of *L. monocytogenes* in all ready-to-eat foods (*584*). He contended that present policy is unrealistic for low-risk foods such as fermented sausages, for which he recommended establishing tolerances for small populations. Greater emphasis should be placed on foods in which the organism is better able to survive and grow and which are likely to be eaten by highly sensitive individuals.

Epidemiology and clinical features

Since the first outbreak of confirmed foodborne listeriosis was reported in 1983, much has been learned about the behavior of *L. monocytogenes* in foods and risk factors for infection (*585–588*). A collaborative study in Oklahoma and parts of California, Georgia, and Tennessee identified 301 cases of listeriosis from November 1988 through December 1990, an annual incidence of 7.4 per 1 million (*586*). There were 67 deaths. One third of the cases were in pregnant women or their newborns. A case–control study of these patients suggested that foodborne transmission accounts for a substantial portion of sporadic cases (*587*). Case-patients were 165 subjects with culture-confirmed listeriosis; 376 controls were matched for age, health-care provider, and immunosuppressive status. Cases were more likely to have eaten soft cheeses [odds ratio (OR) 2.6] or food purchased from delicatessen counters (OR 1.6); one-third of sporadic disease was attributable to these foods. Nearly 70% of cases in men and nonpregnant women were in cancer patients, persons with AIDS, organ transplant recipients, or persons receiving corticosteroid therapy. Among immunosuppressed patients, eating undercooked chicken was also a risk factor (OR 3.3). A companion paper reported the accompanying microbiologic investigation (*588*). Ready-to-eat foods, foods containing *L. monocytogenes* serotype 4b, and foods highly contaminated with *L. monocytogenes* were independently associated with disease. *Listeria* grew from at least one food specimen in the refrigerators of 79 (64%) of 123 patients, representing 11% of >2000 food specimens collected. In order of decreasing percentage of positive samples in the food category, *L. monocytogenes* was isolated from beef > poultry > pork > lunch meat > seafood > vegetables > fruit > dairy products. Bread or pasta, eggs, lamb, and a mixture of food types each yielded one isolate. One third of refrigerators with contaminated foods yielded at least one isolate of the same strain as the isolate from the corresponding patient.

A study of listeriosis in the U.K., 1967–1990, strengthened the conclusion that contaminated paté contributed to the sharp rise in cases that began in 1985 to be followed by an abrupt decline in mid-1989 (*589*). Two strains of *L. monocytogenes* accounted for most of the increase and 30–54% of the annual totals during this period. A survey of patés in July 1989 found them to be frequently contaminated. Products from one manufacturer were more often and more highly contaminated, and the strains involved were the same as those responsible for the increase in listeriosis cases. The beginning of the decline in listeriosis coincided with government warnings about paté consumption and the suspension of products from the implicated manufacturer.

Thirty cases of feto-maternal listeriosis in Denmark, 1981–1988, were reviewed (*590*). A mother and her child were considered a single case. From an incidence of ~1 case per 100,000 live births in the early 1980s the incidence peaked at 25.3/100,000 in 1986; the increase between 1985 and 1987 reflected an outbreak. Details of the individual cases were summarized.

Investigators from Los Angeles, Nashville, and Chicago collaborated in a study of the epidemiological spectrum of listeriosis, 1985–1989 (*591*). More than two-thirds of the 38 Los Angeles cases occurred during the perinatal period and another fifth were late-onset neonatal cases. In contrast, the majority of cases at Vanderbilt University Hospital were in nonpregnant adults who had received organ transplants or were immunocompromised for other reasons; 14 (42%) occurred in the perinatal or neonatal period. Two hospitals in Chicago recorded 15 perinatal and neonatal cases and 33 cases in adults. The most focal infections occurred in the Chicago patients. Ampicillin and penicillin were generally effective as therapeutic agents; cephalosporins were ineffective. The greatest mortality was in fetuses and premature infants.

An outbreak of listeriosis in the Philadelphia area in 1987, which involved multiple strains and implicated no clear source or vehicle of infection, led to the hypothesis that clinical listeriosis may occur in asymptomatic persons with listerial colonization of the intestinal tract if they are subsequently infected by a second gastrointestinal pathogen (*592*; B. Schwartz, *J. Infect. Dis.* 159:680, 1989). In support of this hypothesis, Lorber reported a case of listeriosis following shigellosis (*592*). The patient, a previously healthy farmer at risk for listerial colonization through occupational exposure, was confirmed to be part of a restaurant-associated outbreak of shigellosis due to contaminated water. Shortly thereafter he developed neurologic symptoms and a midbrain listerial abscess.

Investigators in Finland analyzed the clinical presentation and outcome of listeriosis according to whether patients were receiving immunosuppressive therapy (*593*). The study included an estimated 86% of cases in the Helsinki area during 1971–1989. Forty-nine of 74 patients had an underlying disease (most often cancer or diabetes mellitus) or had received renal transplants; 32 had received immunosuppressive therapy within 1 week of the onset of listeriosis. Mortality was not associated with immunosuppression, but 32% of patients with underlying disease died whereas all previously healthy adults survived. The most common manifestation of listeriosis in immunosuppressed patients was bacteremia without known foci, whereas 64% of previously healthy patients had central nervous system infections.

Modulation of the protective response to intravenous challenge with *L. monocytogenes* by a traditional Chinese medicine was demonstrated in mice (*594*). Ren-shen-yang-rong-tang, compounded from spray-dried extracts of 12 medicinal plants, was injected intraperitoneally 2 days before intravenous challenge with the pathogen. Ninety percent of untreated mice died, whereas 90–100% of treated mice survived. The drug appeared to affect the early phase of the protective response, involving nonimmune macrophages. The drug induced interleukin-1 and -6 and granulocyte macrophage–colony stimulating factor, which stimulate proliferation of hematopoietic stem cells and enhance their differentiation to granulocytes or macrophages.

McLauchlin et al. discussed 14 patients who suffered recurrences of listeriosis (*595*). All patients but one had severe underlying disease. In 7, the two episodes were due to the same strain of *L. monocytogenes* and the recurrence was considered a reactivation of the original infection. In one patient, isolates from the two episodes differed, suggesting a reinfection. Twelve of the patients in this series had received inappropriate therapy. A 3- to 4-week treatment with ampicillin plus an aminoglycoside is recommended.

Other authors reported cases of arterial infections due to *L. monocytogenes* (*596*), listerial meningitis in an adult caused by a catalase-negative strain (*597*), and listerial meningitis in an immunocompromised infant (*598*) and an HIV-positive man (*599*). An unusual case of *L. monocytogenes* infection occurred in a 10-year-old girl who had encephalitis involving the brainstem, myelitis, and possible radiculitis (*600*). Cultures of blood and cerebrospinal fluid were negative but blood samples showed an increase in titer to *L. monocytogenes* type 4 from <16 on day 1 to 32 on day 9. This was regarded as seroconversion. An 85-year-old man with well controlled diabetes mellitus but otherwise good health died of a listerial brain abscess (*601*). From their experience with this patient and a literature review the authors concluded that such lesions tend to be subacute and accompanied by bacteremia. Unlike most brain abscesses, those due to *Listeria* can sometimes be diagnosed by blood cultures. One case of listerial pleural fluid infection was reported and 8 others were reviewed (*602*). Eight patients had an underlying malignancy and 6 were receiving immunosuppressive therapy. Four died. Rapid diagnosis, prompt and appropriate antimicrobial therapy, and drainage of the pleural fluid improved chances of survival. Two cases of pleural effusion in patients with listerial pneumonia were also reported (*603*). One patient had recently completed a course of chemotherapy for Hodgkin's disease and one had AIDS and a history of intravenous drug abuse and chronic active hepatitis B. The authors emphasized that although pneumonia due to *L. monocytogenes* is rare it should be considered in severely immunocompromised patients.

Reports of plasmid-mediated antibiotic resistance in *Listeria* are ominous because listeriosis is often fatal even with antibiotic therapy. In a survey of dairy and poultry products, 98 strains of *L. monocytogenes* and 85 of *L. innocua* were isolated (*604*). By disc and agar dilution assays no strains were resistant to ampicillin, vancomycin, chloramphenicol, or cotrimoxazole, but 4 *L. monocytogenes* and 15 *L. innocua* strains were resistant to one or more of the other 7 antibiotics tested. All 4 *L. monocytogenes* strains were resistant to streptomycin, sulphamethoxazole, and kanamycin. A high level of tetracycline resistance in *L. innocua* may be due to the widespread use of this antibiotic in poultry feeding. Thus multiresistant strains are already present in food, and human infection by antibiotic-resistant organisms may stem from that source. The genetic basis of tetracycline resistance in *L. monocytogenes* was studied in 25 clinical isolates (*605*). Evidence was presented that two types of movable genetic elements (transposons and plasmids) in enterococci and streptococci are responsible for the emergence of drug resistance in *L. monocytogenes*.

Occurrence and behavior in foods and the food-system environment

OCCURRENCE. In the aftermath of an Australian outbreak of listeriosis, 342 samples of meat products from delicatessens and butcher shops in Queensland were surveyed to determine the incidence of *Listeria* (*606*). *Listeria monocytogenes* was recovered from 13% of samples, with the following distribution: 15/90 ham, 18/58 bacon, 4/39 corned beef, 5/132 salami, 2/5 roast beef, 1/3 brawn. Serotype 1 accounted for 62% of isolates, 36% were serotype 4, and 2% were serotype 2 or 3. *Listeria innocua* was found in 24% of samples: 18/90 ham, 15/58 bacon, 11/39 corned beef, 35/132 salami, 1/5 roast beef, 1/4 roast pork, 1/1 pickled pork. Seven isolates of *L. welshimeri* and *L. seeligeri* were also recovered. Most of the contaminated products originated from shops where the organisms were introduced from cutting boards and utensils used for raw meat. Another survey of a random selection of processed foods from Australian supermarkets and delicatessens found *L. monocytogenes* in 8 of 50 cooked chicken samples, 5 of 30 chicken liver patés, and none of 20 assorted meat products (*607*). Five isolates of *L. innocua* were recovered, 4 of them from cooked chicken. When contaminated, patés were highly contaminated and could be a serious hazard because they are eaten unheated and may be refrigerated for long periods after being opened. A Welsh survey of 216 patés, most of them imported, found 35% contaminated with *L. monocytogenes*, 5% of samples having counts >10^4/g (*608*). The occurrence of *L. monocytogenes* was not related to the presence of coliforms, and repeated sampling of 7 refrigerated paté loaves over a 21-day period suggested that populations were increasing in 6 of the 7. The predominant serotype was 4b, which is responsible for most cases of human listeriosis but represents a minority of food isolates. Four other serotypes were also identified, and multiple serotypes were isolated from 8 samples. *Listeria innocua,* the only other listeria isolated, was found in 2% of samples.

Listeria species were detected in 53 of 122 samples of frozen food products from retail shops in Berlin (*609*). Twenty-seven products were positive for *L. monocytogenes;* the only serotypes identified were 1/2a and 1/2b. Fish (fingers, fillets) and meat (hamburgers, gyros, meatballs) were most frequently contaminated (52 and 29%, respectively), and raw products were more often contaminated than precooked ones.

Iced cakes and filled doughnuts from four bakeries in Colorado were tested for *L. monocytogenes* (*610*). Icings, fillings, and baked portions were analyzed separately, yielding 55 samples. After a 48-h enrichment, 14 samples yielded grampositive hemolytic bacteria, but none could be identified as *L. monocytogenes* on the basis of other tests.

A survey of 954 hens' eggs from retail markets in Germany found 2 shells and 1 yolk contaminated with *L. innocua* (*611*). No other listerias were isolated. The authors concluded that commercial eggs are not important in the epidemiology of listeriosis.

Retail meats in Beijing were surveyed for contamination with *Listeria* (*612*). Eight of 70 samples were positive for *L. monocytogenes* (7 of 25 pork and 1 of 21 chicken samples); all meats were frozen and all isolates were serotype 1/2. Thirty-nine samples contained other *Listeria* species: 15 of 25 pork, 11 of 21 chicken, 7 of 10 beef, and 6 of 14 lamb samples. The incidence of these species was also greater in frozen meats than in fresh. Palcam medium was more efficient than Oxford medium in recovering listerias. In an Australian study, listerias were found in 93 of 175 samples of vacuum-packed processed meats from retail stores; 76 isolates were *L. monocytogenes*

(*613*). Seven samples contained >1000 cfu/g. Four brands of corned beef and 3 of ham, varying in water, salt, and nitrite content and pH, were inoculated with *L. monocytogenes* and vacuum-packed. Growth rate depended on the composition of the product. High residual nitrite or low a_w reduced growth, particularly when products were stored at 0–5°C. At higher temperatures, growth of *L. monocytogenes* increased more rapidly than growth of lactic acid bacteria and *Brochothrix thermosphacta*. Growth rates were similar in inoculated and naturally contaminated packs, supporting the validity of modeling or predictive studies based on product composition, time, and temperature.

A Canadian study determined the incidence of *L. monocytogenes* in domestic and imported seafood from wholesale and retail outlets (*614*). The organism was found in 8 of 69 shrimp samples, 1 of 12 crab samples, and 10 of 32 salmon samples. Most isolates were from ready-to-eat foods (cooked shrimp and smoked salmon). *Listeria* was not found in surimi, frozen scallops, or other seafood products. *Listeria monocytogenes* grew poorly on naturally contaminated shrimp at 4°C. In inoculation experiments using cooked seafoods, growth occurred on crabmeat, lobster, shrimp, and smoked salmon. The authors concluded that unless temperature abuse occurs, *Listeria*-contaminated cooked seafood is probably not a serious health hazard because only low levels of contamination were found and the shelf life of these products is short.

Because of concern about possible health hazards from illegally produced and marketed soft Hispanic-style cheeses in California, 100 samples were collected from around the state by undercover agents (*615*). Two samples contained *L. monocytogenes* and two contained *L. innocua*. These four samples were phosphatase-positive. Aerobic plate counts were generally high, indicating that the cheeses were processed and handled under unhygienic conditions. In a German survey, listerias were isolated from 311 of 3027 cheese samples (*616*). On biochemical testing, 214 were confirmed as *L. innocua*, 89 as *L. monocytogenes,* and 8 as *L. seeligeri*. The majority of *L. monocytogenes* isolates were serotype 1/2, but 16 isolates of serotype 3 and 5 of serotype 4b were identified. The overall incidence of listerias in raw milk samples from Northern Ireland was 25% (15% for *L. monocytogenes*) (*617*). The incidence was higher in the processing environment (54%) than at dairy farms (9%). *Listeria monocytogenes* was also isolated from 1 of 95 pasteurized milk samples and *L. seeligeri* from 1 of 33 soft cheese samples. The FDA enrichment procedure was much more productive than cold enrichment, and Oxford agar was superior to modified McBride agar. Restriction fragment length polymorphism was more useful than serotyping in discriminating *L. monocytogenes* strains and suggested that specific strains persist in both farm and processing environments. Most strains were not phage-typable.

Investigators in New Zealand determined the incidence of *L. monocytogenes* in a sheep slaughterhouse and the surrounding environment (*618*). The organism was isolated from soil and hay samples in the adjacent paddocks and from 4 of 31 cold-room samples, but not from meat swabs or tissue samples, drain effluents in the evisceration area, or any equipment or surfaces in the processing area (after sanitation) or from the hands or aprons of workers. One isolate of *L. ivanovii* was obtained from a mesh screen in the nearby waste-water treatment plant. The authors concluded that although cold rooms may be a source of listerial contamination and listerias can be found in samples from animal paddocks, it is possible to prepare sheep carcasses free of *L. monocytogenes*.

Of 1315 samples of German meat, poultry, and fish products, 227 (17.3%) contained *Listeria* spp.; more than half of the isolates were *L. monocytogenes* (*619*). However, examination of 186 swabs from 33 plants with substandard hygienic conditions did not detect listerias. Comparable growth occurred on Palcam and Oxford media.

Listeria monocytogenes was isolated from various types of samples from the agricultural environment in Belgium, after enrichment procedures were optimized for each sample type (*620*). Four of 25 samples of fresh pig feces, 5 of 25 samples of fresh cattle feces, and 1 of 15 groundwater samples were positive. The organism was not found in stored liquid manure or manured soil, nor could it be detected in artificially contaminated

liquid pig or cattle manure or soil two months after inoculation. When radishes and carrots were examined 3 months after being sown on artificially contaminated soil, 3 of 6 unwashed radishes were positive but all washed radishes and washed and unwashed carrots were negative. The organism was also found in one sample of manured soil where radishes had previously been cultivated, but 11 other soil samples were negative. The authors concluded that *Listeria* does not survive well in soil or liquid manure and that although manuring practices may introduce the bacterium into the rhizosphere of plants this is probably not the direct cause for listerial contamination of vegetables.

In Japan, 1705 specimens of feces or ileocecal contents of cattle, pigs, dogs, cats, chickens, and rats were examined for *L. monocytogenes* (*621*). The prevalence was 1.9% in cattle, 0.6% in pigs, 0.9% in dogs, and 6.5% in rats; no isolates were obtained from cats or chickens. Of 26 isolates, 8 were serotype 1/2 and 5 were serotype 4b. Because 4 serotype 4b isolates were from dogs or rats, the authors concluded that these animals sharing the human environment may be a dominant source of this pathogenic serotype. The prevalence of all *Listeria* spp. was 5.1% in cattle, 12.2% in pigs, 2.0% in dogs, and 17% in rats. *Listeria innocua* accounted for most isolates that were not *L. monocytogenes*.

GROWTH AND BEHAVIOR. Various sites in food-processing plants, particularly floor drains, support growth of listerias and are consistently found to harbor them. Spurlock and Zottola studied the growth and attachment of *L. monocytogenes* in cast-iron drains (*622*). A culture of *L. monocytogenes* Scott A was inoculated into sterilized free-standing drains containing rich and dilute nutritive media and microbial populations were monitored. During a 28-day growth period the pH was adjusted from an initial level of 6.6–7.0 to 9.0 on day 7, 7.0 on day 14, and 4.5 on day 21—conditions representing the extremes encountered after acid washes and caustic rinses. The organism survived all pH adjustments. Scanning electron micrographs of cast-iron chips incubated in broth cultures of *L. monocytogenes* showed some cells apparently attached to the iron surface, although they attached less readily to cast iron than to stainless steel. The authors concluded that *L. monocytogenes* may attach to walls inside a cast-iron drain and recommended investigation of biofilm formation under these conditions, because such biofilms could be an important reservoir of the pathogen in food-processing plants. Mafu et al. studied the physicochemical forces involved in adhesion of *L. monocytogenes* to surfaces (*623*). In the salt aggregation test, all strains aggregated at very high $(NH_4)_2SO_4$ molarities, indicating that they are hydrophilic. Scott A cells adhered to octyl-Sepharose only at low pH. Zeta potential measurements revealed a net negative surface potential. These and other results indicated that expression of the hydrophobicity of *L. monocytogenes* Scott A is apparent only at low pH and high ionic strength and that other factors are important in the adhesion of this organism to surfaces.

The effect of cleaners and sanitizers on *L. monocytogenes* depends on the surface to which the organism is attached (*624*). Chips of stainless steel, solid polyester, and polyester on a woven polyurethane backing were incubated with a 3-strain culture of *L. monocytogenes* and exposed to cleaners and sanitizers of various types. The most resistance to sanitizers was observed on polyester–polyurethane chips and the least on stainless steel. Similarly, cleaners removed biofilms least effectively from polyester–polyurethane and most easily from stainless steel. The organism was best eliminated when cleaning preceded sanitizing.

To evaluate the survival of *L. monocytogenes* Scott A and V37CE in aerosols, aerosols with populations of 10^3–10^4, 10^5–10^6, and 10^8–10^9 cfu/mL were generated into an enclosed hood from bacterial suspensions in dilute media or distilled water (*625*). At intervals, plates containing nutrient agar were exposed to aerosol fallout. Fallout occurred for 210 min for high-population aerosols of both strains in all media; with low-population aerosols fallout was observed for 5–35 min depending on the medium and strain. These results show the importance of controlling aerosolization of *Listeria* in food-processing plants.

Linton et al. showed that heat resistance of log-phase *L. monocytogenes* Scott A cells was influenced by their physiological condition, the enumeration medium, and the growth environment (*626*). Bacteria were heat-shocked at 48°C for 10 min, then heated at 55°C. D_{55} values were greater for heat-shocked than non-heat-shocked cells and on nonselective than selective enumeration medium. On nonselective medium D_{55} was greater under anaerobic conditions, whereas on selective medium no colonies grew anaerobically under either temperature regimen. When cells were enumerated on nonselective medium, heat-shock more than doubled the D_{55} values. These results underscore the importance of reaching final process temperatures of thermally processed foods as quickly as possible to minimize increased heat resistance due to heat shock.

The ability of *L. monocytogenes* to grow at 4 and 30°C is influenced not only by osmotic conditions (water activity, a_w) but by the type of solute (*627*). At a_w .90, strains Scott A (serotype 4b) and Brie 1 (serotype 1b) grew well in glycerol-supplemented tryptic soy broth but not when sucrose or NaCl was substituted for glycerol. Sucrose was more inhibitory than salt, Brie 1 was more sensitive to sucrose than Scott A, and for both strains and all three solutes, intolerance to low a_w was enhanced at 4°C.

Because temperature fluctuates during the storage and distribution of refrigerated minimally processed foods, Saguy assessed the potential growth of *L. monocytogenes* by mathematical simulation of several temperature scenarios (*628*). Using average times for back-room refrigeration, retail display, transport to the home, and home storage he ran the model assuming average temperatures, the worst 10% found during retail, the average plus one standard deviation during retail, and the average plus one standard deviation during consumer storage. The two-part model accounted for lag time and exponential growth. Under simulated average conditions, the population of *L. monocytogenes* after 7 days was <100 cfu/g. In the "worst 10%" run, the population exceeded 10^9 cfu/g after 7 days. The remaining runs showed populations of roughly 10^3 cfu/g after 7 days—somewhat higher after retail temperature abuse than after home temperature abuse. Due to the influence of lag time, the initial time–temperature conditions of product history significantly affected the final population size. These data demonstrated the dependence of product safety on time–temperature conditions integrated over the product's life-cycle.

"Acid shock" at pH 5.0 induced acid tolerance in *L. monocytogenes* subsequently grown at pH 3.0–3.5 (*629*). Postulated mechanisms for this response include decreased membrane conductivity to protons, increased proton extrusion, and increased buffering capacity of the cytoplasm.

Viable populations of *L. monocytogenes* were monitored in egg fractions during storage at various temperatures (*630*). Commercially dried whole eggs and yolks and liquid whole eggs were inoculated with 10 or 10^5 cfu/g. Dried products were stored at 5 and 20°C for 6 months; liquid eggs were stored at 0°C for 2 weeks and at −18°C for 24 weeks. All products yielded viable listerias throughout storage at both high and low inoculum levels. Some inactivation, more pronounced at 20 than at 5°C, occurred in the dried products.

During fermentation of unacidified horsebean, pea, chickpea, and soybean tempeh inoculated with ~300 cfu/g of *L. monocytogenes*, the *Listeria* population increased to 10^6 cfu/g (*631*). Inoculation with *Lactobacillus plantarum* completely inhibited *L. monocytogenes* growth in fermenting pea, chickpea, and soybean tempeh and retarded growth in horsebean tempeh. Acidification of the beans during soaking had no significant effect on the results. Use of *L. plantarum* was suggested to control undesirable microorganisms during commercial production of tempeh.

Samples of smoked salmon of good and relatively poor microbiological quality were inoculated with 6 or 600 cfu/g of a 3-strain mixture of *L. monocytogenes* and stored for 5 weeks at 4°C (*632*). The *Listeria* grew well in all samples, increasing by as much as a factor of 5. The salmon was still organoleptically acceptable after 4 weeks. Growth of *Listeria* was somewhat faster in fish of better microbiological quality; all three strains were found after 4 weeks in the fish of good quality, whereas only two were recovered from the fish of poorer quality. These results demonstrated the possibility of consumers being exposed to considerable numbers of *L. monocytogenes* in smoked salmon and

emphasized the importance of preventing contamination or recontamination during smoked salmon production. Another study evaluated the survival and growth of *L. monocytogenes* Scott A in refrigerated and frozen shrimp and finfish packaged under conditions supporting different rates of oxygen and water transmission (*633*). During 21 days of storage on ice or 3 months of frozen storage, small decreases in listerial populations were noted. Neither vacuum packaging nor packaging material significantly affected the results.

Evaluation of the effects of modified-atmosphere packaging (MAP) on growth of *Pseudomonas fluorescens* and *L. monocytogenes* Scott A on precooked dark-meat chicken nuggets stored at 3, 7, and 11°C showed that MAP inhibited *P. fluorescens* more than it inhibited *Listeria* (*634*). Even though somewhat inhibited, the *Listeria* could grow at all three temperatures. Comparable results were obtained with an oxygen-free atmosphere and one with 10.7% oxygen. The effectiveness of MAP decreased with increasing temperature.

Because *Listeria* is commonly found in nonfecal habitats and is relatively cold-tolerant, the presence of most indicator organisms in a food has little relationship to the presence of *L. monocytogenes*. Tests of the survival of *Salmonella typhimurium*, *L. monocytogenes*, and several indicator bacteria on vacuum-packaged, cooked, uncured turkey loaf stored at 3°C gave comparable results for *L. monocytogenes* and *Enterococcus faecalis*, suggesting use of enterococci as indicators of possible *L. monocytogenes* contamination of processed refrigerated foods (*635*).

Beaker sausage was made with and without addition of a 1% *Pediococcus* starter culture; 200 ppm of TBHQ or BHA was added to some sausage made without starter culture (*636*). *Listeria monocytogenes* was inoculated to give ~$10^{6.5}$ cfu/g, and pH and listerial populations were monitored during 75 h of fermentation. There was an initial pH increase in sausage without starter culture, followed by a decrease; with *Pediococcus*, pH fell throughout fermentation. The number of *L. monocytogenes* increased by 1.57 log in sausage made with no additives; TBHQ inhibited growth slightly, but BHA had no effect. Starter culture, however, caused a 2.49-log decrease in listerial populations during fermentation. The authors concluded that *L. monocytogenes* can grow during natural fermentation of sausage and eating such a product carries a risk of listeriosis. Addition of a suitable starter culture not only prevents growth of the pathogen but causes its rapid demise.

Samples of sterile cow's milk were inoculated with a yogurt culture and either 10^3 or 10^7 cfu/mL of *L. monocytogenes,* fermented at 42°C for 5 h, and refrigerated at 4°C (*637*). Low inocula survived for 48 h and high inocula survived for 7 days but no cells were detectable after 5 and 15 days, respectively, by either direct-plating or cold-enrichment techniques. Marth's research group inoculated unfiltered skim milk and retentate and permeate from ultrafiltered skim milk with 5.5×10^3–1.5×10^7 cfu/mL of *L. monocytogenes* and 4×10^7–2.3×10^8 cfu/mL of mesophilic lactic acid bacteria (*638*). Bacterial counts were monitored during 36 h of incubation at 30°C. Inactivation of *L. monocytogenes* by lactic acid bacteria ranged from 3.67 log in unfiltered milk to 6.77 log in permeate. The degree of inactivation in retentate was inversely related to the concentration factor. In no case was inactivation complete within 36 h. When fermented products were refrigerated at 4°C, survival ranged from 1 week in permeate to 4–6 weeks in unfiltered milk.

Several investigators have studied the behavior of *L. monocytogenes* in cow's milk under various circumstances (*639–642*). Thermal inactivation of *L. monocytogenes* serotype 4b was monitored in naturally and artificially contaminated milk (*639*). Milk was heated at 71.1°C for 2, 4, 10, 15, 20, and 39 s and survivors were monitored during 4 weeks of storage at 4°C. No survivors were detected in naturally infected milk for any heating time. Survivors were found in inoculated samples with initial titers of 800–7000 from the 2- and 4-s heat treatments, but only after 28 days of cold storage. No survivors were detected for longer heat treatments. Farrag and Marth studied the behavior of *L. monocytogenes* in milk in the presence of other psychrotrophic bacteria (*640,641*). When sterile samples of skim milk were inoculated with *L. monocytogenes* alone or along with *Flavobacterium lutescens* ATCC 27951 or *Flavobacterium* sp. ATCC

21429, listerial growth was significantly enhanced during incubation at 7 or 13°C in mixed culture with *F. lutescens* (*640*). Growth also occurred in mixed culture with *Flavobacterium* sp. ATCC 21429 but was significantly less than in the control. *Listeria* did not affect growth of the flavobacteria, and no marked differences in pH were noted between cultures. *Pseudomonas fluorescens* usually dominates the bacterial flora of refrigerated raw milk (*641*). *Listeria monocytogenes* strains California and V7 were slightly inhibited after extended incubation in the presence of this organism, the degree of inhibition depending on the strain of *Listeria,* incubation temperature, and initial population of *P.fluorescens.* Little or no effect was observed on growth of strain Scott A, other than perhaps a slight stimulation at 7 days. Other investigators have reported that *Pseudomonas* spp. can stimulate the growth of *L. monocytogenes* in milk. Marshall and Schmidt sought a possible physiological mechanism for this (*642*). First they showed that *L. monocytogenes* grew equally well in milk under aerobic and microaerophilic environments, ruling out the microaerophilic hypothesis for *Pseudomonas*-stimulated growth. Then they inoculated milk with *P. fluorescens* and preincubated it for 3 days at 10°C, after which they inoculated it with *L. monocytogenes* and incubated it for 8 days more (*642*). Changes in various milk components were monitored. Both organisms hydrolyzed milk fat but neither could use lactose, showing that neither of these biochemical activities explains *Pseudomonas*-stimulated growth. However, milk protein was hydrolyzed by *P. fluorescens* but not by *Listeria* and the generation time of *L. monocytogenes* was significantly shorter in milk proteolyzed with purified fungal protease. These results provided support for the proteolysis theory of *Pseudomonas*-stimulated growth.

Because soft cheeses are frequently implicated in outbreaks and cases of listeriosis, the survival and growth of five strains of *L. monocytogenes* was determined in 49 artificially contaminated market cheeses stored at 4–30°C (*643*). Eighteen cheeses supported increases in cell numbers of 0.2–3.6 log at at least one temperature. Cheeses that supported growth were soft Hispanic, ricotta, teleme, brie, camembert, and cottage. Except for cottage cheese, all had pH values ≥5.9. In contrast, cheeses that caused gradual death of the pathogen at all temperatures had pH values between 4.3 and 5.6, with the notable exceptions of limburger (pH 7.2) and several process cheeses (pH range 5.7–6.4). There was a highly significant correlation between listerial growth and use of starter cultures during cheese manufacture. The authors concluded that cross-contamination of opened packages of certain cheeses with *L. monocytogenes* could permit significant growth during refrigerated storage. During the manufacture of Swiss cheese from milk artificially contaminated with *L. monocytogenes*, populations of the pathogen increased during initial stages but fell sharply during the brining of cheese blocks and continued to decrease during ripening (*644*). The California strain was no longer detected after 80 days of ripening; two other strains disappeared sooner. The authors concluded that Swiss cheese made according to the procedure described does not support extended survival of *L. monocytogenes* and that ripening for 60 days should result in pathogen-free product if initial contamination is ≤100 cfu/mL of milk. A similar study during manufacture of mozzarella cheese again documented small increases in *L. monocytogenes* populations at early stages but complete disappearance of the pathogen during the stretching procedure (*645*).

Control

NATURAL ANTIMICROBIAL SYSTEMS AND BACTERIOCINS. The lactoperoxidase–thiocyanate–hydrogen peroxide (LP) system in milk is bactericidal against many gram-negative organisms. However, because only bacteriostatic effects had been established against gram-positive organisms, the activity of the LP system against four strains of *L. monocytogenes* was studied in refrigerated raw milk (*646*). The system was activated by adding 0.25 mM sodium thiocyanate and 0.25 mM H_2O_2. A time- and temperature-dependent bactericidal effect that varied with the listerial strain was seen. *D* values in activated LP system milk were 4.1–11.2 days at 4°C and 4.4–9.7 days at 8°C. The lactoperoxidase level fell during the incubation, more at 8 than at 4°C and more in control than in activated milk. The authors

concluded that LP system activation is feasible for temporarily controlling development of *L. monocytogenes* in refrigerated raw milk. Cow's milk also contains lactoferrin, from which the potent antimicrobial peptide lactoferricin has been derived (*647*). In culture media, lactoferricin completely inhibited growth of four strains of *L. monocytogenes*, including clinical isolates, at concentrations of 0.3–9 µg/mL. The bactericidal effect was strong over the pH range of 5.5–7.5, but varied with the listerial strain and medium—particularly its salt composition. The authors concluded that this new peptide deserves further consideration and investigation for control of *Listeria*.

The sensitivity of three strains of *L. monocytogenes* to nisin was determined using a direct-plating method (*648*). At 10 µg/mL, nisin decreased an initial *L. monocytogenes* population of 10^9 cfu/mL by 6–7 log. Sensitivity was enhanced in the presence of 2% NaCl or when the pH of the medium was reduced from 6.5 to 5.5 with HCl or lactic acid. Mutants resistant to 50 µg/mL of nisin occurred at a frequency of 10^{-8}–10^{-6}. The authors warned that nisin-resistant mutants should be expected when nisin is used in food systems. Another study of nisin showed that its activity in foods strongly depends on the chemical composition of the food (*649*). Binding or adsorption to certain food components renders nisin inactive or unavailable for inhibiting microorganisms. In fluid milk, the effectiveness of nisin is inversely related to fat content. Decreases in activity were partially counteracted by the nonionic emulsifier Tween 80, but the anionic emulsifier lecithin had no effect. These results suggest that the usefulness of nisin for listerial control in fat-containing dairy products is limited.

Sulzer and Busse monitored the effects of *Enterococcus faecalis*, *Lactobacillus paracasei*, and *Lactococcus lactis* on growth of listerias on camembert cheese produced in the laboratory and artificially contaminated (*650*). Cheeses having clearly defined bacterial and fungal floras could be produced. Complete inhibition occurred only when the inhibitory strain was used as the sole starter culture, listerial contamination occurred during the early stage of ripening, and the level of contamination was low. In one experiment, there was no inhibitory effect when *Listeria* was added to vat milk, perhaps because rapid multiplication occurred before acidification halted growth. The authors warned against overrating the potential of antilisterial bacteria in cheese-making, although in conjunction with good manufacturing practice, and properly applied, they might provide an added safeguard against low-level contamination with *Listeria* during molding and brining.

Two starter cultures that inhibited *L. monocytogenes* in vitro were tested for inhibitory activity in artificially contaminated mettwurst produced in the laboratory (*651*). No listerial growth occurred during 28 days of storage at 5°C, regardless of whether the inhibitory starter cultures had been added. At 18–22°C, the starter cultures neither reduced colony counts in the raw material nor inhibited listerial growth in the finished product.

Several research groups reported studies of inhibition of *Listeria* in foods by *Pediococcus acidilactici* or its bacteriocin, pediocin (*652–654*). Sterile ground beef, sausage mix, cottage cheese, ice cream, and reconstituted dry milk were suspended in water; *Listeria* cells and pediocin AcH were added, and listerial counts were monitored during storage at 4 and 10°C (*652*). Pediocin AcH exerted its maximal bactericidal effect within 1 h and in this system, food components did not interfere with it. *Listeria ivanovii* ATCC 19119 was extremely sensitive (counts <10 cfu/mL with 1350 AU/mL of pediocin AcH after 1 h at 4°C in all foods, compared to 10^7 cfu/mL without pediocin). The effect on three strains of *L. monocytogenes* was smaller. The reduction in cfu was directly related to pediocin level and inversely related to the size of the *Listeria* inoculum. Surviving listerias multiplied in the presence of residual pediocin during storage at 4 and 10°C. To determine whether pediocin is produced and has antilisterial activity during manufacture of dry fermented sausage, tests were conducted with isogenic pediocin-positive and -negative strains of *P. acidilactici* (*653*). A five-strain composite of *L. monocytogenes* was used to preclude the chance selection of a single unusually sensitive or resistant strain. The production process, involving fermentation, minimal heating, and drying, reduced *L. monocytogenes* populations by 5 log or

more regardless of whether pediocin was produced, although pediocin enhanced the reduction. This effect could be particularly important if fermentation does not sufficiently lower pH. However, emergence of resistant listerial strains is likely after prolonged or repeated exposure to bacteriocins. Other experiments evaluated pediocin AcH–producing and –nonproducing strains of *P. acidilactici* for production of antilisterial compounds in packages of all-beef wieners (*654*). Freshly manufactured commercial wieners were surface-inoculated with *L. monocytogenes, P. acidilactici,* or both, vacuum-packaged, and stored at 4 or 25°C. Both organisms survived 72 days' storage at 4°C but *P. acidilactici* produced neither acid nor pediocin. At 25°C *Listeria* counts increased in the absence of *P. acidilactici,* remained stable with the pediocin-nonproducing strain, and decreased with the pediocin-producing strain. The authors concluded that bacteriocinogenic pediococci can help to control *L. monocytogenes* in temperature-abused cook–chill meats. Another study determined the behavior of *L. monocytogenes* on wieners surface-inoculated with bacteriocin-producing and -nonproducing *P. acidilactici* strains and stored at abuse or refrigeration temperatures (*655*). On wieners refrigerated for 60 days without addition of pediococci, *L. monocytogenes* populations increased from 10^4 to 10^6 cfu/g, with a lag time of 20–30 days. With 10^3–10^4 cfu/g of pediococci lag time was increased and a bacteriocin effect was apparent; 10^7 cfu/g of pediococci prevented growth up to 60 days but no reduction in viable cells occurred. Under anaerobic conditions, high levels of either *Pediococcus* strain prevented growth of *L. monocytogenes* for at least 15 days at 15°C. Some growth occurred during 15 days under aerobic conditions at 15°C; the bacteriocin-producing strain was more inhibitory than the nonproducing strain.

Six strains of *Enterococcus faecalis* were evaluated for antilisterial activity using the agar spot test (*656*). NRIC strains 1143 and 1144 were strongly active against all *L. monocytogenes* strains tested; strain NCFB 2131 was slightly inhibitory. Activity was not affected by addition of catalase but was partially or completely destroyed by pronase, trypsin, or α-chymotrypsin (but not pepsin). This suggests that the inhibitory molecules are proteins.

Lactobacillus sake Lb 706 releases a bacteriocin inhibitory to *L. monocytogenes*. A bacteriocin-negative variant of this strain did not inhibit listerial growth in vitro (*657*). In artificially contaminated pasteurized minced meat, the number of viable *L. monocytogenes* cells increased from 10^5/g to 10^8/g during 6 days at 8°C and to ~10^6/g with the bacteriocin-negative strain, but remained constant in the presence of the bacteriocin-positive strain. Inhibition occurred only during the first week. In model German-type fresh mettwurst at a pH of 6.3, *L. sake* delayed growth of listerias during the first few days but the effect of the bacteriocin-negative strain was small. At a pH of 5.7, listerias did not multiply and the bacteriocin-positive strain of *L. sake* reduced viable counts by about 1 log.

ANTILISTERIAL ACTIVITY IN FOODS. The antilisterial effects of raw egg albumen appear to be caused primarily by lysozyme and enhanced by ovomucoid, conalbumin, and alkaline pH (*658*). At a concentration of 15% in trypticase soy broth, albumen was listeristatic after 24 h at 35°C; at higher concentrations it was listericidal. The activity was heat-labile, but supplementation with iron or biotin had no effect. The antilisterial effect of lysozyme was augmented at pH 9, as was the smaller effect of conalbumin; ovomucoid was inhibitory only at pH 9. Another study of lysozyme showed that *L. monocytogenes* Scott A grown at 37°C was 1.8–2.5 times more resistant to the enzyme's action than cells grown at 5–19°C (*659*). The authors suggested that lysozyme might be used to control *Listeria* in refrigerated foods.

The antilisterial activity of 32 common plant essential oils was evaluated against four strains of *L. monocytogenes* and one of *L. innocua* (*660*). Cinnamon, clove, origanum, pimento, and thyme had considerable activity in a paper disc diffusion test at a 1:5 (v/v) dilution in ethanol. When clove, origanum, and thyme oil were tested at a 1:50 dilution, inhibitory zones were still seen but they were smaller and varied in size among strains. In a saline solution system, pimento oil had marked activity within an hour of exposure; the response to clove, origanum, and thyme oils was slower. Thyme oil incorporated into a minced pork matrix reduced

the *L. monocytogenes* population 100-fold during the first week of storage. The authors concluded that some spices have potential as antilisteric preservatives in food. Experiments with finely ground spices produced slightly different results (*661*). When 13 spices were screened for antilisterial activity at 24°C using a concentration-gradient plate method, cloves and oregano were the most inhibitory, with MICs of 0.5–0.7% (w/v) depending on listerial strain. Sage and rosemary had MICs of 0.7–1.0% and nutmeg, 1.1–1.4%. At a concentration of 0.5% in tryptic soy broth, cloves were bactericidal and oregano was bacteriostatic at 4 and 24°C; sage was bactericidal at the lower temperature and bacteriostatic at the higher. In a sterile meat slurry, however, neither cloves nor oregano had a significant effect on growth of *L. monocytogenes* Scott A.

Shredded or sliced carrots rapidly caused lethal or sublethal damage to *L. monocytogenes* (*662*). Gently macerated carrots were also antilisterial, but vigorous maceration destroyed the activity. All five cultivars tested were active, but to varying degrees, against 9 strains of *L. monocytogenes* and single strains of four other *Listeria* spp. The effect was seen over the pH range of 5.8–7.0 and from 4 to 30°C, but it was heat-labile and unstable, disappearing after a few hours even at 4°C. The authors did not comment on the possible nature of the factor other than to say that antagonism by other microorganisms was extremely unlikely.

CHEMICAL AND PHYSICAL CONTROL. The growth of *L. monocytogenes* on artificially contaminated chicken legs was monitored during buffered lactic acid treatment alone or in conjunction with MAP (*663*). The antimicrobial and antilisterial activity of the pH 3 buffer systems increased as the concentration of lactic acid was increased from 2% to 10%. Combined use of 10% lactic acid–sodium lactate buffer and packaging in an atmosphere of 90% CO_2–10% O_2 produced the best results. This system suppressed growth of both psychrotrophic aerobes and *L. monocytogenes,* prolonging shelf life by 11 days at 6°C; after 13 days of storage, populations of *L. monocytogenes* had just returned to the inoculum level.

Marth and his coworkers investigated the effects of propionate on *L. monocytogenes* (*664,665*). Following up studies suggesting that the limited antilisterial activity of propionate is enhanced at pH 5.0 in the presence of certain other organic acids, El-Shenawy and Marth determined the behavior of *L. monocytogenes* V7 at 13 and 35°C in tryptose broth containing 0–0.3% propionate, when pH was adjusted to 5.0 and 5.6 with acetic, tartaric, citric, or lactic acid or HCl (*664*). Organic acids had some intrinsic antilisterial activity, as manifest by increased lag and generation times. Acetic and tartaric acids were most effective. Effects of all chemical treatments were greater at the higher temperature and the lower pH, and with the highest concentration of propionate. The authors stressed the importance of replicating these studies in food systems. Buazzi and Marth studied the nature of propionate injury to *L. monocytogenes* (*665*). Exposure of bacteria to 8% (w/v) propionate for 60 min injured 87% of the population, as shown by the ability to grow on tryptose agar with no added salt but inability to tolerate addition of 6% NaCl. Repair of injured cells did not require electron transport or synthesis of cell-wall components, mRNA, or protein. Injured cells did not leak protein or nucleotides into the medium. Exogenous cations promoted recovery. The most likely cause of cellular damage appeared to be inhibition of lactic dehydrogenase synthesis or function.

Certain fatty acids are among the natural compounds in foods that inhibit growth of foodborne pathogens. Wang and Johnson studied the sensitivity of *L. monocytogenes* to several fatty acids in bovine milk fat when the compounds were added to brain–heart infusion broth, whole milk, or skim milk (*666*). In brain–heart infusion broth the most active compounds were $C_{12:0}$, $C_{18:3}$, and glyceryl monolaurate (monolaurin); all bactericidal activity was greater at pH 5 than at pH 6. Potassium-conjugated linoleic acid was bacteriostatic in whole and skim milk and prolonged the lag phase, especially at 4°C. Monolaurin was effective only in skim milk. No other acid was effective in milk. These results suggest that potassium-conjugated linoleic acids or monolaurin could be used to inhibit *L. monocytogenes* in dairy foods. Another study showed

that in vitro, the MIC of monolaurin against four strains of *L. monocytogenes* at 35°C was lower than values reported for potassium sorbate, TBH, propyl paraben, and BHA (*667*). Reducing the pH from 7.0 to 5.0 reduced the MIC from 10 to 3 μg/mL.

Marth's group showed that exposure to 8.5% sodium benzoate, pH 7.0, for 1 h injured >99% of *L. monocytogenes* cells, as indicated by their inability to tolerate 6% NaCl in tryptose agar (*668*). Injured cells recovered when they were incubated in tryptose broth containing sublethal amounts of metabolic or synthetic inhibitors. Restoration of salt tolerance required mRNA synthesis but not electron transport, protein synthesis, or cell-wall repair. Injured cells did not leak proteins or nucleotides into the medium, indicating that benzoate did not inflict cell-wall damage. In similar studies, they demonstrated recovery of *L. monocytogenes* cells injured by a 30-min treatment with 1% (w/v) potassium sorbate (*669*). 2,4-Dinitrophenol was the only inhibitor that prevented recovery, suggesting that electron transport, synthesis of high-energy intermediates, and oxidative phosphorylation are involved in the salt tolerance of potassium sorbate–injured *L. monocytogenes* cells. For reasons they discussed, the authors believed the observed phenomena were due to potassium sorbate rather than sorbic acid. In studies similar to those with propionate (*664*), they investigated the interaction of potassium sorbate with other organic acids as a function of temperature and pH (*670*). Again, inhibition was dose-related and greater at higher temperature and lower pH. The greatest antilisterial activity occurred when pH was adjusted with acetic or tartaric acid.

The interactive effects of temperature, pH, NaCl, and $NaNO_2$ on growth of *L. monocytogenes* were clearly demonstrated using an automated turbidimetric system with multiwelled plates (*671*). Combinations that permitted growth were readily apparent when data were presented in tabular form and when pairs of variables were manipulated and results shown as bars in three dimensions. Drawbacks of the turbidimetric system were also discussed.

Because of reports that *L. monocytogenes* has a greater chance to survive heating in cured pork than in fresh pork, the thermal destruction of *L.*

monocytogenes in ground pork was studied in relation to the effects of cooking temperature and added water and curing agents (*672*). At internal product temperatures <65°C, 2.0–2.5% sodium chloride alone or in combination with other curing agents (1% dextrose, 0.055% sodium erythorbate, and 0.156% sodium nitrite) significantly decreased thermal destruction. Added water, sodium phosphates, and sodium erythorbate had no important effect on survival of *L. monocytogenes* in ground pork during heating.

The combined effects of water activity and solute on survival and growth of *L. monocytogenes* were determined at 28°C for a_w values of .99–.80 with glycerol, NaCl, and propylene glycol (*673*). The minimum a_ws for growth for these three solutes were .90, .92, and .97, respectively. Survival time decreased as minimum a_w increased. These results provide quantitative isothermal criteria for estimating the a_w necessary to prevent growth of *L. monocytogenes* in food.

High concentrations of NaCl [6, 16, and 26% (w/v)] were tested for their ability to destroy *L. monocytogenes* at low (10°C), refrigeration (2°C), or freezing (–18°C) temperatures (*674*). No salt concentration was able to reduce numbers during 6 h at 10 or 2°C. Over a 33-day period at low temperatures, the bacterial population grew in 6% NaCl, showed no change in 16% NaCl, and declined in 26% NaCl. The decline was too slow, however, for immersion in 26% brine to be a useful bacteriological treatment. With frozen storage for 33 days there was no significant change in numbers at any NaCl concentration.

The ability of modified atmospheres containing 20, 30, 50, and 80% CO_2 (by volume, remainder as N_2) to inhibit growth of *L. monocytogenes* in sliced brühwurst was determined at 4, 7, and 10°C (*675*). Only 80% CO_2 inhibited growth of the organism at all temperatures. With 50% CO_2 growth was prevented for 3 weeks at 4°C, but there was a 1.5-log increase after 3 weeks at 7°C and a 3-log increase after 2 weeks at 10°C. Decreasing the volume of gas as well as the concentration of CO_2 decreased the inhibitory activity.

Thermal destruction of *L. monocytogenes* was studied in cooked lobster meat (*676*), ice cream mix (*677*), and ground beef and turkey (*678*). In artificially contaminated cooked lobster, D decreased from 97.0 to 1.06 min as temperature increased from 51.6 to 62.7°C; the z value was 5.0°C. Authors of the ice cream study concluded that pasteurization guidelines for ice cream mix are adequate to ensure inactivation of *L. monocytogenes* (*677*). However, the common stabilizer used, which contained guar gum and carrageenan, clearly increased the organism's thermal resistance. Survivor data revealed sigmoidal responses with initial shoulders and tailing. Shoulder values were not significantly affected by high-fructose corn syrup solids or milkfat content, but D and F were affected by high-fructose corn syrup solids, which conferred increasing heat resistance at higher concentrations. *D*- and *z*-values for *L. monocytogenes* strain Scott A were determined in lean and fatty ground beef and attempts were made to determine a $D_{160°F}$ value for ground turkey (*678*). Two recovery media gave similar results, but counts were generally higher on CNA agar base containing sodium pyruvate overlaid with CNA plus horse blood (CBNA) than on *Listeria* plating medium, and z values on CBNA were lower. With the ground turkey emulsion, a discontinuity caused by a phase separation made calculation of $D_{160°F}$ impossible. D was estimated to be ~0.35 min, but the recovery of survivors at 160°F indicated that a few organisms can survive if initial contamination levels are high.

Australian investigators compared the effects of microwave and conventional cooking on temperature profiles and microbial flora of naturally contaminated ground beef cooked in 500-g loaves to the rare, medium, and well-done stages according to procedures recommended for roasts (*679*). All raw samples contained large numbers of bacteria, and low numbers of *L. monocytogenes* occurred in the majority of samples. A substantial proportion of the microflora survived in all microwaved loaves before the recommended 30-min standing period. *Listeria monocytogenes* survived in all samples immediately after microwaving to the rare stage and in 1 of 3 samples after the standing period. It was also detected before the standing period in 1 of 3 samples microwaved to the medium stage. It was not detected in any loaves cooked in a conventional oven. Another study assessed the thermal inactivation of *L. monocytogenes* in culture broth and on chicken skin during a conventional heating process that simulated temperatures achieved during microwave cooking (*680*). In broth, viable bacterial populations were reduced by a factor of $>10^6$ at 70°C. Results on chicken skin were more variable, but no organisms survived at a mean measured temperature of 85°C. When skin was heated in a submerged system to 70°C for 2 min a 10^6- to 10^8-fold reduction in viable cell numbers was achieved. These results suggest that the survival of *L. monocytogenes* during microwave heating is due to uneven heating that leaves cold spots in the food. The heat resistance observed here for *L. monocytogenes* was comparable with that of many other non-spore-forming mesophilic bacteria.

Listeria innocua transformed with an antibiotic resistance plasmid was evaluated as a thermal resistance indicator for *L. monocytogenes* (*681*). It retained the plasmid during heating, was easily selected and enumerated among a large and complex background microflora, and was more heat-resistant between 56 and 66°C than *L. monocytogenes*. It therefore would be a useful indicator to evaluate the lethality of thermal processes with respect to *L. monocytogenes* in a laboratory setting, but might not be appropriate for application in a food-processing environment.

Although MAP and controlled storage are increasingly used to extend the shelf-life of raw chickens, these measures may not prevent proliferation of *Listeria* (*682*). Nor is irradiation certain to destroy *Listeria*. In fact, it may increase the hazard by removing the incentive to practice good husbandry and hygiene. In unirradiated chickens, *L. monocytogenes* proliferated similarly in air- and vacuum-packs, increasing by ~1.5 log after 15 days' storage at 4°C. It was not detected in air-packaged chickens irradiated with 2.5 kGy, but was recovered from vacuum-packaged irradiated chickens after 7 days of cold storage.

Detection and identification

Kerr and Lacey presented general guidelines for isolation and identification of *L. monocytogenes*

from clinical specimens (*683*), and Slade reviewed detection and isolation of *Listeria* in food-processing plants (*684*). No single protocol is ideal for all samples. Slade discussed some useful adjuncts to conventional culture techniques. Resuscitation of stressed *L. monocytogenes* presents special problems, which were addressed. More information is needed on indicators of *L. monocytogenes* in the food-production environment and on the organism's ecology, including its interactions with the normal flora of the processing plant and foods and how these affect its selective recovery.

CULTURE AND BIOCHEMICAL METHODS. During surveillance for sporadic listeriosis, investigators from the CDC and the Listeria Study Group examined 402 food samples collected from refrigerators of listeriosis patients, comparing the cold enrichment and USDA methods (*685*). *Listeria monocytogenes* was isolated from 51 samples (13%). Isolation efficiencies of the USDA and cold-enrichment methods were 96 and 59%, respectively. Cold enrichment failed to detect many positive samples if they contained <0.3 cfu/g. However, the USDA method failed to recover *L. monocytogenes* from two samples that were positive by cold enrichment, and recovery of sublethally injured cells by the USDA procedure may be problematic because of the selective chemicals used for enrichment. Nevertheless, these data convincingly demonstrated the superiority of the USDA method over cold enrichment for isolating *L. monocytogenes* from a broad variety of foods. Eleven Canadian laboratories compared modified FDA and USDA methods in a study designed to establish uniform methodology for regulatory use to detect *L. monocytogenes* in food and environmental samples (*686*). The modified FDA method detected 92% of positive samples after a 24-h enrichment; 10 more samples became positive after 48 h, but 11 that were positive after 24 h became negative. The modified FDA and USDA methods were comparable to within 1% in their ability to isolate *L. moncytogenes*. Modified Fraser broth was a useful screening tool but was not very selective. Oxford agar was slightly better than lithium chloride–phenethanol–moxalactam (LPM) medium and significantly better than modified Oxford agar in isolating the organism. The authors recommended the modified USDA method for all food and environmental samples and offered specific suggestions for the protocol. Another collaborative study compared two enrichment methods (USDA and a modified FDA method) and two isolation media (LPM and Oxford agars) for detecting *L. monocytogenes* in artificially contaminated foods (*687*). Treatment of the enriched culture with KOH before plating was also evaluated. Results from the two enrichment procedures were comparable. Oxford agar was superior to LPM agar. KOH treatment did not significantly increase the detection rate. Fewer than 0.2 cfu/g of *L. monocytogenes* could be detected in cheese; for meat, the detection level was <5 cfu/g. Based on these results, a Nordic Committee on Food Analysis (NMKL) method for detecting *L. monocytogenes* in foods was developed.

Three enrichment media and four selective plating media were compared for isolation of *Listeria* from raw milk (*688*). L-Palcamy broth was slightly more effective in enhancing growth of listerias overall (50 of 300 samples, 16.7%) than University of Vermont medium (UVM) followed by Fraser broth (15.3%) and *Listeria* enrichment broth (14.0%). However, L-Palcamy was far superior in enhancing isolation of *L. monocytogenes*. As plating media, Oxford and Palcam agar were better than LPM and modified McBride agar. The incidence of *Listeria* spp. in the 300 milk samples was 28%; *L. innocua* was isolated from 26.7%, *L. monocytogenes* from 3.0%, and *L. welshimeri* from 1.7%. Milks with high standard plate counts tended to have a high incidence of *Listeria*.

After an enrichment procedure, Oxford agar, Palcam agar, and blood agar with nalidixic acid yielded identical percentages of *Listeria*-positive samples (15.8%) in an examination of 391 samples of meats, fish, and dairy products (*689*). *Listeria monocytogenes* was found in 8.4% of meats and fish and 8.2% of dairy products. Palcam and Oxford agar afforded greater suppression of background microflora and results were easier to read.

Three procedures were compared for isolation and enumeration of *Listeria* spp. in naturally and artificially contaminated fermented sausages (*690*). A double-layer tryptone–soy–yeast extract

agar plus Palcam plating method was slightly more effective than Oxford or Palcam medium, but the difference was not significant. Choice of enrichment broth was more critical. UVM 1 and 2 broths in conjunction with an ELISA or isolation on Oxford medium gave the best results, followed by Palcamy enrichment broth and isolation on Palcam plates; enrichment in *Listeria* enrichment broth with isolation on Oxford agar was least effective. For identification of species, a set of 9 tests was compared with the more extensive Micro-ID Listeria System. The two gave identical results. Although the additional tests in the Micro-ID system are important to distinguish *Listeria* from other genera, they are not necessary to distinguish between species of *Listeria*.

The Rosco system was evaluated by using it to identify previously confirmed isolates of 7 species of *Listeria* from clinical, environmental, and food samples (*691*). The system includes tests for fermentation of trehalose, salicin, mannitol, rhamnose, and xylose and for α-mannosidase activity. All 155 isolates were identified correctly. If heavy inocula were used, results could be obtained in 4 h. Because *L. innocua* and *L. monocytogenes* give identical results in this system, they must be distinguished by the CAMP test and hemolytic activity on sheep-blood agar. Another rapid identification system for *Listeria* spp., Micro-ID, gave results identical to those from the Bacteriological Analytical Manual (BAM) procedure for 73 cultures (63 *Listeria* isolates representing all 7 species and 10 other gram-positive organisms) (*692*). Micro-ID consists of 15 tests and is performed in conjunction with CAMP and hemolysis tests. It yields results after 24 h, compared to 7 days for BAM.

In the Netherlands, 16 laboratories enumerated *L. monocytogenes* in reference samples comparing blood, Palcam, Palcamy, and Oxford agars (*693*). Significant differences were found between laboratories; some consistently obtained counts above or below the average. Blood agar gave significantly higher counts than the other media, and recovery on all media was greater after 48 h of incubation than after 24 h. The egg yolk in Palcamy agar appeared to facilitate recovery of sublethally injured cells.

Busch and Donnelly formulated a *Listeria* repair broth (LRB) by individually testing numerous substances as supplements to trypticase soy broth and selecting those that had the greatest impact on repair of heat-injured *L. monocytogenes* and *L. innocua* cells (*694*). LRB contained trypticase soy broth with glucose, yeast extract, magnesium sulfate, ferrous sulfate, pyruvic acid, and 3-*N*-morpholinepropanesulfonate (as free acid and the sodium salt). Incubated in this medium, heat-injured *Listeria* cells completed repair in 5 h. After repair, acriflavin, nalidixic acid, and cycloheximide were added to the LRB at the concentrations recommended for selective enrichment broths used in FDA and USDA procedures. No repair was observed in FDA, *Listeria*, or University of Vermont enrichment broths. The final *Listeria* populations after 24 h of incubation in these media were 2×10^8–9×10^8 cfu/mL, whereas populations in LRB were consistently in the range of 2×10^{11}–8×10^{11} cfu/mL.

Premaratne et al. modified Welshimer's chemically defined minimal medium to better support growth of *L. monocytogenes* (*695*). The major change was an enhanced buffering capacity and inclusion of ferric citrate. Concentrations of biotin and thioctic acid were increased fivefold, riboflavin was decreased, and L-histidine and L-tryptophan were omitted. Several sugars and amino sugars supported at least some growth in the absence of glucose, but no organic or amino acid tested could replace glucose. Chitin and cell walls of *Lactococcus lactis* supported survival, suggesting that *L. monocytogenes* can obtain carbon and energy during colonization of foods by digesting cell walls of the bacterial flora. The new medium was suggested for use in determining the nutrients involved in food colonization by *L. monocytogenes* and in studies of the organism's survival and resistance properties.

Complete factorial design experiments (5×5×4×5) were conducted to evaluate the interactive effects of atmosphere, listerial strain or species, temperature, and storage time on the probability that one listerial cell would initiate colony formation (*696*). Each variable except strain of *Listeria* had a significant effect. The inhibitory effect of 100% CO_2 was augmented at low temperatures: at ≤8°C it extended the lag phase and at 4°C it also decreased the growth rate. *Listeria ivanovii* was the most sensitive to CO_2.

Thirty-two bacterial isolates from food, chosen for their resistance to the selective agents in *Listeria* enrichment and isolation media, were tested for competition with *L. monocytogenes* LM82 during enrichment (*697*). Competition was rated according to the inoculum size of a test strain required to mask identification of 10 cfu of LM82 inoculated into 10 mL of *Listeria* enrichment broth. Although many strains of food microflora survived in the enrichment and isolation environments, they did not all compete with *Listeria,* and not all strains in a competitive species were necessarily competitive. For example, one strain of *Enterococcus faecium* competed strongly; one was weakly competitive and one noncompetitive.

Even with use of highly selective enrichment and isolation media, the hemolytic phenotype of *Listeria* spp. must be verified. This can be done directly on selective agar by overlaying with an erythrocyte-containing layer. Because the performance of the overlay method is influenced by the choice of selective agar, Fernandez-Garayzabal et al. studied the factors responsible for this effect (*698*). The best performance was achieved on a modified *Listeria* selective agar. Addition of potassium tellurite increased the size of hemolytic zones produced by *L. monocytogenes,* probably by enhancing the cytolytic effect of listeriolysin O. It decreased hemolysis by *L. ivanovii,* apparently by inhibiting sphingomyelinase C. The basal medium also influenced hemolysis: both species displayed bigger zones of hemolysis on brain–heart infusion agar than on Columbia agar base. A new overlay technique for distinguishing between pathogenic and nonpathogenic listerias was based on the presence of phosphatidylinositol-specific phospholipase C (PI-PLC) activity (*699*). A PI-PLC substrate was incorporated into the overlay, and PI-PLC-active colonies had a turbid halo caused by release of insoluble diacylglycerol from the substrate. About 500 well-characterized clinical and food isolates of *Listeria* were tested, and activity was present only in pathogenic strains. PI-PLC activity and listeriolysin are coordinately regulated by the same gene product, and PI-PLC activity was correlated with hemolysis in this study.

Yu and Fung developed a procedure for early determination of listerias in mixed cultures and inoculated meat samples (*700*). They used a U-shaped glass apparatus (the Fung-Yu tube) with Fraser broth for selective enrichment to observe esculin hydrolysis and semisolid modified Oxford agar to detect motility. Oxyrase (membrane fractions of *E. coli*) was incorporated to enhance early growth. A presumptive positive result for 1–100 cfu of *Listeria* per gram of ground beef in the presence of large numbers of competitive microorganisms could be obtained within 10 h. *Listeria* could be isolated from a mixed bacterial culture and from ground beef in 24–48 h. The Oxyrase membrane-bound enzyme system allowed rapid growth of *L. monocytogenes* and other facultative anaerobes in a nonselective broth (*701*). In tests of several selective enrichment broths for *Listeria, Listeria* enrichment broth containing Oxyrase gave the best results. Oxyrase was superior to a variety of nonspecific reducing agents in enhancing growth and resuscitating heat-injured cells. The Fung-Yu tube procedure with Oxyrase was compared with the USDA-FSIS procedure and the GENE-TRAK DNA hybridization system (*702*). The Fung-Yu tube and USDA procedures were equally sensitive but the former provided results in a shorter time. In a survey of 215 retail meat and poultry products, all 48 presumptively positive samples determined by the tube method were confirmed to harbor *Listeria* by biochemical tests. GENE-TRAK missed 11 positive samples, probably because of the enrichment procedure. *Listeria monocytogenes* was isolated from ground beef, pork sausage, smokey links, cooked and uncooked cheese hot dogs, and macaroni and cheese.

Fifteen 4-methylumbelliferyl- and 45 β-naphthylamide-linked fluorogenic substrates were tested for their ability to differentiate *Corynebacterium* spp., *Listeria* spp., and related organisms (*703*). A group of 16 substrates, particularly the glycosidase substrates, were highly discriminatory at the genus level within 6 h of incubation. The authors recommended these tests in conjunction with biochemical tests to achieve precise identifications of coryneforms and listerias.

A microcolony technique combined with an indirect immunofluorescence test was described for the rapid detection of listerias in naturally and artificially contaminated raw meat (*704*). *Listeria monocytogenes* was detected in 5 h if it was initially present at a level $>10^5$ cfu/g. There were no false-positive reactions. The sensitivity of the technique needs to be improved.

IMMUNOLOGICAL METHODS. A polyclonal antibody was used in direct and sandwich ELISAs for detection of *L. monocytogenes* (*705*). The direct ELISA was the more cost-effective method and gave lower readings for non-*Listeria*, permitting easier interpretation of results—especially for low numbers of *Listeria* when other species are present.

Three IgM MAbs specific for *L. monocytogenes* were isolated and tested in an indirect sandwich ELISA (*706*). All MAbs reacted most strongly against *L. monocytogenes* Scott A. One strain of *L. ivanovii* and a few of *L. innocua* showed some cross-reactivity, and one MAb showed some cross-reaction with *Kurthia* spp. The authors did not discuss the nature of the antigen or antigens recognized other than to postulate that they are exposed on the cell surface. Other authors reported isolating an MAb of the IgG2b class with κ light chains (*707*). By dot blot and colony blot analysis, it was reactive with 34 of 34 *L. monocytogenes* strains and 6 of 6 *L. innocua* strains and did not cross-react with any other *Listeria* species or other gram-positive or -negative organisms. In Western blot analyses of crude native cell-surface proteins subjected to PAGE, the MAb reacted with a single protein band that had a molecular mass of 174 kDa in *L. monocytogenes* and 182 kDa in *L. innocua*. It also reacted to several protein bands of lower M_r obtained by SDS-PAGE. It did not react with listeriolysin or invasin proteins. The authors characterized the antigens in several ways, including their distribution among various cell fractions and the epitope's response to several proteolytic enzymes and solvents.

A sandwich ELISA was developed that used whole bacteria (*Listeria* and non-*Listeria* spp.) as solid-phase antigens for evaluating MAbs against flagellar proteins of *L. monocytogenes* (*708*).

Hierarchical cluster analysis of the ELISA extinction values revealed distinct groupings of the 23 supernatants tested. The three MAbs selected using this procedure appeared well suited for recognizing surface epitopes not only by ELISA but also using immunomagnetic separation techniques. A mixture of the three could allow separation of *L. monocytogenes* from foods or other complex matrices. The authors recommended this method for screening supernatants without the need to standardize antibody concentrations or to label established MAbs.

The Listeria-Tek ELISA was compared with a conventional cultural procedure for identifying *Listeria* spp. in cheese and meat products (*709*). The lower limit for detection of four *Listeria* species by ELISA was about 10^4 cfu/mL. The culture method and ELISA gave identical results in tests of 144 cheese samples artificially inoculated with *L. monocytogenes, L. murrayi, L. welshimeri,* or *L. innocua,* although identification by ELISA was possible only after two sequential enrichment steps. In 93 naturally contaminated meat samples, the ELISA gave two false-positive reactions and no false-negatives. Another study compared an ELISA test with the FDA and USDA culture procedures for detecting *Listeria* in artificially contaminated ground beef and naturally contaminated ground beef, pig tonsil, pig feed, and soft cheese (*710*). The USDA method was most sensitive for artificially contaminated meat containing <3 cfu/g of *L. monocytogenes.* At counts higher than 3 cfu/g the ELISA and USDA methods were equally sensitive. For naturally contaminated samples the ELISA had a sensitivity of 92% and a specificity of 80%. The ELISA's detection limit for demonstrating *L. monocytogenes* in pure cultures was ~10^6 cfu/mL, whereas the detection limit for the culture method was ~10^4 cfu/mL. Two commercial ELISA kits, Listeria-Tek and Tecra, were compared with the BAM culture method for detecting *Listeria* in 178 samples of naturally contaminated foods (*711*). *Listeria* was detected and culturally confirmed in 38, 37, and 40 samples by BAM, Listeria-Tek, and Tecra, respectively. As rapid screening methods, both ELISAs qualify as alternatives to the more lengthy cultural method.

POLYMERASE CHAIN REACTION (PCR) AND OTHER GENE-PROBE METHODS. McKee et al. described their procedure for the selective enrichment by the PCR of DNA sequences specific to a particular organism, and its application to the detection of pathogens in food (*712*). They have found that one of the most important problems to be solved is that of sample preparation, to maximize the recovery of bacterial cells and eliminate factors inhibitory to the subsequent enzymic amplification reactions.

Many PCR reactions are based on sequences associated with the listeriolysin O gene, *hly* (also named *hlyA* and *lisA*) (*713–717*). Artificially contaminated food samples were used to develop two PCR procedures for detecting *L. monocytogenes* (*713*). Two pairs of amplification primers were used, representing fragments of the *hly* and *iap* genes. In one procedure, bacteria in the primary or secondary enrichment broth were lysed and the lysate was analyzed by the PCR. This method detected <10 bacteria per 10 g of food. In the other procedure, enrichment cultures were centrifuged once to remove food particles and once to concentrate bacteria; samples were then lysed and analyzed as before. When secondary enrichment cultures from naturally contaminated foods were examined, both methods agreed exactly with the culture method. With the second procedure, primary enrichment cultures also permitted reliable identification. Another PCR reaction, using primers derived from sequences downstream from *hly*, also specifically detected *L. monocytogenes* in soft cheese and mayonnaise-containing salads (*714*). It gave results identical to those with standard microbiological tests, identifying 32 positive samples among the 83 tested. Fragments within the *hly* gene were used for direct enumeration of *L. monocytogenes* in food samples by colony hybridization and also for rapid PCR-based detection in enrichment broth cultures (*715*). The colony hybridization method agreed exactly with standard biochemical methods in identifying positive samples of naturally and artificially contaminated foods; counts of positive colonies were also in near-perfect agreement. In tests of 180 food samples, all positive samples identified by classical culture techniques were also identified by the PCR after a 48-h enrichment; moreover, the PCR detected several positive samples scored as negative by the classical technique initially but as positive after a 7-day enrichment. A PCR based on a primer pair within the listeriolysin O gene could detect a single *L. monocytogenes* cell from the original milk or ground beef samples (0.1 cfu per milliliter or gram, respectively) (*716*). Bacterial DNA was obtained from a two-step selective enrichment procedure; the entire procedure could be completed within 3 days. Two pairs of synthetic oligonucleotide primers were used in a PCR to detect targeted sequences in the *hly* and *lmaA* (*L. monocytogenes* antigen A) genes (*717*). Simultaneous presence of both genes was restricted to serovars 1/2, 3, and 4. Five of 10 *L. innocua* strains and 1 *L. ivanovii* isolate from pork contained *lmaA*. The *hly* gene was found exclusively in *L. monocytogenes*, but some strains of serovar 4c were negative. Strains of *L. seeligeri*, *L. welshimeri*, and *L. grayi* were negative for both genes. Detection limits of the PCR were 10 pg of nucleic acid for *hly* and 1 pg for *lmaA*.

A new oligonucleotide probe associated with a gene specifying production of a cell-surface protein of *L. monocytogenes* was developed for use in a PCR (*718*). The PCR products were visible in agarose gels without an additional DNA hybridization step. The method detected as few as 2 cfu of *L. monocytogenes* in pure cultures and 4–10 cfu in artificially contaminated foods. Base sequence analysis showed the probe to be different from other oligomer probes and gene sequences published for *L. monocytogenes*.

Howard et al. evaluated the use of clamped homogeneous electric field pulsed-field analysis for epidemiologic studies of *Listeria*, using megabase-sized restriction fragments (*719*). The enzyme *Asc*I, not previously employed for pulsed-field gel electrophoresis of listerias, was particularly useful. Like other genomic methods, this one has the advantage of not depending on phenotypic parameters that may not reflect genotype. It reproducibly deciphered the molecular epidemiology of otherwise serologically and phenotypically similar listerias. The study augmented the meager data on pulsed-field gel electrophoretic analysis of foodborne listerias that are otherwise difficult to differentiate from *L. monocytogenes*. In another pulsed-field gel

electrophoretic study, use of the low-frequency cleavage enzymes *Apa*I, *Sma*I, and *Not*I permitted definition of at least 24 groups within 35 strains of *L. monocytogenes* serogroups 1/2 and 3 (*720*). Fourteen human isolates were distributed in 13 groups, 6 animal isolates in 6 groups, and 13 environmental strains in at least 8 groups. Isolates with the same patterns were recovered from different geographic locations. Genetically closely related strains of 42 serovar 4b isolates were also rapidly differentiated by this method (*721*). The authors recommended their method for conventional microbiology laboratories and for epidemiologic studies because of its relative simplicity, cost-effectiveness, and superior discriminatory ability.

From pulsed-field gel electrophoretic patterns of *Apa*I and *Not*I genomic DNA digests, Carriere et al. inferred that strains of serovar 1/2c have emerged only recently (*722*). Strains of this serovar were a homogeneous group showing no restriction fragment length polymorphism; their chromosome was ~15% shorter than the 1/2a, 1/2b, and 4b chromosomes. Electrophoretic patterns varied considerably in 1/2a and 1/2b strains, suggesting the value of this technique in epidemiologic studies—particularly as these serovars frequently cannot be phage-typed. Although restriction polymorphism was less in 4b strains, in most cases it was sufficient to distinguish between strains.

Danish workers showed that *L. monocytogenes* could be divided into two major types based on the nucleotide sequence of the listeriolysin gene (*723*). Overall the gene showed a relatively high level of conservation, particularly at the amino acid level. To analyze the pattern of sequence variability, a 160-base-pair region covering 9 nucleotide differences was sequenced from 36 isolates of different origins. There were two major types, one of which included all epidemic isolates. Oligonucleotide probing of additional *L. monocytogenes* isolates verified that the observed differences could be used to subdivide the species and suggested a relationship between sequence type and flagellar antigens.

Baloga and Harlander compared DNA fingerprinting, ribotyping, serotyping, and multilocus enzyme electrophoresis typing schemes for classifying strains of *Listeria* (*724*). DNA fingerprinting and ribotyping distinguished *L. monocytogenes* from other listerias and from *Lactococcus lactis lactis* and *L. lactis cremoris*. When *L. monocytogenes* isolates from four independent incidents of foodborne illness were typed by all methods, only DNA fingerprinting could differentiate or prove the relatedness of patient–product isolate pairs. The authors recommended DNA fingerprinting in conjunction with ribotyping as a way to provide conclusive evidence for epidemiologic linkage of *L. monocytogenes* strains implicated in foodborne illness.

A simple dried gel hybridization method was described as an alternative to the conventional Southern blot technique for detecting *L. monocytogenes* DNA fragments (*725*). DNA was fractionated on an agarose gel which was then denatured, neutralized, dried, and hybridized with a ^{32}P-labeled DNA probe. This eliminated the necessity for transfer to a nitrocellulose membrane.

A synthetic ^{32}P-labeled listeriolysin O gene probe was evaluated for direct identification of β-hemolytic *L. monocytogenes* in ground beef, using a colony hybridization assay (*726*). Of 118 gram-positive, catalase-positive isolates only 24 gave positive signals with the probe; these same 24 were the only isolates shown by CAMP, tumbling motility, and biochemical tests to be β-hemolytic *L. monocytogenes*. Six of 36 ground beef samples were positive for *Listeria* spp., of which 4 were *L. monocytogenes*. The efficiency of the probe depended on the ability of the media to suppress background colonies and the stringency of the hybridization conditions. In this study, LPM agar complemented the hybridization conditions employed. Another hybridization protocol utilized a digoxigenin-labeled synthetic oligonucleotide probe for rapid confirmation of *L. monocytogenes* isolated from foods (*727*). The specificity of the probe was verified by dot blot assays. When enrichment cultures of 48 food samples were streaked on selective plating medium and tested by conventional methods and DNA colony blot assay, the colony blot method was 100% sensitive and 97% specific and could be completed within 24 h. The method could not be applied directly to enrichment broth cultures.

The gene *prfA*, which positively regulates expression of several virulence factors, was evaluated

in a colony hybridization assay for identification of pathogenic listerias (*728*). The idea was that if the presence of the regulatory gene could be demonstrated in all pathogenic strains, it would be a more attractive target than individual virulence-associated genes for use in identification. A PCR-amplified *prfA* oligonucleotide probe proved to be specific for *L. monocytogenes* of all known serotypes.

A homogeneous protection assay (HPA) was developed for rapid confirmation of presumptive *L. monocytogenes* colonies from blood agar plates (*729*). It used an acridinium ester–labeled chemiluminescent DNA probe in a free-solution hybridization format. After the probe hybridized with the target ribosomal RNA, the label on unhybridized probe was inactivated by chemical differential hydrolysis. A detection reagent was then added and the probe–target hybrid was detected in a luminometer. From 50 to 100 samples could be processed simultaneously and the assay completed in 30–45 min. The assay was 100% specific and 100% sensitive for *L. monocytogenes*, with a lower detection limit of 10^4–10^5 cells.

Wang et al. developed two 16S rRNA–based oligonucleotide probes for *L. monocytogenes* (*730*). Probe RL-1 had one base that differed between *L. monocytogenes* on the one hand and *L. innocua* and *L. ivanovii* on the other; RL-2 differed at two positions. By using a dried gel hybridization protocol (as in reference *725*) in place of Northern (RNA) or dot blot hybridization, the authors showed that RL-2 hybridized with all 36 strains of *L. monocytogenes* tested but with no other species. RL-1 showed some cross reactions with other listerias. An alkaline phosphatase–labeled RL-2 probe gave good results in dot blot hybridization, but a ^{32}P-labeled probe was more sensitive and could be used for as long as 2 months even though much of the radiolabel had decayed. rRNA gene restriction patterns have also been used to identify *Listeria* species (*731,732*). Cleavage of chromosomal DNA by *Eco*RI or *Hind*III and hybridization with a 16S rDNA probe from *Bacillus subtilis* revealed distinct profiles for all *Listeria* species except for *L. grayi* and *L. murrayi*, which shared the same profile (*731*). In a larger study, 94 strains of *L. monocytogenes* of different serovars and phagovars and from various origins were analyzed (*732*). Fourteen ribovars were generated by cleavage with *Eco*RI, whereas *Hin*dIII digestion revealed less important genomic heterogeneity. Ribovar analysis using *Eco*RI yielded a new typing scheme whose results did not match those from routine serotyping and phage typing. However, it strengthened a new view of the species, first inferred from multilocus enzyme analysis (see, for example, reference *733*), as including one clone that encompasses a majority of isolates from human illness.

OTHER METHODS. Multilocus enzyme electrophoresis (MEE) with selective stains for 21 enzymes was employed to type 181 isolates of *L. monocytogenes* from human, animal, food, and environmental sources (*733*). A dendrogram was generated to display genetic relationships among the 50 electrophoretic types identified. A clone responsible for several recent foodborne outbreaks in Switzerland and North America was found frequently among animal strains in Switzerland, suggesting that animals are a major source of this clone. Most food-related isolates of the clone were from milk, cheese, and the environment in which cheese is produced, perhaps indicating its adaptation to milk, cheese, and their production sites. Two different clones (including strains of serovars 1/2b and 1/2c) were frequently isolated from meat but not from animals, suggesting environmental contamination of the meat. An MEE study of 84 Danish *L. monocytogenes* strains found 8 polymorphic enzyme loci having 2–4 alleles per locus (*734*). A dendrogram was constructed, from which 14 electrophoretic types were identified. The dendrogram showed two distinct clusters separated by a genetic distance of .342. One cluster contained only strains belonging to serogroup 1; the other contained strains of serogroups 1 and 4. Only one electrophoretic type contained strains belonging to more than one serogroup. Two types accounted for 77% of human clinical isolates and were the same as those responsible for epidemics in Switzerland and the USA. For strains that could be phage-typed, this method was more discriminatory than MEE. Another MEE study of 29 strains representing 6 serovars also revealed two distinct clusters (*735*). One contained all 10 strains of serovars

1/2a, 1/2c, and 3a; the other contained all 19 strains of serovars 1/2b, 3b, and 4b. Moreover, analysis of restriction fragment length polymorphism of *hly, iap, mpl,* and *prfA* in these strains identified the same two subgroups.

The cellular fatty acids of 22 strains of *Listeria* were analyzed by gas–liquid chromatography (*736*). Differences between strains were quantitative rather than qualitative. When fatty acid ratios were compared by discriminant analysis, two groups of strains were seen: one contained isolates of *L. grayi* and *L. murrayi* and the other contained strains of the remaining five species. Among the latter, *L. monocytogenes* was fairly distinct from *L. seeligeri* and *L. welshimeri* but close to *L. innocua* and *L. ivanovii*. These results agree with recent taxonomic studies of the genus.

Peterkin et al. characterized the plasmids in 132 food, clinical, environmental, and veterinary strains of *L. monocytogenes* and other listerias (*737*). Only 24% harbored plasmids, which ranged in size from 1.3 to 66 MDa. No strain had more than one plasmid. The presence of a plasmid was not related to phenotypic characters known to be inherited extrachromosomally, such as antibiotic resistance.

Listeria monocytogenes isolates from 277 seafood products of 16 varieties were phage-typed using the French International set of *L. monocytogenes* bacteriophages and newly isolated North American phages (*738*). Seventy-six percent of the strains were typable. The phage spectra seen in the different varieties of seafood were discussed.

Virulence

An epidemiologic study in France compared the distribution of *Listeria* species and *L. monocytogenes* serotypes isolated from 496 human and 96 animal cases of listeriosis with that of 103 food isolates (*739*). Serotype 4b accounted for most illness but was rarely isolated from food. Nonpathogenic serotypes 3a and 3b accounted for about half of the food isolates. In virulence studies, some *L. monocytogenes* 1/2a isolates were not virulent and 1/2c strains were considerably less virulent than those of serotype 4b.

Farber et al. determined the infective dose necessary for development of listeriosis in healthy adult cynomolgus monkeys (*Macaca fascicularis*) (*740*). Monkeys that received 10^9 *L. monocytogenes* Scott A or F6861 cells became noticeably ill, with symptoms of septicemia, irritability, loss of appetite, and occasional diarrhea. They developed severe lymphopenia and neutrophilia within 48 h. Monkeys that received 10^7 or 10^9 cells shed the organism in the feces for ~21 days. Doses of 10^5 or 10^7 cells did not produce noticeable signs of infection. Some monkeys were treated with Maalox because of reports that use of antacids is a risk factor for listeriosis. However, no substantial differences were seen between Maalox-treated monkeys and controls. These results were discussed in relation to the little that is known about the infective dose in humans.

Notermans et al. demonstrated that the chick embryo test and the mouse bioassay perform comparably in assessing pathogenicity of *Listeria* species and the chick embryo test is therefore a reliable alternative procedure (*741*). In the mouse test, cells were injected intravenously and survival and growth of the organisms in the spleen were evaluated. *Listeria monocytogenes* strains that grew in the spleen had an LD_{100} of <125 organisms in the chick embryo test; strains that did not grow had an LD_{100} >125. *Listeria seeligeri, L. innocua, L. welshimeri, L. grayi,* and *L. murrayi* did not persist in the spleen and did not kill chick embryos at the levels tested. Another mouse test for virulence involves intraperitoneal injection of known numbers of organisms and counting of bacteria in the spleen and other sites (*742*). *Listeria innocua, L. seeligeri,* and *L. welshimeri* were not pathogenic for mice in this test. *Listeria ivanovii* was detected in liver, spleen, and peritoneal lavage fluid, but in significantly lower numbers than *L. monocytogenes. Listeria monocytogenes* serovars 1/2b and 1/2c, which are frequently isolated from foods, colonized liver and spleen to a significantly lesser extent than serovar 4b. The behavior of serovar 1/2a strains was extremely variable: 2 of 4 strains were strongly hemolytic and as virulent as strains of serovar 4b, whereas the other two were weakly hemolytic and avirulent.

Because immunosuppressed persons are at high risk for listeriosis, the infective dose of nonstressed, heat-stressed, and resuscitated *L. monocytogenes*

1A1 was studied in immunocompromised mice (*743*). Cells were stressed by heating for 20 min at 56°C and resuscitated by incubation in tryptic soy broth at 25°C. The LD_{50} of nonstressed and resuscitated cells was ~10^2, whereas a dose of $10^{4.5}$ heat-stressed cells caused only 12% mortality after 5 days. The decreased virulence was accompanied by loss of hemolytic activity.

Goebel et al. briefly reviewed studies on the pathogenicity of *L. monocytogenes,* especially as revealed by characterization of mutants with reduced virulence (*744*). Reduction in the amount of extracellular protein p60, encoded by the *iap* gene, impairs invasiveness but the mutants are still hemolytic. In contrast, mutants that cannot synthesize listeriolysin remain invasive but are unable to survive within phagocytic cells. One type of listeriolysin-negative mutant is defective in synthesis of the positive regulatory element PrfA, which coordinately regulates a number of virulence-related genes in addition to *hly*. The authors speculated that synthesis of PrfA protein acting alone or with a coregulating factor is induced under stress conditions such as those encountered in the intracellular environment. Another brief review by members of the same research team discussed molecular determinants of *L. monocytogenes* pathogenesis and the cell biology of infection (*745*). The genes *inlA, hly, actA,* and *plcB* are involved, respectively, in internalization of the *Listeria* cell, escape from a vacuole, nucleation of actin filaments, and cell-to-cell spread. These genes were discussed along with others: *plcA,* which encodes a phosphatidylinositol-specific phospholipase C; *mpl,* which occurs with *actA* and *plcB* in the lecithinase operon; *iap; lmaBA;* and *prfA.* The same group reported their study of the coordinate regulation of *L. monocytogenes* virulence genes by the product of *prfA* (*746*). When a site-directed insertion mutation in *prfA* was constructed by chromosomal integration of a novel suicide vector containing a portion of the *prfA* coding region, the mutation not only transcriptionally silenced *hly* but also abolished transcription of the phosphatidylinositol-specific phospholipase C (*plc*) and metalloprotease (*mpl*) genes. The mutant was avirulent in a mice. Studies of *prfA* mutants by Mengaud et al. replicated these findings and characterized the transcription of the gene (*747*). Transcription was not constitutive. During the growth phase, one peak of *prfA* transcription was observed during exponential growth and a second at the beginning of the stationary phase. Early in exponential growth, *prfA* was cotranscribed with *plcA,* which lies upstream, giving rise to a 2.2-kilobase *plcA–prfA* transcript. In late exponential growth and early in the stationary phase, 1-kilobase *prfA* transcripts were predominantly detected. The authors concluded that since *prfA* controls *plcA* transcription it also regulates its own synthesis.

Further study of the expression of virulence genes in *L. monocytogenes* showed that expression of the hemolysis phenotype in wild-type strains is thermoregulated (*748*). An *hly::lacZ* fusion was constructed and its expression studied at various growth temperatures. The fusion β-galactosidase activity was expressed only when cultures were grown at temperatures >37°C. The activity could be specifically repressed or induced depending on growth temperature. No temperature-related change in activity was seen in a strain harboring a control β-galactosidase fusion. Northern blot analysis of *hly*-specific RNA transcripts showed that thermoregulation occurred at the transcription level. Transcription of other PrfA-regulated virulence genes was similarly affected by temperature.

Conlan and North found that virulence factors distinct from listeriolysin are needed for *L. monocytogenes* to survive an early neutrophil-mediated host defense mechanism (*749*). Mutants that did not produce phosphatidylinositol-specific phospholipase C or produced reduced amounts of listeriolysin did not cause progressive infection in normal mice but did grow progressively in MAb 5C6–treated mice, which are unable to focus neutrophils at sites of infection. In treated mice, wild-type strains, phospholipase C–negative mutants, and listeriolysin-deficient mutants gave rise to numerous foci of infected hepatocytes that maintained their morphological integrity during the first 24 h despite a large bacterial burden; listeriolysin-negative mutants were unable to infect even these animals. In normal controls, sites of infection were marked by focal accumulations of neutrophils that lysed infected hepatocytes, releasing the bacteria for ingestion and killing by neutrophils and macrophages. A proportion of wild-type organisms survived this neutrophil defense to initiate progressive infection, but phospholipase C–negative organisms were eliminated.

Strains of *L. monocytogenes* generated by transposon mutagenesis were tested for virulence and ability to induce protective immunity in mice (*750*). The mutants were characterized by decreased listeriolysin production, phospholipase C activity, intracellular growth, and (or) intercellular spread in vitro and reduced virulence for BALB/c mice. Sublethal infection provided protection against challenge with the virulent parent strain. In addition, in vitro infection of J774 macrophages converted the cultured cells to targets of *L. monocytogenes*–immune cytotoxic cells. Listeriolysin-negative strains, however, did not protect mice against challenge with the virulent organism. Nor could these mutants escape phagolysosomes in cultured J774 macrophages or convert them to targets of *L. monocytogenes*–immune cytotoxic cells. This confirms the importance of listeriolysin in the induction of antilisterial immunity and indicates a requirement for a cytoplasmic localization of the pathogen for development of immunity.

Because the fetoplacental unit and the neonate are particularly susceptible to listeriosis and listeriolysin is a virulence factor in *L. monocytogenes* infections of adult mice, McKay and Lu investigated the importance of listeriolysin in perinatal infection (*751*). All neonatal mice injected with 10^4 listeriolysin-positive bacteria died within 12 days, whereas all neonates injected with 10^7 listeriolysin-negative cells survived to the end of the 14-day observation period. The negative strain proliferated poorly in decidual tissue and internal organs, maximum populations being 3 to 5 orders of magnitude lower than populations of the positive strain. The authors concluded that listeriolysin-negative bacteria are not virulent in the neonate and fetoplacental unit despite their poorly developed immune function.

A technique for in vitro construction of mutations in cloned *Listeria* genes and their reintroduction into the *Listeria* chromosome to construct isogenic strains would be useful in studies of virulence and gene regulation. A method using a temperature-sensitive shuttle vector was described for insertional inactivation of *hly* in *L. monocytogenes* (752). The product was a truncated, immunologically cross-reactive listeriolysin protein that resulted in loss of the hemolytic phenotype. The protoplast transformation method of Chang and Cohen was also modified to facilitate genetic manipulation of *Listeria*.

Through production and characterization of neutralizing and nonneutralizing MAbs against listeriolysin O, Nato et al. demonstrated the existence of regions important for hemolytic activity that are unique to *Listeria* hemolysins and showed that regions outside the conserved peptide are important for listeriolysin O activity (753). Three MAbs inhibited hemolytic activity, one inhibited binding to erythrocyte membranes, and two blocked activity at a step subsequent to membrane binding. Two MAbs recognized the hemolysins of *L. ivanovii* and *L. seeligeri*; two recognized seeligerolysin but not ivanolysin. Only two of the nine MAbs recognized other purified thiol-activated toxins. MAbs raised against a specific peptide common to all thiol-activated toxins sequenced so far recognized all the toxins and were not neutralizing. German investigators established the complete DNA sequences for the *ilo* gene encoding ivanolysin and the *lso* gene encoding seeligerolysin and compared them with the sequence for *hly* (754). The *hly* gene shows 78% homology with *ilo* and 77% with *lso*; *ilo* and *lso* are 76% homologous. The corresponding homologies between deduced amino sequences were 80, 82, and 76%. The most interesting finding was a substitution of phenylalanine for alanine within a peptide sequence previously believed to be absolutely conserved among all thiol-activated cytolysins (see reference 753). The implications of this were discussed.

The surface proteins of *Listeria* were analyzed by SDS-PAGE in relation to species, serovar, and pathogenicity (755). Two major protein antigens of 64 and 68 kDa were specific for *L. monocytogenes* and common to all serovars. Others characterized specific serovars, viz., 98 kDa for serovars 1/2 and 3; 76 and 78 kDa for serovars 4b, 4d, and 4e; and 80 and 100 kDa for serovars 4a and 4c. Two of these proteins appeared to be associated with virulence. Overall, the surface-protein profiles of *L. monocytogenes* were very different from those of other *Listeria* species. The results confirmed the classification of *Listeria* derived from genomic studies and should be useful in identifying new virulence factors and developing better methods for detecting and identifying these organisms.

For humans, the virulence of *L. monocytogenes* has been attributed to the presence of hemolysins and oxidative enzymes that facilitate entrance into macrophages and intestinal cells and subsequent intracellular survival. To investigate the effect of iron concentration and food type on production of hemolysin and catalase in *L. monocytogenes*, tests were conducted in various foods and media inoculated with *L. monocytogenes* Scott A (756). High-iron media and aeration enhanced growth and induced production of several catalases. Reduced aeration enhanced hemolysin activity but decreased growth and catalase production. At refrigeration temperatures, the organism grew in milk and culture media but not in meat. This serotype (4b) has seldom been found in meat. The reasons for its poor growth in refrigerated meat in this experiment merit further study.

A new extracellular cytotoxin from virulent (4b) and avirulent (ATCC 15313:1/2a) strains of *L. monocytogenes* was reported (757). Production was first detected in early- to mid-log phase and reached its peak during stationary phase. Production occurred throughout the 4–37°C temperature range tested and the cytotoxin was stable in the growth medium at these temperatures. Both strains also synthesized the cytotoxin at 4 and 10°C in skim and whole milk.

To develop foci of infection and produce systemic disease, *L. monocytogenes* must be able to move within the cytosol of infected cells and to infect adjacent cells. The *actA* gene encodes a 90-kDa polypeptide involved in interactions between the bacterium and host-cell microfilaments (745,758). Cloning of this gene permitted identification of its product and construction of an isogenic mutant defective in production of ActA. In the cytoplasm of infected cells the mutant grew as microcolonies, was unable to accumulate actin after escape from the phagocytic compartment, and could not infect adjacent cells. Its virulence was also greatly reduced, demonstrating that virulence requires the capacity to move intracellularly and spread intercellularly. Like other virulence factors for *L. monocytogenes,* this one's expression is controlled by the PrfA regulator protein, suggesting that these bacteria coordinate their movement in the host cell and that further PrfA-regulated gene products may be involved in polymerization and polarization of host-cell microfilaments, which propels bacteria through the cytoplasm and mediates infection of adjacent cells.

French investigators purified and characterized an extracellular 29-kDa phospholipase C from *L. monocytogenes (759).* It was zinc-dependent, most active at pH 6–7, and expressed both lecithinase and weak sphingomyelinase activity. It hydrolyzed phosphatidylcholine, phosphatidylethanolamine, phosphatidylserine, and sphingomyelin but not phosphatidylinositol. The pure protein had weak, calcium-independent hemolytic activity and was not toxic in mice. All virulent strains of *L. monocytogenes* tested produced an extracellular 29-kDa phospholipase C, whereas no antigenically related proteins were detected in supernatants of other *Listeria* species. Further studies revealed that the virulence of a phospholipase-deficient mutant isolated by transposon insertion was strongly impaired in mice, although the mutant was taken up in vitro by Caco-2 and J774 cells and grew intracellularly *(760).* The transposon insertion occurred within the *mpl* locus, which encodes a zinc metalloprotease. Loss of phospholipase activity coincided with loss of a 29-kDa zinc-dependent phosphatidylcholine-phospholipase C. However, the mutant still synthesized an antigenically closely related protein of ~33 kDa, suggesting that the zinc metalloprotease was involved in maturation of the 29-kDa protein. The same group identified the *L. monocytogenes* lecithinase gene *(plcB),* located immediately downstream of *mpl (761).* Together with four other genes and *mpl* it forms an operon. The lecithinase gene encodes a predicted protein of 289 amino acids homologous to the phosphatidylcholine-specific phospholipases C of *Bacillus cereus* and *Clostridium perfringens.* Mutants produced only small plaques

on fibroblast monolayers. Three other open reading frames identified probably lie outside the *L. monocytogenes* virulence region.

OTHER MICROBIAL PATHOGENS

Legionella

Aerosols from a grocery store mist machine were the source of an outbreak of legionnaires' disease in Bogalusa, Louisiana, in the fall of 1989. An epidemiologic study of this outbreak has now been published *(762).* An increased OR was associated with shopping at that grocery store during the 10 days before illness, shopping at the store for >30 min, and buying produce located close to an ultrasonic mist machine. Employees of the store were more likely than employees of other grocery stores to have elevated antibody titers to *Legionella pneumophila* serogroup 1, which was the organism isolated from the mist machine's water reservoir and from mist. Isolates from the mist machine and two patients had the same MAb subtype. Ultrasonic mist machines produce smaller droplets than other types of misters, increasing the chances of disease transmission. Domestic hot-water systems have also been contaminated by *Legionella,* but the importance of this for public health is unknown *(763).* In a Canadian study, increased risk was associated with electric water heating. Factors that increased this risk were low water temperature, location in an older housing district, and an old water heater. Contamination of peripheral outlets was associated only with contamination of the heater itself.

Brucella

A case–control study examined the etiology of animal-to-human transmission of brucellosis in Saudi Arabia *(764).* The greatest risk was associated with indirect contact with animals, specifically the consumption of unpasteurized dairy products. Milk and buttermilk posed a greater hazard than cheese or uncooked liver, and products derived from sheep and goats were riskier than products derived from camels and cattle. In cases linked to direct contact with animals, assisting in animal parturition bore a high risk but no significant risk was associated with other types of animal contact.

Streptococcus

A foodborne outbreak of group A β–hemolytic streptococcal pharyngitis occurred in an Israeli military base in April 1990 (*765*). Boiled egg salad was the implicated vehicle. Prompt therapy and isolation of the 61 victims prevented secondary respiratory spread of the infection. A symptomatic food handler was considered a primary source of the boiled egg inoculation, through either contaminated hands or sneezing. In Italy, 179 of 300 persons attending wedding banquets in the same restaurant in early July 1986 became ill with group A streptococcal pharyngitis (*766*). In this outbreak, eating a prawn hors-d'oeuvre, squills, or custard cake were associated with illness. Six persons on the restaurant staff, including 4 members of the manager's family, and the manager's three young daughters were colonized by group A streptococci of the same serotype. The suspected route of infection was diffusion of the strain among the staff followed by contamination of the food.

Three infants with group A streptococcal pharyngitis had eaten food prechewed by their parents (*767*). One parent had a history of recent pharyngitis and another had frequent episodes of tonsillitis. The authors suggested that prechewing of babies' food is more common in the USA than is generally recognized, and may be a mode of transmission of streptococcal pharyngitis from parents to infants.

Klebsiella

Antibodies to *Salmonella, Yersinia, Campylobacter jejuni, Borrelia burgdorferi, Klebsiella pneumoniae, Escherichia coli, Proteus mirabilis,* and *Chlamydia trachomatis* were measured by ELISA in sera from 99 patients with ankylosing spondylitis (*768*). Increased antibody levels were most often observed against *K. pneumoniae* (35 patients). Although 54% of patients with elevated titers had antibodies against more than one microbe, there was no clear-cut evidence that this was due to polyclonal stimulation. The only significant differences between patients and controls were that IgA and IgG antibody titers against *Klebsiella* and high IgA titers against *E. coli* were associated with ankylosing spondylitis. *Klebsiella* is an opportunistic foodborne pathogen whose association with ankylosing spondylitis has been disputed (see reference *825*, Chapter 11, *Food Safety 1991*).

Cyanobacteria

Jalaludin and Smith reviewed eight frequently cited studies to evaluate the evidence associating exposure to cyanobacteria with ill health (*769*). The criteria for causality were temporality, strength of association, dose–response, reversibility, biological plausibility, specificity, and analogy. Overall, there was a weak but consistent association between exposure to cyanobacteria and ill health. Long et al. described the morphologic and staining characteristics of a cyanobacterium-like organism isolated from stool specimens (*770*). The spherical organism, 9–10 μm in diameter, was seen in three outbreaks of diarrhea involving >100 patients in Southeast Asia and the USA in 1989 and 1990. The source of the infections was not determined.

Borrelia

In reviewing the literature on *Borrelia burgdorferi,* Farrell and Marth asked whether the emphasis on transmission of *Borrelia* infection by deer ticks deflects attention from other possible modes of transmission—such as food (*771*). There is no obvious necessity for an arthropod vector. The organism is shed in urine for prolonged periods, occurs in the blood of infected food animals, and theoretically could contaminate meat from these animals. Similarly, raw milk could become contaminated from an infected cow or the environment. Experimental oral infection and contact infection have been achieved in laboratory animals. The pathogen's occurrence and behavior in food and the food-processing environment have not been investigated and in vitro cultivation presents many difficulties, but the authors suggested that *B. burgdorferi* be included on any list of foodborne pathogens waiting to "emerge." Interesting and unusual features of the organism were discussed.

Citrobacter

Although a large outbreak of gastroenteritis in the U.S. Air Force Academy was consistent in many respects with illness caused by Norwalk virus, the clinical presentation was not typical (*772*). The implicated food vehicle was chicken salad containing celery that had been washed and soaked in nonpotable water for ~60 min, then refrigerated until its use in the salad, which was eaten the next day. *Citrobacter freundii* was isolated from 22 of 107 stool samples, and was associated with both illness and consumption of chicken salad. Sixteen biotypes of *C. freundii* were isolated from the hose used to wash the celery and from drain water, but none of them showed evidence of enterotoxin production. All food samples were negative for *Citrobacter*. The authors concluded that, based on serologic data, Norwalk virus was most likely responsible for this outbreak and that *C. freundii* was merely a marker linking celery preparation with illness. However, *C. freundii* is an established nonenteric pathogen and there is some evidence supporting its role in gastrointestinal disease. This investigation suggested that point-source cases of acute gastroenteritis associated with nonpotable water be examined for enteric viral agents or multiple etiologic agents.

GENERAL (MULTIPLE PATHOGENS)

The new *Sourcebook of Bacterial Protein Toxins* (*773*) contains much information of interest to food scientists. For example, there are chapters on cytolytic toxins of pathogenic marine vibrios, molecular biology of clostridial neurotoxins, cholesterol-binding thiol-activated cytolytic toxins, Shiga and Shiga-like toxins, carbohydrate receptors for toxins, and genetic analysis of the in vivo role of bacterial toxins.

Lucas and Corthier reviewed the glycolipid and glycoprotein bacterial enterotoxin receptors of the enterocyte brush border and various other types of vertebrate cells (*774*). In general, enterotoxins bind to glucide chains, after which the toxin is usually internalized. Beyond similarities in their binding mechanism enterotoxins are a diverse group of substances; and once inside the cell, they act in a variety of ways, which were reviewed by Lucas et al. (*775*).

Occurrence of food-poisoning bacteria

Sewage discharge to the marine environment has an enormous economic and hygienic impact on shellfish-producing areas. A Brazilian study evaluated the microbiological quality of several growing areas on the northern coast of São Paulo (*776*). Total coliforms, fecal coliforms, and *Salmonella* were enumerated in water and shellfish samples and *Vibrio parahaemolyticus* determinations were made in shellfish. Although coliform counts were high at polluted sites, no *Salmonella* was detected in any sample, reflecting the poor ability of this enteric pathogen to survive in the marine environment. Nor was there a strong relationship between coliform counts and *V. parahaemolyticus,* although the highest frequency of *V. parahaemolyticus* was observed at Ubatuba Bay, the area most polluted by sewage. The percentage of substandard water samples was much greater than that of substandard shellfish samples, suggesting the need to reevaluate Brazilian standards for both shellfish and growing waters.

Contaminated shellfish are purified by placing them in clean seawater for a short time before sale. The effectiveness of this depuration process is related to the pumping rates of shellfish, but other factors are involved and different bacterial species may be eliminated at different rates. Spanish investigators studied the accumulation and elimination of *Escherichia coli, Salmonella typhimurium, V. parahaemolyticus, Aeromonas hydrophila, Streptococcus faecalis, Staphylococcus aureus,* and MS-2 coliphage by the striped venus, *Chamelea gallina* (*777*). Depending on the organism, accumulation occurred for 3–12 h, plateaued, then dropped precipitously by the 24th or 48th hour. These time-courses suggest that microorganisms are eliminated from shellfish in two ways: by simple mechanical pumping action, which results in elimination during the first 12 h, and by a mechanism that depends on the species of microbe and the number accumulated. Microbial size and resistance to molluscan enzymes are probably involved.

Selected bacterial indicators and pathogens were enumerated in pond water and sediment samples and in visceral and surface samples of catfish harvested from the ponds, to determine the relationship between microfloras of ponds and fish (*778*). Channel catfish (*Ictalurus punctatus*) were fed diets containing 26 or 38% protein using restricted and satiety feeding methods. Counts of *A. hydrophila* were significantly higher in viscera than in water or sediment, and viscera had a mean presumptive listerial count of ~100 cfu/g wet weight. The authors concluded that because of the elevated pathogen concentrations in the viscera, cross-contamination could occur during evisceration. Counts of indicator organisms did not differ significantly according to the type of sample, but counts from the fish reflected counts from the pond (in particular, from the sediment). Some influence of feed protein level and feeding method on bacterial populations was seen.

A survey in the Toronto region determined the overall microbiological quality of hot- and cold-smoked ready-to-eat retail fish (*779*). No *E. coli*, *S. aureus*, *Salmonella*, or *Clostridium botulinum* was found in any of the 100 samples, although after 30 days of storage at 4°C roughly one-third of the fish would have been rejected on the basis of their aerobic colony counts.

Japanese boxed meals called "bento" have caused sporadic outbreaks of illness (*780*). Hazard analysis of two bento catering operations found that cooking times and temperatures were usually adequate to kill vegetative bacterial contaminants and meticulous care was taken to avoid contamination during preparation. Despite this, microorganisms were present and multiplied during holding of the meals at ambient temperatures. Aerobic plate counts were high in foods held until midafternoon. *Staphylococcus aureus* was recovered from 4 of 11

samples, *Bacillus cereus* was found in most samples, and *Clostridium perfringens* was isolated from one sample. The critical control point for bento foods was identified as the holding time.

Six milk and four ice cream plants were sampled extensively to determine the occurrence of *Listeria monocytogenes*, *Y. enterocolitica*, and *Salmonella* in the dairy plant environment (*781*). No salmonellas were isolated from any sample. *Yersinia enterocolitica* was isolated from 6.8%, *L. monocytogenes* from 6.5%, and listerias other than *L. monocytogenes* from 9.3% of the 353 samples. The presence of *Y. enterocolitica* was significantly related to high overall bacterial counts. However, routine microbiological measurements had no value in predicting the presence of *L. monocytogenes*. About half of the *Yersinia* isolates came from cooler environments at the dairy plants; other environments harboring the organism included drains and conveyors. Conveyor systems and cooler environments were also favorable sites for *L. monocytogenes*. Other investigators analyzed 292 milk samples from farm bulk tanks in eastern Tennessee and southwestern Virginia for *L. monocytogenes*, *Campylobacter jejuni*, *Y. enterocolitica*, and *Salmonella* (*782*). They found *L. monocytogenes* in 4%, *C. jejuni* in 12%, *Y. enterocolitica* in 15%, and *Salmonella* in 9% of samples. The finding of one or more of these pathogens was not associated with the dairy's size or grade classification, milking hygiene, type of barn, or reported incidence of clinical mastitis in the herd. Sixty-eight of the 195 producers reported consumption of raw bulk milk, and 25% of the bulk tanks from which milk was consumed were contaminated with one or more species of pathogen.

In Mexico, 231 samples of ultrapasteurized and pasteurized milk and whole-milk powder from retail outlets were analyzed for pathogenic and nonpathogenic organisms resistant to multiple antibiotics (*783*). Two-thirds of pasteurized milk samples contained multiply resistant fecal coliforms; 4% contained *Salmonella* that was resistant to penicillin and partially resistant to polymyxin B and chloramphenicol; 3% contained ampicillin- and tetracycline-resistant *S. aureus*. Milk powders and ultrapasteurized samples were relatively pathogen-free, but multiply resistant fecal coliforms were present. These findings uncovered a serious public health hazard, showing not only the incidence of multidrug-resistant pathogens but finding many drug-resistant nonpathogens, which are a reservoir of resistance genes that can be transferred to pathogens.

Zottola and Smith reviewed recent literature on the occurrence of pathogens in cheeses produced commercially and in the home (784). The history of surveillance, establishment of standards, pathogens commonly encountered and their sources, number of outbreaks, and cheeses involved were discussed. Contributing factors in most outbreaks were the use of raw milk in cheese production, faulty pasteurization or equipment, cross-contamination, or postprocessing contamination.

Strains of *S. aureus* and *Salmonella* spp. isolated from beef in Zaire were characterized to evaluate their public health importance (785). The 190 *S. aureus* strains were biotyped, phage-typed, and tested for enterotoxin production; 122 *Salmonella* strains were serotyped and evaluated for drug sensitivity. Eighty-seven percent of the *S. aureus* strains belonged to the human biovar, suggesting that workers were the major source of contamination, and 69% produced staphylococcal enterotoxin A. Most strains responsible for foodborne intoxications belonged to phage group III or to the I+III mixed group. The *Salmonella* strains comprised 16 serotypes. The only antimicrobial drug resistance seen was in a single strain resistant to sulphamethoxazole.

Survival and growth

Michel et al. determined the survival of *C. perfringens*, *S. aureus*, *E. coli*, *S. typhimurium*, and *L. monocytogenes* in precooked roast beef slices (786). Inocula of the pathogens were placed between two slices of beef, which were then vacuum-packaged and stored at 3°C. Pathogens had no effect on aerobic plate counts. Counts of *C. perfringens* decreased steadily throughout the 70 days of storage, whereas most of the decrease in *E. coli* counts occurred in the first 14 days and *S. aureus* counts remained stable. *Listeria monocytogenes* and *S. typhimurium* were isolated from inoculated samples throughout the storage period, but neither was found in uninoculated controls. When locations in the processing sequence of a commercial restructured beef product were tested for *L. monocytogenes*, most sampling locations before heat processing were positive but the pathogen was not detected after heating. Counts of *S. aureus* and total bacteria increased after the cooked product was removed from the package and coated with seasoning mix. Hazard analysis identified the following critical control points: initial bacterial levels on raw products; cooking time and temperature; cooling after cooking; sanitation during opening, seasoning, and rebagging; and temperature control of the final product.

A standardized method for preparing bifidus milk commercially was described (787). The product had substantial antibacterial activity against *E. coli*, *S. aureus*, *B. cereus*, and *Shigella dysenteriae*.

Eckner and Zottola described the behavior of *S. aureus* and *S. typhimurium* during manufacture of high-moisture Monterey Jack cheese from ultrafiltered milk and control whole milk (788). Cheese milk was simultaneously inoculated with starter culture, *Pseudomonas fragi* 4973, and the two pathogens. Cheeses were analyzed monthly during 6 months of storage. Numbers of contaminant microbes increased at a similar rate during manufacture in all cheeses. During ripening, bacterial starter culture populations remained high while psychrotrophs declined slowly, *Staphylococcus* remained stable, and *Salmonella* fell sharply. No staphylococcal enterotoxin was detected by reverse passive latex agglutination assay. Italian investigators studied the growth and survival of *S. aureus* and *S. typhimurium* during the manufacture and ripening of Montasio cheese (789). Raw cheese milk was simultaneously inoculated with ~10^5 cfu/mL of *S. aureus* or ~10^6 cfu/mL of *S. typhimurium* and natural starter culture, with or without *Lactobacillus plantarum*. Without *L. plantarum*, *S. aureus* populations increased slightly early in ripening and then remained stable at about 10^6 cfu/mL, whereas *S. typhimurium* decreased during manufacture and ripening but was detectable throughout the 90-day experiment. Addition of *L. plantarum* caused marked reduction in populations of both *S. aureus* and *S.*

typhimurium in the first 10 days, but no further decrease occurred until late in the experiment. No staphylococcal enterotoxin was detected in the cheese. Further tests suggested that *L. plantarum*'s inhibition of *S. typhimurium* was due to acid production, whereas its inhibition of *S. aureus* was due to production of a bacteriocin. However, when raw skim milk was simply inoculated with 10^6–10^7 cfu/mL of mixed *Lactococcus* strains and artificially contaminated with ~10^4 cfu/mL of *Y. enterocolitica* or ~10^2 cfu/mL of *E. coli* O157:H7, the lactococci had no effect on pathogen populations after 120 h of storage at 4°C (*790*). At this temperature *Lactococcus* did not grow enough to reduce the pH to inhibitory levels; in addition, any H_2O_2 produced by the lactic acid bacteria may have been insufficient to activate the lactoperoxidase system or may have been destroyed by the catalase-positive pathogens.

Milk contains a variety of protective proteins, including several that inhibit bacterial growth. The amounts and specificities of these vary in the milks of different species. In a study of camel milk's protective proteins, the activity of lysozyme, lactoferrin, lactoperoxidase, IgG, and IgA was assayed against *L. lactis* ssp. *cremoris, E. coli, S. aureus, S. typhimurium,* and rotavirus (*791*). The antibacterial spectrum of the lysozyme was more like that of egg white than cow milk; cow and camel milk lactoferrins had similar antibacterial spectra; and camel milk lactoperoxidase had no effect on rotavirus, inhibited gram-positive bacteria, and killed gram-negative bacteria. The immunoglobulins had little effect on bacteria but there were high titers of antibodies against rotavirus.

Turkish sucuk is a nonsmoked dry sausage made from beef or lamb and usually eaten hot (*792*). Possible health risks of quick-ripened sucuk were assessed in model batches inoculated with *S. aureus, S. typhimurium, L. monocytogenes,* and *C. perfringens* in conjunction with a *Staphylococcus carnosis* starter, a *S. carnosus* plus *L. plantarum* starter, or no starter (control). *Clostridium perfringens* did not survive, but the other pathogens grew well in control batches at 25°C and maintained relatively stable populations at 20°C. The *S. carnosus* starter culture inhibited pathogen growth slightly at both temperatures, whereas the mixed starter culture caused a sharp drop in pathogen populations within 4–6 days. This drop was associated with acid production and rapid growth by the starter culture.

In experiments similar to those involving *L. monocytogenes* (*631*), Ashenafi and Busse studied the growth of *Salmonella infantis* and *E. coli* in fermenting tempeh made from various kinds of beans (*793*). An increase in pH brought about by mycelial growth on unacidified beans was always accompanied by a sharp increase in growth of the test organisms, and acidification of the beans during soaking delayed this only until active mycelial growth started. Inoculation of cooked beans with *L. plantarum* decreased growth of the test organisms under all conditions, in some cases completely inhibiting it.

The safety of temperature-abused irradiated pork packaged in 25% CO_2–75% N_2 was evaluated by monitoring growth of pathogens inoculated at levels of 10^3 and 10^6 cfu/g before irradiation with 1.75 kGy (*794*). All pathogens grew well in unirradiated control packages, but at the lower inoculum level only *C. perfringens* was detected in irradiated packages. At both high and low inoculum levels, irradiation produced less than a 1-log reduction in *C. perfringens* populations. With large inocula irradiation produced an initial 2–4 log reduction in populations of *S. typhimurium, E. coli, Y. enterocolitica,* and *L. monocytogenes,* but growth occurred rapidly after a lag of 1–3 days. Whenever large populations of spoilage or pathogenic bacteria were present initially, the meat was organoleptically unacceptable even after irradiation.

Microbial stability and survival of pathogens was evaluated in basturma, an intermediate-moisture product popular in Greece (*795*). During 13 months of refrigerated storage of basturma packaged in air or under vacuum, aerobic counts remained stable and no *Salmonella* or *S. aureus* was detected. When *S. aureus* and *Salmonella abortus ovis* were inoculated into the basturma after salting and pressing but before drying, both pathogens survived the dehydration stage but their populations remained steady during 60 days of refrigerated storage.

Two research groups reported on the fate of *Salmonella* and *L. monocytogenes* in commercial mayonnaise (*796,797*). Glass and Doyle evaluated two reduced-calorie products, one of them cholesterol-free, formulated with different levels of acetic acid (*796*). When formulated with 0.7% acetic acid in the aqueous phase, both products inactivated >10^7 *Salmonella* and >10^4 *L. monocytogenes* per gram within 72 h. The authors concluded that reduced-calorie mayonnaise containing 0.7% acetic acid in the aqueous phase (pH <4.1) is microbiologically safe. Erickson and Jenkins inoculated 10^6 cfu/g of *Salmonella* spp. or *L. monocytogenes* into a commercial sandwich spread, real mayonnaise, reduced-calorie mayonnaise, and reduced-calorie cholesterol-free mayonnaise (*797*). Salmonellas were inactivated within 72 h in all products. Inactivation of *L. monocytogenes,* which was related to aqueous-phase acetic acid concentrations, occurred at relative rates of sandwich spread ≥ real mayonnaise > cholesterol-free reduced-calorie mayonnaise > reduced calorie mayonnaise. Even so, the reduced-calorie products showed a 3–5 log reduction in 72 h, indicating a negligible consumer safety risk. The higher antilisterial activity in the cholesterol-free formulation was attributed to eggwhite lysozyme. The same authors studied the behavior of *L. monocytogenes, Y. enterocolitica,* and *A. hydrophila* in commercially pasteurized liquid egg products held at 2–12.8°C (*798*). Unsalted egg whites and blended whole eggs were visibly spoiled at all temperatures in 4–14 days. At 12.8°C all three pathogens grew well in unsalted whole egg blend. *Aeromonas* grew at 6.7 but not 2°C, *Yersinia* grew well at 6.7 and 2°C after a 4-day lag, and *L. monocytogenes* did not grow at 6.7 or 2°C. *Yersinia*'s growth in unsalted egg white was similar to its growth in whole egg, but *Listeria* did not grow at any temperature and *Aeromonas* grew only at 12.8°C. *Aeromonas* was rapidly inactivated in salted egg blend, whereas *Yersinia* populations were stable and *L. monocytogenes* grew well at 12.8°C.

Droffner and Yamamoto demonstrated that prolonged incubation of *E. coli, S. typhimurium,* or *Pseudomonas aeruginosa* at 48°C with nalidixic acid selected mutants able to grow at 48°C, and a second prolonged incubation of these mutants at 54°C further selected mutants capable of growth at this temperature (*799*). Mutants were susceptible to the same bacteriophages as the original mesophilic strains. *Escherichia coli* and *S. typhimurium* mutants expressed the auxotrophic phenotypic markers of their parents when grown at 48 or 54°C, and the thermophilic alleles were mapped in the *gyrA* chromosomal region. The authors concluded that genetic differences between mesophiles and thermophiles are not as absolute as once thought. These findings have implications for food safety.

Dickson and Daniels studied the effects of cell motility and thickness of the surface moisture film on attachment of *S. typhimurium* and *L. monocytogenes* to glass (*800*). With equal cell densities, surface film thickness did not influence bacterial attachment. However, motile *L. monocytogenes* cells had a greater cell-surface charge than nonmotile cells and generally attached in higher numbers. The authors concluded that although the random motion of motile cells may increase their frequency of contact with surfaces, other factors are also involved in attachment and differences in attachment between motile and nonmotile cells cannot be specifically related to the presence or absence of flagella.

Antibacterial activity in foods

Molan reviewed reports of the antibacterial activity of honey, from ancient to modern times (*801*). Pathogens reportedly sensitive to honey's effects include *E. coli, Klebsiella pneumoniae, B. cereus, S. aureus, L. monocytogenes, Salmonella* and *Shigella* spp., and *Vibrio cholerae.* Honeys vary widely in their antibacterial properties, just as bacteria vary widely in their susceptibility to honey. Although part of honey's bactericidal effect has been attributed to H_2O_2, part of the activity is heat-stable, indicating the presence of other factors as well. Some honeys contain lysozyme at levels approaching that in egg white. Phenolic acids contribute a small part of the activity, and the activity of unidentified volatile constituents and constituents extracted by various organic solvents has been demonstrated. A likely source of antibacterial substances in honey is phytochemicals consumed by the honeybees.

Diallyl thiosulphinate, methyl allyl thiosulphinate, and allyl methyl thiosulphinate from garlic cloves and powders had in vitro antimicrobial activity against *E. coli* and *S. aureus* with MICs of 28–100 µg/mL, whereas neither the polar fraction nor alliin was active (*802*). The nonpolar substances also had strong antifungal activity.

The phenolic compounds of rapeseed were isolated and fractionated and their antioxidative and bactericidal properties were investigated (*803*). In both solid and liquid culture media, sinapic acid was strongly bactericidal against *E. coli, B. cereus,* and representative spoilage bacteria. The free phenolic acid fraction was also active. The authors suggest that these rapeseed compounds be considered as preservatives for food and fodder.

The inhibitory effect of *N*-acylamino fatty acids on gram-positive foodborne pathogens was evaluated (*804*). Test organisms included *B. cereus, S. aureus, L. monocytogenes, E. coli, S. typhimurium,* and *Y. enterocolitica.* Myristoyl (C_{14}) derivatives were most active, followed by lauroyl (C_{12}) and palmitoyl (C_{16}). In terms of the amino acid moiety, aromatic amino acids—particularly phenylalanine—were most active; D-isomers and esters of active derivatives were inactive. Inhibition was greater at pH 6 than at pH 7. *N*-Acylamino fatty acids specifically inhibited production of hemolysin by *L. monocytogenes.* These results suggest that these substances have potential for use as food additives.

Maillard reaction products were prepared by heating a solution of glucose and glycine at pH values of 6.0 and 8.8 (*805*). Both preparations strongly inhibited growth of *A. hydrophila; S. aureus* and *L. monocytogenes* were slightly inhibited by the alkaline preparation; *S. typhimurium* and *Salmonella enteritidis* were resistant to both. Further evaluation of Maillard reaction products for control of *A. hydrophila* in noncured precooked meat was recommended.

Identification

A procedure was described for preenriching food samples to allow simultaneous recovery and detection of *Salmonella* and *Listeria* (*806*). A highly buffered low-carbohydrate "universal preenrichment" (UP) broth enabled injured bacteria to recover and achieve populations high enough that secondary enrichment media could be used to select specific bacteria from the mixed background culture. As few as 10 heat-injured *S. typhimurium* or *L. monocytogenes* cells multiplied to at least 10^6 or 10^5 cfu/mL, respectively, after a 24-h enrichment in UP, even in mixed culture with high levels of known competitive organisms or in the presence of the natural microflora found in chicken, hot dogs, or brie cheese. After the UP broth step, conventional protocols for recovery of *Salmonella* and *Listeria* could be followed.

Investigators in China reported development of a diagnostic phage-typing set for *E. coli, C. freundii, Enterobacter cloacae, Salmonella,* and *Shigella* spp. (*807*). The sensitivity of the set was 84% for *E. cloacae,* 89% for *C. freundii,* 90% for *E. coli,* and >99% for *Salmonella* and *C. freundii.* Bacteriophage lytic patterns were also highly correlated with *Shigella* serotypes. This phage-typing set or a similar one was recommended for routine use in public hygiene and clinical laboratories.

Schraft and Untermann reviewed molecular methods for identifying foodborne bacterial pathogens, with emphasis on analyzing restriction fragment length polymorphisms and PCR techniques (*808*).

PREVENTION AND CONTROL

Food microbiologists and the U.S. FDA continue to rank microbiological hazards as the major food safety issue, and recent surveys suggest that the gap between public concerns and the concerns of the food industry and regulatory agencies is narrowing (*809*; also see reference *1*, this chapter). A major difference is the continuing public concern for the safety of irradiated foods, whereas the safety emphasis of federal regulatory agencies is on microbiological issues, pesticide residues, and new products, processes, and packaging. In a two-part paper, Notermans discussed new problems in food microbiology that have arisen from increased demands on the global food system and rapid changes in consumers' preferences and food technology (*810*). He reviewed the incidence of foodborne illness and its major causes, addressing critical control points in the food system. *Salmonella* contamination of poultry was used as an example. He then discussed emerging pathogens and other health hazards and summarized new methods for their identification and control, including the concept of Hazard Analysis Critical Control Points (HACCP).

Predictive microbiology

The ability to predict microbial growth as a function of the food environment enormously reduces the extent of experimentation and monitoring required to ensure safety. Buchanan reviewed the history of mathematically modeling the effects of multiple variables on growth or survival of foodborne bacteria (*811*). In particular he discussed probability and response-surface models. Data were presented showing the agreement between observed and predicted values for growth of *Salmonella* in culture medium and growth of *Listeria monocytogenes* in various food and culture media. McMeekin et al. reviewed the application of predictive microbiology in the HACCP approach to assure the quality and safety of fish and fish products (*812*). After a mathematical model has been validated under conditions simulating commercial practice, the information obtained must be incorporated into monitoring devices. Not only temperature history but other chemical and physical factors that change during production or storage and influence growth will probably be monitored by the next generation of monitoring devices.

Risk management and the HACCP approach

Total quality management (TQM) and the HACCP system are complementary management philosophies that together can answer the food industry's need to improve quality and productivity while ensuring safety (*813*). The history and philosophy of HACCP were briefly reviewed and requisites and benefits of an effective HACCP program were summarized. The authors argued that to be most useful,

HACCP should focus on food safety, ignoring quality factors. *Critical* control points, where control *must* be exercised and critical limits *must* be met, should be carefully differentiated from control points, where loss of control is not likely to produce an unacceptable risk but correction is nonetheless required. Sperber listed the following HACCP principles: conduct hazard analysis and risk assessment; determine critical control points (CCPs); establish specifications for each CCP; monitor each CCP; establish corrective action to be taken in case of deviation at a CCP; establish a record-keeping system; and establish verification procedures (*814*). The initial risk assessment should consider whether the food will be eaten by at-risk populations, contains a sensitive ingredient, has undergone a process step to eliminate the hazard, has a potential for recontamination before packaging, has potential for product abuse, or is subjected to a terminal heat process. Pillsbury's hazard control plan was described. In a similar discussion of hazard analysis and HACCP, Corlett extended the approach to chemical and physical hazards (*815*). Tisler discussed HACCP from the perspective of a regulatory agency (the FDA) (*816*). The responsibilities of the agency and the food industry were delineated and the FDA's guidelines for an HACCP inspection were presented.

The popularity of the many new "refrigerated pasteurized foods of extended durability" (REPFEDs) has many ramifications for public health (*817*). HACCP allows the design and introduction of longitudinally integrated procedures for manufacture, distribution, handling, and preparation of these foods to insure their safety. This "LISA" strategy (longitudinal integrated safety assurance) was outlined. The colonization of REPFEDs by psychrotrophic pathogens and other microbiological hazards were discussed. Possibilities for providing foods with intrinsic antimicrobial attributes or microbial warning signals were mentioned. The necessity for continuing communication between regulatory agencies, industry, and the public was stressed and some principles of surveillance and inspection were presented.

REPFEDs have provided motivation for extending HACCP systems beyond the manufacture of foods to distribution, retail display, and the home

(818). Temperature audits revealed widespread temperature abuse in display cases and the home. The only options available to the retailer appear to be to use adequate refrigeration and controls or to sell only products that can tolerate the temperature abuse. The ubiquity of temperature abuse may stimulate modifications in manufacturing programs or new retailing approaches. In the home, the problem could be reduced by educating the consumer. A study by Tropicana Products, Inc., audited air and juice temperatures during transit to identify critical control points during the phases of distribution *(819).* Other practices at the warehouse and retail stores were checked, and based on the findings the company was able to implement an HACCP program covering the entire distribution process.

DAIRY PRODUCTS. Abstracts of papers presented at the 78th annual meeting of the International Association of Milk, Food, and Environmental Sanitarians were published in *Journal of Food Protection (820).* Presentations addressed dairy microbiology and sanitation, food microbiology, the spread of foodborne diseases by foodservice workers, microbiological methods, and issues in food processing.

Mettler discussed control of pathogens in the manufacture of spray-dried milk powders in terms of preventing pathogen entry and growth before and after pasteurization, conditions for effective pasteurization, and knowledge of the plant's pathogen status *(821).* Marth discussed raw milk as a source of pathogens and recommended measures for dealing with the problem so that finished products and the environment of the dairy plant are not contaminated *(822).*

MEAT AND MEAT PRODUCTS. Microbial contamination of animal carcasses during slaughter and subsequent processing is probably inevitable but can be minimized by good practices. Dickson and Anderson reviewed the sources of contamination and the process of bacterial attachment to surfaces *(823).* They then discussed washing and sanitizing procedures and equipment. A method patented by Anderson involves an automated high-pressure carcass washer that can remove 90% of the bacteria on

a carcass *(824).* Organic acids are used in the wash. Lactic acid is most effective against *Salmonella,* but no single acid is best against all organisms. Other investigators evaluated the effects of acid-decontamination of beef carcasses after dehiding, after evisceration, or both *(825).* Forty carcasses were sprayed with 1% (v/v) lactic acid, pH 2.8, at 55°C. Surface samples were examined for aerobic plate count, *Salmonella,* and *Listeria.* No salmonellas were detected on any sample. *Listeria* was detected in three samples from unsprayed controls but not in any sprayed sample. Aerobic plate counts of acid-treated carcasses were significantly lower than those of controls, and the reduction was greatest on carcasses receiving two treatments.

A paper on the safety of foods of animal origin emphasized the role and responsibilities of the veterinarian in preventing zoonotic and foodborne disease *(826).* Veterinarians are involved at critical points in live animal production, slaughter and processing, and distribution. Developments in biotechnology, risk assessment, and communications also involve veterinarians *(827).* A recent interdisciplinary workshop at the College of Veterinary Medicine of Texas A&M University addressed the safety of foods of animal origin, judging it to be amenable to scientific management. The biotechnology panel identified advanced diagnostic procedures, use of recombinant proteins, and genetic alteration of animals as approaches for improving food safety. All of these will require careful consideration of risk— the safety of food samples contacted by gene probes, alteration of endogenous biochemical moieties by use of recombinant proteins, and the safety of transgenic animals in dimensions associated with the gene product, the gene construct, and integration of the gene construct. All points of the food-production chain must be considered. The risk assessment panel identified an array of improvements in risk assessment technology that are needed for its maximally effective application in food safety programs. The communications panel analyzed the causes of growing consumer concern and confusion about food-safety issues. It found disagreements among the communicators, contradictions in the messages, and conflicts between the modes in which the audience processes the messages. Emotions, cultural attitudes, economic and policy issues, and historical processes are involved.

The concept of slaughterhouse hygiene was discussed in terms of physical layout, construction, and function; organizational structure and management strategy; the training, personal hygiene, and morale of workers; analysis of the slaughter process; and quality control (828). Another paper identified weak points in the hygiene of slaughtering, cutting, and processing firms (829). The importance of fully trained, knowledgeable workers was emphasized. The appropriate mission and use of a bacteriological factory laboratory in the meat industry were considered, and specifications for designing and equipping such a laboratory were proposed (830). The authors believe that when well integrated into the quality control program, the factory laboratory can make important contributions to food safety.

SEAFOOD. HACCP programs must be tailored to the foods involved, and seafoods present unique problems. Ward reviewed the biological, environmental, and harvesting factors that make seafoods "different" from other muscle protein foods, requiring different strategies for processing, preserving, and packaging (831). Huss reviewed the development and use of the HACCP concept in fish processing (832). Seafoods were ranked in order of decreasing safety risk, from molluscs often eaten with no additional cooking to fresh and frozen fish and crustaceans usually eaten after cooking. Hazards were identified and critical control points were found for most of them. The author argued that while principles of HACCP can be incorporated into national regulations and used by regulatory agencies, the strength of HACCP lies more in its application to individual situations than to general issues. At the regulatory level, Garrett and Hudak-Roos described HACCP applications to seafood inspection in the USA (833,834). The National Marine Fisheries Services is generally credited with designing and implementing the educational and training techniques used to expand the HACCP concept to all products and regulatory issues in the seafood industry, and the authors explained this project (833). Government agencies concerned with seafood safety include the FDA, Department of Commerce, USDA, EPA, Department of Defense, and various state agencies; the activities of these agencies were described (834). HACCP sampling procedures were discussed in some detail.

PUBLIC EDUCATION. The HACCP system was considered as an approach to decreasing consumer complaints about food products (835). Consumer dissatisfaction stems from unfamiliarity with products and unrealistic expectations, price, defects, and consumer mishandling. Most of the unknowns relate to how products are handled by the consumer. Using basic HACCP principles, consumers should check products and containers at the store, handle them properly on the way home, store and prepare them properly, keep the kitchen sanitary and maintain personal hygiene, store prepared foods properly, and carefully manage their pantries. Several avenues for consumer education were suggested. A nationwide survey gathered data on consumers' knowledge of food safety principles and practices (836). Although nearly all consumers would benefit from additional home food-safety education, persons younger than 35 years would benefit most. Knowledge of a term or concept did not necessarily correlate with appropriate food-preparation practice.

A study of knowledge of food-service sanitation among convenience store managers and employees in the Lansing, Michigan, area showed that knowledge of proper food handling procedures was correlated to sanitary conditions in the food-preparation area (837). Overall scores on the questionnaire were ~60% for both managers and employees, but managers' knowledge was more highly correlated with actual conditions than employees' knowledge. The findings suggest that mandatory certification in food service sanitation be recommended for managers of convenience stores and that a certified manager be on duty during all business hours in convenience stores with food-service-type operations.

Food sabotage is an aspect of food safety that may be overlooked in educational programs (838). Perhaps the most notorious example of food sabotage in a food-service establishment occurred in Oregon in 1984, when >750 people became ill with salmonellosis after eating foods, primarily salad bar items, that had been intentionally contaminated by individuals not employed by the establishments. Awareness of the risk is the first step in reducing it, but other factors such as facility design need to be considered.

BIOTECHNOLOGY ISSUES. Pariza considered indirect ramifications of biochemical alterations in foods, whether genetically engineered or modified through processing (*839*). For example, low-acid tomatoes may not inhibit growth of *C. botulinum* and low-caffeine coffee beans may be more susceptible to mold growth and mycotoxin production. Similarly, efforts to reduce use of agricultural chemicals by increasing amounts of natural pesticides in plants may create levels toxic to humans, even by conventional breeding methods. Although the enhancement of food safety through biotechnology appears promising, risks associated with these products must be comprehensively evaluated.

An analysis of the new risks presented by new foods and technologies identified factors in the food environment that favor entry, survival, and growth of foodborne pathogens (*840*). The entire temperature history of the product is important, as are trends toward extended shelf life and reduced salt. Pathogens presenting particular problems in particular settings were considered individually. The role of HACCP and longitudinal risk assessment and control was discussed.

Although the HACCP concept has been widely applied to quality assurance systems in the food industry, implementation in certain areas is hampered by lack of knowledge of critical control points and how to control them (*841*). Traditional microbiological approaches cannot meet the need for highly sensitive and reliable tests at critical control points and rapid, user-friendly tests for monitoring. Future microbiological quality control will probably involve combinations of certified bioanalytical reagents and techniques such as immunoassays, DNA probes and primers, automated culture systems, and flow cytometry. These techniques were discussed as they would apply to highly processed foods, fermented foods, and foods of animal origin. For the last category, the author emphasized that

most of the problems arise and must be controlled in the home. Other authors also emphasized the need for changing the procedures for microbial testing of foods (*842*). Ideally, both incoming ingredients and production lines would be monitored to provide rapid and continuous information on poorly controlled processes. An effective HACCP plan is vital in establishing the safety of new types of foods. Automated versions of traditional microbiological and metabolic tests, bioluminescence, DNA probes and primers, immunoassays, and biosensors were reviewed.

Solberg discussed two high-technology approaches to assuring the microbiological safety of foods with extended shelf life stored under refrigeration or at room temperature (*843*). One is computer-based, involving on-line identification and enumeration of microorganisms, determination of minimum treatment conditions, and choice of end products suitable for processing under these conditions. Existing methods applicable to this approach (predictive mathematical modeling, antibody and hybridization techniques, and bioluminescence) must be improved, particularly in terms of sensitivity. The objective of the second approach is to attack the microorganisms without affecting the food. Targeted energy and interference with microbial membranes are among the possibilities for this approach. The primary target organism is always *C. botulinum*, but *Y. enterocolitica* and *L. monocytogenes* are of concern in refrigerated foods and *Salmonella*, *S. aureus*, *C. perfringens*, *B. cereus*, and *C. jejuni* are important at room temperature. The state of the art of applicable "magic bullet" methods using pulsed lasers, high hydrostatic pressure, and bacteriocins was reviewed.

A volume in the *Bioprocess Technology* series was devoted to biosensors (*844*). It contains chapters on amperometric and potentiometric methods, enzyme thermistors, piezoelectric crystal biosensors, chemically mediated fiberoptic methods, immunosensors, and biosensors based on FET, chromophores, bioluminescence, and chemiluminescence. Needs, trends, and prospects were discussed. The potential role of biosensors in the food and drink industries was discussed in another paper (*845*). Despite the promise of these methods, only a few are used routinely. The advantages and disadvantages of common transducers were summarized, promising amperometric biosensors were described, and the relevance of other methods for the food and drink industries was considered. Problems exist in the distribution and technical support and service of biosensor systems, and in the reliability and production of associated biological materials. Some systems remain too expensive for routine application.

The ability to make microorganisms emit light through the luciferase reaction by introducing the *lux* genes has opened many possibilities in food microbiology and the food industry (*846*). Assays using bacterial luminescence to detect and enumerate microorganisms are rapid, sensitive, and accurate and they can be made specific. The authors reviewed the biochemistry and molecular biology of bioluminescence and the instrumentation involved in measuring it. Applications such as detecting specific pathogens and indicator organisms; monitoring behavior of lactic acid bacteria, starter cultures, and probiotics; and monitoring the recovery of injured cells and the effectiveness of biocides and virucides were discussed.

The status of rapid methods and automation in food microbiology and likely developments were reviewed (*847*). Technologies were considered for detection of biomass and microbial contamination, bioluminescence assays, continuous and segmented flow analyses, and flow-injection analysis (FIA). The incorporation of antigen–antibody reactions into FIA and the combination of FIA with biosensors were discussed.

MICROBIOLOGICAL CRITERIA. The success of an HACCP program and results of microbiological monitoring must be judged against practical goals or criteria. Microbiological criteria for meat products and heat-treated products that can be stored without refrigeration were discussed (*848*). "Hurdle technology" in these products includes use of preservatives and competing flora and manipulations of a_w, pH, and redox potential (Eh). These were considered for specific types of meat products, based on studies with *Clostridium sporogenes* as a model spore-forming bacterium. Recommendations were also presented for enhancing the microbiological

safety of raw molluscan shellfish (*849*). Water classification and restriction of harvest to proper growing water is the first and most essential point of control. Next is strict time/temperature control after harvesting. Introduction and multiplication of bacteria during subsequent distribution is controlled by sanitation and refrigeration. Specific recommendations were made regarding HACCP-based control and revisions to current standards and the National Shellfish Sanitation Program *Manual of Operations.*

A standardized inspection procedure for restaurants was developed to quantitatively assess risks (*850*). Thirty variables based on visual assessment and microbiological sampling were scored as good, satisfactory, poor, or unacceptable. Premises were evaluated for structure and design, cleaning and cleanliness, personal hygiene, risk of contamination, temperature control, and training and knowledge about food hygiene. Microbiological and visual assessments were not highly correlated. Although the inspections were standardized, there was significant variation in scores assigned by different inspectors. This occurred with no clear evidence of bias and in the absence of consistent high or low scoring by particular inspectors. Problem areas revealed by the inspections were discussed.

SANITATION. The attachment of bacteria to food and other surfaces has important consequences in food processing. Pontefract reviewed the phenomenon of attachment and ways of studying it (*851*). Evaluation of the effectiveness of cleaning and sanitation requires methods for enumerating attached organisms. Major problems persist in applying standard bacteriological sampling techniques in a practical time frame for modern food-processing procedures. Possibilities for rapid, accurate assessment of attached bacteria were discussed.

By their nature, new food products and production methods rely more heavily than ever on good in-plant sanitation practices to assure food safety (*852*). Giese reviewed sanitation in terms of plant design and the typical four-step sanitation process. He summarized properties and uses of specific detergents and sanitizers and discussed various equipment and systems.

Natural antimicrobial systems, microbial antagonism, and bacteriocins

A review of intrinsic factors in plants and animals that prevent colonization or reduce proliferation of pathogens in food discussed pH, Eh, moisture content, nutrients, protective structures (e.g., skin, seed coats), antimicrobial substances (e.g., enzymes, fatty acids, organic acids, essential oils, pigments), and microbial antagonism (*853*). All of these have been or could be utilized to enhance the microbiological safety of foods. In general they are less costly than extrinsic factors such as temperature and humidity control, which are used to extend the shelf life of foods.

COLONIZATION OF POULTRY. A monograph in the *Food Science and Technology* series contained papers delivered at a symposium on control of colonization of poultry by human bacterial enteropathogens (*854*). Session I concerned environmental factors involved in colonization. Session II covered studies on competitive exclusion. Session III addressed mechanisms of colonization of chickens by *Salmonella* and *Campylobacter*. Session IV dealt with immunization. It was apparent that only an integrated enteropathogen colonization control program involving all phases of the industry can reduce or eliminate carcass and product contamination. The first line of defense against contamination of poultry meat by enteropathogens is in poultry production; the second involves improvements in processing technology. Beyond that, education is necessary to teach principles of safe handling, cooking, and storage of poultry and poultry products.

Mixed cultures of *Veillonella* and *Enterococcus durans* isolated from the cecal contents of adult broilers inhibited growth of *S. typhimurium* and *E. coli* O157:H7 on culture medium containing 2.5% lactose but not on medium containing 0.25% lactose (*855*). Pure cultures of the two organisms were not effective on either medium. The inhibition apparently was due to production of lactic acid from lactose by *E. durans* and subsequent production of acetic and propionic acids from lactic acid by *Veillonella*. These observations support the theory that the reduction of cecal colonization of young chicks by salmonellas mediated by dietary lactose and anaerobic cecal cultures from mature chickens is related to production of lactic acid and volatile fatty acids from lactose by these bacteria. The same research group reported the effects of an anaerobic gram-positive coccus isolated from the cecal contents of adult chickens (*856*). The organism, a *Streptococcus* sp., was labeled strain CA331. Cultures inhibited growth of *S. typhimurium* and *E. coli* O157:H7 on media containing 0.25 or 2.5% lactose but not on lactose-free medium. Significantly higher concentrations of lactic and acetic acids were produced on media containing lactose and the pH of the medium was significantly lower.

BACTERIOCINS AND ANTIBACTERIAL METABOLITES. Bacteriocins are antimicrobial proteins produced by lactic acid bacteria. These were discussed in a review (*857*). Some are cidal to a narrow range of target organisms, usually closely related to the producer; others, such as nisin and pediocin A, inhibit a broad spectrum of gram-positive organisms including many spoilage and pathogenic bacteria associated with food. The former are generally produced by species of *Lactobacillus* and *Lactococcus* that are used in starter cultures to achieve reliable fermentation through suppression of competing microorganisms. The latter may also have this effect, but in addition they inhibit pathogens such as *L. monocytogenes* and *C. botulinum*. Because they appear to be nontoxic and nonimmunogenic for humans, they have applications as natural preservatives in fermented food products, in conjunction with traditional methods of preservation and proper hygienic control. It may be possible to expand the inhibitory spectrum of bacteriocins or combine them to cover a wider range of target organisms.

Another review discussed both nonpeptide antibacterial substances and bacteriocins produced by lactic acid bacteria (*858*). The nonpeptide inhibitor reuterin, produced by anaerobically grown *Lactobacillus reuteri* in the presence of glycerol, has an exceptionally broad spectrum of activity spanning gram-positive and gram-negative organisms, fungi, and protozoa. Reuterin has been chemically characterized and appears to warrant further study for applications in agriculture and the food industry. In reviewing the bacteriocins, the authors highlighted similarities and differences among these compounds in structure, biochemical properties, nature of their genetic determinants, and activity spectra.

Ten strains of bacteriocin-producing lactic acid bacteria were isolated from retail cuts of beef, lamb, and pork (*859*). The meat isolates were identified as *Lactobacillus bavaricus, L. plantarum, Lactobacillus viridescens, Carnobacterium piscicola, Leuconostoc* sp., and *Streptococcus* sp. These and 11 other bacteriocin-producing lactic acid bacteria were tested for inhibitory activity against *L. monocytogenes, A. hydrophila,* and *S. aureus.* Inhibition due to production of acid or H_2O_2 or to lytic bacteriophages was excluded and sensitivity to proteolytic enzymes confirmed the proteinaceous nature of the inhibitors. Eight meat isolates inhibited all four *L. monocytogenes* strains tested. Most isolates active against *L. monocytogenes* were also active against *A. hydrophila, S. aureus,* or both. One *L. bavaricus* strain was active against *A. hydrophila* and *S. aureus* but not against *L. monocytogenes.* Although the meat strains were isolated on the basis of activity against *L. monocytogenes* Scott A, the *Streptococcus* isolate, on further testing, had lost this characteristic, suggesting the possibility of a plasmidborne determinant. Investigation of bacteriocin S50 (active only against other *Lactococcus* species), strengthened the notion of a plasmidborne determinant (*860*). This bacteriocin is produced by *Lactococcus lactis diacitilactis* S50, an organism containing four plasmids. Plasmid curing abolished bacteriocin production. However, the actual location of the bacteriocin gene(s) was not determined.

Study of the broad-spectrum antibacterial activity of *Pediococcus damnosus* and *Pediococcus pentosaceus* in minced meat confirmed that the activity cannot be explained by acid production and decreased pH in the food matrix, even at high inoculum levels (*861*). All pediococcal strains inhibited growth of *L. monocytogenes, Y. enterocolitica, Pseudomonas fragi,* and *Pseudomonas fluorescens* with inocula of 10^8 cfu/g, but not with smaller inocula. A cell-free extract of the *Pediococcus*

growth medium was much more inhibitory than viable *Pediococcus* cells, possibly because observations were not continued long enough to provide time for maximal bacteriocin production in the meat system. Nevertheless, the authors stressed that the inhibitory potential of bacteriocin-producing organisms may be easier to demonstrate in laboratory media than in food systems, making it imperative that studies in food systems receive high priority.

Traditional direct and deferred antagonism methods and the well diffusion technique for detecting bacteriocins were adapted for use with microdilution wells (*862*). The traditional well diffusion method used to screen lactic acid bacteria for bacteriocin production was a laborious procedure requiring that a number of holes be punched out of the agar with a cork borer. Five strains of *Lactobacillus* were tested in seven variations of the microdilution well method, and the results were compared and discussed. Other authors reported an improved quantitative agar diffusion assay for nisin (*863*). Use of *Lactobacillus sake* ATCC 15521 rather than *Micrococcus luteus* ATCC 10420 greatly increased the sensitivity of the assay, as reflected by the increase in zone size associated with a given increase in nisin concentration, although the minimal detectable level of nisin was the same for both organisms. Preincubation of plates at 3°C further increased sensitivity and gave the greatest assay reproducibility.

Studies in model liposome systems showed that the activity of nisin is enhanced by a membrane potential and/or pH gradient across the membrane (*864*). Liposomes were prepared from *E. coli* phosphatidylethanolamine and egg phosphatidylcholine. The membrane potential and pH gradient were established by artificial ion gradients or by oxidation of ascorbate, *N,N,N',N'*-tetramethyl-*p*-phenylenediamine, and cytochrome *c* by beef-heart cytochrome *c* oxidase incorporated into the liposome membrane. Incorporation of nisin into the membrane made the membrane permeable for ions; it dissipated the membrane potential and pH gradient in both types of liposomes and inhibited oxygen consumption by cytochrome *c* oxidase in the proteoliposomes.

Several new bacteriocins or natural variants have been characterized (*865–867*). *Lactococcus lactis* strain NIZO 22186 produces a 3.5-kDa lanthionine-containing polypeptide highly similar to nisin but not identical (*865*). On biochemical and genetic analysis, it proved to be a natural nisin variant differing from nisin only in a $His_{27}Asn$ substitution, reflected in a C to A transversion at position 148 in the *nisZ* gene. A new bacteriocin, carnocin U149, produced by a *Carnobacterium* species isolated from fish, was purified and partially characterized (*866*). It contains 35–37 amino acids in addition to an unidentified peak migrating at the position of lanthionine, suggesting that like nisin, it belongs to the lantibiotic class of bacteriocins. The sequence of the first 7 amino acid residues was determined, but further sequencing may be hampered by thioether-bridged amino acids and possibly by other modified residues. Lactocin S, produced by *L. sake* L-45, was purified and the major part of its amino acid sequence was determined (*867*). The *N*-terminal amino acid was blocked. Three unidentified residues in the *C*-terminal part were thought to be modified forms of cysteine or amino acids associated with cysteine.

Antibacterial metabolites produced by starter culture bacteria were tested for inhibitory properties against foodborne pathogens able to grow in refrigerated foods (*868*). Three culture preparations containing pediocin AcH, nisin, and sakacin A and four commercial preparations of bacterial metabolites were studied. The four bacteriocins were bactericidal to all strains of *L. monocytogenes, Listeria ivanovii*, and *Listeria innocua* tested, but not to strains of *Salmonella, Y. enterocolitica, E. coli*, or *A. hydrophila*. Diacetyl had some bactericidal effect against *Yersinia, Aeromonas, E. coli*, and *Salmonella anatum*, but not against *Listeria*. Lactate had limited bacteriostatic effect against gram-negative but not gram-positive pathogens. Microgard had no bactericidal or bacteriostatic action against any pathogen tested. These studies were performed in vitro. They should be complemented by testing in food systems.

Processing technology

Many new nonthermal processes for food preservation are being developed. Mertens and Knorr reviewed progress in these technologies (*869*). High electric-field pulses, oscillating magnetic field pulses, microwave irradiation, ionizing irradiation, intense light pulses, high-pressure treatments, CO_2 treatments, antimicrobial chemicals and enzymes, and biological control systems were discussed, with emphasis on the physical methods. Another review considered shelf-life extension and the microbiological safety of fresh meat (*870*). Although the emphasis was on spoilage patterns and combinations of treatments that can enhance the keeping quality of meat during refrigerated storage, the reviewers did address concerns for the safety of fresh meat packaged under modified atmospheres and irradiated—specifically, growth and toxin production by *C. botulinum* and other pathogens in meat under conditions of mild temperature abuse. Pearson and Gray reviewed conventional and new methods for preserving meat and poultry products (*871*). It has been estimated that irradiation of all meat at a level of 4 kGy would virtually eliminate problems from meat and poultry pathogens, so long as subsequent recontamination was prevented. A cost–benefit analysis of such an approach estimated an annual net benefit of $106–$200 million for pork and $186–$498 million for chicken irradiation. A similar rationale could be developed for beef.

The effect of high hydrostatic pressure on survival of *L. monocytogenes* in raw and UHT milk and of *V. parahaemolyticus* in heat-processed canned clam juice was evaluated (*872*). The pressure tolerance of the pathogens was also determined in buffered saline solutions. A population of ~10^6 cfu/mL of *L. monocytogenes* Scott A was killed by exposure to 3400 atm within 80 min at 23°C in UHT milk; killing occurred in 20 min in buffer. A population of ~10^6 cfu/mL of *V. parahaemolyticus* was killed within 10 min by exposure to 1700 atm at 23°C in clam juice or buffer.

El-Gazzar and Marth reviewed applications of ultrafiltration and reverse osmosis in the dairy foods industry (*873*). When milk is processed in this way, calcium phosphate, milk fat, and casein are concentrated in the "retentate." This increases the buffering capacity of the milk and otherwise alters conditions for growth of pathogenic bacteria. The sometimes discrepant results of studies of the growth and survival of specific pathogens in retentate, unconcentrated milk, diluted retentate, retentate plus permeate, and products made from retentate and unconcentrated milk were summarized. The major portion of the review concerned behavior of starter cultures in retentate and characteristics of products made from ultrafiltered milk. A study of membrane processing as a way to eliminate spoilage organisms and pathogens from dairy fluids (rather than as a way to concentrate the fluid) found that no unit or membrane retained all organisms while allowing permeated solids to equal the solids in the original bulk fluid (*874*). Raw milk, reconstituted skim milk, skim milk, sweet whey, and acid whey containing indigenous microorganisms were inoculated with *S. aureus, S. typhimurium,* and/or *Pseudomonas fragi* and processed on units from three manufacturers. Neither the nature of the bulk fluid nor bacterial morphology and size affected the extent of bacterial retention. Moreover, different membranes with the same molecular-weight cut-off had different retention characteristics. Membranes that reduced bacterial loads by 98.9–99.99% allowed 5–6% of the bulk-fluid solids to pass through the membrane.

The safety concerns and risks of packaging fresh seafood products under vacuum or modified atmospheres were reviewed (*875,876*). These methods extend shelf-life and maintain quality by suppressing normal spoilage bacteria but may allow *C. botulinum* to grow and produce toxin, particularly under conditions of temperature abuse. Prepackaging steps such as irradiation or antimicrobial treatment may be necessary to delay clostridial outgrowth and toxin production in fresh fish products beyond their point of spoilage. Mechanisms for the preservative effects of CO_2 were reviewed and Genigeorgis's computer-generated model of the probability of *C. botulinum* outgrowth from one spore was discussed.

The MICs of methyl *p*-hydroxybenzoate (methyl paraben) and potassium sorbate were compared for *L. monocytogenes, Y. enterocolitica, A. hydrophila,* and *Pseudomonas putida* (*877*). Overall, *L. monocytogenes* was the most resistant and *A. hydrophila* the most sensitive. The time for a 3-log decrease in viable counts in medium containing 1000 mg/L methylparaben at 5°C ranged from >4

months for *L. monocytogenes* to a few days for *A. hydrophila.* At pH 5 the preservatives had similar MICs, but at pH 6 the MIC of potassium sorbate was 2.5–10 times that of methyl paraben, except against *A. hydrophila.* MICs were substantially higher at 30 than at 5°C. Concentrations of preservative that permitted growth at 30°C did not lead to resistance to the preservative. Repair of preservative-injured cells was demonstrated. The type of buffer used influenced the MICs and rate of injury of *L. monocytogenes.*

The kinetics of bacterial destruction by microwave irradiation was investigated for an *E. coli* strain that had "average" thermal destruction characteristics (*878*). There were no important differences for microwave exposure and conventional heating, indicating that the destruction profile can be interpreted in terms of thermal effects. From the slope of the Arrhenius plot, the activation energy of thermal destruction was calculated as 4.3×10^5 J/mol for this organism. At low power and short intervals of exposure the survival curve was approximated by a set of three linear segments; with constant exposure at high power, killing was rapid and kinetic analysis was difficult. The effects of container shape, pH, salt, and sucrose were evaluated.

A review of the wholesomeness and safety of irradiated foods found restrictions on the energies of X-rays and fast electrons that can be used if induction of short-lived radioactivity is to be avoided (*879*). Gamma rays, in contrast, are not known to induce radioactivity in foods. Irradiation produces chemical changes (as in polyunsaturated fatty acids) and some nutrient loss (e.g., antioxidants), but these are considered unimportant for persons who eat a balanced diet. However, irradiation does not eliminate risk of foodborne pathogens, particularly in certain foods in which spoilage organisms are most effectively destroyed. Mutations caused by irradiation are considered as unlikely to be dangerous as are mutations caused by other treatments. Another review of the use of ionizing radiation in food preservation gave particular reference to seafood (*880*). Gram-negative bacteria, which include many of the typical seafood spoilage organisms, are generally more sensitive than gram-positive species. However, there is great variation even within a species: for example, among *Salmonella* serotypes. Effects of irradiation also depend strongly on the type of seafood substrate. Because it is relatively sensitive, *E. coli* is a poor indicator of *Salmonella* and enteric viruses in irradiated foods. *Clostridium* and *S. aureus* are among the more radiation-resistant organisms. Vibrios are relatively sensitive. Irradiation at levels needed to inactivate fish parasites may produce an organoleptically unacceptable product, but little research has been done in this area. Evaluation of the microbiological safety and quality of frozen grass prawns irradiated at −10°C suggested this as a practical way to reduce the levels of common pathogens (*881*). The D_{10} values for *V. cholerae, S. aureus, E. coli,* and *Salmonella enteritidis* were, respectively, 0.11, 0.29, 0.39, and 0.48 kGy. The threshold dose for detecting radiation flavor was 4.5 kGy. The greatest nutrient change was a 32% decrease in thiamine with 10 kGy. A study of fresh and frozen irradiated chicken meat suggested that a dose of 2 kGy reduced natural contamination by 3 log but did not eliminate high loads of *Staphylococcus* (*882*). Because of the differing sensitivities of various salmonellas and the protection afforded by natural food components, higher doses also would be necessary to assure eradication of salmonellas.

An interesting application of irradiation technology to shellfish is the irradiation of living shellfish (*883*). Cobalt-60 irradiation of the hard-shelled clam (*Mercenaria mercenaria*) and the oyster (*Crassostrea virginica*) significantly reduced virus carriage without important adverse effects on shellfish survival. Citing evidence for the radiation sensitivity of pathogenic vibrios in shellfish and the reduction of staphylococci by irradiation, the authors concluded that ^{60}Co irradiation is a promising way to improve shellfish sanitation and safety, supplementing the effects of depuration. Another paper reviewed the applications of depuration for removal of viral and bacterial pathogens and various organic and inorganic toxins and contaminants from shellfish (*884*).

Minimal thermal processing of seafoods was reviewed, focusing on impact on the product's microbiology (*885*). Because pasteurization processes are designed to maximize shelf life rather than to destroy *C. botulinum,* this organism was considered in most detail.

The heat resistance of *S. typhimurium* and *L. monocytogenes* was determined in sucrose solutions with various a_w values (*886*). For *S. typhimurium, $D_{65.6°C}$* ranged from 0.29 to 40.2 min as a_w decreased from 0.98 to 0.83. For *L. monocytogenes* in sucrose solutions with a_w ranging from 0.98 to 0.90, $D_{65.6°C}$ ranged from 0.36 to 3.8 min. In four commercial chocolate syrups, the $D_{65.6°C}$ for *S. typhimurium* was 1.2–3.2 min. The a_w of these syrups was between 0.75 and 0.84 but was unrelated to *D.* The influence of the heating menstruum on heat resistance was discussed.

LITERATURE CITED

1. Lechowich, R.V. Current concerns in food safety. In *Food Safety Assessment.* J.W. Finley, S.F. Robinson, and D.J. Armstrong (eds.). Washington, DC, American Chemical Society. *ACS Symp. Ser.* 484:232–242 (1992).

2. Roberts, T., and P.M. Foegeding. Risk assessment for estimating the economic costs of foodborne disease caused by microorganisms. In *Economics of Food Safety.* J.A. Caswell (ed.). New York, Elsevier Sci. Pub. Co., Inc. Pp. 103–129 (1991).

3. Jay, J.M. Microbiological food safety. *Crit. Rev. Food Sci. Nutr.* 31:177–190 (1992).

4. Grossklaus, D., K. Gerigk, H. Kolb, and K.-D. Zastrow. Zur weltweiten Zunahme von Enteritis infectiosa-Fällen—Kritische Anmerkungen. *Arch. Lebensmittelhyg.* 42:136–140 (1991).

5. Schofield, G.M. Emerging food-borne pathogens and their significance in chilled foods. *J. Appl. Bacteriol.* 72:267–273 (1992).

6. Anonymous. Diseases transmitted through the food supply: information taken from the Federal Register. *Food Safety Notebook* 3:94–95 (1992).

7. Guerrant, R.L., and D.A. Bobak. Bacterial and protozoal gastroenteritis. *New Engl. J. Med.* 325:327–340 (1991).

8. Anonymous. *A Review of Foodborne Disease Outbreaks in New York State 1990.* New York State

Department of Health, Bureau of Community Sanitation and Food Protection. April 1992. Summarized in *Food Protect. Rep.* 8(9):1–2 (1992).

9. Todd, E.C.D. Foodborne disease in Canada—a 10-year summary from 1975 to 1984. *J. Food Protect.* 55:123–132 (1992).

10. Herwaldt, B.L., G.F. Craun, S.L. Stokes, and D.D. Juranek. Waterborne-disease outbreaks, 1989–1990. *Morbid. Mortal. Weekly Rep.* 40(SS-3) (1991).

11. Levine, W.C., J.F. Smart, D.L. Archer, et al. Foodborne disease outbreaks in nursing homes, 1975 through 1987. *JAMA* 266:2105–2109 (1991).

12. Zottola, E.A., and L.B. Smith. Pathogenic bacteria in meat and meat products. In *Meat and Health.* A.M. Pearson and T.R. Dutson (eds.). *Adv. Meat Res.* 6:157–183 (1990).

13. Mossel, D.A.A. Management of microbiological health hazards associated with foods of animal origin: contribution of the Plumb strategy. *Arch. Lebensmittelhyg.* 42:27–32 (1991).

14. Anonymous. Seafood safety: highlights of the executive summary of the 1991 report by the Committee on Evaluation of the Safety of Fishery Products of the Food and Nutrition Board, Institute of Medicine, National Academy of Sciences. *Nutr. Rev.* 49:357–363 (1991).

15. Ward, D.R., and C. Hackney (eds.). *Microbiology of Marine Food Products.* New York, Van Nostrand Reinhold (1991).

16. Kvenberg, J.E. Nonindigenous bacterial pathogens. In *Microbiology of Marine Food Products.* D.R. Ward and C. Hackney (eds.). New York, Van Nostrand Reinhold. Pp. 267–284 (1991).

17. Martinez-Manzanares, E., M.A. Moriñigo, R. Cornax, et al. Relationship between classical indicators and several pathogenic microorganisms involved in shellfish-borne diseases. *J. Food Protect.* 54:711–717 (1991).

18. Pancorbo, O.C., and H.M. Barnhart. Microbial pathogens and indicators in estuarine environments and shellfish: critical need for better indicator(s) of human-specific fecal pollution. *J. Environ. Health* 54(5):57–63 (1992).

19. Jeljaszewicz, J., and P. Ciborowski (eds.). *The Staphylococci. Zbl. Bakteriol.* Suppl. 21 (1991).

20. Aronsson, B., H. Hallander, B. Osterman, et al. Fatal outcome in a nosocomial outbreak of *Staphylococ-cus aureus* food-poisoning and foodborn infection. In *The Staphylococci.* J. Jeljaszewicz and P. Ciborowski (eds.). *Zbl. Bakteriol.* Suppl. 21:263–266 (1991).

21. World Health Organization. Suspected food poisoning on flights from Los Angeles to Heathrow. *WHO Surveillance Programme for Control of Foodborne Infections and Intoxications in Europe. Newsletter* No. 30:2 (1991).

22. Maguire, H.C.F., M. Boyle, M.J. Lewis, et al. A large outbreak of food poisoning of unknown aetiology associated with Stilton cheese. *Epidemiol. Infect.* 106:497–505 (1991).

23. Schraft, H., N. Kleinlein, and F. Untermann. Contamination of pig hindquarters with *Staphylococcus aureus. Int. J. Food Microbiol.* 15:191–194 (1992).

24. Isigidi, B.K., A.-M. Mathieu, L.A. Devriese, et al. Enterotoxin production in different *Staphylococcus aureus* biotypes isolated from food and meat plants. *J. Appl. Bacteriol.* 72:16–20 (1992).

25. Marín, M.E, M.d.C. de la Rosa, and I. Cornejo. Enterotoxigenicity of *Staphylococcus* strains isolated from Spanish dry-cured hams. *Appl. Environ. Microbiol.* 58:1067–1069 (1992).

26. Szmanko, T. Entwicklung der Bakterienflora vakuumverpackter, gefriergelagerter Kochschinken. *Fleischwirtschaft* 72:336–338 (1992).

27. Bennett, R.W. The biomolecular temperament of staphylococcal enterotoxin in thermally processed foods. *J. AOAC Int.* 75:6–12 (1992).

28. Domenech, A., F.J. Hernandez, J.A. Orden, et al. Effect of six organic acids on staphylococcal growth and enterotoxin production. *Z. Lebensm. Unters. Forsch.* 194:124–128 (1992).

29. Ashenafi, M., and M. Busse. Growth of *Staphylococcus aureus* in fermenting tempeh made from various beans and its inhibition by *Lactobacillus plantarum. Int. J. Food Sci. Technol.* 27:81–86 (1992).

30. Hamama, A., and S.R. Tatini. Behavior of an enterotoxigenic *Staphylococcus aureus* strain during manufacture of the Moroccan fermented milk "iben." *Lait* 71:589–596 (1991).

31. Gómez-Lucía, E., J. Goyache, J.A. Orden, et al. Growth of *Staphylococcus aureus* and synthesis of enterotoxin during ripening of experimental Manchego-type cheese. *J. Dairy Sci.* 75:9–26 (1992).

32. Gourama, H., W.Y.J. Tsai, and L.B. Bullerman. Growth and production of enterotoxins A and D by

Staphylococcus aureus in salad bar ingredients and clam chowder. *J. Food Protect.* 54:844–847 (1991).

33. Brunner, K.G., and A.C.L. Wong. *Staphylococcus aureus* growth and enterotoxin production in mushrooms. *J. Food Sci.* 57:700–703 (1992).

34. Oh, D., D.L. Marshall, M.W. Moody, and J.D. Bankston. Comparison of forced-air cooling with static-air cooling on the microbiological quality of cooked blue crabs. *J. Food Protect.* 55:104–107 (1992).

35. Pereira, J.L., S.P. Salzberg, and M.S. Bergdoll. Production of staphylococcal enterotoxin D in foods by low-enterotoxin-producing staphylococci. *Int. J. Food Microbiol.* 14:19–26 (1991).

36. Mamo, W., M. Lindahl, and P. Jonsson. Enhanced virulence of *Staphylococcus aureus* from bovine mastitis induced by growth in milk whey. *Vet. Microbiol.* 27:371–384 (1991).

37. Lopes, H.R., A.L.S. Noleto, and M.S. Bergdoll. Production of staphylococcal enterotoxins A, D, and E by sac culture. *J. Food Protect.* 54:650–652 (1991).

38. Shinagawa, K., E. Nishimura, M. Mitsumori, and N. Matsusaka. Production and characterization of murine monoclonal antibodies against staphylococcal enterotoxins A and E. *Can. J. Microbiol.* 37:581–585 (1991).

39. Shinagawa, K., M. Mitsumori, N. Matsusaka, and S. Sugii. Purification of staphylococcal enterotoxins A and E by immunoaffinity chromatography using a murine monoclonal antibody with dual specificity for both of these toxins. *J. Immunol. Meth.* 139:49–53 (1991).

40. Shinagawa, K., K. Omoe, and N. Matsusaka. Immunological studies on staphylococcal enterotoxin D: production of murine monoclonal antibodies and immunopurification. *Can. J. Microbiol.* 37:586–589 (1991).

41. Binek, M., J.R. Newcomb, C.M. Rogers, and T.J. Rogers. Localisation of the mitogenic epitope of staphylococcal enterotoxin B. *J. Med. Microbiol.* 36:156–163 (1992).

42. Bohach, G.A., Y.-I. Chi, and C.V. Stauffacher. Crystallization and preliminary X-ray diffraction analysis of staphylococcal enterotoxin type C. *Proteins Structure Function Genet.* 13:152–157 (1992).

43. Hernandez, F.J., J. Goyache, J.A. Orden, et al. Repair of heat-injured *Staphylococcus aureus* FRI-472 in liquid media. In *The Staphylococci*. J. Jeljaszewicz and P. Ciborowski (eds.). *Zbl. Bakteriol.* Suppl. 21:197–198 (1991).

44. Bergdoll, M.S. *Staphylococcus aureus. J. Assoc. Off. Anal. Chem.* 74:706–710 (1991).

45. Kraatz-Wadsack, G., W. Ahrens, and J. von Stuckrad. ELISA screening of staphylococcal enterotoxins by means of a specially developed test kit. *Int. J. Food Microbiol.* 13:265–272 (1991).

46. Wieneke, A.A. Comparison of four kits for the detection of staphylococcal enterotoxin in foods from outbreaks of food poisoning. *Int. J. Food Microbiol.* 14:305–312 (1991).

47. Notermans S., J. Dufrenne, and P. in 't Veld. Feasibility of a reference material for staphylococcal enterotoxin A. *Int. J. Food Microbiol.* 14:325–331 (1991).

48. Brooks, J.L., B. Mirhabibollahi, and R.G. Kroll. Increased sensitivity of an enzyme-amplified colorimetric immunoassay for protein A–bearing *Staphylococcus aureus* in foods. *J. Immunol. Meth.* 140:79–84 (1991).

49. Rogemond, V., J.M. Da Costa Castro, T. Delaunay, et al. Protein A insensitive ELISA detection of staphylococcal enterotoxin B. *Lett. Appl. Microbiol.* 13:175–178 (1991).

50. Goyache, J., J.A. Orden, J.L. Blanco, et al. Determination of the reactivities and cross-reactivities of monoclonal antibodies against staphylococcal enterotoxin A by indirect ELISA and immunoblot including a semiautomated electrophoresis system. *Lett. Appl. Microbiol.* 14:217–220 (1992).

51. Shinagawa, K., M. Suzuki, N. Matsusaka, and S. Sugii. Detection of staphylococcal enterotoxin A by sandwich enzyme-linked immunosorbent assay with monoclonal antibodies. *J. Vet. Med. Sci.* 53:1093–1095 (1991).

52. Kneifel, W., M. Manafi, and A. Breit. Adaption of two commercially available DNA probes for the detection of *E. coli* and *Staphylococcus aureus* to selected fields of dairy hygiene—an exemplary study. *Zbl. Hyg.* 192:544–553 (1992).

53. Jaulhac, B., M. Bes, N. Bornstein, et al. Synthetic DNA probes for detection of genes for enterotoxins A, B, C, D, E and for TSST-1 in staphylococcal strains. *J. Appl. Bacteriol.* 72:386–392 (1992).

54. Wilson, I.G., J.E. Cooper, and A. Gilmour. Detection of enterotoxigenic *Staphylococcus aureus* in dried skimmed milk: use of the polymerase chain reaction

for amplification and detection of staphylococcal enterotoxin genes *entB* and *entC1* and the thermonuclease gene *nuc*. *Appl. Environ. Microbiol.* 57:1793–1798 (1991).

55. Schantz, E.J., and E.A. Johnson. Properties and use of botulinum toxin and other microbial neurotoxins in medicine. *Microbiol. Rev.* 56:80–99 (1992).

56. Centers for Disease Control. Outbreak of type E botulism associated with an uneviscerated, salt-cured fish product—New Jersey, 1992. *Morbid. Mortal. Weekly Rep.* 41:521–522 (1992).

57. Martínez-Castrillo, J.C., M.A. Del Real, A. Hernandez Gonzalez, et al. Botulism with sensory symptoms: a second case. (Letter.) *J. Neurol. Neurosurg. Psychiat.* 54:844–845 (1991).

58. Lilly, T., Jr., E.J. Rhodehamel, D.A. Kautter, and H.M. Solomon. *Clostridium botulinum* spores in corn syrup and other syrups. *J. Food Protect.* 54:585–586 (1991).

59. Rhodehamel, E.J., H.M. Solomon, T. Lilly, Jr., et al. Incidence and heat resistance of *Clostridium botulinum* type E spores in menhaden surimi. *J. Food Sci.* 56:1562–1563,1592 (1991).

60. Lambert, A.D., J.P. Smith, and K.L. Dodds. Effect of headspace CO_2 concentration on toxin production by *Clostridium botulinum* in MAP, irradiated fresh pork. *J. Food Protect.* 54:588–592 (1991).

61. Lambert, A.D., J.P. Smith, and K.L. Dodds. Effect of initial O_2 and CO_2 and low-dose irradiation on toxin production by *Clostridium botulinum* in MAP fresh pork. *J. Food Protect.* 54:939–944 (1991).

62. Whiting, R.C., and K.A. Naftulin. Effect of headspace oxygen concentration on growth and toxin production by proteolytic strains of *Clostridium botulinum*. *J. Food Protect.* 55:23–27 (1992).

63. Chai, T.J., and K.T. Liang. Thermal resistance of spores from five type E *Clostridium botulinum* strains in eastern oyster homogenates. *J. Food Protect.* 55:18–22 (1992).

64. Hutton, M.T., M.A. Koskinen, and J.H. Hanlin. Interacting effects of pH and NaCl on heat resistance of bacterial spores. *J. Food Sci.* 56:821–822 (1991).

65. Huhtanen, C.N. Gamma radiation resistance of *Clostridium botulinum* 62A and *Bacillus subtilis* spores in honey. *J. Food Protect.* 54:894–896 (1991).

66. Solomon, H.M., D.A. Kautter, E.J. Rhodehamel, and T. Lilly, Jr. Evaluation of unacidified products bottled in oil for outgrowth and toxin production by *Clostridium botulinum*. *J. Food Protect.* 54:648–649 (1991).

67. Montville, T.J., A.M. Rogers, and A. Okereke. Differential sensitivity of *Clostridium botulinum* strains to nisin is not biotype-associated. *J. Food Protect.* 55:444–448 (1992).

68. Hutton, M.T., P.A. Chehak, and J.H. Hanlin. Inhibition of botulinum toxin production by *Pediococcus acidilactici* in temperature abused refrigerated foods. *J. Food Safety* 11:255–267 (1991).

69. Okereke, A., and T.J. Montville. Bacteriocin-mediated inhibition of *Clostridium botulinum* spores by lactic acid bacteria at refrigeration and abuse temperatures. *Appl. Environ. Microbiol.* 57:3423–3428 (1991).

70. Miller, A.J., and D.A. Menichillo. Blood fraction effects on the antibotulinal efficacy of nitrite in model beef sausages. *J. Food Sci.* 1158–1160,1181 (1991).

71. Henning, K., H. Meyer, and J. Cremer. Schnellnachweis der *Clostridium botulinum*–Toxine A und B mittels Enzym-Immuno-Assay (ELISA). *Arch. Lebensmittelhyg.* 42:69–71 (1991).

72. Huhtanen, C.N., R.C. Whiting, A.J. Miller, and J.E. Call. Qualitative correlation of the mouse neurotoxin and enzyme-linked immunoassay for determining *Clostridium botulinum* types A and B toxins. *J. Food Safety* 12:119–127 (1992).

73. Szabo, E.A., J.M. Pemberton, and P.M. Desmarchelier. Specific detection of *Clostridium botulinum* type B by using the polymerase chain reaction. *Appl. Environ. Microbiol.* 58:418–420 (1992).

74. Lin, W.-J., and E.A. Johnson. Transposon Tn*916* mutagenesis in *Clostridium botulinum*. *Appl. Environ. Microbiol.* 57:2946–2950 (1991).

75. Stevens, R.C., M.L. Evenson, W. Tepp, and B.R. DasGupta. Crystallization and preliminary X-ray analysis of botulinum neurotoxin type A. *J. Mol. Biol.* 222:877–880 (1991).

76. Jung, H.H., S.D. Rhee, and K.-H. Yang. Cloning of a *Clostridium botulinum* type B toxin gene fragment encoding the *N*-terminus of the heavy chain. *FEMS Microbiol. Lett.* 91:69–72 (1992).

77. Giménez, J.A., M.A. Giménez, and B.R. DasGupta. Characterization of the neurotoxin isolated from a *Clostridium baratii* strain implicated in infant botulism. *Infect. Immun.* 60:518–522 (1992).

78. Whelan, S.M., M.J. Elmore, N.J. Bodsworth, et al. The complete amino acid sequence of the *Clostridium botulinum* type-E neurotoxin, derived by nucleotide-sequence analysis of the encoding gene. *Eur. J. Biochem.* 204:657–667 (1992).

79. Poulet, S., D. Hauser, M. Quanz, et al. Sequences of the botulinal neurotoxin E derived from *Clostridium botulinum* type E (strain beluga) and *Clostridium butyricum* (strains ATCC 43181 and ATCC 43755). *Biochem. Biophys. Res. Commun.* 183:107–113 (1992).

80. Fujii, N., K. Kimura, T. Yashiki, et al. Cloning and whole nucleotide sequence of the gene for the light chain component of botulinum type E toxin from *Clostridium butyricum* strain BL6340 and *Clostridium botulinum* type E strain Mashike. *Microbiol. Immunol.* 36:213–220 (1992).

81. Haque, A., N. Sugimoto, Y. Horiguchi, et al. Production, purification, and characterization of botulinolysin, a thiol-activated hemolysin of *Clostridium botulinum*. *Infect. Immun.* 60:71–78 (1992).

82. Labbé, R.G. *Clostridium perfringens*. *J. Assoc. Off. Anal. Chem.* 74:711–714 (1991).

83. Mahoney, D.E., R. Ahmed, and S.G. Jackson. Multiple typing techniques applied to a *Clostridium perfringens* food poisoning outbreak. *J. Appl. Bacteriol.* 72:309–314 (1992).

84. Anonymous. Perfringens poisons inmates of county jails. *Food Protect. Rep.* 7(12):3 (1991).

85. Ali, M.S., and D.Y.C. Fung. Occurrence of *Clostridium perfringens* in ground beef and ground turkey evaluated by three methods. *J. Food Safety* 11:197–203 (1991).

86. Tschirdewahn, B., S. Notermans, K. Wernars, and F. Untermann. The presence of enterotoxigenic *Clostridium perfringens* strains in faeces of various animals. *Int. J. Food Microbiol.* 14:175–178 (1991).

87. Nagahama, M., K. Kobayashi, S. Ochi, and J. Sakurai. Enzyme-linked immunosorbent assay for rapid detection of toxins from *Clostridium perfringens*. *FEMS Microbiol. Lett.* 84:41–44 (1991).

88. Ahn, Y.-J., T. Kawamura, M. Kim, et al. Tea polyphenols: selective growth inhibitors of *Clostridium* spp. *Agric. Biol. Chem.* 55:1425–1426 (1991).

89. Sugimoto, N., Y.-M. Chen, S.-Y. Lee, et al. Pathodynamics of intoxication in rats and mice by enterotoxin of *Clostridium perfringens* type A. *Toxicon* 29:751–759 (1991).

90. Granum, P.E., and M. Richardson. Chymotrypsin treatment increases the activity of *Clostridium perfringens* enterotoxin. *Toxicon* 29:898–900 (1991).

91. Gustafson, C., B. Kald, R. Sjödahl, and C. Tagesson. Phospholipase C from *Clostridium perfringens* stimulates formation and release of platelet-activating factor (PAF-acether) in cultured intestinal epithelial cells (INT 407). *Scand. J. Gastroenterol.* 26:1000–1006 (1991).

92. Takumi, K., A. Takeoka, T. Koga, and Y. Endo. Relationships between sporulation, enterotoxin production, and inclusion body formation in *Clostridium perfringens* NCTC 8798. *J. Gen. Appl. Microbiol.* 37:341–353 (1991).

93. Heredia, N.L., R.G. Labbé, M.A. Rodriguez, and J.S. Garcia-Alvarado. Growth, sporulation and enterotoxin production by *Clostridium perfringens* type A in the presence of human bile salts. *FEMS Microbiol. Lett.* 84:15–21 (1991).

94. Garcia-Alvarado, J.S., R.G. Labbé, and M.A. Rodriguez. Sporulation and enterotoxin production by *Clostridium perfringens* type A at 37 and 43°C. *Appl. Environ. Microbiol.* 58:1411–1414 (1992).

95. Rood, J.I., and S.T. Cole. Molecular genetics and pathogenesis of *Clostridium perfringens*. *Microbiol. Rev.* 55:621–648 (1991).

96. Hanna, P.C., T.A. Mietzner, G.K. Schoolnik, and B.A. McClane. Localization of the receptor-binding region of *Clostridium perfringens* enterotoxin utilizing cloned toxin fragments and synthetic peptides. *J. Biol. Chem.* 266:11037–11043 (1991).

97. Hanna, P.C., E.U. Wieckowski, T.A. Mietzner, and B.A. McClane. Mapping of functional regions of *Clostridium perfringens* type A enterotoxin. *Infect. Immun.* 60:2110–2114 (1992).

98. Lewis, E. *Bacillus cereus* food poisoning outbreak, Chinese restaurant, Perth. *Commun. Dis. Environ. Health Scotland Weekly Rep.* 25(42):4–5 (1991).

99. Meer, R.R., J. Baker, F.W. Bodyfelt, and M.W. Griffiths. Psychrotrophic *Bacillus* spp. in fluid milk products: a review. *J. Food Protect.* 54:969–979 (1991).

100. Hostacká, A., A. Kosiarová, V. Majtán, and S. Kohútová. Toxic properties of *Bacillus cereus* strains isolated from different foodstuffs. *Zbl. Bakteriol.* 276:303–312 (1992).

101. Cook, P.E., M.M.-A.L. Themba, and G. Campbell-Platt. Growth of *Bacillus cereus* during rice

tapé fermentation. *Lett. Appl. Microbiol.* 13:78–81 (1991).

102. Malmsten, T., K. Pääkkönen, and L. Hyvönen. Packaging and storage effects on microbiological quality of dried herbs. *J. Food Sci.* 56:873–875 (1991).

103. Kowalksi, E., H. Ludwig, and B. Tauscher. Hydrostatischer Hochdruck zur Sterilisation von Lebensmitteln I: Anwendung bei Pfeffer (*Piper nigrum* L.). *Dtsch. Lebensm.-Rundsch.* 88:74–76 (1992).

104. Shinagawa, K., K. Ichikawa, N. Matsusaka, and S. Sugii. Purification and some properties of a *Bacillus cereus* mouse lethal toxin. *J. Vet. Med. Sci.* 53:469–474 (1991).

105. Shinagawa, K., R. Yokoi, N. Matsusaka, and S. Sugii. Development of murine monoclonal antibodies against an enterotoxin produced by *Bacillus cereus. J. Vet. Med. Sci.* 53:419–422 (1991).

106. Shinagawa, K., T. Takechi, and N. Matsusaka. Purification of an enterotoxin produced by *Bacillus cereus* by immunoaffinity chromatography using a monoclonal antibody. *Can. J. Microbiol.* 38:153–156 (1992).

107. Kamat, A.S., and C.K.K. Nair. Evidence for plasmid-mediated toxin production in *Bacillus cereus* BIS-59. *World J. Microbiol. Biotechnol.* 8:210–211 (1992).

108. Tomita, M., R. Taguchi, and H. Ikezawa. Sphingomyelinase of *Bacillus cereus* as a bacterial hemolysin. *J. Toxicol.—Toxin Rev.* 10:169–207 (1991).

109. Jackson, S.G. *Bacillus cereus. J. Assoc. Off. Anal. Chem.* 74:704–706 (1991).

110. Buchanan, R.L., and F.J. Schultz. Evaluation of the Oxoid BCET-RPLA kit for the detection of *Bacillus cereus* diarrheal enterotoxin as compared to cell culture cytotonicity. *J. Food Protect.* 55:440–443 (1992).

111. Sockett, P.N. The economic implications of human salmonella infection. *J. Appl. Biochem.* 71:289–295 (1991).

112. Sockett, P.N., and J.A. Roberts. The social and economic impact of salmonellosis. A report of a national survey in England and Wales of laboratory-confirmed salmonella infections. *Epidemiol. Infect.* 107:335–347 (1991).

113. Tauxe, R.V. *Salmonella*: a postmodern pathogen. *J. Food Protect.* 54:563–568 (1991).

114. Haddock, R.L., S.N. Cousens, and C.C. Guzman. Infant diet and salmonellosis. *Am. J. Public Health* 81:997–1000 (1991).

115. Telzak, E.E., M.S. Zweig Greenberg, L.D. Budnick, et al. Diabetes mellitus—a newly described risk factor for infection from *Salmonella enteritidis. J. Infect. Dis.* 164:538–541 (1991).

116. Stanley, J., M. Goldsworthy, and E.J. Threlfall. Molecular phylogenetic typing of pandemic isolates of *Salmonella enteritidis. FEMS Microbiol. Lett.* 90:153–160 (1992).

117. Stanley, J., A.P. Burnens, E.J. Threlfall, et al. Genetic relationships among strains of *Salmonella enteritidis* in a national epidemic in Switzerland. *Epidemiol. Infect.* 108:213–220 (1992).

118. Morris, J.G., Jr., D.M. Dwyer, C.W. Hoge, et al. Changing clonal patterns of *Salmonella enteritidis* in Maryland: evaluation of strains isolated between 1985 and 1990. *J. Clin. Microbiol.* 30:1301–1303 (1992).

119. Hickman-Brenner, F.W., A.D. Stubbs, and J.J. Farmer, III. Phage typing of *Salmonella enteritidis* in the United States. *J. Clin. Microbiol.* 29:2817–2823 (1991).

120. Rodrigue, D.C., D.N. Cameron, N.D. Puhr, et al. Comparison of plasmid profiles, phage types, and antimicrobial resistance patterns of *Salmonella enteritidis* isolates in the United States. *J. Clin. Microbiol.* 30:854–857 (1992).

121. Baloda, S.B., and K. Krovacek. Toxin profiles, and cell-surface properties of *Salmonella* strains isolated from Swedish travelers. *Microbiol. Immunol.* 35:1009–1013 (1991).

122. Salmon, R.L., S.R. Palmer, C.D. Ribeiro, et al. How is the source of food poisoning outbreaks established? The example of three consecutive *Salmonella enteritidis* PT4 outbreaks linked to eggs. *J. Epidemiol. Commun. Health* 45:266–269 (1991).

123. Devi, S.J.N., and C.J. Murray. Cockroaches (*Blatta* and *Periplaneta* species) as reservoirs of drug-resistant salmonellas. *Epidemiol. Infect.* 107:357–361 (1991).

124. Threlfall, E.J., M.L.M. Hall, L.R. Ward, and B. Rowe. Plasmid profiles demonstrate that an upsurge in *Salmonella berta* in humans in England and Wales is associated with imported poultry meat. *Eur. J. Epidemiol.* 8:27–33 (1992).

125. Hall, M.L.M., and B. Rowe. *Salmonella arizonae* in the United Kingdom from 1966 to 1990. *Epidemiol. Infect.* 108:59–65 (1992).

126. Centers for Disease Control. Outbreak of *Salmonella enteritidis* infection associated with con-

sumption of raw shell eggs, 1991. *Morbid. Mortal. Weekly Rep.* 41:369–372 (1992).

127. World Health Organization. Lethal salmonellosis in old people's home through pudding with whipped eggs. *WHO Surveillance Programme for Control of Foodborne Infections and Intoxications in Europe. Newsletter* No. 30:1 (1991).

128. Holtby, I., and P. Stenson. Food poisoning in two homes for the elderly. Public Health Laboratory Service, Communicable Disease Surveillance Centre. *Commun. Dis. Rep.* 2(Rev. 11):R125–R126 (1992).

129. Chandrakumar, M., C.A. Joseph, N. Soltanpoor, et al. Food poisoning at a religious event. Public Health Laboratory Service, Communicable Disease Surveillance Centre. *Commun. Dis. Rep.* 2(Rev. 11):R123–R124 (1992).

130. Harrison, C., C. Quigley, E. Kaczmarski, and E. Devlin. An outbreak of gastro-intestinal illness caused by eggs containing *Salmonella enteritidis* phage type 4. *J. Infect.* 24:207–210 (1992).

131. Mishu, B., P.M. Griffin, R.V. Tauxe, et al. *Salmonella enteritidis* gastroenteritis transmitted by intact chicken eggs. *Ann. Intern. Med.* 115:190–194 (1991).

132. Curnow, J. *Salmonella enteritidis* associated with duck egg consumption. *Commun. Dis. Environ. Health Scotland Weekly Rep.* 26(7):4 (1992).

133. Health and Welfare Canada. Hospital outbreak of *Salmonella enteritidis* infection—Ontario. *Can. Commun. Dis. Rep.* 18:57 (1992).

134. Voss, S.N., H.F. Thomas, and K. Kammance. Food poisoning at a wedding reception. Public Health Laboratory Service, Communicable Disease Surveillance Centre. *Commun. Dis. Rep.* 2(Rev. 11):R121–R123 (1992).

135. Hedberg, C.W., K.E. White, J.A. Johnson, et al. An outbreak of *Salmonella enteritidis* infection at a fast-food restaurant: implications of foodhandler-associated transmission. *J. Infect. Dis.* 164:1135–1140 (1991).

136. Wood, J.D., G.A. Chalmers, R.A. Fenton, et al. Persistent shedding of *Salmonella enteritidis* from the udder of a cow. *Can. Vet. J.* 32:738–741 (1991).

137. Glass, W.S. *Salmonella* investigation at a dairy farm in West Lothian. *Commun. Dis. Environ. Health Scotland Weekly Rep.* 26(19):4 (1992).

138. Anonymous. *Salmonella mikawasima.* Public Health Laboratory Service, Communicable Disease Surveillance Centre. *Commun. Dis. Rep.* 2:1 (1992).

139. Centers for Disease Control. *Salmonella hadar* associated with pet ducklings—Connecticut, Maryland, and Pennsylvania, 1991. *Morbid. Mortal. Weekly Rep.* 41:185–187 (1992).

140. Riley, A., M. Hanson, and C. Ramsey. Tropical fish as a source of *Salmonella java* infection. *Commun. Dis. Environ. Health Scotland Weekly Rep.* 26(25):4–5 (1992).

141. Centers for Disease Control. Lizard-associated salmonellosis—Utah. *Morbid. Mortal. Weekly Rep.* 41:610–611 (1992).

142. Renner, F., C. Nimeth, and N. Demmelbauer. High frequency of concomitant pancreatitis in salmonella enteritis. (Letter.) *Lancet* 335:1611 (1991).

143. Murphy, S., N.J. Beeching, S.J. Rogerson, and A.D. Harries. Pancreatitis associated with *Salmonella* enteritis. (Letter.) *Lancet* 338:571 (1991).

144. Gibb, A.P., C.S. Lewin, and O.J. Garden. Development of quinolone resistance and multiple antibiotic resistance in *Salmonella bovismorbificans* in a pancreatic abscess. (Letter.) *J. Antimicrob. Chemother.* 28:318–321 (1991).

145. Nathwani, D., A.J. Morris, R.B.S. Laing, et al. *Salmonella virchow:* abscess former amongst the contemporary invasive salmonellae? *Scand. J. Infect. Dis.* 23:467–471 (1991).

146. Ronald, A.R. Liver abscess due to *Salmonella enteritidis* 19 months after an episode of gastroenteritis in a man who underwent a cholecystectomy. (Letter.) *Rev. Infect. Dis.* 13:1026–1027 (1991).

147. Mäki-Ikola, O., and K. Granfors. *Salmonella*-triggered reactive arthritis. *Lancet* 339:1096–1098 (1992).

148. Mäki-Ikola, O., M. Leirisalo-Repo, A. Kantele, et al. *Salmonella*-specific antibodies in reactive arthritis. *J. Infect. Dis.* 164:1141–1148 (1991).

149. Kraus, A., G. Guerra-Bautista, and D. Alarcón-Segovia. *Salmonella arizona* arthritis and septicemia associated with rattlesnake ingestion by patients with connective tissue diseases. A dangerous complication of folk medicine. *J. Rheumatol.* 18:1328–1331 (1991).

150. Collins, M.A., W.C.G. Peh, and N.S. Evans. Aphthous ulcers in *Salmonella* colitis. (Letter.) *Am. J. Roentgenol.* 158:918 (1992).

151. Scialli, A.R., and T.L. Rarick. *Salmonella* sepsis and second-trimester pregnancy loss. *Obstet. Gynecol.* 79:820–821 (1992).

152. Jones, F.T. A survey of *Salmonella* contamination in modern broiler production. *J. Food Protect.* 54:502–507 (1991).

153. Poppe, C., R.J. Irwin, S. Messier, et al. The prevalence of *Salmonella enteritidis* and other *Salmonella* spp. among Canadian registered commercial chicken broiler flocks. *Epidemiol. Infect.* 107:201–211 (1991).

154. Moll, A., and G. Hildebrandt. Quantitativer Nachweis von Salmonellen in Hühnerklein und -innereien. *Arch. Lebensmittelhyg.* 42:140–144 (1991).

155. James, W.O., W.O. Williams, Jr., J.C. Prucha, et al. Profile of selected bacterial counts and *Salmonella* prevalence on raw poultry in a poultry slaughter establishment. *J. Am. Vet. Med. Assoc.* 200:57–59 (1992).

156. Müller, H., and R. Körber. Zur Epizootologie der *Salmonella-enteritidis*-Infektion bei Legehennen—eine Fallstudie. *Tierärztl. Umschau* 47:257–265 (1992).

157. Barnhart, H.M., D.W. Dreesen, R. Bastien, and O.C. Pancorbo. Prevalence of *Salmonella enteritidis* and other serovars in ovaries of layer hens at time of slaughter. *J. Food Protect.* 54:488–491 (1991).

158. Humphrey, T.J., A. Whitehead, A.L.H. Gawler, et al. Numbers of *Salmonella enteritidis* in the contents of naturally contaminated hens' eggs. *Epidemiol. Infect.* 106:489–496 (1991).

159. Burow, H. Nachweis von *Salmonella enteritidis* bei gewerblich und privat erzeugten Hühnereiern. *Arch. Lebensmittelhyg.* 42:39–41 (1991).

160. Buchner, L., R. Wermter, and S. Henkel. Zum Nachweis von Salmonellen in Hühnereiern unter Berücksichtigung eines Stichprobenplanes. *Arch. Lebensmittelhyg.* 42:86–89 (1991).

161. Ching-Lee, M.R., A.R. Katz, D.M. Sasaki, and H.P. Minette. *Salmonella* egg survey in Hawaii: evidence for routine bacterial surveillance. *Am. J. Public Health* 81:764–766 (1991).

162. Pollan, B., and L. Vasicek. Vorkommen von *Salmonella arizona* bei Puten in Österreich. *Wien. Tierärztl. Mschr.* 78:81–83 (1991).

163. Eld, K., A. Gunnarsson, T. Holmberg, et al. *Salmonella* isolated from animals and feedstuffs in Sweden during 1983–1987. *Acta Vet. Scand.* 32:261–277 (1991).

164. Bhattacharyya, D.K., D.K. Sarma, P. Borah, and B.R. Boro. *Salmonella* in slaughtered pigs: isolation and drug sensitivity. *Indian J. Anim. Sci.* 61:708–709 (1991).

165. Jehl-Pietri, C., J. DuPont, C. Herve, et al. Occurrence of faecal bacteria, *Salmonella* and antigens associated with hepatitis A virus in shellfish. *Zbl. Hyg.* 192:230–237 (1991).

166. Phelps, R.P., and C.L. Stiebel. *Salmonella* in a wastewater–aquaculture system. *Bioresource Technol.* 37:205–210 (1991).

167. Henken, A.M., K. Frankena, J.O. Goelema, et al. Multivariate epidemiological approach to salmonellosis in broiler breeder flocks. *Poult. Sci.* 71:838–843 (1992).

168. Bailey, J.S., L.C. Blankenship, and N.A. Cox. Effect of fructooligosaccharide on *Salmonella* colonization of the chicken intestine. *Poult. Sci.* 70:2433–2438 (1991).

169. McHan, F., and E.B. Shotts. Effect of feeding selected short-chain fatty acids on the in vivo attachment of *Salmonella typhimurium* in chick ceca. *Avian Dis.* 36:139–142 (1992).

170. Waldroup, A.L., W. Yamaguchi, J.T. Skinner, and P.W. Waldroup. Effects of dietary lactose on incidence and levels of salmonellae on carcasses of broiler chickens grown to market age. *Poult. Sci.* 71:288–295 (1992).

171. Waldroup, A.L., J.T. Skinner, R.E. Hierholzer, et al. Effects of bird density on *Salmonella* contamination of prechill carcasses. *Poult. Sci.* 71:844–849 (1992).

172. Goodnough, M.C., and E.A. Johnson. Control of *Salmonella enteritidis* infections in poultry by polymyxin B and trimethoprim. *Appl. Environ. Microbiol.* 57:785–788 (1991).

173. Humbert, F., R. Lalande, R. L'Hospitalier, et al. Effect of four antibiotic additives on the *Salmonella* contamination of chicks protected by an adult caecal flora. *Avian Pathol.* 20:577–584 (1991).

174. Fowler, N.G., and G.C. Mead. *Salmonella enteritidis* PT4: broiler breeder flock breakdowns. *Vet. Rec.* 130:431–432 (1992).

175. Schneitz, C., and L. Nuotio. Efficacy of different microbial preparations for controlling *Salmonella* colonisation in chicks and turkey poults by competitive exclusion. *Br. Poult. Sci.* 33:207–211 (1992).

176. Hinton, M., and G.C. Mead. *Salmonella* control in poultry: the need for the satisfactory evaluation of

probiotics for this purpose. *Lett. Appl. Microbiol.* 13:49–50 (1991).

177. Stavric, S., T.M. Gleeson, B. Buchanan, and B. Blanchfield. Experience of the use of probiotics for *Salmonellae* control in poultry. *Lett. Appl. Microbiol.* 14:69–71 (1992).

178. Cooper, G.L., L.M. Venables, R.A.J. Nicholas, et al. Vaccination of chickens with chicken-derived *Salmonella enteritidis* phage type 4 *aroA* live oral salmonella vaccines. *Vaccine* 10:247–254 (1992).

179. Barrow, P.A., M.A. Lovell, and A. Berchieri. The use of two live attenuated vaccines to immunize egg-laying hens against *Salmonella enteritidis* phage type 4. *Avian Pathol.* 20:681–692 (1991).

180. Ludwig, H.-J., and P. Calsow. Versuche zur Vorbeuge von Salmonelleninfektionen bei Legehennen durch Impfung. *Berl. Münch. Tierärztl. Wochenschr.* 105:96–99 (1992).

181. Alderton, M.R., K.J. Fahey, and P.J. Coloe. Humoral responses and salmonellosis protection in chickens given a vitamin-dependent *Salmonella typhimurium* mutant. *Avian Dis.* 35:435–442 (1991).

182. Nolan, L.K., R.E. Wooley, J. Brown, and J.B. Payeur. Comparison of phenotypic characteristics of *Salmonella* spp. isolated from healthy and ill (infected) chickens. *Am. J. Vet. Res.* 52:1512–1517 (1991).

183. Humphrey, T.J., A. Baskerville, H. Chart, et al. *Salmonella enteritidis* PT4 infection in specific pathogen free hens: influence of infecting dose. *Vet. Rec.* 129:482–485 (1991).

184. Barrow, P.A., and M.A. Lovell. Experimental infection of egg-laying hens with *Salmonella enteritidis* phage type 4. *Avian Pathol.* 20:335–348 (1991).

185. Gorham, S.L., K. Kadavil, H. Lambert, et al. Persistence of *Salmonella enteritidis* in young chickens. *Avian Pathol.* 20:433–437 (1991).

186. Curtin, L., and R. Krystynak. An economic framework for assessing foodborne disease control strategies with an application to *Salmonella* control in poultry. In *Economics of Food Safety*. J.A. Caswell (ed.). New York, Elsevier Sci. Pub. Co., Inc. Pp. 131–151 (1991).

187. McCapes, R.H., B.I. Osburn, and H. Riemann. Safety of foods of animal origin: model for elimination of *Salmonella* contamination of turkey meat. *J. Am. Vet. Med. Assoc.* 199:875–880 (1991).

188. Moye, C.J., and A. Chambers. Poultry processing. An innovative technology for salmonella control and shelf life extension. *Food Aust.* 43:246–249 (1991).

189. Giese, J. Experimental process reduces *Salmonella* on poultry. *Food Technol.* 46(4):112 (1992).

190. Thayer, D.W., S. Songprasertchai, and G. Boyd. Effects of heat and ionizing radiation on *Salmonella typhimurium* in mechanically deboned chicken meat. *J. Food Protect.* 54:718–724 (1991).

191. Szczawinska, M.E., D.W. Thayer, and J.G. Phillips. Fate of unirradiated *Salmonella* in irradiated mechanically deboned chicken meat. *Int. J. Food Microbiol.* 14:313–324 (1991).

192. Slavik, M.F., C. Griffis, Y. Li, and P. Engler. Effect of electrical stimulation on bacterial contamination of chicken legs. *J. Food Protect.* 54:508–513 (1991).

193. Eisgruber, H., and F.A. Stolle. Salmonellen bei luft-sprühgekühlten Hähnchen aus dem Handel. *Z. Ernährungswiss.* 30:214–219 (1991).

194. James, W.O., R.L. Brewer, J.C. Prucha, et al. Effects of chlorination of chill water on the bacteriologic profile of raw chicken carcasses and giblets. *J. Am. Vet. Med. Assoc.* 200:60–63 (1992).

195. D'Aoust, J.-Y. Psychrotrophy and foodborne *Salmonella. Int. J. Food Microbiol.* 13:207–216 (1991).

196. Thomas, L.V., J.W.T. Wimpenny, and A.C. Peters. An investigation of the effects of four variables on the growth of *Salmonella typhimurium* using two types of gradient gel plates. *Int. J. Food Microbiol.* 14:261–275 (1991).

197. Thomas, L.V., J.W.T. Wimpenny, and A.C. Peters. Testing multiple variables on the growth of a mixed inoculum of *Salmonella* strains using gradient plates. *Int. J. Food Microbiol.* 15:165–175 (1992).

198. Humphrey, T.J., N.P. Richardson, A.H.L. Gawler, and M.J. Allen. Heat resistance of *Salmonella enteritidis* PT4: the influence of prior exposure to alkaline conditions. *Lett. Appl. Microbiol.* 12:258–260 (1991).

199. Heddleson, R.A., S. Doores, R.C. Anantheswaran, et al. Survival of *Salmonella* species heated by microwave energy in a liquid menstruum containing food components. *J. Food Protect.* 54:637–642 (1991).

200. Dickson, J.S., and M.E. Anderson. Control of *Salmonella* on beef tissue surfaces in a model system by pre- and post-evisceration washing and sanitizing, with

and without spray chilling. *J. Food Protect.* 54:514–518 (1991).

201. Park, D.L., S.M. Rua, Jr., and R.F. Acker. Direct application of a new hypochlorite sanitizer for reducing bacterial contamination on foods. *J. Food Protect.* 54:960–965 (1991).

202. Lauten, S.D., J. Sarvis, W.B. Wheatley, et al. Efficacies of novel *N*-halamine disinfectants against *Salmonella* and *Pseudomonas* species. *Appl. Environ. Microbiol.* 58:1240–1243 (1992).

203. Stevens, K.A., B.W. Sheldon, N.A. Kalpes, and T.R. Klaenhammer. Nisin treatment for inactivation of *Salmonella* species and other gram-negative bacteria. *Appl. Environ. Microbiol.* 57:3613–3615 (1991).

204. Stevens, K.A., N.A. Klapes, B.W. Sheldon, and T.R. Klaenhammer. Antimicrobial action of nisin against *Salmonella typhimurium* lipopolysaccharide mutants. *Appl. Environ. Microbiol.* 58:1786–1788 (1992).

205. Wood, R.L., and R. Rose. Populations of *Salmonella typhimurium* in internal organs of experimentally infected carrier swine. *Am. J. Vet. Res.* 53:653–658 (1992).

206. Freydiere, A.-M., and Y. Gille. Detection of salmonellae by using Rambach agar and by a C8 esterase spot test. *J. Clin. Microbiol.* 29:2357–2359 (1991).

207. Gruenewald, R., R.W. Henderson, and S. Yappow. Use of Rambach propylene glycol containing agar for identification of *Salmonella* spp. *J. Clin. Microbiol.* 29:2354–2356 (1991).

208. Perales, I., and E. Erkiaga. Comparison between semisolid Rappaport and modified semisolid Rappaport-Vassiliadis media for the isolation of *Salmonella* spp. from foods and feeds. *Int. J. Food Microbiol.* 14:51–58 (1991).

209. Mallinson, E.T., and J.A. Scherrer. Xylose-lysine–tergitol 4: an improved selective agar medium for the isolation of *Salmonella*. *Poult. Sci.* 70:2429–2432 (1991).

210. Poisson, D.M. Novobiocin, brilliant green, glycerol, lactose agar: a new medium for the isolation of *Salmonella* strains. *Res. Microbiol.* 143:211–216 (1992).

211. D'Aoust, J.-Y., A.M. Sewell, and A. Jean. Efficacy of prolonged (48 h) selective enrichment for the detection of foodborne *Salmonella*. *Int. J. Food Microbiol.* 15:121–130 (1992).

212. D'Aoust, J.-Y., A.M. Sewell, and E. Daley. Inadequacy of small transfer volume and short (6 h) selective enrichment for the detection of foodborne *Salmonella*. *J. Food Protect.* 55:326–328 (1992).

213. Allen, G., V.R. Bruce, P. Stephenson, et al. Recovery of *Salmonella* from high-moisture foods by abbreviated selective enrichment. *J. Food Protect.* 54:492–495 (1991).

214. Jetton, J.P., S.F. Bilgili, D.E. Conner, et al. Recovery of salmonellae from chilled broiler carcasses as affected by rinse media and enumeration method. *J. Food Protect.* 55:329–332 (1992).

215. Stephenson, P., R.B. Satchell, G. Allen, and W.H. Andrews. Recovery of *Salmonella* from shell eggs. *J. Assoc. Off. Anal. Chem.* 74:821–826 (1991).

216. Gast, R.K., and C.W. Beard. Detection and enumeration of *Salmonella enteritidis* in fresh and stored eggs laid by experimentally infected hens. *J. Food Protect.* 55:152–156 (1992).

217. Feier, U., and P.-H. Goetsch. Inter-laboratory studies on precision characteristics of analytical methods. Determination of gram-negative bacteria-lipopolysaccharides in raw and heat-treated liquid eggs and products of eggs—*Limulus* microtitre test. *Arch. Lebensmittelhyg.* 42:41–42 (1991).

218. McLeod, S., and P.A. Barrow. Lipopolysaccharide-specific IgG in egg yolk from two chicken flocks infected with *Salmonella enteritidis*. *Lett. Appl. Microbiol.* 13:294–297 (1991).

219. Davda, C., and S.J. Pugh. An improved protocol for the detection and rapid confirmation within 48 h of *Salmonellas* in confectionery products. *Lett. Appl. Microbiol.* 13:287–290 (1991).

220. Fleet, G.H., T. Karalis, A. Hawa, and T. Lukondeh. A rapid method for enumerating *Salmonella* in milk powders. *Lett. Appl. Microbiol.* 13:225–259 (1991).

221. Weber, A., and E. Rackelmann. Zur Erfassung salmonellenhaltiger Lebensmittel mit Hilfe von 1–2 Test®. *Berl. Münch. Tierärztl. Wochenschr.* 104:233–235 (1991).

222. Tsai, H.-C.S., and M.F. Slavik. Rapid method for detection of salmonellae attached to chicken skin. *J. Food Safety* 11:205–214 (1991).

223. Tsen, H.-Y., S.-J. Wang, and S.S. Green. *Salmonella* detection in meat and fish by membrane hybridization with chromogenic/phosphatase/biotin DNA probe. *J. Food Sci.* 56:1519–1523 (1991).

224. Entis, P., and P. Boleszczuk. Rapid detection of *Salmonella* in foods using EF-18 agar in conjunction with the hydrophobic grid membrane filter. *J. Food Protect.* 54:930–934 (1991).

225. Cano, R.J., M.J. Torres, R.E. Klem, et al. Detection of salmonellas by DNA hybridization with a fluorescent alkaline phosphatase substrate. *J. Appl. Bacteriol.* 72:393–399 (1992).

226. Todd, E.C.D., J.M. Mackenzie, L.J. Parrington, et al. Evaluation of *Salmonella* antisera for an optimum enzyme-linked antibody detection of *Salmonella* using hydrophobic grid membrane filters. *Food Microbiol.* 8:311–324 (1991).

227. Dealler, S.F., J. Collins, and A.L. James. A rapid test for *Salmonella* in stools, not requiring refrigeration. *Trans. Roy. Soc. Trop. Med. Hyg.* 85:548 (1991).

228. Dealler, S.F., J. Collins, and A.L. James. A rapid heat-resistant technique for presumptive identification of *Salmonella* on desoxycholate–citrate agar. *Eur. J. Clin. Microbiol. Infect. Dis.* 11:249–252 (1992).

229. Olsson, M., A. Syk, and R. Wollin. Identification of salmonellae with the 4-methylumbelliferyl caprilate fluorescence test. *J. Clin. Microbiol.* 29:2631–2643 (1991).

230. Ruiz, J., M.A. Sempere, M.C. Varela, and J. Gomez. Modification of the methodology of stool culture for *Salmonella* detection. *J. Clin. Microbiol.* 30:525–526 (1992).

231. Manafi, M., and R. Sommer. Comparison of three rapid screening methods for *Salmonella* spp.: 'MUCAP test, MicroScreen[R] latex and Rambach agar'. *Lett. Appl. Microbiol.* 14:163–166 (1992).

232. Kim, C.J., K.V. Nagaraja, and B.S. Pomeroy. Enzyme-linked immunosorbent assay for the detection of *Salmonella enteritidis* infection in chickens. *Am. J. Vet. Res.* 52:1069–1074 (1991).

233. Choi, D., R.S.W. Tsang, and M.H. Ng. Sandwich capture ELISA by a murine monoclonal antibody against a genus-specific LPS epitope for the detection of different common serotypes of salmonellas. *J. Appl. Bacteriol.* 72:134–138 (1992).

234. D'Aoust, J.-Y., A.M. Sewell, and P. Greco. Commercial latex agglutination kits for the detection of foodborne *Salmonella. J. Food Protect.* 54:725–730 (1991).

235. Tsen, H.-Y., S.-J. Wang, B.A. Roe, and S.S. Green. DNA sequence of a *Salmonella*-specific DNA fragment and the use of oligonucleotide probes for *Salmonella* detection. *Appl. Microbiol. Biotechnol.* 35:339–347 (1991).

236. Kerr, S., H.J. Ball, D.P. Mackie, et al. Diagnostic application of monoclonal antibodies to outer membrane protein for rapid detection of salmonella. *J. Appl. Bacteriol.* 72:302–308 (1992).

237. Rahman, H., V.B. Singh, V.D. Sharma, and S.C. Harne. Comparative evaluation of some bioassay models & serological tests for the detection of *Salmonella* enterotoxin. *Indian J. Med. Res. [A]* 93:217–221 (1991).

238. Rahman, H., V.B. Singh, V.D. Sharma, and S.C. Harne. Coagglutination test for rapid detection of *Salmonella* enterotoxin. *Zbl. Bakteriol.* 275:303–311 (1991).

239. Blais, B.W., and H. Yamazaki. Application of polymyxin-coated polyester cloth to the semi-quantitation of *Salmonella* in processed foods. *Int. J. Food Microbiol.* 14:43–50 (1991).

240. Skjerve, E., and Ø. Olsvik. Immunomagnetic separation of *Salmonella* from foods. *Int. J. Food Microbiol.* 14:11–18 (1991).

241. Vermunt, A.E.M., A.A.J.M. Franken, and R.R. Beumer. Isolation of salmonellas by immunomagnetic separation. *J. Appl. Bacteriol.* 72:112–118 (1992).

242. Gibson, D.M., P. Coombs, and D.W. Pimbley. Automated conductance method for the detection of *Salmonella* in foods: collaborative study. *J. AOAC Int.* 75:293–302 (1992).

243. Jones, C., and J. Stanley. *Salmonella* plasmids of the pre-antibiotic era. *J. Gen. Microbiol.* 138:189–197 (1992).

244. D'Aoust, J.-Y., A.M. Sewell, E. Daley, and P. Greco. Antibiotic resistance of agricultural and foodborne *Salmonella* isolates in Canada: 1986–1989. *J. Food Protect.* 55:428–434 (1992).

245. Wray, C., Y.E. Beedell, and I.M. McLaren. A survey of antimicrobial resistance in salmonellae isolated from animals in England and Wales during 1984–1987. *Br. Vet. J.* 147:356–369 (1991).

246. Selabitz, H.-J. Die Virulenz der Salmonellen—Faktoren und Mechanismen. *Prakt. Tierarzt.* 72:589–592 (1991).

247. Chart, H., L.R. Ward, and B. Rowe. Expression of lipopolysaccharide by phage types of *Salmonella enteritidis. Lett. Appl. Microbiol.* 13:39–41 (1991).

248. Vashisht, N., K.D. Sharma, and M. Saxena. Enterotoxigenicity of diarrhoeal isolates of *Salmonella bareilly*. *World J. Microbiol. Biotechnol.* 7:502–504 (1991).

249. Douce, G.R., I.I. Amin, and J. Stephen. Invasion of HEp-2 cells by strains of *Salmonella typhimurium* of different virulence in relation to gastroenteritis. *J. Med. Microbiol.* 35:349–357 (1991).

250. Khurana, S., N.K. Ganguly, M. Khullar, et al. Studies on the mechanism of *Salmonella typhimurium* enterotoxin-induced diarrhoea. *Biochim. Biophys. Acta* 1097:171–176 (1991).

251. Liebold, R., U. Dinjus, and H.-J. Selbitz. Das Vorkommen von zytotonischen und zytotoxischen Enterotoxinen bei Salmonellen. *Berl. Münch. Tierärztl. Wochenschr.* 105:5–10 (1992).

252. Fang, F.C., M. Krause, C. Roudier, et al. Growth regulation of a *Salmonella* plasmid gene essential for virulence. *J. Bacteriol.* 173:6783–6789 (1991).

253. Valone, S.E., and G.K. Chikami. Characterization of three proteins expressed from the virulence region of plasmid pSDL2 in *Salmonella dublin*. *Infect. Immun.* 59:3511–3517 (1991).

254. Taira, S., P. Riikonen, H. Saarilahti, et al. The *mkaC* virulence gene of the *Salmonella* serovar typhimurium 96 kb plasmid encodes a transcriptional activator. *Mol. Gen. Genet.* 228:381–384 (1991).

255. Sizemore, D.R., R.S. Fink, J.T. Ou, et al. Tn5 mutagenesis of the *Salmonella typhimurium* 100 kb plasmid: definition of new virulence regions. *Microb. Pathogen.* 10:493–499 (1991).

256. Lee, C.A., B.D. Jones, and S. Falkow. Identification of a *Salmonella typhimurium* invasion locus by selection for hyperinvasive mutants. *Proc. Natl. Acad. Sci. USA* 89:1847–1851 (1992).

257. Dewanti, R., and M.P. Doyle. Influence of cultural conditions on cytotoxin production by *Salmonella enteritidis*. *J. Food Protect.* 55:28–33 (1992).

258. Aslanzadeh, J., and L.J. Paulissen. Role of type 1 and type 3 fimbriae on the adherence and pathogenesis of *Salmonella enteritidis* in mice. *Microbiol. Immunol.* 36:351–359 (1992).

259. Nascimento, V.P., S. Cranstoun, and S.E. Solomon. Relationship between shell structure and movement of *Salmonella enteritidis* across the eggshell wall. *Br. Poult. Sci.* 33:37–48 (1992).

260. Baskerville, A., T.J. Humphrey, R.B. Fitzgeorge, et al. Airborne infection of laying hens with *Salmonella enteritidis* phage type 4. *Vet. Rec.* 130:395–398 (1992).

261. Lee, L.A., C.N. Shapiro, N. Hargrett-Bean, and R.V. Tauxe. Hyperendemic shigellosis in the United States: a review of surveillance data for 1967–1988. *J. Infect. Dis.* 164:894–900 (1991).

262. Yagupsky, P., M. Loeffelholz, K. Bell, and M.A. Menegus. Use of multiple markers for investigation of an epidemic of *Shigella sonnei* infection in Monroe County, New York. *J. Clin. Microbiol.* 29:2850–2855 (1991).

263. Hyams, K.C., A.L. Bourgeois, B.R. Merrell, et al. Diarrheal disease during Operation Desert Shield. *New Engl. J. Med.* 325:1423–1428 (1991).

264. Levine, O.S., and M.M. Levine. Houseflies (*Musca domestica*) as mechanical vectors of shigellosis. *Rev. Infect. Dis.* 13:688–696 (1991).

265. Bennish, M.L., M.A. Salam, M.A. Hossain, et al. Antimicrobial resistance of *Shigella* isolates in Bangladesh, 1983–1990: increasing frequency of strains multiply resistant to ampicillin, trimethoprim-sulfamethoxazole, and nalidixic acid. *Clin. Infect. Dis.* 14:1055–1060 (1992).

266. Lew, J.F., D.L. Swerdlow, M.E. Dance, et al. An outbreak of shigellosis aboard a cruise ship caused by a multiple-antibiotic-resistant strain of *Shigella flexneri*. *Am. J. Epidemiol.* 134:412–420 (1991).

267. Health and Welfare Canada. Antimicrobial susceptibilities of *Shigella* species isolated in Ontario in 1990. *Can. Dis. Weekly Rep.* 17:275–277 (1991).

268. Health and Welfare Canada. Multiply-resistant *Shigella sonnei* from recent outbreaks in Canada. *Can. Dis. Weekly Rep.* 17:277–279 (1991).

269. Voogd, C.E., C.S. Schot, W.J. van Leeuwen, and B. van Klingeren. Monitoring of antibiotic resistance in shigellae isolated in the Netherlands 1984–1989. *Eur. J. Clin. Microbiol. Infect. Dis.* 11:164–167 (1992).

270. Bennish, M.L., A.K. Azad, and D. Yousefzadeh. Intestinal obstruction during shigellosis: incidence, clinical features, risk factors, and outcome. *Gastroenterology* 101:626–634 (1991).

271. Yoshikawa, M., and C. Sasakawa. Molecular pathogenesis of shigellosis: a review. *Microbiol. Immunol.* 35:809–824 (1991).

272. Hale, T.L. Genetic basis of virulence in *Shigella* species. *Microbiol. Rev.* 55:206–224 (1991).

273. Louise, C.B., and T.G. Obrig. Shiga toxin–associated hemolytic-uremic syndrome: combined cytotoxic effects of Shiga toxin, interleukin-1β, and tumor necrosis factor alpha on human vascular endothelial cells in vitro. *Infect. Immun.* 59:4173–4179 (1991).

274. Sen, A., M.A. Leon, and S. Palchaudhuri. Environmental signals induce major changes in virulence of *Shigella* spp. *FEMS Microbiol. Lett.* 84:231–236 (1991).

275. Soldati, L., and J.C. Piffaretti. Molecular typing of *Shigella* strains using pulsed field gel electrophoresis and genome hybridization with insertion sequences. *Res. Microbiol.* 142:489–498 (1991).

276. Hinojosa-Ahumada, M., B. Swaminathan, S.B. Hunter, et al. Restriction fragment length polymorphisms in rRNA operons for subtyping *Shigella sonnei*. *J. Clin. Microbiol.* 29:2380–2384 (1991).

277. Brook, M.G., and B. Bannister. Verocytotoxin producing *Escherichia coli*. Newish bug on the block. *Br. Med. J.* 303:800–801 (1991).

278. Griffin, P.M., and R.V. Tauxe. The epidemiology of infections caused by *Escherichia coli* O157:H7, other enterohemorrhagic *E. coli*, and the associated hemolytic uremic syndrome. *Epidemiol. Rev.* 13:60–98 (1991).

279. Maher, D.P., and P.J. Stanley. Verotoxin-producing *Escherichia coli* infection in hospitalised patients with acute gastro-enteritis. (Letter.) *J. Infect.* 24:220–221 (1992).

280. Pierard, D., L. Huyghens, and S. Lauwers. Diarrhoea associated with *Escherichia coli* producing porcine oedema disease verotoxin. (Letter.) *Lancet* 338:762 (1991).

281. Bockemühl, J., S. Aleksic, and H. Karch. Serological and biochemical properties of Shiga-like toxin (Verocytotoxin)-producing strains of *Escherichia coli*, other than O-group 157, from patients in Germany. *Zbl. Bakteriol.* 276:189–195 (1992).

282. Rowe, P.C., E. Orrbine, G.A. Wells, et al. Epidemiology of hemolytic-uremic syndrome in Canadian children from 1986 to 1988. *J. Pediatr.* 119:218–224 (1991).

283. Van de Kar, N., P. Reekers, K. van Acker, et al. Association between the epidemic form of hemolytic-uremic syndrome and HLA-B 40 in the Netherlands and Flanders. (Letter.) *Nephron* 59:170 (1991).

284. Bitzan, M., E. Moebius, K. Ludwig, et al. High incidence of serum antibodies to *Escherichia coli* O157 lipopolysaccharide in children with hemolytic-uremic syndrome. *J. Pediatr.* 119:380–385 (1991).

285. Anonymous. *E. coli* in apple cider gives new cause for concern. *Food Protect. Rep.* 8(9):3–4 (1992).

286. Belongia, E.A., K.L. MacDonald, G.L. Parham, et al. An outbreak of *Escherichia coli* O157:H7 colitis associated with consumption of precooked meat patties. *J. Infect. Dis.* 164:338–343 (1991).

287. Bisset, J.G., M.I. Brown, J. Bimson, et al. An outbreak of haemorrhagic colitis due to *E. coli* O157 in two residential homes for the elderly in the Borders. *Commun. Dis. Environ. Health Scotland Weekly Rep.* 26(19):5–6 (1992).

288. Coia, J.E., J. Curnow, and J. Tolland. *Escherichia coli* O157 infection in Scotland, 1991. *Commun. Dis. Environ. Health Scotland Weekly Rep.* 26(39):5–7 (1992).

289. Rowe, P.C., W. Walop, H. Lior, and A.M. MacKenzie. Haemolytic anaemia after childhood *Escherichia coli* O 157.H7 infection: are females at increased risk? *Epidemiol. Infect.* 106:523–530 (1991).

290. Dhuna, A., A. Pascual-Leone, D. Talwar, and F. Torres. EEG and seizures in children with hemolytic–uremic syndrome. *Epilepsia* 33:482–486 (1992).

291. Nagai, T., O. Hasegawa, T. Atsutoshi, et al. Pituitary hemorrhage in hemolytic uremic syndrome. *Pediatr. Neurol.* 8:75–76 (1992).

292. Tarr, P.I., E. Weinberger, E.I. Hatch, Jr., and D.L. Christie. Bacterial ileocecitis caused by *Escherichia coli* O157:H7. *J. Pediatr. Gastroenterol. Nutr.* 14:261–263 (1992).

293. Smith, H.R., T. Cheasty, D. Roberts, et al. Examination of retail chickens and sausages in Britain for Vero cytotoxin-producing *Escherichia coli*. *Appl. Environ. Microbiol.* 57:2091–2093 (1991).

294. Padhye, N.V., and M.P. Doyle. Rapid procedure for detecting enterohemorrhagic *Escherichia coli* O157:H7 in food. *Appl. Environ. Microbiol.* 57:2693–2698 (1991).

295. Kim, M.S., and M.P. Doyle. Dipstick immunoassay to detect enterohemorrhagic *Escherichia coli* O157:H7 in retail ground beef. *Appl. Environ. Microbiol.* 58:1764–1767 (1992).

296. Yassien, N. Enteropathogene *E. coli*–Keime in einem Lebensmittelausgabe-Betrieb. *Fleischwirtschaft* 72:797–798 (1992).

297. Weeratna, R.D., and M.P. Doyle. Detection and production of verotoxin 1 of *Escherichia coli* O157:H7 in food. *Appl. Environ. Microbiol.* 57:2951–2955 (1991).

298. Arocha, M.M., M. McVey, S.D. Loder, et al. Behavior of hemorrhagic *Escherichia coli* O157:H7 during the manufacture of cottage cheese. *J. Food Protect.* 55:379–381 (1992).

299. Farrag, S.A., F.E. El-Gazzar, and E.H. Marth. Use of the lactoperoxidase system to inactivate *Escherichia coli* O157:H7 in a semi-synthetic medium and in raw milk. *Milchwissenschaft* 47:15–17 (1992).

300. Hinton, A., Jr., D.E. Corrier, and J.R. DeLoach. Inhibition of the growth of *Salmonella typhimurium* and *Escherichia coli* O157:H7 on chicken feed media by bacteria isolated from the intestinal microflora of chickens. *J. Food Protect.* 55:419–423 (1992).

301. Stavric, S., B. Buchanan, and T.M. Gleeson. Competitive exclusion of *Escherichia coli* O157:H7 from chicks with anaerobic cultures of faecal microflora. *Lett. Appl. Microbiol.* 14:191–193 (1992).

302. Line, J.E., A.R. Fain, Jr., A.B. Moran, et al. Lethality of heat to *Escherichia coli* O157:H7: *D*-value and *z*-value determinations in ground beef. *J. Food Protect.* 54:762–766 (1991).

303. Murano, E.A., and M.D. Pierson. Effect of heat shock and growth atmosphere on the heat resistance of *Escherichia coli* O157:H7. *J. Food Protect.* 55:171–175 (1992).

304. Lai, X.-H., J.-G. Xu, and B.-Y. Liu. Experimental infection of specific-pathogen-free mice with enterohemorrhagic *Escherichia coli* O157:H7. *Microbiol. Immunol.* 35:515–524 (1991).

305. De Rycke, J. Les colibacilles producteurs de cytotoxines: importance en médecine vétérinaire et en santé publique. *Ann. Rech. Vét.* 22:105–126 (1991).

306. Beutin, L. The different hemolysins of *Escherichia coli*. *Med. Microbiol. Immunol.* 180:167–182 (1991).

307. Haider, K., M.J. Albert, A. Hossain, and S. Nahar. Contact-haemolysin production by entero-invasive *Escherichia coli* and shigellae. *J. Med. Microbiol.* 35:330–337 (1991).

308. Tesh, V.L., and A.D. O'Brien. The pathogenic mechanisms of Shiga toxin and the Shiga-like toxins. *Mol. Microbiol.* 5:1817–1822 (1991).

309. Mainil, J.G. Les vérocytotoxines d'*Escherichia coli* et leur diagnostic par sondes génétiques. *Ann. Méd. Vét.* 135:579–586 (1991).

310. Yamasaki, S., M. Furutani, K. Ito, et al. Importance of arginine at position 170 of the A subunit of Vero toxin 1 produced by enterohemorrhagic *Escherichia coli* for toxin activity. *Microb. Pathogen.* 11:1–9 (1991).

311. Deresiewicz, R.L., S.B. Calderwood, J.D. Robertus, and R.J. Collier. Mutations affecting the activity of the Shiga-like toxin I A-chain. *Biochemistry* 31:3272–3280 (1992).

312. Boodhoo, A., R.J. Read, and J. Brunton. Crystallization and preliminary X-ray crystallographic analysis of verotoxin-1 B-subunit. *J. Mol. Biol.* 221:729–731 (1991).

313. Stein, P.E., A. Boodhoo, G.J. Tyrrell, et al. Crystal structure of the cell-binding B oligomer of verotoxin-1 from *E. coli*. *Nature* 355:748–750 (1992).

314. Meyer, T., H. Karch, J. Hacker, et al. Cloning and sequencing of a Shiga-like toxin II–related gene. *Zbl. Bakteriol.* 276:176–188 (1992).

315. Fujii, Y., M. Hayashi, S. Hitotsubashi, et al. Purification and characterization of *Escherichia coli* heat-stable enterotoxin II. *J. Bacteriol.* 173:5516–5522 (1991).

316. Hitotsubashi, S., M. Akagi, A. Saitou, et al. Action of *Escherichia coli* heat-stable enterotoxin II on isolated sections of mouse ileum. *FEMS Microbiol. Lett.* 90:249–252 (1992).

317. de Sauvage, F.J., T.R. Camerato, and D.V. Goeddel. Primary structure and functional expression of the human receptor for *Escherichia coli* heat-stable enterotoxin. *J. Biol. Chem.* 266:17912–17918 (1991).

318. de Sauvage, F.J., R. Horuk, G. Bennett, et al. Characterization of the recombinant human receptor for *Escherichia coli* heat-stable enterotoxin. *J. Biol. Chem.* 267:6479–6482 (1992).

319. Mezoff, A.G., R.A. Giannella, M.N. Eade, and M.B. Cohen. *Escherichia coli* enterotoxin (ST_a) binds to receptors, stimulates guanyl cyclase, and impairs absorption in rat colon. *Gastroenterology* 102:816–822 (1992).

320. Tsuji, T., T. Inoue, A. Miyama, and M. Noda. Glutamic acid-112 of the A subunit of heat-labile enterotoxin from enterotoxigenic *Escherichia coli* is impor-

tant for ADP-ribosyltransferase activity. *FEBS Lett.* 291:319–321 (1991).

321. Sixma, T.K., A.C.T. van Sheltinga, K.H. Kalk, et al. X-ray studies reveal lanthanide binding sites at the A/B$_5$ interface of *E. coli* heat labile enterotoxin. *FEBS Lett.* 297:179–182 (1992).

322. Qu, Z.-H., M. Boesman-Finkelstein, M. Kazemi, and R.A. Finkelstein. Heterogeneity of immunotypes of heat-labile enterotoxins of enterotoxigenic *Escherichia coli* of human origin. *J. Infect. Dis.* 164:796–799 (1991).

323. Murphy, G.L., and W.S. Dallas. Analysis of two genes encoding heat-labile toxins and located on a single Ent plasmid from *Escherichia coli. Gene* 103:37–43 (1991).

324. Robins-Browne, R.M., and V. Bennett-Wood. Quantitative assessment of the ability of *Escherichia coli* to invade cultured animal cells. *Microb. Pathogen.* 12:159–164 (1992).

325. Winsor, D.K., Jr., S. Ashkenazi, R. Chiovetti, and T.G. Cleary. Adherence of enterohemorrhagic *Escherichia coli* strains to a human colonic epithelial cell line (T$_{84}$). *Infect. Immun.* 60:1613–1617 (1992).

326. Sarvas, H., S. Kurikka, I.J.T. Seppälä, et al. Virulence factors in Shiga-like toxin–producing *Escherichia coli* isolated from humans and cattle. (Letter.) *J. Infect. Dis.* 165:979–980 (1992).

327. Pohl, P. Les *Escherichia coli* verotoxinogénes isolées des bovins. *Ann. Méd. Vét.* 135:569–576 (1991).

328. Beebakhee, G., M. Louie, J. De Azavedo, and J. Brunton. Cloning and nucleotide sequence of the *eae* gene homologue from enterohemorrhagic *Escherichia coli* serotype O157:H7. *FEMS Microbiol. Lett.* 91:63–68 (1992).

329. McConnell, M.M., M.L. Hibberd, M.E. Penny, et al. Surveys of human enterotoxigenic *Escherichia coli* from three different geographical areas for possible colonization factors. *Epidemiol. Infect.* 106:477–484 (1991).

330. Bühler, T., H. Hoschützky, and K. Jann. Analysis of colonization factor antigen I, and adhesin of enterotoxigenic *Escherichia coli* O78:H11: fimbrial morphology and location of the receptor-binding site. *Infect. Immun.* 59:3876–3882 (1991).

331. Singleton, E.R., M.K. Hamdy, S.G. McCay, and F.A. Zapatka. Detection of fimbriae (CFA/I) on enterotoxigenic *Escherichia coli* using antibodies. *J. Food Safety* 11:215–225 (1991).

332. Chauviére, G., M.-H. Coconnier, S. Kerneis, et al. Competitive exclusion of diarrheagenic *Escherichia coli* (ETEC) from human enterocyte-like Caco-2 cells by heat-killed *Lactobacillus. FEMS Microbiol. Lett.* 91:213–217 (1992).

333. Karjalainen, T.K., D.G. Evans, D.J. Evans, Jr., et al. Iron represses the expression of CFA/I fimbriae of enterotoxigenic *E. coli. Microb. Pathogen.* 11:317–323 (1991).

334. Clark, C.A., M.W. Heuzenroeder, and P.A. Manning. Colonization factor antigen CFA/IV (PCF8775) of human enterotoxigenic *Escherichia coli*: nucleotide sequence of the CS5 determinant. *Infect. Immun.* 60:1254–1257 (1992).

335. Yamamoto, T., S. Endo, T. Yokota, and P. Echeverria. Characteristics of adherence of enteroaggregative *Escherichia coli* to human and animal mucosa. *Infect. Immun.* 59:3722–3739 (1991).

336. Benz, I., and M.A. Schmidt. Isolation and serologic characterization of AIDA-I, the adhesin mediating the diffuse adherence phenotype of the diarrhea-associated *Escherichia coli* strain 2787 (O126:H27). *Infect. Immun.* 60:13–18 (1992).

337. Yoh, M., I. Narita, T. Honda, et al. Comparison of preservation methods for enterotoxigenic *Escherichia coli* producing heat-labile enterotoxin. *J. Clin. Microbiol.* 29:2326–2328 (1991).

338. Chapman, P.A., C.A. Siddons, P.M. Zadik, and L. Jewes. An improved selective medium for the isolation of *Escherichia coli* O157. *J. Med. Microbiol.* 35:107–110 (1991).

339. Ritchie, M., S. Partington, J. Jessop, and M.T. Kelly. Comparison of a direct fecal Shiga-like toxin assay and sorbitol–MacConkey agar culture for laboratory diagnosis of enterohemorrhagic *Escherichia coli* infection. *J. Clin. Microbiol.* 30:461–464 (1992).

340. Scotland, S.M., T. Cheasty, A. Thomas, and B. Rowe. Beta-glucuronidase activity of Vero cytotoxin-producing strains of *Escherichia coli*, including serogroup O157, isolated in the United Kingdom. *Lett. Appl. Microbiol.* 13:42–44 (1991).

341. Gordillo, M.E., G.R. Reeve, J. Pappas, et al. Molecular characterization of strains of enteroinvasive *Escherichia coli* O143, including isolates from a large outbreak in Houston, Texas. *J. Clin. Microbiol.* 30:889–893 (1992).

342. Okrend, A.J.G., B.E. Rose, and C.P. Lattuada. Isolation of *Escherichia coli* O157:H7 using O157 specific antibody coated magnetic beads. *J. Food Protect.* 55:214–217 (1992).

343. Lortie, L.-A., J. Harel, J.M. Fairbrother, and J.D. Dubreuil. Immunodot detection of *Escherichia coli* heat-stable enterotoxin b by using enhanced chemiluminescence reaction. *J. Clin. Microbiol.* 29:2250–2252 (1991).

344. Aleksic, S., H. Karch, and J. Bockemühl. A biotyping scheme for Shiga-like (Vero) toxin–producing *Escherichia coli* O157 and a list of serological cross-reactions between O157 and other gram-negative bacteria. *Zbl. Bakteriol.* 276:221–230 (1992).

345. Rice, E.W., E.G. Sowers, C.H. Johnson, et al. Serological cross-reactions between *Escherichia coli* O157 and other species of the genus *Escherichia*. *J. Clin. Microbiol.* 30:1315–1316 (1992).

346. Chart, H., and B. Rowe. Serological identification of infection by Vero cytotoxin producing *Escherichia coli* in patients with haemolytic uraemic syndrome. *Serodiag. Immunother. Infect. Dis.* 4:413–418 (1990).

347. Chart, H., and B. Rowe. Improved detection of infection by *Escherichia coli* O157 in patients with haemolytic uraemic syndrome by means of IgA antibodies to lipopolysaccharide. *J. Infect. Dis.* 24:257–261 (1992).

348. Bitzan, M., and H. Karch. Indirect hemagglutination assay for diagnosis of *Escherichia coli* O157 infection in patients with hemolytic-uremic syndrome. *J. Clin. Microbiol.* 30:1174–1178 (1992).

349. Speirs, J., S. Stavric, and B. Buchanan. Assessment of two commercial agglutination kits for detecting *Escherichia coli* heat-labile enterotoxin. *Can. J. Microbiol.* 37:877–880 (1991).

350. Ram, S., S. Khurana, D.V. Vadehra, et al. ELISA for detection of heat stable enterotoxin producing *Escherichia coli* strains. *Indian J. Med. Res. [A]* 93:286–288 (1991).

351. Germani, Y., H. deRocquigny, and J.L. Guesdon. *Escherichia coli* heat-stable enterotoxin (STa)–biotin conjugates for the titration of STa antisera by an enzyme-linked immunosorbent assay. *J. Immunol. Meth.* 146:25–32 (1992).

352. Drevet, P., and R. Guinet. Comparison of sandwich-ELISA and GM1-ELISA for the detection of *Escherichia coli* thermolabile enterotoxin. *J. Immunoassay* 12:293–304 (1991).

353. Law, D., L.A. Ganguli, A. Donohue-Rolfe, and D.W.K. Acheson. Detection by ELISA of low numbers of Shiga-like toxin–producing *Escherichia coli* in mixed cultures after growth in the presence of mitomycin C. *J. Med. Microbiol.* 36:198–202 (1992).

354. Barrett, T.J., J.H. Green, P.M. Griffin, et al. Enzyme-linked immunosorbent assays for detecting antibodies to Shiga-like toxin I, Shiga-like toxin II, and *Escherichia coli* O157:H7 lipopolysaccharide in human serum. *Curr. Microbiol.* 23:189–195 (1991).

355. Speirs, J.I., and M. Akhtar. Detection of *Escherichia coli* cytotoxins by enzyme-linked immunosorbent assays. *Can. J. Microbiol.* 37:650–653 (1991).

356. Haider, K., S.M. Faruque, M.J. Albert, et al. Comparison of a modified adherence assay with existing assay methods for identification of enteroaggregative *Escherichia coli*. *J. Clin. Microbiol.* 30:1614–1616 (1992).

357. Scotland, S.M., H.R. Smith, B. Said, et al. Identification of enteropathogenic *Escherichia coli* isolated in Britain as enteroaggregative or as members of a subclass of attaching-and-effacing *E. coli* not hybridising with the EPEC adherence-factor probe. *J. Med. Microbiol.* 35:278–283 (1991).

358. Begaud, E., and Y. Germani. Detection of enterotoxigenic *Escherichia coli* in faecal specimens by acetylaminofluorene-labelled DNA probes. *Res. Microbiol.* 143:315–325 (1992).

359. Tamatsukuri, S., K. Yamamoto, S. Shibata, et al. Detection of a heat-labile enterotoxin gene in enterotoxigenic *Escherichia coli* by densitometric evaluation using highly specific enzyme-linked oligonucleotide probes. *Eur. J. Clin. Microbiol. Infect. Dis.* 10:1048–1055 (1991).

360. Rademaker, C.M.A., M.J.H.M. Wolfhagen, M. Jansze, et al. Digoxigenin labelled DNA probes for rapid detection of enterotoxigenic, enteropathogenic and Vero cytotoxin producing *Escherichia coli* in faecal samples. *J. Microbiol. Meth.* 15:121–127 (1992).

361. Jackson, M.P. Detection of Shiga toxin–producing *Shigella dysenteriae* type 1 and *Escherichia coli* by using polymerase chain reaction with incorporation of digoxigenin-11-dUTP. *J. Clin. Microbiol.* 29:1910–1914 (1991).

362. Read, S.C., R.C. Clarke, A. Martin, et al. Polymerase chain reaction for detection of verocytotoxigenic *Escherichia coli* isolated from animal and food sources. *Mol. Cell. Probes* 6:153–161 (1992).

363. Olsvik, Ø., E. Rimstad, E. Hornes, et al. A nested PCR followed by magnetic separation of amplified fragments for detection of *Escherichia coli* Shiga-like toxin genes. *Mol. Cell. Probes* 5:429–435 (1991).

364. Johnson, W.M., S.D. Tyler, G. Wang, and H. Lior. Amplification by the polymerase chain reaction of a specific target sequence in the gene coding for *Escherichia coli* verotoxin (VTe variant). *FEMS Microbiol. Lett.* 84:227–230 (1991).

365. Lortie, L.-A., J. Harel, J.M. Fairbrother, and J.D. Dubreuil. Evaluation of three new techniques for the detection of STb-positive *Escherichia coli* strains. *Mol. Cell. Probes* 5:271–275 (1991).

366. Meyer, R., J. Lüthy, and U. Candrian. Direct detection by polymerase chain reaction (PCR) of *Escherichia coli* in water and soft cheese and identification of enterotoxigenic strains. *Lett. Appl. Microbiol.* 13:268–271 (1991).

367. Wernars, K., E. Delfgou. P.S. Soentoro, and S. Notermans. Successful approach for detection of low numbers of enterotoxigenic *Escherichia coli* in minced meat by using the polymerase chain reaction. *Appl. Environ. Microbiol.* 57:1914–1919 (1991).

368. Keasler, S.P., and W.E. Hill. Polymerase chain reaction identification of enteroinvasive *Escherichia coli* seeded into raw milk. *J. Food Protect.* 55:382–384 (1992).

369. Stavric, S., B. Buchanan, and J. Speirs. Comparison of a competitive enzyme immunoassay kit and the infant mouse assay for detecting *Escherichia coli* heat-stable enterotoxin. *Lett. Appl. Microbiol.* 14:47–50 (1992).

370. El-Shenawy, M.A., M.A. El-Shenawy, and E.H. Marth. *Yersinia*, yersiniosis and food: a review. *Egypt. J. Dairy Sci.* 19:177–193 (1991).

371. Une, T., T. Maruyama, and M. Tsubokura (eds.). *Current Investigations of the Microbiology of Yersiniae.* 5th International Symposium on *Yersinia*. Mt. Fuji, 24–26 September 1990. *Contrib. Microbiol. Immunol.* 12 (1991).

372. Wale, M.C.J., A.J. Liddicoat, and J.V.S. Pether. *Yersinia enterocolitica* biotype 2 serotype O9 septicaemia in a previously fit man, raw goats' milk having been the apparent vehicle of infection: a cautionary tale. *J. Infect.* 23:69–72 (1991).

373. Butt, H.L., D.L. Gordon, T. Lee-Archer, et al. Relationship between clinical and milk isolates of *Yersinia enterocolitica*. *Pathology* 23:153–157 (1991).

374. Blumberg, H.M., J.A. Kiehlbauch, and I.K. Wachsmuth. Molecular epidemiology of *Yersinia enterocolitica* O:3 infections: use of chromosomal DNA restriction fragment length polymorphisms of rRNA genes. *J. Clin. Microbiol.* 29:2368–2374 (1991).

375. Nesbakken, T., G. Kapperud, J. Lassen, and E. Skjerve. *Yersinia enterocolitica* O:3 antibodies in slaughterhouse employees, veterinarians, and military recruits. Occupational exposure to pigs as a risk factor for yersiniosis. In *Current Investigations of the Microbiology of Yersiniae.* T. Une, T. Maruyama, and M. Tsubokura (eds.). *Contrib. Microbiol. Immunol.* 12:32–39 (1991).

376. Morris, J.G., Jr., V. Prado, C. Ferreccio, et al. *Yersinia enterocolitica* isolated from two cohorts of young children in Santiago, Chile: incidence of and lack of correlation between illness and proposed virulence factors. *J. Clin. Microbiol.* 29:2784–2788 (1991).

377. Prentice, M.B., D. Cope, and R.A. Swann. The epidemiology of *Yersinia enterocolitica* infection in the British Isles 1983–1988. In *Current Investigations of the Microbiology of Yersiniae.* T. Une, T. Maruyama, and M. Tsubokura (eds.). *Contrib. Microbiol. Immunol.* 12:17–25 (1991).

378. Verhaegen, J., L. Dancsa, P. Lemmens, et al. *Yersinia enterocolitica* surveillance in Belgium (1979–1989). In *Current Investigations of the Microbiology of Yersiniae.* T. Une, T. Maruyama, and M. Tsubokura (eds.). *Contrib. Microbiol. Immunol.* 12:11–16 (1991).

379. Sæbø, A., and J. Lassen. A survey of acute and chronic disease associated with *Yersinia enterocolitica* infection. A Norwegian 10-year follow-up study on 458 hospitalized patients. *Scand. J. Infect. Dis.* 23:517–527 (1991).

380. Sæbø, A., and J. Lassen. Acute and chronic gastrointestinal manifestations associated with *Yersinia enterocolitica* infection. A Norwegian 10-year follow-up study on 458 hospitalized patients. *Ann. Surg.* 215:250–255 (1992).

381. Wenzel, B.E., J. Heesemann, A. Heufelder, et al. Enteropathogenic *Yersinia enterocolitica* and organ-specific autoimmune diseases in man. In *Current Inves-*

tigations of the Microbiology of Yersiniae. T. Une, T. Maruyama, and M. Tsubokura (eds.). *Contrib. Microbiol. Immunol.* 12:80–88 (1991).

382. Lindholm, H., and R. Visakorpi. Late complications after a *Yersinia enterocolitica* epidemic: a follow up study. *Ann. Rheum. Dis.* 50:694–696 (1991).

383. Abcarian, P.W., and B.E. Demas. Systemic *Yersinia enterocolitica* infection associated with iron overload and deferoxamine therapy. *Am. J. Roentgenol.* 157:773–775 (1991).

384. Mazzoleni, G., D. deSa, H. Gately, and R.H. Riddell. *Yersinia enterocolitica* infection with ileal perforation associated with iron overload and deferoxamine therapy. *Digest. Dis. Sci.* 36:1154–1160 (1991).

385. Van Noyen, R., R. Selderslaghs, J. Bekaert, et al. Causative role of *Yersinia* and other enteric pathogens in the appendicular syndrome. *Eur. J. Clin. Microbiol. Infect. Dis.* 10:735–741 (1991).

386. Viner, N.J., L.C. Bailey, P.F. Life, et al. Isolation of *Yersinia*-specific T cell clones from the synovial membrane and synovial fluid of a patient with reactive arthritis. *Arth. Rheum.* 34:1151–1157 (1991).

387. Pile, K., T. Kwong, J. Fryer, and R. Laurent. Polyarteritis associated with *Yersinia enterocolitica* infection. *Ann. Rheum. Dis.* 51:678–680 (1992).

388. Andersen, J.K., R. Sørensen, and M. Glensbjerg. Aspects of the epidemiology of *Yersinia enterocolitica*: a review. *Int. J. Food Microbiol.* 13:231–238 (1991).

389. Ibrahim, A., and I.C. MacRae. Isolation of *Yersinia enterocolitica* and related species from red meat and milk. *J. Food Sci.* 56:1524–1526 (1991).

390. Falcão, D.P. Occurrence of *Yersinia* spp. in foods in Brazil. *Int. J. Food Microbiol.* 14:179–182 (1991).

391. Tsai, S.-J., and L.-H. Chen. Occurrence of *Yersinia enterocolitica* in pork products from northern Taiwan. In *Current Investigations of the Microbiology of Yersiniae.* T. Une, T. Maruyama, and M. Tsubokura (eds.). *Contrib. Microbiol. Immunol.* 12:56–62 (1991).

392. Shiozawa, K., T. Nishina, Y. Miwa, et al. Colonization in the tonsils of swine by *Yersinia enterocolitica.* In *Current Investigations of the Microbiology of Yersiniae.* T. Une, T. Maruyama, and M. Tsubokura (eds.). *Contrib. Microbiol. Immunol.* 12:63–67 (1991).

393. Bülte, M., G. Klein, and G. Reuter. Schweineschlachtung. Kontamination des Fleisches durch menschen-pathogene *Yersinia enterocolitica*-Stämme? *Fleischwirtschaft* 71:1411–1416 (1991).

394. Kwaga, J.K.P., and J.O. Iversen. Laboratory investigation of virulence among strains of *Yersinia enterocolitica* and related species isolated from pigs and pork products. *Can. J. Microbiol.* 38:92–97 (1992).

395. Larkin, L.L., P.C. Vasavada, and E.H. Marth. Incidence of *Yersinia enterocolitica* in raw milk as related to its quality. *Milchwissenschaft* 46:500–502 (1991).

398. Farrag, S.A., F.E. El-Gazzar, and E.H. Marth. Inactivation of *Yersinia enterocolitica* by the lactoperoxidase system in a semi-synthetic medium and in raw milk. *Milchwissenschaft* 47:95–98 (1992).

397. Klausner, R.B., and C.W. Donnelly. Environmental sources of *Listeria* and *Yersinia* in Vermont dairy plants. *J. Food Protect.* 54:607–611 (1991).

398. Adams, M.R., C.L. Little, and M.C. Easter. Modelling the effect of pH, acidulant and temperature on the growth rate of *Yersinia enterocolitica. J. Appl. Bacteriol.* 71:65–71 (1991).

399. Little, C.L., M.R. Adams, and M.C. Easter. The effect of pH, acidulant and temperature on the survival of *Yersinia enterocolitica. Lett. Appl. Microbiol.* 14:148–152 (1992).

400. Vidon, D.J.M., and A. Ahmedy. Beta-lactamases of strains of *Yersinia enterocolitica* biovar 6 isolated from foods. In *Current Investigations of the Microbiology of Yersiniae.* T. Une, T. Maruyama, and M. Tsubokura (eds.). *Contrib. Microbiol. Immunol.* 12:244–250 (1991).

401. Iinuma, Y., H. Hayashidani, K.-I. Kaneko, et al. Isolation of *Yersinia enterocolitica* serovar O8 from free-living small rodents in Japan. *J. Clin. Microbiol.* 30:240–242 (1992).

402. Fukushima, H., M. Gomyoda, and S. Kaneko. Wild animals as the source of infection with *Yersinia pseudotuberculosis* in Shimane Prefecture, Japan. In *Current Investigations of the Microbiology of Yersiniae.* T. Une, T. Maruyama, and M. Tsubokura (eds.). *Contrib. Microbiol. Immunol.* 12:1–4 (1991).

403. Karapinar, M., and S.A. Gönül. Survival of *Yersinia enterocolitica* and *Escherichia coli* in spring water. *Int. J. Food Microbiol.* 13:315–320 (1991).

404. Bucci, G., P. Maini, L. Pacifico, et al. Direct isolation of *Yersinia enterocolitica* from stool specimens of patients with intestinal disorders. In *Current*

Investigations of the Microbiology of Yersiniae. T. Une, T. Maruyama, and M. Tsubokura (eds.). *Contrib. Microbiol. Immunol.* 12:50–55 (1991).

405. Zheng, X.B., and C. Xie. Comparative evaluation of various media for the detection of pathogenic *Yersinia enterocolitica*. In *Current Investigations of the Microbiology of Yersiniae*. T. Une, T. Maruyama, and M. Tsubokura (eds.). *Contrib. Microbiol. Immunol.* 12:159–163 (1991).

406. Bhaduri, S., C. Turner-Jones, and R.V. Lachica. Convenient agarose medium for simultaneous determination of the low-calcium response and Congo red binding by virulent strains of *Yersinia enterocolitica*. *J. Clin. Microbiol.* 29:2341–2344 (1991).

407. Ibrahim, A., W. Liesack, and E. Stackebrandt. Differentiation between pathogenic and non-pathogenic *Yersinia enterocolitica* strains by colony hybridization with a PCR-mediated digoxigenin-dUTP-labelled probe. *Mol. Cell. Probes* 6:163–171 (1992).

408. Kapperud, G., T. Nesbakken, and K. Dommarsnes. Application of restriction endonuclease analysis and genetic probes in the epidemiology of *Yersinia enterocolitica* infection. In *Current Investigations of the Microbiology of Yersiniae*. T. Une, T. Maruyama, and M. Tsubokura (eds.). *Contrib. Microbiol. Immunol.* 12:68–74 (1991).

409. Pham, J.N., S.M. Bell, and J.Y.M. Lanzarone. Biotype and antibiotic sensitivity of 100 clinical isolates of *Yersinia enterocolitica*. *J. Antimicrob. Chemother.* 28:13–18 (1991).

410. Brubaker, R.R. Factors promoting acute and chronic diseases caused by yersiniae. *Clin. Microbiol. Rev.* 4:309–324 (1991).

411. Chiesa, C., L. Pacifico, A. Guiyoule, et al. Phenotypic characterization and virulence of O8 *Yersinia* strains isolated in Europe. In *Current Investigations of the Microbiology of Yersiniae*. T. Une, T. Maruyama, and M. Tsubokura (eds.). *Contrib. Microbiol. Immunol.* 12:182–191 (1991).

412. Al-Hendy, A., P. Toivanen, and M. Skurnik. Lipopolysaccharide O side chain of *Yersinia enterocolitica* O:3 is an essential virulence factor in an orally infected murine model. *Infect. Immun.* 60:870–875 (1992).

413. Chart, H., T. Cheasty, D. Cope, et al. The serological relationship between *Yersinia enterocolitica* O9 and *Escherichia coli* O157 using sera from patients with yersiniosis and haemolytic uraemic syndrome. *Epidemiol. Infect.* 107:349–356 (1991).

414. Kaneko, S., T. Maruyama, and H. Fukushima. Comparison of plasmid DNA among different serogroups of *Yersinia pseudotuberculosis*. In *Current Investigations of the Microbiology of Yersiniae*. T. Une, T. Maruyama, and M. Tsubokura (eds.). *Contrib. Microbiol. Immunol.* 12:75–79 (1991).

415. Pærregaard, A. Interactions between *Yersinia enterocolitica* and the host with special reference to virulence plasmid encoded adhesion and humoral immunity. *Danish Med. Bull.* 39:155–172 (1992).

416. Naumann, M., C. Hanski, and E.O. Riecken. Expression *in vivo* of additional plasmid-mediated proteins during intestinal infection with *Yersinia enterocolitica* serotype O8. *J. Med. Microbiol.* 35:257–263 (1991).

417. Young, V.B., S. Falkow, and G.K. Schoolnik. The invasin protein of *Yersinia enterocolitica*: internalization of invasin-bearing bacteria by eukaryotic cells is associated with reorganization of the cytoskeleton. *J. Cell Biol.* 116:197–207 (1992).

418. Leong, J.M., R.S. Fournier, and R.R. Isberg. Mapping and topographic localization of epitopes of the *Yersinia pseudotuberculosis* invasin protein. *Infect. Immun.* 59:3424–3433 (1991).

419. Mack, D., M. Pulz, and J. Heesemann. Recognition by peptide mapping of three different structural groups of outer membrane protein YOP-1 of *Yersinia enterocolitica* and *Yersinia pseudotuberculosis*. *Med. Microbiol. Immunol.* 180:205–211 (1991).

420. de Rouvroit, C.L., C. Sluiters, and G.R. Cornelis. Role of the transcriptional activator, VirF, and temperature in the expression of the pYV plasmid genes of *Yersinia enterocolitica*. *Mol. Microbiol.* 6:395–409 (1992).

421. Carniel, E., A. Guiyoule, O. Mercereau-Puijalon, and H.H. Mollaret. Chromosomal marker for the 'high pathogenicity' phenotype in *Yersinia*. In *Current Investigations of the Microbiology of Yersiniae*. T. Une, T. Maruyama, and M. Tsubokura (eds.). *Contrib. Microbiol. Immunol.* 12:192–197 (1991).

422. Carniel, E., A. Guiyoule, I. Guilvout, and O. Mercereau-Puijalon. Molecular cloning, iron-regulation and mutagenesis of the *irp2* gene encoding HMWP2, a protein specific for the highly pathogenic *Yersinia*. *Mol. Microbiol.* 6:379–388 (1992).

423. Rodrick, G.E. Indigenous pathogens: *Vibrionaceae*. In *Microbiology of Marine Food Products*. D.R. Ward and C. Hackney (eds.). New York, Van Nostrand Reinhold. Pp. 285–300 (1991).

424. Kelly, M.T. Pathogenic *Vibrionaceae* in patients and the environment. *Undersea Biomed. Res.* 18:193–196 (1991).

425. World Health Organization. Cholera in the Americas. *Weekly Epidemiol. Rec.* 67:33–39 (1992).

426. World Health Organization. Cholera in 1991. *Weekly Epidemiol. Rec.* 67:253–260 (1992).

427. Tauxe, R.V., and P.A. Blake. Epidemic cholera in Peru. *JAMA* 267:1388–1390 (1992).

428. Anderson, C. Cholera epidemic traced to risk miscalculation. *Nature* 354:255 (1991).

429. Glass, R.I., M. Libel, and A.D. Brandling-Bennett. Epidemic cholera in the Americas. *Science* 256:1524–1525 (1992).

430. Crowley, P. Nicaragua now threatened with cholera. *Br. Med. J.* 304:141 (1992).

431. Glass, R.I., M. Claeson, P.A. Blake, et al. Cholera in Africa: lessons on transmission and control for Latin America. *Lancet* 338:791–795 (1991).

432. Mossel, D.A.A., C.B. Struijk, and J.T. Jansen. Control of the transmission of *Vibrio cholerae* and other enteropathogens by foods originating from endemic areas in South America and elsewhere as a model situation. *Int. J. Food Microbiol.* 15:1–11 (1992).

433. Tamplin, M.L., and C.C. Parodi. Environmental spread of *Vibrio cholerae* in Peru. (Letter.) *Lancet* 338:1216–1217 (1991).

434. Puglielli, L., C. Cattrini, J.J.G. Resa, et al. Symptomless carriage of *Vibrio cholerae* in Peru. *Lancet* 339:1056–1057 (1992).

435. Chen, F., G.M. Evins, W.L. Cook, et al. Genetic diversity among toxigenic and nontoxigenic *Vibrio cholerae* O1 isolated from the Western Hemisphere. *Epidemiol. Infect.* 107:225–233 (1991).

436. Faruque, S.M., and J. Albert. Genetic relation between *Vibrio cholerae* O1 strains in Ecuador and Bangladesh. (Letter.) *Lancet* 339:740–741 (1992).

437. Centers for Disease Control. Cholera associated with an international airline flight, 1992. *Morbid. Mortal. Weekly Rep.* 41:134–135 (1992).

438. World Health Organization. Cholera and international air travel. *Weekly Epidemiol. Rec.* 67:103–104 (1992).

439. Health and Welfare Canada. Cholera associated with international travel, 1992—United States. *Can. Commun. Dis. Rep.* 18:166–168 (1992).

440. Health and Welfare Canada. Non-O1 *Vibrio cholerae* enterocolitis in Quebec tourists returning from the Dominican Republic. *Can. Commun. Dis. Rep.* 18:105–107 (1992).

441. Desenclos, J.-C. A., K.C. Klontz, L.E. Wolfe, and S. Hoecherl. The risk of *Vibrio* illness in the Florida raw oyster eating population, 1981–1988. *Am. J. Epidemiol.* 134:290–297 (1991).

442. Anonymous. Cholera in clams. *New Sci.* 131(1786):18 (1991).

443. DePaola, A., G.M. Capers, M.L. Motes, et al. Isolation of Latin American epidemic strain of *Vibrio cholerae* O1 from US Gulf Coast. (Letter.) *Lancet* 339:624 (1992).

444. McCarthy, S.A., R.M. McPhearson, A.M. Guarino, and J.L. Gaines. Toxigenic *Vibrio cholerae* O1 and cargo ships entering Gulf of Mexico. (Letter.) *Lancet* 339:624–625 (1992).

445. Minami, A., S. Hashimoto, H. Abe, et al. Cholera enterotoxin production in *Vibrio cholerae* O1 strains isolated from the environment and from humans in Japan. *Appl. Environ. Microbiol.* 57:2152–2157 (1991).

446. Visser, I.J.R., E.A. ter Laak, N.W. van Dijk, and W. Wouda. Toxigenic *Vibrio cholerae* non-O:1 isolated from a goat in the Netherlands. *Vet. Q.* 13:114–118 (1991).

447. Kiiyukia, C., H. Nakano, R. Rajendran, et al. Distribution of *Vibrio cholerae* non-O1 in and around the Hiroshima city aquatic environment, Japan. *J. Gen. Appl. Microbiol.* 37:467–477 (1991).

448. Thom, S., D. Warhurst, and B.S. Drasar. Association of *Vibrio cholerae* with fresh water amoebae. *J. Med. Microbiol.* 36:303–306 (1992).

449. Rice, E.W., and C.H. Johnson. Cholera in Peru. (Letter.) *Lancet* 338:455 (1991).

450. Jones, M.V., M.A. Wood, and T.M. Herd. Comparative sensitivity of *Vibrio cholerae* O1 El Tor and *Escherichia coli* to disinfectants. *Lett. Appl. Microbiol.* 14:51–53 (1992).

451. Kitagawa, T., Y. Tsutida, R. Murakami, et al. Detection and quantitative assessment of a *Vibrio cholerae* O1 species in several foods by a novel enzyme immunoassay. *Microbiol. Immunol.* 36:13–20 (1992).

452. Salles, C.A., and H. Momen. Identification of *Vibrio cholerae* by enzyme electrophoresis. *Trans. Roy. Soc. Trop. Med. Hyg.* 85:544–547 (1991).

453. Simonson, J.G., and R.J. Siebeling. Detection of *Vibrio cholerae* O1 serovars in oyster meat homogenate by a dipstick-ELISA method. *Marine Technol. Soc. J.* 25:52–59 (1991).

454. Naka, A., T. Honda, and T. Miwatani. A simple purification method of *Vibrio cholerae* non-O1 hemagglutinin/protease by immunoaffinity column chromatography using a monoclonal antibody. *Microbiol. Immunol.* 36:419–423 (1992).

455. Charania, Z., R. Vanmaele, and G.D. Armstrong. A bioassay for cholera-like toxins using HT29 cells. *J. Microbiol. Meth.* 14:171–176 (1991).

456. Uesaka, Y., Y. Otsuka, M. Kashida, et al. Detection of cholera toxin by a highly sensitive bead–enzyme linked immunosorbent. *Microbiol. Immunol.* 36:43–53 (1992).

457. Miyagi, K., Y. Matsumoto, K. Hayashi, et al. Cholera diagnosed in clinical laboratory by DNA hybridisation. (Letter.) *Lancet* 339:988–989 (1992).

458. Shirai, H., M. Nishibuchi, T. Ramamurthy, et al. Polymerase chain reaction for detection of the cholera enterotoxin operon of *Vibrio cholerae. J. Clin. Microbiol.* 29:2517–2521 (1991).

459. Ramamurthy, T., A. Pal, S.C. Pal, and G.B. Nair. Taxonomical implications of the emergence of high frequency of occurrence of 2,4-diamino-6,7-diisopropylpteridine-resistant strains of *Vibrio cholerae* from clinical cases of cholera in Calcutta, India. *J. Clin. Microbiol.* 30:742–743 (1992).

460. Almeida, R.J., D.N. Cameron, W.L. Cook, and I.K. Wachsmuth. Vibriophage VcA-3 as an epidemic strain marker for the U.S. Gulf Coast *Vibrio cholerae* O1 clone. *J. Clin. Microbiol.* 30:300–304 (1992).

461. Richardson, K. Roles of motility and flagellar structure in pathogenicity of *Vibrio cholerae:* analysis of motility mutants in three animal models. *Infect. Immun.* 59:2727–2736 (1991).

462. Chakrabarti, M.K., S.P. De, A.K. Sinha, and S.C Pal. Toxin production by atypical strains of *Vibrio cholerae* El Tor under different cultural conditions. *Zbl. Bakteriol.* 275:256–263 (1991).

463. Gibbons, A. New 3-D protein structures revealed. The shape of cholera. *Science* 253:382–383 (1991).

464. Pacuszka, T., and P.H. Fishman. Intoxication of cultured cells by cholera toxin: evidence for different pathways when bound to ganglioside G_{M1} or neoganglioproteins. *Biochemistry* 31:4773–4778 (1992).

465. Jonson, G., J. Holmgren, and A.-M. Svennerholm. Epitope differences in toxin-coregulated pili produced by classical and El Tor *Vibrio cholerae* O1. *Microb. Pathogen.* 11:179–188 (1991).

466. DiRita, V.J., C. Parsot, G. Jander, and J.J. Mekalanos. Regulatory cascade controls virulence in *Vibrio cholerae. Proc. Natl. Acad. Sci. USA* 88:5403–5407 (1991).

467. DiRita, V.J. Co-ordinate expression of virulence genes by ToxR in *Vibrio cholerae. Mol. Microbiol.* 6:451–458 (1992).

468. Fasano, A., B. Baudry, D.W. Pumplin, et al. *Vibrio cholerae* produces a second enterotoxin, which affects intestinal tight junctions. *Proc. Natl. Acad. Sci. USA* 88:5242–5246 (1991).

469. Baudry, B., A. Fasano, J. Ketley, and J.B. Kaper. Cloning of a gene (*zot*) encoding a new toxin produced by *Vibrio cholerae. Infect. Immun.* 60:428–434 (1992).

470. Moss, J., and M. Vaughan. Activation of cholera toxin and *Escherichia coli* heat-labile enterotoxins by ADP-ribosylation factors, a family of 20 kDa guanine nucleotide-binding proteins. *Mol. Microbiol.* 5:2621–2627 (1991).

471. Galen, J.E., J.M. Ketley, A. Fasano, et al. Role of *Vibrio cholerae* neuraminidase in the function of cholera toxin. *Infect. Immun.* 60:406–415 (1992).

472. Burnette, W.N., V.L. Mar, B.W. Platler, et al. Site-specific mutagenesis of the catalytic subunit of cholera toxin: substituting lysine for arginine 7 causes loss of activity. *Infect. Immun.* 59:4266–4270 (1991).

473. Jobling, M.G., and R.K. Holmes. Analysis of structure and function of the B subunit of cholera toxin by the use of site-directed mutagenesis. *Mol. Microbiol.* 5:1755–1767 (1991).

474. Kazemi, M., and R.A. Finkelstein. Mapping epitopic regions of cholera toxin B-subunit protein. *Mol. Immunol.* 28:865–876 (1991).

475. Dams, E., M. De Wolf, and W. Dierick. Nucleotide sequence analysis of the CT operon of the *Vibrio cholerae* classical strain 569B. *Biochim. Biophys. Acta* 1090:139–141 (1991).

476. Krasilnikov, O.V., J.N. Muratkhodjaev, S.E. Voronov, and Y.V. Yezepchuk. The ionic channels formed by cholera toxin in planar bilayer lipid membranes are entirely attributable to its B-subunit. *Biochim. Biophys. Acta* 1067:166–170 (1991).

477. Ito, T., Y. Ohshita, K. Hiramatsu, and T. Yokota. Identification and nucleotide sequence determination of the gene responsible for Ogawa serotype specificity of *V. cholerae* O1. *FEBS Lett.* 286:159–162 (1991).

478. Johnson, J.A., P. Panigrahi, and J.G. Morris, Jr. Non-O1 *Vibrio cholerae* NRT36S produces a polysaccharide capsule that determines colony morphology, serum resistance, and virulence in mice. *Infect. Immun.* 60:864–869 (1992).

479. Russell, R.G., B.D. Tall, and J.G. Morris, Jr. Non-O1 *Vibrio cholerae* intestinal pathology and invasion in the removable intestinal tie adult rabbit diarrhea model. *Infect. Immun.* 60:435–442 (1992).

480. Alm, R.A., G. Mayrhofer, I. Kotlarski, and P.A. Manning. Amino-terminal domain of the El Tor haemolysin of *Vibrio cholerae* O1 is expressed in classical strains and is cytotoxic. *Vaccine* 9:588–594 (1991).

481. Williams, S.G., and P.A. Manning. Transcription of the *Vibrio cholerae* haemolysin gene, *hlyA*, and cloning of a positive regulatory locus, *hlyU*. *Mol. Microbiol.* 5:2031–2038 (1991).

482. Häse, C.C., and R.A. Finkelstein. Cloning and nucleotide sequence of the *Vibrio cholerae* hemagglutinin/protease (HA/protease) gene and construction of an HA/protease-negative strain. *J. Bacteriol.* 483:3311–3317 (1991).

483. Finkelstein, R.A., M. Boesman-Finkelstein, Y. Chang, and C.C. Häse. *Vibrio cholerae* hemagglutinin/protease, colonial variation, virulence, and detachment. *Infect. Immun.* 60:472–478 (1992).

484. Chakrabarti, M.K., A.K. Sinha, and T. Biswas. Adherence of *Vibrio parahaemolyticus* to rabbit intestinal epithelial cells in vitro. *FEMS Microbiol. Lett.* 84:113–117 (1991).

485. Nakasone, N., and M. Iwanaga. The role of pili in colonization of the rabbit intestine by *Vibrio parahaemolyticus* Na2. *Microbiol. Immunol.* 36:123–130 (1992).

486. Yoh, M., T. Miwatani, and T. Honda. Comparison of *Vibrio parahaemolyticus* hemolysin (Vp-TRH) produced by environmental and clinical isolates. *FEMS Microbiol. Lett.* 82:157–161 (1992).

487. Nishibuchi, M., K. Kumagai, and J.B. Kaper. Contribution of the *tdh*1 gene of Kanagawa phenomenon–positive *Vibrio parahaemolyticus* to production of extracellular thermostable direct hemolysin. *Microb. Pathogen.* 11:452–460 (1991).

488. Yoh, M., T. Honda, T. Miwatani, and M. Nishibuchi. Characterization of thermostable direct hemolysins encoded by four representative *tdh* genes of *Vibrio parahaemolyticus*. *Microb. Pathogen.* 10:165–172 (1991).

489. Miyoshi, S.-i., H. Matsuoka, H. Taniguchi, et al. The lecithin-dependent hemolysin produced by *Vibrio parahaemolyticus*: characterization as a new type phospholipase. *J. Pharmacobio-Dyn.* 14:s-156 (1991).

490. Lefkowitz, A., G.S. Fout, G. Losonsky, et al. A serosurvey of pathogens associated with shellfish: prevalence of antibodies to *Vibrio* species and Norwalk virus in the Chesapeake Bay region. *Am. J. Epidemiol.* 135:369–380 (1992).

491. Tamplin, M.L., and G.M. Capers. Persistence of *Vibrio vulnificus* in tissues of Gulf Coast oysters, *Crassostrea virginica*, exposed to seawater disinfected with UV light. *Appl. Environ. Microbiol.* 58:1506–1510 (1992).

492. Bullen, J.J., P.B. Spalding, C.G. Ward, and J.M.C. Gutteridge. Hemochromatosis, iron, and septicemia caused by *Vibrio vulnificus*. *Arch. Intern. Med.* 151:1606–1609 (1991).

493. Oliver, J.D., L. Nilsson, and S. Kjelleberg. Formation of nonculturable *Vibrio vulnificus* cells and its relationship to the starvation state. *Appl. Environ. Microbiol.* 57:2640–2644 (1991).

494. Nilsson, L., J.D. Oliver, and S. Kjelleberg. Resuscitation of *Vibrio vulnificus* from the viable but nonculturable state. *J. Bacteriol.* 173:5054–5059 (1991).

495. Oliver, J.D., K. Guthrie, J. Preyer, et al. Use of colistin–polymyxin B–cellobiose agar for isolation of *Vibrio vulnificus* from the environment. *Appl. Environ. Microbiol.* 58:737–739 (1992).

496. Sloan, E.M., C.J. Hagen, G.A. Lancette, et al. Comparison of five selective enrichment broths and two selective agars for recovery of *Vibrio vulnificus* from oysters. *J. Food Protect.* 55:356–359 (1992).

497. Brauns, L.A., M.C. Hudson, and J.D. Oliver. Use of the polymerase chain reaction in detection of culturable and nonculturable *Vibrio vulnificus* cells. *Appl. Environ. Microbiol.* 57:2651–2655 (1991).

498. Martin, S.J., and R.J. Siebeling. Identification of *Vibrio vulnificus* O serovars with antilipopolysaccharide monoclonal antibody. *J. Clin. Microbiol.* 29:1684–1688 (1991).

499. Uchimura, M., and T. Yamamoto. Production of hemagglutinins and pili by *Vibrio mimicus* and its adherence to human and rabbit small intestines in vitro. *FEMS Microbiol. Lett.* 91:73–78 (1992).

500. Yoshida, H., T. Honda, and T. Miwatani. Purification and characterization of a hemolysin of *Vibrio mimicus* that relates to the thermostable direct hemolysin of *Vibrio parahaemolyticus. FEMS Microbiol. Lett.* 84:249–254 (1991).

501. Venkateswaran, K., H. Horiuchi, H. Nakano, et al. *Vibrio* virulence factors and the quantitative analysis of cytotoxicity elaborated by environmental isolates. *Cytobios* 66:143–151 (1991).

502. Ahsan, C.R., M.M. Hoque, Z. Rasul, and M.M. Hoq. Enterotoxicity of *Vibrio furnissii* isolated from eels. *World J. Microbiol. Biotechnol.* 8:187–189 (1992).

503. Buck, J.D. Recovery of *Vibrio metschnikovii* from market seafood. *J. Food Safety* 12:73–78 (1991).

504. Robert, R., G. Grollier, F. Malin, et al. Isolation of *Vibrio alginolyticus* from blood cultures in a leukaemic patient after consumption of oysters. (Letter.) *Eur. J. Clin. Microbiol. Infect. Dis.* 10:987–988 (1991).

505. Yamasaki, S., H. Shirai, Y. Takeda, and M. Nishibuchi. Analysis of the gene of *Vibrio hollisae* encoding the hemolysin similar to the thermostable direct hemolysin of *Vibrio parahaemolyticus. FEMS Microbiol. Lett.* 80:259–263 (1991).

506. Terai, A., K. Baba, H. Shirai, et al. Evidence for insertion sequence–mediated spread of the thermostable direct hemolysin gene among *Vibrio* species. *J. Bacteriol.* 173:5036–5046 (1991).

507. Multi-author review. Research on *Aeromonas* and *Plesiomonas*. Papers presented at the 3rd International Workshop on *Aeromonas* and *Plesiomonas*, Helsingor, 5,6 September 1990. *Experientia* 47:402–446 (1991).

508. Janda, J.M. Recent advances in the study of the taxonomy, pathogenicity, and infectious syndromes associated with the genus *Aeromonas. Clin. Microbiol. Rev.* 4:397–410 (1991).

509. Bergann, T. Bewegliche Aeromonaden und ihre Bedeutung für die Fleischhygiene. *Fleischwirtschaft* 72:786–788 (1992).

510. Hudson, J.A., and K.M. De Lacy. Incidence of motile aeromonads in New Zealand retail foods. *J. Food Protect.* 54:696–699 (1991).

511. Krovacek, K., A. Faris, S.B. Baloda, et al. Prevalence and characterization of *Aeromonas* spp. isolated from foods in Uppsala, Sweden. *Food Microbiol.* 9:29–36 (1992).

512. Barnhart, H.M., and O.C. Pancorbo. Cytotoxicity and antibiotic resistance profiles of *Aeromonas hydrophila* isolates from a broiler processing operation. *J. Food Protect.* 55:108–112 (1992).

513. Noterdaeme, L., S. Bagawa, K.A. Willems, and F. Ollevier. Biochemical and physiological characteristics and plasmid profiles of *Aeromonas hydrophila* strains, isolated from freshwater fish and from fresh water. *J. Fish Dis.* 4:313–321 (1991).

514. Beuchat, L.R. Behavior of *Aeromonas* species at refrigeration temperatures. *Int. J. Food Microbiol.* 13:217–224 (1991).

515. Palumbo, S.A., A.C. Williams, R.L. Buchanan, and J.G. Phillips. Model for the anaerobic growth of *Aeromonas hydrophila* K144. *J. Food Protect.* 55:260–265 (1992).

516. Palumbo, S.A., and A.C. Williams. Growth of *Aeromonas hydrophila* K144 as affected by organic acids. *J. Food Sci.* 57:233–235 (1992).

517. Kaznowski, A., and K. Wlodarczak. Susceptibilities of motile *Aeromonas* sp. to antimicrobial agents. *Zbl. Bakteriol.* 275:85–93 (1991).

518. Carnahan, A.M., S. Behram, and S.W. Joseph. Aerokey II: a flexible key for identifying clinical *Aeromonas* species. *J. Clin. Microbiol.* 29:2843–2849 (1991).

519. Moyer, N.P., G. Martinetti, J. Lüthy-Hottenstein, and M. Altwegg. Value of rRNA gene restriction patterns of *Aeromonas* spp. for epidemiological investigations. *Curr. Microbiol.* 24:15–21 (1992).

520. Husslein, V., T. Chakraborty, A. Carnahan, and S.W. Joseph. Molecular studies on the aerolysin gene of *Aeromonas* species and discovery of a species-specific probe for *Aeromonas trota* species nova. *Clin. Infect. Dis.* 14:1061–1068 (1992).

521. Singh, D.V., and S.C. Sanyal. Enterotoxicity of clinical and environmental isolates of *Aeromonas* spp. *J. Med. Microbiol.* 36:269–272 (1992).

522. Vadivelu, J., S.D. Puthucheary, and P. Navaratnam. Exotoxin profiles of clinical isolates of

Aeromonas hydrophila. J. Med. Microbiol. 35:363–367 (1991).

523. Pal, A., T. Ramamurthy, A.R. Ghosh, et al. Virulence traits of *Aeromonas* strains in relation to species and source of isolation. *Zbl. Bakteriol.* 276:418–428 (1992).

524. Nishikawa, Y., T. Kimura, and T. Kishi. Mannose-resistant adhesion of motile *Aeromonas* to INT407 cells and the differences among isolates from humans, food and water. *Epidemiol. Infect.* 107:171–179 (1991).

525. Hokama, A., and M. Iwanaga. Purification and characterization of *Aeromonas sobria* pili, a possible colonization factor. *Infect. Immun.* 59:3478–3483 (1991).

526. Sibbald, C.J., and J.C.M. Sharp. *Campylobacter* infection in Scotland. *Commun. Dis. Environ. Health Scotland Weekly Rep.* 26(33):7–9 (1992).

527. Hudson, S.J., N.F. Lightfoot, J.C. Coulson, et al. Jackdaws and magpies as vectors of milkborne human campylobacter infection. *Epidemiol. Infect.* 107:363–372 (1991).

528. Allerberger, F., M.J. Kasten, and J.P. Anhalt. *Campylobacter fetus* subspecies *fetus* infection. *Klin. Wochenschr.* 69:813–816 (1991).

529. Chattopadhyay, U.K., R.S. Rathore, D. Pal, and M.S. Das. Incidence of *Campylobacter* species in animal handlers. *Indian J. Med. Res. [A]* 95:31–33 (1992).

530. Söderström, C., C. Schalén, and M. Walder. Septicaemia caused by unusual *Campylobacter* species (*C. laridis* and *C. mucosalis*). *Scand. J. Infect. Dis.* 23:369–371 (1991).

531. Bremell, T., A. Bjelle, and Å. Svedhem. Rheumatic symptoms following an outbreak of campylobacter enteritis: a five year follow up. *Ann. Rheum. Dis.* 50:934–938 (1991).

532. Schieven, B.C., D. Baird, C.L. Leatherdale, and Z. Hussain. *Campylobacter jejuni* infected bursitis. *Diagn. Microbiol. Infect. Dis.* 14:507–508 (1991).

533. v. d. Kruijk, R.A., A.S. Lampe, and H. Ph. Endtz. Bilateral abducens paresis following *Campylobacter jejuni* enteritis. (Letter.) *J. Infect. Dis.* 24:215–216 (1992).

534. Duret, M., A.G. Herbaut, F. Flamme, and J.M. Gerard. Another case of atypical acute axonal polyneuropathy following *Campylobacter* enteritis. *Neurology* 41:2008–2009 (1991).

535. Yuki, N., S. Sato, T. Itoh, and T. Miyatake. HLA-B35 and acute axonal polyneuropathy following *Campylobacter* infection. *Neurology* 41:1561–1563 (1991).

536. Blaser, M.J., A. Olivares, D.N. Taylor, et al. *Campylobacter* serology in patients with Chinese paralytic syndrome. (Letter.) *Lancet* 338:308 (1991).

537. Fujimoto, S., N. Yuki, T. Itoh, and K. Amako. Specific serotype of *Campylobacter jejuni* associated with Guillain-Barré syndrome. (Letter.) *J. Infect. Dis.* 165:183 (1992).

538. Gruenewald, R., A.H. Ropper, H. Lior, et al. Serologic evidence of *Campylobacter jejuni/coli* enteritis in patients with Guillain-Barré syndrome. *Arch. Neurol.* 48:1080–1082 (1991).

539. Denton, K.J., and T. Clarke. Role of *Campylobacter jejuni* as a placental pathogen. *J. Clin. Pathol.* 45:171–172 (1992).

540. Gurgan, T., and K.S. Diker. *In vitro* survival of campylobacters in human amniotic fluid. *Lett. Appl. Microbiol.* 14:140–142 (1992).

541. Park, C.E., and G.W. Sanders. Occurrence of thermotolerant campylobacters in fresh vegetables sold at farmers' outdoor markets and supermarkets. *Can. J. Microbiol.* 38:313–316 (1992).

542. Simango, C., and G. Rukure. Survival of *Campylobacter jejuni* and pathogenic *Escherichia coli* in *mahewu*, a fermented cereal gruel. *Trans. Roy. Soc. Trop. Med. Hyg.* 85:399–400 (1991).

543. Fox, J.G. *Campylobacter* infections and salmonellosis. *Sem. Vet. Med. Surg. (Small Anim.)* 6:212–218 (1991).

544. Chattopadhyay, U.K., R.S. Rathore, M.S. Das, et al. Poultry as a reservoir and source of human campylobacteriosis. *Indian Vet. J.* 68:911–914 (1991).

545. Chen, Y., M.J. Woodburn, and M.W. Kelsey. Microbial and sensory quality of refrigerated market fryers. *J. Food Protect.* 54:704–710 (1991).

546. Castillo-Ayala, A. Comparison of selective enrichment broths for isolation of *Campylobacter jejuni/coli* from freshly deboned market chicken. *J. Food Protect.* 55:333–336 (1992).

547. Berndtson, E., M. Tivemo, and A. Engvall. Distribution and numbers of *Campylobacter* in newly slaughtered broiler chickens and hens. *Int. J. Food Microbiol.* 15:45–50 (1992).

548. Boukraa, L., S. Messier, and Y. Robinson. Isolation of *Campylobacter* from livers of broiler chickens with and without necrotic hepatitis lesions. *Avian Dis.* 35:714–717 (1991).

549. Cudjoe, K.S., and G. Kapperud. The effect of lactic acid sprays on *Campylobacter jejuni* inoculated onto poultry carcasses. *Acta Vet. Scand.* 32:491–498 (1991).

550. Schoeni, J.L., and M.P. Doyle. Reduction of *Campylobacter jejuni* colonization of chicks by cecum-colonizing bacteria producing anti-*C. jejuni* metabolites. *Appl. Environ. Microbiol.* 58:664–670 (1992).

551. Kiehlbauch, J.A., C.N. Baker, and I.K. Wachsmuth. In vitro susceptibilities of aerotolerant *Campylobacter* isolates to 22 antimicrobial agents. *Antimicrob. Agents Chemother.* 36:717–722 (1992).

552. Rautelin, H., O.-V. Renkonen, and T.U. Kosunen. Emergence of fluoroquinolone resistance in *Campylobacter jejuni* and *Campylobacter coli* in subjects from Finland. *Antimicrob. Agents Chemother.* 35:2065–2069 (1991).

553. Adler-Mosca, H., and M. Altwegg. Fluoroquinolone resistance in *Campylobacter jejuni* and *Campylobacter coli* isolated from human faeces in Switzerland. (Letter.) *J. Infect.* 23:341–342 (1991).

554. Rao, G.G. Development of spontaneous resistance to ciprofloxacin in a strain of *Campylobacter jejuni*. (Letter.) *J. Antimicrob. Chemother.* 28:317–318 (1991).

555. Ansary, A., and S. Radyu. Conjugal transfer of antibiotic resistances and plasmids from *Campylobacter jejuni* clinical isolates. *FEMS Microbiol. Lett.* 91:125–128 (1992).

556. Kist, M. Isolierung und Identifizierung von Bakterien der Gattungen *Campylobacter* und *Helicobacter*. *Zbl. Bakteriol.* 276:124–139 (1991).

557. Höller, C. A note on the comparative efficacy of three selective media for isolation of *Campylobacter* species from environmental samples. *Zbl. Hyg.* 192:116–123 (1991).

558. Burnens, A.P., and J. Nicolet. Detection of *Campylobacter upsaliensis* in diarrheic dogs and cats, using a selective medium with cefoperazone. *Am. J. Vet. Res.* 53:48–51 (1992).

559. Goossens, H., and J.-P. Butzler. Isolation of *Campylobacter* spp. from stool specimens with a semisolid medium. (Letter.) *J. Clin. Microbiol.* 29:2681 (1991).

560. Endtz, H.P., and R.P. Mouton. Isolation of *Campylobacter* spp. from stool specimens with a semisolid medium. (Reply.) *J. Clin. Microbiol.* 29:2681–2682 (1991).

561. Uroic-Popovic, T., and N. Sterk-Kuzmanovic. Comparison of two simple microaerobic atmospheres for cultivation of thermophilic campylobacters. *J. Clin. Pathol.* 45:87–88 (1992).

562. Ram, S., S. Khurana, R.P. Singh, and S.B. Khurana. Assessment of the modified internal gas generator system for isolation of *Campylobacter*. *Indian J. Med. Res. [A]* 95:26–30 (1992).

563. On, S.L.W., and B. Holmes. Reproducibility of tolerance tests that are useful in the identification of campylobacteria. *J. Clin. Microbiol.* 29:1785–1788 (1991).

564. On, S.L.W., and B. Holmes. Assessment of enzyme detection tests useful in identification of campylobacteria. *J. Clin. Microbiol.* 30:746–749 (1992).

565. Hazeleger, W.C., R.R. Beumer, and F.M. Rombouts. The use of latex agglutination tests for determining *Campylobacter* species. *Lett. Appl. Microbiol.* 14:181–184 (1992).

566. Hernandez, J., R.J. Owen, and A. Fayos. Biotypes and DNA ribopatterns of thermophilic campylobacters from faeces and seawater in Eastern Spain. *Lett. Appl. Microbiol.* 13:207–211 (1991).

567. Wesley, I.V., R.D. Wesley, M. Cardella, et al. Oligodeoxynucleotide probes for *Campylobacter fetus* and *Campylobacter hyointestinalis* based on 16S rRNA sequences. *J. Clin. Microbiol.* 29:1812–1817 (1991).

568. Fraser, A.D.E., B.W. Brooks, M.M. Garcia, and H. Lior. Molecular discrimination of *Campylobacter coli* serogroup 20 biotype I (Lior) strains. *Vet. Microbiol.* 30:267–280 (1992).

569. Wu, S.-J.L., N.D. Pacheco, J.J. Oprandy, and F.M. Rollwagen. Identification of *Campylobacter jejuni* and *Campylobacter coli* antigens with mucosal and systemic antibodies. *Infect. Immun.* 59:2555–2559 (1991).

570. Mills, S.D., R.V. Congi, J.N. Hennessy, and J.L. Penner. Evaluation of a simplified procedure for serotyping *Campylobacter jejuni* and *Campylobacter coli*. *J. Clin. Microbiol.* 29:2093–2098 (1991).

571. Mills, S.D., B. Kuzniar, B. Shames, et al. Variation of the O antigen of *Campylobacter jejuni* in vivo. *J. Med. Microbiol.* 36:215–219 (1992).

572. Jones, D.M., E.M. Sutcliffe, and A. Curry. Recovery of viable but non-culturable *Campylobacter jejuni*. *J. Gen. Microbiol.* 137:2477–2482 (1991).

573. Beumer, R.R., J. de Vries, and F.M. Rombouts. *Campylobacter jejuni* non-culturable coccoid cells. *Int. J. Food Microbiol.* 15:153–163 (1992).

574. Saha, S.K., S. Saha, and S.C. Sanyal. Recovery of injured *Campylobacter jejuni* cells after animal passage. *Appl. Environ. Microbiol.* 57:3388–3389 (1991).

575. Meinersmann, R.J., W.E. Rigsby, N.J. Stern, et al. Comparative study of colonizing and noncolonizing *Campylobacter jejuni*. *Am. J. Vet. Res.* 52:1518–1522 (1991).

576. McFarland, B.A., and S.D. Neill. Profiles of toxin production by thermophilic *Campylobacter* of animal origin. *Vet. Microbiol.* 30:257–266 (1992).

577. Fendri, C., A. Rosenau, E.N. Moyen, and J.L. Fauchère. Prevalence of virulence markers of enteric *Campylobacter* in France and Tunisia. *Res. Microbiol.* 142:591–596 (1991).

578. Pavlovskis, O.R., D.M. Rollins, R.L. Haberberger, Jr., et al. Significance of flagella in colonization resistance of rabbits immunized with *Campylobacter* spp. *Infect. Immun.* 59:2259–2264 (1991).

579. Wassenaar, T.M., N.M.C. Bleumink-Pluym, and B.A.M. van der Zeijst. Inactivation of *Campylobacter jejuni* flagellin genes by homologous recombination demonstrates that *flaA* but not *flaB* is required for invasion. *EMBO J.* 10:2055–2061 (1991).

580. Khawaja, R., K. Neote, H.L. Bingham, et al. Cloning and sequence analysis of the flagellin gene of *Campylobacter jejuni* TGH9011. *Curr. Microbiol.* 24:213–221 (1992).

581. Farber, J.M., and P.I. Peterkin. *Listeria monocytogenes*, a food-borne pathogen. *Microbiol. Rev.* 55:476–511 (1991).

582. Farber, J.M. *Listeria monocytogenes*. *J. Assoc. Off. Anal. Chem.* 74:701–704 (1991).

583. *Listeria monocytogenes* Working Group. *Listeria monocytogenes:* recommendations by the National Advisory Committee on Microbiological Criteria for Foods. *Int. J. Food Microbiol.* 14:185–246 (1991).

584. Doyle, M.P. Should regulatory agencies reconsider the policy of zero-tolerance of *Listeria monocytogenes* in all ready-to-eat foods? *Food Safety Notebook* 2:98–91 (1991).

585. Schlech, W.F. III. Expanding the horizons of foodborne listeriosis. (Editorial.) *JAMA* 267:2081–2082 (1992).

586. Centers for Disease Control. Update: foodborne listeriosis—United States, 1988–1990. *Morbid. Mortal. Weekly Rep.* 41:251,257 (1992).

587. Schuchat, A., K.A. Deaver, J.D. Wenger, et al. Role of foods in sporadic listeriosis. I. Case–control study of dietary risk factors. *JAMA* 267:2041–2045 (1992).

588. Pinner, R.W., A. Schuchat, B. Swaminathan, et al. Role of foods in sporadic listeriosis. II. Microbiologic and epidemiologic investigation. *JAMA* 267:2046–2050 (1992).

589. McLauchlin, J., S.M. Hall, S.K. Velani, and R.J. Gilbert. Human listeriosis and paté: a possible association. *Br. Med. J.* 303:773–775 (1991).

590. Frederiksen, B., and S. Samuelsson. Fetomaternal listeriosis in Denmark 1981–1988. *J. Infect.* 24:277–287 (1992).

591. Cherubin, C.E., M.D. Appleman, P.N.R. Heseltine, et al. Epidemiological spectrum and current treatment of listeriosis. *Rev. Infect. Dis.* 13:1108–1114 (1991).

592. Lorber, B. Listeriosis following shigellosis. *Rev. Infect. Dis.* 13:865–866 (1991).

593. Skogberg, K., J. Syrjänen, M. Jahkola, et al. Clinical presentation and outcome of listeriosis in patients with and without immunosuppressive therapy. *Clin. Infect. Dis.* 14:815–821 (1992).

594. Yonekura, K., T. Kawakita, Y. Saito, et al. Augmentation of host resistance to *Listeria monocytogenes* infection by a traditional Chinese medicine, ren-shen-yang-rong-tang (Japanese name: ninjin-youei-to). *Immunopharmacol. Immunotoxicol.* 14:154–190 (1992).

595. McLauchlin, J., A. Audurier, and A.G. Taylor. Treatment failure and recurrent human listeriosis. *J. Antimicrob. Chemother.* 27:851–857 (1991).

596. Gauto, A.R., L.A. Cone, D.R. Woodard, et al. Arterial infections due to *Listeria monocytogenes:* report of four cases and review of world literature. *Clin. Infect. Dis.* 14:23–28 (1992).

597. Swartz, M.A., D.F. Welch, R.P. Narayanan, and R.A. Greenfield. Catalase-negative *Listeria monocytogenes* causing meningitis in an adult. *Am. J. Clin. Pathol.* 96:130–133 (1991).

598. Mascola, L., F. Sorvillo, N. Lashley, and E. Steinberg. Fatal listeria meningitis in an immunocompromised infant: therapeutic implications. *J. Infect.* 23:287–291 (1991).

599. France, A.J., V.M. Maclean, G. Phillips, and R.A. Seaton. Listeria meningitis and HIV infection. (Letter.) *J. Infect.* 24:217–218 (1992).

600. Baxter, P., D. Gardner-Medwin, D. Bates, et al. Encephalomyelitis with seroconversion to *Listeria monocytogenes. Arch. Dis. Child.* 66:1080–1081 (1991).

601. Brown, P.H., C.W. Ingram, and C. van der Horst. Brain abscess caused by *Listeria monocytogenes.* (Letter.) *Rev. Infect. Dis.* 13:768–769 (1991).

602. Mazzulli, T., and I.E. Salit. Pleural fluid infection caused by *Listeria monocytogenes:* case report and review. *Rev. Infect. Dis.* 13:564–570 (1991).

603. Hirschhorn, L.R., K. McIntosh, K.G. Anderson, and T.S. Dermody. Pneumonia due to *Listeria monocytogenes.* (Letter.) *Clin. Infect. Dis.* 14:787–789 (1992).

604. Facinelli, B., E. Giovanetti, P.E. Varaldo, et al. Antibiotic resistance in foodborne listeria. (Letter.) *Lancet* 338:1272 (1991).

605. Poyart-Salmeron, C., P. Trieu-Cuot, C. Carlier, et al. Genetic basis of tetracycline resistance in clinical isolates of *Listeria monocytogenes. Antimicrob. Agents Chemother.* 36:463–466 (1992).

606. Varabioff, Y. Incidence of *Listeria* in smallgoods. *Lett. Appl. Microbiol.* 14:167–169 (1992).

607. Trott, D., P. Seneviratna, and J. Robertson. *Listeria* in cooked chicken, paté and mixed smallgoods. *Aust. Vet. J.* 68:249–250 (1991).

608. Morris, I.J., and C.D. Ribeiro. The occurrence of *Listeria* species in pâté: the Cardiff experience 1989. *Epidemiol. Infect.* 107:111–117 (1991).

609. Mangold, S., E. Weise, and G. Hildebrandt. Zum Vorkommen von Listerien in Tiefkühlkost. *Arch. Lebensmittelhyg.* 42:121–124 (1991).

610. Gifford, H., K. Lorenz, and J. Sofos. Analysis of bakery products for presence of *Listeria monocytogenes. Lebensm. Wiss. Technol.* 24:476–477 (1991).

611. Weber, A., and H. Burow. Zum vorkommen von Listerien in Hühnereiern des Handels. *Arch. Lebensmittelhyg.* 42:72–73 (1991).

612. Wang, G.-H., K.-T. Yan, X.-M. Feng, et al. Isolation and identification of *Listeria monocytogenes* from retail meats in Beijing. *J. Food Protect.* 55:56–58 (1992).

613. Grau, F.H., and P.B. Vanderlinde. Occurrence, numbers, and growth of *Listeria monocytogenes* on some vacuum-packaged processed meats. *J. Food Protect.* 55:4–7 (1992).

614. Farber, J.M. *Listeria monocytogenes* in fish products. *J. Food Protect.* 54:922–924 (1991).

615. Genigeorgis, C., J.H. Toledo, and F.J. Garayzabal. Selected microbiological and chemical characteristics of illegally produced and marketed soft Hispanic-style cheeses in California. *J. Food Protect.* 54:598–601 (1991).

616. Neumann, H.-H., H. Konermann, and E.H. Abdel-Hakiem. Zum vorkommen von *Listeria*-Arten und *Listeria*-Serovaren in Käse. *Arch. Lebensmittelhyg.* 42:90–92 (1991).

617. Harvey, J., and A. Gilmour. Occurrence of *Listeria* species in raw milk and dairy products produced in Northern Ireland. *J. Appl. Bacteriol.* 72:119–125 (1992).

618. Pociecha, J.Z., K.R. Smith, and G.J. Manderson. Incidence of *Listeria monocytogenes* in meat production environments of a South Island (New Zealand) mutton slaughterhouse. *Int. J. Food Microbiol.* 13:321–328 (1991).

619. Schullerus, F.R., and H. Stöppler. Listerienbelastung bei Lebensmitteln tierischen Ursprungs unter besonderer Berücksichtigung von Umgebungsuntersuchungen. *Tierärztl. Umschau* 47:27–36 (1992).

620. Van Renterghem, B., F. Huysman, R. Rygole, and W. Verstraete. Detection and prevalence of *Listeria monocytogenes* in the agricultural ecosystem. *J. Appl. Bacteriol.* 71:211–217 (1991).

621. Iida, T., M. Kanzaki, T. Maruyama, et al. Prevalence of *Listeria monocytogenes* in intestinal contents of healthy animals in Japan. *J. Vet. Med. Sci.* 53:873–875 (1991).

622. Spurlock, A., and E.A. Zottola. Growth and attachment of *Listeria monocytogenes* to cast iron. *J. Food Protect.* 54:925–929 (1991).

623. Mafu, A.A., D. Roy, J. Golet, and L. Savoie. Characterization of physicochemical forces involved in adhesion of *Listeria monocytogenes* to surfaces. *Appl. Environ. Microbiol.* 57:1969–1973 (1991).

624. Krysinski, E.P., L.J. Brown, and T.J. Marchisello. Effect of cleaners and sanitizers on *Listeria monocytogenes* attached to product contact surfaces. *J. Food Protect.* 55:246–251 (1992).

625. Spurlock, A.T., and E.A. Zottola. The survival of *Listeria monocytogenes* in aerosols. *J. Food Protect.* 54:910–912 (1991).

626. Linton, R.H., J.B. Webster, M.D. Pierson, et al. The effect of sublethal heat shock and growth atmosphere on the heat resistance of *Listeria monocytogenes* Scott A. *J. Food Protect.* 55:84–87 (1992).

627. de Daza, M.S.T., Y. Villegas, and A. Martinez. Minimal water activity for growth of *Listeria monocytogenes* as affected by solute and temperature. *Int. J. Food Microbiol.* 14:333–337 (1991).

628. Saguy, I. Simulated growth of *Listeria monocytogenes* in refrigerated foods stored at variable temperatures. *Food Technol.* 46(3):69–71 (1992).

629. Kroll, R.G., and R.A. Patchett. Induced acid tolerance in *Listeria monocytogenes. Lett. Appl. Microbiol.* 14:224–227 (1992).

630. Brackett, R.E., and L.R. Beuchat. Survival of *Listeria monocytogenes* in whole egg and egg yolk powders and in liquid whole eggs. *Food Microbiol.* 8:331–337 (1991).

631. Ashenafi, M. Growth of *Listeria monocytogenes* in fermenting tempeh made of various beans and its inhibition by *Lactobacillus plantarum. Food Microbiol.* 8:303–310 (1991).

632. Rørvik, L.M., M. Yndestad, and E. Skjerve. Growth of *Listeria monocytogenes* in vacuum-packed, smoked salmon, during storage at 4°C. *Int. J. Food Microbiol.* 14:111–118 (1991).

633. Harrison, M.A., Y.-W. Huang, C.-H. Chao, and T. Shineman. Fate of *Listeria monocytogenes* on packaged, refrigerated, and frozen seafood. *J. Food Protect.* 54:524–527 (1991).

634. Marshall, D.L., P.L. Wiese-Lehigh, J.H. Wells, and A.J. Farr. Comparative growth of *Listeria monocytogenes* and *Pseudomonas fluorescens* on precooked chicken nuggets stored under modified atmospheres. *J. Food Protect.* 54:841–843,851 (1991).

635. Ingham, S.C., and C.L. Tautorus. Survival of *Salmonella typhimurium, Listeria monocytogenes* and indicator bacteria on cooked uncured turkey loaf stored under vacuum at 3°C. *J. Food Safety* 11:285–292 (1991).

636. Sabel, D., A.E. Yousef, and E.H. Marth. Behavior of *Listeria monocytogenes* during fermentation of beaker sausage made with or without a starter culture and antioxidant food additives. *Lebensm. Wiss. Technol.* 24:252–255 (1991).

637. Massa, S., L.D. Trovatelli, and F. Canganella. Survival of *Listeria monocytogenes* in yogurt during storage at 4°C. *Lett. Appl. Microbiol.* 13:112–114 (1991).

638. El-Gazzar, F.E., H.F. Bohner, and E.H. Marth. Antagonism between *Listeria monocytogenes* and lactococci during fermentation of products from ultrafiltered skim milk. *J. Dairy Sci.* 75:43–50 (1992).

639. Kovincic, I., M. Mrdjen, V. Komnenov-Pupovac, et al. Heat resistance of *Listeria monocytogenes* in naturally infected and inoculated cow's milk. *Acta Microbiol. Hungar.* 38:3–6 (1991).

640. Farrag, S.A., and E.H. Marth. Behavior of *Listeria monocytogenes* in the presence of flavobacteria in skim milk at 7 or 13°C. *J. Food Protect.* 54:677–680 (1991).

641. Farrag, S.A., and E.H. Marth. Variation in initial population of *Pseudomonas fluorescens* affects behavior of *Listeria monocytogenes* in skim milk at 7 or 13°C. *Milchwissenschaft* 46:718–721 (1991).

642. Marshall, D.L., and R.H. Schmidt. Physiological evaluation of stimulated growth of *Listeria monocytogenes* by *Pseudomonas* species in milk. *Can. J. Microbiol.* 37:594–599 (1991).

643. Genigeorgis, C., M. Carniciu, D. Dutulescu, and T.B. Farver. Growth and survival of *Listeria monocytogenes* in market cheeses stored at 4 to 30°C. *J. Food Protect.* 54:662–668 (1991).

644. Buazzi, M.M., M.E. Johnson, and E.H. Marth. Survival of *Listeria monocytogenes* during the manufacture and ripening of Swiss cheese. *J. Dairy Sci.* 75:380–386 (1992).

645. Buazzi, M.M., M.E. Johnson, and E.H. Marth. Fate of *Listeria monocytogenes* during the manufacture of Mozzarella cheese. *J. Food Protect.* 55:80–83 (1992).

646. Gaya, P., M. Medina, and M. Nuñez. Effect of the lactoperoxidase system on *Listeria monocytogenes* behavior in raw milk at refrigeration temperatures. *Appl. Environ. Microbiol.* 57:3355–3360 (1991).

647. Wakabayashi, H., W. Bellamy, M. Takase, and M. Tomita. Inactivation of *Listeria monocytogenes* by lactoferricin, a potent antimicrobial peptide derived from cow's milk. *J. Food Protect.* 55:238–240 (1992).

648. Harris, L.J., H.P. Fleming, and T.R. Klaenhammer. Sensitivity and resistance of *Listeria monocytogenes* ATCC 19115, Scott A, and UAL500 to nisin. *J. Food Protect.* 54:836–840 (1991).

649. Jung, D.-S., F.W. Bodyfelt, and M.A. Daeschel. Influence of fat and emulsifiers on the efficacy of nisin in inhibiting *Listeria monocytogenes* in fluid milk. *J. Dairy Sci.* 75:387–393 (1992).

650. Sulzer, G., and M. Busse. Growth inhibition of *Listeria* spp. on camembert cheese by bacteria producing inhibitory substances. *Int. J. Food Microbiol.* 14:287–296 (1991).

651. Ozari, R. Untersuchungen zur Wirkung von Starterkulturen des Handels auf das Wachstum von *Listeria monocytogenes* in frischen Mettwürsten. *Fleischwirtschaft* 71:1450–1454 (1991).

652. Motlagh, A.M., S. Holla, M.C. Johnson, et al. Inhibition of *Listeria* spp. in sterile food systems by pediocin AcH, a bacteriocin produced by *Pediococcus acidilactici* H. *J. Food Protect.* 55:337–343 (1992).

653. Foegeding, P.M., A.B. Thomas, D.H. Pilkington, and T.R. Klaenhammer. Enhanced control of *Listeria monocytogenes* by in situ–produced pediocin during dry fermented sausage production. *Appl. Environ. Microbiol.* 58:884–890 (1992).

654. Degnan, A.J., A.E. Yousef, and J.B. Luchansky. Use of *Pediococcus acidilactici* to control *Listeria monocytogenes* in temperature-abused vacuum-packaged wieners. *J. Food Protect.* 55:98–103 (1992).

655. Berry, E.D., R.W. Hutkins, and R.W. Mandigo. The use of bacteriocin-producing *Pediococcus acidilactici* to control postprocessing *Listeria monocytogenes* contamination of frankfurters. *J. Food Protect.* 54:681–686 (1991).

656. Arihara, K., S. Ogihara, J. Sakata, et al. Antimicrobial activity of *Enterococcus faecalis* against *Listeria monocytogenes*. *Lett. Appl. Microbiol.* 13:190–192 (1991).

657. Schillinger, U., M. Kaya, and F.-K. Lücke. Behaviour of *Listeria monocytogenes* in meat and its control by a bacteriocin-producing strain of *Lactobacillus sake*. *J. Appl. Bacteriol.* 70:473–478 (1991).

658. Wang, C., and L.A. Shelef. Factors contributing to antilisterial effects of raw egg albumen. *J. Food Sci.* 56:1251–1254 (1991).

659. Smith, J.L., C. McColgan, and B.S. Marmer. Growth temperature and action of lysozyme on *Listeria monocytogenes*. *J. Food Sci.* 56:1101–1103 (1991).

660. Aureli, P., A. Costantini, and S. Zolea. Antimicrobial activity of some plant essential oils against *Listeria monocytogenes*. *J. Food Protect.* 55:344–348 (1992).

661. Ting, W.T.E., and K.E. Deibel. Sensitivity of *Listeria monocytogenes* to spices at two temperatures. *J. Food Safety* 12:129–137 (1992).

662. Nguyen-the, C., and B.M. Lund. The lethal effect of carrot on *Listeria* species. *J. Appl. Bacteriol.* 70:479–488 (1991).

663. Zeitoun, A.A.M., and J.M. Debevere. Inhibition, survival, and growth of *Listeria monocytogenes* on poultry as influenced by buffered lactic acid treatment and modified atmosphere packaging. *Int. J. Food Microbiol.* 14:161–170 (1991).

664. El-Shenawy, M.A., and E.H. Marth. Behavior of *Listeria monocytogenes* in the presence of sodium propionate together with food acids. *J. Food Protect.* 55:241–245 (1992).

665. Buazzi, M.M., and E.H. Marth. Sites of action by propionate on *Listeria monocytogenes*. *Int. J. Food Microbiol.* 15:109–119 (1992).

666. Wang, L.-L., and E.A. Johnson. Inhibition of *Listeria monocytogenes* by fatty acids and monoglycerides. *Appl. Environ. Microbiol.* 58:624–629 (1992).

667. Oh, D.H., and D.L. Marshall. Effect of pH on the minimum inhibitory concentration of monolaurin against *Listeria monocytogenes*. *J. Food Protect.* 55:449–450 (1992).

668. Buazzi, M.M., and E.H. Marth. Characteristics of sodium benzoate injury of *Listeria monocytogenes*. *Microbios* 70:199–207 (1992).

669. Buazzi, M.M., and E.H. Marth. Mechanisms in the inhibition of *Listeria monocytogenes* by potassium sorbate. *Food Microbiol.* 8:249–256 (1991).

670. El-Shenawy, M.A., and E.H. Marth. Organic acids enhance the antilisterial activity of potassium sorbate. *J. Food Protect.* 54:594–597 (1991).

671. McClure, P.J., T.M. Kelly, and T.A. Roberts. The effects of temperature, pH, sodium chloride and

sodium nitrite on the growth of *Listeria monocytogenes*. *Int. J. Food Microbiol.* 14:77–92 (1991).

672. Yen, L.C., J.N. Sofos, and G.R. Schmidt. Thermal destruction of *Listeria monocytogenes* in ground pork with water, sodium chloride and other curing ingredients. *Lebensm. Wiss. Technol.* 25:61–65 (1992).

673. Miller, A.J. Combined water activity and solute effects on growth and survival of *Listeria monocytogenes* Scott A. *J. Food Protect.* 55:414–418 (1992).

674. Hudson, J.A. Efficacy of high sodium chloride concentrations for the destruction of *Listeria monocytogenes. Lett. Microbiol.* 14:178–180 (1992).

675. Krämer, K.-H., and J. Baumgart. Brühwurstaufschnitt. Hemmung von *Listeria monocytogenes* durch eine modifizierte Atmosphäre. *Fleischwirtschaft* 72:666–668 (1992).

676. Budu-Amoako, E., S. Toora, C. Walton, et al. Thermal death times for *Listeria monocytogenes* in lobster meat. *J. Food Protect.* 55:211–213 (1992).

677. Holsinger, V.H., P.W. Smith, J.L. Smith, and S.A. Palumbo. Thermal destruction of *Listeria monocytogenes* in ice cream mix. *J. Food Protect.* 55:234–237 (1992).

678. Fain, A.R., Jr., J.E. Line, A.B. Moran, et al. Lethality of heat to *Listeria monocytogenes* Scott A: *D*-value and *Z*-value determinations in ground beef and turkey. *J. Food Protect.* 54:756–761 (1991).

679. Hollywood, N.W., Y. Varabioff, and G.E. Mitchell. The effect of microwave and conventional cooking on the temperature profiles and microbial flora of minced beef. *Int. J. Food Microbiol.* 14:67–76 (1991).

680. Coote, P.J., C.D. Holyoak and M.B. Cole. Thermal inactivation of *Listeria monocytogenes* during a process simulating temperatures achieved during microwave heating. *J. Appl. Bacteriol.* 70:489–494 (1991).

681. Foegeding, P.M., and N.W. Stanley. *Listeria innocua* transformed with an antibiotic resistance plasmid as a thermal-resistance indicator for *Listeria monocytogenes. J. Food Protect.* 54:519–523 (1991).

682. Varabioff, Y., G.E. Mitchell, and S.M. Nottingham. Effects of irradiation on bacterial load and *Listeria monocytogenes* in raw chicken. *J. Food Protect.* 55:389–391 (1992).

683. Kerr, K.G., and R.W. Lacey. Isolation and identification of *Listeria monocytogenes. J. Clin. Pathol.* 44:624–627 (1991).

684. Slade, P.J. Monitoring *Listeria* in the food production environment. I. Detection of *Listeria* in processing plants and isolation methodology. *Food Res. Int.* 25:45–56 (1992).

685. Hayes, P.S., L.M. Graves, G.W. Ajello, et al. Comparison of cold enrichment and U.S. Department of Agriculture methods for isolating *Listeria monocytogenes* from naturally contaminated foods. *Appl. Environ. Microbiol.* 57:2109–2113 (1991).

686. Warburton, D.W., J.M. Farber, A. Armstrong, et al. A Canadian comparative study of modified versions of the "FDA" and "USDA" methods for the detection of *Listeria monocytogenes. J. Food Protect.* 54:669–676 (1991).

687. Westöö, A., and M. Peterz. Evaluation of methods for detection of *Listeria monocytogenes* in foods: NMKL collaborative study. *J. AOAC Int.* 75:46–52 (1992).

688. Lund, A.M., E.A. Zottola, and D.J. Pusch. Comparison of methods for isolation of *Listeria* from raw milk. *J. Food Protect.* 54:602–606 (1991).

689. Art, D., and P. Andre. Comparison of three selective isolation media for the detection of *L. monocytogenes* in foods. *Zbl. Bakteriol.* 275:79–84 (1991).

690. Rollier, I., Th. Croegaert, A. Verplaetse, and J. van Hoof. Comparison of three plating media for enumeration and three media for isolation of *Listeria* spp. in fermented sausages. *Arch. Lebensmittelhyg.* 42:65–69 (1991).

691. Kerr, K.G., N.A. Rotowa, P.M. Hawkey, and R.W. Lacey. Evaluation of the Rosco system for the identification of *Listeria* species. *J. Med. Microbiol.* 35:193–196 (1991).

692. Robison, B.J., and C.P. Cunningham. Accuracy of Micro-ID® Listeria for identification of members of the genus *Listeria. J. Food Protect.* 54:798–800 (1991).

693. in 't Veld, P.H., and E. de Boer. Recovery of *Listeria monocytogenes* on selective agar media in a collaborative study using reference samples. *Int. J. Food Microbiol.* 13:295–300 (1991).

694. Busch, S.V., and C.W. Donnelly. Development of a repair-enrichment broth for resuscitation of heat-injured *Listeria monocytogenes* and *Listeria innocua. Appl. Environ. Microbiol.* 58:14–20 (1992).

695. Premaratne, R.J., W.-J. Lin, and E.A. Johnson. Development of an improved chemically defined

minimal medium for *Listeria monocytogenes. Appl. Environ. Microbiol.* 57:3046–3048 (1991).

696. Razavilar, V., and C. Genigeorgis. Interactive effect of temperature, atmosphere and storage time on the probability of colony formation on blood agar by four *Listeria* species. *J. Food Protect.* 55:88–92 (1992).

697. Dallas, H.L., T.T. Tran, C.E. Poindexter, and A.D. Hitchins. Competition of food bacteria with *Listeria monocytogenes* during enrichment culture. *J. Food Safety* 11:293–301 (1991).

698. Fernandez-Garayzabal, J.F., C. Delgado, M. Blanco, et al. Role of potassium tellurite and brain heart infusion in expression of the hemolytic phenotype of *Listeria* spp. on agar plates. *Appl. Environ. Microbiol.* 58:434–438 (1992).

699. Notermans, S.H.W., J. Dufrenne, M. Leimeister-Wächter, et al. Phosphatidylinositol-specific phospholipase C activity as a marker to distinguish between pathogenic and nonpathogenic *Listeria* species. *Appl. Environ. Microbiol.* 57:2666–2670 (1991).

700. Yu, L.S.L., and D.Y.C. Fung. Oxyrase enzyme and motility enrichment Fung-Yu tube for rapid detection of *Listeria monocytogenes* and *Listeria* species. *J. Food Safety* 11:149–162 (1991).

701. Yu, L.S.L., and D.Y.C. Fung. Effect of Oxyrase enzyme on *Listeria monocytogenes* and other facultative anaerobes. *J. Food Safety* 11:163–175 (1991).

702. Yu, L.S.L., and D.Y.C. Fung. Comparisons of selected methods with the Fung-Yu tube procedure for determining *Listeria monocytogenes* and other *Listeria* spp. in meats. *J. Food Protect.* 55:349–355 (1992).

703. Kämpfer, P. Differentiation of *Corynebacterium* spp., *Listeria* spp., and related organisms by using fluorogenic substrates. *J. Clin. Microbiol.* 30:1067–1071 (1992).

704. Sheridan, J.J., I. Walls, J. McLauchlin, et al. Use of a microcolony technique combined with an indirect immunofluorescence test for the rapid detection of *Listeria* in raw meat. *Lett. Appl. Microbiol.* 13:140–144 (1991).

705. Oladepo, D.K., A.A.G. Candlish, and W.H. Stimson. Detection of *Listeria monocytogenes* using polyclonal antibody. *Lett. Appl. Microbiol.* 14:26–29 (1992).

706. Gavalchin, J., M.L. Tortorello, R. Malek, et al. Isolation of monoclonal antibodies that react preferen-

tially with *Listeria monocytogenes. Food Microbiol.* 8:325–330 (1991).

707. Bhunia, A.K., P.H. Ball, A.T. Fuad, et al. Development and characterization of a monoclonal antibody specific for *Listeria monocytogenes* and *Listeria innocua. Infect. Immun.* 59:3176–3184 (1991).

708. Skjerve, E., W. Bos, and B. van der Gaag. Evaluation of monoclonal antibodies to *Listeria monocytogenes* flagella by checkerboard ELISA and cluster analysis. *J. Immunol. Meth.* 144:11–17 (1991).

709. Comi, G., M. Valenti, M. Civilini, et al. Evaluation of an enzymatic method for fast identification of *Listeria* spp. in cheese and meat products. *Zbl. Hyg.* 192:134–145 (1991).

710. Nørrung, B., M. Sølve, M. Ovesen, and N. Skovgaard. Evaluation of an ELISA test for detection of *Listeria* spp. *J. Food Protect.* 54:752–755,761 (1991).

711. Noah, C.W., N.C. Ramos, and M.V. Gipson. Efficiency of two commercial ELISA kits compared with the BAM culture method for detecting *Listeria* in naturally contaminated foods. *J. Assoc. Off. Anal. Chem.* 74:819–821 (1991).

712. McKee, R.A., C.M. Gooding, S.D. Garrett, et al. DNA probes and the detection of food-borne pathogens using the polymerase chain reaction. *Biochem. Soc. Trans.* 19:698–701 (1991).

713. Niederhauser, C., U. Candrian, C. Höfelein, et al. Use of polymerase c chain reaction for detection of *Listeria monocytogenes* in food. *Appl. Environ. Microbiol.* 58:1564–1568 (1992).

714. Rossen, L., K. Holmstrøm, J.E. Olsen, and O.F. Rasmussen. A rapid polymerase chain reaction (PCR)-based assay for the identification of *Listeria monocytogenes* in food samples. *Int. J. Food Microbiol.* 14:145–152 (1991).

715. Bohnert, M., F. Dilasser, C. Dalet, et al. Use of specific oligonucleotides for direct enumeration of *Listeria monocytogenes* in food samples by colony hybridization and rapid detection by PCR. *Res. Microbiol.* 143:271–280 (1992).

716. Golsteyn Thomas, E.J., R.K. King, J. Burchak, and V.P.J. Gannon. Sensitive and specific detection of *Listeria monocytogenes* in milk and ground beef with the polymerase chain reaction. *Appl. Environ. Microbiol.* 57:2576–2580 (1991).

717. Johnson, W.M., S.D. Tyler, E.P. Ewan, et al. Detection of genes coding for listeriolysin and *Listeria*

monocytogenes antigen A (lmaA) in *Listeria* spp. by the polymerase chain reaction. *Microb. Pathogen.* 12:79–86 (1992).

718. Wang, R.-F., W.-W. Cao, and M.G. Johnson. Development of cell surface protein associated gene probe specific for *Listeria monocytogenes* and detection of the bacteria in food by PCR. *Mol. Cell. Probes* 6:119–129 (1992).

719. Howard, P.J., K.D. Harsono, and J.B. Luchansky. Differentiation of *Listeria monocytogenes, Listeria innocua, Listeria ivanovii,* and *Listeria seeligeri* by pulsed-field gel electrophoresis. *Appl. Environ. Microbiol.* 58:709–712 (1992).

720. Buchrieser, C., R. Brosch, and J. Rocourt. Use of pulsed field gel electrophoresis to compare large DNA-restriction fragments of *Listeria monocytogenes* strains belonging to serogroups 1/2 and 3. *Int. J. Food Microbiol.* 14:297–304 (1991).

721. Brosch, R. C. Buchrieser, and J. Rocourt. Subtyping of *Listeria monocytogenes* serovar 4b by use of low-frequency-cleavage restriction endonucleases and pulsed-field gel electrophoresis. *Res. Microbiol.* 142:667–675 (1991).

722. Carriere, C., A. Allardet-Servent, G. Bourg, et al. DNA polymorphism in strains of *Listeria monocytogenes. J. Clin. Microbiol.* 29:1351–1355 (1991).

723. Rasmussen, O.F., T. Beck, J.E. Olsen, et al. *Listeria monocytogenes* isolates can be classified into two major types according to the sequence of the listeriolysin gene. *Infect. Immun.* 59:3945–3951 (1991).

724. Baloga, A.O., and S.K. Harlander. Comparison of methods for discrimination between strains of *Listeria monocytogenes* from epidemiological surveys. *Appl. Environ. Microbiol.* 57:2324–2331 (1991).

725. Wang, R.-F., W.-W. Cao, and M.G. Johnson. Dried gel hybridization in place of Southern hybridization for detection of *Listeria monocytogenes* DNA fragments. *Lett. Appl. Microbiol.* 12:224–227 (1991).

726. Mohamood, A., A.R. Datta, and B.E. Eribo. Application of a synthetic listeriolysin O gene probe to the identification of β-hemolytic *Listeria monocytogenes* in retail ground beef. *J. Food Protect.* 55:385–388 (1992).

727. Kim, C., B. Swaminathan, P.K. Cassaday, et al. Rapid confirmation of *Listeria monocytogenes* isolated from foods by a colony blot assay using a digoxigenin-labeled synthetic oligonucleotide probe. *Appl. Environ. Microbiol.* 57:1609–1614 (1991).

728. Wernars, K., K. Heuvelman, S. Notermans, et al. Suitability of the *prfA* gene, which encodes a regulator of virulence genes in *Listeria monocytogenes,* in the identification of pathogenic *Listeria* spp. *Appl. Environ. Microbiol.* 58:765–768 (1992).

729. Okwumabua, O., B. Swaminathan, P. Edmonds, et al. Evaluation of a chemiluminescent DNA probe assay for the rapid confirmation of *Listeria monocytogenes. Res. Microbiol.* 143:183–189 (1992).

730. Wang, R.-F., W.-W. Cao, and M.G. Johnson. Development of a 16S rRNA-based oligomer probe specific for *Listeria monocytogenes. Appl. Environ. Microbiol.* 57:3666–3670 (1991).

731. Jaquet, C., S. Aubert, N. El Solh, and J. Rocourt. Use of rRNA gene restriction patterns for the identification of *Listeria* species. *Syst. Appl. Microbiol.* 15:42–46 (1992).

732. Jacquet, Ch., J. Bille, and J. Rocourt. Typing of *Listeria monocytogenes* by restriction polymorphism of the ribosomal ribonucleic acid gene region. *Zbl. Bakteriol.* 276:356–365 (1992).

733. Boerlin, P., and J.-C. Piffaretti. Typing of human, animal, food, and environmental isolates of *Listeria monocytogenes* by multilocus enzyme electrophoresis. *Appl. Environ. Microbiol.* 57:1624–1629 (1991).

734. Nørrung, B. Characterisation of Danish isolates of *Listeria monocytogenes* by multilocus enzyme electrophoresis. *Int. J. Food Microbiol.* 15:51–59 (1992).

735. Vines, A., M.W. Reeves, S. Hunter, and B. Swaminathan. Restriction fragment length polymorphism in four virulence-associated genes of *Listeria monocytogenes. Res. Microbiol.* 143:281–294 (1992).

736. Ninet, B., H. Traitler, J.-M. Aeschlimann, et al. Quantitative analysis of cellular fatty acids (CFAs) composition of the seven species of *Listeria. Syst. Appl. Microbiol.* 15:76–78 (1992).

737. Peterkin, P.I., M.-A. Gardiner, and N. Malik. Plasmids in *Listeria monocytogenes* and other *Listeria* species. *Can. J. Microbiol.* 38:161–164 (1992).

738. Estela, L.A., J.N. Sofos, and B.B. Flores. Bacteriophage typing of *Listeria monocytogenes* cultures isolated from foods. *J. Food Protect.* 55:13–17 (1992).

739. Bosgiraud, C., A. Menudier, M.P. Champagnol, et al. Étude épidémiologique de la distribution des espèces de *Listeria* et des sérotypes de *Listeria monocytogenes* en pathologie humaine, animale et dans les aliments. *Rev. Méd. Vét.* 142:463–468 (1991).

740. Farber, J.M., E. Daley, F. Coates, et al. Feeding trials of *Listeria monocytogenes* with a nonhuman primate model. *J. Clin. Microbiol.* 29:2606–2608 (1991).

741. Notermans, S., J. Dufrenne, T. Chakraborty, et al. The chick embryo test agrees with the mouse bioassay for assessment of the pathogenicity of *Listeria* species. *Lett. Appl. Microbiol.* 13:161–164 (1991).

742. Menudier, A., C. Bosiraud, and J.-A. Nicolas. Virulence of *Listeria monocytogenes* serovars and *Listeria* spp. in experimental infection in mice. *J. Food Protect.* 54:917–921 (1991).

743. McCarthy, S.A. Pathogenicity of nonstressed, heat-stressed, and resuscitated *Listeria monocytogenes* 1A1 cells. *Appl. Environ. Microbiol.* 57:2389–2391 (1991).

744. Goebel, W., T. Chakraborty, E. Domann, et al. Studies on the pathogenicity of *Listeria monocytogenes*. *Infection* 19(Suppl. 4):S195–S197 (1991).

745. Portnoy, D.A., T. Chakraborty, W. Goebel, P. Cossart. Molecular determinants of *Listeria monocytogenes* pathogenesis. *Infect. Immun.* 60:1263–1267 (1992).

746. Chakraborty, T., M. Leimeister-Wächter, E. Domann, et al. Coordinate regulation of virulence genes in *Listeria monocytogenes* requires the product of the *prfA* gene. *J. Bacteriol.* 174:568–574 (1992).

747. Mengaud, J., S. Dramsi, E. Gouin, et al. Pleiotropic control of *Listeria monocytogenes* virulence factors by a gene that is autoregulated. *Mol. Microbiol.* 5:2273–2283 (1991).

748. Leimeister-Wächter, M., E. Domann, and T. Chakraborty. The expression of virulence genes in *Listeria monocytogenes* is thermoregulated. *J. Bacteriol.* 174:947–952 (1992).

749. Conlan, J.W., and R.J. North. Roles of *Listeria monocytogenes* virulence factors in survival: virulence factors distinct from listeriolysin are needed for the organism to survive an early neutrophil-mediated host defense mechanism. *Infect. Immun.* 60:951–957 (1992).

750. Barry, R.A., H.G.A. Bouwer, D.A. Portnoy, and D.J. Hinrichs. Pathogenicity and immunogenicity of *Listeria monocytogenes* small-plaque mutants defective for intracellular growth and cell-to-cell spread. *Infect. Immun.* 60:1625–1632 (1992).

751. McKay, D.B., and C.Y. Lu. Listeriolysin as a virulence factor in *Listeria monocytogenes* infection of neonatal mice and murine decidual tissue. *Infect. Immun.* 59:4286–4290 (1991).

752. Wuenscher, M.D., S. Köhler, W. Goebel, and T. Chakraborty. Gene disruption by plasmid integration in *Listeria monocytogenes:* insertional activation of the listeriolysin determinant *lisA*. *Mol. Gen. Genet.* 228:177–182 (1991).

753. Nato, F., K. Reich, S. Lhopital, et al. Production and characterization of neutralizing and non-neutralizing monoclonal antibodies against listeriolysin O. *Infect. Immun.* 59:4641–4646 (1991).

754. Haas, A., M. Dumbsky, and J. Kreft. Listeriolysin genes: complete sequence of *ilo* from *Listeria ivanovii* and of *lso* from *Listeria seeligeri*. *Biochim. Biophys. Acta* 1130:81–84 (1992).

755. Tabouret, M., J. de Rycke, and G. Dubray. Analysis of surface proteins of *Listeria* in relation to species, serovar and pathogenicity. *J. Gen. Microbiol.* 138:743–753 (1992).

756. Benedict, R.C., and F.J. Schultz. An effect of iron level and food type on production of hemolysin and catalase of *Listeria monocytogenes* strain Scott A. *J. Food Protect.* 54:528–531 (1991).

757. Van der Kelen, D., and J.A. Lindsay. Production of a new extracellular cytotoxin from *Listeria monocytogenes* serotype 4b and ATCC 15313 serotype 1/2a in relation to growth stage and growth temperature. *J. Food Protect.* 55:252–255 (1992).

758. Domann, E., J. Wehland, M. Rohde, et al. A novel bacterial virulence gene in *Listeria monocytogenes* required for host cell microfilament interaction with homology to the proline-rich region of vinculin. *EMBO J.* 11:1981–1990 (1992).

759. Geoffroy, C., J. Raveneau, J.-L. Beretti, et al. Purification and characterization of an extracellular 20-kilodalton phospholipase C from *Listeria monocytogenes*. *Infect. Immun.* 59:2382–2388 (1991).

760. Raveneau, J., C. Geoffroy, J.-L. Beretti, et al. Reduced virulence of a *Listeria monocytogenes* phospholipase-deficient mutant obtained by transposon insertion into the zinc metalloprotease gene. *Infect. Immun.* 60:916–921 (1992).

761. Vazquez-Boland, J.-A., C. Kocks, S. Dramsi, et al. Nucleotide sequence of the lecithinase operon of *Listeria monocytogenes* and possible role of lecithinase in cell-to-cell spread. *Infect. Immun.* 60:219–230 (1992).

762. Mahoney, F.J., C.W. Hoge, T.A. Farley, et al. Communitywide outbreak of legionnaires' disease associated with a grocery store mist machine. *J. Infect. Dis.* 165:736–739 (1992).

763. Alary, M., and J.R. Joly. Risk factors for contamination of domestic hot water systems by legionellae. *Appl. Environ. Microbiol.* 57:2360–2367 (1991).

764. Cooper, C.W. Risk factors in transmission of brucellosis from animals to humans in Saudi Arabia. *Trans. Roy. Soc. Trop. Med. Hyg.* 86:206–209 (1992).

765. Lossos, I.S., I. Felsenstein, R. Breuer, and D. Engelhard. Foodborne outbreak of group A β-hemolytic streptococcal pharyngitis. *Arch. Intern. Med.* 154:853–855 (1992).

766. Gallo, G., R. Berzero, N. Cattai, et al. An outbreak of group A food-borne streptococcal pharyngitis. *Eur. J. Epidemiol.* 8:292–297 (1992).

767. Steinkuller, J.S., K. Chan, and S.E. Rinehouse. Prechewing of food by adults and streptococcal pharyngitis in infants. *J. Pediatr.* 120:563–564 (1992).

768. Mäki-Ikola, O., K. Lehtinen, K. Granfors, et al. Bacterial antibodies in ankylosing spondylitis. *Clin. Exp. Immunol.* 84:472–475 (1991).

769. Jalaludin, B., and W. Smith. Blue-green algae (cyanobacteria). (Letter.) *Med. J. Aust.* 156:744 (1992).

770. Long, E.G., E.H. White, W.W. Carmichael, et al. Morphologic and staining characteristics of a cyanobacterium-like organism associated with diarrhea. *J. Infect. Dis.* 164:199–202 (1991).

771. Farrell, G.M., and E.H. Marth. *Borrelia burgdorferi:* another cause of foodborne illness? *Int. J. Food Microbiol.* 14:247–260 (1991).

772. Warner, R.D., R.W. Carr, F.K. McCleskey, et al. A large nontypical outbreak of Norwalk virus. Gastroenteritis associated with exposing celery to nonpotable water and with *Citrobacter freundii. Arch. Intern. Med.* 151:2419–2424 (1991).

773. Alouf, J.E., and J.H. Freer (eds.). *Sourcebook of Bacterial Protein Toxins.* San Diego, Academic Press (1991).

774. Lucas, F., and G. Corthier. Les récepteurs aux entérotoxines bactériennes. *Ann. Rech. Vét.* 22:127–145 (1991).

775. Lucas, F., M. Popoff, and G. Corthier. Les entérotoxines bactériennes: structure, mode d'action. *Ann. Rech. Vét.* 22:147–162 (1991).

776. Sato, M.I.Z., C.K. Monteiro, N.C. Stoppe, et al. Shellfish and marine water microbiological quality. *Environ. Toxicol. Water Qual.* 7:95–105 (1992).

777. Martinez-Manzanares, E., F. Egea, D. Castro, et al. Accumulation and depuration of pathogenic and indicator microorganisms by the bivalve mollusc, *Chamelea gallina* L, under controlled laboratory conditions. *J. Food Protect.* 54:612–618 (1991).

778. Leung, C.-K., Y.-W. Huang, and O.C. Pancorbo. Bacterial pathogens and indicators in catfish and pond environments. *J. Food Protect.* 55:424–427 (1992).

779. Dodds, K.L., M.H. Brodsky, and D.W. Warburton. A retail survey of smoked ready-to-eat fish to determine their microbiological quality. *J. Food Protect.* 55:208–210 (1992).

780. Bryan, F.L., I. Fukunaga, S. Tsutsumi, et al. Hazard analysis of Japanese boxed lunches (*Bento*). *J. Environ. Health* 54(1):29–32 (1991).

781. Cotton, L.N., and C.H. White. *Listeria monocytogenes, Yersinia enterocolitica,* and *Salmonella* in dairy plant environments. *J. Dairy Sci.* 75:51–57 (1992).

782. Rohrbach, B.W., F.A. Draughon, P.M. Davidson, and S.P. Oliver. Prevalence of *Listeria monocytogenes, Campylobacter jejuni, Yersinia enterocolitica.* and *Salmonella* in bulk tank milk: risk factors and risk of human exposure. *J. Food Protect.* 55:93–97 (1992).

783. Diaz de Aguayo, M.E., A.B.L. Duarte, and F. Montes de Oca Canastillo. Incidence of multiple antibiotic resistant organisms isolated from retail milk products in Hermosillo, Mexico. *J. Food Protect.* 55:370–373 (1992).

784. Mathieu, A.-M., B.K. Isigidi, L.A. Devriese, et al. Characterization of *Staphylococcus aureus* and *Salmonella* spp. strains isolated from bovine meat in Zaïre. *Int. J. Food Microbiol.* 14:119–126 (1991).

785. Michel, M.E., J.T. Keeton, and G.R. Acuff. Pathogen survival in precooked beef products and determination of critical control points in processing. *J. Food Protect.* 54:767–772 (1991).

786. Zottola, E.A., and L.B. Smith. Pathogens in cheese. *Food Microbiol.* 8:171–182 (1991).

787. Misra, A.K., and R.K. Kuila. Use of *Bifidobacterium bifidum* in the manufacture of bifidus milk and its antibacterial activity. *Lait* 72:213–220 (1992).

788. Eckner, K.F., and E.A. Zottola. The behavior of selected microorganisms during the manufacture of high moisture Jack cheeses from ultrafiltered milk. *J. Dairy Sci.* 74:2820–2830 (1991).

789. Stecchini, M.L., I. Sarais, and M. de Bertoldi. The influence of *Lactobacillus plantarum* culture inoculation on the fate of *Staphylococcus aureus* and *Salmonella typhimurium* in Montasio cheese. *Int. J. Food Microbiol.* 14:99–110 (1991).

790. Farrag, S.A., F.E. El-Gazzar, and E.H. Marth. Behavior of *Escherichia coli* O157:H7 or *Yersinia enterocolitica* at 4 or 7°C in raw milk inoculated with a commercial culture of lactic acid bacteria. *Milchwissenschaft* 47:149–152 (1992).

791. El Agamy, E.S.I., R. Ruppanner, A. Ismail, et al. Antibacterial and antiviral activity of camel milk protective proteins. *J. Dairy Res.* 59:169–175 (1992).

792. Erol, I., and G. Hildebrandt. Einfluß von Starterkulturen auf das Wachstum pathogener Keime in türkischer Rohwurst. *Fleischwirtschaft* 72:90–97 (1992).

793. Ashenafi, M., and M. Busse. Growth potential of *Salmonella infantis* and *Escherichia coli* in fermenting tempeh made from horsebean, pea and chickpea and their inhibition by *Lactobacillus plantarum*. *J. Sci. Food Agric.* 55:607–615 (1991).

794. Grant, I.R., and M.F. Patterson. Effect of irradiation and modified atmosphere packaging on the microbiological safety of minced pork stored under temperature abuse conditions. *Int. J. Food Sci. Technol.* 26:521–533 (1991).

795. Kotzekidou, P., and H.N. Lazarides. Microbial stability and survival of pathogens in an intermediate moisture meat product. *Lebensm. Wiss. Technol.* 24:419–423 (1991).

796. Glass, K.A., and M.P. Doyle. Fate of *Salmonella* and *Listeria monocytogenes* in commercial, reduced-calorie mayonnaise. *J. Food Protect.* 54:691–695 (1991).

797. Erickson, J.P., and P. Jenkins. Comparative *Salmonella* spp. and *Listeria monocytogenes* inactivation rates in four commercial mayonnaise products. *J. Food Protect.* 54:913–916 (1991).

798. Erickson, J.P., and P. Jenkins. Behavior of psychrotropic pathogens *Listeria monocytogenes, Yersinia enterocolitica,* and *Aeromonas hydrophila* in commercially pasteurized eggs held at 2, 6.7, and 12.8°C. *J. Food Protect.* 55:8–12 (1992).

799. Droffner, M.L., and N. Yamamoto. Prolonged environmental stress via a two step process selects mutants of *Escherichia, Salmonella* and *Pseudomonas* that grow at 54°C. *Arch. Microbiol.* 156:307–311 (1991).

800. Dickson, J.S., and E.K. Daniels. Attachment of *Salmonella typhimurium* and *Listeria monocytogenes* to glass as affected by surface film thickness, cell density, and bacterial motility. *J. Ind. Microbiol.* 8:281–284 (1991).

801. Molan, P.C. The antibacterial activity of honey. 1. The nature of the antibacterial activity. *Bee World* 73(1):5–28 (1992).

802. Hughes, B.G., and L.D. Lawson. Antimicrobial effects of *Allium sativum* L. (garlic), *Allium ampeloprasum* L. (elephant garlic), and *Allium cepa* L. (onion), garlic compounds and commercial garlic supplement products. *Phytother. Res.* 5:154–158 (1991).

803. Nowak, H., K. Kujawa, R. Zadernowski, et al. Antioxidative and bactericidal properties of phenolic compounds in rapeseeds. *Fat Sci. Technol.* 94:149–152 (1992).

804. McKellar, R.C., A. Paquet, and C.-Y. Ma. Antimicrobial activity of fatty *N*-acylamino acids against gram-positive foodborne pathogens. *Food Microbiol.* 9:67–76 (1992).

805. Stecchini, M.L., P. Giavedoni, I. Sarais, and C.R. Lerici. Effect of Maillard reaction products on the growth of selected food-poisoning micro-organisms. *Lett. Appl. Microbiol.* 13:93–96 (1991).

806. Bailey, J.S., and N.A. Cox. Universal preenrichment broth for the simultaneous detection of *Salmonella* and *Listeria* in foods. *J. Food Protect.* 55:256–259 (1992).

807. He, X., and R. Pan. Bacteriophage lytic patterns for identification of salmonellae, shigellae, *Escherichia coli, Citrobacter freundii,* and *Enterobacter cloacae. J. Clin. Microbiol.* 30:590–594 (1992).

808. Schraft, H., and F. Untermann. Einsatz molekularbiologischer Methoden zur Differenzierung von Bakterienstämmen in der Lebensmittelmikrobiologie. *Arch. Lebensmittelhyg.* 42:145–149 (1991).

809. Wolf, I.D. Critical issues in food safety, 1991–2000. *Food Technol.* 46(1):64–70 (1992).

810. Notermans, S. Neuzeitliche Probleme in der Lebensmittelmikrobiologie. *Fleischwirtschaft* 71:648–657,770–775 (1991).

811. Buchanan, R.L. Predictive microbiology. Mathematical modeling of microbial growth in foods. In *Food Safety Assessment*. J.W. Finley, S.F. Robinson, and D.J. Armstrong (eds.). *ACS Symp. Ser.* 484:250–260 (1992).

812. McMeekin, T.A., T. Ross, and J. Olley. Application of predictive microbiology to assure the quality and safety of fish and fish products. *Int. J. Food Microbiol.* 15:13–32 (1992).

813. Microbiology and Food Safety Committee of the National Food Processors Association. HACCP and total quality management—winning concepts for the 90's: a review. *J. Food Protect.* 55:459–462 (1992).

814. Sperber, W.H. The modern HACCP system. *Food Technol.* 45(6):116,118,120 (1991).

815. Corlett, D.A., Jr. Importance of the hazard analysis and critical control point system in food safety evaluation and planning. In *Food Safety Assessment*. J.W. Finley, S.F. Robinson, and D.J. Armstrong (eds.). *ACS Symp. Ser.* 484:120–130 (1992).

816. Tisler, J.M. The Food and Drug Administration's perspective on HACCP. *Food Technol.* 45(6):125–127 (1991).

817. Mossel, D.A.A., and C.B. Struijk. Public health implication of refrigerated pasteurized ('sous-vide') foods. *Int. J. Food Microbiol.* 13:187–206 (1991).

818. Daniels, R.W. Applying HACCP to new-generation refrigerated foods at retail and beyond. *Food Technol.* 45(6):122,124 (1991).

819. Kalish, F. Extending the HACCP concept to product distribution. *Food Technol.* 45(6):119–120 (1991).

820. Abstracts of papers presented at the seventy-eighth annual meeting of the IAMFES. *J. Food Protect.* 54:811–827 (1991).

821. Mettler, A.E. Pathogen control in the manufacture of spray dried milk powders. *J. Soc. Dairy Technol.* 45(1):1–2 (1992).

822. Marth, E.H. Raw milk can be a source of disease-causing bacteria. *Cheese Rep.* 116(47):4,21 (1992).

823. Dickson, J.S., and M.E. Anderson. Microbiological decontamination of food animal carcasses by washing and sanitizing systems: a review. *J. Food Protect.* 55:133–140 (1992).

824. Gerrietts, M. Keeping your carcass clean. *Agric. Res.* 40(1):21–22 (1992).

825. Prasai, R.K., G.R. Acuff, L.M. Lucia, et al. Microbiological effects of acid decontamination of beef carcasses at various locations in processing. *J. Food Protect.* 54:868–872 (1991).

826. McCapes, R.H., B.I. Osburn, and H. Riemann. Safety of foods of animal origin: responsibilities of veterinary medicine. *J. Am. Vet. Med. Assoc.* 199:870–874 (1991).

827. Acuff, G.R., R.A. Albanese, C.A. Batt, et al. Implications of biotechnology, risk assessment, and communications for the safety of foods of animal origin. *J. Am. Vet. Med. Assoc.* 199:1714–1721 (1991).

828. Schütz, F. Möglichkeiten und Grenzen eines Hygienekonzepts für den Schlachthofbereich. *Fleischwirtschaft* 71:872–880 (1991).

829. Kasprowiak, R., and H. Hechelmann. Weak points in the hygiene of slaughtering, cutting and processing firms. *Fleischwirtschaft* 72:287–292 (1992).

830. Hechelmann, H., and R. Kasprowiak. Requirements and equipment for a bacteriological factory laboratory in the meat industry. *Fleischwirtschaft* 72:484–488 (1992).

831. Ward, D.R. Seafood microbiology. *Marine Technol. Soc. J.* 25:30–34 (1991).

832. Huss, H.H. Development and use of the HACCP concept in fish processing. *Int. J. Food Microbiol.* 15:33–44 (1992).

833. Garrett, E.S., III, and M. Hudak-Roos. Developing an HACCP-based inspection system for the seafood industry. *Food Technol.* 45(12):53–57 (1991).

834. Garrett, E.S., and M. Hudak-Roos. U.S. seafood inspection and HACCP. In *Microbiology of Marine Food Products*. D.R. Ward and C. Hackney (eds.). New York, Van Nostrand Reinhold. Pp. 111–131 (1991).

835. Beard, T.D., III. HACCP and the home: the need for consumer education. *Food Technol.* 45(6):123–124 (1991).

836. Williamson, D.M., R.B. Gravani, and H.T. Lawless. Correlating food safety knowledge with home food-preparation practices. *Food Technol.* 46(5):94–100 (1992).

837. Burch, N.L., and C.A. Sawyer. Food handling in convenience stores. The impact of personnel knowledge on facility sanitation. *J. Environ. Health* 54(3):23–27 (1991).

838. Look, V.E., and A.M. Messersmith. Is the salad bar safe? *J. Am. Diet. Assoc.* 91:917 (1991).

839. Pariza, M.W. Foods of new biotechnology vs traditional products: microbiological aspects. *Food Technol.* 46(3):100–102 (1992).

840. Tubol, M. Nouvelles technologies et agro-alimentaire: de nouveaux risques biologiques pour la santé humain. *Rev. Méd. Vét.* 142:721–732 (1991).

841. Huis in't Veld, J., and H. Hofstra. Biotechnology and the quality assurance of foods. *Food Biotechnol.* 5:313–322 (1991).

842. Firstenberg-Eden, R., and A.N. Sharpe. Impact of biotechnology and new methodology on microbial testing of foods. In *Biotechnology and Food Ingredients*. I. Goldberg and R. Williams (eds.). New York, Van Nostrand. Pp. 507–535 (1991).

843. Solberg, M. High-technology approaches to microbial safety in foods with extended shelf life. In *Food Safety Assessment*. J.W. Finley, S.F. Robinson, and D.J. Armstrong (eds.). *ACS Symp. Ser.* 484:243–249 (1992).

844. Blum, L.J., and P.R. Coulet (eds.). *Biosensor Principles and Applications.* New York, Marcel Dekker, Inc. *Bioprocess Technol.* 15 (1991).

845. Luong, J.H.T., C.A. Groom, and K.B. Male. The potential role of biosensors in the food and drink industries. *Biosensors Bioelectronics* 6:547–554 (1991).

846. Baker, J.M., M.W. Griffiths, and D.L. Collins-Thompson. Bacterial bioluminescence: applications in food microbiology. *J. Food Protect.* 55:62–70 (1992).

847. Lemieux, L., R. Puchades, and R.E. Simard. Overview of rapid methods and automation in food microbiology with emphasis on flow injection analysis. *Lebensm. Wiss. Technol.* 24:189–197 (1991).

848. Hechelmann, H., and R. Kasprowiak. Microbiological criteria for stable products. *Fleischwirtschaft* 71:1303–1308 (1991).

849. National Advisory Committee on Microbiological Criteria for Foods. Microbiological criteria for raw molluscan shellfish. *J. Food Protect.* 55:463–480 (1992).

850. Tebbutt, G.M. Development of standardized inspections in restaurants using visual assessments and microbiological sampling to quantify the risks. *Epidemiol. Infect.* 107:393–404 (1991).

851. Pontefract, R.D. Bacterial adherence: its consequences in food processing. *Can. Inst. Sci. Technol. J.* 24:113–117 (1991).

852. Giese, J.H. Sanitation: the key to food safety and public health. *Food Technol.* 45(12):74–80 (1991).

853. Chung, K.-T., and C.A. Murdock. Natural systems for preventing contamination and growth of microorganisms in foods. *Food Structure* 10:361–374 (1991).

854. Blankenship, L.C. (ed.). *Colonization Control of Human Bacterial Enteropathogens in Poultry.* San Diego: Academic Press, Inc. *Food Science and Technology Monograph Series* (1991).

855. Hinton, A., Jr., G.E. Spates, D.E. Corrier, et al. In vitro inhibition of the growth of *Salmonella typhimurium* and *Escherichia coli* O157:H7 by bacteria isolated from the cecal contents of adult chickens. *J. Food Protect.* 54:496–501 (1991).

856. Hinton, A., Jr., D.E. Corrier, and J.R. DeLoach. In vitro inhibition of *Salmonella typhimurium* and *Escherichia coli* O157:H7 by an anaerobic gram-positive coccus isolated from the cecal contents of adult chickens. *J. Food Protect.* 55:162–166 (1992).

857. Marugg, J.D. Bacteriocins, their role in developing natural products. *Food Biotechnol.* 5:305–312 (1991).

858. Piard, J.C., and M. Desmazeaud. Inhibiting factors produced by lactic acid bacteria. 2. Bacteriocins and other antibacterial substances. *Lait* 72:113–142 (1992).

859. Lewus, C.B., A. Kaiser, and T.J. Montville. Inhibition of food-borne bacterial pathogens by bacteriocins from lactic acid bacteria isolated from meat. *Appl. Environ. Microbiol.* 57:1683–1688 (1991).

860. Kojic, M., J. Svircevic, A. Banina, and L. Topisirovic. Bacteriocin-producing strain of *Lactococcus lactis* subsp. *diacitilactis* S50. *Appl. Environ. Microbiol.* 57:1835–1837 (1991).

861. Skyttä, E., W. Hereijgers, and T. Mattila-Sandholm. Broad spectrum antibacterial activity of *Pediococcus damnosus* and *Pediococcus pentosaceus* in minced meat. *Food Microbiol.* 8:231–237 (1991).

862. Toba, T., S.K. Samant, and T. Itoh. Assay system for detecting bacteriocin in microdilution wells. *Lett. Appl. Microbiol.* 13:102–104 (1991).

863. Rogers, A.M., and T.J. Montville. Improved agar diffusion assay for nisin quantification. *Food Biotechnol.* 5:161–168 (1991).

864. Gao, F.H., T. Abee, and W.N. Konings. Mechanism of action of the peptide antibiotic nisin in liposomes and cytochrome *c* oxidase-containing proteo-

liposomes. *Appl. Environ. Microbiol.* 57:2164–2170 (1991).

865. Mulders, J.W.M., I.J. Boerrigter, H.S. Rollema, et al. Identification and characterization of the lantibiotic nisin Z, a natural nisin variant. *Eur. J. Biochem.* 201:581–584 (1991).

866. Stoffels, G., J. Nissen-Meyer, A. Gudmundsdottir, et al. Purification and characterization of a new bacteriocin isolated from a *Carnobacterium* sp. *Appl. Environ. Microbiol.* 58:1417–1422 (1992).

867. Mørtvedt, C.I., J. Nissen-Meyer, K. Sletten, and I.F. Nes. Purification and amino acid sequence of lactocin S, a bacteriocin produced by *Lactobacillus sake* L45. *Appl. Environ. Microbiol.* 57:1829–1834 (1991).

868. Motlagh, A.M., M.C. Johnson, and B. Ray. Viability loss of foodborne pathogens by starter culture metabolites. *J. Food Protect.* 54:873–878 (1991).

869. Mertens, B., and D. Knorr. Developments of nonthermal processes for food preservation. *Food Technol.* 46(5):124–133 (1992).

870. Lambert, A.D., J.P. Smith, and K.L. Dodds. Shelf life extension and microbiological safety of fresh meat—a review. *Food Microbiol.* 8:267–297 (1991).

871. Pearson, A.M., and J.I. Gray. New methods of preservation and/or reducing the fat content of meat and poultry products. In *Meat and Health*. A.M. Pearson and T.R. Dutson (eds.). New York, Elsevier. *Adv. Meat Res.* 6:517–542 (1990).

872. Styles, M.F., D.G. Hoover, and D.F. Farkas. Response of *Listeria monocytogenes* and *Vibrio parahaemolyticus* to high hydrostatic pressure. *J. Food Sci.* 56:1404–1407 (1991).

873. El-Gazzar, F.E., and E.H. Marth. Ultrafiltration and reverse osmosis in dairy technology: a review. *J. Food Protect.* 54:801–809 (1991).

874. Eckner, K.F., and E.A. Zottola. Potential for the low-temperature pasteurization of dairy fluids using membrane processing. *J. Food Protect.* 54:793–797 (1991).

875. Reddy, N.R., D.J. Armstrong, E.J. Rhodehamel, and D.A. Kautter. Shelf-life extension and safety concerns about fresh fishery products packaged under modified atmospheres: a review. *J. Food Safety* 12:87–118 (1992).

876. Lampila, L.E. Modified atmosphere packaging. In *Microbiology of Marine Food Products*. D.R. Ward and C. Hackney (eds.). New York, Van Nostrand Reinhold. Pp. 373–393 (1991).

877. Moir, C.J., and M.J. Eyles. Inhibition, injury, and inactivation of four psychrotrophic foodborne bacteria by the preservatives methyl ρ-hydroxybenzoate and potassium sorbate. *J. Food Protect.* 55:360–366 (1992).

878. Fujikawa, H., H. Ushioda, and Y. Kudo. Kinetics of *Escherichia coli* destruction by microwave irradiation. *Appl. Environ. Microbiol.* 58:920–924 (1992).

879. Swallow, A.J. Wholesomeness and safety of irradiated foods. In *Nutritional and Toxicological Consequences of Food Processing*. M. Friedman (ed.). New York, Plenum Press. Pp. 11–31 (1991).

880. Grodner, R.M., and L.S. Andrews. Irradiation. In *Microbiology of Marine Food Products*. D.R. Ward and C. Hackney (eds.). New York, Van Nostrand Reinhold. Pp. 429–440 (1991).

881. Hau, L.-B., M.-H. Liew, and L.-T. Yeh. Preservation of grass prawns by ionizing radiation. *J. Food Protect.* 55:198–202 (1992).

882. Kamat, A.S., M.D. Alur, D.P. Nerkar, and P.M. Nair. Hygienization of Indian chicken meat by ionizing radiation. *J. Food Safety* 12:59–71 (1991).

883. Mallett, J.C., L.E. Beghian, T.G. Metcalf, and J.D. Kaylor. Potential of irradiation technology for improved shellfish sanitation. *J. Food Safety* 11:231–245 (1991).

884. Richards, G.P. Shellfish depuration. In *Microbiology of Marine Food Products*. D.R. Ward and C. Hackney (eds.). New York, Van Nostrand Reinhold. Pp. 395–428 (1991).

885. Hackney, C.R., T.E. Rippen, and D.R. Ward. Principles of pasteurization and minimally processed seafoods. In *Microbiology of Marine Food Products*. D.R. Ward and C. Hackney (eds.). New York, Van Nostrand Reinhold. Pp. 355–371 (1991).

886. Sumner, S.S., T.M. Sandros, M.C. Harmon, et al. Heat resistance of *Salmonella typhimurium* and *Listeria monocytogenes* in sucrose solutions of various water activities. *J. Food Sci.* 56:1741–1743 (1991).

12

Foodborne Parasites

Cryptosporidiosis
Toxoplasmosis
Giardiasis and *Entamoeba histolytica* infection
Cysticercosis and taeniasis
Trichinosis
Anisakiasis
Echinococcosis
Fascioliasis
Opisthorchis viverrini

Parasites were found in 20.1% of 216,275 stool specimens examined by state diagnostic laboratories in 1987 (*1*). Of foodborne pathogens, the protozoans *Giardia lamblia* and *Cryptosporidium* spp. were found in 7.2 and 0.2% of specimens, respectively; trematodes of the genera *Clonorchis* and *Opisthorchis* were found in 0.6% and there were 7 reports each of *Fasciola hepatica* and *Paragonimus* spp.; and *Taenia* spp. (cestodes) were found in 0.1%. *Cryptosporidium* diagnoses were reported by 25 states and showed no regional clustering.

Deardorff and Overstreet discussed the helminths transmitted by seafood in terms of the fishes that harbor infective stages, the specific food dishes that transmit the worms, and characteristics of the worms that cause disease (*2*). Most seafood zoonoses occur where seafood provides a major part of the protein intake, and populations closely associated with marine environments are at greatest risk. Overall, the incidence of seafood zoonoses in the USA is relatively low, probably because of high standards for sanitation and food handling and the tendency to eat products that are effectively processed or cooked.

Two papers from Germany considered the role of manure as a vector for parasites (*3,4*). Hiepe and Buchwalder found that in cattle stables, manure is an important vector for *Eimeria* spp., *Cryptosporidium parvum, Taenia saginata,* and *Fasciola hepatica* (*3*). In pig stables manure is a reservoir for *Toxoplasma gondii*. Eggs of *Ascaris, Taenia,* and *Enterobius* were identified in solid and liquid cattle manure after as much as 20 years of storage, but their infective ability was not determined (*4*).

CRYPTOSPORIDIOSIS

A review of cryptosporidiosis discussed the classification, life cycle, pathogenicity, and cultivation of the pathogen; and the epidemiology, clinical features, diagnosis, treatment, and immunologic aspects of the infection (*5*). Although frequently transmitted by contact with calves or companion animals, the infection may also be spread by human-to-human contact and may be waterborne; through poor sanitary and food-handling practices it can become foodborne. A brief report summarized the illness caused by *C. parvum* in livestock, poultry, and humans (*6*).

TOXOPLASMOSIS

Fishback and Frenkel reviewed the life cycle of *T. gondii* and discussed toxoplasmosis in humans and cats (*7*). The infection is acquired by ingesting oocytes, which may be present in undercooked or raw meat or in soil or feces. In most humans the infection is mild and immunity develops within a few days or weeks. However, women who are infected during pregnancy may transmit the infection to the fetus, with very serious consequences, and toxoplasmosis is also dangerous for immunosuppressed persons. In the USA, 30–50% of adults are seropositive for *Toxoplasma*. Most cases of toxoplasmosis in AIDS patients are relapses of chronic infection rather than new cases of acute infection. Smith's review of toxoplasmosis emphasized foodborne infection (*8*). Earthworms spread oocysts throughout the soil and may transmit infection to earthworm-eating birds and animals, which in turn may infect animals that eat them. Oocysts are also spread by insects that are attracted to feces. Distribution of *T. gondii* in wild and domestic warm-blooded animals was summarized; the organism has not been found in reptiles. Although eating undercooked pork is thought to be the major cause of toxoplasmosis in humans, meat of sheep, goats, deer, elk, horses, and small game may also contain *T. gondii*. Poultry and beef are not considered important sources of infection, although the organism is sometimes found in these foods. Hen's eggs do not appear to contain *T. gondii*. Any nonmeat food that is contaminated by soil or feces may also be a vehicle of infection. Virulence factors in *T. gondii* and the epidemiology and costs of toxoplasmosis were discussed.

In a random sample of 103 sheep farms in Ontario, 102 had some sheep seropositive by an ELISA for *T. gondii* (*9*). The average prevalence within a flock was 58%, with a range of 4–98%. Seropositivity was significantly lower on farms where female cats were neutered and ewes' perineums were clipped before lambing, and higher on farms where sheep were purchased from other flocks, pigs were also raised, sheep shared pasture with other animals, flowing water was available at pasture, or pastured replacements had access to housing. In univariate analyses, prevalence was inversely related to the labor expended on sheep rearing and positively associated with the number of cat litters born during the previous 2 years. These results indicate that kittens can serve as a source of infection for sheep and the neutering of farm cats may be an effective control measure. Nevertheless, associations with the presence of cattle and pigs remained after accounting for the presence of newborn cats. The authors suggested that livestock were also infecting cats.

In the first survey to determine the national prevalence of *T. gondii* in pigs in the USA, serum samples from 23.9% of 11,842 commercial pigs killed in 1983–1984 were seropositive for *T. gondii* by an agglutination test (*10*). The prevalence of anti-*T. gondii* antibodies was 42% in breeder pigs and 23% in market pigs. Results were presented by titer, state or region, and time of year. The data indicate that ~25% of the nation's pigs have been exposed to *T. gondii* and that they may be an important meat source of this parasite for humans. Comparisons of antibody titer with the occurrence of viable *T. gondii* in swine tissues will permit estimates of the number of false-positive and false-negative results given by the agglutination test. With this information, control strategies can be devised.

To study the effect of freezing on infectivity of *T. gondii* tissue cysts, infected mouse and rat brains and tongue, heart, and limb muscles from infected pigs were mixed and thoroughly homogenized (*11*). Rodent brains were added to the pork because they contain roughly a 100-fold higher concentration of tissue cysts. Samples of the homogenized meat were sealed in plastic pouches and frozen at −1 to −171°C for 1 s to 67.2 days, after which their infectivity was assayed in mice. *Toxoplasma gondii* tissue cysts remained viable up to 22.4 days at −1 and −3.9°C and for 11.2 days at −6.7°C, but usually did not survive freezing at −12.4°C. Least squares

linear regression analysis yielded the equation $t^{0.5} = 26.72 + 2.16\,T$, where t is the time for inactivation of *T. gondii* and T is temperature in °C; $r = .77$. Solving the equation for 0 time, a temperature of −12.4°C was calculated as the theoretical temperature at which *T. gondii* would be instantaneously inactivated. The data show that *T. gondii* tissue cysts are more readily inactivated by freezing than are encysted *Trichinella spiralis* larvae.

GIARDIASIS AND *ENTAMOEBA HISTOLYTICA* INFECTION

Of 160 Italian travelers who participated in an organized trip to Thailand and stayed in the same luxury hotel, 17 developed either amebic abscess or colitis (*12*). These patients and 40 asymptomatic travelers responded to a food and beverage questionnaire and provided stool samples. All of the patients' stool samples and 80% of the asymptomatic travelers' stool samples were positive for *Entamoeba histolytica, Giardia lamblia,* or both. No other intestinal parasites were found. No single food or beverage had been consumed by all parasitized patients and by none of the stool-negative patients, but consumption of drinks with ice, ice cream, and raw fruit in ice was significantly associated with parasitic infection (p's = .003–.03).

Clark and Diamond reported that ribosomal RNA genes of pathogenic and nonpathogenic *E. histolytica* differ (*13*). Two forms of the organism can be recognized biochemically, but it was not known whether they represented two morphologically indistinguishable species, one pathogenic and one nonpathogenic, or whether one species existed in two interconvertible forms. The finding of distinct ribosomal RNA genes supports the hypothesis that "*E. histolytica*" is two species. Further evidence was provided by Tachibana et al., who used a polymerase chain reaction to reveal differences between pathogenic and nonpathogenic isolates in the genomic DNA encoding the 30-kDa antigen (*14*). No products were amplified from nonpathogenic isolates or from other parasitic amoebas. The results agreed perfectly with results of zymodeme analysis and reactivity with the MAb 4G6, which is specific for pathogenic isolates regardless of culture conditions, geographic origin, or host symptoms.

CYSTICERCOSIS AND TAENIASIS

Three cases of locally acquired neurocysticercosis were reported in North Carolina, South Carolina, and Massachusetts from 1989 to 1991 (15). This infection is caused by the tissue-invading larval stages of the pork tapeworm, *Taenia solium,* but is acquired by ingesting tapeworm eggs shed in human feces, not by eating pork. Although the cysticerci may appear throughout the body, most symptoms stem from their presence in the central nervous system. In the case acquired in North Carolina, the patient had no personal or family history of neurologic illness or tapeworm infection but some seasonal workers on the family farm came from countries with endemic cysticercosis. Three of four family members of the Massachusetts patient, who had emigrated from the Cape Verde Islands, were positive for cysticercosis in the immunoblot assay and stool specimens from the patient's father contained *Taenia* sp. eggs. The South Carolina patient had contact with cysticercosis-seropositive Mexican immigrants at the home of a neighbor.

The prevalence of cysticercosis in pigs and risk factors associated with infection were studied in a rural Mexican community (16). Prevalence increased with the pig's age and was higher in males than females. The most important risk factors for the pigs were access to human feces at a public washing area, presence of an indoor latrine, and indiscriminate disposal of human feces around the pig owner's household. Two regular visitors to the public washing area were diagnosed with intestinal taeniasis by stool examination. Because the pig is the obligatory natural intermediate host of *T. solium* this study helped document the role of the scavenging pig in the pig–human cycle.

Two papers reported ELISAs for detecting *Taenia* antigens in stool samples (17,18). In the first, 85% of 34 samples from 23 untreated persons with *Taenia saginata* infection (previously demonstrated by detection of proglottids or eggs) were positive by ELISA, whereas *Taenia* eggs were detected in only 62% of this set of samples (17). A high concentration of *T. saginata* coproantigens persisted for 1–4 days after niclosamide or praziquantel. Moreover, the antigens could be detected after storage of untreated feces at 25°C for 5 days. There was ~40% cross-reactivity with *Taenia hydatigena* in this ELISA. The second ELISA detected *T. solium* antigens in supernatants of stool samples preserved in merthiolate-formalin, distinguishing all 9 *T. solium* carriers from 41 negative controls (18). However, there was cross-reactivity with the single sample from a patient with *T. saginata* infection.

TRICHINOSIS

The number of cases of trichinosis reported by state health departments annually has declined steadily since the Public Health Service began recording statistics on this infection in 1947 (19). The earliest reports showed an average of 400 cases and 10–15 deaths per year; the years 1982–1986 averaged 57 cases, with only three deaths; from 1987 through 1990 there were 206 cases, but 106 of these occurred in 1990 during two outbreaks associated with commercial pork. In recent years the frequently observed December–January peak related to eating homemade pork sausage during the Christmas holidays has not been seen. Although pork (and particularly sausage) is the most frequently implicated food source, infected walrus and bear meat have also caused some outbreaks. The decrease in cases has been attributed to increased use of home freezers, success of public awareness programs, and laws prohibiting the feeding of garbage to pigs. Twenty-six cases of travel-associated trichinosis were reported to the CDC from 1975 to 1989 (20). Increased risk was associated with travel to Mexico or Asia, consumption of undercooked pork products, use of unsanitary cooking practices, and importing potentially contaminated meat products into the USA.

In November and December 1990, the Central Shenandoah Health District, Virginia Department of Health, identified 15 cases of trichinosis due to eating raw or undercooked commercial pork sausage produced by a local processing plant (*21*). Nine patients required hospitalization. Thirteen patients reported eating pork sausage 4–21 days before onset of symptoms, and 10 had tasted or eaten the sausage uncooked. During the 6 weeks before the outbreak the processing plant purchased sows from two brokers, who obtained them from many producers in Virginia and surrounding states. The plant produces 1500 pounds of sausage weekly and distributes it throughout 8 counties in the Shenandoah Valley. Most cases of trichinosis reported in Virginia have occurred in this area during the past decade. This review prompted the *Food Safety Notebook* to publish a short review of trichinosis from commercial pork (*22*). The time–temperature relationships for destruction of *T. spiralis* larvae were summarized and recommendations for conventional and microwave cooking of fresh pork were reviewed.

An outbreak of trichinosis in central Italy at the end of 1988 involved 48 persons (*23*). It was caused by eating sausages recently made with wild boar meat, and the victims were mostly friends and relatives of hunters. *Trichinella* larvae were found in samples of the sausage and in household cats that had eaten raw leftover sausage.

Study of a trichinosis outbreak in northern Québec in 1987 identified two distinct clinical syndromes (*24*). The outbreak occurred in an Inuit community and was caused by eating the uncooked meat of a walrus. Patients with the myopathic syndrome were much younger, had much lower IgG anti-*Trichinella* titers, a higher IgM:IgG ratio, higher creatinine kinase levels, a higher hospitalization rate, and lower albumin levels than patients with the diarrheic syndrome. These findings are consistent with the idea that the myopathic form represented a primary *T. nativa* infection, whereas the diarrheic form represented a secondary infection in previously sensitized persons.

An outbreak of trichinosis affected three members of a rural Mexican family who habitually ate raw pork prepared with lemon juice (*25*). All three patients first experienced diarrhea, vomiting, and abdominal pain, which were followed by myalgias and severe proximal muscle weakness

that mimicked polymyositis. This unusual clinical manifestation of trichinosis was discussed.

To establish the value of ELISA for diagnosing trichinosis in humans, sera were collected from proved cases of trichinosis and other helminthic infections and examined for IgG and IgM antibodies (*26*). On the 23rd, 50th, and 57th day of infection the IgG ELISA was positive in 69, 100, and 100% of cases, respectively, whereas the IgM ELISA was positive in 12, 86, and 93%. The IgG ELISA showed 21% cross-reactivity with parasitic infections other than trichinosis; there were 9% false-positive reactions in the IgM ELISA. Maximum sensitivity for serodiagnosis of human trichinosis apparently does not occur before 1 month after infection. For diagnosis of trichinosis in pigs, the histamine-release test was compared with an ELISA (*27*). Six pigs were inoculated with 200 *T. spiralis* larvae and 6 with 5000 larvae; 6 controls were not infected. Forty days after inoculation all pigs in the high-inoculum group and 5 of 6 in the low inoculum group were antibody-positive by ELISA with all three coating antigens used. Four pigs in the high-dose group and only one in the low-dose group were positive in the histamine-release test. The earliest ELISA seroconversions took place 15 days after inoculation, but pigs varied with respect to which test was more sensitive for early detection of infection. A modified enhanced chemiluminescent enzyme assay was developed to rapidly screen pigs for trichinosis in slaughterhouses (*28*). Optimum conditions for the assay were described. The method was evaluated by testing serum samples from 73 pigs at a slaughterhouse in a region where trichinosis was not endemic. All samples were negative. The assay was judged satisfactory for this application provided that chemicals and antigen coating are already prepared. The major drawback of the assay is the cost of magnetic beads.

ANISAKIASIS

Numerous anisakidae larvae were found in marine fishes and squids caught in the Gulf of Tongking, East China Sea, and Yellow Sea (*29*). About 30%

of animals caught in the Gulf of Tongking and 60% of those caught in the other areas contained *Anisakis simplex* larvae. Larvae of *Raphidascaris* (or *Raphidascaroides*), *Hysterothylacium,* and *Terranova* were also detected. No larvae of *Pseudoterranova decipiens* were found. Infection rates varied widely among species. For the first time, infection was confirmed in squids of the genus *Sepia*. Although anisakiasis has not been a problem in China, the authors warned that the high infection rate in fishes and squids and the recently acquired taste for sushi and sashimi will likely lead to identification of cases of anisakiasis in China in the near future.

In Japan, a woman complained of severe epigastric pain and nausea about 8 h after eating sashimi prepared from raw bonito (*30*). A gastrocamera examination revealed that numerous worms had penetrated the posterior gastric walls; 56 larvae were removed with a biopsy clipper and identified as *Anisakis simplex*. This case was unusual in the high multiplicity of infection. Usually only one larva is found in patients suffering from gastric anisakiasis. Symptoms from mild infections do not appear to differ from those in heavy infection.

A German study found that *Anisakis* larvae are killed by carbon dioxide–shock freezing at –60°C, obviating the need for additional frozen storage (*31*). The time required for elimination of infective worms depends on the size and type of fish. In herring fillets nematodes were killed within 10 min; 20 min was required to kill all larvae in unfilleted herring.

ECHINOCOCCOSIS

Echinococcus granulosus infection in people can cause cystic hydatid disease, particularly of the lungs and liver. In northwest Scotland a dog–sheep life cycle of the parasite has been identified and exposure of humans is recognized. Three new cases of hydatid disease were discovered in Scotland during 1987–1991 (*32*). Two of the three cases were in young children in whom ELISAs were initially negative but became positive after surgery. The third

case was in a 59-year-old woman, whose ELISA was positive from the beginning but the indirect hemagglutination test and confirmatory immunoelectrophoresis test were negative. The inadequacy of diagnostic tests was discussed.

FASCIOLIASIS

Fasciola hepatica is a common parasite of cattle, sheep, and goats and may infect a variety of other wild and domestic animals as well. Although infection is not common in humans, it can severely damage the liver and bile ducts, sometimes causing death. The worldwide incidence and epidemiology of fascioliasis was recently reviewed (*33*). In Europe, most cases have occurred in France, Spain, Portugal, the U.K., and the former USSR. Most African cases have been reported from Egypt and are probably due to *Fasciola gigantica*. In the Americas, the infection is most prevalent in Bolivia (>5000 cases in the last 30 years); Cuba and Peru have each reported >100 cases. Fewer cases have been described in Asia and the Western Pacific. The occurrence of the infection is determined by the presence of the intermediate snail hosts, herbivorous animals, and human dietary habits. Persistent high temperatures and dry conditions adversely influence snail populations and impair larval development of the fluke, whereas both snails and flukes are relatively resistant to low temperatures if there is sufficient moisture. In France, human infections are more frequent in years of heavy rainfall. Watercress and other aquatic vegetables are vehicles of human infection. In China, where vegetables are nearly always eaten cooked, infection may occur through cross-contamination of kitchen utensils or consumption of unboiled water. Most clinical cases are diagnosed during cooler seasons of the year. Familial clusters are common because the family shares contaminated food. Fascioliasis is predominantly a rural disease, and sheep- and cattle-herders are most frequently infected. The first two Australian cases of migratory ectopic fascioliasis were reported (*34*). Neither patient had eaten watercress, although one "thought" he may have occasionally chewed grass blades or drunk water from a pond or stream. The other patient ate raw meat, but it is not known whether she ate raw liver. No ova were recovered from fecal samples from either patient. The spread of snail vectors throughout grazing districts of Australia may lead to greater numbers of human infections in the future.

OPISTHORCHIS VIVERRINI

In Thailand, incidence of cholangiocarcinoma shows striking regional variation and is closely correlated with markers of exposure to the liver fluke *Opisthorchis viverrini* (35). Hepatocellular carcinoma, in contrast, shows little geographic variation in incidence and no correlation with exposure to the fluke. The authors concluded that long-term infection with *O. viverrini* is the overwhelming etiological factor for development of cholangiocarcinoma in Thailand. The infection is acquired by ingesting raw or improperly cooked fish containing *O. viverrini* metacercaria cysts. The life cycle of the fluke was reviewed.

LITERATURE CITED

1. Kappus, K.K., D.D. Juranek, and J.M. Roberts. Results of testing for intestinal parasites by state diagnostic laboratories, United States, 1987. *Morbid. Mortal. Weekly Rep.* 40(SS-4):25–47 (1991).

2. Deardorff, T.L., and R.M. Overstreet. Seafood-transmitted zoonoses in the United States: the fishes, the dishes, and the worms. In *Microbiology of Marine Food Products*. D.R. Ward and C. Hackney (eds.). New York, Van Nostrand Reinhold. Pp. 211–265 (1991).

3. Hiepe, Th., and R. Buchwalder. Wirtschaftsdünger also Vektor für Parasiten—ein Erfahrungsbericht. *Dtsch. Tierärztl. Wochenschr.* 98:245–292 (1991).

4. Deutrich, V., and G. Pioch. Infektionsrisiko für Mensch und Tier durch langjährig gelagerte Rindergülle. *Mh. Vet. Med.* 46:651–655 (1991).

5. Current, W.L., and L.S. Garcia. Cryptosporidiosis. *Clin. Microbiol. Rev.* 4:325–358 (1991).

6. Anonymous. Cryptosporidium & cryptosporidiosis. *Commun. Dis. Environ. Health Scotland Weekly Rep.* 26(15):4–5 (1992).

7. Fishback, J.L., and J.K. Frenkel. Toxoplasmosis. *Sem. Vet. Med. Surg. (Small Anim.)* 6:219–226 (1991).

8. Smith, J.L. Foodborne toxoplasmosis. *J. Food Safety* 12:17–57 (1991).

9. Waltner-Toews, D., R. Mondesire, and P. Menzies. The seroprevalence of *Toxoplasma gondii* in Ontario sheep flocks. *Can. Vet. J.* 32:734–737 (1991).

10. Dubey, J.P., J.C. Leighty, V.C. Beal, et al. National seroprevalence of *Toxoplasma gondii* in pigs. *J. Parasitol.* 77:517–521 (1991).

11. Kotula, A.W., J.P. Dubey, A.K. Sharar, et al. Effect of freezing on infectivity of *Toxoplasma gondii* tissue cysts in pork. *J. Food Protect.* 54:687–690 (1991).

12. de Lalla, F., E. Rinaldi, D. Santoro, et al. Outbreak of *Entamoeba histolytica* and *Giardia lamblia* infections in travellers returning from the tropics. *Infection* 20:78–82 (1992).

13. Clark, C.G., and L.S. Diamond. Ribosomal RNA genes of 'pathogenic' and 'nonpathogenic' *Entamoeba histolytica* are distinct. *Mol. Biochem. Parasitol.* 49:297–302 (1991).

14. Tachibana, H., S. Kobayashi, M. Takekoshi, and S. Ihara. Distinguishing pathogenic isolates of *Entamoeba histolytica* by polymerase chain reaction. *J. Infect. Dis.* 164:825–826 (1991).

15. Centers for Disease Control. Locally acquired neurocysticercosis—North Carolina, Massachusetts, and South Carolina, 1989–1991. *Morbid. Mortal. Weekly Rep.* 41:1–4 (1992).

16. Sarti-G., E., P.M. Schantz, J. Aguilera, and A. Lopez. Epidemiologic observations on porcine cysticercosis in a rural community of Michoacan State, Mexico. *Vet. Parasitol.* 41:195–201 (1992).

17. Deplazes, P., J. Eckert, Z.S. Pawlowski, et al. An enzyme-linked immunosorbent assay for diagnostic detection of *Taenia saginata* copro-antigens in humans. *Trans. Roy. Soc. Trop. Med. Hyg.* 85:391–396 (1991).

18. Maass, M., E. Delgado, and J. Knobloch. Detection of *Taenia solium* antigens in merthiolate-formalin preserved stool samples. *Trop. Med. Parasitol.* 42:112–114 (1991).

19. McAuley, J.B., M.K. Michelson, and P.M. Schantz. Trichinosis surveillance, United States, 1987–

1990. *Morbid. Mortal. Weekly Rep.* 40(SS-3):35–42 (1991).

20. McAuley, J.B., M.K. Michelson, and P.M. Schantz. *Trichinella* infection in travelers. *J. Infect. Dis.* 164:1013–1016 (1991).

21. Landry, S.M., D. Kiser, T. Overby, et al. Trichinosis: common source outbreak related to commercial pork. *South. Med. J.* 85:428–429 (1992).

22. Hall, K.N. Trichinosis from commercial pork: a review. *Food Safety Notebook* 3:76–77 (1992).

23. Frongillo, R.F., B. Baldelli, E. Pozio, et al. Report on an outbreak of trichinellosis in central Italy. *Eur. J. Epidemiol.* 8:283–288 (1992).

24. MacLean, J.D., L. Poirier, T.W. Gyorkos, et al. Epidemiologic and serologic definition of primary and secondary trichinosis in the Arctic. *J. Infect. Dis.* 165:908–912 (1992).

25. Durán-Ortiz, I. García-de la Torre, G. Orozco-Barocio, et al. Trichinosis with severe myopathic involvement mimicking polymyositis. Report of a family outbreak. *J. Rheumatol.* 19:310–312 (1992).

26. Morakote, N., C. Khamboonruang, V. Siriprasert, et al. The value of enzyme-linked immunosorbent assay (ELISA) for diagnosis of human trichinosis. *Trop. Med. Parasitol.* 42:172–174 (1991).

27. Lind, P., L. Eriksen, Sv.Aa. Henricksen, et al. Diagnostic tests for *Trichinella spiralis* infection in pigs. A comparative study of ELISA for specific antibody and histamine release from blood cells in experimental infections. *Vet. Parasitol.* 39:241–252 (1991).

28. Ko, R.C., and M.H.F. Yeung. Enhanced chemiluminescent enzyme immunoassay for the detection of trichinellosis antibodies in pigs. *Vet. Parasitol.* 42:101–110 (1992).

29. Sun, S., T. Koyama, and N. Kagei. Anisakidae larvae found in marine fishes and squids from the Gulf of Tongking, the East China Sea and the Yellow Sea. *Jpn. J. Med. Sci. Biol.* 44:99–108 (1991).

30. Kagei, N., and H. Isogaki. A case of abdominal syndrome caused by the presence of a large number of *Anisakis* larvae. *Int. J. Parasitol.* 22:251–253 (1992).

31. Karl, H., and K. Priebe. Abtötung von juvenilen Nematoden (*Anisakis sp.*) in Seefischen. *Arch. Lebensmittelhyg.* 42:46–48 (1991).

32. Evans, R., W.J. Reilly, and D.O. Ho-Yen. Scottish hydatid infections: 1987–1991. *Commun. Dis. Environ. Health Scotland Weekly Rep.* 26(17):4–6 (1992).

33. World Health Organization. Fascioliasis. *Weekly Epidemiol. Rec.* 67:326–329 (1992).

34. Prociv, P., J.C. Walker, and M. Whitby. Human ectopic fascioliasis in Australia: first case reports. *Med. J. Aust.* 156:349–351 (1992).

35. Srivatanakul, P., D.M. Parkin, Y.-Z. Jiang, et al. The role of infection by *Opisthorchis viverrini*, hepatitis B virus, and aflatoxin exposure in the etiology of liver cancer in Thailand. *Cancer* 68:2411–2417 (1991).

Food- and Water-Associated Viruses

Contributed by Dean O. Cliver

Food virology
Water and soil virology
Viral hepatitis
Viral gastroenteritis

FOOD VIROLOGY

Although transmission of viruses via foods is increasingly being recognized as a problem in the USA, several European countries have reported no foodborne viral disease during the period 1985–1989 (*1*).

Foodborne viral disease

An "ice slush" beverage sold at a convenience store in a suburb of Anchorage, Alaska, was the evident vehicle in an outbreak of hepatitis A (*2*). A worker who reportedly was eventually jaundiced prepared the beverage under unsanitary conditions and led to 32 primary (consumed the contaminated beverage), 23 secondary (infected through household or other contact with the primary cases), and 2 tertiary cases (infected through household or other contact with secondary cases). Administration of immune serum globulin prevented further transmission of the disease to household contacts of those who were ill.

An outbreak of severe gastroenteritis occurred at the U.S. Air Force Academy in Colorado Springs in July of 1988 (*3*). Serologic testing implicated the Norwalk virus as the cause; transmission was via celery stalks that were washed with water from an unsafe source and then included in a chicken salad.

A moderate-sized (38 cases, including 8 food handlers) food-associated outbreak of hepatitis A in the area of Denver late in 1992 received so much publicity that 10,000 people requested and received immune serum globulin prophylaxis (*4*). The apparent source was one or more workers for a catering and baking business that dealt principally with the more affluent segment of Denver society.

There are indications that food- and waterborne hepatitis A is on the rise in the USA or that reporting of vehicle-associated transmission is becoming more efficient (*5*). In contrast to data from earlier years, in which only about 1% of hepatitis A cases in the USA were associated with vehicular transmission, 3.3% of illnesses in 1989 were described as "suspected food- or waterborne

outbreak." Among cases reported within 6 weeks of illness, this figure rose to 6.2%.

The relatively low incidence of reported food-associated virus disease in Canada—only two incidents of hepatitis A comprising seven cases in 1983, for the entire 1975–1984 decade—may be because "shellfish in Canada tends to be harvested from non-industrial areas" (*6*). However, shellfish are by no means the only food by which viruses are transmitted: incidence of antibody to the frequently foodborne Norwalk virus was not significantly correlated with shellfish consumption or contact in a recent survey of people in the area of the Chesapeake Bay, eastern USA (*7*).

At the end of 1992, there were six outbreaks, some of which are likely to have been food-associated, attributed to small round structured viruses (SRSV) in the U.K.—three in hospitals, one in a nursing home, one from a restaurant, and one from a wedding reception (*8*). A 1991 outbreak of gastroenteritis among those who ate a gourmet dinner in St. Andrews, Scotland, was thought to have been caused by viruses in oysters harvested and depurated in County Cork, Ireland (*9*). Orange juice from a supplier in Melbourne was the apparent vehicle of SRSV that caused more than 3000 illnesses among air travelers in Australia (*10*).

In a larger compilation of foodborne disease in Europe from 1985 to 1989 by the WHO Surveillance Programme (*1*), England and Wales reported 48 incidents of virus transmission via food during 1986–1988: 25 of hepatitis (3 general outbreaks, 2 family outbreaks, and 19 sporadic cases); 1 general outbreak of rotavirus gastroenteritis; and 22 incidents of SRSV gastroenteritis (14 general outbreaks, 2 family outbreaks, and 6 sporadic cases). During the stated 5-year period, (the then Federal Republic of) Germany reported 29,717 foodborne cases of hepatitis A, but only three food-associated outbreaks of hepatitis A, three of rotavirus gastroenteritis, and three of Norfolk [sic] virus gastroenteritis, comprising 3% of foodborne disease outbreaks for which a cause was determined.

The 1985–1989 report (*1*) shows that systems of recording foodborne disease outbreaks and individual outbreaks differ greatly among countries. Malta reports 27 foodborne cases of hepatitis A but

148 cases of food-associated gastroenteritis of apparently undetermined etiology. The Netherlands says there were 639 outbreaks of foodborne disease of unknown etiology versus 132 outbreaks of known etiology, yet 6 outbreaks (4.5% of the 5-year total) are reported as "Viral/unknown" in the "Total known" category. In contrast, only 0.7% of foodborne disease outbreaks in the Netherlands for the 11-year period 1979–1989 were attributed to viruses, but it was pointed out that the causative agent was not identified in 70% of reported illnesses during that period (*11*). Norway reports (*1*) 2586 cases of foodborne rotavirus gastroenteritis from 1980 to 1989, but no other foodborne viral disease (which contradicts some of their earlier reports). Romania reports 256,675 cases of foodborne/waterborne hepatitis A for the 1985–1989 period, but no foodborne viral disease *outbreaks* during the period. Scotland attributed four outbreaks of foodborne disease to "virus" during 1985–1989.

Detection

Methods for detecting viruses of fecal origin in shellfish have been extensively reviewed by Williams and Fout (*12*). After an epidemiologic history of virus transmission via shellfish, both methods for extracting the virus from the molluscs and for final detection are addressed.

Prevention of foodborne viral disease

To prevent transmission of viruses via foods, one might either undertake to prevent contamination of foods by viruses infectious for humans or to heat (or otherwise process) food that might be contaminated, so as to inactivate the virus. Because most viruses transmitted to humans via foods come from human feces, sanitation is an important aspect of prevention, as it is for many foodborne diseases. Prevention of virus infections in food handlers may also be important.

Hepatitis A has been described as an "occupational hazard" among food handlers working in hospitals in southwest Germany (*13*). The study reports that these workers are disproportionately likely to have antibody against the hepatitis A virus, suggesting that they have been infected at some time with the virus. The authors point out that these jobs are often held by workers from "south Europe," so the findings do not necessarily suggest that working in hospital food service puts one at risk of hepatitis A. Rather, it is possible that the workers in this category had been infected and were immune for life before they came to work in Germany.

An inactivated-virus vaccine against hepatitis A has been developed—it requires three injections (and perhaps later boosters) to induce durable immunity (*14*). The vaccine has now been licensed in several European countries and will be used for pre-exposure immunization of people at especially high risk (health care workers and those traveling to high-endemicity areas) and perhaps for early post-exposure immunization (together with immune serum globulin) where an outbreak threatens (*15*). The World Health Organization has recently suggested that the vaccine be administered to food handlers, to diminish the risk that they will become infected and shed the virus while handling food (*16*). Clearly, immunization is not a substitute for sanitation, but food handlers have been sources in enough food-associated outbreaks of hepatitis A to suggest that this "ounce of prevention" is worthwhile. Fingers have been shown to be a potential carrier of hepatitis A virus that could contaminate food, though attempts to disinfect contaminated fingers are not described in this first report (*17*).

Another approach to preventing viral contamination of foods would be to find better means of avoiding waters and conditions that are conducive to contamination of shellfish. Monitoring in the USA is presently based on levels of "fecal coliform" bacteria in water and shellfish, but studies with the eastern hard clam (*Mercenaria mercenaria*) have shown that "male-specific bacteriophages" (viruses that infect *Escherichia coli* bacteria which have F-pili) are more efficiently accumulated than fecal coliforms by clams, especially during the spring, when risk of transmitting gastroenteritis via these molluscs is high (*18*). The bacteriophages could only multiply at temperatures above 25°C (highly inappropriate for shellfish storage) in the presence of susceptible bacteria, but would persist up to 7 days in clams held below 25°C—temperatures typical of seawater (*19*).

If food does become contaminated with virus, transmission of the virus can be prevented by inactivating the virus in the food. Weaning foods based on rice gruel, which might be used in developing countries, were evaluated as vehicles for rotavirus—a major cause of infant diarrhea in these countries (*20*). Lactic fermentation of these foods to near pH 4, which confers some protection against bacterial disease agents, was found to be ineffective against rotavirus unless the acidified food was also heated above 40°C.

Tissues (blood clots, bone marrow, and lymph nodes) from animals infected with foot-and-mouth disease virus (an important animal health agent that generally does not infect humans) were inserted into muscle and subjected to aging (1°C, 2 or 7 days), curing (0.5 or 5% NaCl), heat (78°C, 20 min), and irradiation (1.5 or 2.5 Mrad) with cobalt-60 gamma rays (*21*). Among these treatments, said not to alter the sensory characteristics of the product, only the combination of heat and irradiation eliminated the virus completely.

Bovine spongiform encephalopathy (BSE), often called "mad cow disease," has had a disastrous impact on the cattle industry in the United Kingdom. It was first reported in 1986, and the U.K. total had risen to 44,482 cases by the end of 1992 (*22*). The slow-onset brain deterioration is characterized by aggregates of "PrP" proteins in the brain, as in scrapie of sheep and a few other encephalopathies. The disease has not been reported in the USA, and the U.S. Department of Agriculture has banned imports of ruminants and associated products from the U.K. and other countries where BSE is known to occur. Diagnosis had been based on histopathologic examination of the brain, but a serologic test for the PrP protein has recently been developed (*23*). BSE has now been transmitted to mice, as has scrapie; the syndrome resulting in mice is not identical for the two diseases (*24*). A captive puma in the U.K. has been diagnosed with spongiform encephalopathy that may have resulted from feeding the animal portions of uncooked cattle carcasses that had been declared unfit for human consumption (*25*). Despite this apparent instance of interspecies transfer, BSE is still not known to be transmissible to humans.

WATER AND SOIL VIROLOGY

Drinking water

The U.S. Centers for Disease control have issued a very brief report of waterborne disease in the USA during 1989 and 1990 (*26*). Of 26 outbreaks associated with drinking water, 2 of hepatitis A and 1 of gastroenteritis due to a Norwalk-like agent were attributed to use of well water. Details of the outbreaks are not provided. An outbreak of hepatitis E in several college dormitories in Sargodha, Pakistan, resulted from contamination of drinking water with raw sewage (*27*). Stool specimens from the patients were shown by electron microscopy to contain the virus as early as 9 days before the onset of jaundice and no later than 7 days after onset. Levels of fecal virus were found to be lower than those seen with other enteric viruses. An outbreak of drinking water–associated hepatitis E in Kanpur, India, is estimated to have affected 79,000 people, perhaps as a result of drinking water that derived from the Ganges River and was not adequately chlorinated (*28*). Remarkably, a quest for secondary (transmitted by contact from those infected by drinking the contaminated water), intrafamilial illnesses revealed none.

Wastewater and surface waters

Among 30 outbreaks of illness due to recreational use of water in the USA during 1989 and 1990, one outbreak of hepatitis A was associated with a swimming pool (*26*). In what may be the first documented outbreak of hepatitis A associated with swimming (*29*), 20 of 822 persons who camped at a public campground in Louisiana were affected. Though the attack rate was highest for children aged 5 to 9 years, an "adult" swimming pool and a jacuzzi pool were the deduced sites of exposure. The water may have been contaminated with feces, or by sewage through improper operation of a water filtration apparatus.

Tests of 10-L samples of recreational waters in Northern Ireland revealed enteroviruses in 53 of 153 samples from coastal waters and 33 of 39 from inland waters during 1986 and 1987 (*30*). The enterovirus-positive samples often met one or both coliform standards specified by the European Economic Community for recreational waters. The Safo River in Japan yielded monthly average levels of enteric viruses ranging from 13 to 192 plaque-forming units/L during the period January 1988 to December 1989 (*31*). Adenoviruses, coxsackieviruses B, echoviruses, polioviruses, and reoviruses were detected under various circumstances. Studies of marine bacteriophages in coastal seawater from the Gulf of Mexico indicated that inactivation resulted from ultraviolet irradiation (from sunlight) and from the action of flagellate protozoa, but perhaps not of bacteria (*32*).

The genome of human immunodeficiency virus type 1 [HIV-1, the principal cause of acquired immunodeficiency syndrome (AIDS)] has been detected in some wastewater samples by nucleic acid techniques, notably the polymerase chain reaction (*33*). Although AIDS is not known to be waterborne, the authors suggest further studies to determine whether the virus is being inactivated in the situations in which it is detected. Monochloramine disinfection of wastewater for reuse as drinking water in Denver was found not always to inactivate coliphages that were followed as indicators of the antiviral effectiveness of the water recycling process (*34*). When septic tank effluent was added (20% v/v) to swine manure slurry, bacteria in the swine manure were shown to play a significant role in inactivating experimentally added poliovirus 1 (*35*). Bacterial proteases appeared to be at least partly responsible for the viral inactivation.

Soil and groundwater

Recovery of experimentally added poliovirus 1 from sludge-amended soils with 3% beef extract buffered at pH 9.5 has been shown to increase significantly as ratios (v/v) of soil to eluent increased from 1:1 to 1:10 (*36*). Then, it was shown that poliovirus 1 and two bacteriophages were more rapidly inactivated in sludge-amended desert soils by desiccation and by high temperature (40°C) over the range of 15 to 40°C (*37*).

VIRAL HEPATITIS

Epidemiology of hepatitis A

After the peak in 1989, hepatitis A in the USA has continued its dramatic decline (*38*). Unexplained cycles in hepatitis A incidence have long been known, but their periodicity has become less predictable in recent decades. Although there is only one serotype of hepatitis A, strains detected in endemic and outbreak contexts show significant genetic individuality (*39*). These genetic specificities can be used epidemiologically to differentiate between endemic infections and those imported from outside a community.

Hepatitis A immunity

Passive immunization against hepatitis A with pooled human immunoglobulin has been reviewed in the light of recent findings (*40*). Now that antigen preparations (candidate vaccines) are available to evoke active immunity to hepatitis A, the effectiveness of the two means—passive and active—of immunization is being compared (*41*). Active immunity is, of course, more durable, with antibody still present at significant levels after 3 years or more (*42*). Antigenic variants of the hepatitis A virus are numerous (*43*), but this variation has not precluded development of vaccines that will protect most of the world's population against almost all infections with the virus (*44*).

Hepatitis A in cell culture

Adaptation of hepatitis A virus to replicate in cell culture has had an important role in studies on transmission and inactivation of the virus, as well as in development of vaccines to prevent transmission of the virus. Three mutation sites in the viral genome, not involving structural proteins, have been shown to relate to adaptation to cell culture—at least two of these must be changed to permit the virus to replicate in cell cultures (*45*).

Hepatitis E

The hepatitis E virus continues to attract attention as an agent of waterborne and sporadic disease. A survey with a new serologic method showed that antibody against the virus occurs only in areas of the world where outbreaks of hepatitis E have occurred (*46*). Hepatitis E virus has been associated with acute, sporadic illness in Cairo, Egypt (*47*), and in the Netherlands (*48*). Sequencing of the hepatitis E virus RNA genome has shown that homology is greatest in isolates from nearby sources (*49,50*). Fecal shedding of the virus for up to 14 days after onset of jaundice has now been demonstrated (*51*). A strain of hepatitis E virus isolated in Mexico has been shown to infect owl monkeys (*Aotus trivirgatus*) and cynomolgus monkeys (*Macaca fascicularis; 52*), and another from Xinjiang, China, has replicated and caused cytopathic effects in a diploid cell culture line from human embryo lung (*53*).

VIRAL GASTROENTERITIS

Recent findings regarding diarrhea caused by rotaviruses, the Norwalk virus, and others have been reviewed (*54*). The Norwalk virus and related agents, as well as the virus of hepatitis E, have recently been classified as members of the family *Caliciviridae* (*55*). A reverse transcription polymerase chain reaction test has been developed for detecting Norwalk virus in stools and is proposed for detecting the virus in food and environmental samples (*56*). Recombinant Norwalk virus protein that self-assembles into empty viral coats has been used in an ELISA test to demonstrate anti-Norwalk antibody in patient sera (*57*).

Rotaviruses are frequent causes of diarrhea in children but less often affect adults. Coproantibody develops after infection in children and may significantly protect against reinfection in children (*58*). Susceptibility to rotavirus in adults may be further diminished by gastric acid and pepsin secretion (*59*).

LITERATURE CITED

1. World Health Organization. *WHO Surveillance Programme for Control of Foodborne Infections and Intoxications in Europe*. Fifth Report. 1985–1989. Institute of Veterinary Medicine—Robert von Ostertag-Institute (FAO/WHO Collaborating Centre for Research and Training in Food Hygiene and Zoonoses), Berlin (1992).

2. Beller, M. Hepatitis A outbreak in Anchorage, Alaska, traced to ice slush beverages. *West. J. Med.* 156:624–627 (1992).

3. Warner, R.D., R.W. Carr, F.K. McCleskey, et al. A large nontypical outbreak of Norwalk virus: gastroenteritis associated with exposing celery to nonpotable water and with *Citrobacter freundii. Arch. Intern. Med.* 151:2419–2424 (1991).

4. Anonymous. Foodhandlers implicated in Denver hepatitis outbreak. *Food Protect. Rep.* 9(1):1–3 (1993).

5. Centers for Disease Control. *Hepatitis Surveillance Report No. 54*. Centers for Disease Control, Atlanta (1992).

6. Todd, E.C.D. Foodborne disease in Canada—a 10-year summary from 1975 to 1984. *J. Food Protect.* 55:123–132 (1992).

7. Lefkowitz, A., G.S. Fout, G. Losonsky, et al. A serosurvey of pathogens associated with shellfish: prevalence of antibodies to *Vibrio* species and Norwalk virus in the Chesapeake Bay region. *Am. J. Epidemiol.* 135:369–380 (1992).

8. Anonymous. Gastrointestinal virus infections, England and Wales: laboratory reports, weeks 92/52–93/01. *Commun. Dis. Rep.* 3(3):10 (1993).

9. Malcolm, R. Food poisoning outbreak following gourmet function held at a hotel in St. Andrews. *Commun. Dis. Environ. Health Scotland Weekly Rep.* 26(4):4–6 (1992).

10. World Health Organization. Air travel-associated foodborne illness. *WHO Surveillance Programme for Control of Foodborne Infections and Intoxications in Europe. Newsletter* 31:1 (1992).

11. Notermans, S., and A. Hoogenboom-Verdegaal. Existing and emerging foodborne diseases. *Int. J. Food Microbiol.* 15:197–205 (1992).

12. Williams, F.P., Jr., and G.S. Fout. Contamination of shellfish by stool-shed viruses: methods of detection. *Environ. Sci. Technol.* 26:689–696 (1992).

13. Hofmann, F., G. Wehrle, H. Berthold, and D. Köster. Hepatitis A as an occupational hazard. *Vaccine* 10(Suppl. 1):S82–S84 (1992).

14. Gust, I.D. A vaccine against hepatitis A—at last. *Med. J. Aust.* 157:345–346 (1992).

15. World Health Organization. Inactivated hepatitis A vaccine. *Weekly Epidemiol. Rec.* 67:261–264 (1992).

16. World Health Organization. Prevention of foodborne hepatitis A. Considerations on the vaccination of food handlers. *Weekly Epidemiol. Rec.* 68:25–32 (1993).

17. Mbithi, J.N., V.S. Springthorpe, J.R. Boulet, and S.A. Sattar. Survival of hepatitis A virus on human hands and its transfer on contact with animate and inanimate surfaces. *J. Clin. Microbiol.* 30:757–763 (1992).

18. Burkhardt, W., III, W.D. Watkins, and S.R. Rippey. Seasonal effects on accumulation of microbial indicator organisms by *Mercenaria mercenaria. Appl. Environ. Microbiol.* 58:826–831 (1992).

19. Burkhardt, W., III, W.D. Watkins, and S.R. Rippey. Survival and replication of male-specific bacteriophages in molluscan shellfish. *Appl. Environ. Microbiol.* 48:1371–1373 (1992).

20. Wood, G.W., and M.R. Adams. Effects of acidification, bacterial fermentation, and temperature on the survival of rotavirus in a model weaning food. *J. Food Protect.* 55:52–55 (1992).

21. Lasta, J., J.H. Blackwell, A. Sadir, et al. Combined treatments of heat, irradiation, and pH effects on infectivity of foot-and-mouth disease virus in bovine tissues. *J. Food Sci.* 57:36–39 (1992).

22. Weaver, A. Bovine spongiform encephalopathy: its clinical features and epidemiology in the United Kingdom and significance for the United States. *Compendium on Continuing Education for Practicing Veterinarians* 14:1647-1656 (1992).

23. Mohri, S., C. Farquhar, R. Somerville, et al. Immunodetection of a disease specific PrP fraction in scrapie-affected sheep and BSE-affected cattle. *Vet. Rec.* 131:537-539 (1992).

24. Fraser, H., M. Bruce, A. Chree, et al. Transmission of bovine spongiform encephalopathy and scrapie to mice. *J. Gen. Virol.* 73:1891-1897 (1992).

25. Willoughby, K., D. Kelly, D. Lyon, and G. Wells. Spongiform encephalopathy in a captive puma. *Vet. Rec.* 131:431-434 (1992).

26. Centers for Disease Control. Waterborne-disease outbreaks, 1989–1990. *Morbid. Mortal. Weekly Rep.* 41:86 (1992).

27. Ticehurst, J., T.J. Popkin, J.P. Bryan, et al. Association of hepatitis E virus with an outbreak of hepatitis in Pakistan: serologic responses and pattern of virus excretion. *J. Med. Virol.* 36:84–92 (1992).

28. Naik, S.R., R. Aggarwal, P.N. Salunke, and N.N. Mehrotra. A large waterborne viral hepatitis E epidemic in Kanpur, India. *Bull. WHO* 70:597–604 (1992).

29. Mahoney, F.J., T.A. Farley, K.Y. Kelso, et al. An outbreak of hepatitis A associated with swimming in a public pool. *J. Infect. Dis.* 165:613–618 (1992).

30. Hughes, M.S., P.V. Coyle, and J.H. Connolly. Enteroviruses in recreational waters of Northern Ireland. *Epidemiol. Infect.* 108:529–536 (1992).

31. Tani, N., K. Shimamoto, K. Ichimura, et al. Enteric virus levels in river water. *Water Res.* 26:45–48 (1992).

32. Suttle, C.A., and F. Chen. Mechanisms and rates of decay of marine viruses in seawater. *Appl. Environ. Microbiol.* 58:3721–3729 (1992).

33. Ansari, S.A., S.R. Farrah, and G.R. Chaudhry. Presence of human immunodeficiency virus nucleic acids in wastewater and their detection by polymerase chain reaction. *Appl. Environ. Microbiol.* 58:3984–3990 (1992).

34. Dee, S.W., and J.C. Fogleman. Rates of inactivation of waterborne coliphages by monochloramine. *Appl. Environ. Microbiol.* 58:3136–3141 (1992).

35. Deng, M.Y., and D.O. Cliver. Inactivation of poliovirus type 1 in mixed human and swine wastes and by bacteria from swine manure. *Appl. Environ. Microbiol.* 58:2016–2021 (1992).

36. Soares, A.C., I.L. Pepper, and C.P. Gerba. Recovery of poliovirus from sludge-amended soils. *J. Environ. Sci. Health* A27:999–1005 (1992).

37. Straub, T.M., I.L. Pepper, and C.P. Gerba. Persistence of viruses in desert soils amended with anaerobically digested sewage sludge. *Appl. Environ. Microbiol.* 58:636–641 (1992).

38. Centers for Disease Control. Summary of notifiable diseases, United States, 1991. *Morbid. Mortal. Weekly Rep.* 40(53):1–64 (1991).

39. Robertson, B.H., R.W. Jansen, B. Khanna, et al. Genetic relatedness of hepatitis A virus strains recovered from different geographical regions. *J. Gen. Virol.* 73:1365–1377 (1992).

40. Winokur, P.L., and J.T. Stapleton. Immunoglobulin prophylaxis for hepatitis A. *Clin. Infect. Dis.* 14:580–586 (1992).

41. Fujiyama, S., S. Iino, K. Odoh, et al. Time course of hepatitis A virus antibody titer after active and passive immunization. *Hepatology* 15:983–988 (1992).

42. Berger, R., and M. Just. Vaccination against hepatitis A: control 3 years after the first vaccination. *Vaccination* 10:295 (1992).

43. Ping, L.-H., and S.M. Lemon. Antigenic structure of human hepatitis A virus defined by analysis of escape mutants selected against murine monoclonal antibodies. *J. Virol.* 66:2208–2216 (1992).

44. Lemon, S.M. Hepatitis A virus: current concepts of the molecular virology, immunobiology and approaches to vaccine development. *Rev. Med. Virol.* 2:73–87 (1992).

45. Emerson, S.U., Y.K. Huang, C. McRill, et al. Mutations in both the 2B and 2C genes of hepatitis A virus are involved in adaptation to growth in cell culture. *J. Virol.* 66:650–654 (1992).

46. Favorov, M.O., H.A. Fields, M.A. Purdy, et al. Serologic identification of hepatitis E virus infections in epidemic and endemic settings. *J. Med. Virol.* 36:246–250 (1992).

47. Hyams, K.C., M.C. McCarthy, M. Kaur, et al. Acute sporadic hepatitis E in children living in Cairo, Egypt. *J. Med. Virol.* 37:274–277 (1992).

48. Zaaijer, H.L., M.F. Yin, and P.N. Lelie. Seroprevalence of hepatitis E in the Netherlands. *Lancet* 340:681 (1992).

49. Aye, T.T., T. Uchida, X. Ma, et al. Sequence comparison of the capsid region of hepatitis E viruses isolated from Myanmar and China. *Microbiol. Immunol.* 36:615–621 (1992).

50. Tsarev, S.A., S.U. Emerson, G.R. Reyes, et al. Characterization of a prototype strain of hepatitis E virus. *Proc. Natl. Acad. Sci. USA* 89:559–563 (1992).

51. Aggarwal, R., and S.R. Naik. Faecal excretion of hepatitis E virus. *Lancet* 340:787 (1992).

52. Ticehurst, J., L.L. Rhodes, Jr., K. Krawczynski, et al. Infection of owl monkeys (*Aotus trivirgatus*) and cynomolgus monkeys (*Macaca fascicularis*) with hepatitis E virus from Mexico. *J. Infect. Dis.* 165:835–845 (1992).

53. Huang, R.T., D.R. Li, J. Wei, et al. Isolation and identification of hepatitis E virus in Xinjiang, China. *J. Gen. Virol.* 73:1143–1148 (1992).

54. Bricout, F. Viral diarrhoea. *Presse Méd.* 21:309–314 (1992).

55. Pringle, C.R. Committee pursues medley of virus taxonomic issues. *Am. Soc. Microbiol. News* 58:475–476 (1992).

56. Jiang, X., J. Wang, D.Y. Graham, and M.K. Estes. Detection of Norwalk virus in stool by polymerase chain reaction. *J. Clin. Microbiol.* 30:2529–2534 (1992).

57. Jiang, X., M. Wang, D.Y. Graham, and M.K. Estes. Expression, self-assembly, and antigenicity of the Norwalk virus capsid protein. *J. Virol.* 66:6527–6532 (1992).

58. Coulson, B.S., K. Grimwood, I.L. Hudson, et al. Role of coproantibody in clinical protection of children during reinfection with rotavirus. *J. Clin. Microbiol.* 30:1678–1684 (1992).

59. Bass, D.M., M. Baylor, R. Broome, and H.B. Greenberg. Molecular basis of age-dependent gastric inactivation of rhesus rotavirus in the mouse. *J. Clin. Invest.* 89:1741–1745 (1992).

Index